Sports Injury Management

SECOND EDITION

Sports Injury Management

SECOND EDITION

MARCIA K. ANDERSON, PhD, LATC
Professor and Director, Athletic Training Program
Department of Movement Arts, Health Promotion, and Leisure Studies
Bridgewater State College
Bridgewater, Massachusetts

SUSAN J. HALL, PhD
Professor and Chair
Department of Health and Exercise Sciences
University of Delaware
Newark, Delaware

MALISSA MARTIN, EdD, ATC
Assistant Professor
Director, Athletic Training Educational Program
Department of Health, Physical Education, and Recreation
Middle Tennessee State University
Murfreesboro, Tennessee

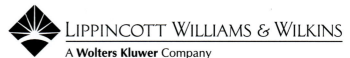
LIPPINCOTT WILLIAMS & WILKINS
A **Wolters Kluwer** Company
Philadelphia • Baltimore • New York • London
Buenos Aires • Hong Kong • Sydney • Tokyo

Editor: Eric Johnson
Managing Editor: Linda S. Napora
Marketing Manager: Christen DeMarco
Production Manager: Susan Rockwell

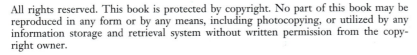

351 West Camden Street
Baltimore, Maryland 21201-2436 USA

530 Walnut Street
Philadelphia, Pennsylvania 19106 USA

First Edition, 1995

Printed in the United States of America

Library of Congress Cataloging-in-Publication Data

Anderson, Marcia K.
 Sports injury management/Marcia K. Anderson, Susan J. Hall, Malissa Martin.—2nd
  ed. p. ; cm.
 Includes bibliographical references and index.
 ISBN 0-683-30602-2
 1. Sports injuries. I. Hall, Susan J. (Susan Jean) 1953- II. Title.
 [DNLM: 1. Athletic Injuries—therapy. QT 261 A548s 2000]
RD97.A53 2000
617.1′027—dc21
                                                              00-023235

The publishers have made every effort to trace the copyright holders for borrowed material. If they have inadvertently overlooked any, they will be pleased to make the necessary arrangements at the first opportunity.

To purchase additional copies of this book call our customer service department at **(800) 638-3030** or fax orders to **(301) 824-7390**. International customers should call **(301) 714-2324**.

                                    00 01 02
                          1 2 3 4 5 6 7 8 9 10

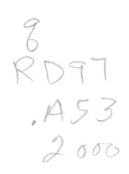

The second edition of *Sports Injury Management* by Marcia Anderson, Susan Hall, and Malissa Martin fulfills a significant need in the athletic training profession by providing a text for upper level students and practicing colleagues as it addresses current and relevant information in the discipline. The book provides a unifying theme and focus on specific joint kinematics, as well as prevention, assessment, management, and rehabilitation of the most common conditions found in an athletic training environment.

In addition to citing current literature, the Appendix of Medical Terminology includes abbreviations and symbols, prefixes, suffixes, and combined word forms. Together with the text glossary, this information will provide the student with easy access to critical medical documentation language and a source of immediate and convenient reference material for understanding textual content.

Upper level students and athletic training educators will find *Sports Injury Management*, second edition, to be an excellent resource that includes all aspects of athletic training. It will be of value both as a core text and later during clinical practice. The book can also serve as a reference for the preparticipation examination, emergency procedure management, modalities, and therapeutic exercise.

The authors have organized the material by anatomical structure and conditions. The chapters have been significantly expanded by the addition of management information, diagnostic testing, psychological aspects of the injured participant, sport-specific functional testing, and vascular and neural disorders.

Special features of the second edition provide detailed information regarding conditions athletic trainers commonly observe and manage that go beyond everyday musculoskeletal injuries—respiratory tract, gastrointestinal, and dermatological conditions; common infectious diseases; blood pressure disorders; and the diabetic athlete. The information provided on senior and disabled athletes will assist the athletic trainer in providing quality care for the physically active person across the lifespan.

The second edition of *Sports Injury Management* has numerous outstanding features that enhance the pedagogical structure for the reader. In addition to goals and objectives, chapters include case-based critical thinking questions and answers, management algorithms, and field strategies. Carefully selected and expanded illustrations, figures, color plates, and succinct chapter summaries complement the narrative and provide a functional and pleasing visual environment for the student. The content is presented in a concise, integrated approach that can assist synthesis and enhance individual student needs and cognitive learning styles. This timely revision updates common practices, clarifies content, and places greater emphasis on concepts and practical application.

To facilitate learning and retention, text material presents challenging content in a user-friendly format for the student. It also allows the athletic training educator flexibility in altering the sequence of material to meet teaching preferences, level of the learner, time constraints, and course requirements. This comprehensive text is well positioned to meet the needs of upper level athletic training students and educators as our discipline continues to address reforms in athletic training education and the ongoing changes in healthcare delivery.

Karen R. Toburen, EdD, ATC
Professor and Department Head
Sports Medicine and Athletic Training
Southwest Missouri State University
Springfield, Missouri

I t was exciting to prepare the second edition of *Sports Injury Management*, particularly in light of the rapidly changing profession of athletic training and its impact on the academic and clinical expectations placed on entry-level professionals. Our primary goal with this edition was to continue our commitment to provide the most comprehensive, challenging content in a "user-friendly" format to help facilitate student learning and retention as they prepare to enter the athletic training profession. In addition, this text can serve as a resource book for practicing athletic trainers who want to remain current in the profession. This text, more than any other text on the market, sets the standard for a concise, integrated approach to learning using the most current research available in athletic training and related fields.

Following the publication of the first edition of *Fundamentals in Sports Injury Management*, an introductory text, the second edition of *Sports Injury Management* was developed to address the needs of the more advanced athletic training student. Our intent was to construct a strong foundation of general athletic training practices, and then branch into greater detail on advanced conditions or injuries seen in the physically active population across the lifespan. This text can be used in a general upper-level athletic training class or integrated into a specific injury assessment or evaluation class. Because of the detailed content, it is advisable that the student complete prerequisite coursework in an applied musculoskeletal anatomy class and an introductory athletic training class.

NEW FEATURES IN THIS EDITION

Sports Injury Management has undergone extensive review from leaders in the athletic training field, leading to the most comprehensive text available to the athletic training educator. Expanded illustrations, figures, color plates, and succinct critical information boxes, tables, field strategies, and management algorithms highlight each chapter to enhance the learning process. Many chapters have been expanded and new chapters have been added to reflect the ever-increasing body of knowledge in the athletic training profession. Many of the highlighted changes and additions include:

- Highlighted medical terms are defined within the text and in the glossary.
- Chapter 1, *Sports Injury Management and the Athletic Trainer*, presents up-to-date information on certification standards of the athletic trainer, and legal concerns of the profession.
- Chapter 2, *Preparticipation Examination*, presents current standards for the administration of a preparticipation exam (PPE), including goals for the PPE, setting up the exam utilizing a group format, taking a medical history, conducting the physical exam, standards for determining the physical fitness profile, and finally, the criteria used to determine if the individual should be allowed to participate and at what level of intensity.
- Chapter 3, *Protective Equipment*, describes the most popular materials used to design protective pads, discusses liability issues associated with protective equipment, provides a weekly helmet inspection checklist, and summarizes the proper fitting of protective equipment with an expanded section on the selection and fit of athletic footwear.
- Chapter 4, *Sport Injury Assessment*, details the injury evaluation process using the SOAP note format. This is continued throughout Part III, The Axial Region; Part IV, The Upper Extremity; and Part V, The Lower Extremity. In addition, four new sections have been added to the chapter. Preseason preparation and the responsibility of medical personnel are highlighted in light of the emergency medical services (EMS) system. Specific on-the-field assessment procedures and techniques to move the injured participant are then followed by coverage of various diagnostic testing techniques used to help the physician diagnose the injury.
- Chapter 5, *Tissue Healing and Wound Care*, seeks to simplify the complex process of soft tissue healing, and discusses the role of growth factors in facilitating the process. New information is presented on soft tissue wound care, including current universal precautions and infection control standards. A new section has been added on bone injury management, nerve injury classifications, and general management of nerve injuries.
- Chapter 6, *Therapeutic Modalities*, explains the electromagnetic spectrum and clinical use of cryotherapy, thermotherapy, ultrasound, diathermy, electrotherapy, and other treatment modalities. An added section includes medications used in the rehabilitation of athletic training injuries.
- Chapter 7, *Therapeutic Exercise*, now includes extensive coverage of the psychological aspects of the injured participant and explains the athletic trainer's role in recognizing, intervening, and referring the injured athlete to an appropriate professional if psychological problems hinder the rehabilitation process. Also covered is information on the effects of immobilization and remobilization, general principles of joint mobilization, detailed discussion on the principles of proprioception, and the functional application of exercise.
- Expanded joint Chapters 8–16 cover specific injuries or conditions organized by body regions. Each chapter has been expanded to include the most current, com-

prehensive coverage of each condition. The organization of body regions has also been changed to reflect a better flow through the body, beginning at the head and face; moving down the spine, thorax, and abdomen; then moving to the shoulder, elbow, wrist, and hand; and finally moving to the hip, knee, lower leg, ankle, and foot.

- Each chapter opens with an expanded coverage of joint anatomy with detailed illustrations drawn by a medical illustrationist. Kinematics and major muscle actions, kinetics of the region, and injury prevention strategies are also presented.
- Chapters are organized to provide information on contusions, sprains, strains, overuse conditions, fractures, and nerve entrapment syndromes. Each condition is explained, signs and symptoms are identified, and management protocols are provided. Conditions that warrant immediate transportation to the nearest medical facility are highlighted by the icon

  . This is intended to visually identify critical conditions that demand priority management.
- Assessment in each chapter has been expanded to include more comprehensive and complex tests for a wider range of conditions.
- Finally, general rehabilitation exercises are included to offer the student a consistent format in rehabilitating the various body regions.

- Chapter 8, *Head and Facial Conditions*, now includes a comparison of the different classifications used to define the various degrees of brain dysfunction in cerebral concussions, and provides the more current techniques used to determine the history of a head injury, mental status testing, external provocative testing, and standardized criteria used to return an athlete to competition.
- Chapter 9, *Spinal Conditions*, now includes detailed discussion and illustrations of the brachial plexus, lumbar plexus, and sacral plexus. New information is presented on cervical spinal stenosis, spear tackler's spine, classification of burners, suprascapular nerve injury, and sacroiliac joint sprains. Multiple special tests have been added to provide a more comprehensive assessment section.
- Chapter 10, *Throat, Thorax, and Visceral Conditions*, provides information on the anatomy of the genitalia and associated conditions. New information is presented on pulmonary contusions, hernias, liver contusion and rupture, kidney injuries, and common nonmusculoskeletal sources of abdominal pain.
- Chapter 11, *Shoulder Conditions*, now includes expanded coverage of the kinematics of the throwing motion, and thoracic outlet compression syndrome. New information is presented on the classification of acromioclavicular sprains, and on glenohumeral instabilities and glenoid labrum tears. Multiple special tests have

been added to provide a more comprehensive assessment section.
- Chapter 12, *Upper Arm, Elbow, and Forearm Conditions*, includes expanded coverage of bursitis and neural entrapment injuries.
- Chapter 13, *Wrist and Hand Conditions*, includes expanded coverage of joint anatomy of the wrist articulations, retinacula of the wrist, and tendon sheaths, along with new information on dislocations of the wrist and fingers, intersection syndrome, anterior interosseous nerve syndrome, carpal tunnel syndrome, ulnar tunnel syndrome, distal posterior interosseous nerve syndrome, superficial radial nerve entrapment, and Kienbock's disease.
- Chapter 14, *Pelvis, Hip, and Thigh Conditions*, includes new information on the sacroiliac joint, sacrococcygeal joint, pubic symphysis, bony structure of the thigh, Q-angle, toxic synovitis, and obturator nerve entrapment. Expanded coverage is provided on hip pointers, quadriceps contusions, acute compartment syndrome, ischial bursitis, hamstrings strains, Legg-Calvé-Perthes disease, and osteitis pubis. Multiple special tests have been added to provide a more comprehensive assessment section.
- Chapter 15, *Knee Conditions*, now includes expanded coverage of the joint capsule and bursae, anterior cruciate ligament, patellofemoral joint, Q-angle, A-angle, bursitis, multidirectional instabilities, knee dislocations, patellar instability and dislocations, Sinding-Larsen-Johansson's disease, and stress fractures. Multiple special tests have been added to provide a more comprehensive assessment section.
- Chapter 16, *Lower Leg, Ankle, and Foot Conditions*, includes expanded anatomical coverage of the talocrural joint, subtalar joint, and plantar fascia, along with new information on lateral ankle sprains, Achilles tendinitis, exertional compartment syndrome, and venous disorders. New sections have been added on hallus rigidus, hallus valgus, mallet toe, reverse turf toe (soccer toe), bunions, retrocalcaneal bursitis, syndesmosis sprains, subtalar sprains, subtalar dislocations, tarsal tunnel syndrome, sural nerve entrapment, and a LisFranc injury. Multiple special tests have been added to provide a more comprehensive assessment section.
- Chapter 17, *Environmental Conditions*, includes more information on air pollution and exercise, and new information on exercising in thunderstorms.
- Chapter 18, *Respiratory Tract Conditions*, explains how to use a metered-dose inhaler, and a peak flowmeter, in the management of asthma.
- Chapter 19, *Gastrointestinal Conditions*, includes information on dysphagia, gastroesophageal reflux, dyspepsia, peptic ulcers, gastritis, gastroenteritis, diarrhea, constipation, and hemorrhoids.
- Chapter 20, *The Diabetic Athlete*, discusses the physiological basis of diabetes, explains the four types of dia-

betes mellitus and complications that may arise from the disease, and provides nutrition and exercise recommendations.

- Chapter 21, *Common Infectious Diseases*, presents current information on common childhood diseases, infectious mononucleosis, viral meningitis, sexually transmitted diseases, hepatitis, and acquired immunodeficiency syndrome.
- Chapter 22, *Seizure Disorders*, explains the difference between seizure disorders and epilepsy, details the causes of epilepsy, classification of seizures, seizure management, discusses medications and epilepsy, and suggests physical activity guidelines.
- Chapter 23, *Blood Pressure Disorders*, presents a major section on hypertension, including causes, risk factors for developing it, categories and classifications, and management of the condition through lifestyle modification, exercise, and pharmaceutical medications. Hypotension is also presented along with nonneurogenic causes and nonpharmacologic treatment of orthostatic hypotension.
- Chapter 24, *Sudden Death*, discusses cardiac and noncardiac causes of sudden death, details ACSM coronary artery disease risk factors, explains screening techniques for Marfan's syndrome, recommendations for screening for sudden death during the cardiovascular preparticipation examination, and diagnostic tests used to identify individuals at risk for sudden death.
- Chapter 25, *Conditions of the Female Athlete, Disabled Athlete, and Senior Athlete*, highlights injuries and conditions that can affect special populations across the lifespan. The section on the Female Athlete includes discussion on the menstrual cycle, menstrual irregularities, endometriosis, premenstrual syndrome, birth control and sport participation, pregnancy and sport participation, anemia, eating disorders, osteoporosis, and the Female Triad. The section on the Disabled Athlete covers common injuries and conditions associated with wheelchair, amputee, cerebral palsy, and the visually impaired athlete. Common upper and lower extremity considerations are discussed for the Senior Athlete.
- Chapter 26, *Pharmacology*, introduces the student athletic trainer to pharmacokinetics, the study of how a drug moves through the body to produce the desired effects. Factors that contribute to the therapeutic effect of a drug are followed by discussion on drug interactions and adverse drug reactions. Students are then introduced to drug names, guidelines for the use of therapeutic medications, and finally, common medications used to treat sport-related injuries.
- Chapter 27, *Dermatology*, illustrates the common types of skin lesions, and discusses the more common bacterial, fungal, and viral skin conditions. The chapter also includes discussion on common skin irritations not related to a skin infection. Color plates illustrate the more common skin conditions.

- Two new Appendices of Medical Terminology include: (1) a glossary of prefixes, suffixes, and combining words; and (2) abbreviations and symbols used frequently in writing SOAP notes.

PEDAGOGICAL FEATURES

As educators, we have highlighted and summarized information in the text by incorporating several pedagogical features to enhance the text's usefulness as a teaching tool. This is designed to increase readability and retention of relevant and critical information. These in-text features include:

Learning Objectives

Each chapter opens with a series of learning objectives. These objectives list the most important concepts in the chapter that the student should focus on during reading.

Critical Thinking Questions

Critical thinking questions, identified by the icon, are found at the beginning of most of the major sections in each chapters. Their role is to encourage the student to critically analyze information in the text to solve the opening scenario. The answer to each critically thinking question is given at the end of that section within the text, and is identified by the icon.

Medical Terminology

New and difficult medical terminology is bolded and defined in the text, and can also be found in the glossary.

Critical Information Boxes

A unique feature of this edition is the use of boxes interspersed throughout each chapter to list or summarize critical information to supplement material in the text. In Parts III, IV, and V, for example, these boxes summarize signs and symptoms of specific conditions.

Tables

Several chapters have tables that expand upon pertinent information discussed in the text. This allows a large amount of didactic knowledge to be organized in an easy-to-read summary of information.

Field Strategies and Management Algorithms

Another unique feature of this book is the use of Field Strategies and Management Algorithms to clinically apply cognitive knowledge. In Parts III, IV, and V, for example, the charts move step by step through the specific condition, listing immediate management, and in many instances, provide several rehabilitation exercises for the specific condition.

Art and Photography Program

Art plays a major role in facilitating the learning process for visual learners. The editor and authors worked very hard to incorporate appropriate, detailed illustrations and photographs to supplement material presented in the text. The medical illustrator worked tirelessly to provide realistic and accurate figures to depict anatomical structures, and has devised innovative approaches to illustrate injury mechanisms.

Summary

Each chapter has a summary of key concepts discussed in the text. Several chapters also contain a list of injuries or conditions that necessitate immediate referral to a physician for further care.

References

Any valuable teaching tool must include a listing of cited references used to gather information for the text. We have tried to limit the references to a 5-year period, except where the reference is considered to be the original groundbreaking research. With an accurate bibliography, the instructor or student can refer to additional information on the topic if needed.

Appendices

Two appendices have been included to supplement the text. Appendix A provides abbreviations and symbols that are used frequently in writing SOAP notes; Appendix B provides prefixes, suffixes, and combining forms to help the athletic training student understand the construction of a medical term.

Glossary and Index

At the end of the book, the student will find an extensive glossary of terms gathered from the highlighted words in the individual chapters. Furthermore, the comprehensive index contains cross-referencing information to locate specific information within the text.

Instructor's Resource Manual

Written by Dr. Malissa Martin, Director of the Undergraduate Athletic Training Curriculum Program at Middle Tennessee State, the Instructor's Manual provides suggestions and exercises to supplement material presented in each chapter. The modules include chapter objectives, vocabulary terms, and laboratory exercises with injury scenarios to facilitate the learning process. These exercises can be photocopied for student use. They are designed to move the student step by step through the SOAP note format, emphasizing proper vocabulary skills, and techniques to thoroughly assess and manage each injury. At the end of the Manual are more than 1,000 sample test questions that cover pertinent information in each of the chapters.

Marcia K. Anderson
Bridgewater, Massachusetts

Susan J. Hall
Wilmington, Delaware

Malissa Martin
Murfreesboro, Tennessee

ACKNOWLEDGMENTS

The authors would like to thank several friends and colleagues, many of whom assisted in the development of the text through their critical analysis and review of the initial drafts. These individuals include:

Lori Dewald, EdD, Shippensburg University, Shippensburg, Pennsylvania

Dan Foster, PhD, The University of Iowa, Iowa City, Iowa

Donald Fuller, PhD, East Tennessee State University, Johnson City, Tennessee

Mark H. Gibson, MSEd, LaCrosse, Wisconsin

David A. Kaiser, EdD, Central Michigan University, Mt. Pleasant, Michigan

Randy Meador, MS, West Virginia University, Morgantown, West Virginia

Gail Parr, PhD, Towson University, Towson, Maryland

Stephen G. Rice, MD, PhD, MPH, Jersey Shore Medical Center, Neptune, New Jersey

Cynthia Trowbridge, MS, Ithaca College, Ithaca, New York

Benito Velasquez, DA, The University of Southern Mississippi, Hattiesburg, Mississippi.

We would also like to thank the many athletic training students at Bridgewater State College and the University of South Carolina who reviewed several of the chapters and student exercises included in the Instructor's Manual.

Their ability to analyze the information and raise the standard of learning was exceptional. These individuals will certainly be welcome colleagues in the field of athletic training.

We would like to thank the hard-working and talented staff of Lippincott Williams & Wilkins: Eric Johnson, Linda Napora, Nancy Peterson, and Susan Rockwell; Loren Marshall of the Treeline Writers Group; and Lydia V. Kibiuk, medical illustrator. Their patience and attention to detail were paramount in producing a text of quality and depth.

A special thanks to Victoria Bacon and Kim Shibinski for their support and encouragement to stick with the project and see it to its completion. I would also like to acknowledge all the help, direction, and guidance of my good friends and colleagues Cheryl Hitchings and Kathy Laquale, who assumed additional tasks within the department and athletic training program so that I could have time to complete this contribution to the profession.

And, finally, a very special thanks to Demeter, who was my ever-faithful companion for more than 14 years. She provided a solid foundation of love and support, and never once complained about waiting to go for her walk in the woods. I miss her.

Marcia K. Anderson
Susan J. Hall
Malissa Martin

CONTENTS

Comprehensive Contents

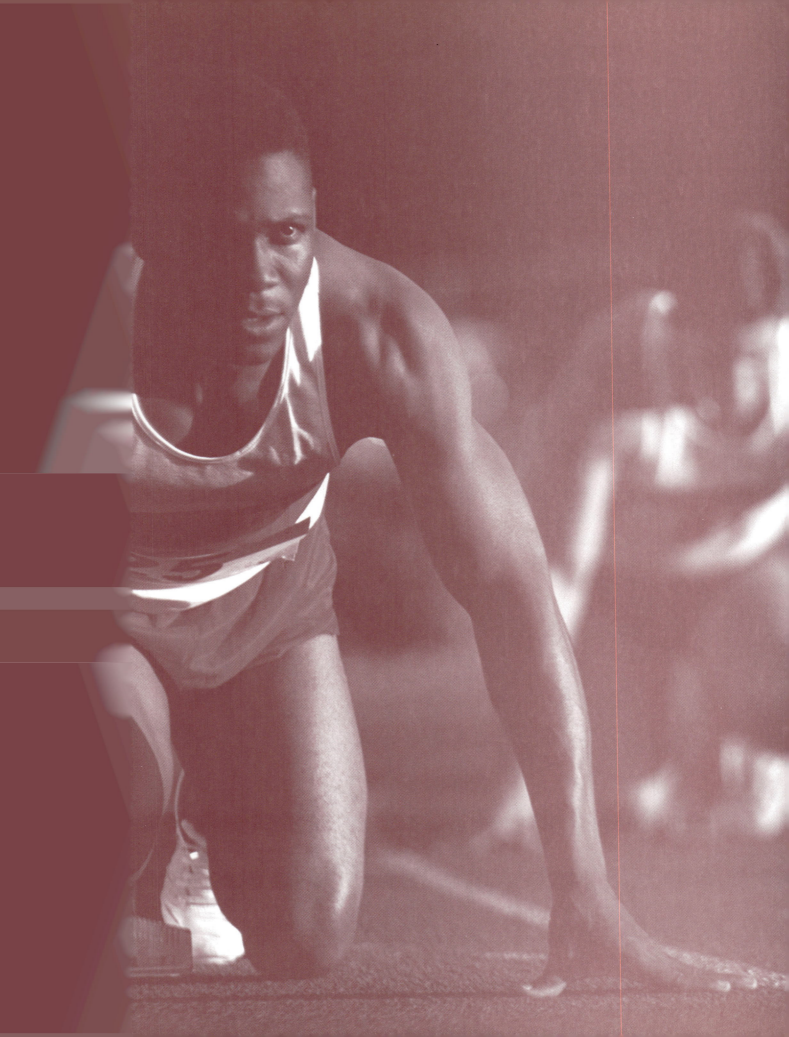

SECTION I

1

Sports Injury Management and the Athletic Trainer

OBJECTIVES

1. Define sports medicine.
2. Identify members of the primary sports medicine team and describe their roles and responsibilities in sports injury management.
3. Explain the basic parameters of ethical conduct and standards of professional practice for athletic trainers.
4. Specify academic and clinical requirements necessary to become a NATA certified athletic trainer.
5. Describe the continuing education requirements needed to maintain certification and how to report CEUs once they are fulfilled.
6. Describe potential job opportunities for an individual interested in athletic training as a career.
7. Explain standard of care and what factors must be proven to show legal breach of that duty of care.
8. Describe measures that can reduce the risk of litigation.

Sport, with the inherent risks involved, leads to injury at one time or another for nearly all participants. Physicians and athletic trainers responsible for the health and safety of sport participants are called sports medicine specialists. These individuals are essential in the prevention, recognition, assessment, management, and rehabilitation of sport injuries. Furthermore, these individuals educate and counsel sport participants to prevent chronic degenerative injuries and diseases through life-long activity-related fitness and health education.

This chapter examines the role of the team physician and athletic trainer within the primary sports medicine team. In the absence of an athletic trainer, the coach or designated supervisor of the sport-related activity must assume the role of the immediate health care provider. Standards of professional practice and criteria for national certification as an athletic trainer are presented along with potential job opportunities. Finally, legal liability surrounding sports injury care will be presented relative to reducing the risk of possible litigation.

THE PRIMARY SPORTS MEDICINE TEAM

 Many health care professionals refer to themselves as sports medicine specialists. Think for a minute about what this term implies. Which professionals provide on-site immediate medical care to physically active individuals? What duties do you think each member of this team should be responsible for?

Sports medicine is a broad and complex branch of health care encompassing several disciplines. Essentially it is an area of health care and special services that applies medical and scientific knowledge to prevent, recognize, assess, manage, and rehabilitate injuries or illnesses related to sport, exercise, or recreational activity, and in doing so, enhances health fitness and performance of the participant (1). No single profession can provide the expertise to carry out this enormous responsibility. As such, the team approach has proven to be the most successful method of addressing health care for sport participants (2).

The primary sports medicine team is the pivotal group of individuals with specialized training and expertise in their chosen fields to provide immediate on-site health care. This team includes the team physician or primary care physician, certified athletic trainer, coach or sport supervisor in the absence of an athletic trainer, and the sport participant **(Figure 1.1)**. Of these, the certified athletic trainer is the primary individual responsible for daily on-site health care. In the absence of a certified athletic trainer, the coach will assume this role. Other professionals, not necessarily on-site but readily accessible to the primary sports medicine team, also contribute their knowledge and expertise. These individuals may include orthopedic physicians, physical therapists, emergency medical technicians

(EMTs), podiatrists, radiologists, nutritionists, exercise physiologists, and sport psychologists.

Team Physician

In organized sport, such as interscholastic, intercollegiate, or professional athletic programs, a team physician may be hired or may volunteer his or her services to direct the primary sports medicine team. This individual supervises the various aspects of health care and is the final authority to determine the mental and physical fitness of athletes in organized programs (2).

In an athletic program, the team physician should administer and review preseason physical exams; review preseason conditioning programs; assess the quality, effectiveness, and maintenance of protective equipment; diagnose injuries; dispense medications; direct rehabilitation programs; educate the athletic staff on emergency policies, procedures, health care insurance coverage, and legal liability; and review all medical forms, policies and procedures to ensure compliance with school and athletic association guidelines **(Box 1.1)** (1,2). This individual may also serve as a valuable resource on current therapeutic techniques, facilitate referrals to other medical specialists, and provide educational counseling to sport participants, parents, athletic trainers, coaches, and sport supervisors.

➤➤ **BOX 1.1**

Duties of the Team Physician
- Know the common risk factors associated with sports injuries and the physical demands of specific sports
- Plan and organize the preparticipation examination (PPE)
- Review PPE results and determine readiness for sport participation
- Review preseason conditioning programs
- Assess the quality, effectiveness, and maintenance of protective equipment
- Provide on-site medical coverage at athletic events, particularly involving collision and contact sports
- Diagnose injuries and direct rehabilitation programs
- Dispense medications
- Facilitate referrals to other medical specialists
- Provide educational counseling to sport participants, parents, athletic trainers and coaches
- After rehabilitation, determine readiness to return to competition
- Protect confidentiality of medical history
- Review all medical forms, policies and procedures to ensure compliance with school and athletic association guidelines
- Educate the athletic staff on emergency policies, procedures, health care insurance coverage, and legal liability
- Provide in-service training on current therapeutic methods, problems, and techniques

---

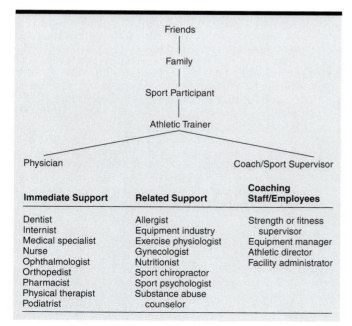

➤ **FIGURE 1.1 Sports medicine team.**

In many high school and collegiate settings, financial constraints may prevent hiring a full-time team physician. Instead, several physicians may rotate the responsibility of being present at competitions and are paid a per-game stipend. Primary care physicians, orthopedists, and other specialists, such as osteopaths, internists, general surgeons, and pediatricians who have a broad and thorough understanding of sport injuries may serve as a team physician. The team physician should be present at competitions, particularly with high-risk sports, such as football, hockey, or lacrosse to assess emergency injury and treat any injury or illness.

Primary Care Physician

In the absence of a team physician, the primary care physician or family physician assumes a more pivotal role in providing health care to the sport participant. This individual can provide information on the growth and development of an adolescent, immunization records, and a comprehensive medical history. In addition, they may administer preparticipation exams, provide initial clearance for sport participation, diagnose sport injuries, prescribe medications, and clear individuals for sport participation after an injury (2).

Athletic Trainer

Athletic trainers are the critical link between the sport program and medical community and are certified by the National Athletic Trainers' Association Board of Certification (NATABOC). They provide a broad range of direct services to the sport participant on a daily basis and serve as the liaison between the physician and athlete, and physician and coach. An athletic trainer must have a strong background in human anatomy, human physiology, kinesiology or biomechanics, exercise physiology, psychology, nutrition, pharmacology, physics, general medical conditions and disabilities, risk management and injury prevention, acute care of injury and illness, injury assessment and evaluation, therapeutic exercise, therapeutic modalities, and health care administration. The primary duties and responsibilities of the certified athletic trainer are outlined in the 1999 Role Delineation Study **(Box 1.2)**. The major domains include (3):

- Prevention
- Recognition, evaluation and assessment
- Immediate care
- Treatment, rehabilitation, and reconditioning
- Organization and administration
- Professional development and responsibility

Prevention

Injury prevention may occur with preparticipation physical exams (see Chapter 2); regular safety checks of equipment, facilities and field areas; designing and implementing year-round conditioning programs to develop and maintain

---

➤➤ **B O X 1.2**

Duties of the Athletic Trainer

PREVENTION

- Educate individual(s) about risks associated with participation to minimize risk of injury.
- Review pre-participation screening information by applying accepted guidelines.
- Instruct individual(s) about required standard protective equipment.
- Apply appropriate prophylactic/protective measures using commercial products or custom-made devices.
- Identify safety hazards in activity areas and equipment and make appropriate recommendations.
- Monitor participants and environmental conditions following accepted guidelines to make recommendations regarding safe participation.
- Facilitate physical conditioning by designing and implementing appropriate programs.
- Maintain clinical and treatment areas by complying with safety and sanitation standards.
- Promote sound nutritional practices by encouraging adherence to accepted guidelines.

RECOGNITION, EVALUATION AND ASSESSMENT

- Obtain a history through observation, interview, and/or review of relevant records to assess the pathology and extent of the condition.
- Inspect the involved area(s) visually to assess the pathology and extent of the condition.
- Palpate the involved area(s) using standard techniques to assess the pathology and extent of the condition.
- Perform specific tests systematically to assess the pathology and extent of the condition.
- Formulate a clinical impression by interpreting the signs and symptoms of the condition to determine the appropriate course of action.
- Educate the appropriate individual(s) about the assessment to encourage compliance with recommended care.
- Inform members of the health care team about your assessment through direct communication to facilitate appropriate care.

IMMEDIATE CARE

- Initiate and/or execute techniques to mitigate life-threatening and other emergency conditions through the use of standard emergency care procedures.
- Initiate care for medical or musculoskeletal conditions to stabilize and/or prevent exacerbation of the condition through the use of standard techniques.
- Facilitate referral or guidance for psychosocial crises by implementing established intervention strategies to match services to the need.
- Educate appropriate individuals in standard immediate care procedures to facilitate immediate care.

TREATMENT, REHABILITATION AND RECONDITIONING

- Administer therapeutic exercise and therapeutic modalities using standard techniques and procedures to facilitate recovery, function and/or performance.

Continued

BOX 1.2   **Duties of the Athletic Trainer**
Continued

- Administer treatment for general illnesses and/or conditions using standard techniques and procedures to facilitate recovery.
- Reassess the status of the condition to determine appropriate treatment, rehabilitation and/or reconditioning to evaluate readiness to return to a desired level of activity.
- Educate the individual(s) in the treatment, rehabilitation and reconditioning of the condition to facilitate recovery.
- Provide guidance for the individual(s) in the treatment, rehabilitation and reconditioning of injuries, illnesses and/or condition to facilitate recovery.

ORGANIZATION AND ADMINISTRATION

- Establish a plan of action using available resources to provide routine and emergency health care services for individuals, athletic activities and events.
- Write policies and procedures for individuals to promote safe participation, timely care and legal compliance.
- Write policies and procedures for facilities, treatment and activity areas to promote safety and legal compliance.
- Comply with safety and sanitation standards for treatment and activity areas by establishing policies and procedures to meet the current standard of care.
- Manage resources by constructing and monitoring an annual budget and time management plan to provide for appropriate health care services.
- Maintain records using an appropriate system to document the services rendered and provide for continuity of care.

PROFESSIONAL DEVELOPMENT AND RESPONSIBILITY

- Demonstrate appropriate professional conduct by complying with applicable standards to provide quality athletic training services.
- Maintain competence through continuing education to provide quality athletic training services.
- Educate the public about the role and standards of practice of the athletic trainer through informal and formal means to improve the public's ability to make informed decisions about the use of athletic training services.
- Adhere to statutory, regulatory and case law relating to the practice of athletic training by maintaining an understanding of these requirements to contribute to the safety and welfare of the public and the profession.

such as temperature, humidity, or lightning during thunderstorms can help the athletic trainer adhere to guidelines for safe participation in adverse weather, thus further reducing the potential for injury.

Recognition, Evaluation, and Assessment

The athletic trainer is responsible for recognizing, evaluating, and providing immediate treatment for an injury that occurs during sport participation. To do so, the athletic trainer needs a strong background in human anatomy and physiology, joint biomechanics, neuroanatomy, and tissue healing and repair. With this knowledge, the athletic trainer can recognize the body's normal physiologic response to trauma, evaluate common soft tissue injuries, such as contusions, sprains, strains, dislocations, and fractures and determine the extent or seriousness of injury. Injury evaluation follows a systematic format including the history, observation and inspection of the injury site, palpation of soft tissues and bony structures, and special tests (i.e., testing range-of-motion, muscle strength, sensory and motor neurologic function, ligamentous/capsular integrity, and functional status). Once a clear understanding of the extent and seriousness of injury is determined, the athletic trainer must interpret the signs and symptoms of the injury and decide what actions are appropriate to prevent additional pain or discomfort for the individual.

Immediate Care

Once a clear understanding of the extent of injury has been determined, the athletic trainer must initiate or execute techniques to mitigate life-threatening and other emergency conditions through the use of standard emergency care procedures. These actions may include activating the emergency medical plan to summon an ambulance and emergency medical technicians (EMTs) for transportation to the nearest medical facility. In less serious cases, immediate care may involve stabilizing the medical or musculoskeletal condition to prevent exacerbation of the condition, such as immobilizing a possible fracture, applying appropriate protective and prophylactic equipment, or removing the individual from participation **(Figure 1.2)**. The athletic trainer would then communicate with the appropriate medical personnel to make the necessary referral. In some cases, this referral may involve a referral for a psychosocial/emotional crisis. Established intervention protocols can then be used to match the needs of the individual with the appropriate professionals.

Rehabilitation and Reconditioning Treatment

After acute inflammation has subsided, usually within 24 to 72 hours, the athletic trainer can design and implement a rehabilitation program to help the individual return to their pre-injury status. In consultation with a physician, a

strength, flexibility, agility, and endurance; promoting proper lifting technique and safety in the weight room; and following universal safety precautions to prevent the spread of infectious diseases. With a working knowledge of joint mechanics and injury mechanisms, the athletic trainer can design and apply appropriate taping, wrappings, protective devices, or braces to prevent injury or re-injury from occurring. Monitoring environmental conditions,

➤ FIGURE 1.2 **Injury management**. After evaluating an injury, the athletic trainer can determine what action is appropriate to manage the situation. This may include sideline treatment to control inflammation or immediate referral to a physician.

comprehensive rehabilitation program is developed including therapeutic goals and objectives, selection of appropriate therapeutic **modalities** and exercise, use of pharmacological agents, methods to assess and document progress, and criteria for return to participation. Information gathered and documented during rehabilitation will assist the physician in determining when the individual may be cleared for participation.

Organization and Administration

The athletic trainer is responsible for documenting and maintaining all health care records of the athlete, including those pertaining to health services (i.e., preparticipation exams, injury evaluations, immediate treatment of injuries/ illnesses, rehabilitation progress, and medical clearance to participate); other services rendered to an injured party (counseling, educational programs, referrals to specialists); financial management; training room management; personnel management; and public relations. Regular inspection records of athletic training facilities, therapeutic modalities and equipment, gymnasiums, pools, and fields verify compliance with mandated safety and sanitation standards. The purchase of equipment and supplies, equipment reconditioning records, policies and procedures for drug testing and screening programs can verify compliance with safety standards established by national governing athletic associations. Written policies and procedures, such as the supervision of student athletic trainers, emergency care protocols, confidentiality of medical records, and normal operating procedures should also be documented (3).

Professional Development and Responsibility

Participating in continuing education activities is critical to staying informed on contemporary sports medicine issues.

Many athletic trainers work closely with physicians, physical therapists, coaches, and parents and must be prepared to counsel sport participants on health related topics, such as nutrition, weight management, disordered eating patterns, exercise protocols for individuals with special conditions, alcohol or other chemical substance abuse, infectious diseases, personal hygiene, depression, family problems, or school-related stress. Because of the athletic trainer's unique working relationship, they can serve as an important resource to refer an individual to an appropriate specialist for further care or counseling.

The Coach or Sport Supervisor

A coach is responsible for teaching skills and strategies of a sport. A sport supervisor may not necessarily be a coach, but instead may be responsible for administering and supervising recreational sport activities or activity areas within health club facilities. Both individuals are responsible for encouraging good sportsmanship and developing an overall awareness of safety and injury prevention. For brevity, coaches and sport supervisors will be jointly referred to as coaches.

In the absence of an athletic trainer, the coach must assume a more active role in providing health care to sport participants. When compared to the academic preparation of a certified athletic trainer, coaches do not typically have the background in human anatomy and physiology, health and nutrition, injury prevention, assessment, management, and rehabilitation, or first aid and emergency care. Because of this, all coaches should maintain current certification in cardiopulmonary resuscitation (CPR) and emergency first aid. In the absence of an athletic trainer, coaches are also expected to evaluate the daily status of sport participants prior to any activity, properly fit and use quality safety equipment, teach proper skill development and technique, and constantly reinforce the importance of safety and injury prevention throughout the year (2).

Concern for safety and injury prevention must be communicated during the preseason team meeting with players and parents. Each player and parent should be informed of the risk of injury, how to prevent injuries, and what to do if an injury occurs. Conditioning programs should be based on sound physiologic principles and training techniques, and be properly supervised. Activities should be planned so as not to predispose the participants to excessive fatigue or heat injury. Coaches should meet with their respective staff to develop an emergency plan and should periodically practice implementing that plan. Periodic in-service training can provide an opportunity to practice emergency skills, techniques, and use of emergency equipment. If possible, at least one staff person should have advanced training in emergency care.

Sport Participant

Sport participants play an essential role in working with the athletic trainer and coach to maximize injury prevention.

Participants are responsible for maintaining a high level of fitness, eating nutritious foods, and playing within the rules of the sport. All sport participants should refrain from ingesting alcohol and other chemical substances, such as anabolic steroids, human growth hormones, and amphetamines to enhance performance. Each can impair judgment, alter coordination, and place the individual at risk for injury. The participant should be responsible for maintaining and wearing safety equipment at all times during activity. In the event of an injury, the individual should know where to seek immediate health care and follow medical advice from the physician or athletic trainer. If sport participants understand and practice safety and preventive measures, the number of injuries or illnesses can be reduced.

Student Athletic Trainer

Student athletic trainers provide the work force in organized sport programs to implement the policies and procedures of daily health care at team practices and games **(Figure 1.3)**. Many students gain practical experience on the high school level and enroll in a college to pursue a degree program in athletic training, human performance, physical education, or a health related area. At the college or university, NATA certified athletic trainers supervise and guide the student athletic trainer through the clinical application of sports injury care. Initially, the student athletic trainer may only observe the staff athletic trainers and assist when needed. As the student's skills and knowledge improve, the athletic trainers will help the student learn the NATA competencies in athletic training and prepare the student athletic trainer to meet the NATA Board of Certification standards. Student athletic trainers can view first hand the contributions athletic trainers provide in the total health care of sport participants.

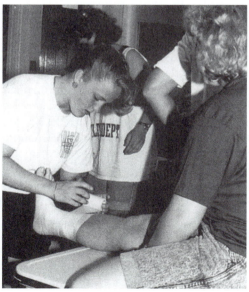

➤ **FIGURE 1.3 Student athletic trainers**. Student athletic trainers provide the work force to implement the policies and procedures of daily health care to sport participants.

Physical Therapist

Physical therapists are not a part of the on-site primary sports medicine team, yet they provide a unique and valuable resource in the overall rehabilitation of a sport participant. Whereas the athletic trainer typically works with healthy athletes, the physical therapist has a broader background in treating patients of all ages and with a wider variety of physical conditions. Physical therapists often supervise the rehabilitation of an injured sport participant in a hospital setting, or in an industrial or sports medicine clinic. In many cases, athletic trainers are also registered physical therapists. Likewise, many physical therapists are also working toward certification as an athletic trainer. Dual certification is a strong asset in the job market.

 Sports medicine refers to the combined health care and special services that applies medical and scientific knowledge to prevent, recognize, assess, manage, and rehabilitate injuries or illnesses related to sport participation. The primary sports medicine involves the team physician, athletic trainer, coach, and athlete. Of these, the athletic trainer is the primary individual responsible for daily on-site health care.

STANDARDS OF PROFESSIONAL PRACTICE

 What parameters establish the level of care and professional conduct that athletic trainers should provide to their clients?

Standards of professional practice are ethical responsibilities that guide one's actions and promote high standards of conduct and integrity to assure high quality health care (4). A certified athletic trainer should never compromise the health of any sport participant. Decisions concerning whether or not a sport participant should be allowed to participate must be based on sound medical consideration. Individuals should be informed of the risks for injury, protected from injury whenever possible, and if an injury occurs, should receive expedient health care and rehabilitation. Participants have a right to confidentiality about their health status. Athletic trainers, coaches, and physicians should be sensitive about dissemination of health information and should honor the wishes of an individual not to make the information public.

The National Athletic Trainers' Association (NATA) has established 5 basic ethical principles for athletic trainers to abide by. These include (5):

- Members shall respect the rights, welfare, and dignity of all individuals.
- Members shall comply with the laws and regulations governing the practice of athletic training.
- Members shall accept responsibility for the exercise of sound judgment.
- Members shall maintain and promote high standards in the provision of services.

- Members shall not engage in any form of conduct that constitutes a conflict of interest or that adversely reflects on the profession.

NATA Certification for the Athletic Trainer

Individuals seeking to become NATA certified athletic trainers must complete the following core requirements (6):

1. Clinical athletic training hours may not begin to accumulate until after the high school degree has been completed
2. Proof of graduation (an official transcript) at the baccalaureate level at an accredited college or university in the United States. Graduates of foreign universities may petition for a substitution of the degree requirement. Such a request will be evaluated at the candidate's expense by an independent consultant selected by the NATABOC
3. Proof of current American National Red Cross Standard First Aid Certification and current Basic CPR (American Red Cross or American Heart Association), or EMT equivalent. Both cards must be current at the time of application
4. At least 25% of all clinical athletic training experience hours must be attained in actual (on location) practice and/or game coverage with one or more of the following sports: football, soccer, hockey, wrestling, basketball, gymnastics, lacrosse, volleyball, and rugby
5. Endorsement of certification application by a NATA certified athletic trainer
6. Subsequently passing the certification examination (written, oral-practical, and written simulation sections)

Currently, an individual may qualify for application through two options: (1) by graduating from an undergraduate or graduate college that has an educational program accredited through the American Medical Association's (AMA) Commission on Accreditation of Allied Health Education Programs (CAAHEP), or (2) by completing an internship. However, as of January 1, 2004, graduation from a CAAHEP accredited athletic training program will become the only recognized route to certification.

Students in CAAHEP-accredited entry-level programs must complete formal instruction in the following core curriculum subject matter (6):

> Human anatomy
> Human physiology
> Psychology
> Kinesiology/biomechanics
> Exercise physiology
> Prevention of athletic injuries/illnesses
> Evaluation of athletic injuries/illnesses
> First aid and emergency care

> Therapeutic modalities
> Therapeutic exercise
> Personal/community health
> Nutrition
> Administration of athletic training programs

In addition to core subject matter, additional coursework is highly recommended in chemistry, physics, pharmacology, statistics and research design. Students are also required to complete 800 clinical hours under the supervision of a NATA certified athletic trainer at the college or affiliated site (i.e., an area high school or local college) (6). Students who do not attend a college with a CAAHEP-accredited entry-level program may currently complete requirements for certification through internship. Requirements for this option are established by the NATA Board of Certification (NATABOC). Individuals must complete at least one formal, single *course* in each of the following areas (6):

> Health (i.e., nutrition, drugs/substance abuse, health education)
> Human anatomy
> Human physiology
> Kinesiology/biomechanics
> Physiology of exercise
> Basic athletic training
> Advanced athletic training (The only acceptable alternative for advanced athletic training is *one course each* in therapeutic modalities and rehabilitative exercise.)

Beginning January 1, 2001 the classes Basic and Advanced Athletic Training should incorporate content in the following areas: prevention of athletic injuries, recognition and management of acute athletic injuries, rehabilitation of athletic injuries, therapeutic modalities and evaluation of injury. The basic and advanced athletic training courses (or the acceptable alternative) must be successfully completed in a college or university in the United States, or taught by a NATABOC-certified athletic trainer in a foreign college or university for academic credit. The remaining core courses may be accepted from foreign universities as deemed acceptable by the consultant.

If seeking certification via the internship route, the NATABOC requires 1500 hours of athletic training experience under the supervision of a NATA certified athletic trainer. Of these, at least 1000 hours must be attained in an athletic training facility at the interscholastic, intercollegiate, or professional sports level. The remaining 500 hours may be completed at an allied clinical setting, such as in a sports medicine clinic, campus health center, industrial health facility, other health care facility, and/or sport camp setting under the supervision of a NATA certified athletic trainer. These hours must be accumulated in no less than two, nor more than five years (6). As noted, this route to certification will cease to exist as of January 1, 2004. Candidates wishing to pursue eligibility for the examination via the internship route must have done so by December 31, 2003.

Students taking the NATABOC examination will be evaluated on entry-level competencies as identified in the current Role Delineation Study. The performance domains contain several elements or subject areas that transcend the six domains. These content areas, called universal competencies, encompass the knowledge and psychomotor skills for each task.

Continuing Education Requirements

Continuing education programs provide an opportunity for athletic trainers to acquire new innovative skills and techniques and learn about current research within the profession. Once certified as a NATA athletic trainer, the NATABOC requires eight continuing education units (CEUs) over a three-year period. These may be accumulated by attending workshops, seminars, conferences, and conventions, speaking at a clinical symposium, publishing professional articles, enrolling in related correspondence or postgraduate education courses, or becoming involved in the NATA certification exam testing program. In addition, current proof of CPR certification is required at least once during the CEU requirement period (7). For current standards of certification and continuing education requirements write to: NATABOC, 1512 South 60th Street, Omaha, NE 68106-2102, or call (402) 559-0091.

Registration and Licensure

States regulate professions to protect the public from harm by unqualified individuals. Without some type of regulation, there is no legal foundation to assure quality of care because there is no legal definition as to what an athletic trainer can and cannot do. Licensure is the strictest form of state regulation and is therefore the most effective means of protecting the public. Licensure is necessary to protect the general public, insure public safety, maintain minimum standards in the practice of athletic training, and promote the highest degree of professional conduct on the part of the athletic trainer (8). Athletic trainers, through their state associations, have worked very hard over the past two decades to secure recognition and establish some type of regulation of the practice of athletic training within their respective states. To date there are 36 of the 50 states that now require athletic trainers to meet specific standards of practice within the individual state, referred to as state licensure, certification, or registration (**Box 1.3**) (9). These laws define the role of the athletic trainer and set the legal parameters under which the athletic trainer can operate within that state. These laws may delineate the specific clientele and services that can be provided in the various work settings.

Although standards vary, in most states athletic trainers provide services to athletes or physically active individuals under the direct supervision of a physician licensed in that state. Nearly all states accept the successful completion

---

> ➤ ➤ **Box 1.3**

State Regulation of Athletic Trainers as of January 1998

Alabama†	Kansas‡	North Carolina†
Arkansas†	Kentucky§	North Dakota†
Airzona*	Louisiana§	Ohio†
Colorado*	Maine†	Oklahoma†
Connecticut*	Massachusetts†	Oregon‡
Delaware†	Minnesota‡	Pennsylvania§
Florida†	Mississippi†	Rhode Island†
Georgia†	Missouri‡	South Carolina§
Hawaii*	Nebraska†	Tennessee§
Idaho‡	New Hampshire†	Texas†
Illinois§	New Jersey‡	Virginia§
Indiana§	New Mexico†	
Iowa†	New York§	

_____
* States that are exempt from existing licensure standards that limit other related professions.
† States with licensure
‡ States with registration
§ States with certification
Note: For information on individual state licensure laws or an up-date on states regulating the practice of athletic training contact: Government Affairs Committee, The National Athletic Trainers Association, 2952 Stemmons, Dallas, TX 75247

---

of the NATA examination as a basis for obtaining licensure, although there may or may not be any mechanism for assessing continued competency (10). In nontraditional settings or in states that do not have licensure laws, athletic trainers may be restricted in the services they provide. Being properly licensed and practicing within the established standards of practice are two of the strongest safeguards against litigation.

 Standards of professional practice reflect what the profession believes the standard of care and professional conduct should be for an athletic trainer. These standards are often used by state regulatory agencies to protect the public from harm by unqualified individuals.

CAREER OPPORTUNITIES IN ATHLETIC TRAINING

 Career opportunities for athletic trainers are becoming increasingly available in both the public and private sectors. Envision yourself 10 years from now as a certified athletic trainer. Where would you like to be working at that time?

Many women and men select athletic training as a career choice because they want to work with children, interscholastic, intercollegiate, recreational, and professional athletes in a health care environment. This allied health profession provides a challenging and valuable service needed at all levels of sport participation. Athletic trainers are generally employed in secondary school, intercollegiate, or professional athletic programs, sports medicine clinics, clinical and industrial health care programs, health and fitness clubs, or a combination of any of the above. The more common employment sites will be discussed.

High School and Collegiate Settings

High school and collegiate settings are often referred to as traditional athletic training settings. In high schools, the athletic trainer is often hired as a faculty member and given a reduced teaching load, or paid additional moneys for athletic training duties. The individual begins work 2 to 3 weeks prior to the start of school with preseason practice sessions and provides health care coverage to athletes throughout the academic school year.

At the college level, athletic training responsibilities vary. At most colleges the athletic trainer is hired to provide services only to intercollegiate athletes. The individual is placed on a 10 or 12 month work schedule depending on the demands of the job. In smaller schools the athletic trainer may teach part-time in the physical education or health department and provide athletic training services to athletes. The athletic trainers may also be asked to work in the campus health center supervising rehabilitation programs or educating students on health issues.

Working in a school setting allows the athletic trainer to see a variety of injuries and illnesses and often contributes to general self-satisfaction in helping competitive athletes stay healthy. Many individuals also enjoy the prestige of working in a highly visible high school or college program. Depending on the number of athletic trainers working at the school, however, long work hours and excessive travel responsibilities may lead to premature burnout.

Sports Medicine Clinics

Privately owned sports medicine clinics and related clinics provide another career opportunity for athletic trainers **(Figure 1.4)**. Patients vary in age and level of performance and have a variety of conditions needing treatment. Under the direction of a physician, the athletic trainer provides activity related health care services. Some clinics specialize in only sport-related injuries, others deal in cardiac rehabilitation, exercise physiology, biomechanical analysis, workman's compensation injuries, or they may serve the general population. Athletic trainers working in a sports medicine clinic can expect to work a standardized workday; however in some states, direct billing or licensure standards may restrict them from providing certain services, such as initial patient evaluation or using electrical modalities.

Dual High School/Clinic Athletic Trainer

Many sports medicine clinics are subcontracting athletic training services to area high schools. The clinic hires the

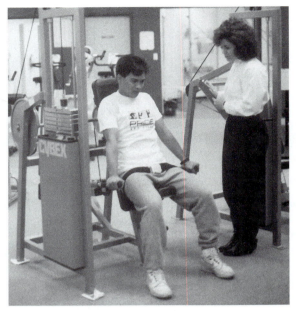

➤ FIGURE 1.4 **Sports medicine clinics.** Patients at a sports medicine clinic vary in age, level of performance, and have a wider variety of conditions needing treatment. This site is a growing source of employment for athletic trainers.

athletic trainer full-time, but splits their time between the clinic in the morning and high school in the afternoon or evening. As mentioned earlier, direct billing or licensure laws may restrict some services provided by the athletic trainer in a clinic setting. This arrangement is growing in popularity throughout the United States. As licensure laws begin to adapt to the changing athletic training profession, the clinical setting may provide an excellent career option.

Industrial Health Care Programs

Many companies hire athletic trainers to provide employees with in-house athletic training services. Working under the direction of a physician, the athletic trainer can perform injury assessment, management, rehabilitation, develop wellness and fitness programs, and provide education and counseling for employees. Not only is this cost effective, it is also time efficient, as employees do not need to leave work for these services.

Professional Sport Teams

Athletic trainers for professional sport teams are usually hired by a single sport team to perform athletic training services throughout the year. During the competitive season the athletic trainer will concentrate on traditional duties, but during the remainder of the year the athletic trainer may be asked to develop and supervise general reconditioning programs, recruit players, do scouting, manage equipment, or make travel arrangements for the team. Salaries vary considerably depending on the length of the playing season, revenues from television, and potential moneys from playoffs and championships.

Have you determined what setting you would like to be working in as an athletic trainer? What advantages and disadvantages exist in each setting?

LEGAL LIABILITY

 A first-year college athlete missed the preseason physical examination. The earliest an exam could be scheduled with the team physician was for the second day of pre-season camp. The coach insists that the athlete be allowed to participate the first day of camp, since they will only be doing basic conditioning and technique drills, but no contact drills. What implications exist concerning your legal responsibility to this athlete, and would you allow the athlete to participate?

Prevention of injuries and reducing further injury or harm are major responsibilities for all athletic trainers and coaches. Regardless of providing the best possible care, accidents do happen, some of which may result in legal action against the coach, athletic trainer, or team physician. Legal action involving the practice of athletic training is typically tried under tort law. A **tort** is a wrong done to an individual whereby the injured party seeks a remedy for damages suffered. In lawsuits, actions are measured against a standard of care provided to those individuals for whom you are directly responsible. **Standard of care** is defined as what another minimally competent individual educated and practicing in that profession would have done in the same or similar circumstance to protect an individual from harm or further harm. This standard of care is dictated by the profession's **scope of care**, which outlines the role and responsibilities of an individual in that profession and delineates what should be learned in the professional preparation of that individual. In athletic training, the Education Council of the NATA determined the competencies, which defines the educational content that students enrolled in a CAAHEP-accredited athletic training program must master. These include twelve major domains **(Box 1.4)**, each of which includes the following method of classifying behavioral objectives:

- Cognitive domain (knowledge and intellectual skills)
- Psychomotor domain (manipulative and motor skills)
- Affective domain (attitudes and values)
- Clinical proficiencies (decision-making and skill application)

By delineating the scope of care for entry-level athletic trainers, the NATA establishes the standard of care that the public can expect to receive from a certified athletic trainer. As such, an individual responsible for providing athletic training services would be held to a standard of care expected of a NATA certified athletic trainer. Therefore, in states with specific registration, certification, or

> ➤➤ Box 1.4

NATA Athletic Training Domains
- Risk management and injury prevention for the physically active
- Pathology of injuries and illnesses
- Assessment and evaluation
- Acute care of injury and illness
- Pharmacology
- Therapeutic modalities
- Therapeutic exercise for the physically active
- General medical conditions and disabilities
- Nutritional aspects of injury and illnesses
- Psychosocial intervention and referral
- Health care administration
- Professional development and responsibilities

licensure laws, valid NATA certification and registration or licensure would be essential to protect ones' self against litigation.

The question may arise as to who is the final authority to clear an individual for play. Because this falls outside the scope of care of a certified athletic trainer, the final authority in measuring an individual's status for participation rests with the supervising team physician, regardless of the age of the participant. In the absence of a team physician, the final authority rests with the family physician. Parents of minors cannot assume the risk involved in sport for their child (1).

Negligence

Athletic trainers and coaches are expected to teach, supervise, inspect and provide quality equipment, ensure a safe environment, and provide a duty of care to all sport participants (12). Failure to provide this care can result in liability, or **negligence**. Negligent torts may occur as a result of **malfeasance**, **misfeasance**, **nonfeasance**, **malpractice**, or **gross negligence (Box 1.5)**.

To find an individual liable, the injured person must prove that 1) there was a duty of care, 2) there was a breach of that duty, 3) there was harm (e.g., pain and suffering, permanent disability, or loss of wages), and 4) the resulting harm was a direct cause from that breach of duty (10). If a spectator notices a large hole in the field prior to a game, and a player steps into the hole and fractures an ankle, the spectator is not liable because that individual has no duty of care for the player. However, an athletic trainer or coach does have a duty of care to check the field for hazards prior to competition. As such, the athletic trainer or coach could be held liable for the injury sustained by the participant.

Although a sport participant does assume some risk inherent in any activity, the individual does not assume the risk that the professional will breach their duty of care. Fortunately, the number of lawsuits brought against ath-

Box 1.5

Definition of Negligent Torts

Malfeasance occurs when an individual commits an act that is not their responsibility to perform. If you suspect a neck injury and remove the football helmet, you could be liable

Misfeasance occurs when an individual commits an act that is their responsibility to perform, but uses the wrong procedure, or does the right procedure in an improper manner. If you suspect a neck injury and improperly secure the head and neck region to the rigid spine board, you could be held liable

Nonfeasance occurs when an individual fails to perform their legal duty of care. If you suspect, or should have suspected, a neck injury and failed to use a rigid back board to stabilize the individual, you could be held liable

Malpractice occurs when an individual commits a negligent act while providing care

Gross negligence occurs when an individual has total disregard for the safety of others

letic trainers in the performance of their duties is rare (10). Negligence may occur as a result of an action, or lack of action. Situations that can result in litigation are listed in **Box 1.6**.

Box 1.6

Actions that Can Result in Litigation

- Failing to warn an individual about the risks involved in sport participation
- Treating an injured party without their consent
- Failing to provide medical information concerning alternative treatments or the risks involved with the treatment to an athlete
- Failing to provide safe facilities, fields, and equipment
- Being aware of a potentially dangerous situation and failing to do anything about it
- Failing to provide an adequate injury prevention program
- Allowing an injured or unfit player to participate resulting in further injury or harm
- Failing to provide quality training, instruction, and supervision
- Using unsafe equipment
- Negligently moving an injured athlete before properly immobilizing the injured area
- Failing to employ qualified medical personnel
- Failing to have a written emergency care plan
- Failing to properly recognize an injury or illness, both as immediate acute care and as long-term treatment
- Failing to immediately refer an injured party to the proper physician
- Failing to keep adequate records
- Treating an injury that did not occur within the school athletic environment

Failure to Warn

Athletic trainers and coaches should inform potential athletes of the risks for injury during sport participation. Participants and parents of minor children should learn that risk for injury exists and must understand the nature of that risk so informed judgments may be made about participation. Understanding and comprehending the nature of the risk is determined by the participant's age, experience, and knowledge of pertinent information about the risk. An advanced gymnast, for example, would know of and appreciate the risk of injury much more than a novice gymnast. Therefore, it is crucial to warn the novice of any inherent dangers in the activity and continually reinforce that information throughout the entire sport season. Warnings may be communicated at the preseason meeting with parents and participants, posting visible warning signs around equipment, requiring protective equipment, and discouraging dangerous techniques. Other methods that may be used are discussed later in the chapter.

Informed Consent

Informed consent implies that an injured party has been reasonably informed of needed treatment, possible alternative treatment, and advantages and disadvantages of each course of action. To be valid, consent can only be obtained from one who is competent to grant it, that is, an adult who is physically and mentally competent, or, in the case of children under 18, only the parent can grant consent on behalf of the minor. For minors, exceptions exist in emergency situations when parents are unavailable. Authorization to treat in the absence of the parent, or in the event the individual is physically unable to consent to treatment, should be obtained in writing prior to the beginning of sport participation. This consent may be obtained during preparticipation meetings as part of the documentation depicting consent to participate in that activity.

It may also be wise to include an exclusionary clause on the consent form that identifies what will not be treated by the athletic trainer (e.g., injuries not associated with direct participation in sport). This can protect the athletic trainer from litigation if they refuse to treat a non-athletic related injury. For example, let's say that an athlete is injured in a recreational bicycling accident (not related to competitive sport participation) and fails to seek immediate treatment from an emergency room or physician. The individual comes to the athletic training room 2 days later with an infected open wound. In this instance, the athletic trainer should immediately refer this individual to a physician for treatment. In most states, if the athletic trainer attempted to clean the wound and complications arose, the athletic trainer could be held liable for practicing medicine outside the scope of the athletic training profession.

As the sport population continues to attract a diverse multicultural pool of participants, informed consent must be granted prior to any treatment. Athletic trainers must be sensitive to cultural and religious beliefs and practices, and honor those practices by providing appropriate care consistent with the wishes of the athlete. For example, in some cultures, a woman may be taught not to undress or bare skin in the presence of a man other than her husband. Therefore, if a male athletic trainer was assigned to treat a woman with a thoracic injury, and she did not feel comfortable in that situation, it would be better to refer the athlete to another female athletic trainer.

Failure to receive informed consent may constitute **battery**, which is any unpermitted or intentional contact with another individual without their consent. Although many courts require that intent to harm be present in an allegation of battery, written documentation of informed consent should be obtained from an individual, or parents of minor children prior to treatment to avoid litigation.

Foreseeability of Harm

To recognize the potential for injury first, then remove that danger before an injury occurs, is another duty of care for athletic trainers and coaches. **Foreseeability of harm** exists when danger is apparent, or should have been apparent, resulting in an unreasonably unsafe condition. This potential for injury can be identified during regular inspections of gymnasiums, field areas, swimming pools, safety equipment, and athletic training facilities. For example, unpadded walls under the basketball hoops, glass or potholes on playing fields, slippery floors near a whirlpool, exposed wiring, and failure to follow universal safety precautions against the spread of infectious diseases all pose a threat to safety. Unsafe conditions should be identified, reported in writing to appropriate personnel, restricted from use, and repaired or replaced as soon as possible.

Product Liability

Athletes, parents, coaches, and athletic trainers place a high degree of faith in the quality and safety of equipment used in sport participation. Manufacturers have a duty of care to design, manufacture, and package safe equipment that will not cause injury to an individual when the equipment is used as it was intended (10,11). This is called an **implied warranty**. An **expressed warranty** is a written guarantee that the product is safe for use. In football there is an implied warranty that if fitted and used properly, the helmet can protect the head and brain from certain injuries. The National Operating Committee on Standards for Athletic Equipment (NOCSAE) has established minimum standards for football helmets to tolerate certain forces when applied to different areas of the helmet. Manufacturers and reconditioners of helmets place a visible expressed warranty on all helmets that meet NOCSAE standards. This statement informs players that the helmet is not intended to be used to butt, ram or spear an opposing player, and that use in this manner could result in serious head, brain, or neck injuries, paralysis, or death for the player or opposing player. **Strict liability** makes the manufacturer liable for any and all defective or hazardous equipment that unduly threatens an individual's personal safety (10,11).

Teachers, coaches, athletic trainers, fitness specialists, and sport supervisors should know the dangers involved in using sport equipment, and have a duty to properly supervise its fitting and intended use. For example, the practice of cutting down mouth guards to cover only the front teeth should be strongly prohibited. Supervisors also have a duty to warn participants of the dangers inherent in using the equipment.

Confidentiality

A major concern of all individuals involved in providing health care is the athlete's right to privacy. If the individual is older than 18 years of age, release of any medical information must be acknowledged in writing by the sport participant. For individuals younger than 18 years of age, parents or legal guardians must provide consent for the dissemination of this information. This permission should identify what, if any, information can be shared with an individual other than the patient's physician. In many cases, schools and professional teams have the athlete give consent that all medical information can be shared between the athletic trainers and the supervising physician (12). Information provided to coaches and parents should be on a need to know basis only, and given with the full knowledge and consent of the athlete, supervising physician, and athletic trainer. Confidentiality should also extend to all medical records kept within the confines of the athletic training room, and may include:

- Consent to treat form
- Release of medical information form
- Emergency information
- Treatment documentation including:
  Injury report forms
  Medical referrals
  Physician evaluations
  Laboratory reports
  Surgical reports
  Progress notes
- Living will
- Counseling

Preventing Litigation

All members of the sports medicine team should be aware of their duty of care consistent with current state law and complete that duty of care within established policies and standards of practice. Several steps can reduce the risk of subsequent litigation and include: regular inspection of athletic fields and facility design, safety checks of equipment and facilities, hiring qualified personnel, proper su-

➤➤ BOX 1.7

Strategies to Avoid Litigation

- Ensure that all personnel are properly licensed for practicing within the laws of the state, particularly in providing athletic training services
- Hire qualified coaches, athletic trainers, and fitness instructors and establish strict rules for supervision and use of the facility
- Have an established preparticipation plan including:
  - Annual preparticipation health examination
  - Insurance verification
  - Medical data information cards
  - Physician's clearance to participate
- Hold a preseason/preparticipation meeting to:
  - Inform participants and parents of the risks involved in sport participation
  - Obtain written informed consent from the parents of minor children before participation
  - Document what was said at the preseason or preparticipation meeting
- Have a well-established primary sports medicine team to:
  - Develop a total health care plan including staff responsibilities during emergency situations
  - Obtain adequate secondary health insurance for participants and liability insurance for the staff
  - Establish a communication system at each field or gymnasium station
  - Maintain appropriate standard injury documentation and referral forms
  - Develop criteria to return an injured player to participation
  - Select and purchase quality safety equipment from a reputable dealer
  - Inspect safety equipment and supervise proper fitting, adjustment, and repair of equipment
  - Inspect equipment, facilities and fields for hazards and prohibit their use if found to be dangerous
  - Establish policies for documentation, confidentiality, and storage of medical records
  - Keep accurate records of equipment purchases, reconditioning, and repairs
- Post warning signs in plain sight on and around equipment to inform of the risks involved in abuse of equipment, and to describe proper use of the equipment
- Post visible signs in the swimming pool area giving the depth of the pool and prohibiting diving in the shallow area
- Post warning signs in the whirlpool area to inform individuals not to touch the turbine device while standing or sitting in water
- Require participants to wear protective equipment regularly, including protective eyewear in appropriate racquet sports
- Issue only those helmets that meet standards established by the National Operating Commission on Standards for Athletic Equipment (NOCSAE). Inform players the helmet cannot prevent all injuries and the possibility exists that serious head and neck injuries may occur in the sport
- Provide continuing education for coaches and athletic trainers through in-service workshops and programs
- Act as a reasonably prudent professional in caring for all sport participants

pervision and instruction, purchasing quality equipment, posting appropriate warning signs, maintaining accurate and complete health care records, and having a well organized emergency care plan. Other steps may be seen in **Box 1.7**.

 The college athlete was unable to re-schedule the preparticipation examination until the second day of preseason practice. If you determined that the athlete should not participate in any physical activity until he or she completes the examination and is cleared by the team physician, you are correct.

Summary

1. Sports medicine is a branch of medicine that applies medical and scientific knowledge to improve sport performance.
2. The primary sports medicine team provides immediate on-site supervision to prevent injury and deliver immediate health care, and includes the team physician, primary care physician in the absence of a team physician, athletic trainer, coach, and sport participant.
3. Athletic trainers are the essential link between the sport program and medical community, and are responsible for:
   - Prevention
   - Recognition, evaluation, and assessment
   - Immediate care
   - Treatment, rehabilitation and reconditioning
   - Organization and administration
   - Professional development and responsibility
4. Athletic trainers are usually employed in secondary schools, intercollegiate, or professional athletic programs, sports medicine clinics, clinical and industrial health care programs, at research facilities, health clubs, or a combination of any of the above.
5. Standards of professional practice are ethical judgments that guide your actions and promote high standards of conduct and integrity.
6. For an athletic trainer, NATA certification and state licensure can help meet one's duty of care in providing health care to sport participants.
7. Decisions concerning whether an individual should participate in an activity should be made by the physician based on sound medical consideration and should never compromise the health of the individual.
8. To find an individual liable, the injured person must prove that there was:
   - A duty of care
   - A breach of that duty
   - Harm caused by that breach
   - Harm as a direct cause of the breach of duty

9. Steps to reduce the risk of injury and subsequent litigation should include:
   - Obtaining informed consent
   - Recognizing the potential for injury and correcting it
   - Warning participants of the risk of injury
   - Hiring qualified personnel
   - Providing proper supervision and instruction
   - Purchasing, fitting, and maintaining quality equipment
   - Posting appropriate warning signs
   - Maintaining accurate and complete health care records
   - Protecting confidentiality of medical history
   - Having a well-organized emergency care system.

References

1. Herbert DL. Legal Aspects of Sports Medicine. Canton, OH: Professional Reports Corporation, 1994.
2. Mellion MB, Walsh WM. The team physician. In: Mellion MB, Walsh WM, Shelton GL, eds. The Team Physician's Handbook. Philadelphia: Hanley & Belfus, 1997.
3. The National Athletic Trainers' Association Board of Certification, Inc. Role Delineation Study. Omaha, NE: National Athletic Trainers' Association Board of Certification, 1999.
4. National Athletic Trainers' Association. New NATA code of ethics approved. NATA News 1992;4(7):15-16.
5. National Athletic Trainers' Association. NATA Code of Ethics. Approved at the annual meeting of the National Athletic Trainers' Association, Kansas City, June, 1993.
6. National Athletic Trainers' Association Board of Certification. Credentialing information and Professional Practice and Discipline, Standards for the Practice of Athletic Training. Omaha: NATABOC, 1998.
7. NATA Board of Certification Continuing Education Office. Continuing education file 1997-1999. Dallas: NATA Board of Certification, Inc., 1997.
8. Rello MN. The importance of state regulation to the promulgation of the athletic training profession. J Ath Tr 1996;31(2):160-164.
9. Governmental Affairs Committee, National Athletic Trainers' Association. Personal communication with author, 13 November, 1997.
10. Leverenz LJ, Helms LB. Suing athletic trainers: Part I, A review of the case law involving athletic trainers. Ath Train (JNATA) 1990;25(3):212-216.
11. Leverenz LJ, Helms LB. Suing athletic trainers: Part II, Implications for the NATA competencies. Ath Train (JNATA) 1990;25(3):219-226.
12. Arendt E. What every health care professional should know. NATA News 1996;8(1): 20-21.

2

Preparticipation Examination

OBJECTIVES

1. Identify the goals and objectives of a preparticipation examination (PPE).

2. Design a preparticipation examination.

3. Identify the specific areas in a PPE that should be examined using a mass station screening process.

4. List follow-up questions to validate information on a medical history questionnaire.

5. Demonstrate the ability to take vital signs, and identify criteria used to denote abnormal pulse and blood pressure rates.

6. Identify specific questions that should be asked at the various stations utilizing a group format to elicit a history of the athlete's physical condition.

7. Explain the importance of completing a physical fitness profile as part of the preparticipation examination.

8. Demonstrate skinfold measurement at the various sites used to determine body composition.

9. Describe the various stages of maturation using the Tanner Scale.

10. Contrast the criteria used to categorize hypermobility and hypomobility.

11. Describe specific methods of measuring strength, power, speed, cardiovascular endurance, agility, balance, and reaction time.

12. Identify specific conditions that could exclude an athlete from participating in physical activity or sport.

The preparticipation examination (PPE), often performed annually, helps to ensure a physically active individual's health and safety while participating in sport. Physicians and athletic trainers are responsible for conducting the PPE, and by doing so, can identify pre-existing conditions that may place the individual at risk for injury or illness. This chapter examines the entire process of the PPE. After introducing the general principles and goals of the PPE, information will be presented on how to organize the PPE using a group format. This will include setting up the exam, gathering a medical history, conducting the physical examination, and finally, the criteria used to determine if the individual should be allowed to participate and at what level of intensity.

GOALS OF THE PREPARTICIPATION EXAMINATION

 Why is it important to do a thorough preparticipation examination? What objectives can be gained by completing the examination?

The basic objective of the PPE is to ensure the health and safety of a physically active individual. This can be accomplished by gathering information on the individual's general health, maturity, and fitness level. Those at risk for injury, or those who have conditions that may limit participation, can be identified and counseled on health-related issues and steered into participating in appropriate activities (1-3). Many states and sport governing bodies require some type of PPE for competitive athletes; however, states differ greatly regarding specific requirements. Although the frequency and depth of PPEs may vary, most examinations share common goals **(Box 2.1)**.

Because sport participants range in age from the very young to the very old, the focus of the PPE is dependent on the specific age group. For example, in the prepubescent child (6 to 10 years of age), the focus may be on identifying previously undiagnosed congenital abnormalities. In the pubescent child (11 to 15 years of age), the examination

should center on maturation and establishing good health practices for safe participation. In the postpubescent or young adult group (16 to 30 years of age), the history of previous injuries and sport-specific examinations are critical. The more strenuous activities and those involving contact or collision sports for this age group require a more extensive examination **(Table 2.1)**. The adult population (30 to 65 years of age) has a high incidence of overuse injuries. These individuals need an examination based on the nature of the activity in which they intend to engage. The final group, those older than 65 years of age, often begins or increases activity to prevent a major medical illness. These individuals need an extensive examination based on individual needs, taking into consideration not only their physical needs, but also possible medications they may be taking and possible side effects (4).

 A PPE can establish a positive working relationship between the athletic trainer, team physician, and athlete. The exam can also evaluate the level of physical fitness and detect conditions that may limit participation or predispose an individual to a specific injury or illness.

SETTING UP THE EXAMINATION

 Should the PPE be performed by the family physician? What advantages or disadvantages does this practice entail? What other option is available?

Preparticipation examinations may be set up in a variety of ways. Much will depend on the level of competition (i.e., athlete in an organized competitive sport or recreational athlete), the community, the availability of personnel and facilities, the number of athletes being screened, and the personal preference of the evaluator. Because certified athletic trainers tend to be more involved in screening an athlete who is competing in an organized sport program (e.g., interscholastic or intercollegiate athletics), this chapter will focus on the process used for evaluating those individuals.

Examination Format

The primary care physician usually does preparticipation examinations. Physically active adults, whether competitive or recreational athletes, depend solely on this individual for medical clearance to participate in sport. The primary care physician is more knowledgeable about the athlete's and family's medical history, congenital or developmental deficiencies, immunization status, and recent injuries or illnesses that could limit sport participation. There is a closer examiner-athlete relationship, and when done in the physician's office, a more thorough and comprehensive exam can be completed. This setting provides greater pri-

---

➤➤ BOX 2.1

Goals of the Preparticipation Exam
- Determine general health and current immunization status
- Establish rapport with the sport participant
- Detect medical conditions that are not healed or may predispose the individual to injury or illness so medical treatment can start prior to the exercise program
- Identify health risk behaviors that may be corrected through informed counseling
- Establish baseline parameters for determining when an injured athlete may return to play
- Assess physical maturity
- Evaluate level of physical fitness
- Classify the athlete as to readiness for participation
- Recommend appropriate levels of participation of individuals with medical contraindications to exercise
- Meet legal and insurance requirements related to athletic participation

TABLE 2.1   CLASSIFICATION OF SPORTS BASED ON PEAK DYNAMIC AND STATIC COMPONENTS DURING COMPETITION

	Low Dynamic	Moderate Dynamic	High Dynamic
I. Low static	Billiards Bowling Cricket Curling Golf Riflery	Baseball Softball Table tennis Tennis (doubles) Volleyball	Badminton Cross-country skiing Field hockey* Orienteering Race walking Racquetball Running (long-distance) Soccer* Squash Tennis (singles)
II. Moderate static	Archery Auto racing*† Diving*† Equestrian*† Motorcycling*†	Fencing Field events (jumping) Figure skating* Football (American) Rodeo*† Rugby* Running (sprint) Surfing*† Synchronized swimming†	Basketball* Ice hockey* Cross-country skiing (skating technique) Football (Australian rules)* Lacrosse* Running (middle-distance) Swimming Team handball
III. High static	Bobsledding*† Field events (throwing) Gymnastics*† Karate/judo* Luge*† Sailing Rock climbing*† Water skiing*† Weight lifting*† Wind surfing*†	Body building*† Downhill skiing*† Wrestling*	Boxing Canoeing/kayaking Cycling*† Decathlon Rowing Speed skating

*Danger of bodily collision.
†Increased risk if syncope occurs.
Reprinted with permission from Mitchell J, Haskell WL, Raven PB. Classification of sports. Med Sci Sports Exerc 1994;26(10):S244.

vacy and a more optimal environment for counseling. The cost, however, is higher and the time commitment on the part of the physician is more significant.

Because some individuals may have a physician who does not understand the physical demands of a particular sport activity, organized competitive sport programs often utilize a group or station format to examine a large number of athletes during a limited time span. The team physician and several different health care providers perform a series of examinations at different stations. At the conclusion of the examination, the team physician determines the athlete's readiness for sport participation. This format is more time efficient, reduces costs significantly, and allows coaches, athletic trainers, and area medical specialists to be involved. There are, however, several disadvantages of this format, including the organizational coordination needed to execute such a comprehensive examination, the decreased privacy, the time spent with each athlete is usually brief and often impersonal, the difficulty in following up on any medical concerns that may arise, and the inability to have essential communication with parents of young and middle-age adolescents after the examination.

Timing of the Examination

Ideally, the examination is completed at least 6 weeks before the start of any practice session. This allows time to evaluate and correct minor problems, such as limited flexibility, muscle weakness, or minor illnesses without interfering with the athlete and team as they prepare for the competitive season. It also allows sufficient time for an athlete with a potential medical problem to be referred to a specialist (e.g., cardiologist, neurologist, ophthalmologist). Although many high schools and colleges do PPEs in late July or early August for fall sports, PPEs can also be completed during the spring, provided there is some mechanism to report and evaluate any injury or illness that may have occurred during the summer.

Frequency of the Examination

Although the annual complete examination is common, it is probably unnecessary unless there is a change in physician or the records are not available. A joint publication prepared by the American Academy of Family Physicians, the American Academy of Pediatrics, the American Medical

Society of Sports Medicine, and the American Osteopathic Academy of Sports Medicine recommends that an entry-level complete physical examination be performed, followed by a limited annual re-evaluation. Many physicians also complete an entry-level examination at each level of participation (e.g., middle school, high school, collegiate level). The entry-level examination is discussed in detail in this chapter. The re-evaluation should focus on the medical history and a limited physical examination, including height, weight, blood pressure, pulse, visual acuity, cardiac auscultation, and examination of the skin (5).

 Although an examination by a primary care physician can be more thorough due to their knowledge of the competitive athlete and the athlete's family, some individuals may not have a primary care physician who understands the demands of sport participation. Utilizing the team physician and other health care providers in a mass station format is another valid option for completing a detailed physical examination.

MEDICAL HISTORY

 Why is the medical history such a key component of the preparticipation exam? What general areas should be focused on? How can an athletic trainer ensure its accuracy?

A comprehensive medical history can identify nearly 60 to 75% of the problems affecting a sport participant (6). Typically, a written form is completed by the individual answering in a "yes-no" format **(Figure 2.1)**. To ensure accuracy, this information should be confirmed by the athlete or the parents of minor children. A supplemental health history questionnaire can be provided for female participants to gather information on menstrual history, as well as menstrual or vaginal irregularities, eating habits, urinary tract disorders, and use of birth control pills or hormones **(Figure 2.2)** (7).

One option to gather a medical history is to have a separate station at the start of the mass station screening. This station should have a knowledgeable examiner who can go through each questionnaire and ask detailed follow-up questions. These questions might explore current immunization status; past episodes of infectious diseases, loss of consciousness, recurrent headaches, musculoskeletal injuries, heat stroke, chest pains during or after exercise, seizures, breathing difficulties, eating disorders, and chronic medical problems; medication and drug use; allergies; heart murmurs or unusual heart palpitations; use of contact lenses, corrective lenses, dentures, prosthetic devices, or special equipment (pads, braces, neck rolls, eye guards); and family history of cardiac, vascular problems, such as sickle cell anemia, diabetes, high blood pressure, sudden death, or neurologic problems. Underweight indi-

viduals can be questioned about weight loss, eating patterns, body image, and, in the case of females, menses dysfunction.

When utilizing the group/station format, two avenues of cross-referencing can address specific responses on the medical questionnaire. One option is to "red flag" certain answers and inform the examiner at a specific station to further investigate the athlete's condition. For example, if an individual identifies that he or she has a history of exercise-induced asthma, the individual doing the pulmonary exam can question the athlete further as to the onset, extent, and severity of the condition. This option allows for the examiner who is more knowledgeable about the condition to do a more complete examination on the body system most affected by the condition. For matters of organizational brevity, specific questions related to medical history are included with each of the specific areas of the physical examination.

 The medical history is undoubtedly the most important tool of the PPE because it builds a foundation of the athlete's medical history. This information can reveal possible congenital, hereditary, or acquired conditions that may put the athlete at risk for future problems. It also offers an opportunity for counseling on issues such as substance abuse, STDs, and disordered eating habits.

THE PHYSICAL EXAMINATION

 In a comprehensive physical examination, what body systems should be fully evaluated to determine their potential impact on the athlete's readiness to participate?

The preparticipation physical examination is not intended to be all-encompassing. Rather, it is intended to focus on body systems that are of most concern to the athlete depending on the activity or sport of choice. Particular attention should be paid to any red flags identified during the medical history.

Vital Signs

The PPE should establish the athlete's baseline physiological parameters and vital statistics. Height and weight should be taken and compared to standard growth charts for prepubescent adolescents. Information such as pulse rate, blood pressure, and body temperature may be recorded at this station by an athletic trainer or other allied health professional **(Box 2.2)**.

Pulse is usually taken at the carotid artery by doubling the pulse rate during a 30-second time period. When taking blood pressure, it is important that a proper cuff size be used. The bladder should encircle the mid-arm and cover two-thirds of the length of the arm. A small cuff on a

---

Medical History Form

This evaluation is only to determine readiness for sports participation. It should not be used as a substitute for regular health maintenance examinations.

Name_____ Age (Yr)_____ Grade_____ Date_____
Address_____ Phone_____
Sports_____

The Health History (Part A) and Physical Examination (Part C [table 3]) must both be completed, at least every 24 months, before sports participation. The Interim Health History (Part B) must be completed at least annually.

Part A: Health History
To be completed by athlete and parent.

	Yes	No
1. Have you ever had an illness that:		
a. required you to stay in the hospital?	☐	☐
b. lasted longer than a week?	☐	☐
c. caused you to miss 3 days of practice or competition?	☐	☐
d. is related to allergies (e.g., hay fever, hives, asthma, insect sting reactions)?	☐	☐
e. required an operation?	☐	☐
f. is chronic (e.g., asthma, diabetes)?	☐	☐
2. Have you ever had an injury that:		
a. required you to go to an emergency room or see a doctor?	☐	☐
b. required you to stay in the hospital?	☐	☐
c. required x-rays?	☐	☐
d. caused you to miss 3 days of practice or a competition?	☐	☐
e. required an operation?	☐	☐
3. Do you take any medication or pills?	☐	☐
4. Have any members of your family under age 50 had a heart attack, had a heart problem, or died unexpectedly?	☐	☐
5. Have you ever:		
a. been dizzy or passed out during or after exercise?	☐	☐
b. been unconscious or had a concussion?	☐	☐
6. Are you able to run ½ mile (2 times around the track) without stopping?	☐	☐
7. Do you:		
a. wear glasses or contacts?	☐	☐
b. wear dental bridges, plates, or braces?	☐	☐
8. Have you ever had a heart murmur, high blood pressure, or a heart abnormality?	☐	☐
9. Do you have any allergies to any medicine?	☐	☐
10. Are you missing a kidney?	☐	☐

11. When was your last tetanus booster? _____

12. For women.
   a. At what age did you experience your first menstrual period?_____
   b. In the last year, what is the longest time you have gone between periods?_____

Explain any "yes" answers. _____
_____
_____

➤ **FIGURE 2.1 Medical history form.** A medical history should be confirmed by the athlete or the parents of minor children to ensure accuracy.

I hereby state that, to the best of my knowledge, my answers to the above questions are correct.

Date _____

Signature of athlete _____

Signature of parent _____

Part B: Interim Health History
The form should be used during the interval between preparticipation evaluations. Positive responses should prompt a medical evaluation.

1. Over the next 12 months, I wish to participate in the following sports:
    a. _____
    b. _____
    c. _____
    d. _____

                                                                        Yes   **No**
2. Have you missed more than 3 consecutive days of participation in
    usual activities because of any injury this past year?   ☐   ☐
    If yes, please indicate:
    a. Site of injury _____
    b. Type of injury _____

3. Have you missed more than 5 consecutive days of participation in
    usual activities because of an illness, or have you had a medical illness
    diagnosed that has not been resolved in the past year?   ☐   ☐
    If yes, please indicate:
    a. Type of illness_____

4. Have you had a seizure or a concussion or been unconscious for
    any reason in the last year?   ☐   ☐

5. Have you had surgery or been hospitalized in this past year?
    If yes, please indicate: ☐   ☐
    a. Reason for hospitalization_____
    b. Type of surgery_____

6. List all medications you are currently taking and what condition the medication is for.
    a. _____
    b. _____
    c. _____

7. Are you worried about any problem or condition at this time?   ☐   ☐
    If yes, please explain: _____
    _____

I hereby state that, to the best of my knowledge, my answers to the above questions are correct.

Date _____

Signature of athlete _____

Signature of parent _____

➤ FIGURE 2.1 *Continued.*

large athlete who requires a thigh cuff could cause a falsely elevated reading (11). To measure blood pressure accurately, the guidelines listed in **Field Strategy 2.1** should be followed. Individuals with abnormal heart rates or high blood pressure should be rechecked several times at 15- to 20-minute intervals, with the athlete lying down between measurements to determine if the high reading is accurate or due to anxiety ("white coat syndrome"). If three consec-utive readings are high, the athlete is identified as having hypertension (high blood pressure). **Table 2.2** shows hypertension standards by age in children, adolescents, and adults.

Athletes with severe degrees of hypertension (Stages 3 and 4) should be further examined by a physician and restricted from high static sports until the condition is controlled by lifestyle modification or drug therapy (8).

Medical History Form Questionnaire for the Female Participant

Name _____ Age _____

Directions: Please answer the following questions to the best of your ability.

1. How old were you when you had your first menstrual period? _____
2. How often do you have a period? _____
3. How long do your periods last? _____
4. How many periods have you had in the last 12 months? _____
5. When was your last period? _____
6. Do you ever have trouble with heavy bleeding? _____
7. Do you have questions about tampoon use? _____
8. Do you ever experience cramps during your period? _____
   If so, how do you treat them? _____
9. Do you take birth control pills or hormones? _____
10. Do you have any unusual discharge from your vagina? _____
11. When was your last pelvic exam? _____
12. Have you ever had an abnormal PAP smear? _____
13. How many urinary tract infections (bladder or kidney) have you had? _____
14. Have you ever been treated for anemia? _____
15. How many meals do you eat each day? How many snacks? _____
16. What have you eaten in the last 24 hours? _____
17. Are there certain food groups you refuse to eat (e.g., meats, breads)? _____
18. Have you ever been on a diet? _____
19. What is your present weight? _____
20. Are you happy with this weight? If not, what would you like to weigh? _____
21. Have you ever tried to control your weight by vomiting? _____
    Using laxatives? _____ Diuretics? _____ Diet pills?_____
22. Have you ever been diagnosed as having an eating disorder? _____
23. Do you have questions about healthy ways to control weight? _____

➤ FIGURE 2.2 **Medical history for the female participant**. Additional questions should be asked of a female athlete concerning menstrual history, eating habits, urinary tract disorders, and use of birth control pills or hormones.

Mild to moderate hypertension in the absence of organ disease or heart disease does not preclude sport participation, but this condition should be noted and evaluated on an individual basis (2,11). Once beginning a training program, the hypertensive athlete should have blood pressure remeasured every 2 to 4 months, or more frequently if indicated, to monitor the impact of exercise.

Body temperature is measured by a thermometer placed under the tongue, in the ear, or under the armpit. Additionally, infrared tympanic thermometers (ITTs) measure infrared energy emitted by the tympanic membrane, and provide a rapid, efficient, and noninvasive method of measuring body temperature.

General Medical Problems

General systemic problems should be investigated early in the PPE to allow for follow-up evaluation on any "red flags" that are noted. Information about past surgery or hospitalizations may lead to facts about a previous injury or an attempt to control a chronic disease. If a previous injury exists, it is necessary to determine if there has been an adequate amount of time for optimal healing and if subsequent rehabilitation must be completed prior to clear-

➤➤ **BOX 2.2**

Normal Vital Statistics
- Pulse

Males	60 to 100 bpm
Females	60 to 100 bpm (may increase 10 to 15 bpm during pregnancy
Children	120 to 140 bpm
Well-conditioned athletes	Can be as low as 50 bpm

- Blood pressure

Adults	120/80 mg HG
Children (age: 10 years)	105/70 mm Hg

FIELD STRATEGY 2.1 MEASURING BLOOD PRESSURE

GENERAL GUIDELINES

- No caffeine during the hour prior to the reading; no smoking 30 minutes prior to the reading
- Take the measurement in a quiet, warm setting
- Subject should sit quietly for 5 minutes with the back supported and the arm supported at the level of the heart before recording blood pressure
- The air bladder should encircle and cover two-thirds of the length of the arm. If it does not, place the bladder over the brachial artery. If the bladder is too short, misleadingly high readings can result
- Manomet: aneroid gauges should be calibrated every 6 months against a mercury manometer

TECHNIQUE

- Inflate the bladder quickly to about 200 mm Hg
- Place the stethoscope over the brachial artery in the cubital fossa
- Deflate the bladder 3 mm Hg/second and listen for the first soft beating sounds (systolic pressure)
- As pressure is reduced, the sound will become louder and more distinct, but will gradually disappear as blood no longer becomes constricted
- The pressure at which the sound disappears is the diastolic pressure
- If the sounds are weak, ask the patient to raise the arm, open and close the hand 5 to 10 times, and then reinflate the bladder quickly
- Record blood pressure, patient position, arm, and cuff size

NUMBER OF READINGS AND SITES

- Take at least two readings, separated by as much time as is practical. If readings vary by more than 5 mm Hg, take additional readings until two consecutive readings are close
- If the initial values are elevated, obtain two other sets of readings at least 1 week apart
- Initially, measure pressure in both arms; if the pressures differ, use the arm with the higher pressure
- If arm pressure is elevated, take the pressure in one leg (particularly in patients younger than 30)

---

ing the individual for sport participation. Recurrent visits to a doctor and/or hospitalization for a chronic disease suggest a poorly controlled chronic condition, such as asthma, diabetes, hypertrophic cardiomyopathy, anemia, or a seizure disorder (5). General questions on these disorders might ascertain the presence, severity, frequency, and control of these chronic disorders. This information is necessary so the condition can be adequately managed throughout the season.

Inquire about over-the-counter (OTC) medications, such as antihistamines, which may predispose the athlete to certain conditions or illnesses, such as decreased alertness, drowsiness, or heat illness. The use of birth control pills, or illicit drugs, such as anabolic steroids, amphetamines, and cocaine may lead to hypertension (8). In addition, the use of alcohol, tobacco, caffeine, ergogenic aids, or illegal substances should be identified through direct inquiry. Ask questions on general medical conditions such as:

1. Are you currently seeing a doctor for a medical problem?

2. Have you ever been diagnosed with a disease or been hospitalized overnight for a disease (e.g., diabetes, epilepsy, anemia, sickle-cell anemia, mononucleosis, hepatitis)?

3. Have you ever been diagnosed with a progressive disease (e.g., muscular dystrophy, multiple sclerosis, tuberculosis)?

4. Have you ever been hospitalized for a chronic disease or illness?

5. Have you even been told you have cancer?

6. Are you on any medications or allergic to any medications?

7. Have you ever had surgery or an operation?

8. Do you tend to bleed excessively?

9. Are you missing, or have function of only one organ (eye, kidney, lung, testicle)?

The presence of a chronic condition does not preclude activity, but the condition should be well controlled. An appropriate sport should be selected so the extent or intensity of activity does not pose a threat to the athlete's physical

TABLE 2.2   HYPERTENSION STANDARDS BY AGE IN CHILDREN AND ADOLESCENTS

	Mild Stage 1	Moderate Stage 2	Severe Stage 3	Very Severe Stage 4
Children (6 to 9 years)†				
Systolic	120-124	125-129	130-139	≥140
Diastolic	75-79	80-84	85-89	≥90
Children (10 to 12 years)†				
Systolic	125-129	130-134	135-144	≥145
Diastolic	80-84	85-89	90-94	≥95
Children (13 to 15 years)†				
Systolic	135-139	140-149	150-159	≥160
Diastolic	85-89	90-94	95-99	≥100
Adolescent (16 to 18 years)				
Systolic	140-149	150-159	160-179	≥180
Diastolic	90-94	95-99	100-109	≥110
Adult (>18 years)‡				
Systolic	140-159	160-179	180-209	≥210
Diastolic	90-99	100-109	110-119	≥120

*These definitions apply to individuals who are not taking antihypertensive drugs and are not acutely ill. When the systolic and diastolic blood pressures fall into different categories, the higher category is used to classify blood pressure status. In adults, isolated systolic hypertension is defined as a systolic blood pressure greater or equal to 140 mm Hg and a diastolic blood pressure of less than 90 mm Hg and stage appropriate. Blood pressure values are based on the average of three or more readings taken at each of two or more visits after the initial screening.

†These levels are adapted from the recommendations of the Second Task Force on Blood Pressure Control, in Children (Pediatrics 1987;79:1-25.) to be consistent with the classification in adults.

‡Reprinted with permission from the Fifth Report of the Joint National Committee on Detection, Evaluation, and Treatment of High Blood Pressure (JNC V). Arch Intern Med 1993;153:154-83.

condition. If an individual has a history of severe allergic symptoms (i.e., throat edema and airway constriction from anaphylaxis) and requires use of an Epipen, the athletic trainer should take appropriate steps to ensure one is always available should the athlete need immediate treatment for an allergic reaction. The examiner should also be concerned about problems such as acute infection, malignancy, and progressive diseases such as multiple sclerosis.

Acute illnesses (gastritis, flu, fever, diarrhea, colds, etc.) tend to be self limiting and usually require only temporary withdrawal from activity, often to prevent spread to other teammates. Many of these conditions can lead to increased dehydration, which could, in certain circumstances, increase the risk of heat disorders.

Cardiovascular Examination

The cardiovascular examination should be completed in a quiet area so outside noise will not interfere with **auscultation** of heart sounds. The physician should check for cardiac abnormalities to identify those individuals at risk for sudden death. More than 90% of sudden deaths in exercise and sports involve the cardiovascular system in participants

younger than 30 years of age; hypertrophic cardiomyopathy is the leading cause. Questions evaluating the cardiovascular system should focus on a history of loss of consciousness, **syncope** or near syncope, dizziness, shortness of breath, heart palpitations and chest pain during or after exercise, as well as sudden death occurring in a family member under 50 years of age, which may indicate a predisposition to cardiac anomalies, such as a prolonged QT syndrome, Marfan's syndrome, or mitral valve prolapse (5,9,10). Questions that should be asked of sport participants include:

1. Have you ever experienced pain or discomfort in the chest, neck, jaw, or arms during or after sport participation?
2. Have you ever experienced dizziness or passed out during or after sport participation?
3. Have you ever experienced shortness of breath at rest or with mild exercise?
4. When participating, do you tire more quickly than your teammates?
5. Have you ever had rheumatic fever, high or low blood pressure, or been told you have diabetes?
6. Have you ever noticed rapid heart palpitations or felt like your heart "raced"?
7. Have you ever been told you have a heart murmur, an irregular heart beat, or any heart disease?
8. Do you have persistent ankle swelling?
9. Has anyone in your family had any heart problems, had a heart attack, or died suddenly before the age of 50?

If the answer to any of these questions is yes, the individual should be fully evaluated by a cardiologist to determine possible conditions such as hypertrophic cardiomyopathy, conduction abnormalities, **dysarrhythmias**, valvular problems, and coronary artery defects **(Box 2.3)** (10). Hypertrophic cardiomyopathy is the most common cause of sudden death in young athletes, followed by congenital coronary artery anomalies, aortic rupture associated with Marfan's syndrome, mitral valve prolapse, and cardiac conduction disorders. In the older athlete, arteriosclerosis is almost always the cause of sudden death (10,12,13). If any of these conditions are present, strenuous activity is precluded until an electrocardiogram (ECG) or stress ECG is completed.

Pulmonary Examination

The pulmonary examination may be done in conjunction with the cardiovascular examination. The physician will auscultate for clear breath sounds and watch for symmetric movement of the diaphragm. A history of coughing spells or difficulty breathing may indicate exercise-induced bronchospasm. Although easily treated, this condition often goes undetected. In addition, up to 40% of athletes with environmental allergies or seasonal **rhinitis** will experience exercise-induced bronchospasm. Up to 80% of asthmatics will be similarly affected. Prolonged symptoms may also

➤➤ BOX 2.3

Cardiovascular Red Flags Requiring Further Examination
- Chest pain during exertion
- Unusual fatigue or shortness of breath at rest or with mild exertion
- Dizziness or syncope with activity
- Breathing difficulty while lying down
- Ankle edema
- Heart palpitations or tachycardia
- Known heart murmur
- Abnormal heart rate or arrhythmias
- Uncontrolled hypertension
- Hypertrophic cardiomyopathy
- Congenital coronary artery anomalies
- Marfan's syndrome or aortic coarctation
- Mitral valve prolapse
- Conduction abnormalities
- Arteriosclerotic coronary artery disease
- Anemia
- Enlarged spleen
- Dextrocardia (heart located on right side of chest rather than left)
- Family history of heart problems or sudden death in family

➤➤ BOX 2.4

Pulmonary Red Flags Requiring Further Examination
- Abnormal coughing
- Abnormal shortness of breath at rest or with minimal exertion
- Abnormal breath sounds (wheezing, rhonchi, rubs, or rales)
- Abnormal or prolonged expiratory phase
- Asthma (uncontrolled or exertional)
- Exercise-induced bronchospasm
- Pulmonary insufficiency
- Pneumothorax
- Severe allergies

indicate possible congenital heart defects, cardiomyopathy, or valvular dysfunction (5). The ears, nose, and mouth may also be checked at this exam station. If any hearing problems are suspected, the athlete should be referred to a specialist. Questions include:

1. Have you ever experienced excessive coughing during or after sport participation?
2. Have you ever experienced breathing difficulties or been told you have asthma, bronchitis, or allergies?
3. Have you ever had shortness of breath, or heard unusual breath sounds during or after sport participation?
4. Have you ever had a collapsed lung?

If any abnormalities are found (wheezing, rhonchi, rubs, or rales), appropriate lung function tests may be ordered. Concerns, such as tuberculosis, uncontrolled asthma, exertional asthma, exercise-induced bronchospasm, pulmonary insufficiency resulting from a collapsed lung, or chronic bronchial asthma, should be checked by the physician and discussed with the athlete (Box 2.4) (14).

Musculoskeletal Examination

The musculoskeletal examination is critical to the sport participant. A history of previous fractures, strains, tendinitis, sprains, and dislocations may suggest potential arthritis. Questions should focus on the nature of the injury, when it occurred, who evaluated it, what the duration of the treatment and rehabilitation was, and if surgical intervention was necessary. Information on wearing special protective equipment may identify injuries or conditions that

might otherwise have gone undetected. For example, the use of an ankle brace may indicate a chronic lateral ankle sprain. The use of a neck roll may indicate previous neurologic impairment of the cervical region. Questions that might be asked in this phase of the exam include:

1. Have you ever sprained or dislocated a joint?
2. Have you ever had repeated backaches or strained (pulled) a muscle?
3. Have you ever fractured any bone?
4. Do you experience any persistent swelling of a joint or body region?
5. Have you ever experienced pain in any muscle or joint when you first wake up in the morning?
6. Have you ever been awakened at night due to pain in any joint or muscle?
7. Do you ever have pain during or after activity?
8. What special protective equipment do you regularly use?

The physical examination involves a basic musculoskeletal examination (Field Strategy 2.2) (5). If red flags are noted, a more comprehensive examination of the specific body part should be completed (Box 2.5). It is also recommended to perform the apprehension test for possible glenohumeral anterior instability; the patellar grind test to

➤➤ BOX 2.5

Musculoskeletal Red Flags Requiring Further Examination
- Chronic joint or spinal instability
- Unhealed fracture, ligament, or muscular injury
- Muscle weakness
- Inflammation or infection of a joint
- Unusual hypomobility or hypermobility
- Growth or maturation disorders
- Symptomatic spondylolysis or spondylolisthesis
- Spear tackler's spine
- Herniated disc with spinal cord compression
- Repetitive stress disorders

FIELD STRATEGY 2.2 **MUSCULOSKELETAL EXAMINATION**

OBSERVE:

- Postural symmetry: Note unusual swelling or asymmetry of body segments, including scapular asymmetry, pelvic tilting, and hamstring and calf atrophy
- Back and spine: Place athlete in a forward flexed/knee extended position to detect scoliosis and assess hamstring flexibility
- Lower extremities: Note quadriceps symmetry during contraction and relaxation, genu valgus or varus, pes cavus or pes planus, and excessively pronated or supinated feet
- Squatting and duck walking to assess functional movement of the hip, knee, and ankle
- Heel standing and toe standing to assess strength and range of motion in dorsiflexion and plantar flexion, respectively

ASSESS RESISTED:

- Cervical flexion, extension, lateral flexion, and rotation
- Shoulder abduction (shrug) to determine trapezius strength
- Shoulder abduction in the neutral position and in 30 degrees of forward flexion (plane of scapula) with medial (internal) rotation to determine deltoid and supraspinatus strength, respectively
- Glenohumeral medial and lateral rotation
- Elbow flexion and extension
- Wrist flexion, extension, pronation, and supination
- Finger flexion, extension, abduction, and adduction
- Hip flexion, extension, abduction, adduction, and internal and external rotation
- Knee flexion and extension
- Ankle dorsiflexion, plantar flexion, inversion, and eversion

assess patellofemoral function; Lachman's test for anterior cruciate ligament (ACL) integrity; and the anterior drawer and talar tilt test for ankle stability (14).

When determining whether or not an individual should be limited in his or her activity, consideration must be given to the demands of the sport and the needs of the individual. For example, limited range of motion or instability in the cervical or lumbar region may preclude the athlete from participating in a collision or contact sport. An athlete with a chronic hamstring strain may need to complete a rehabilitation program prior to being cleared for participation.

Neurologic Examination

The neurologic examination need not be overly complicated. The responses to the questions will give a clear indication if the individual is at risk for serious head or nerve injuries. The neurological history should include questions on past head injuries, loss of consciousness, amnesia, or seizures. A history of seizures requires detailed information on frequency, treatment, and whether adequate control has been achieved with prescribed medication. Any episodes of brachial plexus injuries (burners or stingers) or pinched nerves should be documented if there is a history of transient **paresthesia**, loss of sensation, or motor function anywhere in the body. In addition, if an athlete has a pre-existing narrow cervical spinal canal, a straightened or reversed cervical lordotic curve, and a his-

tory of using a spear-tackling technique (**spear tackler's spine**), the individual should be fully evaluated by a neurosurgeon. A detailed examination of the neurologic system, including cervical radiographs, may be warranted before considering athletic participation. Questions may include:

1. Have you ever had a head injury or neck injury?
2. Have you ever been knocked out or been unconscious?
3. Do you have frequent or repeated headaches?
4. Have you ever had a seizure or been told you have epilepsy?
5. Have you ever had a burner stinger, or had one of your limbs feel numb or fall "asleep" during activity?
6. Have you ever had unexplained muscle weakness?

The assessment should involve pupillary examination and reaction to light (PEARL), cranial nerve assessment **(Table 2.3)**, a brief motor-sensory examination of the upper and lower extremities (see **Field Strategy 2.2**), and testing of the deep tendon reflexes **(Table 2.4)**. If problems are identified, such as recurrent concussions, headaches, or nerve palsies, the athlete should be seen by a specialist prior to being cleared for participation **(Box 2.6)**.

If seizure disorders are reported, the examiner should document the initial onset, frequency and duration of the episodes, use of medications to control the disorder, and whether the athlete is informed of the condition, its side effects, and predisposing factors (14). Individuals with epilepsy should be discouraged from activities that may involve

TABLE 2.3	CRANIAL NERVE ASSESSMENT
I. Olfactory	Identify familiar odors (chocolate, coffee)
II. Optic	Test acuity—Snellen chart (blurring or double vision)
III. Oculomotor	Test pupillary reaction to light Perform up- and downward gaze
IV. Trochlear	Perform downward and lateral gaze
V. Trigeminal	Touch face to note difference in sensation Clench teeth; push down on chin to separate jaws
VI. Abducens	Perform lateral and medial gaze
VII. Facial	Close eyes tight Smile and show the teeth
VIII. Vestibulocochlear (acoustic nerve)	Identify the sound of fingers snapping near the ear Balance and coordination (stand on one foot)
IX. Glossopharyngeal	Gag reflex; ability to swallow
X. Vagus	Gag reflex; ask athlete to swallow or say "Ahhh"
XI. Accessory	Resisted shoulder shrug
XII. Hypoglossal	Stick out the tongue

recurrent head trauma or the risk of falling, such as rock climbing, football, skiing, scuba diving, or parachuting.

Eye Examination

Visual acuity is best tested using the Snellen or common eye chart **(Figure 2.3)**. For sport activities, however, peripheral vision and depth perception may also be tested. The exam-

TABLE 2.4	DEEP TENDON REFLEX TESTING		
Reflex	Site of Stimulation	Normal Response	Nerve Segment
Jaw	Mandible	Mouth closure	Cranial nerve V
Biceps	Biceps tendon	Biceps contraction	C5-C6
Brachio-radialis	Brachioradialis tendon	Elbow flexion and/or pronation	C5-C6
Triceps	Triceps tendon	Elbow extension	C7-C8
Patellar	Quadriceps tendon	Knee extension	L3-L4
Medial hamstrings	Semimembranosus tendon	Knee flexion	L5-S1
Lateral hamstrings	Biceps femoris tendon	Knee flexion	S1-S2
Tibialis posterior	Tibialis posterior tendon behind medial malleolus	Plantar flexion with inversion	L4-L5
Achilles	Achilles tendon	Plantar flexion	S1-S2

iner should also note the presence of involuntary cyclical movement of the eyes (**nystagmus**). Although it may be normal for the individual, its presence should be documented in the athlete's medical file, especially if the individual participates in a contact or collision sport in case head trauma occurs during the season. Pupil size should also be noted. Normally the pupils are equal in size and shape. However, some individuals may have a congenital slight difference in pupil size (**anisocoria**). Again, this should be documented in case the athlete is evaluated later for a head injury. Questions related to the eye examination might include:

1. Have you ever had problems with blurring or double vision?

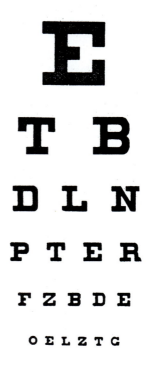

➤ **FIGURE 2.3 Snellen eye chart**. Visual acuity is measured by the Snellen or common eye chart.

▶▶ Box 2.7

Ocular Red Flags Requiring Further Examination
- Corrected vision greater than 20/50
- Vision in one eye only
- Severely limited peripheral vision
- Severe myopia (nearsightedness)
- Retinal detachment or tear

2. Have you ever injured your eyes or the area around your eyes?
3. Do you wear glasses, contact lenses, or protective eyewear on a regular basis? What type?
4. Are you visually impaired or partially impaired in either eye?
5. Are you color blind?
6. Do you have good peripheral vision?

Any positive responses to the questions, or corrected vision poorer than 20/50 (this means the athlete can read at 20 feet what the average person can read at 50 feet), or the absence of one eye will require further evaluation by an ophthalmologist (**Box 2.7**). Athletes with sight in only one eye or limited sight in both eyes may continue to participate in physical activities only if they are informed of the risks involved and understand the dangers associated with loss of depth perception, and the potential for an eye injury to the remaining good eye. These individuals should not participate in activities in which the eyes cannot be protected (e.g., boxing, wrestling, martial arts). An additional consent form specific to eye injuries should be obtained from the athlete that outlines the risks involved and the acceptance of those risks (6,14).

If the individual wears glasses, the lenses should be made of plastic, polycarbonate, or heat-treated (safety) glass to prevent them from shattering during activity. When possible, contact lenses should be of the soft type; the hard type often become dislodged, are associated more frequently with irritation from foreign bodies, and may shatter.

Myopia, or near-sightedness, should be noted, as such individuals tend to have retinal degeneration, which increases the possibility of retinal detachment. Individuals with retinal detachment may be excluded from contact sports. Those with a healed retinal tear may be allowed to participate in strenuous activity only after being examined and cleared by an ophthalmologist.

Dental Examination

A dental examination is usually done by a dentist. It is important to determine how many teeth the athlete has and the last time they were seen by a dentist. This is critical because of potential liability if teeth are avulsed (knocked out) during sport participation. Questions that can be asked include:

1. When did you last see a dentist?
2. Have you ever had any problems with your teeth or gums?
3. Have you ever experienced bleeding gums after brushing or flossing your teeth?
4. Have you ever had any teeth knocked out, damaged, or extracted?
5. Do you wear dentures, crowns, caps, or have a partial plate?
6. Do you wear a mouthguard?
7. Do you smoke cigarettes or chew tobacco?
8. Have you ever had an injury to the jaw or face?

During the examination, the dentist can assess gum condition and the presence of cavities. Dental appliance work should be checked to ensure it is in good condition. The importance of using properly fitted mouthguards and the safety and legal issues stemming from cutting down a mouthguard can be stressed. Dental red flags requiring further examination are listed in **Box 2.8**.

Gastrointestinal Examination

This examination involves evaluating the digestive system, eating habits, and nutrition. General questions on the gastrointestinal system may center on bouts of heartburn, indigestion, diarrhea, or constipation. Questions that may be asked include:

1. Do you eat regularly and have a balanced diet?
2. Do you skip meals?
3. Are there any foods groups that you predominantly eat?
4. Do you view yourself as too thin, too fat, or just right?
5. Have you ever tried to control your weight? How was this done?
6. Have you ever had excessive heartburn or indigestion?
7. Have you ever had an ulcer or vomited blood?
8. Have you ever been constipated or had diarrhea?
9. Have you ever had mononucleosis or hepatitis?

Any positive responses to the questions should be further investigated (**Box 2.9**). During the examination, the athlete

▶▶ Box 2.8

Dental Red Flags Requiring Further Examination
- Bleeding gums
- Lesions in the mouth
- Loose or displaced teeth
- Loose caps or crowns
- Dental appliances in poor condition

> ➤➤ **Box 2.9**

Gastrointestinal Red Flags Requiring Further Examination
- Organomegaly (e.g., enlarged liver or spleen)
- History of hepatitis or infectious mononucleosis
- History of repeated episodes of diarrhea or constipation
- History of gastritis or burning sensation in the stomach (ulcers)
- Extreme tenderness (e.g., over appendix, liver, or spleen)
- Suspicion of anorexia or bulimia

should be supine with the lower ribs exposed to the anterior superior iliac spines (ASIS). The examiner palpates for tenderness, masses, or **organomegaly** (enlarged organs) to ensure there is no inflammation of the liver (hepatitis, enlarged liver) or spleen, especially for individuals involved in contact sports.

In sports in which weight control is particularly important (e.g., gymnastics, ballet, crew, boxing, wrestling), it is advisable to investigate the athlete's nutritional status to determine a tendency toward anorexia or bulimia (15). This can be completed by having the athlete record his or her food intake for at least 3 days and have the record analyzed by a nutritionist.

Genitourinary Examination

Information gained at this station will vary depending on the sex of the athlete. For female athletes, a complete menstrual history should be gathered. Any responses related to **oligomenorrhea** (long cycles with 35 to 150 days between bleeding) and **amenorrhea** (no bleeding) should necessitate further assessment and counseling about the increased risk of bone demineralization (**osteopenia**), stress fractures, and potential **osteoporosis**. Gynecological symptoms that may need further evaluation include **dysmenorrhea** (painful cramps), lower abdominal pain, unusual vaginal discharge, pain during urination, and use of birth control medication. Oral contraceptives may alter the pH of the vagina and increase the risk of pelvic inflammatory disease (PID) and hypertension. Discussion surrounding the use of birth control may also promote discussion of safe sexual practices, sexually transmitted diseases, and pregnancy. Common questions that may be asked in this examination include:

1. Have you ever had problems with your kidneys or genitourinary organs?
2. Have you ever had a kidney or bladder infection?
3. Does it hurt to urinate?
4. Have you ever had a sexually transmitted disease (STD)? When? What medication was prescribed?
5. Have you noticed any skin lesions on the genitalia, or any vaginal or penile discharge?

6. Have you ever been diagnosed as having sugar, albumin, or blood in the urine?
7. Females: Have you ever been, or are you now pregnant? At what age were you when menarche first occurred? How many periods have you had in the last 6 months? When was your last menstrual period? What is the usual length of time between periods? Are the cycles fairly constant or irregular? Do you have a history of abnormal heavy bleeding (**menorrhagia**), scant bleeding, or intermittent bleeding?
8. Males: Are you missing a testicle or do you have an undescended testicle? Have you ever had a history of testicular pain or a testicular abnormality, such as a hydrocele or varicocele?

The examiner should check the kidney for CVA (costovertebral angle) tenderness. Generally, an athlete with one kidney should be warned of the risks involved in participating in contact sports, especially if the remaining kidney is abnormally positioned or is diseased (5). Males will be given a genital examination looking for hernias, testicular torsion, or an absent, undescended, or atrophied testicle. Although not necessarily required in the PPE, a urinalysis should be carried out if diabetes or kidney disease is suspected. Conditions such as **albuminuria** (protein in the urine), **hematuria** (blood in the urine), and **hemoglobinuria** (hemoglobin in the urine) can indicate problems with the urogenital system. These conditions do not preclude activity, but should be evaluated. The athlete and athletic trainer should be informed of potential dangers caused by these conditions. See **Box 2.10** for genitourinary red flags requiring further examination.

Dermatological Examination

Examination of the skin can identify contagious lesions, such as herpes simplex (cold sores), molluscum contagiosum, tinea capitis or corporis, furuncles, impetigo, scabies, and secondary syphilis, which can preclude participation in sports. Skin infections that may be contagious to other participants should be identified and treated. In contrast,

> ➤➤ **Box 2.10**

Genitourinary Red Flags Requiring Further Examination
- One kidney or diseased kidney
- Absent or undescended testicle
- Hernia (femoral or inguinal)
- Pain with urination
- Possible exercise amenorrhea or pregnancy
- Endometriosis and pelvic inflammatory disease
- Possible sexually transmitted disease
- Hematuria
- Albuminuria
- Hemoglobinuria
- Nephroptosis

➤➤ BOX 2.11

Dermatological Red Flags Requiring Further Examination

- Herpes (e.g., simplex, gladiatorum)
- Impetigo
- Molluscum contagiosum
- Tinea capitis or corporis
- Furuncles
- Secondary syphilis
- Severe acne
- Dermatitis (e.g., contact, clothes)
- Warts
- Fungal infections
- Psoriasis

➤➤ BOX 2.12

Heat-Related Red Flags Requiring Further Examination

- Cardiac disease
- Uncontrolled diabetes
- Hypertension
- Drug use (e.g., amphetamines, cocaine, hallucinogens, laxatives, narcotics)
- Medications (e.g., anticholinergics, diuretics, antihistamines, beta blockers)
- Excessive muscle cramps in heat
- Heat exhaustion
- Heat stroke

other lesions such as warts, fungal infections, contact dermatitis, psoriasis, seborrhea, and nevi (birthmarks) require further evaluation but do not necessarily mean exclusion from participation. With acne, certain medications may induce sun sensitivity or other organ toxicity (8). Early treatment can take care of the condition prior to the start of the season. Questions that might be asked include:

1. Have you ever had problems with acne?
2. Have you ever had any skin rashes, itching, or scaling in areas covered by clothing, equipment, or footwear?
3. Do you have any unusual blemishes (e.g., warts or moles) that have changed in size or color over the year?

Any skin lesion associated with a contagious or sexually transmitted disease should have immediate referral to a physician for treatment and appropriate counseling. See **Box 2.11** for dermatologic red flags requiring further examination. Chapter 27 provides more detail and photographs of dermatologic conditions.

Examination for Heat Disorders

In activities that may take place under conditions of high temperature, high humidity, or a combination of the two, a history should include questions about cramping, syncope, exhaustion, and heat stroke. Individuals taking certain medications may impair the body's ability to release heat (e.g., antihistamines), and place an individual at risk for heat illness (see Chapter 17—Environmental Conditions). Specific questions related to heat disorders might include:

1. Have you ever suffered from heat illness or heat cramps?
2. Have you ever participated in an activity in a high-temperature, high-humidity environment?
3. Have you ever passed out or become dizzy in the heat?
4. Do you have a heart problem, uncontrolled diabetes, hypertension, or poor eating habits?
5. Are you on any medications such as diuretics, antihistamines, or beta blockers?

6. Do you drink more than two alcoholic or caffeinated beverages (cola, coffee, tea) per day?

Intake of antihistamines or excessive caffeine, as well as lack of fluid and/or metabolites, can increase the risk for heat disorders. In addition, individuals at risk for heat-related disorders include poorly acclimated or poorly conditioned athletes, children, overweight or large individuals, and individuals with excessive muscle mass. If an athlete has a history of heat-related disorders or chronic illnesses, the condition should be more thoroughly investigated **(Box 2.12)**.

Laboratory Tests

Laboratory tests are not recommended by the American Academy of Pediatrics as part of a routine PPE. When used, the most frequently employed screening test has been the urine dipstick analysis for protein, glucose, and blood. However, urine testing has not proven to be effective in detecting renal disease in children (5). The cost involved, coupled with the low incidence of true renal pathology, do not bear out its use in the PPE.

Similarly, there is no evidence to support the routine use of blood work such as hemoglobin and hematocrit, complete blood count, and blood chemistries (8). However, a few states do require particular laboratory tests as a component of the PPE. If certain problems are suspected, then specific laboratory tests should be ordered. For example, if concerns exist relative to the heart, then an electrocardiogram (ECG) or stress ECG may be necessary. These tests should be reserved only for athletes with suggestive positive historical or clinical findings. In addition, in some institutions and at certain levels of competition, drug screening must be performed.

 The physical examination should focus on general systemic conditions and conditions of the cardiovascular, pulmonary, musculoskeletal, neurologic, gastrointestinal, genitourinary, and dermatological systems. In addition, the eyes and teeth should be evaluated, and the athlete's risk for heat-related illness should be identified.

PHYSICAL FITNESS PROFILE

 After the physical examination of the body is complete, what advantages can be realized from testing the physical fitness of athletes?

It is critical to assess the physical fitness status of an athlete prior to the start of physical activity to determine whether the individual possesses the attributes, skills, and abilities necessary to meet the demands of the sport. Data from the examination can identify weaknesses that may hinder athletic performance or predispose the athlete to injury, and establishes a baseline of data in the event an injury does occur (16). A physical fitness profile can assess body composition; maturation and growth; flexibility, strength, power, and speed; agility, balance, and reaction time; and cardiovascular endurance. To be effective, the parameters of the test must be relevant and specific to the selected sport. The test must be easy to perform, measure, reproduce, and be inexpensive. The test should be standardized and controlled, and should be repeated during the season to assess improvement. Results should be explained to the athletes in a meaningful way so they can understand the significance of the results (14).

Body Composition

Body composition refers to the relative percentage of body weight comprised of fat and fat-free body tissues. For the data to be accurate and reliable, the examiner must be well-trained, routinely practice the techniques, and demonstrate reliability in his/her measurements before collecting actual data. Two methods are often used to measure body composition: skinfold measurements and hydrostatic weighing. Of the two, hydrostatic weighing is more accurate, but skinfold measurement is easier and faster, and nearly as reliable.

Seven to nine skinfold sites are typically used (**Field Strategy 2.3**), although many professionals believe measurement at three sites is adequate (i.e., a different three for males and females) (9,17). Most men and women athletes should fall between 12 to 17% body fat, although these percentages are only guidelines. Some male athletes may compete at 3 to 5%, while other male and female athletes perform very well at higher body fat percentages. Additional methods of body composition measurement include girth measurements, bone diameter measurements, ultrasound measurement, arm radiograph measurement, and computed tomography (CT) assessment of fat (18).

 FIELD STRATEGY 2.3 STANDARDIZED DESCRIPTION OF SKINFOLD SITES AND PROCEDURES

Skinfold Site	Description
Abdominal	Vertical fold; 2 cm to the right side of the umbilicus
Triceps	Vertical fold; on the posterior midline of the upper arm, halfway between the acromion and olecranon processes, with the arm held freely to the side of the body
Biceps	Vertical fold; on the anterior aspect of the arm over the belly of the biceps muscle, 1 cm
Chest/Pectoral	Diagonal fold; one-half the distance between the anterior axillary line and the nipple (men) or one-third of the distance between the anterior axillary line and the nipple (women)
Medial calf	Vertical fold; at the maximum circumference of the calf on the midline of its medial border
Midaxillary	Vertical fold; on midaxillary line at the level of the xiphoid process. (An alternate method is a horizontal fold taken at the level of the xiphoid/sternal border in the midaxillary line.)
Subscapular	Diagonal fold (at a 45-degree angle); 1 to 2 cm below the inferior angle of the scapula
Suprailiac	Diagonal fold; in line with the natural angle of the iliac crest taken in the anterior axillary line immediately superior to the iliac crest
Thigh	Vertical fold; on the anterior midline of the thigh, midway between the proximal border of the patella and the inguinal crease (hip)

GENERAL GUIDELINES

- All measurements should be made on the right side of the body
- Caliper should be placed 1 cm away from the thumb and forefinger, perpendicular to the skinfold, and halfway between the crest and base of the fold
- Pinch should be maintained while reading the caliper
- Wait only 1 to 2 seconds before reading caliper
- Take duplicate measures at each site and retest if measurements are not within 1 to 2 mm
- Rotate through measurement sites or allow time for skin to regain normal texture and thickness before retesting

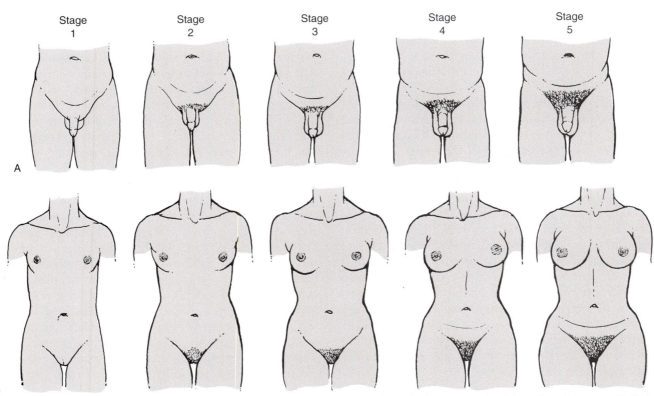

Stage 1   Stage 2   Stage 3   Stage 4   Stage 5

A

B

➤ FIGURE 2.4 **Tanner Scale of Maturity**. This scale measures breast and pubic hair development in girls and genital and pubic hair development in boys to determine the appropriate stage of maturity.

Maturation and Growth

Physical maturation refers to the developmental stage of an individual. In adolescents, growth spurts can affect sport participation and may play a role in certain injuries. The growth spurt in girls usually occurs at about age 12; in boys, it occurs around age 14. For example, a growth spurt in a gymnast may adversely affect balance and flexibility. A growth spurt in the bones of the foot may predispose a young athlete to toe deformities if shoes are not repeatedly fitted to the growing foot. Pubertal growth accounts for 20 to 25% of final adult height, and pubertal weight gain accounts for 50% of ideal adult weight (7).

The most common method of measuring maturation in males and females is the Tanner scale (4,19). The five stages of the scale are based on pictorial standards of breast development and pubic hair for females and genitalia and pubic hair for males **(Figure 2.4)**. The primary care physician is typically the individual who would conduct this examination in the privacy of the physician's office and in the presence of a parent. The adolescent is usually given a gown to avoid embarrassment in front of the parent.

Flexibility

Flexibility is the total range of motion at a joint that occurs pain-free in each of the planes of motion. In most cases, less flexibility is better than too much. However, in certain

sports (e.g., gymnastics, wrestling) excessive flexibility is a necessity. Several factors can limit flexibility and range of motion **(Box 2.13)**.

Flexibility can be measured with a goniometer, flexometer, or tape measure. Measurements can be taken to assess flexibility of the hamstrings, quadriceps, gastrocne-

---

➤➤ **BOX 2.13**

Factors Affecting Flexibility and Range of Motion
- Bony block
- Joint adhesions
- Muscle tightness
- Tight skin or an inelastic, dense scar tissue
- Muscle bulk
- Swelling
- Pain
- Presence of fat or other soft tissues that block normal motion
- Gender (women tend to be more flexible than men)
- Dominant limb tends to be less mobile than the nondominant limb
- Age (flexibility decreases with age)
- Race (Native Americans are more mobile than blacks, who are more mobile than Caucasians)
- Genetic makeup

> ➤➤ **Box 2.14**
>
> ## Hypermobile Traits
> * Passive opposition of the thumb can reach the flexor aspect of the forearm
> * Passive hyperextension of the fingers so they lie parallel with the extensor aspect of the forearm
> * Ability to hyperextend the elbow at least 10°
> * Ability to hyperextend the knee at least 10°
> * Excessive passive dorsiflexion of the ankle and eversion of the foot

mius, shoulder, and low back. **Hypermobility** (laxity in a joint) should be noted and recorded (**Box 2.14**). Laxity in one joint does not necessarily mean hypermobility in all joints or in all directions, nor does it identify a pathological state. Total range of motion can be related to genetic makeup or the stresses placed on individual joints. Loose-jointed individuals tend to do poorly in strength events and are more susceptible to ligament sprains, dislocations, chronic back pain, disc prolapse, spondylolisthesis, pes planus (flat feet), joint effusion, and tendinitis (14). If strength and endurance are not at the appropriate level in hypermobile individuals, the joints cannot be supported and may become unstable and subject to injury. These individuals should avoid further stretching exercises, and support the joint through proper positioning, balance, and strengthening programs.

In contrast, tight-jointed or **hypomobile** individuals tend to be more susceptible to muscle strains, nerve pinch syndromes, and overstress tendinitis. If a person is hypomobile, mobilization or manipulation of the affected joint in the direction of tightness may be helpful. Tight supporting structures should be stretched and active exercises are used to maintain the restored range of motion. It is important that these individuals retrain their kinesthetic sense so that the acquired range of motion can be maintained or improved (14).

Strength, Power, and Speed

Strength is the ability of a muscle or group of muscles to produce resulting force in one maximal resistance (1 RM) effort, either statically or dynamically. The demands of a particular sport or activity will dictate the level of strength needed to perform the necessary skills of that sport. Strength measures can involve isometric, isotonic, or isokinetic testing through manual muscle testing, grip strength, sit-ups, push-ups, pull-ups, or using a bench press or leg press. Power is the ability of a muscle to produce force in a given time (e.g., move the body over a distance). Power activities can be measured by throwing a medicine ball, vertical jump and reach, single- or two-legged hop for distance, and stair climbing. As with strength, power measurement should be related to the activity in which the athlete will be participating. Speed is the ability to move

body mass over time and can be assessed by timed sprints (e.g., 40-, 100-, or 400-meter run).

Agility, Balance, and Reaction Time

Agility is the ability to change directions rapidly when moving at a high rate of speed. Balance is the body's coordinated neuromuscular response to maintain a defined position of equilibrium in response to changing visual, tactile, or kinesthetic stimuli (16). Agility and balance tests are often measured by time or accuracy (e.g., correct two out of three), and should be developed to be sport specific. Reaction time is measured by the ability to respond to a stimulus. Examples of agility, balance, and reaction tests include run-and-cut drills, carioca steps, shuttle runs, pivoting drills, front-to-back and side-to-side hops, figure-of-eight running drills, kicking a stationary or moving target, and beam-walking tests.

Cardiovascular Endurance

Cardiovascular endurance, commonly called aerobic capacity, is the body's ability to sustain submaximal exercise over an extended period, and depends on the efficiency of the pulmonary and cardiovascular systems. Several tests may be used; however, selection should be dependent on the specific demands of the sport. The Harvard step test is commonly used in a physical fitness profile. The athlete is instructed to step up onto an 18-inch platform using a four step cadence "up-up-down-down" at a rate of about 30 times per minute (a metronome is used for cadence). At the conclusion of 3.5 minutes at a pace of 2 seconds per step, the athlete then sprints as fast as possible for 30 seconds (total time: 4 minutes). The athlete then immediately sits down in a chair and relaxes for 3 minutes while the pulse is determined. The pulse is taken at 30, 60, 120, and 180 seconds after the exercise. The index formula for the pulse is (14):

$$\text{Index} = \frac{\text{duration of exercise (in seconds)} \times 100}{2 \times \text{the sum of any three pulse counts}}$$

The higher the index, the better the person's fitness. If the index is less than 65, the athlete is not ready for sports activity. Other examples of common endurance tests include the 12-minute walk-run, 1.5-mile run, submaximal ergometer test, and a treadmill test. Although anaerobic fitness is not directly related to the cardiovascular system, if the proposed activity is primarily anaerobic, this measurement will involve the ability to move large muscle groups for at least 1 minute, but not more than 2 minutes (16).

 Testing the physical fitness of athletes prior to the start of the competitive season can identify poorly conditioned individuals who may be at risk for certain injuries. By identifying deficits (i.e., excessive body fat percentage, hypermobile joints, lack of flexibility, strength, power, agility, or endur-

ance), individuals can be started on a corrective program to reduce their risk of injury during the season.

CLEARANCE FOR PARTICIPATION

 What conditions might preclude an athlete from being cleared to participate in sport? Can you think of examples in which an athlete might be excluded from participating in a contact or colli-sion sport, but could be cleared to participate in other sports?

At the conclusion of the PPE, the physician must determine the level of participation based on conditions identified during the examination and knowledge of the physical demands of the sport activity. The physician must ask:

1. Will the condition increase the risk of injury to the athlete or to other participants?

TABLE **2.5**　**D**ISQUALIFYING **C**ONDITIONS FOR **S**PORT **P**ARTICIPATION					
Physical condition	**Contact/ collision**	**Limited contact/ impact**	**Noncontact— strenuous**	**Noncontact— moderately strenuous**	**Noncontact— nonstrenuous**
Atlantoaxial instability	No	No	Yes; in swimming, no butterfly, breast stroke, or diving starts	Yes	Yes
Acute illness	Requires individual assessment (e.g., contagiousness, exacerbation of illness)				
Cardiovascular Carditis	No	No	No	No	No
Hypertension Mild	Yes	Yes	Yes	Yes	Yes
Moderate	Requires individual assessment				
Severe	Requires individual assessment				
Congenital heart disease	Patients with mild forms can be allowed a full range of physical activities; patients with moderate or severe forms or those who are postoperative should be evaluated by a cardiologist before athletic participation				
Absence or loss of function in one eye	Eye guards may allow the athlete to participant in most sports, but this must be judged on an individual basis				
Detached retina	Consult an ophthalmologist				
Inguinal hernia	Yes	Yes	Yes	Yes	Yes
Absence of one kidney	No	Yes	Yes	Yes	Yes
Enlarged liver	No	No	Yes	Yes	Yes
Musculoskeletal disorders	Requires individual assessment				
History of serious head or spine trauma, repeated concussions, or craniotomy	Requires individual assessment		Yes	Yes	Yes
Convulsion disorder Poorly controlled	No	No	Yes	Yes	Yes
Well controlled	Yes	Yes	Yes; no swimming or weight lifting	Yes	Yes; no archery or riflery
Absence of one ovary	Yes	Yes	Yes	Yes	Yes
Pulmonary insufficiency	May be allowed to compete if oxygenation remains satisfactory during a graded stress test			Yes	
Asthma	Yes	Yes	Yes	Yes	Yes
Sickle cell trait	Yes	Yes	Yes	Yes	Yes
Skin: boils, herpes, impetigo, scabies	While contagious, no contact sports or gymnastics using mats		Yes	Yes	Yes
Enlarged spleen	No	No	No	Yes	Yes
Absent or undescended testicle	Yes; certain sports may require a protective cup		Yes	Yes	Yes

From American Academy of Pediatrics, Committee on Sports Medicine: Pediatrics 1988;81:737-739, with permission.

2. Can participation be allowed if medication, rehabilitation, or protective bracing or padding is used? If so, can limited participation be allowed in the interim?

3. If clearance is denied for a particular sport, are there other sports or activities in which the individual can safely participate?

Recent interpretations of the federal Rehabilitation Act and Americans with Disabilities Act have stated that individuals have the legal right to participate in any competitive sport regardless of a pre-existing medical condition. For this reason, physicians cannot totally exclude an athlete from participation, but rather can only recommend that the athlete not participate due to a medical condition that increases the risk of further injury and/or death as a result of participation (20). In these situations, an **exculpatory waiver** may be used. An exculpatory waiver is based on the athlete's assumption of risk and is a release signed by the athlete or parent of an athlete under the age of 18 that releases the physician from liability of negligence.

Most physicians base their recommendations on the American Academy of Pediatrics Committee on Sports Medicine guidelines. These conditions include atlantoaxial instability, severe hypertension, aortic disorders, tuberculosis, severe pulmonary insufficiency, uncontrolled diabetes or convulsive disorders, serious bleeding tendencies, acute infections, enlarged liver or spleen, hernias, symptomatic abnormalities or inflammations, functional instability, previous serious head trauma or surgery, renal disease, or absence of one kidney (17). In general, any athlete with a solitary paired organ, such as an eye, kidney, or testicle should be recommended not to participate in contact sports, especially if the remaining organ is abnormal. **Table 2.5** provides a more complete list of disqualifying conditions for sport participation.

 Several serious conditions can preclude an individual from participation in a contact or collision sport, including congenital glaucoma, retinal detachment, severe musculoskeletal abnormalities, repeated concussions or head trauma, certain heart abnormalities, and uncontrolled asthma, diabetes, jaundice, and acute infections. However, even with some of these conditions, a recommendation of alternative acceptable activities may exist.

Summary

1. The basic objective of the preparticipation examination is to determine the general health and fitness level of a physically active individual to ensure safe athletic participation.

2. A medical history questionnaire should be completed prior to the examination, and then validated for accuracy during the actual examination.

3. The physical examination involves assessing the vital signs, general medical conditions, cardiovascular, pulmonary, musculoskeletal, neurologic, gastrointestinal, genitourinary, and dermatologic systems. In addition, the eyes and teeth should be evaluated, and athletes at risk for heat-related illness should be identified.

4. The physical fitness of the athlete should be assessed by measuring body composition, maturation, flexibility, strength, power, speed, agility, balance, reaction time, and cardiovascular endurance.

5. At the conclusion of the examination, the physician must ask:
   - Will the abnormality increase the risk of injury to the athlete or to other participants?
   - Can participation be allowed if medication, rehabilitation, or protective bracing or padding is used? If so, can limited participation be allowed in the interim?
   - If clearance is denied for a particular sport, are there other sports or activities in which the individual can safely participate?

References

1. Smith DM. The preparticipation physical evaluation. In: The Team Physician's Handbook. Edited by Mellion MB, Walsh M, Shelton GL. Philadelphia: Hanley & Belfus, 1997.

2. Sanders B, Nemeth WC. Preparticipation physical examination. JOSPT 1996;23(2):144-163.

3. Kibler WB. The preparticipation examination. In: ACSM's handbook for the team physician. Edited by Kibler WB. Baltimore: Williams & Wilkins, 1996.

4. McKeag DB. Preparticipation screening of the potential athlete. Clin Sports Med 1989;8(3):373-397.

5. Bergfeld J, Lombardo JA, Nelson M. Pre-participation physical examination. Chicago: Joint publication by the American Academy of Family Physicians, the American Academy of Pediatrics, the American Medical Society for Sports Medicine, and the American Osteopathic Academy of Sports Medicine, 1992.

6. Hunter SC. Preparticipation physical examination. In: Orthopedic Knowledge Update: Sports Medicine. Edited by Griffin LY. Rosemont, Illinois: American Academy of Orthopaedic Surgeons, 1994.

7. Johnson MD. Tailoring the preparticipation exam to female athletes. Phys Sportsmed 1992;20(7):61-72.

8. Halpern B, Blackburn T, Incremona B, Weintraub S. Preparticipation sports physicals. In: Athletic Injuries and Rehabilitation. Edited by Zachazewski JE, Magee DJ, and Quillen WS. Philadelphia: WB Saunders, 1996.

9. American College of Sports Medicine. ACSM's Guidelines for Exercise Testing and Prescription, 5th Ed. Baltimore: Williams & Wilkins, 1995.

10. Van Camp SP. Sudden death. Clin Sports Med 1992;11(2):291-302.

11. Kaplan NM, Deveraux RB, Miller HS. Systemic hypertension. Med Sci Sports Exerc 1994;26(10):S268-S270.

12. Maron BJ. Hypertrophic cardiomyopathy in athletes: Catching a killer. Phys Sportsmed 1993;21(9):83-91.

13. Allison TB. Counseling athletes at risk for sudden death. Phys Sportsmed 1992;20(6):140-149.

14. Magee DJ. Orthopedic Physical Assessment. Philadelphia: WB Saunders, 1997.

15. Slavin J. Assessing athletes' nutritional status: Making it part of the sports medicine physical. Phys Sportsmed 1991;19(11):79-97.

16. Baker CL (ed.) The Hughston Clinic Sports Medicine Field Manual. Baltimore: William & Wilkins, 1996.

17. Magnes SA, Henderson JM, Hunter SC. What conditions limit sports participation: Experience with 10,540 athletes. Phys Sportsmed 1992;20(5):143-160.

18. McArdle WD, Katch JI, Katch VL. Exercise Physiology: Energy, Nutrition, and Human Performance, 4th Ed. Baltimore: Williams & Wilkins, 1996.

19. Tanner JM. Growth of Adolescence. Oxford, England: Blackwell Scientific Publications, 1962.

20. Mellion MB. Office Sports Medicine. Philadelphia: Hanley & Belfus, 1996.

3

Protective Equipment

OBJECTIVES

1. Describe the forces that produce focal and diffuse injuries.

2. Specify the principles used to design protective equipment.

3. Identify the different types of soft and hard materials used to make protective pads.

4. Explain the athletic trainer's legal duty of care in selecting and fitting protective equipment.

5. List the agencies responsible for establishing material standards for protective devices.

6. Describe what information should be documented to support the organization's legal duty to provide safe equipment.

7. Correctly select and fit equipment (e.g., football helmets, mouth guards, and shoulder pads).

8. Identify and describe common protective equipment for the head and face, torso, and the upper and lower body.

Protective equipment, when properly used, can protect the sport participant from accidental or routine injuries associated with a particular sport. There are, however, limitations to its effectiveness. Today's players are faster, stronger, and more skilled. A natural outcome of wearing protective equipment is to feel more secure. Unfortunately, this often leads to more aggressive play, which can result in injury to the participant or an opponent. It is the responsibility of the certified athletic trainer to ensure that protective equipment meets minimum standards of protection, is in good condition, clean, properly fitted, used routinely, and used as it was intended.

In this chapter, principles of protective equipment and materials used in the development of padding are discussed first. Secondly, protective equipment for the head and face is followed by equipment commonly used to protect the upper body and lower body. Where appropriate, guidelines for fitting specific equipment are listed in field strategies. Although several commercial braces and support devices are illustrated, these are intended to only demonstrate the variety of products available to protect a body region.

PRINCIPLES OF PROTECTIVE EQUIPMENT

 What type of protective equipment might be barred during competition? Why?

In athletic events involving impact and collisions, the sport participant must be protected from high-velocity, low-mass forces, and low-velocity, high-mass forces. High-velocity, low-mass forces occur, for example, when an individual is struck by a ball, puck, bat, or hockey stick. The low mass and high speed of impact can lead to forces concentrated in a smaller area, causing **focal injuries** (injuries concentrated in a small area, such as a bruise). Low-velocity, high-mass forces occur when an individual, for example, falls on the ground or ice, or is checked into the sideboards of an ice hockey rink, thereby absorbing the forces over a larger area, leading to **diffuse injuries** (injuries spread over a larger area, such as a concussion). The function of protective equipment is to prevent injury or protect an existing injury through the use of **prophylactic** or preventative braces.

Sport-related injuries can result from a variety of factors, including:

- Illegal play
- Poor technique
- Inadequate conditioning
- Poorly matched player levels
- A previously injured area that is now vulnerable to re-injury
- Low tolerance of a player to injury
- Inability to adequately protect an area without restricting motion
- Poor quality, maintenance, or cleanliness of protective equipment

Protective equipment can protect an area from accidental or routine injuries associated with a particular sport. This is accomplished through several means, many of which are listed in **Box 3.1**. Equipment design extends beyond the physical protective properties to include size, comfort, style, tradition, and initial and long-term maintenance costs. Individuals responsible for the selection and purchase of equipment should be less concerned about appearance, style, and cost, and most concerned about the ability of the equipment to prevent injury.

Materials Used

The design and selection of protective equipment is based on the optimal level of impact intensity afforded by the given thickness, density, and temperature of energy-absorbing material. Soft, **low-density material** is light and comfortable to wear, but only effective at low levels of impact intensity. Examples of low-density material include gauze padding, foam, neoprene, Sorbothane™, felt, and moleskin. In contrast, firmer, **high-density material** of the same thickness tends to be less comfortable, offers less cushioning of low-level impact, but can absorb more energy by deformation and thus, transfers less stress to an area at

---

> ➤➤ **Box 3.1**

Equipment Design Factors That Can Reduce Potential Injury

- Increase the impact area
- Transfer or disperse the impact area to another body part
- Limit the relative motion of a body part
- Add mass to the body part to limit deformation and displacement
- Reduce friction between contacting surfaces
- Absorb energy
- Resist the absorption of bacteria, fungus, and viruses

---

higher impact intensity levels. Examples of high-density material include thermomoldable plastics, such as orthoplast and thermoplast, and casting materials, such as fiberglass or plaster. Many of these materials are shown in **Figure 3.1**.

Another factor to consider in energy-absorbing material is **resilience** to impact forces. Highly resilient materials regain their shape after impact and are commonly used over areas subject to repeated impact. Nonresilient or slow-recovery resilient material offers the best protection, and is used over areas that are subject to one-time or occasional impact. It is important to select equipment that will absorb impact and disperse it before injury occurs to the underlying body part.

Soft Materials

Soft materials are light because of the incorporation of air into the material. Examples include gauze padding, neoprene, Sorbothane™, felt, moleskin, and foam. Gauze padding comes in a variety of widths and thicknesses, and is used as an absorbent or protective pad. Neoprene sleeves provide uniform compression, therapeutic warmth, and support for a chronic injury, such as a quadriceps or hamstrings strain. The nylon-coated rubber material is comfortable, allows full mobility, better absorption of sweat, less skin breakdown, and provides the athlete with proprioceptive feedback in the affected area (1). Sorbothane™ is often used for shoe insoles to absorb and dissipate impact forces during walking and running. Felt is made from matted wool fibers and is pressed into several thicknesses ranging from 1/4 to 1 inch thick. Felt can absorb perspiration, but in doing so, has less tendency to move under stress, but often times must be replaced daily. Moleskin is a thin felt product with an adhesive bonding on one side that prevents any movement once applied to the skin. This product is used over friction spots to reduce skin irritation or blisters.

Foam, like felt, comes in a variety of thicknesses ranging from 1/8 inch to 1 inch and ranges in density from a very soft open-cell foam to a more dense closed-cell foam. **Open-cell foam** has cells that are connected to allow air passage from cell to cell. Similar to a sponge, this material

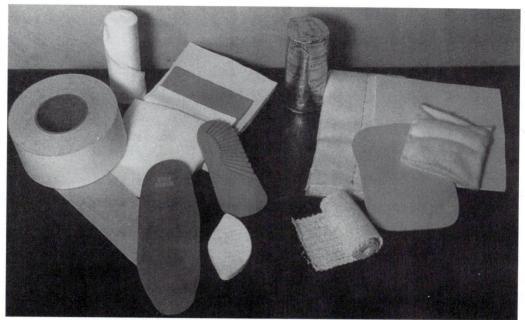

➤ FIGURE 3.1 **Materials used in protective padding**. On the left are examples of low-density material used to cushion low-level impact forces. These include moleskin, gauze padding, foam materials, neoprene, Sorbothane™, and felt. On the right are high-density materials, such as thermomoldable plastics and casting materials that can absorb more energy by deformation and thus transfer less stress to an injured area.

can absorb fluids and is commonly used to pad bony prominences or to protect the skin under hard edges of protective equipment or custom fabricated pads. Open-cell foams deform quickly under stress and, therefore, do not have good shock-absorbing qualities. **Closed-cell foam** is used primarily for protection because air cannot pass from one cell to another. The material rebounds and returns to its original shape quickly, but offers less cushioning at low levels of impact and is not as comfortable next to the skin.

To address this factor, many equipment designers layer materials of varying density. Air management pads combine open- and closed-cell foam encased in polyurethane or nylon to provide maximal shock absorption. Soft, lower density material is placed next to the skin covered by increasingly more dense, closed-cell material away from the skin to absorb and disperse higher-intensity blows. The pad is airtight, which prevents quick deformation of the foam so the energy can be dissipated over the entire surface of the pad. Air management pads are often used in football shoulder pads, but are more expensive and require extensive maintenance if the nylon covering is torn. Once torn, air can pass into the pads, reducing their effectiveness. The liners must be patched or replaced. Nylon prevents the absorption of perspiration or water, which can help avoid additional weight, and is easily cleaned with a weak bleach solution (1).

Some dense foams are thermomoldable; that is, when heated, they can be molded and shaped to fit any body part. When cooled, they retain their shape. These pads can be used repeatedly to immobilize a body structure, deflect impact, and absorb shock. The pad is secured to the body part with elastic or non-elastic tape.

Hard Materials

Hard materials include thermomoldable plastics, such as orthoplast and thermoplast, and casting materials, such as fiberglass or plaster, that can be used to splint or protect an area. Thermoplastics are divided into two categories: plastic and rubber. The plastic group uses a polycaprolactone base with varying amounts of inorganic filler, resins, and elastomers to affect the memory, stiffness, and durability of the material. The plastic category tends to conform better than the rubber-type and is more appropriate for small splints, such as on the hand. Plastics include materials such as Aquaplast Bluestripe™ (WFR/Aquaplast), Multiform I and II™ (Alimed), Orfit™ (North Coast Medical), and Orthoplast II™ (Johnson & Johnson). Rubber-like materials use a polyisoprene base and include Aquaplast Greenstrip™ (WFR/Aquaplast), Orthoplast™ (Johnson & Johnson), Synergy™ (Roylan), and Ultraform Traditions™ (Sammons) (1).

Most of these materials are heated while lying flat for about 1 minute at temperatures between 150° to 180°F. The material is then shaped for 3 to 4 minutes before returning to a hardened form. Minor changes can be made with a heat gun, but should never be performed while the splint is on the athlete.

Casting materials, such as fiberglass or plaster, are used to splint a body part, but conditions such as macerations, ulcerations, infections, burns, blisters, rashes, and allergic contact dermatitis can result from extended use. Individuals often report that such casts itch, smell, and are difficult to keep dry. Although fiberglass casts with a stockinette or cast padding can limit moisture, they must be dried (usually with a hair dryer) to prevent maceration, odor, and itching.

A new Gore-Tex™ liner developed to be used under fiberglass repels water and permits evaporation, and allows bathing, swimming, sweating, and hydrotherapy without any special drying of the cast or skin. The liner comes in 2-, 3-, and 4-inch widths and is applied directly to the skin. Fiberglass casting material is then applied over the liner. Although slightly more expensive than traditional casts, they do not have to be changed as often because they stay more comfortable throughout the immobilization period (2).

Rules Regarding Protective Pads

The National Federation of State High School Associations (NFSHSA) and the National Collegiate Athletic Association (NCAA) have specific rules regarding the use of soft and hard materials to protect a body area. The on-site referee must determine that specific fabricated pads are made of soft materials or meet the standards for hard materials established by the NFSHSA or NCAA. Hard, abrasive, or unyielding substances may be used on the hand, wrist, forearm, or elbow if the substance is covered on all exterior surfaces with no less than 1/2 inch thick, high density, closed-cell polyurethane, or a material of the same minimum thickness and similar physical properties. In addition, there must be a written authorization form signed by a licensed medical physician that indicates the cast or splint is necessary to protect the body part. This form must be available to the referee prior to the start of competition. The referee must verify that the hard material is properly padded according to the guidelines, and has the right to eject the player if he or she uses the cast or splint as a weapon.

Although protective equipment made from a hard, abrasive substance may be legally worn on the hand, wrist, forearm or elbow, it can be barred from competition if the substance is not covered on all exterior surfaces with at least 1/2 inch thick, closed-cell foam. This is designed to protect other players from injury should they be struck by the protective equipment.

LIABILITY AND EQUIPMENT STANDARDS

After fitting the kicker with a football helmet and double bar guard, the athletic trainer notices that he has come to the practice field with a single face guard. What legal ramifications may exist if the athlete sustains a facial or head injury during a practice or game?

Legal issues concerning protective equipment are a major concern for every athletic trainer and organized sport program. An organization's duty to ensure the proper use of protective equipment is usually a shared responsibility among the members of the athletic staff. For example, the head coach may be responsible for recommending specific equipment for his or her sport. The athletic director may be responsible for purchasing this recommended equipment. The equipment manager or athletic trainer may then be responsible for properly fitting the equipment based on the manufacturer's guidelines, instructing and warning the athlete about proper use of the equipment, regularly inspecting the protective equipment, and keeping accurate records of any repair or reconditioning of the equipment.

In Chapter 1, negligence and standard of care for the certified athletic trainer were discussed in broad terms. When focusing on protective equipment, the athletic trainer has a duty to select the most appropriate equipment, properly fit it to the individual athlete, instruct the athlete in its care, warn the athlete of any danger in using the equipment inappropriately, and supervise and monitor its proper use. Again, manufacturers have a duty to design, manufacture, and package safe equipment that will not cause injury to an individual when the equipment is used as it was intended.

To protect the sport participant from ineffective and poorly constructed athletic equipment, several agencies have developed standards of quality to ensure that equipment does not fail under normal athletic circumstances or contribute to injury. The National Operating Committee on Standards for Athletic Equipment (NOCSAE) sets the standards for football helmets to tolerate certain forces when applied to different areas of the helmet. Currently, baseball, softball, and lacrosse helmets and facemasks must also be NOCSAE certified. Other testing agencies for protective equipment include the American Society for Testing and Materials (ASTM) and the Hockey Equipment Certification Council (HECC) of the Canadian Standards Association (CSA). These agencies have established material standards for equipment such as protective eye wear, ice hockey helmets, and facemasks.

In addition to agencies that establish standards for the manufacture of equipment, athletic governing bodies establish rules for the mandatory use of specific protective equipment and determine rules governing special protective equipment. These governing bodies include the National Federation of State High School Associations (NFSHSA), the National Association of Intercollegiate Athletics (NAIA), the National Collegiate Athletic Association (NCAA), and the United States Olympic Committee (USOC). For example in football, the NCAA requires the use of a facemask and helmet with a secured, four-point chin strap. All players must wear helmets that carry a warning label regarding the risk of injury and a manufacturer's or reconditioner's certification indicating the equipment meets the NOCSAE test standards (3).

After equipment has been purchased, the manufacturer's information materials, such as brochures and warranties used in the selection process, should be cataloged for reference in the event an injury occurs. This information can document the selection process and particular attributes of the equipment ultimately chosen. When an athlete provides his or her own protective equipment, the responsibilities of the athletic trainer do not change. The athletic trainer still must ensure that the equipment meets safety standards and is fitted correctly, properly maintained and cleaned, and used appropriately. Athletic trainers and coaches should know the dangers involved in using sport equipment and have a duty to properly supervise its fitting and intended use. Athletes should not be allowed to wear any equipment or alter any equipment that may endanger the individual or other team members.

 Interscholastic and collegiate athletic governing bodies require helmet face protection to be no less than two bars. As such, the single bar does not meet minimum protection standards and should not be allowed on the helmet. The athletic trainer must inform the player of the safety concerns with only one bar, then replace it with an appropriate legal face guard.

PROTECTIVE EQUIPMENT FOR THE HEAD AND FACE

 What standards exist for eye protective wear? Do spectacles or contact lenses protect the eyes from injury?

Many head and facial injuries can be prevented with regular use of properly fitted helmets and facial protective devices, such as face guards, eye wear, ear wear, mouthguards, and throat protectors. Helmets, in particular, are required in football, ice hockey, men's lacrosse, baseball, softball, whitewater sports (kayaking), amateur boxing and bicycling, and must be fitted properly to disperse impact forces.

Football Helmets

Football helmet designs are typically a single or double air bladder, closed-cell padded, or a combination of the two. Air bladders are excellent at absorbing shock, but must be inspected daily by the players to ensure that adequate inflation is maintained for a proper fit. Helmet shells can be constructed of plastic or a polycarbonate alloy. Polycarbonate is a plastic used in making jet canopies and police riot gear, and is lightweight, scratch- and impact-resistant. Helmets vary in life expectancy. The polycarbonate alloy shell has a 5-year warranty; the ABS plastic shell has a 2-year warranty; the Athletic Helmets, Inc., helmet should be retired after 6 years; and Riddell recommends retiring their helmet after 10 years (2).

Helmets must be NOCSAE approved. Heat, as an environmental factor, can alter the effectiveness of shock absorption in the liner and some shell materials. As a result, materials compress more easily and absorb less shock at higher temperatures than lower. To compensate, NOCSAE drops the helmet twice within 1 minute from a height of 152 cm (60 inches) on the right frontal boss in ambient temperature. The process is repeated after soaking the helmet for 4 hours at 49°C (120°F). The helmet must meet the same criterion at both temperatures (4). The NOCSAE mark on a helmet indicates it meets minimum impact standards and can tolerate forces applied to several different areas of the helmet. NOCSAE also includes a warning label regarding risk of injury on each helmet that states:

> **Warning**: Do not strike an opponent with any part of this helmet or face mask. This is a violation of football rules and may cause you to suffer severe brain or neck injury, including paralysis or death. Severe brain or neck injury may also occur accidentally while playing football. NO HELMET CAN PREVENT ALL SUCH INJURIES. USE THIS HELMET AT YOUR OWN RISK.

This warning label must be clearly visible on the exterior shell of all new and reconditioned helmets. In addition, the athletic trainer and coach should continually warn athletes of the risks involved in football and ensure that the helmet is properly used within the guidelines and rules of the game.

Always follow manufacturers' guidelines when fitting a football helmet. Prior to fitting, the athletes should have haircuts in the style that will be worn during the athletic season, and wet their heads to simulate game conditions. **Field Strategy 3.1** lists the general steps in fitting a football helmet. Once fitted, the helmet should be checked daily for proper fit, which can be altered by hair length, deterioration of internal padding, loss of air from cells, and spread of the facemask. This is performed by inserting a tongue depressor between the pads and face. When moved back and forth, a firm resistance should be felt. A snug-fitting helmet should not move in one direction when the head moves in another. In addition, the helmet should be checked weekly by the athletic trainer to ensure proper fit and compliance with safety standards **(Box 3.2)**.

➤➤ **BOX 3.2**

Weekly Helmet Inspection Checklist
- Check proper fit according to manufacturer's guidelines.
- Examine the shell for cracks, particularly around the holes. Replace the shell if any cracks are detected.
- Examine all mounting rivets, screws, Velcro®, and snaps for breakage, sharp edges, and/or looseness. Repair or replace as necessary.
- Replace the face guard if bare metal is visible, has a broken weld, or is grossly misshapen.
- Examine and replace any parts that are damaged, such as jaw pads, sweatbands, nose snubbers, and chin straps.
- Examine the chin strap for proper shape and fit; inspect the hardware to see if it needs replacement.
- Inspect shell according to NOCSAE and the manufacturer's standards: only approved paints, waxes, decals, or cleaning agents are to be used on any helmet. Severe or delayed reaction to the substances may permanently damage the shell and affect its safety performance.
- If air- and fluid-filled helmets are used, and the team travels to a different altitude, recheck the fit prior to use.

FIELD STRATEGY 3.1   **PROPER FITTING OF A FOOTBALL HELMET**

1. The player should have a haircut in the style that will be worn during the competitive season and should wet his hair to simulate game conditions. Measure the circumference of the head above the ears, using the tape measure supplied by the manufacturer. The suggested helmet size is listed on the reverse side of the tape.

2. Select the proper sized shell, and adjust the front and back sizers and jaw pads for a proper fit.

3. Inflate the air bladder by holding the bulb with an arch in the hose; to deflate, the hose is in a straight position.

4. Ensure that the helmet fits snugly around the player's head and covers the base of the skull, but does not impinge the cervical spine when the neck is extended. The ear holes should match up with the external auditory ear canal.
   - Check that the four-point chin strap is of equal tension and length on both sides, placing the chin pad an equal distance from each side of the helmet (**Figure A**).
   - Check that the facemask allows for a complete field of vision and the helmet is one to two finger widths above the eyebrows and extends two finger widths away from the forehead and nose (**Figure B**).
   - Check that the helmet does not move when the athlete presses forward on the rear of the helmet and when he presses straight down on top of the helmet (**Figure C**).
   - Check that the helmet does not slip when the athlete is asked to "bull" their neck while you grasp the facemask pulling left then right (**Figure D**).

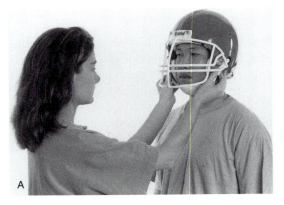

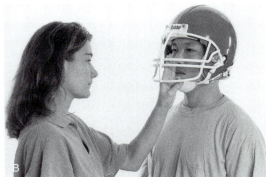

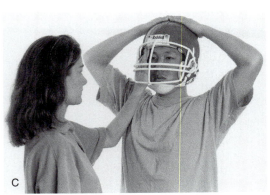

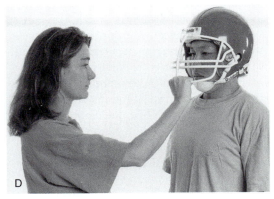

Each helmet should have the purchase date and tracking number engraved on the inside. Detailed records should be kept that identify the purchase date, use, reconditioning history, and certification seals. Each athlete should also be instructed on the proper use, fit, and care of the helmet. In addition, each athlete should sign a statement that confirms he or she has read the NOCSAE seal and been informed of the risks of injury through improper use of the helmet or facemask when striking an opponent. This statement should be signed, dated, and kept as part of the player's medical files.

Ice Hockey Helmets

Ice hockey helmets must absorb and disperse high-velocity, low-mass forces, e.g., being struck by a stick or puck, and

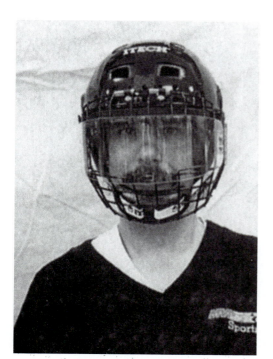

➤ FIGURE 3.2 **Ice hockey helmet.** Helmets used in ice hockey must absorb and disperse high velocity–low-mass forces (being hit by a high stick or puck), and low velocity–high-mass forces (being checked into the boards). Full face guards may be clear or wire mesh.

low-velocity, high-mass forces, e.g., being checked into the sideboard or falling on the ice. As with football helmets, ice hockey helmets reduce head injuries; however, they do not prevent neck injuries due to axial loading, (force of impact is exerted along the long axis of a structure). The use of head protection with a facemask seems to have given many players a sense of invulnerability to injury. Studies have shown that the risk of spinal cord injury, and in particular quadriplegia, may be as high as three times greater in hockey than in American football (5). The major mechanism for this injury is head-first contact with the boards secondary to a push, or a check from behind.

Ice hockey helmet standards are monitored by the American Society for Testing and Materials (ASTM) and the Hockey Equipment Certification Council (HECC) and are required to carry the stamp of approval from the Canadian Standards Association (CSA) **(Figure 3.2)**. Proper fit is achieved when a snug-fitting helmet does not move in one direction when the head is turned in the other.

Batting Helmets

Batting helmets used in baseball and softball require the NOCSAE mark and must be a double ear-flap design. It is best to have a thick layer of foam between the primary energy absorber and head to allow the shell to move slightly and deform. This maximizes its ability to absorb missile kinetic energy from a ball or bat and prevents excessive pressure on the cranium. The helmet should be snug enough so it does not move or fall off during batting and running bases.

Other Helmets

Lacrosse helmets are mandatory in the men's game, optional in the women's game, and are also worn by field hockey goalies. The helmet is made of a high-resistant plastic or fiberglass shell, and must meet NOCSAE standards. The helmet, wire face guard, and chin pad are secured with a four-point chin strap **(Figure 3.3)**. The helmet should not move in one direction when the head moves in another.

An effective bicycle helmet has a plastic or fiberglass rigid shell with a chin strap and an energy-absorbing foam liner. Regardless of the type, the helmet can provide substantial protection against head injuries and injuries to the upper and midface region (6). A stiffer shell results in better diffusion and resilience to impact. A firmer, dense foam liner is more effective at higher velocities, whereas a less stiff foam provides more protection at lower velocities. Increasing the thickness of the liner may lead to a more effective level of protection, but the increased mass and weight of the helmet may make it more uncomfortable. In addition, helmets today have more ventilation ports and are more lightweight and aerodynamic than ever before. Wearing a cycling helmet does not increase thermal discomfort to the head or body and has no additional impact on core temperature, head skin temperature, thermal sensation, heart rate, sweat rate, and overall perceived exertion (7). As in other helmets, a snug fit is necessary for a proper fit.

Face Guards

Face guards vary in size and style and protect and shield the facial region from flying projectiles. NOCSAE has set standards for strength and deflection for football face guards worn at the high school and college levels. Football

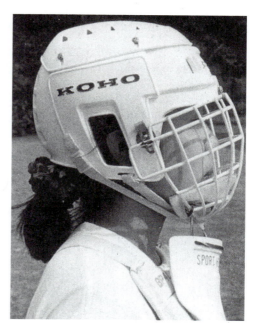

➤ FIGURE 3.3 **Lacrosse helmet.** Lacrosse helmets provide full face and neck protection.

face guards are made of heavy-gauge, plastic-coated steel rod, designed to withstand impacts from blunt surfaces, such as the turf or another player's knee or elbow. The effectiveness of a football face guard depends on the strength of the guard itself, the helmet attachments, and the four-point chin strap on the helmet. When properly fitted, the facemask should extend two finger widths away from the forehead and allow for complete field of vision (see **Field Strategy 3.1**). No face protection should be less than two bars. If needed, eye shields made of Plexiglas or polycarbonate can be attached to the facemask.

Ice hockey face guards are made of clear plastic (polycarbonate), steel wire, or a combination of the two, and must meet HECC and ASTM standards **(Figure 3.2)**. Hockey face guards primarily prevent penetration of the hockey stick, but are also effective against flying pucks and collisions with helmets, elbows, side boards, and the ice. The use of full-coverage facemasks in amateur ice hockey has greatly reduced facial trauma. The use of a single chin strap, however, still allows the helmet to ride back on the head when a force is directed to the frontal region, thus exposing the chin to lacerations. The guard stands away from the nose approximately 1 to 1 1/2 inches. If a wire mesh is used, the holes should be small enough to prevent penetration by a hockey stick.

Lacrosse face guards must meet NOCSAE standards. The wire mesh guard stands away from the face, but the four-point chin strap has a padded chin region in case the guard is driven back during a collision with another player (see **Figure 3.3**). Face masks used by catchers and the home plate umpire in baseball and softball should fit snugly to the cheeks and forehead, but should not impair vision **(Figure 3.4)**. These devices can be used on players in the field and must meet ASTM standards. Men's and women's fencing masks have an adjustable spring to prevent the mask from moving during competition.

Eye Wear

Eye injuries are relatively frequent and almost always preventable, yet no interscholastic or intercollegiate sport re-

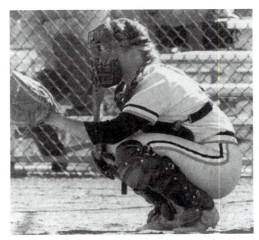

➤ FIGURE 3.4 **Facial protection**. Baseball and softball catchers must wear full face and neck protection.

quires protective eye wear. There are three types of protective eye wear: goggles, faceshields, and spectacles. Goggles have two designs. One is the eyecup design seen in swimming, whereby the eye socket is completely covered. They are made of hard, impact-resistant plastic that is water tight. Because of the streamlined shape and design, contact lenses may be worn during competition. Vision may be slightly distorted, however, enhanced vision with the goggles could be a great advantage during flip-turns. The other style can be worn over spectacles, such as a ski goggle. These are usually well ventilated to allow air currents to minimize fogging. Faceshields are secondary protective devices that can be attached to specific helmets. Athletes who wear contact lenses often prefer the shield because there is less chance that a finger or hand can hit the eye. The shield can be tinted to reduce glare from the sun; however, the plastic can become scratched and may fog up in cold weather.

Spectacles (eye glasses) contain the lenses, frame, and side shields commonly seen in industrial eye protective wear. The lenses should be 3 mm thick and be made from CR 39 plastic or polycarbonate, both of which can be incorporated with prescription lenses. CR 39 plastic lenses are less expensive, but scratch more easily, are often thicker and heavier than polycarbonate, and are not impact resistant. In contrast, polycarbonate is lightweight, scratch-resistant, and can have an antifog and ultraviolet inhibitor incorporated into the lens (1). Polycarbonate has the greatest impact resistance of the clear materials developed for protective equipment. A disadvantage of the polycarbonate is that static charges will cause dust to cling to the lenses more readily than glass lenses.

The frame should be constructed of a resilient plastic, with reinforced temples, hinges, and nose piece. Adequate cushioning should protect the eyebrow and nasal bridge from sharp edges. Only polycarbonate eye protectors and eye frames that meet ASTM and parallel CSA standards, offer enough protection for a sport participant. Approved eye guards protect the eye when impacted with a racquet ball traveling at 90 mph (40 meters per second) or a racquet going 50 mph (22.2 meters per second). Approved eye guards will state so on the package **(Figure 3.5)**.

Regardless of the type of protection used, the lenses should be cleaned with warm soapy water and rinsed with clean water, or a commercially available eye glass cleaner should be used. A soft cloth is used to blot dry the lenses. You should never wipe or rub a dry lens, because of the possibility of scratching the lens by moving foreign particles across the surface. The frames and elastic straps may also be cleaned with soap and water and air dried. Lenses should be replaced when scratches affect vision or cracks appear at the edges. Always store protective eye wear in a hard case to protect the polycarbonate lenses from being scratched.

Any individual with monocular vision or vision in only one eye should consult an ophthalmologist prior to participation in any sport because of the reduced visual fields and depth perception. If a decision is made to participate, the

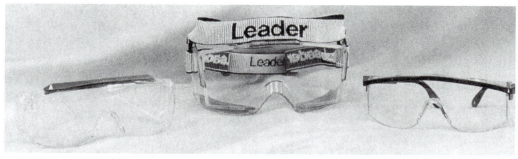

➤ FIGURE 3.5 **Eye protectors**. Protective eyewear should be made from polycarbonate, which is lightweight, scratch- and impact-resistant, and meet ASTM or CSA standards.

individual should wear maximum eye protection during all practices and competitions. Sport participants should wear a sweatband to keep sweat out of the eye guard and should remove the eye guard when not participating.

Although sport participants often wear contact lenses because they improve peripheral vision and astigmatism, and do not normally cloud during temperature changes, they do not protect against eye injury. Contact lenses come in two types: hard, or corneal type lens, which covers only the iris of the eye; and soft, or scleral type, which covers the entire front of the eye. Hard contact lenses often become dislodged, and are associated more frequently with irritation from foreign bodies (corneal abrasions). Dust and other foreign matter may get underneath the lens and damage the cornea, or the cornea may be scratched while inserting or removing the lens.

Soft contact lenses can protect the eye from irritation by chlorine in pools. Although research has shown that pool water causes soft lenses to adhere to the cornea, reducing the risk of loss, wearing soft lenses while swimming is not recommended. Micro-organisms found in pool water, especially *Acanthamoeba*, are responsible for a rare, but serious, corneal infection, *Acanthamoeba* keratitis. It is recommended that goggles should always be worn in water, with or without contact lenses, to protect against organisms in the water and irritation from chlorine. Swimmers should wait 20 to 30 minutes after leaving the water to remove the contact lenses or use saline drops if the lenses must be removed earlier. This allows time for the lenses to stop sticking to the cornea. Lenses should then be immediately disinfected. Removing the lenses too soon may cause corneal abrasions, leaving the cornea susceptible to infection.

Ear Wear

With the exception of boxing, wrestling, and water polo, few sports have specialized ear protection **(Figure 3.6)**. Repeated friction and trauma to the ear can lead to a permanent deformity, called hematoma auris or cauliflower ear (see Chapter 8). For this reason, ear protection should be worn regularly in these sports. Proper fit is achieved when the chin strap is snug and the head gear does not move during contact with another player. The protective ear cup should be deep enough so as not to compress the external ear.

Mouthguards

An intraoral readily visible mouthguard is required in all interscholastic and intercollegiate football, ice hockey, field hockey, and men's and women's lacrosse. Properly fitted across the upper teeth, a mouthguard can absorb energy, disperse impact, cushion contact between the upper and lower teeth, and keep the upper lip away from the incisal edges of the teeth. This action significantly reduces dental and oral soft-tissue injuries, and to a lesser extent jaw fractures, cerebral concussions, and temporomandibular joint (TMJ) injuries. The practice of cutting down mouthguards to cover only the front four teeth invalidates the manufacturer's warranty, cannot prevent many dental injuries, and can lead to airway obstruction, should the mouthguard become dislodged. Although players may complain that use of a mouthguard interferes with speech and can reduce forced expiratory air volume and peak expiratory flow rates, the benefits of preventing oral injuries far outweigh the disadvantages (8).

The most frequently used mouthguard is the thermal set, mouth-formed mouthguard, which consists of a firm

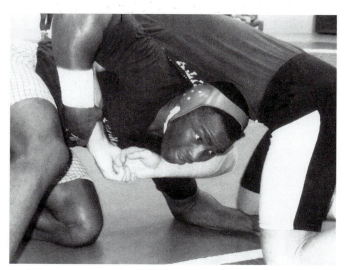

➤ FIGURE 3.6 **Ear protectors**. Protective ear wear can prevent friction and trauma to the ear that may lead to permanent deformity.

outer shell, fitted with a softer inner material. The softer material is thermally or chemically set after being molded to the player's teeth. When properly fitted, the mouth-formed guard can virtually match the efficacy and comfort of the custom-made guard. This type of guard is readily available, inexpensive, and has a loop strap for attachment to a facemask. The loop strap has two advantages in that it prevents individuals from choking on the mouthguard, and prevents the individual from losing the mouthguard when it is ejected from the mouth. These mouthguards often lack full extension into the labial and buccal vestibules. Therefore, they do not provide adequate protection against oral soft-tissue injuries. Furthermore, the thermoplastic inner material loses its elasticity at mouth temperature and may cause the protector to loosen. **Field Strategy 3.2** demonstrates how to fit a thermoplastic mouth-formed mouthguard.

The most effective type of mouth protector is the pressure-formed laminated type. This protector is expensive and requires special training to obtain the best results. In addition, the cost of the basic materials is higher than vacuum-formed mouthguards. The laminated mouthguard uses high heat and pressure to form the material leading to less deformation of the material when worn for a long period of time. In addition, the mouthguard can be thickened in selected areas as needed and may have inserts added for additional wearer protection. Vacuum-formed mouthguards, on the other hand, are less expensive and easier to design. Because of the low heat used in the construction, their fit, however, can be compromised by an elastic memory. After a few minutes of wearing the mouthguard, the warmth from the mouth can trigger the elastic memory leading to adaptations in the design making speaking and unrestricted breathing more difficult (8).

The recommended care of mouthguards is to thoroughly rinse the guard with water after each use and place it in a plastic mouthguard retainer box to air dry. Periodically, the mouthguard should be soaked over night in a weak bleach solution (1 quart water to 1 tablespoon of bleach).

Throat and Neck Protectors

Blows to the anterior throat can cause serious airway compromise as a result of a crushed larynx and/or upper trachea, edema of the glottic structures, vocal cord disarticulation, hemorrhage, or laryngospasm. The NCAA requires that

---

 FIELD STRATEGY 3.2   FITTING MOUTH-FORMED MOUTHGUARDS

1. Submerge the mouthguard (not the loop strap) in boiling water for 20 to 25 seconds. Shake off excess water but do not rinse the mouthguard in cold water as this decreases pliability.
2. Place the mouthguard directly in the mouth over the upper dental arch. Center the mouthguard with the thumbs using the loop strap as a guide **(Figure A)**.
3. Close the mouth, but do not bring the teeth together or bite down on the mouthguard. Place the tongue on the roof of the mouth and *suck* as hard as possible for 15 to 25 seconds. The sucking mechanism acts as a vacuum to mold the mouthguard around the teeth and gums **(Figure B)**.
4. Rinse the mouthguard in cold water to harden the material. Check the finished product for any significant indentations. If any imperfections or errors are noted, do not reheat the mouthguard as this decreases its effectiveness. Select a new mouthguard and repeat the process.

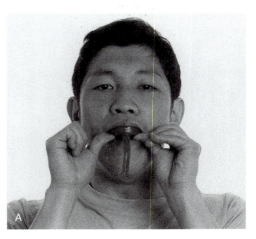

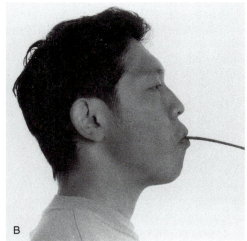

catchers in baseball and softball wear a built-in or attach-able throat guard on their masks (see **Figure 3.4**) (4). Fencing masks and helmets used in field hockey, lacrosse, and ice hockey also provide anterior neck protectors to protect this vulnerable area.

Cervical neck rolls and collars are designed to limit motion of the cervical spine and are effective in protecting players with a history of repetitive burners or stingers. Properly fitted shoulder pads are perhaps the most critical factor, however, in preventing brachial plexus injuries. Several commercial collars can be added to the shoulder pads, including the Cowboy collar™ (McDavid), Long Horn neck roll™, LaPorta collar™, and numerous others of similar design.

The Cowboy collar is a closed-cell polyethylene foam that fits underneath the shoulder pads **(Figure 3.7)**. This collar can be further reinforced by adding a plastic back plate along the posterior aspect of the support. The Long Horn neck roll is larger in diameter than conventional foam collars and can further restrict motion by attaching auxiliary pads over the collar at specific sites. The LaPorta collar is a more rigid plastic shell secured directly to the shoulder-pad arch. The helmet wedges into the collar, further restricting cervical motion (1). Cervical collars, however, do not decrease axial loading on the cervical spine when the neck is flexed during a tackle.

 Protective eyewear should be 3 mm thick and be made from CR 39 plastic or polycarbonate. CR 39 plastic lenses are generally less expensive, but scratch more easily and are not impact resistant. In contrast, polycarbonate is lightweight, scratch-resistant, impact-resistant, and can have an antifog and ultraviolet inhibitor incorpo-

 rated into the lens. Although contact lenses improve peripheral vision and astigmatism, and do not normally cloud during temperature changes, they do not protect against eye injury.

PROTECTIVE EQUIPMENT FOR THE UPPER BODY

What is the basis behind a cantilevered system of protection in football shoulder pads? Is this superior to flat shoulder pads?

In the upper body, special pads and braces are often used to protect the shoulder region, ribs, thorax, breasts, arms, elbows, wrists, and hands. Depending on the sport, special design modifications are needed to allow maximum protection while providing maximal performance.

Shoulder Protection

Shoulder pads should protect the soft and bony tissue structures in the shoulder, upper back, and chest. The external shell is generally made of a lightweight, yet hard plastic. The inner lining may be composed of closed-cell or open-cell padding to absorb and disperse the shock; however, use of open-cell padding reduces peak impact forces when compared with closed-cell pads.

Football shoulder pads are available in two general types: cantilevered and flat. A channel system, incorporated into both types, utilizes a series of long, thinner pads attached by Velcro® in the shoulder pads. The pads can be individually fitted so there is an air space at the acromioclavicular (AC) joint. The impact forces are placed entirely on the anterior and posterior aspect, of the shoulder.

Cantilever pads have a hard plastic bridge over the superior aspect of the shoulder to protect the AC joint. These bridges are lightweight, allow maximal range of motion at the shoulder, and can distribute the impact forces throughout the entire shoulder girdle. The cantilevers come in three types: inside, outside, and double cantilever. The inside cantilever fits under the arch of the pads and rests against the shoulder. It is more commonly used because it is less bulky than the outside cantilever, which sits on top of the pad, outside of the arch. The outside cantilever is preferred by linemen because it provides a larger blocking surface and more protection to the shoulder region. The double cantilever is a combination of the inside and outside cantilever. It provides the greatest amount of protection, but is not feasible for all players because of its bulk.

Flat shoulder pads are lightweight, provide less protection to the shoulder region, but allow more glenohumeral joint motion. These pads are often used by the quarterback or receivers who must raise their arms above the head to

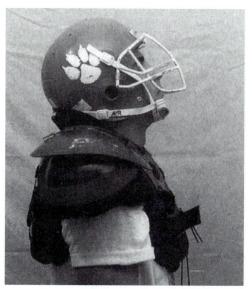

➤ **FIGURE 3.7 Cervical collars.** A high, thick stiff posterolateral pad at the base of the neck can provide added protection to the cervical spine, but cannot reduce axial loading during a tackle when the head is lowered.

throw or catch a pass. The flat pads often use a belt buckle strapping to prevent pad displacement, since the elastic webbing straps typically seen in most shoulder pads are inadequate in maintaining proper positioning of the flat pads.

In addition to cantilevers, football shoulder pads consist of an arch, two sets of epaulets (shoulder flaps), shoulder cups, and anterior and posterior pads. The arch is shaped to fit the contour of the upper body. The epaulets extend from the edge of the arch and cover the shoulder cups to protect the top of the entire shoulder region. The shoulder cups attach to the arch, run under the epaulets, and should cover the entire deltoid. The anterior pads cover the pectoral muscles and protect the sternum and clavicles. The posterior pads cover the trapezius and protect the scapula and spine.

Football shoulder pads should be selected based on the player's position, body type, and medical history. Linemen need more protection against constant contact and use larger cantilevers. Quarterbacks, offensive backs, and receivers require smaller shoulder cups and flaps to allow greater range of motion in passing and catching. **Field Strategy 3.3** lists the general steps used in fitting football shoulder pads.

 FIELD STRATEGY 3.3   FITTING FOOTBALL SHOULDER PADS

1. Determine the chest girth measurement at the nipple line or measure the distance between shoulder tips. Select pads based on the player's position. Place the pads on the shoulders and tighten all straps and laces. The laces should be pulled together until touching. The straps should have equal tension and be as tight as functionally tolerable to ensure proper force distribution over the pads. Tension on the straps should prevent no more than two fingers from being inserted under the strap. The entire clavicle should be covered and protected by the pads. If the clavicles can be palpated without moving the pads, refit with a smaller pad **(Figure A)**.
2. Anterior view: The laces should be centered over the sternum with no gap between the two halves. There should be full coverage of the acromioclavicular joint, clavicles, and pectoral muscles. Caps should cover the upper portion of the arch and entire deltoid muscle **(Figure B)**.
3. Posterior view: The entire scapula and trapezius should be covered with the lower pad arch extending below the inferior angle of the scapula to adequately protect the latissimus dorsi. The laces should be pulled tight and be centered over the spine **(Figure C)**.
4. With the arms abducted, the neck opening should not be uncomfortable or pinch the neck. Finally, inspection should include the shoulder pads with the helmet and jersey in place to ensure that no impingement of the cervical region is present **(Figure D)**.

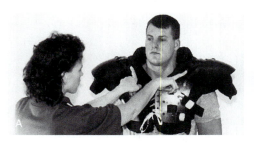

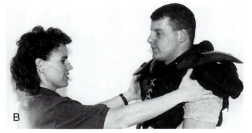

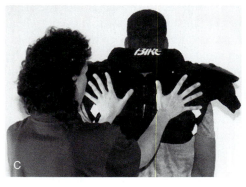

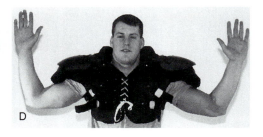

Elbow, Forearm, Wrist, and Hand Protection

The entire arm is constantly subjected to compressive and shearing forces, such as those seen in blocking and tackling an opponent, deflecting projectiles, pushing opponents away to prevent collisions, or breaking a fall. Goalies and field players in many sports are required to have arm, elbow, wrist, and hand protection. However, in high school and collegiate play, no rigid material can be worn at the elbow or below unless covered on all sides by closed-cell foam padding (3). A counterforce forearm brace may be worn by certain individuals with lateral epicondylitis to reduce tensile forces in the wrist extensors, particularly the extensor carpi radialis brevis. Although these braces may relieve pain upon return to activity, debate continues about the effectiveness of counterforce forearm straps. These straps should not be used for other causes of elbow pain, such as growth plate problems in children and adolescents, or medial elbow instability in adults. The forearm, wrist, and hand are especially vulnerable to external forces and often neglected when considering protective equipment. In collision and contact sports, this area should be protected with specialized gloves and pads, such as those seen in **Figure 3.8**.

Thorax, Rib, and Abdominal Protection

Many collision and contact sports require special protection of the thorax, rib, and abdominal areas. Catchers in baseball and softball wear full thoracic and abdominal protectors to prevent high-speed blows from a bat or ball. Individuals in fencing, and goalies in many sports, also wear full thoracic protectors **(Figure 3.9A)**. Quarterbacks and wide receivers in football often wear rib protectors composed of air-inflated, interconnected cylinders to absorb impact forces caused during tackling **(Figure 3.9B)**. These protectors should be fitted according to the manufacturer's instructions.

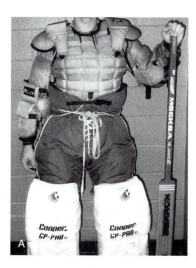

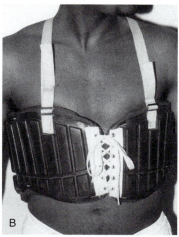

➤ FIGURE 3.9 **Chest and rib protection**. A, Several sports require extensive chest protection (ice hockey). B, Rib protectors absorb impact forces caused during tackling.

Sport Bras

Sport bras provide added support to prevent excessive vertical and horizontal breast motion during exercise **(Figure 3.10)**. Although sport bras are designed to limit motion, few bras on the market actually do so, and as a result, many women continue to experience sore or tender breasts after exercise. Sport bras fall into two categories:

1. Bras made from nonelastic material with wide shoulder straps and wide bands under the breasts to provide upward support. Waist-length designs can prevent cutting in below the breasts.
2. Compressive bras that bind the breasts to the chest wall. Women with medium-sized breasts prefer this type.

Girls and women with small breasts may not need a special bra. Women with a size C cup or larger need a firm, supportive bra. The bra should have nonslip straps and no irritating seams or fasteners next to the skin, and should be firm and durable. Choice of fabric will depend on the

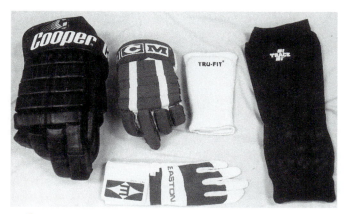

➤ FIGURE 3.8 **Forearm and hand protection**. Specialized gloves can protect the forearm and hand from blunt trauma and friction forces.

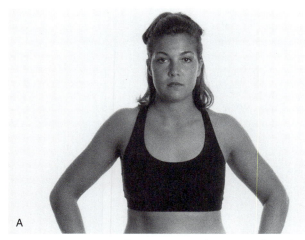
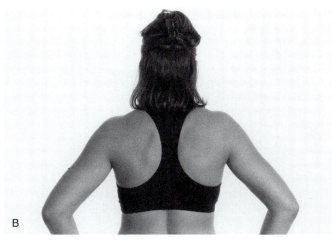

➤ FIGURE 3.10 **Sport bras**. Sport bras made from a nonelastic material with wide shoulder straps and wide bands under the breasts provide upward support by compressing the breasts against the rib cage. A, Anterior view. B, Posterior view.

intensity of activity, support needs, sensitivity to fiber, and climatic and seasonal conditions. A cotton/poly/lycra fabric is a popular blend seen in sport bras. In hot weather, an additional outer layer of textured nylon mesh can promote natural cooling of the skin. In sports requiring significant overhead motion, bra straps should stretch to prevent the bra from riding up over the breasts. In activities in which overhead motion is not a significant part of the activity, nonstretch straps connected directly to a nonelastic cup are preferable.

Lumbar/Sacral Protection

Lumbar/sacral protection includes weight-training belts used during heavy weight lifting, abdominal binders, and other similar supportive devices **(Figure 3.11)**. Each should support the abdominal contents, stabilize the trunk, and prevent spinal deformity or injury during heavy lifting. Use of belts or binders can significantly increase intra-abdominal pressure to reduce compressive forces in the vertebral bodies and lessen the risk of low back trauma.

 Cantilever pads have a hard plastic bridge over the superior aspect of the shoulder to protect the AC joint. These lightweight bridges allow maximal range of motion at the shoulder and can distribute the impact forces throughout the entire shoulder girdle. As such, they provide the greatest amount of protection to the shoulder region, but is not feasible for all players because of its bulk.

PROTECTIVE EQUIPMENT FOR THE LOWER BODY

 A field hockey player had an anterior cruciate ligament (ACL) reconstruction during the off sea-

son. After completing an extensive rehabilitation program, what method of support might be used to protect the knee from further injury?

In the lower body, commercial braces are commonly used to protect the knee and ankle. In addition, special pads are used to protect bony and soft-tissue structures in the hip and thigh region. Depending on the sport, special design modifications are needed to allow maximum protection while providing maximal performance.

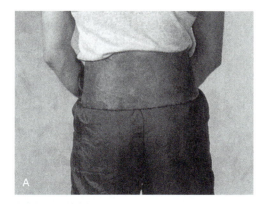
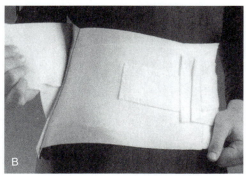

➤ FIGURE 3.11 **Lumbar/sacral protection**. Weight training belts (A) and abdominal binders (B) support the abdominal contents, stabilize the trunk, and prevent spinal deformity or injury.

Hip and Buttock Protection

In collision and contact sports, the hip and buttock region require special pads typically composed of hard polyethylene covered with layers of Ensolite™ to protect the iliac crest, sacrum, coccyx, and genital region. A girdle with special pockets can effectively hold the pads in place (**Figure 3.12A**). The male genital region is best protected by a protective cup placed in the athletic supporter (**Figure 3.12B**).

Thigh Protection

Thigh and upper leg pads, such as those illustrated in **Figure 3.12,** slip into ready-made pockets in the girdle to prevent injury to the quadriceps area. Thigh pads should

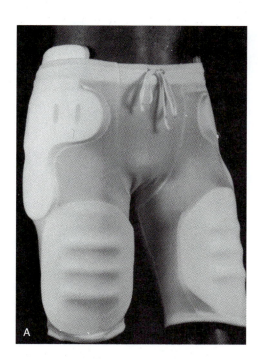

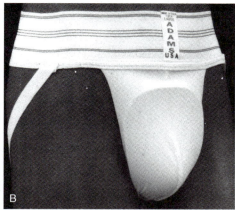

➤ FIGURE 3.12 **Hip protection**. A, Girdle pads protect the gluteal and sacral area from high-velocity forces. Thigh pads can also be inserted to protect the quadriceps area. B, Protective cups placed inside an athletic supporter reduce trauma to the male genital region.

be placed over the quadriceps muscle group, approximately 6 to 7 inches proximal to the patella. When using asymmetrical thigh pads, the larger flare should be placed on the lateral aspect of the thigh to avoid injury to the genitalia (1). In addition to thigh pads, neoprene sleeves can provide uniform compression, therapeutic warmth, and support for a quadriceps or hamstring strain.

Knee and Patella Protection

The knee is second only to the ankle and foot in incidence of injury. Knee pads can protect the area from impact during a collision or fall, and in wrestling can protect the prepatellar and infrapatellar bursa from friction injuries. In football, knee pads reduce contusion and abrasions when falling on turf.

Knee braces fall into three broad functional categories: prophylactic, functional, and rehabilitative (**Figure 3.13**). Prophylactic knee braces (PKBs) are designed to protect the medial collateral ligament (MCL) by redirecting a lateral valgus force away from the joint itself to points more distal on the tibia and femur. Functional knee braces are widely used to protect moderate anterior cruciate ligament (ACL) injuries, or in postsurgical ACL ligament repair or reconstruction cases. Rehabilitative braces provide absolute immobilization at a selected angle after surgery, permit controlled range of motion through predetermined arcs, and prevent accidental loading in non–weight-bearing patients.

PROPHYLACTIC KNEE BRACES

Two general types of PKBs are the lateral and bilateral bar designs. The lateral bar PKBs are constructed with single, dual, or polycentric hinge designs. Each model has a knee hyperextension stop, and is applied using a combination of neoprene wraps, Velcro® straps, and/or adhesive tape. The bilateral bar PKB has a medial and lateral upright bar with biaxial hinges. One study concluded that certain PKBs made from graphite and aluminum showed a marked reduction in force and impulse transference to the MCL during low-energy impacts (9). Other studies have shown that PKBs have little impact on running gait or proprioceptive feedback mechanisms, yet can inhibit isokinetic muscular strength parameters and sprint speed in players unaccustomed to wearing the brace (10-12).

After comprehensive review of available research, the American Academy of Orthopedic Surgeons (AAOS) concluded that the routine use of available PKBs has not been proven effective in reducing either the number or severity of knee injuries, and in some instances may have been a contributing factor to the injury. As future innovations and design modifications are made in PKBs, benefits in injury prevention may become more cost effective. Until then, clinicians should base decisions on PKB use on the individual needs of the athlete.

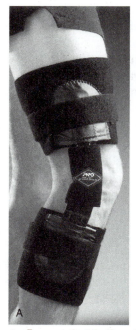
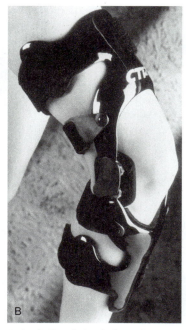
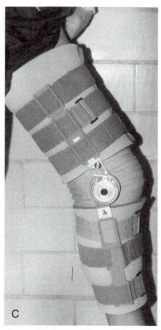

➤ **FIGURE 3.13 Knee braces**. A, Prophylactic knee braces may be a single or bilateral bar design and are used to protect the MCL. B, Functional knee braces control tibial translation and rotational stress relative to the femur, and can provide extension limitations to protect the ACL. C, Rehabilitative braces provide absolute or relative immobilization following surgery.

FUNCTIONAL KNEE BRACES

Functional knee braces, commonly called derotation or ACL braces, are designed to control tibial translation and rotational stress relative to the femur with a rigid snug fit, and extension limitations. There are two basic styles of ACL braces: hinge-post-strap and the hinge-post-shell. Performance of either brace depends on the magnitude of anterior shear load, and the internal torque applied across the tibiofemoral joint, and may be affected by several factors **(Box 3.3)**.

Derotation braces may be prescribed by a physician in individuals with a mild to moderate degree of instability who participate in activities with low or moderate load potential. Functional knee braces do not guarantee in-creased stability in those sports requiring cutting, pivoting, or other quick changes in direction (13).

REHABILITATIVE BRACES

Rehabilitative braces come in two distinct designs: a straight immobilizer made of foam with two metal rods running down the side that is secured with Velcro to prevent all motion, and a hinged brace that allows range of motion to be set by tightening a screw control. Early motion prevents joint adhesions from forming, enhances proprioception, and increases synovial nutrient flow to promote healing of cartilage and collagen tissue. The braces are lighter in weight, adjustable for optimal fit, and can be easily removed and reapplied for wound inspection and rehabilitation. As the individual progresses in the rehabilitation program, the allowable range of motion is adjusted periodically by the clinician.

Decisions to use any of the three major categories of knee braces should rest with the supervising physician or surgeon. Selection should be based on the projected objectives, needs of the sport participant relative to sport demands, cost effectiveness, durability, fit, and comfort.

PATELLOFEMORAL PROTECTION

Patella braces are designed to dissipate force, maintain patellar alignment, and improve patellar tracking. A horseshoe-type silicone or felt pad is sewn into an elastic or neoprene sleeve to relieve tension in recurring patellofemoral subluxation or dislocations **(Figure 3.14A)**. These

---

➤➤ **BOX 3.3**

Factors Affecting Functional Knee Braces

The technique of attachment
The design of the brace, including:
- Hinge design
- Materials of fabrication
- Geometry of the attachment interface
- Mechanism of attachment

Variables in the attachment interface, including:
- How the interface molds around the soft-tissue contours of the limb
- How much displacement occurs between the rigid brace and compliant soft tissues surrounding the distal femur and proximal tibia while loads are applied across the knee

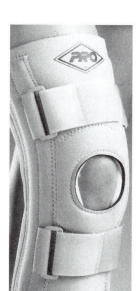

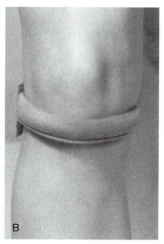

➤ FIGURE 3.14 **Patellofemoral braces**. A, A horseshoe type silicone or felt pad sewn into a sleeve can relieve chronic patella pain. B, A strap worn over the infrapatellar ligament may also relieve patellar pain.

braces relieve anterior knee pain syndrome (14). An alternative brace for treating patellar pain is a strap worn over the infrapatellar ligament (**Figure 3.14B**).

Lower Leg Protection

Pads for the anterior tibia area should consist of a hard, deflective outer layer and an inner layer of thin foam. Velcro straps and stirrups help stabilize the pad inside the sock. Many styles also incorporate padding or plastic shells over the ankle malleoli, which is often subject to repeated contusions. Several commercial designs are available (**Figure 3.15**).

Ankle and Foot Protection

Commercial ankle braces can be used to prevent or support a postinjury ankle sprain and come in three categories: lace-up brace, semirigid orthrosis, or air bladder brace (**Figure 3.16**). A lace-up brace can limit all ankle motions, whereas a semirigid orthrosis and air bladder brace limit only inversion and eversion. Ankle braces have often been compared with ankle strapping. It is fairly well accepted that maximal loss in taping restriction for both inversion and eversion occurs after 20 minutes or more of exercise. Ankle braces are more effective in reducing ankle injuries, are easier for the wearer to apply independently, do not produce some of the skin irritation associated with adhesive tape, provide better comfort and fit, are more cost effective and comfortable to wear (15,16).

Specific foot conditions, such as fallen arches, pronated feet, or medial tibial stress syndrome can be padded and supported with innersoles, semirigid orthotics, and rigid orthotics (**Figure 3.17A**). Research has found that a 6.5 mm thick polymetric foam rubber material is more effective in absorbing heel-strike impact than a viscoelastic polymetric shoe insert (17). Antishock heel lifts use a dense silicone mixture to cushion heel impact to relieve strain on the Achilles tendon, and heel cups reduce tissue shearing and shock in the calcaneal region (**Figure 3.17B**). Other commercially available pads may be used to protect the forefoot region, bunions, and toes, or adhesive felt (moleskin), felt, and foam can be cut to construct similar pads.

Selection and fit of shoes may also affect injuries to the lower extremity. Shoes should adequately cushion impact forces and support and guide the foot during the stance and final push-off phase of running. In sports requiring repeated heel impact, additional heel cushioning should be present. Length should be sufficient to allow all toes to be fully extended. Individuals with toe abnormalities or bunions may also require a wider toe box. **Field Strategy 3.4** identifies factors to keep in mind when selecting and fitting athletic shoes.

In field sports, shoes may have a flat-sole, long cleat, short cleat, or a multicleated design (**Figure 3.18**). The cleats should be properly positioned under the major weight-bearing joints of the foot, and should not be felt through the sole of the shoe. Shoes with the longer irregular cleats placed at the peripheral margin of the sole with a number of smaller pointed cleats positioned in the middle of the sole produce significantly higher torsional resistance

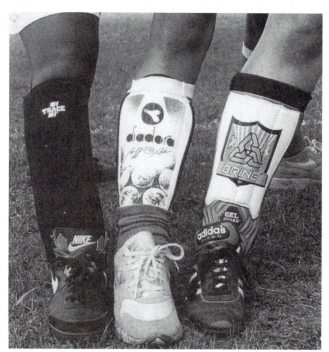

➤ FIGURE 3.15 **Shin guards**.

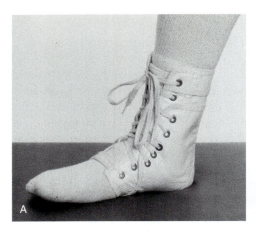

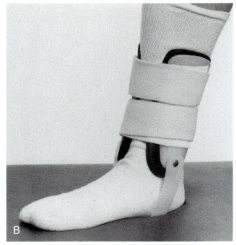

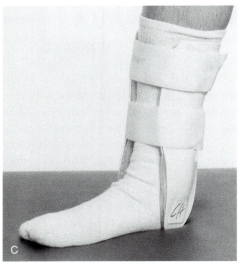

➤ FIGURE 3.16 **Ankle protectors**. Commercial designs include the lace-up brace (A), semirigid orthrosis (B), and air bladder brace (C).

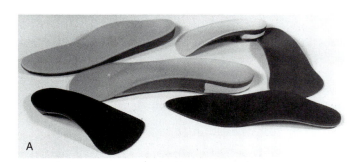

➤ FIGURE 3.17 **Foot and heel protection**. A, Semirigid orthotics provide stability and support to the intrinsic structures of the foot. B, Heel cups are used to reduce tissue shearing and shock in the calcaneal region.

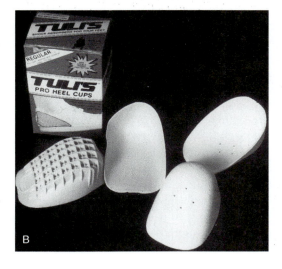

FIELD STRATEGY 3.4   FACTORS IN THE SELECTION AND FIT OF ATHLETIC SHOES

- Fit shoes toward late afternoon or evening, preferably after a workout, and wear socks typically worn during sport participation.
- Fit shoes to the longest toe of the largest foot, providing one thumb's width to the end of the toe box.
- The widest part of the shoe should coincide with the widest part of the foot. Eyelets should be at least 1 inch apart with normal lacing. Women with big or wider feet should consider purchasing boy's or men's shoes.
- The sole of the shoe should provide moderate support but should not be too rigid. Sole tread typically comes in a horizontal bar (commonly used on asphalt or concrete), or waffle design (used on off-road terrain).
- The midsole may be composed of ethylene vinyl acetate (EVA), polyurethane, or preferably, a combination of the two. EVA provides good cushioning, but will break down over time. Polyurethane has minimal compressibility, and provides good durability and stability.
- A thermoplastic heel counter maintains its shape and firmness even in adverse weather conditions.
- Running shoes should position the heel at least $\frac{1}{2}$ inch above the outsole to minimize stretch on the Achilles tendon.
- While wearing the shoes, approximate athletic skills (walking, running, jumping, and changing directions).
- Individuals with specific conditions need special shoes, such as:
  - Runners with normal feet—more forefoot and toe flexibility
  - Overpronation—greater control on the medial side
  - Achilles tendinitis—at least a 15-mm heel wedge
  - Court sports—added side-to-side stability
  - High, rigid arches—soft midsoles, curved lasts, and low or moderate hindfoot stability
  - Normal arches—firm midsole, semicurved lasts, and moderate hindfoot stability
  - Flexible low arch—very firm midsole, straight last, and strong hindfoot stability
- After purchasing the shoes, walk in the shoes for two to three days to allow them to adapt to the feet. Then begin running or practicing in the shoes for about 25 to 30% of the workout. To prevent blisters, gradually extend the length of time the shoes are worn.
- Avid runners should replace shoes every three months, recreational runners every six months.

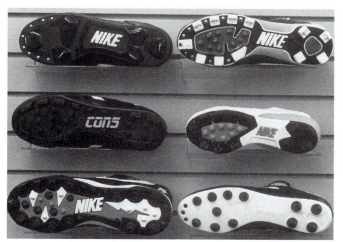

➤ FIGURE 3.18 **Cleated shoes.** Athletic shoes may have long cleats, short cleats, or a multicleated design. Selection will depend on the surface and weather conditions.

and are associated with a significantly higher anterior cruciate ligament injury rate when compared with shoe models with flat cleats, screw-in cleats, or pivot disk models (18). When increased temperature is a factor, such as when playing on turf, only the flat-soled basketball-style turf shoe had low-release coefficients at varying elevated temperatures (19). This may lead to a lower incidence of lower leg injuries. In individuals with arch problems, the shoe should include adequate forefoot, arch, and heel support. In all cases, individuals should select shoes based on the demands of the activity.

 Did you determine that the field hockey player could benefit from a derotation or functional knee brace? Several custom-made braces and commercial braces are available; however, the athletic trainer should consult the orthopedic surgeon to determine which one is best for the athlete.

Summary

1. Protective equipment is only effective when it is:
   - Properly fitted and maintained
   - Periodically cleaned and disinfected
   - Used as intended
2. The sport participant must be protected from high-velocity, low mass forces to prevent focal injuries, and low-velocity, high mass forces to prevent diffuse injuries.
3. Design and selection of protective equipment is based on the following energy-absorbing material factors:
   - Thickness
   - Density
   - Resilience
   - Temperature
4. The National Operating Committee on Standards for Athletic Equipment (NOCSAE) establishes standards for football, baseball, softball, and lacrosse helmets and facemasks.
5. The Hockey Equipment Certification Council (HECC) of the Canadian Standards Association establishes standards for ice hockey helmets and facemasks.
6. The American Society for Testing and Materials (ASTM) establishes standards for protective eye wear, ice hockey helmets and facemasks, and other protective equipment.
7. The athletic trainer is ultimately responsible for knowing the rules and standards governing the selection and fitting of protective equipment for each sport.

References

1. Saliba E, Foreman S, Abadie RT, Jr. Protective equipment considerations. In: Athletic Injuries and Rehabilitation. Edited by Zachazewski JE, Magee DJ, and Quillen WS. Philadelphia: WB Saunders, 1996.

2. Selesnick H, Griffiths G. A waterproof cast line earns high marks. Phys Sportsmed 1997;25(9):67-74.

3. Benson M (ed.). Protective equipment. In: 1997-1998 NCAA Sports Medicine Handbook. Overland Park, KS: The National Collegiate Athletic Association, 1997.

4. Hodgson VR. Impact standards for protective equipment. In: Athletic Injuries to the Head, Neck, and Face. Edited by Torg JS. St. Louis: Mosby-Year Book, 1991.

5. Reynan PD, Clancy WG, Jr. Cervical spine injury, hockey helmets, and face masks. Am J Sports Med 1994;22(2):167-170.

6. Thompson DC, et al. Effectiveness of bicycle safety helmets in preventing serious facial injury. JAMA 1996;276(24):1974-1975.

7. Sheffield-Moore M, et al. Thermoregulatory responses to cycling with and without a helmet. Med Sci Sports Exerc 1997;29(6):755-761.

8. Stenger JM, Lawson EA, Wright JM, Ricketts J. Mouthguards: Protection against shock to head, neck and teeth. J Am Dental Assoc 1994;69(3):273-281.

9. Patterson PE, Eason J. The effects of prophylactic brace construction materials on the reactive responses of the MCL during repetitive impacts. J Ath Tr 1996;31(4):329-333.

10. Kaminski TW, Perrin DH. Effect of prophylactic knee bracing on balance and joint position sense. J Ath Tr 1996;31(2):131-136.

11. Liggett CL, Tandy RD, Young JC. The effects of prophylactic knee bracing on running gait. J Ath Tr 1995;30(2):159-161.

12. Borsa PA, Lephart SM, Fu FH. Muscular and functional performance characteristics of individuals wearing prophylactic knee braces. Ath Train (JNATA) 1993;28(4):336-342.

13. Wichman S, Martin DR. Bracing for activity. Phys Sportsmed 1996; 24(9):88-94.

14. BenGal S, et al. The role of the knee brace in the prevention of anterior knee pain syndrome. Am J Sports Med 1997;25(1):118-122.

15. Metcalfe RC, et al. A comparison of moleskin tape, linen tape, and lace-up brace on joint restriction and movement performance. J Ath Tr 1997;32(2):136-140.

16. Gross MT, et al. Effect of ankle orthoses on functional performance for individuals with recurrent lateral ankle sprains. JOSPT 1997; 25(4):245-252.

17. Shiba N, et al. Shock-absorbing effect of shoe insert materials commonly used in management of lower extremity disorders. Clin Orthop 1995;310(1):130-136.

18. Lambson RB, Barnhill BS, Higgins RW. Football cleat design and its effect on anterior cruciate ligament injuries: A three year prospective study. Am J Sports Med 1996;24(2):155-159.

19. Torg JS, Stilwell G, Rogers K. The effect of ambient temperature on the shoe-surface interface release coefficient. Am J Sports Med 1996;24(1):79-82.

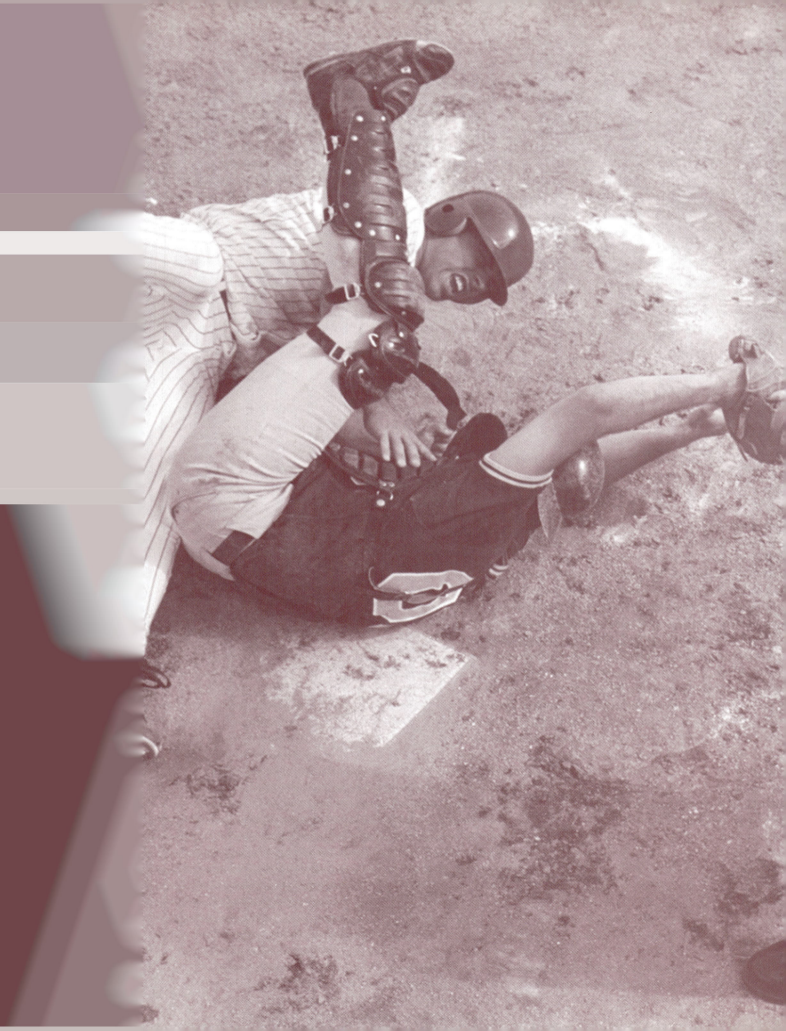

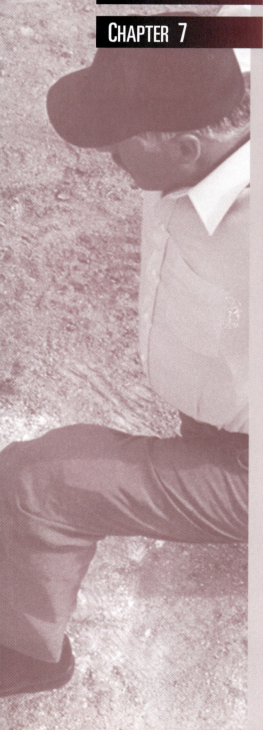

SECTION II

4

Sports Injury Assessment

OBJECTIVES

1. Differentiate between the HOPS injury assessment format and the SOAP note format used to assess and manage a sports-related injury.

2. Name and explain the general components that comprise a complete history of an athletic-related injury or illness.

3. Differentiate between visual observation and inspection at the primary injury site.

4. Describe the various tests included in the physical examination of an injury.

5. Develop an emergency medical systems plan for an athletic training facility.

6. Identify the responsibilities of each member of the on-site sports medicine team in providing emergency care at an athletic event.

7. List supplies and emergency equipment that should be present at an athletic event.

8. Explain the procedures used in an "on-the-field" sports injury assessment.

9. Identify emergency conditions that warrant immediate activation of the emergency medical services (EMS) system.

10. Demonstrate proper procedures for transporting an injured individual.

11. Describe testing techniques used by medical specialists to make an accurate diagnosis.

Accurate injury assessment is critical to successfully evaluate and render proper care for any sports-related injury or illness. Although the evaluation process is often thought of in terms of acute injuries, chronic injuries make up a majority of all evaluations. As the individual responsible for doing injury evaluations, the athletic trainer must have a sound background in human anatomy, human physiology, and biomechanics. This is because the injury evaluation process is nothing more than searching for atypical or dysfunctional anatomy, physiology, or biomechanics. Without a strong understanding of these areas, the execution of the evaluation techniques and the implications for their results will not lead the athletic trainer to correct conclusions concerning the potential injury. This can have a devastating effect on proper treatment and development of appropriate rehabilitation protocols.

This chapter describes two popular methods of injury assessment: the HOPS format and the SOAP note format. Information is then presented on the various components of the injury assessment process. The principles for developing and implementing an emergency medical system (EMS) plan will be presented along with the responsibilities of each member of the sports medicine team. The components of an "on-the-field" emergency assessment will then be presented with a list of conditions that warrant activation of EMS. Details on transporting an injured player from the scene are followed by information on several tests and procedures used by the physician to diagnose an injury. As it is impossible to include basic first aid techniques in this book, athletic trainers must maintain current certification in first aid and cardiopulmonary resuscitation (CPR). For the purposes of this athletic training text, the authors assume that students have already completed a basic athletic training course or a first aid course and hold current certification in CPR or its equivalent.

THE INJURY EVALUATION PROCESS

 What components are essential in any injury evaluation process? When working with several colleagues, why is it important for each employee to be consistent and thorough in all injury evaluations and keep accurate records?

When evaluating any injury or condition, symptoms and diagnostic signs are gathered to determine the extent of injury. A **symptom** is information provided by the injured individual regarding his or her perception of the problem. Examples of these subjective feelings include blurred vision, ringing in the ears, fatigue, dizziness, nausea, headache, pain, weakness, and the inability to move a body part. A diagnostic **sign** is an objective, measurable physical finding regarding the individual's condition. A sign is what the athletic trainer hears, feels, sees, or smells when assessing the individual. Interpreting the symptoms and signs is the foundation used to recognize and identify the injury or condition.

The injury assessment process must include several key components. They include taking a history of the current condition, visually inspecting the area for noticeable abnormalities, physically palpating the region for abnormalities, and completing functional and stress tests. Although several models may be used, each follows a consistent, sequential order to ensure that no essential component is omitted, unless there is sufficient reason.

Two popular methods are the HOPS format and SOAP note format. Each has its advantages, but the SOAP note format is much more inclusive of the entire injury management process.

HOPS Format

HOPS is an acronym for: **H**istory of the injury, **O**bservation and inspection, **P**alpation, and **S**pecial tests. This format uses both subjective information (history of the injury) and objective information (observation and inspection, palpation, and special tests) to recognize and identify problems contributing to the condition. This format is easy to use and follows a basic consistent format. Often used in the beginning steps of injury assessment, the HOPS format has one major disadvantage: it focuses on only the evaluation component of sports injury management and excludes the rehabilitation process.

SUBJECTIVE EVALUATION

The subjective evaluation (history of the injury) includes the primary complaint, mechanism of injury, characteristics of the symptoms, and related medical history. This information comes from the individual and reflects his or her attitude, mental condition, and perceived physical state.

OBJECTIVE EVALUATION

The objective evaluation (observation and inspection, palpation, and special tests) provides appropriate, measurable documentation relative to the individual's condition. This information can be repeatedly measured to track progress from the initial evaluation through final clearance for discharge and return to sport participation. Measurable factors may include edema, ecchymosis, atrophy, range of motion, strength, joint instability, functional disability, motor and sensory function, and cardiovascular endurance. A detailed postural assessment and gait analysis may also be documented in this section.

SOAP Note Format

The SOAP note format provides a more detailed and advanced structure for decision making and problem solving in sports injury management. Used in many physical therapy clinics, sports medicine clinics, and athletic training facilities, these notes document patient care and serve as a vehicle of communication between the on-site clinicians and other health care professionals. The records provide information to avoid duplication of services, and state the present status and tolerance of that individual to the care being rendered by a given health care provider.

SOAP is an acronym for the following sections: **S**ubjective evaluation, **O**bjective evaluation, **A**ssessment, and **P**lan. The supervising physician determines the diagnosis of the patient and may note the results of any diagnostic testing, including x-rays, magnetic resonance imaging (MRI), computed tomography (CT) scans, laboratory testing, or personal notes. When appropriate, the patient is referred to an athletic trainer or physical therapist for detailed evaluation to determine an appropriate treatment and rehabilitation program. The subjective and objective evaluation is identical to that used in the HOPS format; however, two additional components are added to the documentation: **A**ssessment and **P**lan. Abbreviations are used throughout the notes for brevity. Although abbreviations vary from facility to facility, commonly used abbreviations can be seen in **Table 4.1**.

TABLE 4.1	COMMON ABBREVIATIONS		
abnor.	abnormal	MAEEW	moves all extremities equally well
AC	acute; before meals; acromioclavicular	mm	muscle; millimeter; mucous membrane
ADL	activities of daily living	MMT	manual muscle test
ant.	anterior	MOD	moderate
ante	before	N	normal; never; no; not
A&O	alert & oriented	NC	neurologic check; no complaints; not completed
AOAP	as often as possible		
AP	anterior-posterior; assessment and plans	NEG	negative
AROM	active range of motion	NP	no pain; not pregnant; not present
ASAP	as soon as possible	NPT	normal pressure and temperature
B	bilateral	NSA	no significant abnormality
BID	twice daily	NSAID	nonsteroidal anti-inflammatory drug
c	with	NT	not tried
CC	chief complaint; chronic complainer	NWB	non-weight bearing
ck.	check	o	negative; without
C/O	complained of; complaints; under care of	O	objective finding; oral; open; obvious; often; other
CP	cerebral palsy; chest pain; chronic pain		
d/c, DC	discharged; discontinue; decrease	OH	occupational history
DF	dorsiflexion	P&A	percussion and auscultation
DOB	date of birth	PA	posterior-anterior (x-ray); physician assistant; presents again
DTR	deep tendon reflexes		
Dx	diagnosis	PE	physical examination
E	edema	PF	plantar flexion
EENT	eyes, ears, nose, throat	PH	past history; poor health
ELOP	estimated length of program	PMH	past medical history
EMS	emergency medical services	PNS	peripheral nervous system
EMT	emergency medical technician	PPPBL	peripheral pulses palpable both legs
EOA	examine, opinion, and advice; esophageal obturator airway	prog.	prognosis
		PROM	passive range of motion
EV	eversion	PWB	partial weight bearing
exam.	examination	Px	physical exam; pneumothorax
FH	family history	R	right
FROM	full range of movement	rehab	rehabilitation
Fx	fracture	R/O	rule out
G1–4	grades 1 to 4	ROM	range of motion
GA	general appearance	RTP	return to play
HA	headache	Rx	therapy; drug; medication; treatment; take
H/O	history of	s	without
H&P	history and physical	S	subjective findings
HPI	history of present illness	stat	immediately
ht.	height; heart	STG	short-term goals
Hx	history	Sx	signs, symptom
IC	individual counseling	T	temperature
IN	inversion	UK	unknown
IPPA	inspection, percussion, palpation, and auscultation	w	white; with
		WNL	within normal limits
L	left; liter	W/O	without
LAT	lateral	y.o.	year old
LOM	limitation of motion	1tive	positive

ASSESSMENT

Following the objective evaluation, the clinician will analyze and assess the individual's status and prognosis. Although a definitive diagnosis may not be known, the suspected injury site, damaged structures involved, and severity of injury is documented. Long-term goals are then established to accurately reflect the individual's status after a period of rehabilitation. These long-term goals might include pain-free range of motion, bilateral strength, power, and muscular endurance, cardiovascular endurance, and return to full functional status. Short-term goals are then developed to outline the expected progress within a week or two of the initial injury. These might include immediate protection of the injured area and control of inflammation, hemorrhage, muscle spasm, or pain. Short-term goals are updated with each progress note. Progress notes may be written daily, weekly, or biweekly to document progress (**Figure 4.1**).

PLAN

The final section of the note lists the modalities, therapeutic exercises, educational consultations, and functional activities utilized to achieve the short-term goals. The action plan includes the following information:

1. The immediate treatment given to the injured individual
2. The frequency and duration of treatments, therapeutic exercises, therapeutic modalities, and evaluation standards to determine progress toward the goals
3. On-going patient education
4. Criteria for discharge

Physical Therapy	Daily Treatment/Progress Report	
Patient Name:	Physician:	Diagnosis:
Date:	Date:	Date:
S:	S:	S:
O:	O:	O:
A:	A:	A:
STG'S:	STG'S:	STG'S:
P:	P:	P:
Initials/Treatment Time:	Initials/Treatment Time:	Initials/Treatment Time:

Signature 1 _____

Signature 2 _____

➤ **FIGURE 4.1** Progress notes are added to the patient's file daily, weekly, or biweekly to document progress.

As the short-term goals are achieved and updated, periodic "in-house review" of the individual's records permits the facility and clinicians to evaluate joint range of motion, flexibility, muscular strength, power, endurance, balance or proprioception, and functional status. These reviews also allow the clinicians to discuss the continuity of documentation, efficacy of treatment, average time to discharge the individuals, as well as other parameters that may reflect quality of care. As the individual progresses in the treatment plan, gradual return to activity may help motivate them to work even harder to return to full functional status. When it is determined the individual can be discharged and cleared for participation, a discharge note is written to close the file. All information included within the file is confidential, and cannot be released to anyone without written approval from the patient.

In a clinical setting, SOAP notes are the sole means of documenting what was done or not done for the patient. It is the ethical responsibility of all clinicians to keep accurate and factual records. This information verifies specific services rendered, evaluates patient progress, and efficacy of the treatment plan. Insurance companies use this information to determine if services are being appropriately rendered and therefore, qualify for reimbursement. More importantly, this comprehensive record-keeping system can minimize the ever-present threat of malpractice and litigation. In general, the primary error in writing SOAP notes is the error of omission, whereby clinicians fail to adequately document the nature and extent of care provided to the patient. Formal documentation and regular review of records can reduce this threat, and minimize the likelihood that inappropriate or inadequate care is being rendered to a patient.

Using the process listed above, each component of the subjective and objective assessment will be described in detail in the following sections and repeated throughout each chapter on the various body regions. A brief outline of the steps can be seen in **Field Strategy 4.1**. Because of the vast amount of detailed information necessary to cover the treatment plan, students should enroll in separate classes on therapeutic modalities and therapeutic exercise to see how all components of the SOAP note relate to the total care provided to an injured athlete.

 Essential components in any injury evaluation process are the subjective evaluation (history of the injury), and the objective evaluation (observation and inspection, palpation, and functional/ stress tests). In addition, the assessment and treatment plan should be documented to follow the athlete throughout the rehabilitation program until the criteria to return to participation are met. Clinicians should uniformly document patient assessment findings, identify specific services rendered, and record rehabilitation progression to evaluate patient progress and efficacy of the treatment plan.

HISTORY OF THE INJURY

 A high school football player is complaining of a sharp, aching pain in the posterior ankle region. Pain increases when he goes up on his toes, during sprints, and when going up and down the stairs. What questions should be asked to identify the cause and extent of this injury?

Identifying the history of the injury can be the most important step in injury assessment. A complete history includes information on the primary complaint; cause, or mechanism, of injury; characteristics of the symptoms; and related medical history that may have a bearing on this specific condition **(Figure 4.2)**. This information can provide possible reasons for the symptoms and identify possible injured structures prior to initiating the physical examination. An individual's medical history file can be an excellent resource for identifying past injuries, subsequent rehabilitation programs, and any factors that may predispose the athlete to further injury. The National Collegiate Athletic Association (NCAA) has identified primary components that should be in the athlete's medical record and readily accessible to the athletic trainer **(Box 4.1)** (1).

History taking involves asking the right questions, but also requires establishing a professional and comfortable atmosphere. In taking a history, the athletic trainer should present a competent manner, listening attentively and maintaining eye contact in an effort to establish rapport with the injured individual. Ideally, this will encourage the

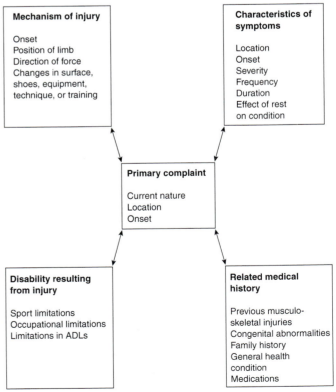

➤ **FIGURE 4.2** Components to explore in taking a history of an injury.

FIELD STRATEGY 4.1 **INJURY ASSESSMENT PROTOCOL**

HISTORY OF THE INJURY

Primary complaint
  Current nature, location, and onset of the condition
Mechanism of injury
  Cause of stress, position of limb, and direction of force
  Changes in running surface, shoes, equipment, techniques, or conditioning modes
Characteristics of the symptoms
  Evolution of the onset, nature, location, severity and duration of symptoms
Disability resulting from the injury
  Limitations in occupation and activities of daily living
Related medical history
  Past musculoskeletal injuries, congenital abnormalities, family history, childhood dis-
    eases, allergies, or cardiac, respiratory, vascular, or neurologic problems

OBSERVATION AND INSPECTION

Observation should analyze
  Overall appearance
  Body symmetry
  General motor function
  Posture and gait
Inspection at the injury site
  Observe for deformity, swelling, discoloration, scars, and general skin condition

PALPATION

Bony structures: determine a possible fracture first
Soft-tissue structures: skin temperature, swelling, point tenderness, crepitus, deformity,
  muscle spasm, cutaneous sensation, and pulse

FUNCTIONAL TESTS

Active movement
Passive movement and end feel
Resisted manual muscle testing

STRESS TESTS

Ligamentous instability tests
Special tests

NEUROLOGIC TESTS

Dermatomes
Myotomes
Reflexes
Peripheral nerve testing

SPORT-SPECIFIC FUNCTIONAL TESTING

Proprioception and motor coordination

SPORT-SPECIFIC SKILL PERFORMANCE

---

individual to respond more accurately to questions and instructions. Gather information, such as the individual's name, sex, age, date of birth, occupation, and what activity the individual was participating in when the injury occurred. Notes regarding body size, body type, and general physical condition are also appropriate.

Although information provided by the individual is subjective, it should still be gathered and recorded as quantitatively as possible. This can be accomplished by recording a number correlating with the described symptoms. For example, when asking about pain, the individual

can rate the severity of pain using a scale from 1 to 10 with 10 being the most severe pain. Ask the individual how long the pain lasts. In using such measures, the progress of the injury can be determined. If the individual reports that pain begins immediately after activity and lasts for three or four hours, a baseline of information has been established. As the individual undergoes treatment and rehabilitation for the injury, a comparison with baseline information can determine if the condition is getting better, worse, or has remained the same. Although the intent of taking a history is to narrow the possibilities of conditions

>> BOX 4.1

National Collegiate Athletic Association (NCAA) Guideline 1B: Medical Evaluations, Immunizations and Records

The following primary components should be included in the athlete's medical record:

- History of injuries, illnesses, pregnancies and operations both athletic and nonathletic
- Physician referral for and feedback from, treatment, rehabilitation, disposition, or consultation
- Preparticipation and preseason medical health questionnaire including:
  - Illnesses suffered (acute and chronic); previous hospitalization and surgery
  - Allergies, including hypersensitivity to drugs, foods, and insect bites/stings
  - Medications taken on a regular basis
  - Conditioning status
  - Musculoskeletal injuries (previous and current)
  - Concussions or loss of consciousness
  - Syncope or near syncope with exercise

  - Exercise-induced asthma or bronchospasm
  - Loss of paired-organs
  - Heat related illness
  - Cardiac conditions and family history of cardiac disease including sudden death in a family member under 50 years of age and Marfan syndrome
  - Menstrual history
  - Exposure to tuberculosis
- Immunization records
  - Measles, mumps, rubella (MMR)
  - Hepatitis B
  - Diphtheria and tetanus
- Written permission signed by the athlete and parent if the athlete is under 18 years of age
  - Release of medical records
  - Consent to treatment

Adapted with permission from the National Collegiate Athletic Association. *1997–1998 NCAA sports medicine handbook.* Overland Park, KS: NCAA Sport Sciences, 1997:8–9.

causing the injury, the history should always be taken with an open mind. If too few factors are considered, the athletic trainer may reach premature conclusions and fail to adequately address the severity of injury. It is essential to document in writing the information obtained during the history.

Primary Complaint

The primary complaint focuses on what the injured individual believes is the current injury. Questions should be phrased to allow the individual to describe the current nature, location, and onset of the condition. The following questions could be asked:

- Why are you here?
- What is the problem?
- Where does it hurt?
- What activities or motions are weak or painful?

It is important to realize that the individual may not wish to carry on a lengthy discussion about the injury or may trivialize the extent of pain or disability. The athletic trainer must be patient and keep questions simple and open-ended. It is advantageous to pay close attention to words and gestures used to describe the condition, as they may provide clues to the quality and intensity of the symptoms.

Mechanism of Injury

After identifying the primary complaint, attempt to determine the mechanism of injury. This is probably the most important information gained in the history. Questions that might be asked include:

- How did the injury occur?
- Did you fall? If so, how did you land?
- Were you struck by an object or another individual? If so, in what position was the involved body part, and what direction was the force?
- Did you hear or feel anything?
- How long has the injury been a problem?
- Have there been recent changes in running surface, shoes, equipment, techniques, or conditioning modes?

It is important to visualize how the injury occurred to identify possible injured structures. This directs the objective evaluation.

Characteristics of the Symptoms

The primary complaint must be explored in detail to discover the evolution of symptoms, including the location, onset, severity, frequency, duration, and limitations due to the pain or disability. The individual's pain perception, for example, can indicate what structures may be injured. There are two categories of pain: somatic and visceral. **Somatic pain** arises from the skin, ligaments, muscles, bones, and joints, and is the most common type of pain encountered in sport injuries. It is classified into two major types: deep and superficial. Deep somatic pain is described as diffuse or nagging, as if intense pressure is being exerted on the structures, and may be complicated by stabbing pain. Deep somatic pain is longer lasting and usually indicates significant tissue damage either to bone, internal joint structures, or muscles. Superficial somatic pain results from injury to the epidermis or dermis, and is usually a sharp, prickly type of pain that tends to be brief (2).

Visceral pain results from disease or injury to an organ in the thoracic or abdominal cavity, such as compression, tension, or distention of the viscera. Similar to deep somatic pain, it is perceived as deeply located, nagging, and pressing, and it is often accompanied by nausea and vomiting (2). **Referred pain** is a type of visceral pain that travels along the same nerve pathways as somatic pain. It is perceived by the brain as somatic in origin. In other words, the injury is in one region but the brain considers it in another. Referred pain, for example, occurs when an individual has a heart attack and feels pain in the chest, left arm, and sometimes the neck. **Figure 4.3** illustrates cutaneous areas where pain from visceral organs can be referred.

Pain can travel up or down the length of any nerve and be referred to another region. An individual who has a low back problem may feel the pain down the gluteal region into the back of the leg. If a nerve is injured, pain or a change in sensation, such as a numbing or burning sensation, can be felt along the length of the nerve. In assessing the injury, the athletic trainer should ask detailed questions about the location, onset, severity, frequency, and duration of the pain. For example, ask:

- Where does it hurt the most?
- Can you point to a specific spot?
- Is the pain limited to that area, or does it radiate into other parts of the leg or foot?
- On a scale from 1 to 10 with 10 being most severe, how bad is the pain?

In chronic conditions, the following questions should be asked:

- When does the pain begin (when you get out of bed, while sitting, while walking, during exercise, or at night)?
- How long does the pain last?
- Is the pain worse before, during, or after activity?
- What activities aggravate or alleviate the symptoms?

- Does it wake you up at night?
- How long has the condition been present?
- Has the pain changed or stayed the same?
- In the past, what medications, treatments, or exercise programs have improved the situation?

If pain is localized, it suggests limited bony or soft-tissue structures may be involved. Diffuse pain around the entire joint may indicate inflammation of the joint capsule or injury to several structures. If pain radiates into other areas of the limb or body, it may be traveling up or down the length of a nerve. Obtaining information about the symptoms can determine if the individual has an **acute injury** resulting from a specific event leading to a sudden onset of symptoms, or a **chronic injury** characterized by a slow, sustained development of symptoms that culminate in a painful inflammatory condition. These answers can also determine if the condition is disabling enough to require a physician referral. **Table 4.2** provides more detailed information on pain characteristics and probable causes.

Disability Resulting from the Injury

The athletic trainer should attempt to determine the limitations of the individual due to pain, weakness, or disability from the injury. Questions should not be limited to sport participation, but should inquire if the injury has affected his or her job, school, or daily activities. Activities of daily living (**ADLs**) are actions most people perform without thinking, such as combing the hair, brushing the teeth, and walking up or down stairs.

Related Medical History

Obtain information regarding other problems or conditions that might have affected this injury. Information extrapolated from the individual's preseason physical examination may verify past childhood diseases; allergies; cardiac, respiratory, vascular, musculoskeletal, or neurological problems; use of contact lenses, dentures, or prosthetic

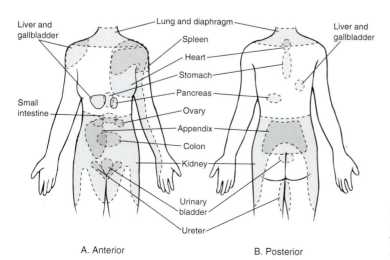

Liver and gallbladder — Lung and diaphragm — Liver and gallbladder
Spleen
Heart
Stomach
Pancreas
Small intestine — Ovary
Appendix
Colon
Kidney
Urinary bladder
Ureter

A. Anterior   B. Posterior

➤ **FIGURE 4.3** Certain visceral organs can refer pain to specific cutaneous areas. Keep this in mind if all special tests are negative, yet the individual continues to feel pain at a specific site.

TABLE 4.2	PAIN CHARACTERISTICS AND WHAT MAY BE INDICATED
Characteristics	**Possible Causes**
Morning pain with stiffness that improves with activity	Chronic inflammation with edema, or arthritis
Pain increasing as the day progresses	Increased congestion in a joint
Sharp, stabbing pain during activity	Acute injury, such as ligament sprain or muscular strain
Dull, aching pain aggravated by muscle contraction	Chronic muscular strain
Pain that subsides during activity	Chronic condition or inflammation
Pain on activity relieved by rest	Soft-tissue damage
Pain not affected by rest or activity	Injury to bone
Night pain	Compression of a nerve or bursa
Dull, aching, and hard to localize; aggravated by passive stretching of the muscle and resisted muscle contractions	Muscular pain
Deeply located, nagging, and very localized	Bone pain
Sharp, burning, or numbing sensation that may run the length of the nerve	Nerve pain
Aching over a large area that may be referred to another area of the body	Vascular pain

devices; and past episodes of infectious diseases, loss of consciousness, recurrent headaches, heat stroke, seizures, eating disorders, or chronic medical problems. Previous musculoskeletal injuries or congenital abnormalities may place additional stress on joints and predispose the individual to certain injuries. The athletic trainer should ask if the individual is taking any medication. The type, frequency,

dosage, and effect of a medication may mask some symptoms.

 The varsity football player is 17 years old. His primary complaint is a sharp, aching pain in the region of the Achilles tendon. He rates the pain as a 6 on a 10-point scale when he is walking, and a 9 when he does wind sprints. Pain is reduced when he ices the region after practice. He cannot recall injuring the ankle, but the pain has been present for a week and seems to be getting worse. A physician has not been consulted about this injury.

OBSERVATION AND INSPECTION

 A detailed history of the injury has been gathered from the football player. The next step is to observe the individual and inspect the injury site. What observable factors might indicate the seriousness of injury?

Observation and inspection begins the objective evaluation in an injury assessment. Although explained as a separate step, observation begins the moment the injured person is seen and continues throughout the assessment. **Observation** refers to the visual analysis of overall appearance, symmetry, general motor function, posture, and gait (**Figure 4.4**). **Inspection** refers to factors seen at the actual injury site, such as redness, bruising, swelling, cuts, or scars.

Observation

Occasionally, the athletic trainer actually sees an acute injury occur. In many instances, however, the individual will come to the sideline, office, athletic training room, or clinic complaining of pain or discomfort. The athletic trainer should immediately assess the individual's state of

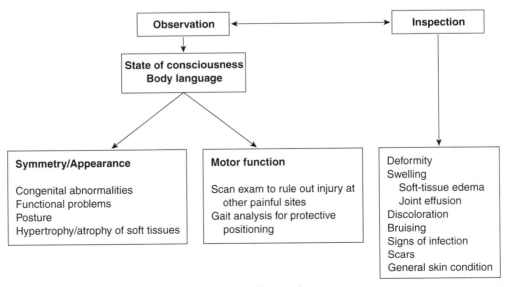

➤ **FIGURE 4.4** Components of observation and inspection.

consciousness and body language that may indicate pain, disability, fracture, dislocation, or other conditions. It is also important to note the individual's general posture, willingness and ability to move, ease in motion, and general overall attitude. Using discretion in safeguarding the athlete's privacy, the injured area should be fully exposed. This may require the removal of protective equipment and clothing.

SYMMETRY AND APPEARANCE

The body should be scanned visually to detect **congenital** (exiting at birth) or functional problems that may be contributing to the injury. This includes observing any abnormalities in the spinal curves, general symmetry of the various body parts, and general posture of the body from an anterior, lateral, and posterior view. General questions that should be answered include those listed in **(Field Strategy 4.2)**.

If it is not **contraindicated**, the athletic trainer should observe the normal swing of the individual's arms and legs during walking. Stand behind, in front, and to the side of the individual to observe from all angles. A shoulder injury may be evident in a limited arm swing, or by holding the arm close to the body in a splinted position. A lower extremity injury may produce a noticeable limp, or **antalgic gait**. Running on a treadmill may show functional problems that may have contributed to a lower extremity injury.

 FIELD STRATEGY 4.2   POSTURAL ASSESSMENT

ANTERIOR VIEW

- Are the head and neck in the midline of the body? Is the nose centered? Does the jaw appear well shaped and normal?
- Is the slope of the shoulder muscles bilaterally equal? The level of the shoulder on the dominant side will usually be lower than the non-dominant side.
- Do both shoulders have a well-rounded deltoid musculature with no prominent bony structures?
- Are any scars or muscular atrophy present in the arm?
- Is the space between the arms and body the same on both sides?
- Are both hands held in the same position?
- Does the rib cage look symmetrical with no bony protrusions?
- Are the folds of the waist at the same height?
- Are the kneecaps level and facing forward? The knees should be straight with the heads of the fibula level.
- Are the distal bony prominences of the lower leg bilaterally level?
- Are arches present on both feet? When standing in a comfortable position, the feet should angle equally.

SIDE VIEW

- Can you draw an imaginary, straight plumb line from the ear through the middle of the shoulder, hip, knee, and ankle?
- Does the back have any excessive curves?
- Are the elbows held near full extension?
- Do the chest, back, and abdominal muscles have good tone with no obvious chest deformities?
- Does the pelvis appear to be level?
- Are the knees straight, flexed, or hyperextended? Normally they should be slightly flexed.

POSTERIOR VIEW

- Are the head and neck centered? Note any abnormal prominence of bony structures or muscle atrophy.
- Are the scapula at the same height and resting at the same angle? Are both scapula lying flat against the rib cage?
- Does the spine appear to be straight?
- Is there any atrophy in the muscle groups of the shoulder and arm?
- Is the posterior side of the elbow at the same height bilaterally? Is the space between the body and elbow the same on both sides?
- Do the ribs protrude?
- Are the waist folds level? Are the posterior gluteal folds level?
- Are the skin creases on the posterior knee level?
- Do both Achilles tendons descend straight to the floor? Are the heels straight, angled in (varus), or angled out (valgus)?

Scan Exam to Assess General Motor Function

Ask the athlete to:
- Extend, flex, laterally flex, and rotate the neck
- Bend forward to touch the toes
- Stand and rotate the trunk to the right and left
- Bring the palms together above the head and then behind the back
- Straight leg raise in hip flexion, extension, and abduction
- Flex the knees
- Walk on the heels and toes

MOTOR FUNCTION

Many individuals begin observation in the examination room with a scan exam to assess general motor function. This exam rules out injury at other joints that may be overlooked due to intense pain or discomfort at the primary injury site. In addition, pain in one area may be referred from another area. The injured person is observed doing gross motor movements in the neck, trunk, and extremities **(Box 4.2)**. Note if there is any hesitation to move a body part, or if the individual favors one side over the other.

Inspection of the Injury Site

The localized injury site is inspected for any deformity, swelling (edema or joint effusion), discoloration (redness, bruising, or ecchymosis), signs of infection (redness, swelling, pus, or red streaks), scars that might indicate previous surgery, and general skin condition (oily, dry, blotchy with red spots, sores, or hives). Swelling inside the joint is called localized intra-articular swelling, or joint **effusion**, and makes the joint appear enlarged, red, and puffy.

Ecchymosis is discoloration or swelling outside the joint in the surrounding soft tissue due to a bruise or injury under the skin. The injured area should be compared to the opposite side if possible. This bilateral comparison helps to establish what is normal for this individual.

 Although the football player appeared to have good body symmetry, he was unable to raise up on his toes or walk without an antalgic gait. Visual inspection of the Achilles tendon demonstrated redness and slight swelling on the posterior aspect of the tendon.

PALPATION

 The Achilles tendon is red, swollen, and painful. How can the area be palpated to determine the extent and severity of injury without causing additional pain?

Bilateral palpation of paired anatomical structures can detect eight physical findings: temperature, swelling, point tenderness, crepitus, deformity, muscle spasm, cutaneous sensation, and pulse **(Figure 4.5)**. Before touching the individual, the athletic trainer should have clean, warm

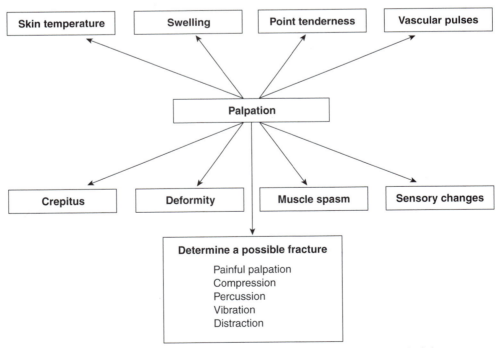

➤ **FIGURE 4.5** Begin palpation with gentle circular pressure followed by gradual deeper pressure. Feel for skin temperature, swelling, point tenderness, crepitus, deformity, muscle spasm, cutaneous sensation, and pulse.

hands. Latex examination gloves should be worn as a precaution against disease and infection. Palpation should begin with gentle, circular pressure followed by gradual, deeper pressure. Begin on structures away from the injury site and progress toward the injured area. Palpating the most painful area last avoids any carry over of pain into noninjured areas.

When the fingers first touch the skin, skin temperature should be noted. Increased temperature at the injury site could indicate inflammation or infection, whereas decreased temperature could indicate a reduction in circulation. Swelling can be diffuse or localized in a small area. If swelling is inside the joint, motion will often be limited because of congestion caused by extra fluid.

Palpation of the bones and bony landmarks can determine the possibility of fractures, crepitus, or loose bony or cartilaginous fragments. Possible fractures can be assessed with percussion, vibrations through use of a tuning fork, compression, and distraction (**Figure 4.6**). If test results

indicate a possible fracture, the region should be immobilized.

Point tenderness and **crepitus** (crackling sensation) indicate damage to bony or soft-tissue structures and should be palpated with as little pressure as possible. Cutaneous sensation can be tested by running your fingers along both sides of the body part and asking the individual if it feels the same on both sides. This technique can determine possible nerve involvement, particularly if the individual has numbness or tingling in the limb. Peripheral pulses are taken distal to an injury to rule out damage to a major artery. Common sites are the radial pulse at the wrist and dorsalis pedis pulse on the dorsum of the foot (**Figure 4.7**).

 Palpation reveals warmth and slight swelling over the distal Achilles tendon. Sharp pain was elicited directly over the tendon, approximately 1 inch proximal to its distal insertion into the calcaneus. All fracture tests were negative.

PHYSICAL EXAMINATION TESTS

 There is little risk of a fracture present. How will you proceed to test the integrity of the soft-tissue structures to determine the extent and severity of injury? What factors might limit range of motion at the joint?

After fractures and/or dislocations have been ruled out, soft-tissue structures, such as muscles, ligaments, the joint capsule, and bursae are assessed using special tests. Although more extensive explanations are given in the individual chapters, general principles are discussed here. Special tests include functional tests (active, passive, and resisted range of motion), ligamentous and capsular testing, special tests, neurologic testing, and sport-specific functional testing (**Figure 4.8**).

Functional Testing

Functional tests identify the athlete's ability to move a body part through the range of motion (ROM) actively, passively, and against resistance. As with all tests, the uninjured side should be evaluated first to establish **normative data**. All motions common to each joint should be tested. Occasionally, it may also be necessary to test the joints proximal and distal to the injury to rule out any referred pain. The available active and passive ROM can be objectively measured with the use of a **goniometer** (**Figure 4.9**). The goniometer is a protractor with two rigid arms that intersect at a hinge joint. It is used to measure both joint position and available joint motion, and can determine when the individual has regained normal motion at a joint. The arms of the goniometer measure from 0 to 180° of motion, or 0 to 360° of motion. Measurements are obtained

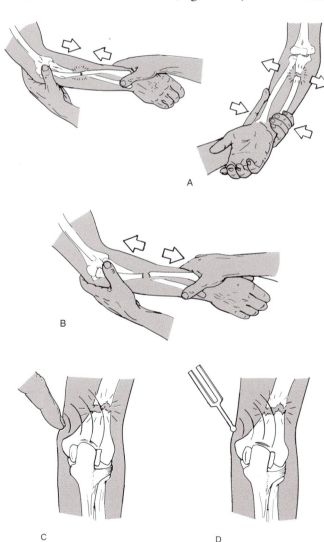

➤ **FIGURE 4.6 Determining a possible fracture.** A, Compression (axial and circular). B, Distraction. C, Percussion. D, Vibration.

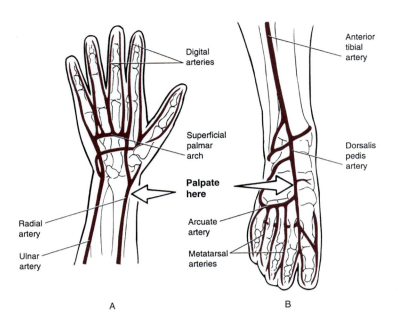

A   B

➤ **FIGURE 4.7** Pulses can be taken at the radial pulse in the wrist (A) or the dorsalis pedis on the dorsum of the foot (B).

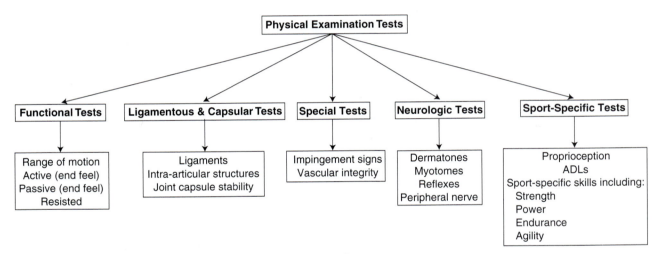

➤ **FIGURE 4.8** Components of physical examination tests.

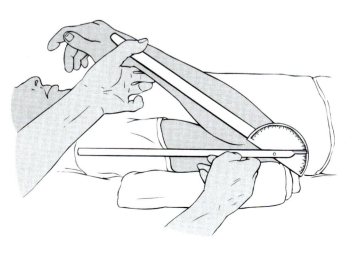

➤ **FIGURE 4.9 Goniometry measurement at the elbow.** In anatomical position, the elbow is flexed. The goniometer axis is placed over the lateral epicondyle of the humerus. To accommodate using a goniometer that ranges from 0° to 180°, the stationary arm is held parallel to the longitudinal axis of the radius, pointing toward the styloid process of the radius. The moving arm is held parallel to the longitudinal axis of the humerus, pointing toward the tip of the acromion process. Range of motion is measured where the pointer intersects the scale.

by placing the goniometer's stationary arm parallel to the proximal bone. The axis of the goniometer should coincide with the joint axis of motion. The goniometer's moving arm is then placed parallel to the distal bone, utilizing specific anatomical landmarks as points of reference. Normal ROM for selected joints is listed in **Table 4.3** and in the individual joint chapters.

ACTIVE RANGE OF MOTION

Active range of motion (AROM) is joint motion performed voluntarily by the individual through muscular contraction. Unless contraindicated, AROM should always be performed before passive range of motion (PROM). This indicates the individual's willingness and ability to move the injured body part. Active movement determines possible damage to contractile tissue (muscle, muscle-tendon junction, tendon, and tendon-periosteal union), and measures muscle strength and movement coordination. Measuring all motions, except rotation, starts with the body in anatomical position. For rotation, the starting body position is midway between internal (medial) and external (lateral) rotation. Starting position is measured as 0°. Maximal movement away from the 0° point is the total available range of motion. For example, to subjectively measure plantar flexion against gravity, place the individual prone on a table with the knees flexed. Stabilize both thighs against the table, and ask the athlete to plantar flex both ankles. Comparison of movement in both legs will indicate if plantar flexion is bilaterally equal.

Note the individual's willingness to perform the movement, the fluidity, and extent of movement (joint ROM). Note the location in the arc of movement when symptoms occur. Any increase in intensity or quality of symptoms should also be noted. Limitation in motion may be due to pain, swelling, muscle spasm, muscle tightness, joint contractures, nerve damage, or mechanical blocks, such as a loose body. If the individual has pain or other symptoms on motion, it is difficult to determine at this time if the joint, muscle, or both are injured. It is important to assess the following: if motion causes pain, at what point in the motion does pain begin? Does pain appear only in a limited range of motion (painful arc)? Is the pain the same type of pain associated with the primary complaint? Perform any painful movements last to avoid any carryover of pain from testing one motion to the next.

TABLE 4.3   NORMAL RANGES OF MOTION AT SELECTED JOINTS

Joint	Motion	Range of Motion	Joint	Motion	Range of Motion
Cervical	Flexion	0–80°	Digit 2–5		
	Extension	0–70°	MCP	Flexion	0–90°
	Lateral flexion	0–45°		Extension	0–45°
	Rotation	0–80°		Abduction	0–20°
Lumbar	Forward flexion	0–60°	PIP	Flexion	0–100°
	Extension	0–35°	DIP	Flexion	0–90°
	Lateral flexion	0–20°	Hip	Flexion	0–120
	Rotation	0–50°		Extension	0–30°
Shoulder	Flexion	0–180°		Abduction	0–40°
	Extension	0–60°		Adduction	0–30°
	Abduction	0–180°		Internal rotation	0–40°
	Internal rotation	0–70°		External rotation	0–50°
	External rotation	0–90°	Knee	Flexion	0–135°
	Horizontal abduction/ adduction	0–130°		Extension	0–15°
				Medial rotation with knee flexed	0–25°
Elbow	Flexion	0–150°		Lateral rotation with knee flexed	0–35°
	Extension	0–10°			
Forearm	Pronation	0–80°	Ankle	Dorsiflexion	0–20°
	Supination	0–80°		Plantar flexion	0–50°
Wrist	Flexion	0–80°		Pronation	0–30°
	Extension	0–70°		Supination	0–50°
	Ulnar deviation	0–30°	Subtalar	Inversion	0–5°
	Radial deviation	0–20°		Eversion	0–5°
Thumb			Toes		
CMC	Abduction	0–70°	1st MTP	Flexion	0–45°
	Flexion	0–15°		Extension	0–75°
	Extension	0–20°	1st IP	Flexion	0–90°
	Opposition	Tip of thumb to tip of 5th finger	2–5 MTP	Flexion	0–40°
				Extension	0–40°
MCP	Flexion	0–50°	PIP	Flexion	0–35°
	IP	Flexion 0–80°	DIP	Flexion	0–30°
				Extension	0–60°

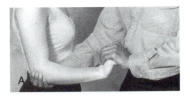

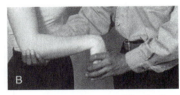

➤ FIGURE 4.10 **Passive movement.** The body part is moved through the range of motion with no assistance from the injured individual. Any limitation of movement or presence of pain is documented. A, Starting position. B, End position.

PASSIVE RANGE OF MOTION

If the individual is unable to perform all active movements at the injured joint because of pain or spasm, passive movement can be performed. In **passive movement**, the injured limb or body part is moved through the ROM with no assistance from the injured individual **(Figure 4.10)**. As PROM is performed, the individual should be positioned to allow the muscles to be in a relaxed state. PROM distinguishes injury to contractile tissues from noncontractile or inert tissues (bone, ligament, bursae, joint capsule, fascia, duramater, and nerve roots). If no pain is present during passive motion but is present during active motion, injury to contractile tissue is involved. If noncontractile tissue is injured, passive movement is painful and limitation of movement may be seen. Again, any painful motions should be performed last to avoid any carry over of pain from one motion to the next. At the end of the range of motion, a gentle overpressure is applied to determine **end feel**. Overpressure is repeated several times to determine whether pain increases, which signifies damage to noncontractile joint structures. The end feel can determine the type of disorder. There are three normal end feel sensations and four abnormal end feel sensations **(Table 4.4)** (3).

Differences in ROM between active and passive movements can be due to muscle spasm, muscle deficiency, neurologic deficit, contractures, or pain (4). If pain occurs before the end of the available ROM, it may indicate an acute injury. Stretching and manipulation of the joint are contraindicated. If pain occurs simultaneously at the end of the ROM, a subacute injury may be present, and a mild stretching program may be started cautiously. If no pain is felt as the available ROM is stretched, a chronic injury is present. An appropriate treatment and rehabilitation program should be initiated immediately (4).

Accessory movements are movements within the joint that accompany traditional active and passive ROM, but cannot be voluntarily performed by the individual. Joint play motions, for example, allow the joint capsule to "give" so bones can move to absorb an external force. These

TABLE 4.4	NORMAL AND ABNORMAL JOINT END FEELS

Normal End Feel Sensations

End Feel	Structure	Example
Soft	Soft tissue approximation	Elbow flexion (contact between soft tissue of the forearm with anterior arm)
Firm	Muscular stretch	Hip extension (passive stretch of iliopsoas muscle)
	Capsular stretch	External rotation at the shoulder (passive stretch of anterior glenohumeral joint capsule)
	Ligamentous stretch	Forearm supination (tension in the palmar radioulnar ligament of the inferior radioulnar joint, interosseous membrane, oblique cord)
Hard	Bone to bone	Elbow extension (contact between olecranon process and olecranon fossa)

Abnormal End Feel Sensations

End Feel	Description	Example
Soft	Occurs sooner or later in the ROM than is usual or in a joint that normally has a firm or hard end feel; feels boggy	Soft-tissue edema Synovitis Ligamentous stretch or tear
Firm	Occurs sooner or later in the ROM than is usual; or in a joint that normally has a soft or hard end feel	Increased muscular tonus Capsular, muscular, ligamentous shortening
Hard	Occurs sooner or later in the ROM than is usual; or in a joint that normally has a soft or firm end feel; a bony grating or bony block is felt	Chondromalacia Osteoarthritis Loose bodies in joint Myositis ossificans Fracture
Empty	No end feel because end of ROM is never reached due to pain. No resistance is felt except for patient's protective muscle splinting or muscle spasm	Acute joint inflammation Bursitis Fracture Psychogenic in origin

movements include distraction, sliding, compression, rolling, and spinning of joint surfaces. These motions occur within the joint, but only as a response to an outside force, and not as a result of any voluntary movement. These movements aid the healing process, relieve pain, reduce disability, and restore full normal range of motion. If any joint play movement is found to be absent or decreased, this movement must be restored before functional voluntary movement can be fully accomplished (5).

The presence of accessory movement can be determined by manipulating the joint in a position of least strain, called the **loose packed**, or resting **position (Table 4.5)**. The resting position is the position in the joint's ROM in which the joint is under the least amount of stress, and is also the position in which the joint capsule has its greatest capacity. The advantage of testing accessory movements in the loose packed position is that the joint surface contact areas are reduced, proper joint lubrication is enhanced, and friction and erosion in the joints is decreased.

In contrast, a **close packed position** is the position in which two joint surfaces fit precisely together. The ligaments and joint capsule are maximally taut, and joint surfaces are maximally compressed and cannot be separated by distractive forces, nor can accessory movements occur. Therefore, if a bone or ligament is injured, pain will increase as the joint moves into the close packed position. If swelling is present within the joint, the close packed position cannot be achieved. **Table 4.6** lists the close packed positions of the major joints of the body.

TABLE 4.5   **LOOSE PACKED POSITION OF SELECTED JOINTS**

Joint(s)	Position
Glenohumeral	55° abduction, 30° horizontal adduction
Elbow (ulnohumeral)	70° elbow flexion, 10° forearm supination
Radiohumeral	Full extension, full forearm supination
Proximal radioulnar	70° elbow flexion, 35° supination
Distal radioulnar	10° forearm supination
Wrist (radiocarpal)	Neutral with slight ulnar deviation
Carpometacarpal	Midway between abduction-adduction and flexion-extension
Metacarpophalangeal	Slight flexion
Interphalangeal	Slight flexion
Hip	30° flexion, 30° abduction, slight lateral rotation
Knee	25° flexion
Ankle (talocrural)	10° plantar flexion, midway between maximum inversion and eversion
Subtalar	Midway between extremes of inversion and eversion
Tarsometatarsal	Midway between extremes of range of motion
Metatarsophalangeal	Neutral
Interphalangeal	Slight flexion

TABLE 4.6   **CLOSE PACKED POSITION OF SELECTED JOINTS**

Joint(s)	Position
Glenohumeral	Abduction and lateral rotation
Elbow (ulnohumeral)	Extension
Radiohumeral	Elbow flexed 90°, 5° forearm supination
Proximal radioulnar	5° forearm supination
Distal radioulnar	5° forearm supination
Wrist (radiocarpal)	Extension with radial deviation
Metacarpophalangeal (fingers)	Full flexion
Metacarpophalangeal (thumb)	Full opposition
Interphalangeal	Full extension
Hip	Full extension, medial rotation and abduction
Knee	Full extension, lateral rotation of tibia
Ankle (talocrural)	Maximum dorsiflexion
Subtalar	Full supination
Midtarsal	Full supination
Tarsometatarsal	Full supination
Metatarsophalangeal	Full extension
Interphalangeal	Full extension

RESISTED MANUAL MUSCLE TESTING

Resisted manual muscle testing can assess muscle strength and detect injury to the nervous system. To test resistance, an overload pressure is applied in a stationary or static position, sometimes referred to as a **break test**, or may be applied throughout the full range of motion. Muscle weakness and pain indicate a muscular strain. Muscle weakness in the absence of pain may indicate nerve damage.

In performing a break test, overload pressure is applied with the joint in a neutral or relaxed position to relax joint structures and reduce joint stress. As such, contractile tissues (muscles) are more effectively stressed. The limb is stabilized proximal to the joint to prevent other motions from compensating for weakness in the involved muscle. Resistance is provided distally on the bone to which the muscle or muscle group attaches, and should not be distal to a second joint. In a fixed position, the individual is asked to elicit a maximal contraction while the body part is stabilized to prevent little or no joint movement. For example, to test strength in the elbow flexors, flex the elbow at 90° and stabilize the upper arm against the body. Apply downward overpressure on the distal forearm and tell the individual not to allow the arm to move **(Figure 4.11)**. Contractions are held for at least 5 seconds and repeated 5 to 6 times to indicate muscle weakening and the presence or absence of pain (5). A standardized grading system can be used to measure muscle contraction, but the results are negated if the contraction causes pain **(Table 4.7)**.

Two advantages of testing throughout the full range of motion are: 1) a better overall assessment of weakness

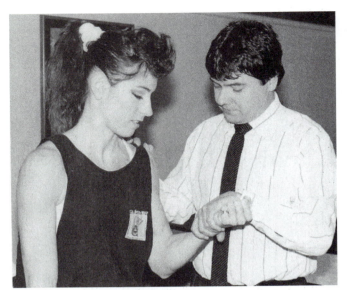

▶ FIGURE 4.11 **Resisted manual muscle testing in a static position**. Stabilize the arm against the body. Apply downward pressure on the distal forearm, and ask the individual to prevent any movement.

can be determined, and 2) a **painful arc** of motion can be located, which might otherwise go undetected if the test is only performed in the mid-range. In performing resisted testing, the body segment is placed in a specific position to isolate the muscle(s). The muscle(s) to be tested is placed in a stretched or elongated position. This position prevents other muscles in the area from performing the movement. Manual pressure is exerted throughout the full range of motion, and is repeated several times to reveal weakness or pain. The presence of pain during motion should be noted. In this manner, both subjective (what the individual feels) and objective information (weakness) is gathered.

TABLE 4.7		GRADING SYSTEM FOR MANUAL MUSCLE TESTING
Numerical	**Verbal**	**Clinical Findings**
5	Normal	Complete range of motion (ROM) against gravity with maximal overload
4	Good	Complete ROM against gravity with moderate overload
3+	Fair +	Complete ROM against gravity with minimal overload
3	Fair	Complete ROM against gravity with no overload
3−	Fair −	Some, but not complete ROM against gravity
2+	Poor +	Initiates motion against gravity
2	Poor	Complete ROM with some assistance and gravity eliminated
2−	Poor −	Initiates motion if gravity is eliminated
1	Trace	Evidence of slight muscular contraction, no joint motion
0	Zero	No muscle contraction palpated

TABLE 4.8		GRADING SYSTEM FOR LIGAMENTOUS LAXITY
Grade	**Ligamentous End Feel**	**Damage**
I	Firm (normal)	Slight stretching of the ligament with little to no tearing of the fibers. Pain is present, but the degree of stability roughly compares with that of the opposite extremity.
II	Soft	Partial tearing of the fibers. The joint line "opens up" significantly when compared with the opposite side.
III	Empty	Complete tearing of the ligament. The motion is restricted by other joint structures, such as tendons.

Ligamentous and Capsular Testing

Each body segment has a series of tests to assess joint function and integrity of joint structures. These tests assess noncontractile tissues (e.g., ligaments, intra-articular structures, joint capsule stability), impingement signs, muscle balance, and vascular integrity (6). For examples, sprains of ligamentous tissue are generally graded on a three-degree scale after a specific stress is applied to a ligament to test its laxity **(Table 4.8)**. **Laxity** describes the amount of "give" within a joint's supportive tissue. **Instability** is a joint's inability to function under the stresses encountered during functional activities. All ligamentous testing should be done bilaterally and compared with baseline measures. It is essential to perform the test at the proper angle, because a seemingly minor change in the joint angle can significantly alter the laxity of the tissue being stressed (6). **Figure 4.12** demonstrates a **valgus** stress test on the elbow joint to assess the integrity of the joint medial collateral ligaments. During an on-the-field assessment, tests to determine a possible fracture and major ligament damage at a joint should always be performed before moving an injured indi-

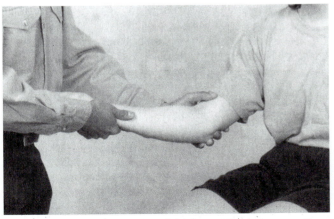

▶ FIGURE 4.12 **Stress tests**. Applying a valgus stress on the elbow joint can assess the integrity of the joint medial collateral ligaments.

vidual. Only the specific tests deemed necessary for the injury should be used. Because of the wide variety of stress tests, each is discussed within subsequent chapters.

Neurologic Testing

A segmental nerve is the portion of a nerve that originates in the spinal cord and is referred to as a nerve root. Most nerve roots share two components: 1) a somatic portion, which innervates a series of skeletal muscles and provides sensory input from the skin, fascia, muscles, and joints; and 2) a visceral component, which is part of the autonomic nervous system. The autonomic system supplies the blood vessels, dura mater, periosteum, ligaments, and intervertebral discs, among many other structures.

Nerves are commonly injured by tensile or compressive forces and will be reflected in both motor and sensory deficits. The motor component of a segmental nerve is tested using a **myotome**, a group of muscles primarily innervated by a single nerve root. The sensory component is tested using a **dermatome**, an area of skin supplied by a single nerve root. An injury to a segmental nerve root will often affect more than one peripheral nerve and will not demonstrate the same motor loss or sensory deficit as an injury to a single peripheral nerve. Dermatomes, myotomes, and reflexes are used to assess the integrity of the central nervous system. Peripheral nerves are assessed using manual muscle testing and noting cutaneous sensory changes in peripheral nerve patterns. Neurologic testing is only necessary in orthopedic injuries when an athlete complains of numbness, tingling, or a burning sensation, or suffers from unexplained muscular weakness.

DERMATOMES

The sensitivity of a dermatome can be assessed by touching the person with a cotton ball, paper clip, pads of the fingers, and fingernails. In doing so, the clinician should ask the individual about the sensations being experienced. It is important to determine the nature of the sensation (e.g., a sharp or dull sensation) and to assess whether the same sensation was experienced in testing the uninjured body segment. Abnormal responses may be decreased tactile sensation (**hypoesthesia**), excessive tactile sensation (**hyperesthesia**), or loss of sensation (**anesthesia**). **Paresthesia** is another abnormal sensation characterized by a numbness, tingling, or burning sensation. **Figure 4.13** illustrates dermatome patterns for the segmental nerves.

MYOTOMES

The majority of muscles receive segmental innervation from two or more nerve roots. However, selected motions may be innervated predominantly by a single nerve root (myotome). Resisted muscle testing of a selected motion can determine the status of the nerve root that supplies that myotome **(Table 4.9)**. Muscle contractions must be held at least 5 seconds (5). Weakness in the myotome

TABLE 4.9	MYOTOMES USED TO TEST SELECTED NERVE ROOT SEGMENTS
Nerve Root Segment	**Action Tested**
C_1–C_2	Neck flexion*
C_3	Neck lateral flexion*
C_4	Shoulder elevation
C_5	Shoulder abduction
C_6	Elbow flexion and wrist extension
C_7	Elbow extension and wrist flexion
C_8	Thumb extension and ulnar deviation
T_1	Intrinsic muscles of the hand (finer abduction and adduction)
L_1–L_2	Hip flexion
L_3	Knee extension
L_4	Ankle dorsiflexion
L_5	Toe extension
S_1	Ankle plantar flexion, foot eversion, hip extension
S_2	Knee flexion

*These myotomes should not be performed in an individual with a suspected cervical fracture or dislocation, as they may cause serious damage or possible death.

indicates a possible spinal cord nerve root injury. In testing a myotome, a normal response is a strong muscle contraction. A weakened muscle contraction may indicate partial paralysis (**paresis**) of the muscles innervated by the nerve root being tested. In a peripheral nerve injury, there is complete paralysis of the muscles supplied by that nerve. For example, the L_3 myotome is tested with knee extension. If the L_3 nerve root is damaged at its origin in the spine, there is a weak muscle contraction. This is because the quadriceps muscle also receives nerve root innervation from L_2 and L_4 segmental nerves. If, however, the peripheral femoral nerve, which contains segments of L_2, L_3, and L_4, is damaged proximal to the quadriceps muscle, the muscle cannot receive any nerve impulses and, therefore, will be unable to contract to execute knee extension.

REFLEXES

Damage to the central nervous system can also be detected by stimulation of the reflexes. Exaggerated, distorted, or absent reflexes indicate degeneration or injury in specific regions of the nervous system. This may be demonstrated before other signs are apparent. The most familiar deep tendon reflex is the patellar, or knee-jerk, reflex elicited by striking the patellar tendon with a reflex hammer, causing a rapid contraction of the quadriceps muscle **(Figure 4.14)**. Deep tendon reflexes tend to be diminished or absent if the specific nerve root being tested is damaged **(Table 4.10)**.

PERIPHERAL NERVE TESTING

Motor function in peripheral nerves is assessed with resisted manual muscle testing throughout the full range of motion. Sensory deficits are assessed in a manner identical to dermatome testing, except the cutaneous patterns differ

Spinal dermatomes   Peripheral nerves   Spinal dermatomes

Ophthalmic
Maxillary   Divisions of
Mandibular   trigeminal
Branches from cervical plexus

Posterior
cervical rami

Anterior thoracic   Axillary
rami   Posterior thoracic
                           rami
Lateral thoracic rami
Branches from medial
cord of brachial plexus
Radial
Posterior lumbar rami
Lateral antebrachial cutaneous
Median antebrachial cutaneous
Posterior sacral
rami
Iliohypogastric
Radial
Ulnar
Median
Posterior femoral
cutaneous
Ilioinguinal
Lateral femoral cutaneous
Obturator
Anterior femoral cutaneous
Common peroneal
Saphenous
Superficial peroneal
Deep peroneal

Anterior   Posterior

➤ FIGURE 4.13 **Cutaneous sensation**. The cutaneous sensation patterns of the spinal nerves (*dermatomes*) differ from the patterns innervated by the peripheral nerves.

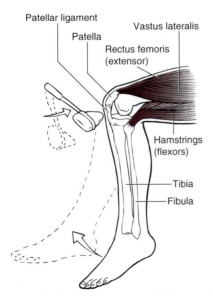

Patellar ligament
Patella
Vastus lateralis
Rectus femoris
(extensor)
Hamstrings
(flexors)
Tibia
Fibula

➤ FIGURE 4.14 **Reflexes**. Reflexes can indicate if there is nerve root damage. The most familiar stretch reflex is the knee jerk, or patellar reflex, performed by tapping the patellar tendon with a reflex hammer, causing involuntary knee extension.

(see **Figure 4.13**). Special compression tests may also be used on nerves close to the skin surface, such as the ulnar and median nerves. The "Tinel sign" test is performed by tapping the skin directly over a superficial nerve (see **Figure 12.23**). A positive sign, indicating irritation or compression of the nerve, would result in a tingling sensation traveling into the muscles and skin supplied by the nerve.

Sport-Specific Functional Testing

Before permitting an individual to return to sport participation after an injury, the individual's condition must be fully

TABLE 4.10	COMMONLY TESTED DEEP TENDON REFLEXES
Deep Tendon Reflexes	**Segmental Levels**
Biceps	Cervical **5**, 6
Brachioradialis	Cervical 5, **6**
Triceps	Cervical **7**, 8
Patellar	Lumbar 2, **3**, 4
Medial hamstrings	Lumbar **5**
Lateral hamstrings	Sacral **1**
Achilles	Sacral **1**

evaluated so risk of reinjury is minimal. Sport-specific tests involve the performance of active movements typical of the movements executed by the individual during sport participation. These movements should assess strength, agility, flexibility, joint stability, endurance, coordination, balance, and sport-specific skill performance. In the rehabilitation process, the individual initially performs these skills at low intensity and increases intensity as the individual's condition improves. For example, in a lower leg injury, testing should begin by assessing walking, jogging, and then running forward and backward. If these skills are performed pain-free and without a limp, the individual might then be asked to run in a figure-8 or zigzag pattern. Again, each test must be performed pain-free and without a limp. An individual's balance can be tested by performing tasks with the eyes closed, such as walking a straight line on the toes and heels, balancing on a wobble board, or walking sideways on the hands while in a push-up position. Any individual who has been discharged from rehabilitation should also pass the functional tests and be cleared by a physician for participation.

Special tests were completed on the football player. Active plantar flexion and passive dorsiflexion were painful. Resisted plantar flexion was weak and caused sharp pain in the distal Achilles tendon. Joint stability tests were negative and did not produce an increase in pain. The individual has normal bilateral sensation on the feet and a good distal pulse. After reviewing the subjective and objective evaluation, did you determine that this athlete has a strain of the Achilles tendon? If so, you are correct.

THE EMERGENCY MEDICAL SERVICES SYSTEM

A basketball player goes up for a lay-up shot, gets tangled with another player, and falls onto his back striking his head on the floor. The athlete is not moving. As you approach the player, think for a minute or two about how you will handle this situation, and what actions should be performed if his condition requires immediate transportation to a local medical facility.

Serious injuries can be frightening, particularly if breathing or circulation is impaired. As the first responder on the scene, the athletic trainer is expected to evaluate the situation, assess the severity of injury, recognize life-threatening conditions, provide immediate emergency care, and initiate any emergency procedures to ensure the athlete is transported to the nearest medical facility without delay. Although few sport-related injuries are serious enough to require immediate transportation to the nearest medical facility, these injuries do occur. An **emergency**

medical services (EMS) system is a well-developed process that activates the emergency health care services of the athletic training facility and community to provide immediate health care to an injured individual. As discussed in Chapter 1, the team physician, athletic trainer, and coach have a legal duty to develop and implement an emergency plan to provide health care to their athletes.

Preseason Preparation

Prior to the start of the sport season, the emergency response team should meet with representatives from local EMS agencies to discuss, develop, and evaluate the emergency procedures plan. This is an excellent opportunity to review individual responsibilities and protocols for an emergency situation at an athletic event. Questions to be answered include:

- What emergency equipment must be available at each event, particularly at contact and collision sporting events?
- What equipment will be provided by the local EMS agency (spine board, splints, blankets) if in attendance at the event?
- Who will be responsible for ensuring that all emergency equipment is operational prior to the event?
- What type of communication will be used to contact emergency personnel, and who will activate EMS?
- Who will assess the injured athlete on the field, and under what circumstances will EMS be called onto the field?
- If a physician is present, what will the athletic trainer(s) and EMS be responsible for?
- If a physician is not present and the athletic trainer is evaluating the situation, what will the EMS be responsible for?
- Who will remain on the sideline to bring necessary supplies or equipment on the field if summoned by the athletic trainer or team physician?
- If it becomes necessary to stabilize and transport the individual to a medical facility, who will direct the stabilization and what protocol will be followed for the removal of protective equipment?

A written emergency plan should be developed for each activity site to address these questions, as well as who will render emergency care and control the situation, what type of care will be initiated, what care will be provided while EMS is en route to the facility, who will supervise the other sport participants if the athletic trainer is assessing an injured athlete, and the proper use and disposal of items and equipment exposed to blood or other bodily fluids. It is critical during emergencies that everyone work together to ensure medical attention is not delayed. **Field Strategy 4.3** summarizes several important issues in developing an emergency care plan.

The emergency response team, along with local EMTs or paramedics, should practice the emergency plan through

FIELD STRATEGY 4.3   DEVELOPING AN EMERGENCY CARE PLAN

Personnel:
- All medical and staff members working with sport participants must be currently certified in emergency first aid and CPR.
- Appoint one individual as the medical liaison or "captain." Ensure that this individual has advanced first aid training.

Preseason Planning:
- Have all sport participants been medically cleared to participate? Are appropriate documents completed (e.g., physical examination, permission to participate, informed consent, and emergency information)? Have the athletic trainers and coaches been informed of any orthopedic or health problems that might affect participation?
- Do you have emergency cards for each participant with family phone numbers, physicians' names and phone numbers, special instructions/considerations, and who to contact when parents/guardians are unavailable?
- Is the athletic training facility and activity areas checked regularly for safety hazards? Does everyone know the location and have easy access to first-aid kits, splints, stretchers, fire extinguishers, and a phone? Are emergency numbers posted in clear view near each phone (e.g., EMS, hospital, athletic training room, school nurse, facility medical liaison, fire and police departments)?
- Are all medical staff including local EMS agencies familiar with the activity areas and informed of the most accessible routes to the athletic training room, fields, gymnasia, and pool?
- Do you have different emergency procedures for the various facilities (pool, gymnasia, weight room, training room, and fields)? If so, is the staff aware of them?
- What type of communication will be used by the entire medical staff (e.g., hand signals, two-way radios, cellular phones)?
- At what events will the team physician and EMS providers be present?
- If EMS is in attendance, what emergency equipment will be available through them? Who will ensure that it is operational? What other emergency equipment will be needed on the field/court? Who will ensure that it is available and operational?
- Who will contact the visiting team and inform them of what emergency equipment and services will be available on-site?
- What procedures will be followed if a head or neck injury is suspected and protective equipment is worn by the athlete? Who will direct the stabilization of the athlete and removal of any protective equipment?

In the Event of an Emergency:
- Do all medical staff understand their roles during an emergency situation?
    - Who will complete the initial injury assessment?
    - Who will activate EMS for additional assistance?
    - Who will be on the sideline to bring additional supplies onto the field?
    - Who has access to locked gates or doors?
    - Who will direct the ambulance to the accident scene?
- Under what conditions will the team physician go onto the field?
- Under what conditions will the EMS providers be summoned onto the field?
- If the team physician or EMS must be summoned, what information should be provided over the phone or radio (e.g., type of emergency situation, possible injury/condition, current status of the injured party, type of assistance being given to the injured party, exact location of the facility or injured individual [give cross streets to assist EMS] and specific point of entry to the facility, telephone number of phone being used)?
- Who will decide the best method with which to transport the individual off the field?

After an Emergency:
- Who will be responsible for informing the individual's parents/guardians that an emergency has occurred?
- Are proper injury records completed after the injury and kept on file in a central, secure location?

regular educational workshops and training exercises. These workshops can provide continuing education in emergency care management and recertification in first aid and cardiopulmonary resuscitation protocols. This will help prepare individuals to assume their roles in rendering emergency care to an injured sport participant.

Responsibilities of Medical Personnel

The emergency response team consists of the team physician, athletic trainer, student athletic trainers, coaching staff, and EMS providers from the local EMS agency. Each has specific responsibilities associated with emergency medical care of sport participants. Prior to a sport event, the emergency response team should meet to review emergency procedures. Everyone should know the location and proper use of medical supplies and equipment, and they must be operational and easily accessible. A method of communication on the field should be established, e.g., hand signals or two-way radios to summon the team physician, the EMS providers, and equipment and supplies. For example, a right hand on the head may summon the team physician onto the field, and crossed arms may indicate the need for a spine board; both hands on the head may indicate the need to summon EMS.

TEAM PHYSICIAN

Prior to the season, the team physician should delineate the responsibilities for all personnel so there is no confusion about treatment decisions. It must be clearly understood what events the team physician will attend, what role he or she will play in the assessment of injuries, and what, if any, responsibility he or she will have in providing emergency medical services to bystanders and spectators.

Although present at the event, the team physician is not always the "first responder" to an injured athlete; the most experienced certified athletic trainer assigned to cover that sport will usually be the first individual to assess the athlete. Once called onto the field, however, the team physician should evaluate any serious injury (e.g., head, neck, or spinal injuries, cardiac emergencies, joint injuries) and determine the level of severity. If needed, the team physician will summon additional supplies or assistance and direct the athletic trainer to assist as needed. When appropriate, the physician will also direct the stabilization and immobilization of the athlete in preparation for transportation to the nearest medical facility. If transportation is not necessary, the team physician will decide whether to return the athlete to competition.

ATHLETIC TRAINER

The athletic trainer is responsible for setting up the event area with appropriate equipment and supplies for the medical kit (**Box 4.3**) and emergency "crash" kit (**Box 4.4**), and providing a method of communication (e.g., telephone,

Continued

➤➤ **BOX 4.3**

Checklist for Athletic Training Medical Kit

- ☐ Adhesive bandages (assorted sizes)
- ☐ Adhesive tape
  - ☐ 1/2 inch
  - ☐ 1 inch
  - ☐ 1/2 inch
  - ☐ 2 inch
- ☐ Airway (pocket mask and oropharyngeal)
- ☐ Alcohol (isopropyl)
- ☐ Antacid tablets or liquid
- ☐ Antifungal powder or spray
- ☐ Antiseptic/antibiotic ointment
- ☐ Antiseptic soap
- ☐ Aspirin tablets
- ☐ Blister tape (Dermiclear®)
- ☐ Butterfly bandage and Steri–strips
- ☐ Cloth ankle wraps
- ☐ Contact lens case and solution
- ☐ Cotton balls
- ☐ Cotton-tipped applicators
- ☐ Elastic tape (Elastikon® or Conform®)
  - ☐ 1 inch
  - ☐ 2 inch
  - ☐ 3 inch
- ☐ Elastic wraps
  - ☐ 4 inch
  - ☐ 6 inch
  - ☐ Double-length 6 inch
- ☐ Emergency kit
  - ☐ Coins for pay phone
  - ☐ Emergency telephone numbers
  - ☐ Location of nearest trauma center
  - ☐ Health information cards
  - ☐ Injury reports
  - ☐ Insurance information
- ☐ Eyepatchs (sterile)
- ☐ Eyewash and eye cup
- ☐ Felt (compression/horseshoe pads)
  - ☐ 1/4 inch
  - ☐ 1/2 inch
- ☐ Fingernail clipper
- ☐ Flexible collodion
- ☐ Foam padding
  - ☐ 1/8 inch
  - ☐ 1/4 inch
  - ☐ 1/2 inch
  - ☐ 1 inch
- ☐ Forceps (tweezers)
- ☐ Fungicide cream
- ☐ Gauze pads (sterile and nonsterile)
- ☐ Germicide solution
- ☐ Heel and lace pads
- ☐ Heel cups
- ☐ Hydrogen peroxide
- ☐ Latex gloves
- ☐ Mirror (handheld)
- ☐ Moleskin
- ☐ Nasal pledget (plug)
- ☐ Nonadhering sterile pads
- ☐ Nonocclusive dressing
- ☐ Oral thermometer
- ☐ Paper, pen or pencil
- ☐ Penlight

BOX 4.3 Checklist for Athletic Training Medical Kit *Continued*

☐ Plastic bags for ice
☐ Ring cutter
☐ Scalpel and blades, disposable
☐ Scissors
   ☐ Bandage
   ☐ Heavy duty
   ☐ Surgical
   ☐ Taping
   ☐ Trainer's Angel®
☐ Second skin
☐ Skin lubricant (petroleum jelly)
☐ Sling or triangular bandages
☐ Stethoscope and blood pressure cuff
☐ Suntan lotion or sunblock
☐ Tape adherent
☐ Tape cutter
☐ Tape remover
☐ Tongue depressors
☐ Towlettes, moist
☐ Underwrap

➤➤ **BOX 4.5**

Duties of the Athletic Trainer

- Stock medical kit and emergency "crash" kit
- Gather emergency supplies and equipment and make sure all equipment is operational
- Provide method of communication
- Contact visiting team's athletic trainer and communicate regarding available on-site medical services and emergency procedures
- Meet the visiting team's athletic trainer upon arrival and address any concerns
- Assess on-the-field injuries
- Summon additional supplies and assistance as needed
- Assist team physician as needed
- In the absence of the team physician.
   Assess severity of all injuries
   Direct stabilization and immobilization of the injured athlete
   Determine mode for removing injured player from the field or court
   Determine when the athlete may return to competition
   Refer the athlete to a physician or medical facility as needed

two-way radio, or cellular phone). The equipment must meet the needs, size, and age of the athletes, and be compatible with equipment used by other health professionals.

For home events, the host athletic trainer should contact the visiting team's athletic trainer to inform him or her of services and supplies that will be made available to the visiting team. Emergency procedures can also be explained at this time. When the team arrives, the host athletic trainer should immediately introduce himself or herself to the visiting athletic trainer and answer any questions concerning access to the athletic training facilities,

emergency equipment, emergency procedures, and location of the nearest medical facility. For an away event, if the team physician does not travel with the team, the athletic trainer should be informed of what services will be provided by the on-site team physician.

If the team physician is present at the sporting event, the certified athletic trainer will assist as needed. He or she may be responsible for giving hand signals to summon additional equipment or supplies and will assist in stabilizing an injury site and removing the athlete from the field. If the team physician is not present, the certified athletic trainer directs the on-the-field management of all injuries **(Box 4.5)**. It is his or her responsibility to stabilize and calm the athlete, assess severity of all injuries, summon additional resources or equipment if necessary, manage the injury if appropriate, direct the stabilization and immobilization of the athlete in preparation for transport if appropriate, and determine when an injured athlete may return to competition.

➤➤ **BOX 4.4**

Checklist for Emergency Crash Kit

On the Sideline or Court
☐ Blood pressure cuff
☐ Stethoscope
☐ Immoblizer splints and slings
☐ Crutches
☐ Cervical collars (soft and Philadelphia®)
☐ Spine board, stretcher, cart, and chair
☐ Oropharyngeal airway
☐ Biohazard equipment
   ☐ Hazardous waste disposal containers with labels
   ☐ Spill kits
   ☐ Personal protective equipment
☐ Water and cups
☐ Ice bags
☐ Towels
Carried by the Athletic Trainer
☐ Latex gloves
☐ Sterile gauze
☐ Penlight
☐ CPR pocket mask
☐ Device for removing facemasks (e.g., Trainer's Angel)

STUDENT ATHLETIC TRAINERS

Student athletic trainers must follow the direction of the athletic trainer or team physician. In the absence of a team physician or athletic trainer, the student athletic trainer should follow the responsibilities and duties as delineated (in writing) by the athletic trainer in accordance with applicable state licensure or registration laws. If student athletic trainers travel in the absence of the athletic trainer or team physician, the athletic trainer should contact the on-site host to notify them that a student athletic trainer is traveling with the team and inquire about what services will be provided to the athletes by the on-site medical staff.

COACHING STAFF

As a member of the emergency response team, the coach will follow the direction of the team physician or athletic trainer. The specific responsibilities of the coach should be stated in the emergency plan and reviewed prior to the start of the season. For example, the emergency plan may dictate that the coach remain on the sideline to supervise the team or it may dictate that the coach take a more active role in the management of the injured player. It is essential that the coach be familiar with the role he or she is expected to assume. The coach must understand that the team physician, or in the absence of the team physician, the athletic trainer, is the final authority with regard to medical decisions. The coach should not attempt to intervene in decisions regarding the playing status of an athlete.

EMS PERSONNEL

EMS personnel include certified emergency medical technicians (EMTs) or paramedics trained in emergency care. Sports injuries and clinical training are not typically emphasized in EMS education so confusion can result during the emergency care of an athlete. It is the responsibility of the team physician or athletic trainer to specify the circumstances warranting the services of an EMT and to ensure that EMTs are instructed on the management and protocol to be followed in handling athletic injuries. For example, the removal of protective equipment and stabilization of an athlete onto a spine board must be addressed. This information should be documented in the emergency care plan and agreed upon by all parties prior to the start of the sport season. Workshops or seminars may be conducted with area EMS providers and athletic trainers so there is no confusion about emergency care protocol for an injured athlete.

 As you approach the injured basketball player, look for any signs of movement or breathing and mentally review the facility's EMS plan in case you need to direct your colleagues to summon additional supplies or assistance.

EMERGENCY INJURY ASSESSMENT

 In beginning to evaluate the injured basketball player, what sequential process can be used to determine if the central nervous system and/or cardiorespiratory systems are critically injured? What diagnostic tests can help determine the severity of the injury, and under what conditions would EMS be activated for immediate transport to the nearest medical facility?

Injuries or conditions that impair, or have the potential to impair, vital function of the central nervous system and cardiorespiratory system are considered emergency situations. In many cases, serious injuries are clearly evident and recognizable, such as lack of breathing, absence of pulse, or massive hemorrhage (bleeding). This assessment, called a **primary survey**, determines level of responsiveness, recognizes and identifies immediate life-threatening situations (ABCs), and dictates what actions are needed to care for the individual. Because the authors assume that students at this level should already have received instruction in their first aid class on cardiopulmonary resuscitation (CPR), techniques associated with the primary survey will not be discussed.

Occasionally, collisions occur in sport activities in which more than one player is injured. **Triage** refers to the rapid assessment of all injured individuals followed by return to the most seriously injured to give them immediate treatment. If possible, at least two medically trained individuals should be present during the initial assessment. The athletic trainer responsible for the team is designated as the **charge person**, or person in control. This individual controls the scene in part by not allowing the athlete to be moved until some type of assessment is completed. The assistant, or **call person**, is responsible for providing assistance, relaying messages to the sideline, and obtaining additional help if necessary (5). If at anytime during the assessment "red flags" are noted **(Box 4.6)**, the assessment process should be terminated and EMS activated.

During the on-the-field assessment, the athletic trainer must ascertain whether a serious or moderate injury is present. In order of priority, the on-the-field evaluation should address (6):

- Life-threatening trauma to the head
- Spinal cord injury with abnormal or absent neurologic signs
- Massive hemorrhage
- Fractures with gross deformity
- Joint dislocations
- Other soft-tissue injuries

When identified, appropriate immobilization and transportation should be utilized in removing the individual from the field. Once off the field, a more thorough exam can be conducted. Decisions on the extent of injury, treatment, and playing status must be based on sound medical assessment despite external influencing factors. Regardless of where the assessment occurs, all protocols should con-

---

➤➤ **Box 4.6**

"Red Flags" Indicating Serious Emergency and Activation of EMS

- Airway obstruction
- Respiratory failure
- Severe shock
- Severe chest or abdominal pains
- Excessive bleeding
- Suspected spinal injury
- Head injury with loss of consciousness
- Severe heat illness
- Fractures involving several ribs, the femur, or pelvis

FIELD STRATEGY 4.4   **DETERMINING THE HISTORY OF INJURY AND LEVEL OF RESPONSIVENESS**

Stabilize the head and neck. Do not move individual unnecessarily until a spinal injury is ruled out. If nonresponsive:

- Call the person's name loudly and gently tap the sternum or touch the arm. If no response, rap the sternum more forcibly with a knuckle or pinch the soft tissue in the armpit (axillary fold). Note if there is a withdrawal from the painful stimuli. If no response, immediately initiate the primary survey.
- If ABCs are adequate, gather a history of the injury. If you did not see what happened, question other players, supervisors, officials, and bystanders. Ask:

  What happened?

  Did you see the individual get hit, or did the individual just collapse?

  How long has the individual been unresponsive?

  Did the individual suddenly become unresponsive or deteriorate gradually?

  If it was gradual, did anyone talk to the individual before you arrived?

  What did the person say? Was it coherent? Did the person moan, groan, or mumble?

  Has this ever happened before to this individual?

If conscious, ask:

- What happened? If the individual is lying down, find out if he or she was knocked down, fell, or rolled voluntarily into that position.
- Are you in pain? Where is the pain? Is it localized or does it radiate into other areas?
- Did you hear any sounds or any unusual sensations when the injury occurred? Note if the individual is alert and aware of his or her surroundings, or has any short- or long-term memory loss.
- Have you ever injured this body part before, or experienced a similar injury?
- Do you have a headache? Are you nauseous or sick to your stomach? Are you dizzy? Can you see clearly?
- Are you taking any medication (prescription, over-the-counter, vitamins, birth control pills, etc.)?
- Do not lead the individual. Let him or her describe what happened and *listen attentively* for clues to the nature of the injury. Be professional and reassuring.

---

tain the same basic components that are relevant, accurate, and measurable.

On-the-Field History

When the athletic trainer reaches the individual, a position close to the injured athlete should be taken. Place one hand on the forehead to stabilize the head and neck to prevent any unnecessary movement. The history of the injury can be obtained from the athlete or, if the athlete is unconscious, from bystanders who may have witnessed the injury. Questions should be open-ended to allow the person to provide as much information as possible about the injury. Listen attentively for clues that may indicate the nature of the injury. On-the-field history taking should be relatively brief as compared to a more comprehensive clinical evaluation. Critical areas of information include:

- **Location of pain**. Be as specific as possible, but be aware that other areas may also be injured.
- **Presence of abnormal neurologic signs**. Identify if there is any tingling, numbness, or loss of sensation.
- **Mechanism of injury**. Identify the position of the injured body part at the point of impact and the direction of force.

- **Associated sounds**. A "snap" or "pop" may indicate a fracture or rupture of a ligament or tendon.

The athletic trainer can then determine the possibility of an associated head or spinal injury, calm the athlete down, and then rule out injury to other body areas while summoning assistance to appropriately manage the condition. If the individual cannot open the eyes on verbal command or does not demonstrate withdrawal from painful stimulus, a serious "red flag" injury exists. **Field Strategy 4.4** lists several questions to determine a history of the injury and assess the level of responsiveness.

On-the-Field Observation and Inspection

In an on-the-field evaluation, much of the observation process is completed en route to the injured athlete, and therefore, occurs prior to the history taking. Critical areas to observe include:

- **Check the surrounding area**. Determine if any equipment or apparatus may have contributed to the injury.
- **Body position**. Is the athlete prone, supine, or side-lying? Is there a gross deformity in one of the limbs?

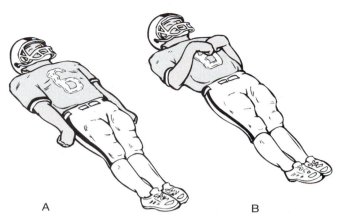

➤ FIGURE 4.15 **Body posturing.** A, Decerebrate rigidity is characterized by extension in all four extremities. B, Decorticate rigidity is characterized by extension of the legs and flexion of the elbows, wrist, and fingers. Both conditions indicate a severe brain injury.

In severe brain injuries, a neurological sign called "posturing" of the extremities can occur **(Figure 4.15)**. **Decerebrate rigidity** is characterized by extension in all four extremities. **Decorticate rigidity** is characterized by extension of the legs and marked flexion in the elbows, wrists, and fingers.

- **Movement of the athlete**. Is the athlete holding the injured body part and in pain? This indicates the athlete is conscious and has an intact central nervous system (CNS) and cardiovascular system. If the athlete is not moving or is having a seizure, suspect possible systemic, psychological, or neurological dysfunction.
- **Level of responsiveness**. Sometimes referred to the "shake and shout" stage, the athletic trainer tries to arouse the unconscious athlete by gently shaking (without moving the head or neck) and by shouting into each ear. Is the person alert, restless, lethargic, or nonresponsive? Does he or she moan, groan, or mumble?
- **Primary survey**. Employ the ABC technique to ensure an open **A**irway, adequate **B**reathing, and **C**irculation.
- **Inspection for head trauma**. Do the pupils of the eyes appear normal or dilated? Is there redness, bruising, or discoloration in the facial area or behind the ears? Note any clear fluid or bloody discharge from the ears or nose. This could be cerebrospinal fluid leaking from the cranial area as a result of a skull fracture.
- **Inspection of the injured body part**. Check for joint alignment, redness, swelling, bruising, or cuts. These observations should always be compared to the uninjured body part.

On-the-Field Palpation

A general head-to-toe assessment should be performed by the athletic trainer. This is done by using a gentle squeezing motion to palpate methodically down the trunk of the body to the fingers and toes. The purpose of the palpation is to detect the following:

- **Abnormal joint angulation**. Identifies a possible joint dislocation.
- **Bony palpation**. Possible fractures can be detected with palpation, percussion, vibration, compression, and distraction (see **Figure 4.6**). Crepitus is associated with fracture, swelling, or inflammation.
- **Soft tissue palpation**. Swelling may indicate diffuse hemorrhage or inflammation in a muscle, ligament, bursa, or joint capsule. Deformity, such as an indentation, may indicate a rupture in a musculotendinous unit. A protruding firm bulge may indicate a joint dislocation, ruptured bursa, muscle spasm, or hematoma.
- **Skin temperature**. Normally the skin is dry, but certain conditions, such as cold, shock, or fever can alter surface blood vessels. Skin temperature is assessed by placing the back of the hand against the individual's forehead or by palpating appendages bilaterally.

On-the-Field Functional Testing

When not contraindicated, the athletic trainer should identify the athlete's willingness to move the injured body part. For a lower extremity injury, this should be expanded to include the willingness to bear weight. Movement, however, is contraindicated in the presence of a possible head or spinal injury, fracture, dislocation, or muscle/tendon rupture.

- **Active range of motion**. The athlete is asked to move the injured body part through the available range of motion. The athletic trainer should note quantity and quality of movement in the absence of pain.
- **Passive range of motion**. The athletic trainer should attempt to move the athlete to a stretcher and try to move the injured extremity through the available pain-free range of motion, noting any painful arc of motion.
- **Resisted range of motion**. The athletic trainer should apply an overpressure (break pressure) to the involved muscle(s) to determine the muscle's ability to sustain a forceful contraction.
- **Weight bearing**. If the athlete successfully completes active, passive, and resisted motion, he or she may be permitted to walk off the field. If, however, the athlete is unable to perform these tests, or if critical signs and symptoms are apparent, the athlete should be removed from the field in a non–weight-bearing manner.

On-the-Field Stress Testing

Testing for ligamentous integrity is performed prior to any muscle guarding or swelling to prevent obscuring the extent of injury. Typically, only single-plane tests are performed and then compared with the noninjured limb (6).

On-the-Field Neurologic Testing

Neurologic testing is critical to prevent a catastrophic injury. Although listed as a separate testing phase, this evaluation may be done earlier in the evaluation, if warranted. Critical areas to include are:

- **Cutaneous sensation**. This can be done by running the fingernails along both sides of the injured athlete's arms and legs to determine if the individual experiences the same feeling on both sides of the body part. Pain perception can also be tested by applying a sharp and dull point to the skin. Note whether the individual can distinguish the difference.
- **Motor function**. The athletic trainer should complete a cranial nerve assessment (see Chapter 8) or ask the athlete to wiggle the fingers and toes on both hands and feet. Compare grip strength in both hands.

Vital Signs

When warranted, the athletic trainer should assess the vital signs to establish a baseline of information about the health status of the individual. Vital signs indicate the status of the cardiovascular and central nervous system. These signs include the pulse, respiratory rate and quality, blood pressure, and temperature. Although not specifically cited as vital signs, skin color, pupillary response to light, and eye movement may also be assessed to determine neurologic function. Abnormal vital signs indicate a serious injury or illness **(Table 4.11)**.

TABLE 4.11   ABNORMAL VITAL SIGNS AND POSSIBLE CAUSES

Pulse

Rapid, weak	Shock, internal hemorrhage, hypoglycemia, heat exhaustion, or hyperventilation
Rapid, bounding	Heat stroke, fright, fever, hypertension, apprehension, hyperglycemia, or normal exertion
Slow, bounding	Skull fracture, stroke, drug use (barbiturates and narcotics), certain cardiac problems or some poisons
No pulse	Blocked artery, low blood pressure, or cardiac arrest

Respiratory Rate and Quality

Shallow breathing	Shock, heat exhaustion, insulin shock, chest injury, or cardiac problems
Irregular breathing	Airway obstruction, chest injury, diabetic coma, asthma, or cardiac problems
Rapid, deep	Diabetic coma, hyperventilation, some lung diseases
Frothy blood	Lung damage, such as a puncture wound to the lung from a fractured rib or other penetrating object
Slowed breathing	Stroke, head injury, chest injury, or use of certain drugs
Wheezing	Asthma
Crowing	Spasms of the larynx
Apnea	Hypoxia (lack of oxygen), congestive heart failure, head injuries
No breathing	Cardiac arrest, poisoning, drug abuse, drowning, head injury, or intrathoracic injuries with death imminent if action is not taken to correct condition

Blood Pressure

Systolic is <100 mm	Hypotension caused by shock, hemorrhage, heart attack, internal injury, or poor nutrition
Systolic is >140 mm	Hypertension caused by certain medications, oral contraceptives, anabolic steroids, amphetamines, chronic alcohol use, and obesity

Skin Temperature

Dry, cool	Exposure to cold or cervical, thoracic, or lumbar spine injuries
Cool, clammy	Shock, internal hemorrhage, trauma, anxiety, or heat exhaustion
Hot, dry	Disease, infection, high fever, heat stroke, or overexposure to environmental heat
Hot, moist	High fever
Isolated hot spot	Localized infection
Cold appendage	Circulatory problem
"Goose pimples"	Chills, communicable disease, exposure to cold, pain, or fear

Skin Color

Red	Embarrassment, fever, hypertension, heat stroke, carbon monoxide poisoning, diabetic coma, alcohol abuse, infectious disease, inflammation, or allergy
White or ashen	Emotional stress (fright, anger, etc.), anemia, shock, heart attack, hypotension, heat exhaustion, insulin shock, or insufficient circulation
Blue or cyanotic	Heart failure, some severe respiratory disorders, and some poisoning. In dark-skinned individuals, a bluish cast can be seen in the mucous membranes (mouth, tongue, and inner eyelids), the lips, and nail beds
Yellow	Liver disease or jaundice

Pupils

Constricted	Individual is using opiate-based drug, or has ingested a poison
Unequal	Head injury or stroke
Dilated	Shock, hemorrhage, heat stroke, use of a stimulant drug, coma, cardiac arrest, or death

PULSE

Factors such as age, gender, aerobic physical condition, degree of physical exertion, medications or chemical substances being taken, blood loss, and stress all influence pulse rate and strength. Pulse is usually taken at the carotid artery because a pulse at that site is not normally obstructed by clothing, equipment, or strappings. Normal adult resting rates range between 60 and 90 beats a minute; children from 80 to 100 beats per minute. Aerobically conditioned athletes may have a pulse rate as low as 40 beats a minute. Pulse is assessed by counting the pulse rate for a 30-second period and then doubling it.

RESPIRATORY RATE

Breathing rate also varies with the gender and age, but averages between 10 to 25 breaths per minute in an adult and between 20 to 25 breaths per minute in a child. Breathing rate is assessed by counting the number of respirations in 30 seconds and then doubling it.

BLOOD PRESSURE

Blood pressure is the pressure or tension of the blood within the systemic arteries, generally considered to be the aorta. As one of the most important vital signs, blood pressure reflects the effectiveness of the circulatory system. Changes in blood pressure are very significant. **Systolic blood pressure** is measured when the left ventricle contracts and expels blood into the aorta. It is approximately 120 mm Hg for a healthy adult and 125 to 140 for healthy children aged 10 to 18. **Diastolic blood pressure** is the residual pressure present in the aorta between heart beats and averages 70 to 80 mm Hg in healthy adults and 80 to 90 in healthy children aged 10 to 18. Blood pressure may be affected by gender, weight, race, lifestyle, and diet. Blood pressure is measured in the brachial artery with a sphygmomanometer and stethoscope (see **Field Strategy 2.1**).

TEMPERATURE

Core temperature can be measured by a thermometer placed under the tongue, in the ear, armpit, or, in case of unconsciousness, in the rectum. Rectal temperature, usually 0.5° higher than oral temperatures, is considered to be a more accurate measurement of core temperature (skull, thoracic and abdominal regions) (5,8). Infrared tympanic thermometers (ITTs) measure infrared energy emitted by the tympanic membrane, and provide a rapid, efficient, and noninvasive method of measuring body temperature. ITTs have failed to detect fever in some patients with AIDS, neonates, infants, and children, and are not useful in hypothermic or significantly hyperthermic individuals (9).

SKIN COLOR

Skin color can indicate abnormal blood flow and low blood oxygen concentration in a particular body part or area. Three colors are commonly used to describe light-skinned individuals: red, white or ashen, and blue. The colors, and what they indicate, can be seen in **Table 4.11**. In dark-skinned individuals, skin pigments mask cyanosis. A bluish cast, however, can be seen in mucous membranes (mouth, tongue, and inner eyelids), the lips, and nail beds. Fever in these individuals can be seen by a red flush at the tips of the ears.

PUPILS

The pupils respond to situations affecting the CNS. Rapid constriction of pupils when the eyes are exposed to intense light is called the **pupillary light reflex**. The pupillary response to light can be assessed by holding one hand over one eye and then moving the hand away quickly, or shining the light from a penlight into one eye and observing the pupil's reaction. A normal response would be constriction with the light shining in the eye, and dilation as the light is removed. The pupillary reaction is classified as brisk (normal), sluggish, nonreactive, or fixed. The eyes may appear normal, constricted, unequal, or dilated.

Eye movement is tested by asking the individual to focus on a single object. If the individual sees two images instead of one, it is called **diplopia**, or double vision. This condition occurs when the external eye muscles fail to work in a coordinated manner. The tracking ability of the eyes can be assessed by asking the individual to watch your fingers move through the six cardinal fields of vision (**Figure 4.16**). Test the individual's depth perception by placing a finger several inches in front of the individual and ask the person to reach out and touch the finger. Move the finger to several different locations.

Disposition

The final decision in any injury assessment is often very difficult. Information gathered during the assessment must be analyzed and decisions made based on what is best for the injured individual. Can the situation be handled on-site or should the individual be referred to a physician? As a general rule, the individual should always be referred to the nearest trauma center or emergency clinic if any life-threatening situation is present, if the injury results in loss of normal function, or if no improvement is seen in an injury's status after a reasonable amount of time. Examples

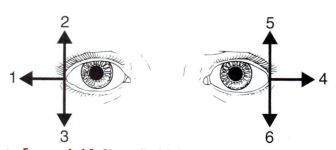

➤ FIGURE 4.16 **Six cardinal fields of vision.**

➤➤ Box 4.7

Non–life-threatening Conditions That Require Immediate Referral to a Physician

- Eye injuries
- Dental injuries in which a tooth has been knocked loose or knocked out
- Minor or simple fractures
- Lacerations that may require suturing
- Injuries in which a functional deficit is noticeable
- Loss of normal sensation or diminished or absent reflexes
- Noticeable muscular weakness in the extremities
- Any injury if you may have doubts about its severity or nature

of these injuries were provided in **Box 4.6**. Other conditions, not necessarily life-threatening, but serious enough to warrant referral to a physician for immediate care include those listed in **Box 4.7**.

When evaluating the injured basketball player, a primary survey should have been conducted to assess the level of responsiveness, airway, breathing, and circulation. Measurement of the vital signs, along with a list of signs and symptoms gathered during the on-the-field assessment, can determine if EMS should be activated.

MOVING THE INJURED PARTICIPANT

What criteria should be used to determine whether or not an injured athlete should be allowed to walk off the field? What is the safest method to transport an injured athlete with a lower extremity injury?

Once the athletic trainer has determined the extent and severity of the injury, a decision must be made on the manner to safely remove the athlete off the field. These include ambulatory assistance, manual conveyance, and transporting by a stretcher or spine board.

Ambulatory Assistance

Ambulatory assistance is used to provide support or aid an injured athlete who is able to walk. This implies that the injury is minor, and no further harm will occur if the individual is ambulatory. In performing this technique, two individuals of equal or near equal height should support both sides of the athlete. The athlete drapes his or her arms across the shoulders of the assistants while their arms encircle the injured player's back. The assistants then escort the player off the field.

Manual Conveyance

If the individual is unable to walk or the distance is too great to walk, manual conveyance may be used. The athlete continues to drape his or her arms across the assistants' shoulders, while one arm from each assistant is placed behind the athlete's back and the other arm is placed under the athlete's thigh. Both assistants lift the legs up, placing the athlete in a seated position. The athlete is then carried off the field. Again, it is essential that the injury be fully evaluated prior to moving the individual in this manner.

Transporting by Spine Board

The safest method to move an individual is with a spine board or stretcher. Ideally, five trained individuals should roll, lift, and carry an injured person. The captain (the more medically trained) will stabilize the head and give commands for each person to slowly lift the injured individual onto the stretcher. The individual is then secured onto the stretcher. On command the stretcher is raised to waist level. The individual should be carried feet first so the captain can constantly monitor the individual's condition. **Field Strategy 4.5** describes how to secure and move an individual on a stretcher.

Pool Extrication

Serious injuries can also occur in a swimming pool environment. If a head or neck injury is suspected, the individual must be placed on a spine board prior to being removed from the water. Although the principles are the same, carrying the tasks out in water requires practice. **Field Strategy 4.6** describes how to move and secure an individual in the water onto a spine board.

An injured athlete may walk off the field if the injury is minor and no further harm will occur if the individual is ambulatory. If the injury is more serious, however, then the individual should be non-weight bearing. Manual conveyance or removal by a spine board, stretcher, or chair may be necessary to avoid any additional pain or injury to the athlete.

DIAGNOSTIC TESTING

In the initial injury assessment, you determined that the athlete had a moderate strain of the Achilles tendon. Does the individual need to see a physician? Are there special imaging techniques that may be used to help the physician reach an accurate diagnosis?

Injury recognition is the final step in assessment. A fine line is drawn between recognition of a sports-related

FIELD STRATEGY 4.5   TRANSPORTING AN INJURED INDIVIDUAL ON A SPINE BOARD

A. *Unless ruled out, assume the presence of a spinal injury.* The "captain" of the team stabilizes the head and neck in the exact position in which they were found, regardless of the angle. Place the arms next to the body and legs straight. If the individual is lying face down, roll the individual supine. Four or five people are required to "log roll" the individual. The captain should position the arms in the cross arm technique so that during the log roll, the arms will end in the proper position.

B. Place the spine board as close as possible beside the individual. Each person is responsible for one body segment: one at the shoulder, one at the hip, one at the knees, and if needed, one at the feet. On command, roll the individual on the board in a single motion.

C. Once on the board, the captain continues to stabilize the head and neck while another person applies support around the cervical region. The chest is secured to the board first, then the feet. With a football player, *do not* remove the helmet.

D. When secured, four people lift the stretcher while the captain continues to monitor the individual's condition. Transport the individual feet first.

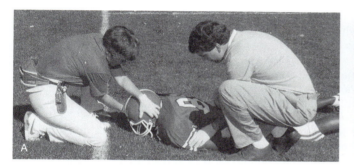

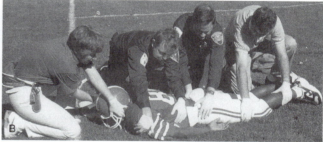

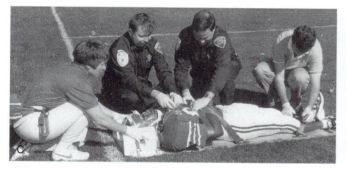

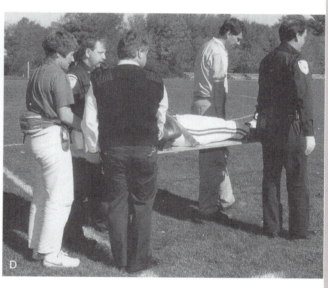

injury and establishment of a diagnosis. A **diagnosis**, the definitive determination of the nature of the injury or illness, can only be made by medical professionals, such as physicians, orthopedists, chiropractors, neurologists, and dentists. Athletic trainers recognize a possible injury or illness based on their assessment and, as needed, refer the individual for a diagnosis. Various forms of laboratory tests and imaging techniques may be used by the physician to make a diagnosis. Although the team physician or medical specialist orders tests and interprets the results, the athletic trainer should have a basic understanding of what the tests are used for.

Laboratory Tests

A variety of laboratory tests can be used by physicians (**Box 4.8**). For example, if an athlete has a grossly swollen knee, the physician may draw fluid out of the joint with a hypo-

FIELD STRATEGY 4.6   POOL EXTRICATION

A. Ease yourself into the water near the individual to avoid any additional wave movement.

B. Face the individual's side, and place one forearm along the length of the individual's sternum. Support the chin by placing the thumb on one side of the chin and the fingers on the other.

C. Place the other forearm along the length of the individual's back; cradle the head near the base of the skull. Lock both wrists. Press the forearms inward and upward to provide mild traction and stabilization of the neck.

D. Turn the individual supine by slowly rotating the person toward you as you submerge and go under the individual. Avoid any unnecessary movement of the individual's trunk or legs. Slowly tow the individual to the shallow end of the pool. [*Note: In diving pools without a shallow end, move the individual to the side of the tank. The "captain" lies prone on the deck with arms in the water and takes over the in-line stabilization of the neck.*]

E. Approach the individual from the side with the backboard. Glide the foot of the board diagonally under the individual, making sure the board extends beyond the head. Allow the board to rise under the individual.

F. Maintain in-line stabilization while a rigid cervical collar is applied. Secure the individual to the backboard beginning at the chest, then moving to the hips, thighs, and shins.

G. Before securing the head, it may be necessary to place padding under the head to fill the space between the board and head to maintain stabilization. Place a towel or blanket roll in a horseshoe configuration around the head and neck, and secure to the board.

H. Place the board perpendicular to the pool side and maintain the board in a horizontal position. Remove the board, head first. Tip the board at the head to break the initial suction holding it in the water. Two people should be on the deck to lift and slide the board onto the pool deck. Once on the deck, check vital signs and assess the individual's condition. Treat for shock and transport.

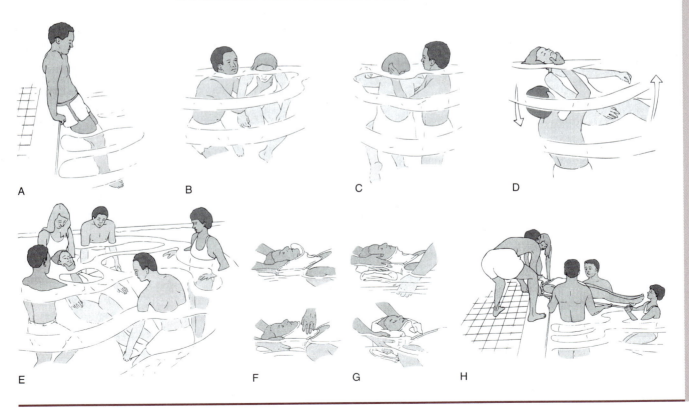

A   B   C   D

E   F   G   H

➤➤ BOX 4.8

Laboratory Blood Testing

- Red blood cell (RBC) count determines the approximate number of circulating red blood cells (erythrocytes). A decreased count indicates possible anemia, chronic infection, internal hemorrhage, certain types of cancers, or deficiencies in iron, B_{12} or folic acid.
- White blood cell (WBC) count determines approximate number of circulating white blood cells (leukocytes). A decreased count indicates an inability to fight infections.
- Hemoglobin gives the red color to erythrocytes and transports oxygen to the tissues and carries away the carbon dioxide. A decreased count indicates possible anemia or carbon monoxide poisoning.
- Hematocrit measures the volume of erythrocytes packed by centrifugation in a given volume of blood and is expressed as a percent. A decreased value indicates anemia.
- Platelets aid in blood clotting. A decreased value indicates a decreased clotting ability, internal bleeding, or possible bleeding disorder.

TABLE 4.13 NORMAL RANGES FOR SELECTED BLOOD VARIABLE IN ADULTS

Laboratory Test	Men	Gender Neutral	Women
Hemoglobin (g/dL)	13–18		12–16
Hematocrit (%)	42–52		37–48
Red blood cell count ($\times 10^{12}$/L)	4.5–6.5		3.9–5.6
White blood cell count		4.3–10.8 ($\times 10^9$/L)	
Platelet count		150–350 ($\times 10^9$/L)	
Iron, total (μg/dL)		50–100	

TABLE 4.14 NORMAL URINE VALUES

Color	Yellow to amber
Transparency	Clear
Specific gravity	1.010 to 1.025
pH	6
Creatinine	1.5–2.5 g/day
Protein	<165 mg/day
Glucose	Negative
Ketone	Negative
Bilirubin	Negative
Blood	Negative
Urobilinogen	0.1–1.0 EU/dL
Bacteria (nitrite)	Negative

dermic needle to examine the synovial fluid **(Table 4.12)** (5). If the athlete reports a sore throat, feeling lethargic, and somewhat feverish, a throat culture and blood test may be ordered. A complete blood count (CBC) may address several factors; however, the more common factors tested and normal values are listed in **Table 4.13** (10,11). An athlete who has blood in the urine would likewise require a urinalysis. The more common factors assessed in this laboratory test and normal values can be seen in **Table 4.14** (11).

Radiographs

The most common imaging technique is the radiograph or x-ray **(Figure 4.17)**. An x-ray provides an image of

TABLE 4.12 SYNOVIAL FLUID CLASSIFICATIONS

Type	Appearance	Significance
Group 1	Clear yellow	Noninflammatory state, no trauma
Group 2*	Cloudy	Inflammatory, arthritis, excludes most patients with osteoarthritis
Group 3	Thick exudate, brownish	Septic arthritis; occasionally seen in gout
Group 4	Hemorrhagic	Trauma, bleeding disorders, tumors, fractures

*Inflammatory fluids will clot and should be collected in heparin-containing tubes. All group 2 or 3 fluids should be cultured if the diagnosis is uncertain.

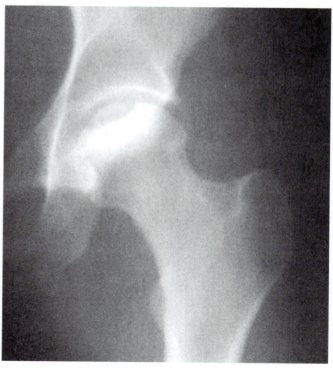

➤ **FIGURE 4.17 Radiograph.** Bone absorbs the x-rays and therefore appears white on the radiograph.

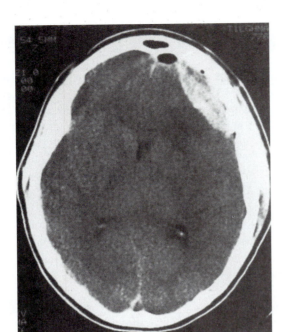

➤ FIGURE 4.18 **Computed tomography**. In this CT scan, you can see an epidural hematoma on the right frontal lobe of the brain.

certain body structures, and can rule out fractures, infections, and **neoplasms**. The image is formed when a minute amount of radiation passes through the body to expose sensitive film placed on the other side. The ability to penetrate tissues depends on the tissue composition and mass. For example, bones (calcium) restrict rays from passing through. Therefore, the images appear white on the film. Lungs or other air-filled structures allow most x-rays to pass through, resulting in the images appearing black. Soft tissues, (e.g., heart, kidneys, liver), allow varying degrees of penetration and are difficult to identify on the x-ray. Images are preserved on sheets of film. As film quality and electronic technology advance, better imaging has been achieved while the dose of radiation to the patient has been decreased. Contraindications for the use of radiographs include over the thyroid gland, pregnant abdomen, and reproductive organs. However, if the information gained outweighs the risk, these areas can be shielded with a lead drape.

Some forms of radiographs use radio-opaque dyes that are absorbed by the tissues, allowing them to be visualized by x-ray examination. A **myelogram** uses an opaque dye that is introduced into the spinal canal through a lumbar puncture. The patient is then tilted, allowing the dye to flow to different levels of the spinal cord. In viewing the contrasts, physicians can identify pathologies of the spinal canal (e.g., tumors, nerve root compression, and disc disease). Another form of radiographic testing is the **arthrogram**. Again, an opaque dye, air, or a combination of the two are injected into a joint space. The visual study of the joint can detect capsular tissue tears and articular cartilage lesions.

Computed Tomography (CT Scan)

A CT scan is a form of radiography that produces a "3-D" cross-sectional picture of a body part **(Figure 4.18)**. This test is used to reveal abnormalities in bone, fat, and soft tissue, such as in head and abdominal trauma and is excellent at detecting tendinous and ligamentous injuries in varying joint positions. Scanners use a beam of light across a "slice" or layer of the body. A special receptor located opposite the beam detects the number of rays passing through the body. The tube emitting the beams of light rotates around the body, and thousands of readings are taken by the receptors. The computer determines the density of the underlying tissues based on the absorption of x-rays by the body, allowing for more precision in viewing soft tissues. The computer records the data, analyses the receptor readings, and calculates the absorption of the light beams at thousands of different points. This information is then converted into a two-dimensional image, or slice, of the body and stored on a video screen and/or radiographic film. These slices can be obtained at varying positions and thicknesses, allowing the radiologist or physician to study the area and its surroundings. A CT scan is relatively safe, since there is little radiation exposure during the procedure, and yields highly detailed results.

Magnetic Resonance Imaging (MRI)

Magnetic resonance imaging is an excellent tool for visualizing the central nervous system (CNS), spine and musculoskeletal and cardiovascular systems **(Figure 4.19)**. One of its greatest assets is its ability to do soft tissue differentiation (i.e., ligamentous disruption, such as an anterior cruciate ligament tear). It is also used to demonstrate space-occupying lesions in the brain (tumor or hematoma), joint damage (meniscal tears, osteochondral fracture), and view

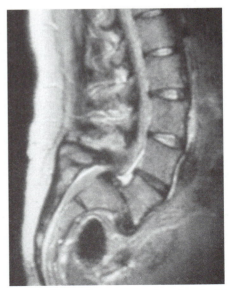

➤ FIGURE 4.19 **Magnetic resonance imaging**. In this MRI scan of spondylolisthesis, you can see the anterior shift of the L5 vertebra.

blood vessels and blood flow without the use of a contrast medium (e.g., cardiac function). In many cases, the MRI has replaced the myelogram and arthrography.

Images are obtained by placing the patient in an MRI tube that produces the magnetic field. This causes the body's hydrogen nuclei to align with the magnetic axis. The tissues are then bombarded by radio waves, which causes the nuclei to resonate as they absorb the energy. When the energy from the radio waves ceases, the nuclei return to their state of equilibrium by releasing energy, which is then detected by the MRI unit and transformed by a computer into visible images.

Radionuclide Scintigraph (Bone Scan)

A bone scan is used to detect stress fractures of the long bones and vertebrae, degenerative diseases, infections, or tumors of the bone. A **radionucleotide** material, Tc-99m, is injected into a vein and is slowly absorbed by areas of bone undergoing remodeling. Several hours later, the patient returns for evaluation. The patient is placed under a recording device that scans radioactive signals and records the images on film. In some scans, active images will be recorded on videotape. A total body scan or a localized scan can take close to an hour. Any areas subject to stress, e.g., fractures or increases of metabolic activity such as bone marrow centers or tumors, will show as areas of greatest uptake and will appear darker on the film **(Figure 4.20)**. Bone scans may be clinically correlated to plain x-rays or

other diagnostic tests. No special preparation is needed prior to the bone scan, and the risk to the patient is minimal. The body will excrete the radioactive material over a 24-hour period.

Ultrasonic Imaging

Sonography, as it is sometimes called, uses sound waves to view the various internal organs and certain soft-tissue structures, such as tendons. The energy produced is similar to that used during therapeutic ultrasound treatments, but has a frequency of less than 0.8 MHz. Although it is commonly used to monitor development of the fetus during pregnancy, in an athletic population it can be used to view tendon and other soft-tissue imaging. Similar to a sonar device on a submarine, a piezoelectric crystal is used to convert electrical pulses into vibrations that penetrate the body structures. The sound waves are reflected away from the tissues and create a two-dimensional image of the subcutaneous structures (6).

Electromyography

Certain muscular conditions can be detected by using electromyography. This diagnostic tool consists of a thin electrode needle that is inserted into the muscle to determine the level of muscular contraction following an electrical stimulation. Motor unit potentials can be observed on an oscilloscope screen or recorded on an electromyogram. Electromyography is used to detect denervated muscles, nerve root compression injuries, and other muscle diseases.

 If the team physician needed additional imaging techniques to determine the extent of damage to the football player's Achilles tendon, an MRI or ultrasound image may be ordered. Each can demonstrate damage to soft-tissue structures far superiorly than a radiograph.

Summary

1. In a sports injury assessment, a problem-solving process incorporates subjective and objective information about an injury that is reliable, accurate, and measurable.
2. The HOPS format includes history, observation and inspection, palpation, and special tests.
3. A more popular method of injury management is the SOAP note format because the format:
   • Documents the injury evaluation.
   • Assesses the individual's status and prognosis.
   • Establishes short- and long-term goals for recovery.
   • Outline the treatment plan, such as the frequency and duration of treatments, rehabilitation exercises, on-going patient education, evaluation standards to determine progress, and criteria for discharge.

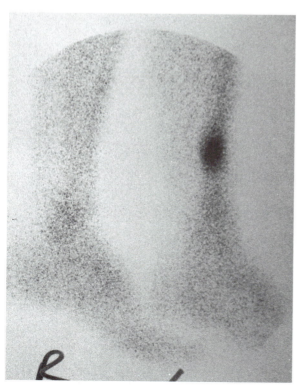

➤ **FIGURE 4.20 Radionuclide scinitigraph.** Bone scans can detect stress fractures long before the fracture becomes visible on traditional x-rays.

4. The subjective information gathered during the history taking should include:
   - The primary complaint
   - Mechanism of injury
   - Characteristics of the symptoms
   - Disabilities resulting from the injury
   - Related medical history
5. The objective assessment should include:
   - Observation and inspection.
   - Palpation. Bony and soft-tissue palpation to determine a possible fracture or dislocation, and abnormal temperature, swelling, point tenderness, crepitus, deformity, muscle spasm, cutaneous sensation, and pulse
   - Functional tests. Active, passive, and resisted range of motion to detect available range of motion and distinguish injuries to contractile tissue versus noncontractile tissue
   - Stress tests for specific joints or structures
   - Neurological testing through resisted manual muscle testing, dermatomes, myotomes, and reflexes
   - Sport-specific functional tests
6. The sports medicine team should develop and implement an emergency procedures plan in consultation with local EMS agencies to ensure rapid and complete emergency care to an injured athlete. The plan should be evaluated annually and practiced by all parties on a regular basis. In addition, members of the medical staff should hold current certification in standard first aid and CPR or its equivalent.
7. In an emergency injury assessment, assume that a head or spinal cord injury is present and stabilize the head and neck before proceeding. Assessment of all injuries, no matter how minor, should include a primary injury assessment to determine unresponsiveness and assess the ABCs. Further assessment will determine the presence of moderate to severe injuries.
8. As a general rule, an individual should always be referred to the nearest trauma center or emergency clinic if any life-threatening situation is present, or if the injury results in loss of normal function. Information provided by the athletic trainer, along with any laboratory or imaging techniques, can help the team physician accurately diagnose the problem, and provide a basis for treatment and rehabilitation programs.

References

1. The National Collegiate Athletic Association. 1997–1998 NCAA Sports Medicine Handbook. Overland Park, KS: NCAA Sport Sciences, 1997.
2. Cailliet R. Pain: Mechanisms and Management. Philadelphia: FA Davis, 1993.
3. Norkin CC, White DJ. Measurement of Joint Motion: A Guide to Goniometry. Philadelphia: FA Davis, 1995.
4. Nitz AJ, Bellew JW Jr, Hazle CR. Evaluation of the Musculoskeletal Disorders. In: Orthopaedic and Sports Physical Therapy. Edited by Malone TR, McPoil TG, Nitz AJ. St. Louis: Mosby-Year Book, 1997.
5. Magee DJ. Orthopedic Physical Assessment. Philadelphia: WB Saunders, 1997.
6. Starkey C, Ryan JL. Evaluation of Orthopedic and Athletic Injuries. Philadelphia: FA Davis, 1996.
7. Grant HD, Murray RH, Bergeron D. Brady Emergency Care. Englewood Cliffs, NJ: Prentice Hall, 1993.
8. McArdle WD, Katch FI, Katch VL. Exercise Physiology: Energy, Nutrition, and Human Performance. Baltimore: Williams & Wilkins, 1996.
9. Guertler AT. The clinical practice of emergency medicine. Emer Med Clin North Am 1997;15(2):303-313.
10. Normal reference laboratory values. Massachusetts General Hospital, January 1977.
11. Estridge BH. Basic Medical Laboratory Techniques. Albany: Delmar Publishing, 1996.

5

Tissue Healing and Wound Care

OBJECTIVES

1. Define compression, tension, shear, stress, strain, bending, and torsion, and explain how each can play a role in injury to biological tissues.

2. Explain how the material constituents and structural organization of skin, tendon, ligament, muscle, and bone affect the ability of these structures to withstand the mechanical loads to which each is subjected.

3. List and describe common injuries of skin, tendons, ligaments, muscles, and bone.

4. Describe the processes by which tissue healing occurs in skin, tendons, ligaments, muscles, and bone.

5. Explain wound care for both superficial and deep soft-tissues injuries.

6. Explain the mechanisms by which nerves are injured and the processes by which nerves can heal.

7. Describe the types of altered sensation that can result from a nerve injury.

8. Outline immediate management of bone and nerve injuries.

9. Describe the neurological basis of pain and identify factors that mediate pain.

Human movement during sport and exercise is typically faster and produces greater force than during activities of daily living. As a result, the potential for injury is also heightened. Understanding the different ways in which forces act upon the body is necessary in comprehending how to prevent injuries. Likewise, knowing the material and structural properties of skin, tendon, ligament, muscle, bone, and nerve can lay a foundation for understanding how these tissues respond to applied forces, and can facilitate the athlete's safe return to sport participation.

This chapter begins with a general discussion of injury mechanisms, including descriptions of force and torque and their effects. Next, sections on soft tissues, bone, and nerve address the mechanical characteristics of these tissues, the types of injuries one might see, the processes by which the specific tissues heal, and finally, how to provide general wound care for these injuries. A more detailed explanation of wound care for specific injuries is discussed throughout Chapters 8 to 27.

INJURY MECHANISMS

 Athletes routinely sustain unusually large forces during both physical training and competition. What factors determine whether a given force results in injury?

Analyzing the mechanics of injuries to the human body is complicated by several factors. First, potentially injurious forces applied to the body act at different angles, over different surface areas, and over different periods of time. Second, the human body is composed of many different types of tissue, which respond differently to applied forces. Finally, injury to the human body is not an all-or-none phenomenon. That is, injuries range in severity. This section introduces the types of mechanical loading that can cause injury and describes the basic mechanical responses of biological tissues to these forms of loading.

Force and Its Effects

Force may be thought of as a push or a pull acting on a body. A multitude of forces act on our bodies routinely during the day. The forces of gravity and friction enable us to move about in predictable ways when muscles produce internal forces. During sport participation, we apply forces to balls, bats, racquets, and clubs, and we absorb forces from impacts with the ball used in the sport, the ground or floor, and our opponents in contact sports.

When a force acts, there are two potential effects on the target object. The first is acceleration, or change in velocity, and the second is deformation, or change in shape. For example, when a racquetball is struck with a racquet, the ball is both accelerated (put in motion in the direction of the racquet swing) and deformed (flattened on the side struck). The greater the stiffness of the material to which a force is applied, the greater the likelihood that the deformation will be too small to be easily seen. The more elastic the material to which a force is applied, the greater the likelihood that the deformation will be temporary, with the body springing back to regain its original shape.

When tissues sustain a force, two primary factors will dictate whether injury occurs **(Box 5.1)**. The first is the size, or magnitude, of the force, and the second is the material properties of the involved tissues. **Figure 5.1** is a load-deformation curve, which shows the deformation of a structure in response to progressive loading, or force application. With relatively small loads, the response of the structure is elastic, meaning that when the load is removed, the material will return to its original size and

shape. Within the elastic region of the load-deformation curve, the greater the stiffness of the material, the steeper the slope of the line. Greater stiffness, therefore, translates to less deformation in response to a given load. With loads exceeding the material's **yield point**, or **elastic limit**, however, the response of the structure is plastic, meaning that when the load is removed, some amount of deformation will remain. Loads exceeding the ultimate failure point on the load-deformation curve result in mechanical **failure** of the structure, which translates to fracturing of bone or rupturing of soft tissues.

The direction in which force is applied also has important implications for injury potential. Many tissues are **anisotropic**, meaning that the structure is stronger in resisting force from certain directions than from others. The anatomical makeup of many of the joints of the human body also makes them more susceptible to injury from a given direction. For example, lateral ankle sprains are much more common than medial ankle sprains because ligamentous support of the ankle is much stronger on the medial side. Consequently, in discussing injury mechanisms, force is commonly categorized according to the direction from which the force acts on the affected structure.

Force acting along the long axis of a structure is termed **axial force**. When the opponent in fencing is touched with the foil, the foil is loaded axially. When the human body is in an upright standing position, body weight creates axial loads on the femur and the tibia, the major weight-bearing bones of the lower extremity.

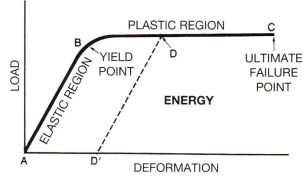

➤ **FIGURE 5.1 Load-deformation curve.** Load-deformation curve for a structure composed of pliable material.

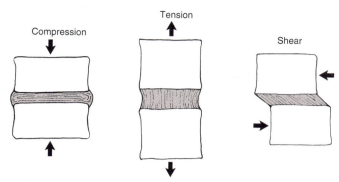

▶ **FIGURE 5.2 Mechanisms of injury**. Compression and tension are directed along the longitudinal axis of a structure, whereas shear acts parallel to a surface.

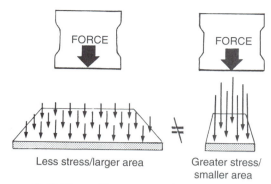

▶ **FIGURE 5.3 Stress**. The stress produced by a force depends on the area over which the force is spread.

Axial loading that produces a squeezing or crushing effect is termed **compressive force**, or compression (**Figure 5.2A**). The weight of the human body constantly produces compression on the bones that support it. The 5th lumbar vertebra must support the weight of the head, trunk, and arms when the body is erect, producing compression on the intervertebral disc below it. When a football player is sandwiched between two opposing players, the force acting on the player is compressive. In the absence of sufficient padding, compressive forces often result in bruises, or contusions.

Axial loading in the direction opposite that of compression is called **tensile force**, or tension (**Figure 5.2B**). Tension is a pulling force that tends to stretch the object to which it is applied. Muscle contraction produces tensile force on the attached bone, enabling movement of that bone. When the foot and ankle are inverted, the tensile forces applied to the lateral ligaments may result in an ankle sprain.

Whereas compressive and tensile forces are directed toward and away from an object, a third category of force, termed **shear force**, acts parallel or tangent to a plane passing through the object (**Figure 5.2C**). Shear force tends to cause one part of the object to slide or displace with respect to another part of the object. Shear forces acting on the spine can cause spondylolisthesis, a condition involving anterior slippage of a vertebra with respect to the vertebra below it.

When the human body sustains force, another important factor related to the likelihood of injury is the magnitude of the **stress** produced by that force. Mechanical stress is defined as force divided by the surface area over which the force is applied (**Figure 5.3**). When a given force is distributed over a large area, the resulting stress is less than if the force were distributed over a smaller area. Alternatively, if a force is concentrated over a small area, the mechanical stress is relatively high. It is a high magnitude of stress, rather than a high magnitude of force, that tends to result in injury to biological tissues. One of the reasons that football and ice hockey players wear pads is that a pad dissipates the force across the entire pad, thereby reducing the stress acting on the player.

Strain may be thought of as the amount of deformation an object undergoes in response to an applied force. Application of compressive force to an object produces shortening and widening of the structure, whereas tensile force produces lengthening and narrowing of the structure. Shear results in internal changes in the structure acted upon. The ultimate strength of biological tissues determines the amount of strain that a structure can withstand without fracturing or rupturing.

Injury to biological tissues can result from a single traumatic force of relatively large magnitude, or from repeated forces of relatively smaller magnitude. When a single force produces an injury, the injury is called an **acute injury** and the causative force is termed **macrotrauma**. An acute injury, such as a ruptured anterior cruciate ligament or a fractured humerus, is characterized by a definitive moment of onset followed by a relatively predictable process of healing. When repeated or chronic loading over a period of time produces an injury, the injury is called a **chronic injury** or **stress injury**, and the causative mechanism is termed **microtrauma**. A chronic injury, such as glenohumeral bursitis or a metatarsal stress fracture, develops and worsens gradually over time, typically culminating in a threshold episode in which pain and inflammation become evident. Chronic injuries may persist for months or years.

Many tissues, including tendon, ligament, muscle, and bone, tend to respond to gradually increased mechanical stress by becoming larger and stronger. When a runner's training protocol incorporates progressively increasing mileage, it is important that this occur in a gradual fashion so the body can adapt to the increased mechanical stress to prevent a stress injury. Overuse syndromes and stress fractures result from the body's inability to adapt to an increased training regimen.

Torque and Its Effects

Consider what happens when a swinging door is opened. A hand applies force to the door, causing it to rotate about its hinges (**Figure 5.4**). Two factors influence whether the door will swing in response to the force. One factor is the force's magnitude. Equally important, however, is the

Top view

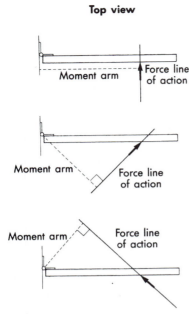

> ➤ **FIGURE 5.4 Torque**. Torque created at the hinges of a door is the product of force and the force's moment arm.

force's moment arm. The moment arm is the perpendicular distance from the force's line of action to the axis of rotation. The product of a force and its moment arm is called **torque**, or moment. Torque may be thought of as a rotary force. It is the amount of torque acting on an object that determines whether a rotating body such as a door will move.

In the human body, torque produces rotation of a body segment about a joint. When a muscle develops tension, it produces torque at the joint that it crosses. The amount of torque produced is the product of muscle force and the muscle's moment arm with respect to the joint center **(Figure 5.5)**. For example, the torque produced by the biceps brachii is the product of the tension developed by the muscle and the distance between its attachment on the radius and the center of rotation at the elbow.

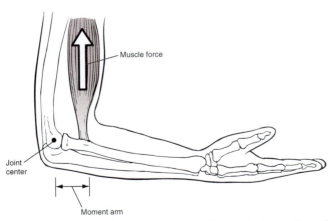

> ➤ **FIGURE 5.5 Movement and torque**. Torque is the product of the magnitude of muscle force and the muscle's moment arm (perpendicular distance of the muscle's line of action to the axis of rotation at the joint center).

Excessive torque can produce injury. Such torque is usually generated by forces external to the body rather than by the muscles. The simultaneous application of forces from opposite directions at different points along a structure such as a long bone generates a torque known as a bending moment, which can cause **bending** and ultimately fracture of the bone. If a football player's leg is anchored to the ground and he is tackled on that leg from the front while being pushed into the tackle from behind, a bending moment is created on the leg. When bending is present, the structure is loaded in tension on one side and in compression on the opposite side **(Figure 5.6A)**. Because bone is stronger in resisting compression than tension, the side of the bone loaded in tension will fracture if the bending moment is sufficiently large.

The application of torque about the long axis of a structure such as a long bone can cause **torsion**, or twisting of the structure **(Figure 5.6B)**. Torsion results in the creation of shear stress throughout the structure. In skiing accidents where one boot and ski are firmly planted and the skier rotates during a fall, torsional loads can cause a spiral fracture of the tibia.

> 💡 *Factors that influence the likelihood of injury when a force is sustained include force magnitude and direction, the area over which the force acts, the force's moment arm (which determines the amount of torque generated), and the type(s) of tissue affected.*

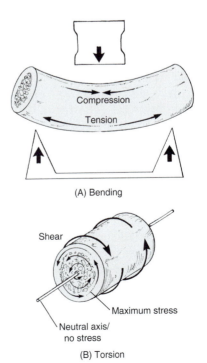

> ➤ **FIGURE 5.6 Bone injury mechanisms**. Bones loaded in bending are subject to compression on one side and tension on the other. Bones loaded in torsion develop internal shear stress, with maximal stress at the periphery and no stress at the neutral axis.

SOFT TISSUE INJURIES

 Tendon and ligament are both collagenous connective tissues, yet they are somewhat different in both structure and function. Based on these differences, what are the implications for injury?

Skin, tendon, ligament, and muscle are soft (nonbony) tissues that behave in characteristic ways when subjected to different forms of loading. Anatomic structure and material composition influence the mechanical behavior of each tissue.

Anatomical Properties of Soft Tissue

Skin, tendon, and ligament are known as collagenous tissues after their major building block: collagen. Collagen is a protein that is strong in resisting tension. Collagen fibers have a wavy configuration in a tissue that is not under tension **(Figure 5.7)**. This enables collagenous tissues to stretch slightly under tensile loading as these fibers straighten. Thus, collagen fibers provide strength and flexibility to tissues, but are relatively inelastic. Elastin, another protein, provides added elasticity to some connective tissue structures, such as the ligamentum flavum of the spine.

SKIN

The skin is composed of two major regions. The outer region, known as the epidermis, has multiple layers containing the pigment melanin, along with the hair, nails, sebaceous glands, and sweat glands **(Figure 5.8)**. Beneath the epidermis is the dermis, containing blood vessels, nerve endings, hair follicles, sebaceous glands, and sweat glands.

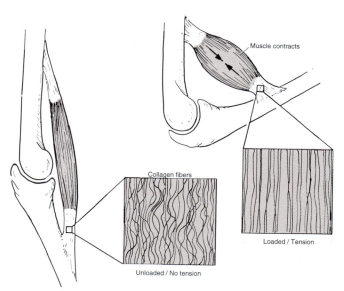

➤ **FIGURE 5.7 Collagen fibers.** Collagen fibers are a wavy configuration when unloaded, and straightened when loaded in tension.

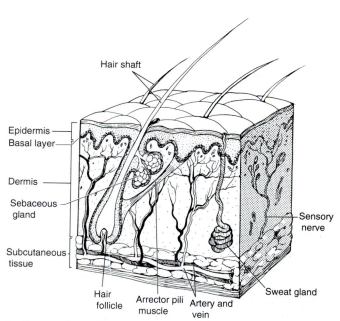

➤ **FIGURE 5.8 Skin.** The structures contained in the epidermis and dermis.

The dermis is composed of dense, irregular connective tissue, characterized by a loose, multidirectional arrangement of collagen fibers. This fiber arrangement enables resistance to multidirectional loads, including compression, tension, and shear. This type of tissue also forms fascia, fibrous sheets of connective tissue that surround muscles. Dense, irregular connective tissue also covers internal structures such as the liver, lymph nodes, and testes, as well as bone, cartilage, and nerves.

Other components of the skin are elastic fibers and reticular fibers. Elastic fibers provide the skin with some elasticity. Reticular fibers are composed of a type of collagen known as reticulin. These fibers function like collagen fibers, but are much thinner, and provide support for internal structures such as the lymph nodes, spleen, bone marrow, and liver.

TENDONS, LIGAMENTS, AND APONEUROSES

Tendons connect muscle to bone, whereas ligaments connect bone to bone. Both structures are composed of dense, regular connective tissue, consisting of tightly packed bundles of unidirectional collagen fibers **(Figure 5.9)**. In tendons, the collagen fibers are arranged in a parallel pattern, enabling resistance to high, unidirectional tensile loads when the attached muscle contracts. In ligaments, the collagen fibers are largely parallel, but are also interwoven. This arrangement is well-suited to ligament function, providing resistance to large tensile loads along the long axis of the ligament, but also providing resistance to smaller tensile loads from other directions.

Ligaments contain more elastin than tendons, and so are somewhat more elastic. From a functional standpoint this is critical, because ligaments are connected at both ends to bones, while tendons attach on one end to muscle,

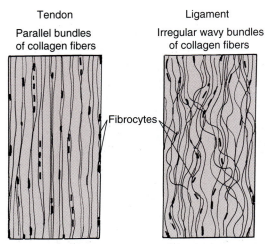

Tendon
Parallel bundles
of collagen fibers

Ligament
Irregular wavy bundles
of collagen fibers

Fibrocytes

➤ **FIGURE 5.9 Collagen arrangements in tendon and ligament tissue.**

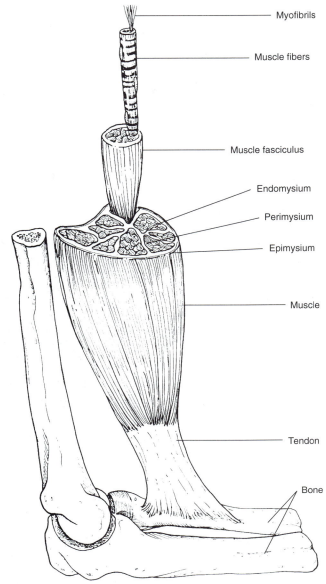

Myofibrils

Muscle fibers

Muscle fasciculus

Endomysium

Perimysium

Epimysium

Muscle

Tendon

Bone

➤ **FIGURE 5.10 Muscle tissue.**

a tissue with some elasticity. Although most ligaments contain only small amounts of elastin, the ligamentum flavum of the spine is composed of approximately two-thirds elastic fibers and one-third collagen fibers. This ligament has a specialized role in providing stability to the multi-segmented spine; it stretches to allow spinal flexion, but remains taut when the spine is in a neutral position.

The aponeuroses are another set of structures formed by dense, regular connective tissue. These are strong, flat, sheet-like tissues that attach muscles to other muscles or to bones.

MUSCLE

Muscle is a highly organized structure. A sheath known as the endomysium surrounds each muscle cell, or fiber. Small numbers of fibers are bound up into fascicles by a dense connective tissue sheath called the perimysium. A muscle is composed of several fascicles surrounded by the epimysium **(Figure 5.10)**.

The structure and composition of muscle enable it to function in a **viscoelastic** fashion—that is, with both elasticity and time-dependent extensibility **(Box 5.2)**. Extensibility is the ability to be stretched or to increase in length, whereas elasticity is the ability to return to normal length after either lengthening or shortening has taken place. The viscoelastic aspect of muscle extensibility enables muscle to stretch to greater lengths over time in response to a sustained tensile force. This means that a static stretch maintained for 30 seconds is more effective in increasing muscle length than a series of short, ballistic stretches.

Another of muscle's characteristic properties, irritability, is the ability to respond to a stimulus. Stimuli affecting muscles can be either electrochemical, such as an action potential from the attaching nerve, or mechanical, as with an external blow to the muscle. If the stimulus is of sufficient magnitude, muscle responds by developing tension.

The ability to develop tension is a property unique to muscle. Although some sources refer to this ability as *contractility*, a muscle may or may not contract (shorten) when tension is developed. For example, isometric "contraction" involves no joint movement and no change in muscle length, and eccentric "contraction" actually involves lengthening of the muscle developing tension. Only when a muscle develops tension concentrically does it also shorten. When a stimulated muscle develops tension, the amount of tension present is the same throughout the muscle and tendon, and at the site of the tendon attachment to bone.

Skin Injury Classifications

Forces applied to the body in different ways and from different directions result in different types of injury. Because the skin is the body's first layer of defense against injury, it is the most frequently injured body tissue.

Abrasions are common minor skin injuries caused by shear when the skin is scraped with sufficient force, usually in one direction, against a rough surface. The greater the applied force, the more layers of skin that are scraped away.

Blisters are minor skin injuries caused by repeated application of shear in one or more directions, as happens when a shoe rubs back and forth against the foot. The result is the formation of a pocket of fluid between the epidermis and dermis as fluid migrates to the site of injury.

Skin bruises are injuries resulting from compression sustained during a blow. Damage to the underlying capillaries causes the accumulation of blood within the skin.

Incisions, lacerations, avulsions, and punctures are breaks in the skin resulting from injury. An incision is a clean cut, produced by the application of a tensile force to the skin as it is stretched along a sharp edge. A laceration is an irregular tear in the skin that typically results from a combination of tension and shear. An avulsion is a severe laceration that results in complete separation of the skin from the underlying tissues. A puncture wound results when a sharp, cylindrical object penetrates the skin and underlying tissues with tensile loading.

Other Soft Tissue Injury Classifications

Injuries to the soft tissues below the skin are also dependent upon the nature of the causative force, as well as the location (superficial versus deep) and the material properties of the involved tissues. Muscle **contusions** or bruises result from a direct compressive force sustained from a heavy blow. Such injuries vary in severity in accordance with the area and depth over which blood vessels are ruptured (**Box 5.3**). **Ecchymosis**, or tissue discoloration, may be present if the

TABLE 5.1	CLASSIFICATIONS OF CONTUSIONS		
	First Degree	**Second Degree**	**Third Degree**
Damage to tissue	Superficial tissues are crushed	Superficial and some deep tissues are crushed	Deeper tissues are crushed (fascia surrounding muscle may rupture, allowing swollen tissues to protrude)
Weakness	None	Mild to moderate	Moderate to severe
Muscle spasm	None	None	Possibility
Loss of function	Mild	Moderate	Severe
Ecchymosis	Mild	Moderate	Severe
Swelling	Mild	Moderate	Severe
Range of motion	No restriction	Decreased	Significantly decreased due to swelling

hemorrhage is superficial. As blood and lymph flow into the damaged area, swelling occurs, often resulting in the formation of a hard mass composed of blood and dead tissue called a **hematoma**. This mass may restrict joint motion. Nerve compression usually accompanies such injuries, leading to pain and sometimes temporary paralysis.

Muscle contusions are rated in accordance with the extent to which associated joint range of motion is impaired (**Table 5.1**). A first-degree contusion causes little or no range of movement restriction, a second-degree contusion causes a noticeable reduction in range of motion, and a third-degree contusion causes severe restriction of motion. With a third-degree contusion, the fascia surrounding the muscle may also be ruptured, causing swollen muscle tissues to protrude.

Traumatic injury to muscles and tendons (strains) and ligaments (sprains) are caused by indirect forces (i.e., abnormally high tensile forces) that produce rupturing of the tissue and subsequent hemorrhage and swelling (**Box 5.4**).

➤➤ **Box 5.3**

Signs and Symptoms of Contusions
- History of acute onset
- Mechanism is usually a compressive force
- Pain is localized over the injury site
- Ecchymosis may be present if hemorrhage is superficial
- Range of motion may be limited due to swelling and hemorrhage
- Swelling may compress nerves, leading to pain and temporary paralysis
- If compressive force is great enough, injury may also occur in muscle tissue (strain)

➤➤ **Box 5.4**

Signs and Symptoms of Strains and Sprains
Strains
- History of acute onset
- Mechanism of injury in due to overstretch or overload
- Pain is localized over the injury site, which tends to be at or near a musculotendinous junction
- Discoloration, in severe cases, is caused by blood pooling distal to the site of trauma
- If moderate, muscle weakness is evident

Sprains
- History of acute onset
- Mechanism may be due to overstretch or overload
- Pain is localized over the injury site
- Detectable joint instability, if assessed prior to joint effusion
- If severe, injury may result in subluxation or dislocation of the joint

The likelihood of strains and sprains depends on the magnitude of the force and the structure's cross-sectional area. The greater the cross-sectional area of a muscle, the greater its strength, meaning it can produce more force and translate that force to the attached tendon. The larger the cross-sectional area of the tendon, however, the greater the force it can withstand, because increased cross-sectional area translates to reduced stress. It is almost always the muscle portion of the musculotendinous unit that ruptures first, because tendons, by virtue of their collagenous composition, are about twice as strong as the muscles to which they attach. Muscle strains tend to be located near the musculotendinous junction, where muscle cross-sectional area is smallest. Tendon begins to develop tears when it is stretched to approximately 5 to 8% beyond normal length (1).

Strains and sprains are categorized as first, second, and third degree **(Tables 5.2 and 5.3)**. First-degree strains or sprains are accompanied by some pain, but may involve only microtearing of the collagen fibers, with no readily observable symptoms. There may be mild discomfort, local tenderness, mild swelling, and ecchymosis, but no loss of function. Second-degree tensile injuries of these tissues are characterized by more severe pain, more extensive rupturing of the tissue, detectable joint instability, and/or muscle weakness. Third-degree injuries of this nature produce severe pain, a major loss of tissue continuity, loss of range of motion, and complete instability of the joint.

Although typically not associated with injury, muscle **cramps** and **spasms** are painful, involuntary muscle contractions common to the sport setting. A cramp is a painful involuntary contraction that may be clonic, with alternating contraction and relaxation, or tonic, with continued contraction over a period of time. Cramps appear to be brought on by a biochemical imbalance, sometimes associated with muscle fatigue. A muscle spasm is an involuntary contraction of short duration caused by reflex action that can be biochemically derived or initiated by a mechanical blow to a nerve or muscle.

Myositis and **fasciitis** refer respectively to inflammation of a muscle's connective tissues and inflammation of the sheaths of fascia surrounding portions of muscle. These are chronic conditions that develop over time as the result of repeated body movements that irritate these tissues.

Tendinitis and **tenosynovitis** involve inflammation within the tendon itself, or of the tendon sheath, respectively. Tendinitis is closely related to the process of normal aging and degenerative changes within tendons (tendonosis), and is characterized by pain and swelling with tendon movement **(Box 5.5)**. Tenosynovitis may be either acute or chronic. Acute tenosynovitis is characterized by a snapping sound (crepitus) with movement, inflammation, and local swelling. Chronic tenosynovitis has the additional symptom of nodule formation in the tendon sheath.

Prolonged chronic inflammation of muscle or tendon can result in the accumulation of mineral deposits resembling bone in the affected tissues, a process known as ectopic calcification. Accumulation of mineral deposits in muscle is known as **myositis ossificans**. A common site is

TABLE 5.3	CLASSIFICATIONS OF SPRAINS		
	First Degree	**Second Degree**	**Third Degree**
Damage to ligament	Few fibers of ligament are torn	Nearly half of fibers are torn	All ligament fibers are torn (rupture)
Distraction with stress tests	<5 mm distraction	5–10 mm distraction	>10 mm distraction
Weakness	Mild	Mild to moderate	Mild to moderate
Muscle spasm	None	None to minor	None to minor
Loss of function	Mild	Moderate to severe	Severe (instability)
Swelling	Mild	Moderate	Moderate to severe
Pain on contraction	None	None	None
Pain with stretching	Yes	Yes	No
Range of motion	Decreased	Decreased	May increase or decrease depending on swelling; dislocation or subluxation possible

TABLE 5.2	CLASSIFICATIONS OF STRAINS		
	First Degree	**Second Degree**	**Third Degree**
Damage to muscle fibers	Few fibers of muscle are torn	Nearly half of muscle fibers are torn	All muscle fibers are torn (rupture)
Weakness	Mild	Moderate to severe (reflex inhibition)	Moderate to severe
Muscle spasm	Mild	Moderate to severe	Moderate to severe
Loss of function	Mild	Moderate to severe	Severe (reflex inhibition)
Swelling	Mild	Moderate to severe	Moderate to severe
Palpable defect	No	No	Yes (if early)
Pain on contraction	Mild	Moderate to severe	None to mild
Pain with stretching	Yes	Yes	No
Range of motion	Decreased	Decreased	May increase or decrease depending on swelling

➤➤ **BOX 5.5**

Signs and Symptoms of Tendinitis

- History of chronic onset
- Mechanism of injury is due to overuse, or repetitive overstretch or overload
- Pain exists throughout the length of the tendon and increases during palpation
- Swelling may be minor to major and thickening of the tendon may be present
- Crepitus may be present
- Pain occurs at the extremes of motion during passive range of motion (PROM) and active range of motion (AROM)
- Pain increases during stretching and resisted range of motion (RROM); strength decreases with pain

the quadriceps region. With this condition, a superficial bruise may be present and effusion of the distal joint closest to the injury site occurs. The muscle is typically very tender, and as the ossificans develops, a hardened mass can be palpated within the muscle mass. In tendons, the condition is called **calcific tendinitis.**

Overuse injuries may be due to either intrinsic factors (e.g., malalignment of limbs, muscular imbalances, other anatomical factors) or extrinsic factors (e.g., training errors, faulty technique, incorrect surfaces and equipment, poor environmental conditions)—characterized by pain and dysfunction. Typically, overuse injuries are classified in four stages:

Stage 1 Pain after activity only

Stage 2 Pain during activity, does not restrict performance

Stage 3 Pain during activity, restricts performance

Stage 4 Chronic, unremitting pain, even at rest

Bursitis involves irritation of one or more bursae, the fluid-filled sacs that serve to reduce friction in the tissues surrounding joints. Bursitis may also be either acute or chronic, depending on whether it is brought on by a single traumatic compression, or by repeated compressions associated with overuse of the joint. Local swelling of a bursa can be very pronounced, particularly at the elbow (olecranon bursa) and patella (prepatellar bursa). The area is point tender and can be warm to the touch.

 Earlier, a question was posed relative to the injury potential of tendons and ligaments based on their anatomical structure and function. Because tendons are stronger than the muscles to which they attach, the muscle typically ruptures rather than the tendon when the musculotendinous unit is overloaded. Although ligaments have more elasticity than tendons because they attach at both ends to bone, they tend to rupture or become permanently stretched when bones displace at a joint.

Soft Tissue Healing

The reparative process for injured soft tissues involves a complex series of interrelated physical and chemical activities. Because the normal healing process takes place in a regular and predictable fashion, the knowledgeable athletic trainer can follow the various signs and symptoms exhibited at the injury site to monitor how healing is progressing. This will determine when it is appropriate to begin rehabilitation and when to return an athlete to participation.

Healing of soft tissues is a three-phase process involving inflammation, proliferation, and maturation. Although it is useful to discuss the healing phenomenon in terms of these different stages, it should be recognized that within

a wound there is usually overlap of these processes, both spatially and temporally.

INFLAMMATORY PHASE (0–6 DAYS)

The familiar symptoms of inflammation have long been recognized and, in fact, were documented by early Greek and Roman physicians as rubor (redness), calor (local heat), tumor (swelling), dolar (pain), and in severe cases, functio laesa (loss of function). Although inflammation can be produced by adverse response to chemical, thermal, and infectious agents, our focus will be on the characteristic course of the inflammatory response following injury. Depending on the nature of the causative forces, inflammation can be acute or chronic. Acute inflammatory response is of relatively brief duration and involves a characteristic hemodynamic activity that generates **exudate**, a plasma-like fluid that exudes out of tissue or its capillaries and is composed of protein and granular leukocytes (white blood cells). Chronic inflammatory response, alternatively, is of prolonged duration and is characterized by the presence of nongranular leukocytes and the production of scar tissue.

The beginning of the acute inflammatory phase involves the activation of three mechanisms that act to stop blood loss from the wound. First, local vasoconstriction occurs, lasting from a few seconds to as long as 10 minutes. Larger blood vessels constrict in response to signals from neurotransmitters, and the capillaries and smaller arterioles and venules constrict due to the influence of serotonin and catecholamines released from the platelets and serum during injury. The resulting reduction in the volume of blood flow in the region promotes increased blood viscosity or resistance to the flow, which further reduces blood loss at the injury site.

A second response to the loss of blood is the platelet reaction. The platelet reaction provokes clotting as individual cells irreversibly combine with each other and with fibrin to form a mechanical plug that occludes the end of a ruptured blood vessel. The platelets also produce an array of chemical mediators that play significant roles in the inflammatory and proliferation phases of healing. Included are serotonin, adrenaline, noradrenaline, and histamine, all of which are primary agents in the inflammatory response. Also found in platelets is the enzyme adenosine triphosphotase (ATP'ASE), which is central in supplying the energy needed for healing.

The third response is the activation of the coagulation cascade. A cascade is a heightened physiological response consisting of several different, interrelated processes. Fibrinogen molecules are converted into fibrin for clot formation through two different pathways. The extrinsic pathway is activated by thromboplastin, which is released from damaged tissue. The intrinsic pathway, inside the blood vessels, is enabled by the interaction between platelets and the Hageman factor. Both paths result in the formation of prothrombin activator that converts prothrombin into thrombin.

Following vasoconstriction, vasodilation is brought on by a local axon reflex and the complement and kinin cascades. In the complement cascade, approximately 20 proteins that normally circulate in the blood in inactive form become active to promote a variety of activities essential for healing. One process activated is the attraction of neutrophils and macrophages to rid the injury site of debris and infectious agents through **phagocytosis**. As blood flow to the injured area slows, these cells are redistributed to the periphery, where they begin to adhere to the endothelial lining. Mast cells and basophils are also stimulated to release histamine, further promoting vasodilation. The kinin cascade provokes the conversion of the inactive enzyme kallikrein to the activated bradykinin in both blood and tissue. Bradykinin promotes vasodilation and increases blood vessel wall permeability, contributing to the formation of tissue exudate.

In conjunction with this, increased blood flow to the region causes swelling. Blood from the broken vessels and damaged tissues forms a hematoma, which, in combination with necrotic tissue, forms the **zone of primary injury**.

Approximately 1 hour postinjury, swelling, or **edema**, occurs as the vascular walls become more permeable and increased pressure within the vessels forces a plasma exudate out into the interstitial tissues **(Figure 5.11)**. This increased permeability or porosity of the blood vessel walls typically exists for only a few minutes in cases of mild trauma, with a return to normal permeability in 20 to 30 minutes. More severe traumas can result in a prolonged state of increased permeability, and sometimes result in delayed onset of increased permeability, with swelling not apparent until some time has elapsed since the original injury. The tissue exudate provides a critically important part of the body's defense, both by diluting toxins present in the wound and by enabling delivery of the cells that remove damaged tissue and enable reconstruction.

The complement and kinin cascades act to speed the arrival of reparative cells in the exudate. **Mast cells** are connective tissue cells that carry heparin, which prolongs clotting, and histamine. Platelets and basophil leukocytes also transport histamine, which serves as a vasodilator and increases blood vessel permeability. The leukocytes release enzymes that interact with phospholipids in the cell membranes to produce arachidonic acid. Arachidonic acid activates further inflammation of the affected cells through production of chemical mediators, including prostaglan-dins and leukotrienes. Bradykinin, a major plasma protease present during inflammation, increases vessel permeability and stimulates nerve endings to cause pain. This chain of chemical activity produces the **zone of secondary injury**, which includes all of the tissues affected by inflammation, edema, and hypoxia. After the debris and waste products from the damaged tissues are ingested through phagocytosis, the leukocytes re-enter the blood stream and the acute inflammatory reaction subsides.

THE PROLIFERATIVE PHASE (3–21 DAYS)

The proliferative phase involves repair and regeneration of the injured tissue and takes place from approximately 3 days following the injury through the next 3 to 6 weeks, overlapping the later part of the inflammatory phase. The proliferative processes include the development of new blood vessels (angiogenesis), the process of fibrous tissue formation (fibroplasia), the generation of new epithelial tissue (re-epithelialization), and wound contraction.

This stage begins when the hematoma's size is sufficiently diminished to allow room for the growth of new tissue. Although the skin has the ability to regenerate new skin tissue, the other soft tissues replace damaged cells with scar tissue.

Healing through scar formation begins with the accumulation of exuded fluid containing a large concentration of protein and damaged cellular tissues. This accumulation forms the foundation for a highly vascularized mass of immature connective tissues that include fibroblasts, which are cells capable of generating collagen. The fibroblasts begin to produce immature collagen through the process known as fibroplasia.

Fibroplasia and angiogenesis are interdependent processes, with the deposition of the new connective tissue matrix fueled by nutrients from the blood supply, and the newly forming blood vessels reliant on mechanical support and protection from the matrix. The developing connective tissue at the wound site is primarily Types I and III collagen, cells, blood vessels, and a matrix containing glycoproteins and proteoglycans. Type III collagen is particularly useful at this stage because of its ability to rapidly form crosslinks that contribute to stabilization of the wound site. It is fibroblasts that have been chemically drawn to the region that secrete the collagen. The enzymatic reactions involved in collagen production are dependent on specific

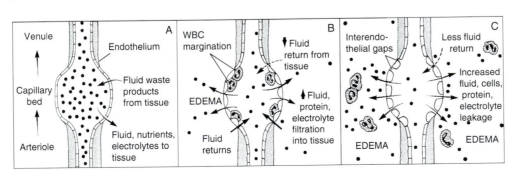

▶ **FIGURE 5.11 Acute inflammatory process.** Edema forms when histochemical agents open the pores in the vascular walls, allowing plasma to migrate into the interstitial space.

concentrations of oxygen, ascorbate, ferrous ions, and lactate within the microenvironment of the wound.

Fibroblasts also produce attachment factors that promote angiogenesis by helping the growing vessels attach to basement membrane collagen. The primary driving force for angiogenesis, however, comes from the platelet response and the hypoxic wound environment. New vessel formation begins with activation of enzymes by a potent growth factor, which act on the existing vessels to dissolve their basement membranes and liberate endothelial cells. These cells are then chemically drawn to hypoxic sites within a wound, where they fuse and form new vessels.

Other characteristics of the proliferation stage include an increase in the number of blood vessels present, increased water content in the injury zone, and re-epithelialization at the surface caused by epithelial cells migrating from the periphery toward the center of the wound.

MATURATION PHASE (UP TO 1+ YEAR)

The final phase of soft tissue wound repair is known as the maturation, or remodeling, phase. This period involves maturation of the newly formed tissue into scar tissue. The associated processes include decreased fibroblast activity, increased organization of the extracellular matrix, decreased tissue water content, reduced vascularity, and a return to normal histochemical activity. In soft tissue, these processes begin about 3 weeks postinjury, overlapping the proliferative phase. Types I and III collagen continue to increase, replacing immature collagen resulting in contraction of the wound.

Although the epithelium has typically completely regenerated by 3 to 4 weeks post-injury, the tensile strength of the wound at this time is only approximately 25% of normal (2). After several more months, strength may still be as much as 30% below preinjury strength (3). This is partly due to the orientation of the collagen fibers, which tends to be more vertical during this time period than in normal tissue, where their orientation is usually horizontal. The collagen turnover rate in a newly healed scar is also very high, so that failure to provide appropriate support for the wound site can result in a larger scar.

Because scar tissue is fibrous, inelastic, and nonvascular, it is less strong and less functional than the original tissues. The development of the scar also typically causes the wound to shrink, resulting in decreased flexibility of the affected tissues following the injury.

Remodeling continues for a year or more as collagen fibers become oriented along the lines of mechanical stress to which the tissue is usually subjected. The tensile strength of scar tissue may continue to increase for as long as 2 years postinjury. **Box 5.6** summarizes the three stages of the healing process.

Muscle fibers are permanent cells that do not reproduce or proliferate in response to either injury or training. There are, however, reserve cells in the basement membrane of each muscle fiber that are able to regenerate mus-

> ## ➤➤ BOX 5.6
>
> ## Phases of Soft Tissue Wound Healing
>
> ### INFLAMMATION (0–6 DAYS):
>
> - Vasoconstriction promotes increased blood viscosity (thickness), reducing blood loss through bleeding.
> - The platelet reaction initiates clotting and releases growth factors that attract reparative cells to the site.
> - The coagulation cascade affects clot formation.
> - The complement and kinin cascades provoke vasodilation and increase blood vessel wall permeability, facilitating the migration of neutrophils and macrophages in plasma exudate to cleanse the site through phagocytosis.
>
> ### PROLIFERATION (3–21 DAYS):
>
> - Fibroblasts produce a supportive network of Types I and III collagen.
> - The platelet response and the hypoxic wound environment stimulate angiogenesis.
> - Epithelial cells migrate from the periphery toward the center of the wound to enact re-epithelialization.
>
> ### MATURATION (UP TO 1+ YEARS):
>
> - Fibroblast activity decreases and habitual loading produces increased organization of the extracellular matrix.
> - A return to normal histochemical activity allows for reduced vascularity and water content.
> - Types I and III collagen continue to proliferate, replacing immature collagen precursors and resulting in contracture of the wound.
> - Scar tissue formation results in decreased size and flexibility of the involved tissues.
> - Remodeling causes collagen fiber alignment along lines of habitual stress, with tensile strength increasing for up to 2 years post-injury.

cle fiber following injury. Severe muscle injury can result in scarring or the formation of **adhesions** within the muscle, which inhibits the potential for fiber regeneration from the reserve cells. Consequently, following severe injury, muscle may regain only about 50% of its preinjury strength (1).

Because tendons and ligaments have few reparative cells, healing of these structures is a slow process that can take more than a year. Regeneration is enhanced by proximity to other soft tissues that can assist with supply of the chemical mediators and building blocks required. For this reason, isolated ligaments such as the anterior cruciate have poor chances for healing (4). If tendons and ligaments undergo abnormally high tensile stress before scar formation is complete, the newly forming tissues can be elongated. If this occurs in ligaments, joint instability may result.

Because tendons, ligaments, and muscles **hypertrophy** (increase in size) and **atrophy** (decrease in size) in response to levels of mechanical stress, complete immobilization of the injury leads to atrophy, loss of strength, and decreased rate of healing in these tissues. The amount of atrophy is generally proportional to the time of immobilization. Thus, although immobilization may be necessary to protect the injured tissues during the early stages of recovery, strengthening exercises should be implemented as soon as appropriate during rehabilitation of the injury. The sport participant is at increased risk for reinjury as long as the affected tissues are below preinjury strength.

THE ROLE OF GROWTH FACTORS

Growth factors are proteins that play crucial roles during all three phases of the healing process. Their functions include attracting cells to the wound, stimulating their proliferation, and directing the deposition of the extracellular matrix.

First discovered in the α granules of platelets, platelet-derived growth factor (PDGF) is also released from macrophages, endothelial cells, vascular smooth cells, and fibroblasts. The presence of PDGF is one of the most important factors in the success of the first two stages of healing. PDGF acts as a chemical attractant for fibroblasts, neutrophils, and macrophages and also promotes the replication of fibroblasts and vascular smooth muscle cells. It also activates macrophages and stimulates fibroblasts to secrete Types I and III collagen.

Another important growth factor, transforming growth factor-β (TGF-β), is actually a group of several different proteins with similar structural and chemical properties. TGF-β is produced by platelets, macrophages, bone cells, monocytes, and lymphocytes, and is capable of both stimulating and inhibiting fibroblasts. TGF-β also stimulates angiogenesis and accelerates collagen deposition.

Another group of proteins with a common high affinity for heparin is termed basic fibroblast growth factor (bFGF). The platelet-derived enzyme heparitinase chemically separates bFGF from heparin. The bFGFs stimulate proliferation of endothelial cells, and are distributed in endothelial cells, macrophages, and fibroblasts. They are also critically important in angiogenesis, releasing the basement membrane-degrading enzymes that separate endothelial cells prior to new vessel formation.

Two closely related growth factors are epidermal growth factor (EGF) and transforming growth factor-α (TGF-α). Both originate from transmembrane proteins and both act on the EGF receptor. Whereas both of these growth factors facilitate the development of granulation tissue, TGF-α also regulates angiogenesis and promotes epidermal regrowth (5).

Soft Tissue Wound Care

As previously discussed, soft tissue injuries may involve open wounds (abrasions, blisters, lacerations, puncture wounds) or closed wounds (contusion, strains, sprains, bursitis). This section will explain immediate care of both broad categories of soft tissue injuries.

OPEN SOFT TISSUE INJURY CARE

In providing wound care for open soft tissue injuries, it is critical to follow universal precautions and infection control standards (**Field Strategy 5.1**). In addition to using safety equipment, disinfecting equipment and materials used during wound care, and properly discarding contaminated materials, several steps in general wound care should be followed by the athletic trainer:

- If possible, wash hands before beginning treatment.
- Apply gloves and apply direct pressure to the wound with sterile gauze or a nonstick material.
- Cleanse the wound and the area around the wound (at least twice its size) with saline water or a similar antiseptic agent, such as povidine-iodine (Betadine).
- Dress and bandage the wound site securely for continued play.
- Creams or ointments may or may not be used with occlusive dressings. If used, cover dressings beyond their borders with underwrap and elastic adhesive tape where possible.
- Change dressings as necessary and look for signs of infection (local heat, swelling, redness, pain, pus, elevated body temperature).

For specific injuries, **Field Strategy 5.2** explains the basic care for common skin injuries. It is assumed that the athletic trainer is already gloved. These techniques can be adapted for other open wounds.

CLOSED SOFT TISSUE INJURY CARE

Closed wound care focuses on immediately reducing inflammation, pain, and secondary hypoxia. Several initial steps should be followed by the athletic trainer in providing general acute care:

- Apply crushed ice packs directly to the skin as quickly as possible following the injury.
- Do not place a towel or elastic wrap (dry or wet) between the crushed ice pack and skin. This will reduce the effectiveness of the treatment.
- Apply the crushed ice cold pack for 30 minutes (40 minutes for a large muscle mass such as the quadriceps).
- Elevate the body part at least 6 to 10 inches above the level of the heart.
- After the initial ice treatment, remove the ice pack, replace the compression wrap, and continue elevation.
- Reapply the crushed ice pack every 2 hours (every hour if the athlete is active between applications, i.e., walking on crutches or showering) until the athlete goes to bed.

FIELD STRATEGY 5.1   GENERAL GUIDELINES FOR PREVENTING SPREAD OF BLOODBORNE PATHOGENS

- Latex gloves should always be worn. Other protective equipment that should be worn when blood and/or other bodily fluids could be splashed, spurted, or sprayed include:
  - Eye wear/face guards
  - Masks and/or protective guards
  - Gowns or aprons
- Following any exposure to potentially infectious material, immediately wash and disinfect hands and other skin surfaces.
- Clean large spills of bodily fluids and bloodborne pathogens by flooding the contaminated area with disinfectant prior to removing the spill. Following removal, the area should be disinfected again and thoroughly scrubbed.
- Disinfect all horizontal surfaces (i.e., treatment tables, taping tables, workspace, and floors) regularly, after each use, and immediately after spills or soiling occurs. Use a scrubbing process.
- Disinfect with a cleaning solution of 1:10 to 1:100 solution (bleach to water). Caution should be used when using this solution near therapeutic modalities or skin due to caustic and corrosive properties of bleach. The solution must be mixed daily to be effective.
- Soiled linens and towels should be separated from regular laundry, handled with gloves, and placed in a leak-proof bag that is visibly designated for biohazard items.
- All items should be washed with detergent and water for 25 minutes, at a minimum of 71°C (160°F). Disinfectant solution should be added to water that is heavily contaminated.
- All disposable contaminated products (e.g., gauze, paper towels, cotton) should be handled with gloves and placed in leak-proof biohazard bags.
- Sharps containers should be readily available, leak proof, puncture resistant, red in color, and visibly designated with a biohazard sign. Reusable sharps, such as pointed scissors or tweezers, should be sterilized after each use.
- Disposal of contaminated items and sharps containers should be in compliance with OSHA standards.

- The compression wrap should be worn throughout the night.

Field Strategy 5.3 discusses the basic care of closed soft tissue injuries after the acute protocol has been followed. Because the severity of injuries can range from mild to severe, these guidelines are provided as a general guide. Each injury must be assessed and treated on an individual basis.

BONE INJURIES

 A soccer player is complaining of localized pain on the lateral side of the lower leg about 3 inches proximal to the ankle joint. The pain has been present for 3 weeks and is particularly noticeable during weight bearing activities. What injury might you suspect? What are the implications for the athlete's continued training?

Bone behaves predictably in response to stress, in keeping with its material constituents and structural organization. The composition and structure of bone make it strong for its relatively light weight.

Anatomical Properties of Bone

The primary constituents of bone are calcium carbonate, calcium phosphate, collagen, and water. The minerals, making up 60 to 70% of bone weight, provide stiffness and strength in resisting compression. Collagen provides bone with some degree of flexibility and strength in resisting tension. Aging causes a progressive loss of collagen and increase in bone brittleness. Thus, children's bones are more pliable than adults' bones.

As bones develop, longitudinal bone growth continues only as long as the bone's epiphyseal plates, or growth plates, continue to exist **(Figure 5.12)**. Epiphyseal plates are cartilaginous discs found near the ends of the long bones. These are the sites where longitudinal bone growth takes place on the diaphysis (central) side of the plates. During or shortly after adolescence, the plate disappears and the bone fuses, terminating longitudinal growth. Most epiphyses close around age 18, but some may be present until about age 25.

Although the most rapid bone growth occurs prior to adulthood, bones continue to grow in diameter throughout most of the lifespan. The internal layer of the periosteum

FIELD STRATEGY 5.2   CARE OF OPEN WOUNDS

ABRASIONS

1. Clean and remove visible contaminants with a fluid flush with water and sweeps of gauze.
2. Clean the wound site and area around the wound with antiseptic solution.
3. Dress and bandage the wound securely for continued play.
4. For dirty abrasions, or when it has been at least 5 years since a tetanus booster, refer for medical care.

BLISTERS

1. Clean both the wound site and area around the wound with antiseptic solution.
2. Leave the roof of the blister intact for at least 24 hours, and cover the area with a topical antibiotic and dry sterile dressing. Do *not* aspirate a blood-filled blister.
3. If the blister is large and subject to continued compression, use a small, sterile needle to aspirate the clear fluid, or incise the skin of clear blisters according to physician protocol.
4. Once the fluid is removed, cleanse the area again with an antiseptic solution.
5. Pad the nontender skin around the blister with an adhesive soft foam material (donut pad), New Skin®, or 2nd Skin®.
6. Dress and bandage the wound site securely for continued play.

INCISIONS AND LACERATIONS

1. Clean both the wound site and area around the wound with antiseptic solution.
2. Spray tape adherent on a cotton-tipped applicator and apply above and below the wound.
3. Beginning in the middle of the wound, bring the edges together and secure the Steri-Strip® below the wound. Lift up and secure above the wound. Make sure the edges of the wound are approximated.

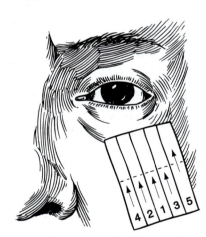

4. Apply the second Steri-Strip® in a similar manner immediately adjacent to one side of the original strip. Apply the third strip on the other side. Alternate sides until the entire wound is covered.
5. Dress the wound with an adhesive tincture base covered with an occlusive or non-stick sterile dressing.
6. Sutures may be desirable for any depth of laceration, especially around the face. However, any wound open to the full-thickness of the dermis should be sutured within 10 hours of the injury.
7. Refer for medical care if more than 5 years since a tetanus booster, or if signs of infection appear.

FIELD STRATEGY 5.3   CARE OF CLOSED WOUNDS

CONTUSIONS

For superficial contusions:
1. Pad with soft (open-celled) material next to the skin and more dense (closed-cell) material as an external covering.
2. Cut a hole that matches the contused area in the soft material, or keep it solid.
3. Secure the pad with elastic athletic tape or an elastic wrap.
4. Following play, and periodically during the next few days, apply ice, compression, and elevation to the site.
5. Repeat until pain and swelling are gone.

For deep contusions, determine disability after temporary paralysis subsides:
1. In moderate and severe cases, follow acute protocol for at least 24 hours with the muscle in a stretched position.
2. If an antalgic gait is present, fit for crutches and instruct the athlete to use a partial- or non-weight-bearing gait.
3. Seek medical advice for complications.

MUSCLE STRAINS

Mild strains:
1. Apply a compression wrap (elastic, stockinette, or athletic tape) to muscle belly and tendon.
2. If cold is applied immediately before return to play, use a mild warm-up with a compression wrap before allowing return.
3. Apply heat after 72 hours.

Moderate to severe cases are treated by acute care protocol and referred for medical care:
1. Maintain joints above and below the strain in a neutral, lengthened position.
2. Immobilize, if necessary, and modify daily activity.
3. Apply heat when no increase in swelling has occurred within 1 to 2 days, and point tenderness and pain is minimal during active motion.

TENDON INJURIES

Mild injuries:
1. Use cold and isometric or eccentric exercise as tolerated.
2. Apply heat after 72 hours; combine strengthening with stretching.

Moderate to severe cases are treated by acute care protocol and referred for medical care:
1. Maintain joints above and below the affected tendon in a neutral, lengthened position.
2. Immobilize, if necessary, and modify daily activities.
3. Apply heat when no increase in swelling has occurred within 1 to 2 days, and point tenderness and pain are minimal during active motion.

LIGAMENT SPRAINS

Mild injury:
1. Use protective device (brace) or athletic tape to limit joint laxity and motion at end range.
2. If ice is applied immediately before return, use a mild warm-up before allowing return to play.
3. Heat may be applied when swelling has subsided, and palpable pain upon movement is minimal.

Moderate to severe cases are treated by acute care protocol and referred for medical care:
1. In a neutral stable position, follow general guidelines for ice application and immobilize, if necessary.
2. Modify daily activity, sport activity level, or equipment.

Dislocations:
1. Splint using standard first aid procedures, and refer for medical care.
2. Assess the distal pulse, sensation, and movement; treat for shock and activate EMS, if necessary.

 Activate EMS

Continued

FIELD STRATEGY 5.3   CARE OF CLOSED WOUNDS *Continued*   *continued from page 111*

BURSITIS

Mild cases:
1. Pad (donut pad) the area surrounding the bursitis.
2. Apply heat after 72 hours; continue to pad until pain free.

Moderate to severe cases:
1. Limit movement by placing a compression pad over the bursa using a compression wrap.
2. Immobilize, if necessary, and modify daily activities.
3. When pain and inflammation are under control, apply heat.

Infected bursa:
1. Immobilize the joint and apply hot packs.
2. Refer to a physician for medical care. Antibiotics may need to be prescribed.

builds new concentric layers of bone tissue on top of the existing ones. At the same time, bone is resorbed or eliminated around the sides of the medullary cavity, so that the diameter of the cavity is continually enlarged. The bone cells that form new bone tissue are called osteoblasts, and those that resorb bone are known as osteoclasts. In healthy adult bone, the activity of osteoblasts and osteoclasts, referred to as bone turnover, is largely balanced. The total amount of bone remains approximately constant until women reach their forties and men reach their sixties, when a gradual decline in bone mass begins. Sport participants past these ages may be at increased risk for bone fractures. Regular participation in weight-bearing exercise, however, has been shown to be effective in reducing age-related bone loss.

No matter what the athlete's age, some bones are also more susceptible to fracture as a result of their internal composition. Bone tissue is categorized as either **cortical**, if the porosity is low—with 5 to 30% nonmineralized tissue, or as **cancellous**, if the porosity is high—with 30 to more than 90% of nonmineralized tissue (**Figure 5.13**). Most human bones have outer shells of cortical bone, with cancellous bone underneath. Cortical bone is stiffer, which means that it can withstand greater stress but less strain than cancellous bone. Cancellous bone, however, has the advantage of being spongier than cortical bone, which means that it can undergo more strain before fracturing. The mineralization of cancellous bone varies with the individual's age and location of the bone in the body. Both cortical and cancellous bone are anisotropic, which means that they exhibit different strengths and stiffnesses in response to forces applied from different directions. Bone is strongest in resisting compressive stress, and weakest in resisting shear stress.

Bone size and shape also influence the likelihood of fracture. The direction and magnitude of the forces to which they are habitually subjected largely determine the shape and size of the bone. The direction in which new bone tissue is formed has been found to be adapted to best resist the loads encountered, particularly in regions of high stress such as the femoral neck. The mineralization and girth of bone increase in response to increased stress levels. For example, the bones of the dominant arm of professional tennis players and professional baseball players have been found to be larger and stronger than the bones of their nondominant arms (6,7).

Bone Injury Classifications

A **fracture** is a disruption in the continuity of a bone (**Figure 5.14**). The type of fracture sustained depends on

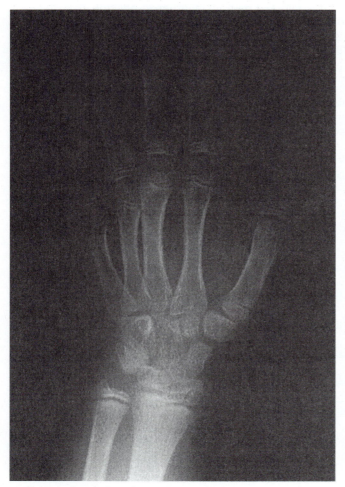

➤ FIGURE 5.12 **Epiphyseal growth plate.**

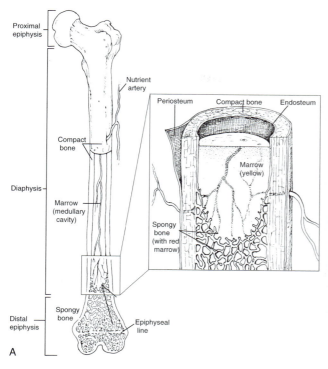

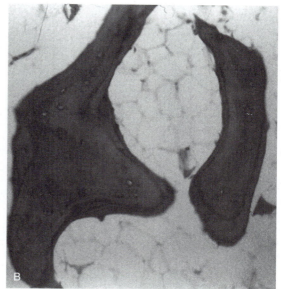

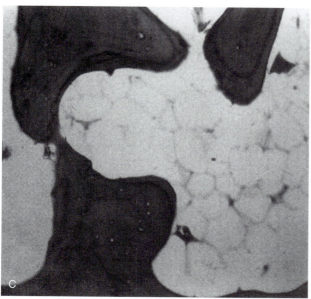

➤ **FIGURE 5.13 Bone macrostructure**. Note the epiphyseal growth lines at either end of the bone (A). The cortical bone surrounds the cancellous bone and medullary cavity. Cancellous bone is more porous than cortical bone, as can be seen in the electron micrograph photo above (B,C).

the type of mechanical loading that caused it, as well as the health and maturity of the bone at the time of injury. Fractures are considered to be closed when the bone ends remain intact within the surrounding soft tissues, and open or compound when one or both bone ends protrude from the skin.

Excessive torsional and bending loads, as exemplified by tibial fractures resulting from skiing accidents, often produce spiral fractures of the long bones. Such fractures are the result of a combined loading pattern of shear and tension, producing failure at an oblique angle to the long axis of the bone.

Because bone is stronger in resisting compression than both tension and shear, acute compression fractures of bone are rare. Under combined loading, however, a fracture resulting from a torsional load may be affected by the presence of a compressive load. An impacted fracture is one in which the opposite sides of the fracture are compressed together. Fractures that result in depression of bone fragments into the underlying tissues are termed depressed.

Because the bones of children contain relatively larger amounts of collagen than adult bones, they are more flexible and more resistant to fracture under day-to-day loading

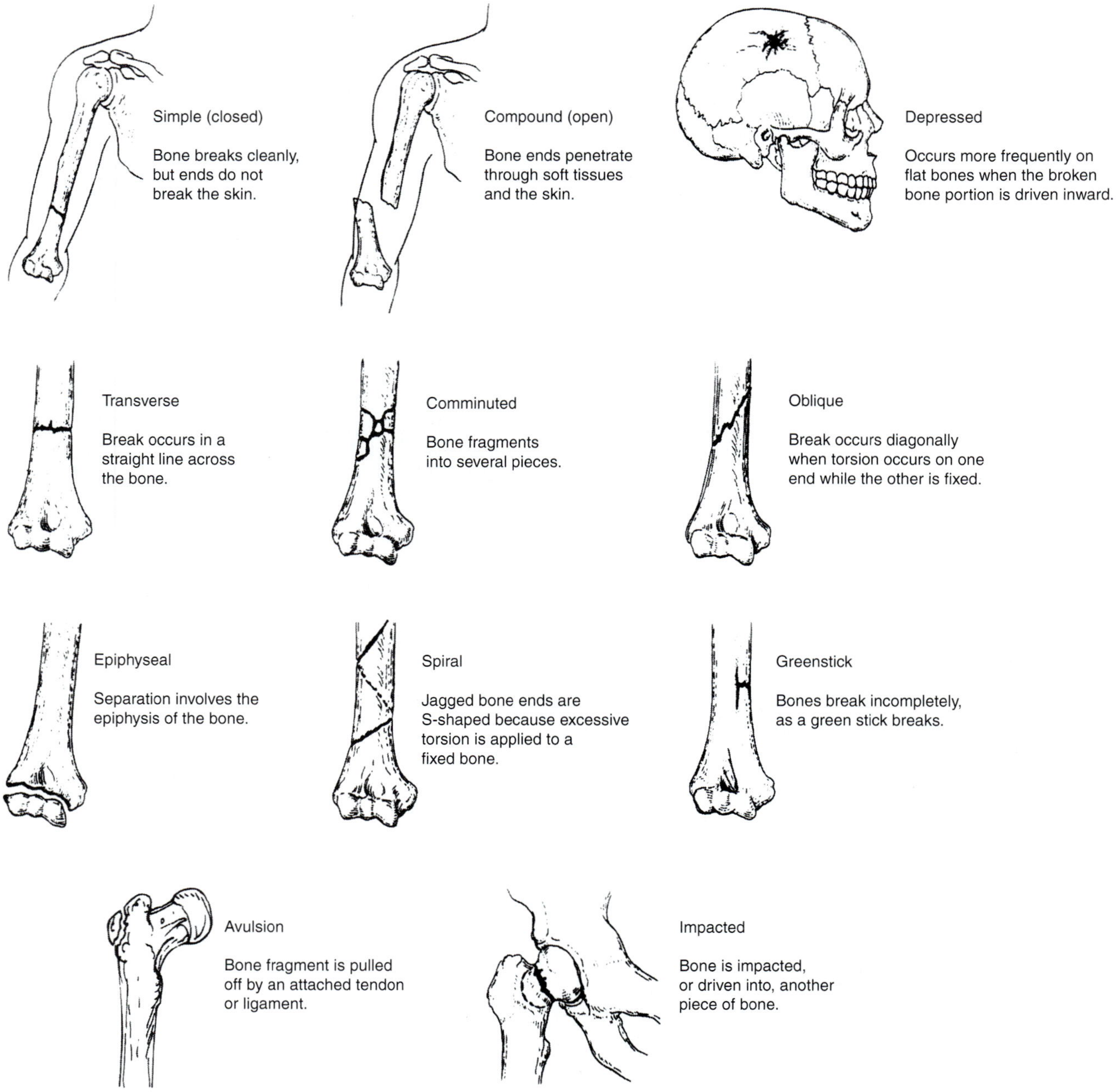

Simple (closed)

Bone breaks cleanly, but ends do not break the skin.

Compound (open)

Bone ends penetrate through soft tissues and the skin.

Depressed

Occurs more frequently on flat bones when the broken bone portion is driven inward.

Transverse

Break occurs in a straight line across the bone.

Comminuted

Bone fragments into several pieces.

Oblique

Break occurs diagonally when torsion occurs on one end while the other is fixed.

Epiphyseal

Separation involves the epiphysis of the bone.

Spiral

Jagged bone ends are S-shaped because excessive torsion is applied to a fixed bone.

Greenstick

Bones break incompletely, as a green stick breaks.

Avulsion

Bone fragment is pulled off by an attached tendon or ligament.

Impacted

Bone is impacted, or driven into, another piece of bone.

➤ FIGURE 5.14 **Types of fractures**.

than adult bones. Consequently, greenstick fractures, or incomplete fractures, are more common in children than in adults. A greenstick fracture is an incomplete fracture typically caused by bending or torsional loads.

Avulsions are another type of fracture caused by tensile loading that involve a tendon or ligament pulling a small chip of bone away from the rest of the bone. Explosive throwing and jumping movements may result in avulsion fractures. When loading is very rapid, a fracture is more likely to be comminuted, meaning it contains multiple fragments.

Stress fractures, also known as fatigue fractures, result from repeated low-magnitude forces. Stress fractures differ from acute fractures in that they can worsen over time, beginning as a small disruption in the continuity of the outer layers of cortical bone and ending as complete cortical fracture with possible displacement of the bone ends. Stress fractures of the metatarsals, the femoral neck, and the pubis have been reported among runners who have apparently overtrained. Stress fractures of the pars interarticularis region of the lumbar vertebrae occur in higher-than-normal frequencies among football linemen and female gymnasts.

Osteopenia, a condition of reduced bone mineral density, predisposes the athlete to fractures of all kinds, but particularly to stress fractures. The condition is primarily found among adolescent female athletes, especially distance runners, who are amenorrheic. Although **amenorrhea**

(cessation of menses) among this group is not well understood, it appears to be related to a low percentage of body fat and/or high training mileage. The link between cessation of menses and osteopenia is also not well understood. Possible contributing factors include hyperactivity of osteoclasts, hypoactivity of osteoblasts, hormonal factors, and insufficiencies of dietary calcium or other minerals or nutrients.

Epiphyseal Injury Classifications

The bones of children and adolescents are vulnerable to epiphyseal injuries, including injuries to the cartilaginous epiphyseal plate, articular cartilage, and apophysis. The apophyses are sites of tendon attachments to bone, where bone shape is influenced by the tensile loads to which these sites are subjected. Both acute and repetitive loading can injure the growth plate, potentially resulting in premature closure of the epiphyseal junction and termination of bone growth. "Little League elbow," for example, is a stress injury to the medial epicondylar epiphysis of the humerus. Salter (8) has categorized acute epiphyseal injuries into five distinct types **(Figure 5.15)**.

Type I Complete separation of the epiphysis from the metaphysis with no fracture to the bone

Type II Separation of the epiphysis and a small portion of the metaphysis

Type III Fracture of the epiphysis

Type IV Fracture of a part of the epiphysis and metaphysis

Type V Compression of the epiphysis without fracture, resulting in compromised epiphyseal function

Type I
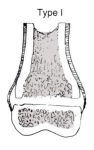

Type II
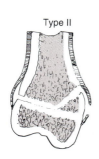

Type III
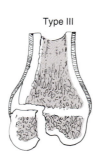

Type IV
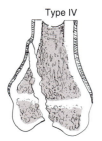

Type V
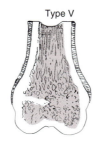

➤ **FIGURE 5.15 Epiphyseal injuries**.

Another category of epiphyseal injuries is referred to collectively as **osteochondrosis**. Osteochondrosis results from disruption of blood supply to an epiphysis, with associated tissue necrosis and potential deformation of the epiphysis. Because the cause of the condition is poorly understood, it is typically termed idiopathic osteochondrosis. The osteochondroses occur most commonly between the ages of 3 and 10, and are more prevalent among boys than girls (8). Specific disease names have been given to sites where osteochondrosis is common, such as Legg-Calvé-Perthes disease, which is osteochondrosis of the femoral head.

The apophyses are also subject to osteochondrosis, particularly among children and adolescents. These conditions, referred to as apophysitis, may be idiopathic. They are also often associated with traumatic avulsion-type fractures. Common sites for apophysitis are the calcaneus (Sever's disease) and the tibial tubercle at the site of the patellar tendon attachment (Osgood-Schlatter's disease).

Bony Tissue Healing

Healing of acute bone fractures is a three-phase process, as is soft tissue healing. The acute inflammatory phase lasts approximately 4 days. Damage to the periosteum and surrounding soft tissues results in the formation of a hematoma in the medullary canal and surrounding tissues. The ensuing inflammatory response involves vasodilation, edema formation, and the histochemical changes associated with soft tissue inflammation.

During repair and regeneration, osteoclasts resorb damaged bone tissues, whereas osteoblasts build new bone. Between the fractured bone ends, a fibrous, vascularized tissue known as a **callus** is formed **(Figure 5.16)**. The callus contains weak, immature bone tissue that strengthens with time through bone remodeling. The process of callus formation is known as enchondral bone healing. An alternative process, known as direct bone healing, can occur when the fractured bone ends are immobilized in direct contact with one another. This enables new, interwoven bone tissue to be deposited without the formation of a callus. Unless a fracture is fixed by metal plates, screens, or rods, healing normally takes place through the enchondral process. Because noninvasive treatment is generally preferred, a fixation device is only implanted when it appears unlikely that the fracture will heal acceptably without one.

Maturation and remodeling of bone tissue involves osteoblast activity on the concave side of the fracture, which is loaded in compression, and osteoclast activity on the convex side of the fracture, which is loaded in tension. The process continues until normal shape is restored and bone strength is commensurate with the loads to which the bone is routinely subjected.

Because stress fractures continue to worsen as long as the site is overloaded, it is important to recognize these injuries as early as possible. Elimination or reduction of the repetitive mechanical stress causing the fracture is the

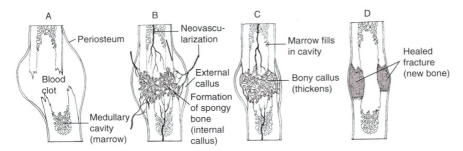

➤ FIGURE 5.16 **Bone healing**. The process of endochondral bone healing through callus formation.

primary factor necessary for healing. This allows a gradual restoration of the proper balance of osteoblast and osteoclast activity present in the bone.

Bone Injury Management

Possible fractures can be detected with palpation, percussion, use of a tuning fork (vibrations), compression, and distraction (see **Figure 4.6**). Palpation can detect deformity, crepitus, swelling, or increased pain at the fracture site. Percussion uses a tapping motion of the finger over a bony structure. A tuning fork works in the same manner. Vibrations travel through the bone and cause increased pain at a fracture site. Compression is performed by gently compressing the distal end of the bone toward the proximal end, or by encircling the body part, such as a foot or hand, and gently squeezing, thereby compressing the heads of the bones together. Again, if a fracture is present pain will increase at the fracture site. Distraction employs a tensile force, whereby the application of traction to both ends of the fractured bone will help relieve pain. Signs of fracture include swelling and bruising (discoloration), deformity or shortening of the limb, point tenderness, grating or crepitus, guarding or disability, and exposed bone ends.

A suspected fractured should be splinted before the individual is moved to avoid damage to surrounding ligaments, tendons, blood vessels, and nerves. **Field Strategy 5.4** explains the immediate management of fractures.

 Pain localized over a bone that is particularly painful during weight-bearing activities is a classic symptom of a stress injury. The soccer player should be referred to a physician. If a fracture is present, activity should be curtailed until the injury has healed.

NERVE INJURIES

 A swimmer is complaining of numbness and tingling radiating down the medial aspect of the right arm, particularly when the arm is raised over the head. She has also noticed that fatigue seems to be setting in earlier during the practice sessions. What soft tissue structure might be injured? Is medical referral necessary?

The nervous system is divided into the central nervous system, consisting of the brain and spinal cord, and the peripheral nervous system, which includes 12 pairs of cranial nerves and 31 pairs of spinal nerves, along with their branches **(Figure 5.17)**. There are 8 pairs of cervical spinal nerves (C_1–C_8), 12 pairs of thoracic nerves (T_1–T_{12}), 5 pairs of lumbar nerves (L_1–L_5), 5 pairs of sacral nerves (S_1–S_5) and 1 pair of tiny coccygeal nerves (designated C_0). Injuries to any of these nerves can be devastating to the individual, potentially resulting in temporary or permanent disability.

Anatomical Properties of Nerves

Each spinal nerve is formed from anterior and posterior roots on the spinal cord that unite at the intervertebral foramen. The posterior branches are the **afferent** (sensory) **nerves** that transmit information from sensory receptors in the skin, tendons, ligaments, and muscles to the central nervous system. The anterior branches are

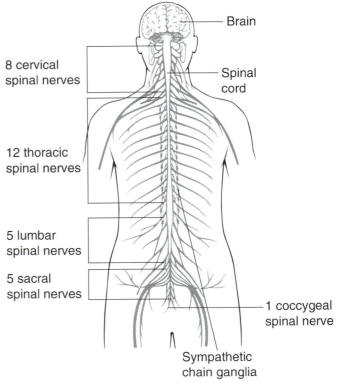

➤ FIGURE 5.17 **Spinal nerves**.

FIELD STRATEGY 5.4 MANAGEMENT ALGORITHM FOR BONE INJURIES

Remove clothing and jewelry from around the injury site
(Cut clothing away with scissors to avoid moving the injured area)

↓

Activate EMS

Check distal pulse and sensation
If either is abnormal, activate EMS

↓

Cover all wounds, including open fractures,
with sterile dressings, and secure them

↓

Do not attempt to push bone ends back underneath the skin

↓

Pad the splint to prevent local pressure

↓

Apply minimal in-line traction and maintain
it until the splint is in place and secured

↓

Immobilize the joints above and below the fracture site

↓

Splint in the position found if:

↙　　　　　　↘

*Pain increases with gentle traction
or the limb resists positioning*

The fracture is severely angulated

↓

Do **not** straighten **unless** it is
absolutely necessary to incorporate
the limb into the splint; move as
little as possible

Splint firmly, but do not impair circulation

↓

Recheck distal pulse and sensation after applying splint

↓

Check vital signs, treat for shock, and transport to a medical facility

---

the **efferent** (motor) **nerves** that transmit control signals to the muscles. The nerve fibers are heavily vascularized and encased in a multilayered, segmental protective sheath called the myelin sheath. Myelin protects and electrically insulates fibers from one another, and it increases the speed of transmission of nerve impulses. Myelinated fibers (axons bearing a myelin sheath) conduct nerve impulses rapidly,

whereas unmyelinated fibers tend to conduct impulses quite slowly.

Nerve Injury Classifications

Tensile or compressive forces most commonly injure nerves. Tensile injuries typically occur during severe high-speed accidents, such as automobile accidents or impact collisions in contact sports. When a nerve is loaded in tension, the nerve fibers tend to rupture prior to the rupturing of the surrounding connective tissue sheath. Because the nerve roots on the spinal cord are not protected by connective tissue, they are particularly susceptible to tensile injury, especially in response to stretching of the brachial plexus or cervical nerve roots.

Nerve injuries due to tensile forces are typically graded in three levels. *Grade I* injuries represent **neurapraxia**, the mildest lesion. A neuropraxia is a localized conduction block that causes temporary loss of sensation and/or motor function from selective demyelination of the axon sheath without true axonal disruption. Recovery usually occurs within days to a few weeks. *Grade II* injuries are called **axonotmesis injuries** that produce significant motor and mild sensory deficits that last at least 2 weeks. Axonotmesis disrupts the axon and myelin sheath but leaves the epineurium intact. The epineurium is the connective tissue that encapsulates the nerve trunk and binds the fascicles together. Axonal regrowth occurs at a rate of 1 to 2 mm per day; full or normal function is usually restored. *Grade III* injuries represent **neurotmesis injuries**, which disrupt the endoneurium. These severe injuries have a poor prognosis, with motor and sensory deficit persisting for up to 1 year. Surgical intervention is often necessary to avoid poor or imperfect regeneration

Compressive injuries of nerves are more complex because their severity depends on the magnitude and duration of loading, and on whether the applied pressure is direct or indirect. Because nerve function is highly dependent on oxygen provided by the associated blood vessels, damage to the blood supply caused by a compressive injury results in damage to the nerve.

Nerve injuries can result in a range of afferent symptoms, from severe pain through complete loss of sensation. Terms used to describe altered sensation include **hypoesthesia**, a reduction in sensation; **hyperesthesia**, heightened sensation; and **paresthesia**, a sense of numbness, prickling, or tingling. Pinching of a nerve can result in a sharp wave of pain that is transmitted through a body segment. Irritation or inflammation of a nerve can result in chronic pain along the nerve's course, known as **neuralgia**.

Nerve Healing

When a nerve is completely severed, healing does not occur and loss of function is typically permanent. Unless such injuries are surgically repaired, random regrowth of the nerve occurs, resulting in the formation of a **neuroma**, or nerve tumor.

When nerve fibers are ruptured in a tensile injury, but the surrounding myelin sheath remains intact, it is sometimes possible for a nerve to regenerate along the pathway provided by the sheath. Such regeneration is rela-

tively slow, however, proceeding at a rate of less than 1 mm per day or about 2.5 cm per month (1).

Management of Nerve Injuries

If nerves are injured, cutaneous sensation or muscle movement may become impaired. In Chapter 4, neurologic testing was explained and demonstrated. To assess sensitivity, touch the person with a cotton ball, paper clip, pads of the fingers, and fingernails. Ask the individual if each feels sharp or dull. Does the sensation feel the same on the injured body segment as it does on the uninjured body segment? The motor component can be tested with manual muscle testing. In testing a myotome, a normal response is a strong muscle contraction. A weakened muscle contraction may indicate partial paralysis of the muscles innervated by the nerve root being tested. With a peripheral nerve injury, there is complete paralysis of the muscles supplied by that nerve. If a muscle strain is present, a weakened muscle contraction will be accompanied by pain.

It is critical to identify a possible nerve injury and immediately refer the individual to a physician for advanced evaluation and care. For this reason, **Field Strategy 5.5** explains only basic principles used in the management of nerve injuries.

 The swimmer complained of numbness and tingling radiating down the medial aspect of the arm with early muscle fatigue. Radiating pain is a symptom of nerve pathology. The athlete should be immediately referred to her primary care physician for evaluation.

PAIN

 You notice that, in two individuals who are working to rehabilitate ankles that were sprained at about the same time, one shirks exercises because of excessive pain while the other performs workouts without complaint. What variables may be at work here?

Pain is a negative sensory and emotional experience associated with actual or potential tissue damage. It is also a universal symptom common to most injuries. The individual's perception of pain is influenced by various physical, chemical, social, and psychological factors.

The Neurological Basis of Pain

Pain can originate from somatic, visceral, and psychogenic sources. Somatic pain originates in the skin, as well as in internal structures in the musculoskeletal system. Visceral pain originates from the internal organs, which is often diffuse or referred rather than localized to the problem

FIELD STRATEGY 5.5 **MANAGEMENT OF NERVE INJURIES**

Mild cases — rest the extremity

1. Ice, transcutaneous electrical nerve stimulation (TENS), ultrasound, and nonsteroidal anti-inflammatory drugs (NSAIDs) may be used to address persistent pain and tenderness.
2. Use protective padding or bracing to decrease repetitive compression or excessive tension forces.
3. Athlete may participate when motor and sensory nerve function return to normal.

Moderate to severe cases need to be referred to a physician. After appropriate acute care protocol:

1. Perform gentle mobilization of neural tissues, beginning away from the site of the lesion and applying only gentle movement or tensile loads across the injured nerve.
2. Include strengthening exercises of the injured region, and carefully monitor proper technique.
3. Instruct the athlete on appropriate posture, muscle tension, and joint stability.
4. Correct any biomechanical factors that may have contributed to the injury.
5. No return to activity until asymptomatic.

site. With psychogenic pain, no physical cause of the pain is apparent, although the sensation of pain is felt.

Stimulation of specialized afferent nerve endings called **nociceptors** produces the pain sensation. The name *nociceptor* is derived from the word noxious, meaning physically harmful or destructive. Nociceptors are prevalent in the skin, the meninges, the periosteum, the teeth, and some internal organs.

With most acute sport-related injuries, pain is initiated by **mechanosensitive** nociceptors responding to the traumatic force that caused the injury. With chronic injuries and during the early stages of healing of acute injuries, pain persists due to the activation of **chemosensitive** nociceptors. Bradykinin, serotonin, histamines, and prostaglandins are all chemicals transported to the injury site during inflammation that activate the chemosensitive nociceptors. Thermal extremes can also stimulate other specialized nociceptors to produce pain.

Two types of afferent nerves transmit the sensation of pain to the spinal cord. Small-diameter, slow-transmission, unmyelinated C fibers transmit low-level pain that might be described as dull or aching. Sharp, piercing types of pain are transmitted by larger, faster, thinly myelinated A fibers. Pain can be transmitted along both types of afferent nerves from somatic and visceral sources. Activity in A and C fibers from the visceral organs can also provoke autonomic responses such as changes in blood pressure, heart rate, and respiration.

Afferent nerves carrying pain impulses, along with those transporting sensations such as touch, temperature, and proprioception, all articulate with the spinal cord through the substantia gelatinosa (SG) of the cord's dorsal horn. Specialized T cells then transmit impulses from all of the afferent fibers up the spinal cord to the brain, with each T cell carrying a single impulse. Within the brain, the pain impulses are transmitted to the thalamus, primarily

its ventral posterior lateral nucleus (VPL), as well as to the somatosensory cortex, where pain is perceived.

According to the gate control theory of pain proposed by Melzack and Wall in 1965, the SG acts as a gate keeper by allowing either a pain response or one of the other afferent sensations to be transported by each T cell (9). The theory is substantiated by the observation that increased sensory input can reduce the sensation of pain. For example, extreme cold can often numb pain. Because hundreds or thousands of "gates" are in operation, however, it is more common that added sensory input reduces rather than eliminates the feeling of pain because pain impulses get through to some of the T cells.

Factors That Mediate Pain

Some brain cells have the ability to produce narcotic-like, pain-killing compounds known as opioid peptides, including beta-endorphin and methionine enkephalin. Both work by blocking neural receptor sites that transmit pain. Several different sites in the brain produce endorphins. Stressors such as physical exercise, mental stress, and electrical stimulation provoke the release of endorphins into the cerebrospinal fluid. A phenomenon called "runner's high," a feeling of euphoria that occurs among long distance runners, has been attributed to endorphin release. The brain stem and pituitary gland produce enkephalins. Enkephalins block pain neurotransmitters in the dorsal horn of the spinal cord.

The central nervous system also imposes a set of **cognitive** (quality of knowing or perceiving) and **affective** (pertaining to feelings or a mental state) filters on both the perception of pain and the subsequent expression of perceived pain. Social and cultural factors can be powerful influences on pain tolerance level. In American society, for example, it is much more acceptable for females than for males to express feelings of pain. Individual personality and a state of mental preoccupation can also be significant modifiers of pain.

Referred Pain and Radiating Pain

Referred pain is perceived at a location remote from the site of the tissues actually causing the pain. A proposed explanation for referred pain begins with the fact that neurons carrying pain impulses split into several branches within the spinal cord. Although some of these branches connect with other pain-transmitting fibers, some also connect with afferent nerve pathways from the skin. This cross-branching can cause the brain to misinterpret the true location of the pain. In at least some instances, referred pain behaves in a logical and predictable fashion. For example, pain from the internal organs is typically projected outward to corresponding **dermatomes** of the skin. Heart attacks, for example, can produce a sensation of pain in the superior thoracic wall and the medial aspect of the left arm. In most cases, the affected internal organ and corresponding dermatome receive innervation from the same spinal nerve roots.

Referred pain should not be confused with radiating pain, which is pain that is felt both at its source and along a nerve. Pinching of the sciatic nerve at its root may cause pain that radiates along the nerve's course down the posterior aspect of the leg.

 Differences in pain perception and tolerance can be caused by differences in chemical, social, and psychological influences, as well as by differences in the severity of the original injury and the progression of the healing process.

Summary

1. When a force acts, two effects occur on the target tissue: acceleration, or change in velocity, and deformation, or change in shape.
2. Two factors determine if injury occurs to a tissue: the magnitude of the force and the material properties of the involved tissues.
3. Biological tissues are strongest in resisting the form of loading to which they are most commonly subjected.
4. Force exceeding a structure's yield point causes rupture or fracture.
5. The most common mechanisms of injury include:
   - Compressive force from axial loading, which compresses or crushes an object.
   - Tensile force from tension or traction on an object.
   - Shearing force, which acts parallel or tangent to a plane passing through the object.

6. In tendons, the collagen fibers are arranged in a parallel pattern, enabling resistance to high, unidirectional tensile loads when the attached muscle contracts.
7. In ligaments, the collagen fibers are largely parallel, but also interwoven, providing resistance to large tensile loads along the long axis of the ligament, and to smaller tensile loads from other directions.
8. The viscoelastic aspect of muscle extensibility enables muscles to stretch to greater lengths over time in response to a sustained tensile force.
9. Wound healing entails three overlapping phases: inflammation, proliferation, and maturation (remodeling).
   - During the inflammatory phase, blood loss is curtailed, clotting takes place, and histochemical cascades promote coagulation, vasodilation, and attraction of specialized cells to rid the wound site of foreign or infectious agents.
   - The proliferative phase includes angiogenesis, fibroplasia, re-epithelialization, and wound contraction.
   - The maturation phase involves remodeling of the newly formed tissue.
10. Growth factors are proteins that attract cells to the wound, stimulate their proliferation, and direct the deposition of the extracellular matrix.
11. The mineralization and girth of bone increases in response to increased stress levels.
12. Because bone is stronger in resisting compressive forces than both tension and shear forces, acute compression fractures are rare. Most fractures occur on the side of the bone placed in tension.
13. Maturation of bone tissue involves osteoblast activity on the concave side of the fracture, which is loaded in compression, and osteoclast activity on the convex side of the fracture, which is loaded in tension.
14. Nerve injuries due to tensile forces are graded in three levels:
    - Neurapraxia injury, with temporary loss of sensation or motor function.
    - Axonotmesis injury, with significant motor and sensory deficits that last at least 2 weeks.
    - Neurotmesis injury, with significant motor and sensory deficits persisting for up to 1 year.
15. Pain associated with injury is transmitted by specialized afferent nerve endings called nociceptors.
    - Mechanosensitive nociceptors respond to traumatic forces that cause the injury.
    - Chemosensitive nociceptors respond to chronic injuries and during the early states of healing in acute injuries.
16. Pain is transmitted along two types of afferent nerves:
    - Small-diameter, slow-transmission unmyelinated C fibers, which transmit low-level pain.

- Larger, faster, finely myelinated A fibers, which transmit sharp, piercing types of pain.

17. Afferent nerves carry nerve impulses to the spinal cord through the substantia gelatinosa (SG) of the cord's dorsal horn up to the thalamus, as well as to the somatosensory cortex, where pain is perceived.

18. Stressors, such as physical exercise, mental stress, and electrical stimulation, provoke the release of endorphins into the cerebrospinal fluid and can mediate pain perception.

References

1. American Academy of Orthopaedic Surgeons. Athletic Training and Sports Medicine. Park Ridge, IL: American Academy of Orthopaedic Surgeons, 1991.

2. Wong ME, Hollinger JO, Pinero GJ. Integrated processes responsible for soft tissue healing. Oral Surg Oral Med Oral Pathol 1996; 82(5):475-492.

3. Orgill D, Demling RH. Current concepts and approaches to wound healing. Crit Care Med 1988;16:899.

4. Hefti F, Stoll TM. Healing of ligaments and tendons. Orthopedics 1995;24(3):237-245.

5. Rappolee DA, et al. Wound macrophages express TGF-alpha and other growth factors in vivo: analysis by mRNA phenotyping. Science 1988;241:708.

6. Jones HH, et al. Humeral hypertrophy in response to exercise. J Bone Joint Surg Am 1977;59:204-208.

7. Watson RC. Bone growth and physical activity. In: International Conference on Bone Measurements. Edited by Mazess RB. DHEW Pub No. NIH 75-683, Washington, DC, 1973.

8. Salter RB. Textbook of Disorders and Injuries of the Musculoskeletal System. Baltimore: Williams & Wilkins, 1999.

9. Melzack R, Wall PD. Pain mechanisms: a new theory. Science 1965;150(699):971-979.

6

Therapeutic Modalities

OBJECTIVES

1. Explain the principles behind the electromagnetic spectrum and identify the different types of energy found in the non-ionizing range of the spectrum.

2. Explain how energy is transferred from one object to another and identify the factors that may affect that transfer.

3. Describe the physiologic effects of cryotherapy and thermotherapy.

4. List the indications and contraindications for the various methods of cold and heat treatments, including ultrasound and diathermy.

5. Describe the principles behind ultrasound and explain the physiological effects and mode of application.

6. Explain the principles of electricity and describe the different types of current.

7. Describe the various parameters that can be manipulated in electrotherapy to produce the desired effects.

8. Explain the various types of electrical stimulating units and the use of each.

9. Describe the benefits attained in each of the five basic massage strokes and explain their application.

10. Identify the principles behind traction and continuous passive motion.

11. List the various categories of therapeutic medications used to promote healing, and give examples of common drugs in each category.

The ultimate goal of rehabilitation is to return the injured sport participant to activity, pain-free and fully functional. To accomplish this, attention must focus on controlling pain and inflammation, and regaining normal joint range of motion, flexibility, muscular strength, muscular endurance, coordination, and power. Therapeutic modalities and medications are used to create an optimal

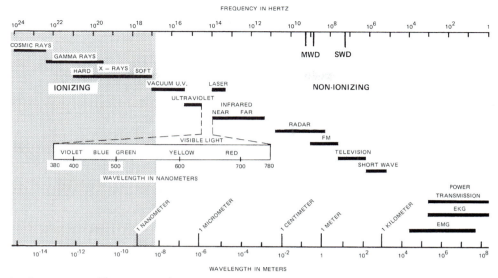

➤ FIGURE 6.1 Electromagnetic spectrum.

environment for injury repair by limiting the inflammatory process and breaking the pain-spasm cycle. Use of any modality depends on the supervising physician's exercise prescription, and on the injury site, type of injury, and severity of injury. An **indication** is a condition that could benefit from a specific modality, whereas a **contraindication** is a condition that could be adversely affected if a particular modality is used. In some cases, a modality may be indicated and contraindicated for the same condition. For example, thermotherapy (heat therapy) may be contraindicated for tendinitis during the initial phase of the exercise program. However, once acute inflammation is controlled, heat therapy may be indicated. Frequent evaluation of the individual's progress can indicate whether the appropriate modality is being used.

In this chapter, the initial material addresses the basic principles associated with the electromagnetic spectrum, and the factors affecting the transfer of energy. The more common therapeutic modalities used in sports injury management will then be discussed. The material presented in this chapter is a general overview of the various modalities. Because of the extensive information and clinical skills needed to adequately comprehend and apply therapeutic modalities in a clinical setting, this chapter should not be used in lieu of a specialized course on therapeutic techniques. It is essential that a separate course in therapeutic modalities be a part of any student's professional preparation to become an entry-level athletic trainer.

ELECTROMAGNETIC SPECTRUM

 After practice, a sprinter is complaining of a sore right lateral hamstring muscle. Following an assessment, you determine that the individual has a biceps femoris strain, and following acute care protocol, you decide to apply ice, compression,

and elevation. How is the energy transmitted between the ice and underlying soft tissues?

There are various forms of energy in the environment that bombard us each day: the light from the sun, radio waves, heat from an oven, or cold from ice cubes. Each form of energy falls under the category of **electromagnetic radiation**, and can be located on an **electromagnetic spectrum** based on its wavelength or frequency **(Figure 6.1)**. Electrical therapeutic modalities are part of the electromagnetic spectrum. The spectrum is divided into two major zones: ionizing range and non-ionizing range. Regardless of the range, electromagnetic energy has several common characteristics **(Box 6.1)**.

Ionizing Range

Energy in the ionizing range can readily alter the components of atoms (electrons, protons, and neutrons). This radiation can easily penetrate tissue to deposit energy within the cells. If the energy level is high enough, the cell losses its ability to regenerate, leading to cell death. Used diagnostically in x-rays (in dosages below that required for cell death) and therapeutically to treat certain cancers (above the threshold), the level is strictly controlled and

---

➤➤ **BOX 6.1**

Characteristics of Electromagnetic Energy
- Electromagnetic energy is composed of pure energy and does not have a mass
- Energy travels at the speed of light (300 million meters per second)
- Energy waveforms travel in a straight line and can travel in a vacuum

monitored to prevent injury to the patient. It is not used by athletic trainers or physical therapists.

Non-ionizing Range

Energy in the non-ionizing range is commonly used in the management of sports injuries. This portion of the spectrum incorporates ultraviolet, visible, and infrared light. Electromagnetic waves are produced when temperature rises and electron activity increases. Ultraviolet light has a shorter wavelength than visible light, and is therefore undetectable by the human eye. This energy source causes superficial chemical changes in the skin and is used to treat certain skin conditions. Sunburns are an example of excessive exposure to ultraviolet rays. Wavelengths greater than visible light are called infrared light, or infrared energy. Infrared wavelengths closest to visible light are called near infrared and can produce thermal effects 5- to 10-mm deep in tissue. Far infrared energy results in more superficial heating of the skin (less than 2-mm deep). Energy forms with much longer wavelengths are collectively known as diathermy, and can increase tissue temperature through a process called conversion. Microwave and short-wave diathermy are examples of this energy source.

Transfer of Energy

Electromagnetic energy can travel through a vacuum with no transfer medium. Energy moves from an area of high concentration to an area of lower concentration by energy carriers, such as mechanical waves, electrons, photons, and molecules. This energy flow in the form of heat involves the exchange of kinetic energy, or energy possessed by an object by virtue of its motion, and is transferred via radiation, conduction, convection, conversion, or evaporation.

RADIATION

Radiation is the transfer of energy in the form of infrared waves (radiant energy) without physical contact. All matter radiates energy in the form of heat. Usually, body heat is warmer than the environment, and radiant heat energy is dissipated through the air to surrounding solid, cooler objects. When the temperature of surrounding objects in the environment exceed skin temperature, radiant heat is absorbed. Shortwave and microwave diathermy are examples of both radiant energy transfer, but can also heat by conversion.

CONDUCTION

Conduction is the direct transfer of energy between two objects in physical contact with each other. A difference in temperature is necessary to initiate the movement of kinetic energy from one molecule to another, and the energy moves from an area of high temperature to an area of lower temperature. Examples of conductive thermal agents are ice bags, ice packs, moist hot packs, and paraffin.

CONVECTION

Convection, a more rapid process than conduction, occurs when a medium, such as air or water, moves across the body, creating temperature variations. The effectiveness of heat loss or heat gain by conduction depends on how fast the air (or water) next to the body is moved away once it becomes warmed. For example, if air movement is slow, air molecules next to the skin are warmed and act as an insulation. In contrast, if warmer air molecules are continually replaced by cooler molecules, such as on a breezy day or in a room with a fan, heat loss increases as the air currents carry heat away. Fluidotherapy and whirlpools are examples of therapeutic modalities that exchange energy by convection.

CONVERSION

Conversion involves the changing of another energy form (e.g., sound, electricity, or a chemical agent) into heat. In ultrasound therapy, mechanical energy produced by high-frequency sound waves is converted to heat energy at tissue interfaces. In microwave diathermy, high electromagnetic energy is converted into heat, which can heat deep tissues. Chemical agents, such as liniments or balms, create heat by acting as a counterirritant to superficial sensory nerve endings, thus reducing the transmission of pain from underlying nerves.

EVAPORATION

Heat loss can also occur during evaporation. Vapocoolant sprays, for example, spread a liquid over the skin surface. The heat absorbed by the liquid cools the skin surface as the liquid changes into a gaseous state. Evaporation is also the means by which the body cools itself on a hot day through the evaporation of sweat.

Factors Affecting Energy Transfer

When electromagnetic energy is transmitted in a vacuum, it travels in a straight line. When traveling through a physical medium, however, the path is influenced by the density of the medium and the energy may be reflected, refracted, or absorbed by the material, or it may continue to pass through the material, unaffected by its density **(Figure 6.2)**. **Reflection** occurs when the wave strikes an object and is bent back away from the material. An echo is an example of a reflected sound. The reflection itself may be complete or partial. **Refraction** is the deflection of waves due to a change in the speed of absorption as the wave passes between mediums of different densities. If energy passes through a high-density layer and enters a low-

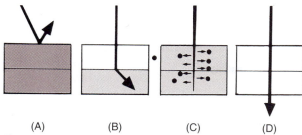

(A)　　　　(B)　　　　(C)　　　　(D)

➤ FIGURE 6.2 **Factors affecting the transmission of energy.** A, Reflection. The energy wave may be partially or fully reflected by the tissue layer. B, Refraction. The energy wave is bent as it strikes an interface between two different tissue layer densities. C, Absorption. Energy can be absorbed by one layer reducing the energy available to deeper tissues. D, Transmission. Any energy that is not reflected or absorbed by a tissue layer will continue to pass through the medium to the next layer where it can again be reflected, refracted, absorbed, or transmitted through the tissue.

density layer, its speed increases. In contrast, if energy passes through a less dense layer to a more dense layer, its speed decreases. **Absorption** occurs when the wave passes through a medium and its kinetic energy is partially or totally assimilated by the tissue. Any energy that is not reflected or absorbed by a tissue layer will pass through the layer until it strikes another density layer. It may again be reflected, refracted, absorbed, or transmitted through the medium. Each time the wave is partially reflected, refracted, or absorbed, the remaining energy available to the deeper tissues is reduced. This inverse relationship is called the **law of Grotthus-Draper**: the more energy absorbed by superficial tissues, the less is available to be transmitted to the underlying tissues.

Energy's Effect on Tissue

To be effective, therapeutic modalities must be capable of producing the desired effects at the intended tissue depth. When energy is applied to the body, the maximal effect occurs when energy rays strike the body at a right angle (90°). As the angle deviates from 90°, some the energy is reflected away from the target site, thereby reducing the level of absorption. The **cosine law** states that, as the angle deviates from 90°, the energy varies with the cosine of the angle:

Effective energy
= Energy × cosine of the angle of incidence

With radiant energy, a difference of ±10° from the right angle is considered to be within acceptable limits (1). Another law that affects energy absorption is the **inverse square law**. This law states that the intensity of radiant energy striking the tissues is directly proportional to the square of the distance between the source of the energy and the tissues: $E = E_S/D^2$.

E_S = amount of energy produced by the source
D^2 = square of the distance between the target and the source
E = resulting energy absorbed by the tissue

This means that each time the distance between the energy and the tissue is doubled, the intensity of the energy received by the tissue is reduced by a factor of four.

 The sprinter had an acute biceps femoris strain. If a crushed-ice bag is used, thermal energy would be transferred from the skin surface to the ice pack via conduction.

CRYOTHERAPY

 If you decided to use an ice pack on the sprinter, how long should you apply the ice? What contraindications may prohibit you from using this modality on the athlete?

Cryotherapy describes multiple types of cold application that use the type of electromagnetic energy classified as infrared radiation. When cold is applied to skin (warmer object), heat is removed or lost. This is referred to as heat abstraction. The most common modes of heat transfer with cold application are conduction and evaporation. Cold application for less than 15 minutes causes immediate skin cooling, cooling of subcutaneous tissue after a slight delay, and a longer delay in cooling muscle tissue (2). Depth of cold penetration can reach 5 cm (1). The magnitude of temperature change will depend on:

1. Type of cooling agent (e.g., ice versus water)
2. Temperature difference between the cold object and the tissue
3. Amount of subcutaneous insulation (fat)
4. Thermal conductivity of the area being cooled
5. Limb circumference
6. Duration of the application (2)

The greater the temperature gradient between the skin and the cooling source, the greater the resulting tissue temperature change. Likewise, the deeper the tissue, the longer the time required to lower the temperature. Adipose (fat) tissue acts as an insulator and resists heat transfer, both heat gain and heat loss. The amount of adipose tissue will influence the degree and rate at which muscle is cooled, and conversely, returns to its precooled temperature.

Cold application leads to vasoconstriction at the cellular level and decreases tissue metabolism (i.e., decreases the need for oxygen), which reduces secondary hypoxia. Capillary permeability and pain are decreased, and the release of inflammatory mediators and prostaglandin synthesis is inhibited. As the temperature of peripheral nerves decreases, a corresponding decrease is seen in nerve conduction velocity across the nerve synapse, thus increasing the threshold required to fire the nerves. The gate theory of pain hypothesizes that cold inhibits pain transmission by stimulating large-diameter neurons in the spinal cord, acting as a counterirritant, which blocks pain perception. With nerve impulses inhibited and muscle spindle activity decreased, muscles in spasm are relaxed, breaking the pain-spasm cycle, leading to an **analgesic**, or pain-free, effect. Recent research has also shown that during ice application, a decline in fast-twitch muscle fiber tension occurs, resulting in a more significant recruitment of slow-twitch muscle fibers and thereby increasing muscle endurance (3).

Because vasoconstriction leads to a decrease in metabolic rate, inflammation, and pain, cryotherapy is the modality of choice during the acute phase of an injury. According to Starkey, the therapeutic application of cold ranges in temperature from 0 to 18.3°C (32 to 65°F) (1). Other researchers, however, have identified that maximal decreases in localized blood flow can occur at temperatures ranging from 12.83° to 15°C (55 to 59°F) (4,5). To accomplish the desired therapeutic range of cooling, many athletic trainers use ice bags (crushed or cubed), commercial ice packs, ice cups (ice massage), cold water baths (immersion or whirlpool), and vapocoolant sprays. Recent technology has also provided new forms of cold application such as the Cryo Cuff or controlled cold therapy (CCT) units.

Cryotherapy is usually applied for 20 to 30 minutes for maximum cooling of both superficial and deep tissues. Barriers used between the ice application and skin can affect heat abstraction. Research has shown that a dry towel or dry elastic wrap should not be used in treatment times of 30 minutes or less. Rather, the cold agent should be applied directly to the skin for optimal therapeutic effects (6,7). Ice application is continued during the first 24 to 72 hours after injury, or until acute bleeding and capillary leakage have stopped, whichever is longer. Another consideration is the length of time it takes to rewarm the injured area. Knight has shown that except for the fingers, the rewarming time to approach normal body temperature is at least 90 minutes (7). This results in a treatment protocol of applying an ice pack for 20 to 30 minutes, followed by 90 minutes of rewarming. Fingers can rewarm more quickly, even following a 20- to 30-minute ice treatment, presumably due to their increased circulation. Fingers need only 20 to 30 minutes to rewarm.

Cold therapy has long been used after arthroscopic knee surgery. Although some researchers have found that the addition of cryotherapy to a regime of exercises following arthroscopic knee surgery did produce some benefits of increased compliance, improved weight-bearing status, and lower prescription medication consumption (8), other researchers have shown that this use of cold therapy is questionable (9,10).

Certain methods of cryotherapy may also be used prior to range of motion exercises and at the conclusion of an exercise bout (see **Box 6.2**). Use of cold treatments prior to exercise is called **cryokinetics**. Cryokinetics alternates several bouts of cold using ice massage, ice packs, ice immersion, or iced towels with active exercise. The injured body part is numbed (generally 10 to 20 minutes of immersion), and the athlete is instructed to perform various progressive exercises. These exercises may begin with simple, non–weight-bearing range of motion activities and prog-

> ▶▶ **Box 6.2**

Cryotherapy Application

Indications	Contraindications
Acute or chronic pain	Decreased cold sensitivity and/or hypersensitivity
Acute or chronic muscle spasm/guarding	
Acute inflammation or injury	Cold allergy
Postsurgical pain and edema	Circulatory or sensory impairment
Superficial first-degree burns	Raynaud's disease or cold urticaria
Used with exercises to:	Hypertension
Facilitate mobilization	Uncovered open wounds
Relieve pain	Cardiac or respiratory disorders
Decrease muscle spasticity	Nerve palsy
	Arthritis

ress to more complex, weight-bearing activities. All exercise bouts must be pain free. As the mild anesthesia from the cold wears off, the body part is renumbed with a 3- to 5-minute cold treatment. The exercise bout is repeated 3 to 4 times each session. The session then ends with exercise if the athlete is able to participate, or with cold if the athlete is not able to participate in practice.

Methods of cryotherapy include ice massage, ice and cryo packs, ice immersion and cold whirlpools, commercial gel and chemical packs, controlled cold compression units, and vapocoolant sprays. With each method, the individual will experience four progressive sensations: cold, burning, aching, and finally **analgesia**.

Ice Massage

Ice massage is an inexpensive and effective method of cold application. Performed over a relatively small area, such as a muscle belly, tendon, bursa, or trigger point (localized area of spasm within a muscle), it produces significant cooling of the skin and a large reactive **hyperemia**, or increase of blood flow into the region, once the treatment has ended. As such, it is not the treatment of choice in acute injuries. Ice massage is particularly useful for its analgesic effect in relieving pain that may inhibit stretching of a muscle, and has been shown to decrease muscle soreness when combined with stretching (2). It is commonly used prior to range of motion exercises and deep friction massage when treating chronic tendinitis and muscle strains.

Treatment consists of water frozen in a cup, then rubbed over an area 10 cm × 15 cm in small, overlapping circular motions for 5 to 10 minutes. A continuous motion is used to prevent tissue damage. If done properly, skin temperature should not decrease below 15°C (59°F) (2). A wooden tongue depressor frozen in the cup provides a handle for easy application. With ice massage, the stages of cold, burning, and aching pass rapidly within about 1

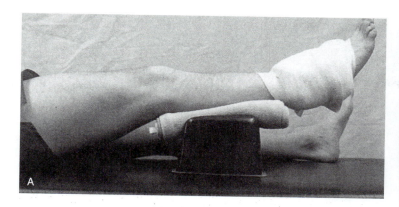

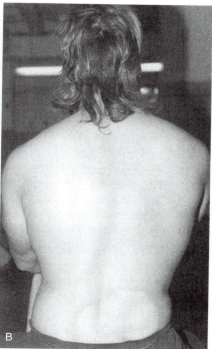

➤ FIGURE 6.3 **Ice treatments**. A, Ice, compression, and elevation can reduce acute inflammation. B, A slightly raised wheal formation may appear shortly after cold application in individuals who are sensitive to cold or have cold allergies.

to 2 minutes. A prolonged aching or burning sensation may result if the area covered is too large, or if a hypersensitive response occurs.

Ice Packs and Contoured Cryo Cuffs

Ice packs are inexpensive and maintain a constant temperature, making them very effective in cooling tissue. When filled with flaked ice or small cubes, the ice packs can be safely applied to the skin for 30 to 40 minutes without danger of frostbite. Furthermore, ice packs can be molded to the body's contours, held in place by a cold compression wrap, and elevated above the heart to minimize swelling and pooling of fluids in the interstitial tissue spaces (**Figure 6.3A**). During the initial treatments, the skin should be checked frequently for **wheal** or blister formation (**Figure 6.3B**).

Contoured Cryo Cuffs use ice water placed in an insulated thermos. When the thermos is raised above the body part, water flows into the Cryo Pack, maintaining cold compression for 5 to 7 hours (**Figure 6.4**). Although more expensive than ice packs, these devices combine ice and compression over a longer period without threat of frostbite.

Ice Immersion

Ice immersion is used to reduce temperature quickly over the entire surface of a distal extremity (forearm, hand, ankle, or foot). A variety of containers or basins may be used. Because of the analgesic effect and buoyancy of water, ice immersion and cold whirlpools are often used during the inflammatory phase to reduce edema formation after

blunt injury (see **Field Strategy 6.1**). Cold whirlpool baths also provide a hydromassaging effect. This is controlled by the amount of air emitted through the electrical turbine. The turbine can be moved up and down, or directed at a specific angle and locked in place. The whirlpool turbine should not be operated unless water totally covers the impeller. In addition to controlling acute inflammation, cold

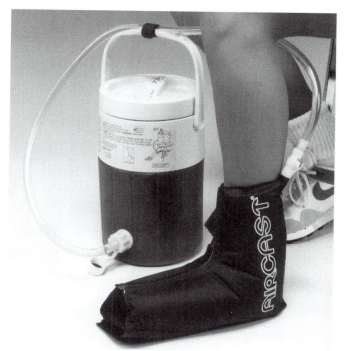

➤ FIGURE 6.4 **Contoured Cryo Cuffs**. When the thermos is raised above the body part, water flows into the Cryo pack, maintaining cold compression for 5 to 7 hours.

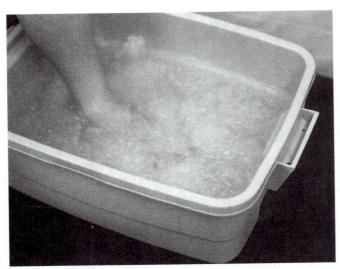

➤ FIGURE 6.5 **Ice immersion**. This technique quickly reduces temperature over the entire surface area of a distal extremity. Toe caps may be used to prevent frostbite of the toes during the treatment.

whirlpools can be used to decrease soft tissue trauma and increase active range of motion after prolonged immobilization.

If the goal is to reduce edema, placing the body part in a stationary position below the level of the heart keeps fluid in the body segment and is contraindicated. This can be avoided by placing a compression wrap over the body part prior to submersion and doing active muscle contractions. Neoprene toe caps may be used to reduce discomfort on the toes.

A bucket or cold whirlpool is filled with water and ice, and maintained at a temperature between 13 and 18°C (55 and 65°F) (**Figure 6.5**). The lower the temperature, the shorter the duration of immersion. Treatment lasts from 5 to 15 minutes. When pain is relieved, the part is removed from the water and functional movement patterns

are performed. As pain returns, the area is reimmersed. The cycle continues three to four times.

Contrast Bath

A contrast bath alternates cold and hot tubs or whirlpools. This elicits a local vasoconstriction-vasodilation fluctuation to reduce edema and restore range of motion in subacute or chronic injuries. Two whirlpools or containers are placed next to each other. One is filled with cold water and ice at 10 to 18°C (50 to 65°F), and the other is filled with hot water at 38 to 44°C (100 to 111°F) (11). The injured extremity is alternated between the two tubs. Some athletic trainers use a 3:1 or 4:1 ratio (hot water to cold water) for approximately 20 minutes. In subacute conditions, the treatment begins and ends in cold water prior to starting therapeutic exercise. In chronic conditions, treatment is more often concluded in warm immersion. A second method is to use a variable time frame: during the first cycle, 75% of the time is in cold water and 25% of the time is in hot water. The second cycle moves to 50% in cold water and 50% in hot water, with the third cycle moving to 25% in cold and 75% in hot water. Research, however, has failed to demonstrate any significant physiologic effect on intramuscular tissue temperature 1 cm below the skin and subcutaneous fat (12,13). Therefore, contrast therapy may need to be reconsidered as a viable therapeutic modality.

Commercial Gel and Chemical Packs

Commercial gel packs are composed of a flexible gelatinous substance enclosed in a strong vinyl or plastic case, and come in a variety of sizes to conform to the body's natural contours (**Figure 6.6A**). Used with compression and elevation, they are an effective cold application. The packs are stored at a temperature of about −5°C (−23°F) for at least 2 hours prior to application (2). Because the packs are

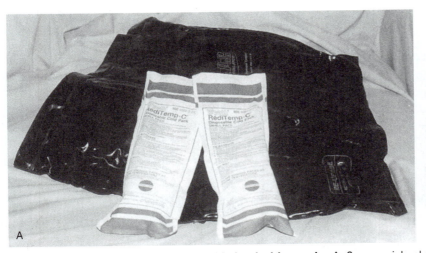
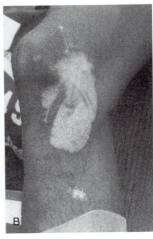

➤ FIGURE 6.6 **Commercial and chemical ice packs**. A, Commercial gel packs come in a variety of sizes to conform to the body's natural contours. Chemical ice packs are convenient to carry in a training kit, disposable after a single use, and can also conform to the body part. B, Chemical ice packs, however, can leak and burn the skin.

stored at sub-zero temperatures, they may cause frostbite if used improperly. A wet towel or cloth should be placed between the pack and skin to prevent frostbite and maintain a hygienic surface for the reusable packs. Treatment time is 15 to 20 minutes.

Chemical packs can be advantageous because they are convenient to carry in a training kit, disposable after a single use, and conform to the body part. A disadvantage of the packs is their expense. The packs are activated by squeezing or hitting the pack against a hard area. The chemical substance has an alkaline pH and can cause skin burns if the package breaks and the contents spill (**Figure 6.6B**). As such, the packs should never be squeezed or used in front of the face, and if possible, should be placed inside another plastic bag. Treatment ranges from 15 to 20 minutes. In longer treatments, the pack warms and becomes ineffective. Some commercial packs can be refrozen and reused.

Controlled Cold-Compression Units

Controlled cold-compression units like the Cryotemp use compression and elevation to decrease blood flow to an extremity and assist venous return, thus decreasing edema. A boot or sleeve is applied around the injured extremity. Cooled water is circulated through the sleeve. Compression is formed when the sleeve is inflated intermittently. This is done for 20 to 30 minutes, several times a day, to pump edema fluid from the extremity (**Figure 6.7**). During deflation, the patient can do active range of motion exercises to enhance blood flow to the injured area. The unit can be used several times a day, but should never be used with a suspected compartment syndrome or fracture, or in an individual with a peripheral vascular disease or impaired circulation.

Vapocoolant Sprays

Fluori-methane is a nonflammable, nontoxic spray that uses rapid evaporation of chemicals on the skin area to cool the skin prior to stretching a muscle (**Figure 6.8**). The effects are temporary and superficial. When using a vapocoolant spray to increase range of motion in an area

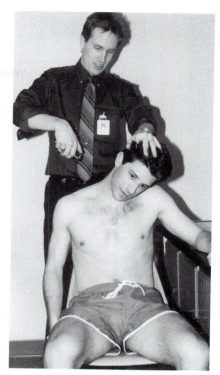

➤ **FIGURE 6.8 Vapocoolant sprays.** These sprays temporarily freeze superficial tissues and can reduce the pain-spasm cycle prior to stretching exercises.

where no trigger point is present, the patient is comfortably positioned with the muscle passively stretched. The bottle of vapocoolant spray is then inverted and held at a 30 to 45° angle and sprayed from approximately 12 to 18 inches away from the skin. The entire length of the muscle is sprayed two to three times in a unidirectional, parallel sweeping pattern as a gradual stretch is applied by the athletic trainer.

When using this spray to treat trigger points and myofascial pain, the athletic trainer must first determine the presence of an active trigger point. The muscle is put under moderate tension. The athletic trainer then applies firm pressure over the painful site for 5 to 10 seconds. Another technique involves eliciting a jump response, again, by placing the muscle under moderate tension. Firm pressure is applied over the tense muscle, and a finger is pulled across the tight band of muscle. If the athlete winces or cries out, an active trigger point is present. The athlete is then placed in a relaxed, but well-supported position with the involved muscle placed on stretch. The vapocoolant spray is sprayed from about 12 inches above the skin at an acute angle to the painful site. The entire length of the muscle is sprayed, including the painful site, while the athletic trainer begins a mild passive stretch of the involved muscle, within the patient's tolerance. After several parallel sweeps of the muscle and continued passive stretching, the muscle should be warmed with a hot pack or with vigorous massage. The athlete should be encouraged to actively but gently move the body part throughout the full range of motion. The process may need to be repeated; however,

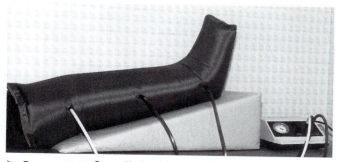

➤ **FIGURE 6.7 Controlled cold compression unit.** An air- or water-filled boot or sleeve can provide pressure or intermittent compression to an injured area to decrease edema.

it is critical not to overload the muscle with strenuous exercise immediately after the session.

 In applying an ice pack to the posterior thigh of the sprinter, treatment time should range between 20 to 30 minutes. A maximum of 90 minutes should be allowed to rewarm the tissues, followed by another cold treatment. If the individual experiences any skin blanching, numbness, burning, or tingling sensations, the cold treatment should be stopped.

THERMOTHERAPY

 The sprinter demonstrates a marked improvement in swelling, tenderness, and range of motion over the next 5 days, although strength has not totally returned to normal. Is it safe at this time to move to a heat modality, or is there a risk that swelling and edema may return to the region?

Thermotherapy, or heat application, is typically used in the second phase of rehabilitation to increase blood flow and promote healing in the injured area (see **Box 6.3**). If used during the acute inflammatory stage, heat application may overwhelm the injured blood and lymphatic vessels, leading to increased hemorrhage and edema. When applied at the appropriate time, however, heat can increase circulation and cellular metabolism; produce an analgesic, or sedative effect; and assist in the resolution of pain and muscle-guarding spasms. Vasodilation and increased circulation result in an influx of oxygen and nutrients into the area to promote healing of damaged tissues. Debris and waste products are removed from the injury site. Used prior to stretching exercises, joint mobilization, or active exercise, thermotherapy can increase extensibility of connective tissue, leading to increased range of motion. In the same manner as cold application, heat flow through tissue also varies with the type of tissue, and is called thermal conductivity. Changes in surface tissue temperature caused by superficial heating agents depend on:

• Intensity of heat applied
• Time of heat exposure
• Thermal medium for surface heat

The greatest degree of elevated temperature occurs in the skin and subcutaneous tissues within 0.5 cm of the skin surface. In areas with adequate circulation, temperature will increase to its maximum within 6 to 8 minutes of exposure. Muscle temperature at depths of 1 to 2 cm will increase to a lesser degree and require a longer duration of exposure (15 to 30 minutes) to reach peak values (14). After peak temperatures are reached, a plateauing effect or slight decrease in skin temperature is seen over the rest of the heat application. As mentioned earlier, fat is an insulator and has a low thermal conductivity value. Therefore, tissues under a large amount of fat will be minimally affected by superficial heating agents. To elevate deep tissues to the desired thermal levels without burning the skin and subcutaneous tissue, a deep-heating agent such as continuous ultrasound or shortwave diathermy should be selected.

With superficial heating agents, heat is transferred by conduction, convection, and radiation. Common examples of superficial thermotherapy are whirlpools, hot tubs and jacuzzis, moist hot packs, and paraffin baths. Penetrating thermotherapy, including ultrasound, phonophoresis, and diathermy heat, will be discussed in more detail later in the chapter.

Whirlpool and Immersion Baths

Whirlpool and immersion baths combine warm or hot water with a hydromassaging effect to increase superficial skin temperature (**Figure 6.9**). Tanks may be portable or

---

➤ ➤ **BOX 6.3**

Thermotherapy Application

Indications	**Contraindications**
Subacute or chronic injuries, to:	Acute inflammation or injuries
Reduce swelling, edema, and ecchymosis	Impaired or poor circulation
Reduce muscle spasm/guarding	Subacute or chronic pain
Increase blood flow, to:	Impaired or poor sensation
Increase ROM prior to activity	Impaired thermal regulation
Resolve hematoma	Malignancy
Facilitate tissue healing	
Relieve joint contractures	
Fight infection	

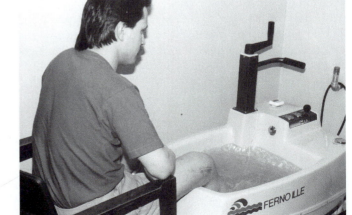

➤ **FIGURE 6.9 Whirlpools.** Hot whirlpools increase superficial skin temperatures, leading to an analgesic effect that can reduce muscle spasm and pain, facilitate range of motion exercises, and promote healing.

fixed, and include the more common extremity tanks and the full-body therapeutic tubs, such as the Hubbard tank or walk tank.

Physiologically, warm or hot whirlpools are analgesic agents that relax muscle spasms, relieve joint pain and stiffness, provide mechanical debridement, and facilitate range of motion exercises after prolonged immobilization. As with cold whirlpools and immersion baths, buoyancy facilitates increased range of motion, and the hydromassaging effect is controlled by the amount of air emitted through the electrical turbine. The more agitation, the greater the water movement. The turbine can be moved up and down, or directed at a specific angle and locked in place. Treatment time ranges from 20 to 30 minutes. Total body immersion exceeding 20 to 30 minutes can dehydrate the athlete, leading to dizziness and high body core temperature. Only the body parts being treated should be immersed. **Field Strategy 6.1** explains how to use this modality.

For safety reasons, ground-fault circuit interrupters (GFCI) should be installed in all receptacles or in the circuit, breaker box in the hydrotherapy area, and should be no more than 1.5 m away from the tanks. A sensor located within the GFCI monitors current in the hot and neutral lines that feed the receptacle. Because the maximum safe transthoracic current (through intact skin) is deemed to be 5 mA, the GFCI will activate at this level and immediately trip the circuit to disconnect all current to the receptacle. These receptacles should be inspected annually to ensure that they are operating properly.

Hot Tubs and Jacuzzis

Although not a common modality in the athletic training room, many athletes have access to hot tubs and jacuzzis. Because organic contaminates, high water temperature, and turbulence reduce the effectiveness of chlorine as a bacterial agent, infection with *Pseudomonas aeruginosa*, causing folliculitis is an alarming and increasing problem. To prevent infection, these tubs must have a good filtration and chlorination system. Chlorine and pH levels should be monitored hourly during periods of heavy use, and calcium hardness should be evaluated weekly (11). The water should be drained, superchlorinated, and refilled once every 3 months. The water temperature should not exceed 38.9°C (102°F).

Moist Hot Packs

Moist hot packs provide superficial heat, transferring energy to the athlete's skin by way of conduction. Each subsequent underlying tissue layer is heated through conduction from the overlying tissue, reaching a slightly deeper tissue level than a whirlpool. Like other forms of superficial heating, deeper tissues, including the musculature, are usually not significantly heated. The heat transfer is inhibited by subcutaneous fat, which acts as a thermal insulator, and by the increased blood flow through the area that carries away externally applied heat. Moist hot packs are used most often to reduce pain and superficial muscle spasm, and to improve tissue extensibility.

FIELD STRATEGY 6.1   TECHNIQUES FOR USING A WHIRLPOOL BATH

1. Inspect the electrical system. To avoid electrical surges, make sure that ground-fault circuit breakers are used in the electrical outlet or in the circuit-breaker box.
2. Apply a povidone-iodine (Betadine) additive, or chloramine-T (Chlorazene) in concentrations of 100 to 200 parts per million (ppm) to the water as an antibacterial agent, especially if the athlete has an open wound.
3. Recommended temperature and treatment time include:

Cold whirlpools	55–65° F	5–15 min
Hot whirlpools		
Extremity	98–110° F	20–30 min
Full body	98–102° F	10–12 min

4. Assist the patient into the water and provide towels for padding and drying off.
5. Turn the turbine on and adjust the height to direct the water flow 6 to 8 inches away from the injury site.
6. Instruct the patient to move the body part through the available range of motion. This will increase blood flow to the area, aid in removal of debris, and improve balance and proprioception.
7. Turn the turbine off and remove the patient from the water. Dry the treated area and assist the individual from the whirlpool area.
8. Drain and cleanse the whirlpool tub after each use. Disinfect the hard-to-reach places with glutaraldehyde, formalin alcohol, ethylene oxide, or beta propiolactone to kill sport-forming bacteria. A solution of sodium hypochlorite (chlorine bleach), in concentrations ranging from 500 ppm (1:100 dilution) to 5000 ppm (1:10 dilution) is effective in cleaning surface organic material (blood, mucus).
9. Cultures for bacterial and fungal agents should be conducted monthly from water samples in the whirlpool turbine and drain.

➤ FIGURE 6.10 **Moist hot packs.** Moist heat treatments can burn sensitive skin. To avoid this, place the pack in a commercial padded towel, or six to eight layers of towel, and periodically check the skin surface for redness or signs of burning.

The pack consists of a canvas or nylon case filled with a hydrophilic silicate or other hydrophilic substance, or with sand. The packs are stored in a hot water unit at a temperature ranging from 70 to 75°C (158 to 170°F) (**Figure 6.10**) (14). When removed from the water, the pack is wrapped in a commercial padded cover, or in six to eight layers of toweling, and placed directly over the injury site for 20 minutes. Commercial hot-pack covers may need another layer or two of toweling to ensure adequate insulation for the hot pack.

The pack should be secured and completely cover the area being treated. As with other forms of heat application, the patient should only feel a mild to moderate sensation of heat. The patient should never lie on top of the pack, as this may accelerate the rate of heat transfer leading to burns on sensitive skin. After 5 minutes of treatment, the area should be checked for any redness or signs of burning.

The hot packs should also be checked regularly for leaks, and should be discarded if any leaking occurs. This may become evident when cleaning the unit on a monthly basis. Hydrophilic silicate may accumulate on the bottom of the unit, and should be removed so as not to interfere with the heating element.

Paraffin Baths

Paraffin baths provide heat to contoured bony areas of the body (e.g., feet, hands, or wrists). They are used to treat subacute or chronic rheumatoid arthritis associated with joint stiffness and decreased range of motion, as well as other common chronic injuries. A paraffin and mineral oil mixture (6:1 or 7:1 ratio) is heated in a unit at 48 to 52°C (118 to 126°F).

There are two principal methods of application: 1) dip and wrap, and 2) dip and reimmerse. For both methods, the body part is thoroughly cleansed and dried, and all

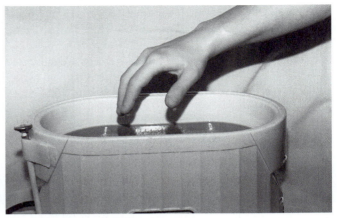

➤ FIGURE 6.11 **Paraffin bath.** The limb is thoroughly cleansed and dipped several times into the paraffin solution. The body part is then wrapped in plastic and a towel to maintain heat, or it can be reimmersed into the solution and held motionless for the duration of the treatment.

jewelry is removed. The body part is placed in a relaxed position, then dipped into the bath several times, each time allowing the previous coat to dry (**Figure 6.11**). The patient should not move the fingers or toes, so as not to break the seal of the glove being formed. In addition, outer layers of paraffin should not extend over new skin, as burning may occur. When completed, the body part is wrapped in a plastic bag and towel to maintain heat, then elevated for 15 to 20 minutes or until heat is no longer generated.

With the dip and reimmerse method, after the wax glove is formed, the body part covered by the glove is put back into the wax container for 15 to 20 minutes without moving it. This method will result in a more vigorous response relative to temperature elevation and blood flow changes. However, this technique should not be used in individuals predisposed to edema, or those who cannot sit in the position required for treatment.

When the treatment is completed, the wax is peeled off and returned to the bath where it can be reused. The mineral oil in the wax helps keep skin soft and pliable during massage when treating a variety of hand and foot conditions. In comparison with other heat modalities, paraffin wax is not significantly better at decreasing pain or increasing joint range of motion. It should not be used in patients with decreased sensation, open wounds, thin scars, skin rashes, or peripheral vascular disease.

Fluidotherapy

Fluidotherapy is a dry heat modality used to treat acute injuries and wounds, decrease pain and swelling, and increase range of motion and inadequate blood flow. The unit contains fine cellulose particles that become suspended when a stream of dry hot air is forced between them, making the fluidized bed behave with properties similar to that of liquids. Both temperature and the amount of particle agitation can be varied. Treatment temperature ranges from 38.8 to 47.8°C (102 to 118°F). An advantage of this superficial heating modality is that exercise can be performed during the treatment, and higher treatment temperatures can be tolerated. If a body part has an open wound, a plastic barrier or bag can be placed over the wound to prevent any fine cellulose particles from becoming embedded in the wound and to minimize the risk of cross-contamination. Treatment duration ranges from 15 to 20 minutes.

 The sprinter showed marked improvement after 5 days of ice treatments. As long as the athlete does not complain of tenderness to touch, it is probably safe to move to a heat treatment. Heat can increase the local circulation, promote healing, and can be used in conjunction with stretching and mild exercise to strengthen the injured muscle.

ULTRASOUND

 After 2 weeks, the sprinter is no longer point tender on palpation, but there is still a small, palpable swollen area in the region of the short head of the biceps femoris. What type of heat treatment would be most effective at this point of the injury process?

In the previous section, superficial heating agents were discussed. These agents produce temperature elevations in skin and underlying subcutaneous tissues to a depth of 1 to 2 cm. Ultrasound uses high-frequency acoustic (sound) waves, rather than electromagnetic energy, to elicit thermal and nonthermal effects in deep tissue to depths of 3 cm or more. This transfer of energy takes place in the deep structures without causing excessive heating of the overlying superficial structures. The actual mechanism of ultrasound, produced via the **reverse piezoelectric effect**, converts electrical current to mechanical energy as is passes through a piezoelectric crystal (e.g., quartz, barium titanate, lead zirconate or titanate) housed in the transducer head. The vibration of the crystal results in organic molecules moving in longitudinal waves that move the energy into the deep tissues to produce temperature increases (thermal effects), and mechanical and chemical alterations (nonthermal effects). Thermal effects increase collagen tissue extensibility, blood flow, sensory and motor neuron velocity, and enzymatic activity, and decrease muscle spasm, joint stiffness, inflammation, and pain. Nonthermal effects decrease edema by increasing cell membrane and vascular wall permeability, blood flow, protein synthesis, tissue regeneration, thus promoting the healing process.

The Ultrasound Wave

Unlike electromagnetic energy, sound cannot travel in a vacuum. Sound waves, such as those produced by a human voice, diverge in all directions. This principles allows you to hear someone talking behind you. As the frequency

increases, the level of divergence decreases. Like sound waves, the frequencies used in therapeutic ultrasound produce collimated cylindrical beams, similar to a light beam leaving a flashlight, that have a width slightly smaller than the diameter of the transducer head. The **effective radiating area** (ERA) is the portion of the transducer's surface area that actually produces the ultrasound wave.

Frequency and Attenuation

The frequency of ultrasound is measured in megahertz (MHz) and represents the number of waves (in millions) occurring in 1 second. Frequencies range between 0.75 MHz and 3.3 MHz. For a given sound source, the higher the frequency, the less the emerging sound beam diverges. For example, low-frequency ultrasound produces a more widely diverging beam than high-frequency ultrasound, which produces a collimated beam. The more commonly used 1.0-MHz generator is transmitted through superficial tissues and absorbed primarily in deeper tissues at depths of 3 to 5 cm or greater.

Energy contained within a sound beam decreases as it travels through tissue. The level of absorption depends on the type of tissues to which it is applied. Tissues with a high protein content (e.g., nerve and muscle tissue) absorb ultrasound readily. Deflection (reflection or refraction) is greater at heterogeneous (different or unrelated) tissue interfaces, especially at the bone-muscle interface. This deflection creates standing waves that increase heat. Ultrasound that is not absorbed or deflected is transmitted through the tissue.

Absorption of sound, and therefore attenuation, increases as the frequency increases. The higher the frequency, the more rapidly the molecules are forced to move against this friction. As the absorption increases, there is less sound energy available to move through the tissue. The 1-MHz machine is most often used on individuals with a high subcutaneous body fat percentage, and whenever the desired effects are in the deeper structures. This ultrasound unit has also been used to stimulate collagen synthesis in tendon fibroblasts after an injury, and to stimulate cell division during periods of rapid cell proliferation (15). It has also been used on tendons on the 2nd and 4th days after surgery to increase tensile strength. However, after the 5th day, application decreases tensile strength (16).

The high-frequency 3.0-MHz machine provides treatment to superficial tissues and tendons. The low penetration depth is associated with limited transmission of energy, a rapid absorption of energy, and a higher heating rate in a relatively limited tissue depth.

Types of Waves

Sound waves can be produced as a continuous wave or a pulsed wave. A continuous wave is one in which the sound intensity remains constant, whereas a pulsed wave is intermittently interrupted. Pulsed waves are further delineated by the fraction of time the sound is present over one pulse period, or duty cycle. This is calculated with the following equation:

$$\text{Duty cycle} = \frac{\text{duration of pulse (time on)} \times 100}{\text{pulse period (time on + time off)}}$$

Typical duty cycles in the pulse mode range from 0.05 (5%) to 0.5 (50%), with the most commonly used duty cycle being that of 0.02 (20%) (17). Continuous ultrasound waves provide both thermal and nonthermal effects, and are used when a deep, elevated tissue temperature is advisable. Pulsed ultrasound and low-intensity, continuous ultrasound produce primarily nonthermal effects and are used to facilitate repair and soft tissue healing when a high increase in tissue temperature is not desired.

Intensity

Therapeutic intensities are expressed in watts per square centimeter (W/cm^2), and range from 0.25 to 2.0 W/cm^2. The greater the intensity, the greater the resulting temperature elevation. Thermal temperature can increase 7 to 8° F up to a depth of 5 cm (1). As mentioned earlier, ultrasound waves are absorbed in tissues highest in collagen content, and they are reflected at tissue interfaces, particularly between bone and muscle.

Clinical Uses of Ultrasound

Ultrasound is used to manage several soft tissue conditions, such as tendinitis, bursitis, and muscle spasm; to reabsorb calcium deposits in soft tissue; and to reduce joint contractures, pain, and scar tissue (see **Box 6.4**). Wound healing is enhanced with low-intensity, pulsed ultrasound. It is recommended that ultrasound treatment begin 2 weeks after injury during the proliferative phase of healing. Earlier treatment may increase inflammation and delay healing time. Tissue healing is thought to occur predominantly through nonthermal effects. An intensity of 0.5 to 1.0 W/cm^2 pulsed at 20% is recommended for superficial wounds. For skin lesions and ulcers, a frequency of 3 MHz or higher is recommended (17).

> ➤➤ **Box 6.4**

Ultrasound Application

Indications
Increase deep tissue heating
Decrease inflammation and resolve hematomas
Decrease muscle spasm/ spasticity
Decrease pain
Increase extensibility of collagen tissue
Decrease pain of neuromas
Decrease joint adhesions and/or joint contractures
Treat postacute myositis ossificans

Contraindications
Acute and postacute hemorrhage
Infection
Thrombophlebitis
Over suspected malignancy/cancer
Areas of impaired circulation or sensation
Over stress fracture sites
Over epiphyseal growth plates
Over the eyes, heart, spine, or genitals

Application

Because ultrasound waves cannot travel through air, a coupling agent is used between the transducer head and skin to facilitate passage of the waves. Coupling gels are applied liberally over the area to be treated. The transducer head is then stroked slowly over the area (**Figure 6.12**). Strokes are applied in small continuous circles or longitudinal patterns to distribute the energy as evenly as possible at a rate of 4 cm/s to prevent **cavitation** (gas bubble formation) in deep tissues (17). The total area covered is usually 2 to 3 times the size of the transducer head for every 5 minutes of exposure. If a larger area is covered, the effective dosage and elevated temperature changes delivered to any one region decrease. A firm, uniform amount of pressure exerted on the transducer head maximizes the transmission of acoustic energy between the sound head and tissue interface.

A common alternate method for irregularly shaped areas (e.g., wrist, hand, ankle, or foot) is application under

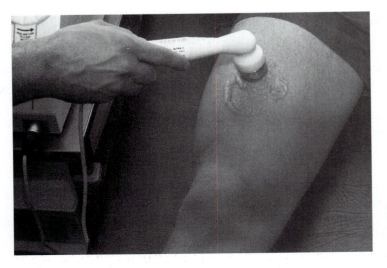

> ➤ **FIGURE 6.12 Ultrasound.** A coupling agent is used between the transducer head and area being treated. The head is then moved in small circles or longitudinal strokes to distribute the energy as evenly as possible to prevent damage to the underlying tissues.

water. If the treatment is given in a metal basin or whirl-pool, some of the ultrasound energy will be reflected off the metal, thus increasing intensity in certain areas near the metal. In addition, water in a whirlpool often has a large number of air bubbles, which tend to reduce the transmission of ultrasound. This problem is even more pronounced if the turbine was used prior to the ultrasound treatment. For these reasons, metal containers and whirl-pools should not be used for underwater treatments. Water treatments are indirect and generally have a 0.5 to 3 cm space between the patient and the sound head. Intensity is increased .5 W/cm² to compensate for air and minerals in the water (1). Small air bubbles tend to accumulate on the face of the transducer head and the skin surface when this method is used. The athletic trainer should quickly wipe off the accumulated bubbles during the treatment. No jewelry should be worn under the water surface. In addition, the athletic trainer should hold the transducer head so his or her hand is out of the water.

Research has shown that ultrasound treatments using gel in direct contact with the patient produced more heat than did ultrasound administered indirectly underwater (18,19). A more recent method of application over bony protuberances or irregular surfaces is use of a reusable gel pad. These pads, when used with ultrasound gel, have been found to be more effective than using the traditional water bath immersion method (20). Intensity for both gel and underwater treatment is determined by the stage of injury, mode used (pulsed or continuous), desired depth of penetration, and patient tolerance. The patient may feel a mild, warm sensation.

When the treatment goal is to elevate tissue temperature over a large quantity of soft tissue (hip or back), a continuous-wave mode with intensities as high as 1.5 to 2.0 W/cm² is typically used. A lower intensity (0.5 to 1.0 W/cm²) and a higher frequency are used over areas where there is less soft tissue coverage and where bone is closer to the skin surface. At tissue-bone interfaces, about 35% of the ultrasound beam is reflected, resulting in increased intensity in the soft tissue overlying the bone, particularly the periosteum (18). Elevated temperatures should be maintained at least 5 minutes after the patient reports the sensation of gentle heat, to allow for an increase in extensibility. If heat production in tissues greater than 3 cm deep is the desired effect, 8 minutes of treatment after the patient reports the sensation of heat is the minimum (21).

Phonophoresis

Phonophoresis is a technique whereby the mechanical effects of ultrasound are used to enhance percutaneous absorption of anti-inflammatory drugs (cortisol, dexameth-asone, **salicylates**) and local analgesics (lidocaine), through the skin to the underlying tissues. One advantage of this modality is that the drug is delivered directly to the site where the effect is sought. High intensities of ultrasound have been used to deliver these medications to depths of 5

to 6 cm subcutaneously into skeletal muscle and peripheral nerves (18).

This technique is used in the postacute stage in conditions to treat painful trigger points, bursitis, contusions, or other chronic soft tissue conditions. The standard coupling gel is replaced by a gel or cream containing the medication. Commercial chem-pads impregnated with the medication are also readily available, and may be used in lieu of the traditional medicated ointment applicators. Continuous ultrasound is used because tissue permeability is increased by the thermal effects, so the medication is more easily absorbed. Treatment occurs at a lower intensity (1 to 1.5 W/cm²) for 5 to 15 minutes.

 Ultrasound would be an excellent choice in treating the biceps femoris strain. This modality can provide both thermal and nonthermal effects to increase circulation, blood flow, and tissue extensibility, and to reduce hematoma formation and enhance the healing process.

DIATHERMY

 Diathermy is another form of heat treatment that could be used to treat the sprinter's biceps femoris strain. What type of tissues more readily absorb the heat produced by this modality? Are there any tissues that can limit the absorption rate?

Diathermy, which literally means to heat through, uses electromagnetic energy from the nonionizing radio frequency (RF) part of the spectrum. Because the duration of the impulses is so short, no ion movement occurs; thus there is no stimulation of motor or sensory nerves. Rapid vibration of the continuous shortwave diathermy (CSWD) waves is absorbed by the body and converted into heat by the resisting tissues. This elicits deep, penetrating thermal effects. When these waves are interrupted at regular intervals, pulses or bursts of RF energy are delivered to the tissues, and are referred to as pulsed radio-frequency radiation (PRFR). PRFR may produce either thermal or nonthermal effects on tissues; low power produces nonthermal effects, and high power produces thermal effects.

Therapeutic devices that deliver CSWD and PRFR use high-frequency alternating currents to oscillate at specified radio frequencies between 10 and 50 MHz. The most commonly used RF is 27.12 MHz. Microwave diathermy, another form of electromagnetic radiation, can be directed toward the body and reflected from the skin, and uses ultra-high frequencies (UHF) at 2450 MHz. Microwave diathermy is seldom used today, and will not be discussed in this section.

Continuous Shortwave Diathermy

The goal of CSWD is to raise tissue temperature to within the physiologically effective range of 37.5 to 44°C (99.5 to

111.2°F) in deeper tissues (2.5 to 5 cm). This is done by introducing a high-frequency electrical current with a power output of 80 to 120 W. The depth of penetration and extent of heat production depends on wave frequency, the electrical properties of the tissue(s) receiving the electromagnetic energy, and the type of applicator used.

The physiological effects known to occur with other therapeutic heat treatments are also produced with CSWD. Mild heating is usually desired in acute musculoskeletal conditions, whereas vigorous heating may be needed in chronic conditions. Because the effects occur in deeper tissue, CSWD is used to increase extensibility of deep collagen tissue, decrease joint stiffness, relieve deep pain and muscle spasm, increase blood flow, assist in the resolution of inflammation, and facilitate healing of soft tissue injuries in the postacute stage (see **Box 6.5**).

There are two methods for heating. One places two condensor plates on either side of the injured area, thus placing the patient in the electrical circuit. The other method uses an induction coil wrapped around the body part that places the patient in an electromagnetic field. Heating is uneven because different tissues resist energy at different levels, an application of **Joule's law**, which states that the greater the resistance or impedance, the more heat will be developed. Tissues with a high fluid content, such as skeletal muscle and areas surrounding joints, absorb more of the energy and are heated to a greater extent, whereas fat is not heated as much. Because the applicators are not in contact with the skin, CSWD can be used for heating skeletal muscle when the skin is abraded, as long as edema is not present.

Pulsed Shortwave Diathermy

Pulsed shortwave diathermy (PSWD), a relatively new type of diathermy, uses a timing circuit to electrically interrupt the 27.12 MHz waves and produce bursts or pulse trains containing a series of high-frequency, sine wave oscillations. Each pulse train has a preset "time on" and is separated from successive pulse trains by a "time off" that is determined by the pulse repetition rate, or frequency. The pulse frequency can be varied from 1 to 700 pulses per second by turning the pulse-frequency control on the equipment operation panel.

The production of heat in tissues depends on the manipulation of peak pulse power, pulse frequency, and pulse duration. The measure of heat production is the mean power, which is lower than the power delivered (80 to 120 W) during most CSWD treatments. Nonthermal effects may be produced at mean power values less than 38 W; thermal effects are produced when mean power values exceed 38 W. Mean powers between 38 and 80 W would be appropriate to treat acute and subacute inflammatory conditions, and have been shown to assist in the absorption of hematomas, reduce ankle swelling, and stimulate collagen formation. PSWD is applied to the patient in the same manner as CSWD. Most PSWD devices have the drum type of inductive applicator. Therefore, one could expect less heating of superficial fat and more heating of tissues like superficial muscle, which has a high electrolyte level. Indications and contradictions are the same for PSWD as for CSWD.

 Although shortwave diathermy can provide deep heating to tissues with a higher water content, such as muscle, the extent of muscle heating can be inhibited by the thickness of the subcutaneous fat layer. Therefore, when dealing with a biceps femoris muscle strain, other modalities may be more effective in providing a deep heat treatment.

ELECTROTHERAPY

 If the athletic trainer wanted to elicit a muscle contraction in the strained biceps femoris muscle to decrease muscle guarding and atrophy in conjunction with a heat treatment, what type of electrotherapy might be used?

Electrical therapy is a popular therapeutic modality that can be applied to injured or immobilized muscles in the early stages of exercise when the muscle is at its weakest. The various forms of electrotherapy are used to decrease pain; increase blood flow, range of motion, and muscle strength; re-educate muscle; facilitate absorption of anti-inflammatory, analgesic, or anesthetic drugs to the injured area; and promote wound healing. To understand how electrical stimulation is used clinically, the basic principles of electricity must be addressed.

➤➤ Box 6.5

Diathermy Applications

Indications	Contraindications
Bursitis	Over internally and externally worn metallic objects
Joint capsule contractures	Over metal surgical implants
Degenerative joint disease	Over the lumbar, pelvic, or abdominal areas in women with metallic intrauterine devices
Sacroiliac strains	Metal objects within the immediate treatment area
Deep muscles spasms	Unshielded cardiac pacemaker
Ankylosing spondylitis	Over the eyes, testes, and fluid-filled joints
Osteoarthritis	Over ischemic, hemorrhagic, malignant, and acutely inflamed tissues
Chronic pelvic inflammatory disease	Over moist wound dressings, clothing, or perspiration
Epicondylitis	Pregnant abdomen
Subacute inflammation	Patients with hemophilia
	Over epiphyses

Principles of Electricity

Electrical energy flows between two points. In an atom, protons are positively charged, electrons are negatively charged, and neutrons have no charge. Equal numbers of protons and electrons produce a balanced neutrality in the atom. To transfer energy from one atom to the next, only electrons are moved from the nucleus, creating an electrical imbalance. This subtraction and addition of electrons causes atoms to become electrically charged, and such atoms are then called ions. An ion that has more electrons is said to be negatively charged; an ion with more protons is positively charged. Ions of similar charge repel each another, whereas ions of dissimilar charge attract one another. The strength of the force and the distance between ions determine how quickly the transfer of energy occurs.

Types of Currents

Four types of electrical current can be applied to tissues (**Figure 6.13**). Two types fall under the category of continuous current: direct and alternating. Direct current (DC) is a continuous one-directional flow of ions, and is used for pain modulation, to elicit a muscle contraction, or to produce ion movement. Alternating current (AC) is a continuous two-directional flow of ions used for pain modulation or muscle contraction. Pulsed current is a flow of ions in direct or alternating current that is briefly interrupted. It may be one-directional (monophasic) or two-directional (biphasic) depending on the type of current used. Pulsed currents are used in interferential and so-called Russian currents. In therapeutic use, each current can be manipulated by altering the frequency, intensity, and duration of the wave or pulse.

Current Modifications

Once the basic current type is known, there are several parameters that can be manipulated for the desired effects. The more common parameters include the amplitude, frequency, pulse duration, pulse charge, electrode setup, polarity, mode, duty cycle, and duration of treatment. **Table 6.1** provides some guidelines for parameter modifications to achieve certain therapeutic effects. An electrical unit with the prescribed current type should be selected, and then the modifications indicated for the desired effect should be applied.

AMPLITUDE

Amplitude is a measure of the force, or intensity, that drives the current, the maximum amplitude being the top or highest point of each phase. The term is synonymous with **voltage** and is measured in millivolts (mV), although some units use milliamperage (mA) as a measure of amplitude. Voltage causes the ions to move, but the actual movement is called **current.** If the current is graphically presented, the voltage is represented by the magnitude of the wave. If resistance remains the same, an increase in voltage will increase the amperage (rate of current flow). Average current can be increased by either increasing pulse duration or increasing pulse frequency or by some combination of the two.

Mediums that facilitate movement of the ions are called **conductors** and include water, blood, and electrolyte solutions such as sweat. Mediums that inhibit movement of the ions are called **resistors**, such as skin, fat, and lotion. The combination of voltage, current, and resistance is measured in ohms (Ω). **Ohm's law** ($I = V/R$) states that current (I) in a conductor increases as the driving force (V) becomes larger, or resistance (R) is decreased. For example, 1 V is the amount of electrical force required to send a current of 1 amp through a resistance of 1 ohm.

FREQUENCY

Frequency refers to the number of waveform cycles per second (cps) or hertz (Hz) with alternating current, the number of pulses per second (pps) with monophasic or biphasic current, or the number of bursts per second (bps) with Russian stimulation. One purpose in altering

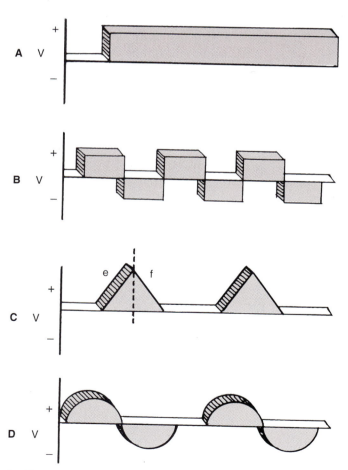

➤ **FIGURE 6.13 Four basic currents.** The shape of the waveforms can be altered by changing the rate of rise and rate of decay. A, Direct current (DC) with square wave; B, alternating current (AC) with square wave; C, monophasic with triangular wave e = rate of rise; f = rate of decay; D, biphasic with sine wave.

TABLE 6.1   PARAMETER MODIFICATION FOR ELECTROTHERAPY

Desired Effect	Current Type	Intensity	Frequency	Pulse Duration	Electrodes	Mode
Muscle contraction	Biphasic	Motor	<15 pps twitch 15–25 pps sum >40 pps tetany	300–500 µs	Ends of muscle motor points	Duty cycle
	Monophasic	Motor	<15 pps twitch 15–25 pps sum >40 pps tetany	300–500 µs	Negative/ends of muscle or motor points	Alternate or reciprocate duty cycle
Pain control Gate	Biphasic	Sensory	110 pps	30–200 µs	Direct contiguous nerve root dermatomes	Modulated
	Monophasic	Sensory	100–150 pps	Short	Positive/over pain site	Continuous
Opiate release	Biphasic	Motor	1–5 pps	300–500 µs	Trigger points	Burst
	Monophasic	Motor	1–5 pps	300–500 µs	+ (acute) – (chronic)/ over pain site	Continuous
Central biasing	Biphsic	Noxious	100–150 pps	250–500 µs	Trigger points	Modulated
Edema reduction	Monophasic	Sensory	80–150 pps	20–200 µs	Negative/over edema	Continuous

Note: Interferential stimulation can be used for muscle contraction, gate, and opiate pain control by using similar parameters. Russian current can be used for muscle contraction by substituting bps for pps. (Printed with permission from Holcomb WR. J Sport Rehab 1997;6(3):280.)

frequency is to control the force of muscle contractions during neuromuscular stimulation. A low-frequency stimulation will cause the muscle to twitch with each pulse, cycle, or burst. As frequency increases, stimulation will minimize the relaxation phase of the muscle contraction. At still higher frequencies, the stimulation is so fast that no relaxation occurs and a sustained, maximal contraction (tetany) is generated. Therefore, if the intent is to bring about fatigue in a muscle, the athletic trainer can choose the appropriate frequency to bring about this effect.

PULSE DURATION

Phase duration, or current duration as it is sometimes called, refers to the length of time that current is flowing. Pulse duration is the length of a single pulse of monophasic or biphasic current. With biphasic current, the sum of the two phases represents the pulse duration, whereas in monophasic current, the phase and pulse duration are synonymous. The time between each subsequent pulse is called the interpulse interval. The combined time of the pulse duration and the interpulse interval is referred to as the pulse period. More powerful muscle contractions are generated with a pulse duration of 300 to 400 µs.

PULSE CHARGE

In a single phase, the pulse charge, or quantity of an electrical current, is the product of the phase duration and amplitude, and represents the total amount of electricity being delivered to the athlete during each pulse. Amplitude, pulse duration, the interpulse interval, phase duration, and phase charge are illustrated in **Figure 6.14**.

ELECTRODE SETUP

Electrical currents are introduced into the body through electrodes and a conducting medium. The smaller active pad has the greatest current density and brings the

current into the body. The active electrode ranges from a very small pad to 4 inches square. Water or an electrolyte gel is used to obtain high conductivity. The arrangement of the pads depends on the polarity of the active pad, and not on the number or size. If only one active electrode is used, or if the active electrodes are of the same charge, the arrangement is monopolar. With this pattern, a large dispersal pad is needed to take on the opposite charge of the active pad to complete the circuit. The dispersal pad, from which the electrons leave the body, should be as large as possible to reduce current density. With the low current density, no sensation should be felt beneath the dispersal pad. When the active pads are of opposite charges, the arrangement is bipolar. Because this arrangement provides a complete circuit, no dispersal pad is necessary. Interferential stimulation requires a quadripolar electrode arrangement. This is nothing more than a bipolar arrangement from two channels where the currents cross at the treatment site. This electrode arrangement can be seen in **Figure 6.17**.

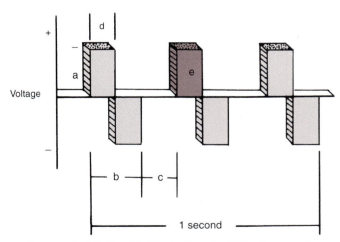

▶ **FIGURE 6.14 Graphic illustration of a biphasic current.** a = amplitude (intensity); b = pulse duration; c = interpulse interval; d = phase duration; e = phase charge. Frequency = 3 pps.

The pads should be placed at least one pad width apart. The closer the pads are, the shallower and more isolated the contraction; the farther apart they are, the deeper and more generalized the contraction. The physiological effects can occur anywhere between the pads, but usually occur at the active electrode because current density is greatest at this point.

POLARITY

Polarity refers to the direction of current flow, and can be toward either a positive or negative pole. During direct current and monophasic stimulation, the active electrode(s) can be either positive or negative, and current will flow in a predetermined direction (away from the negative electrode). During AC or biphasic stimulation, the polarity of the active pads alternates between positive and negative with each phase of the current.

MODE

In a monopolar arrangement, mode refers to the alternating (reciprocating) or continuous flow of current through the active electrodes. Alternating means that the active electrodes receive current on an alternating basis, whereas with continuous flow, each electrode receives current throughout the treatment period. In neuromuscular stimulation, another popular mode is a ramped or surge amplitude. The amplitude gradually builds to the desired level, which improves patient comfort and safety by preventing sudden, powerful muscle contractions.

DUTY CYCLE

Duty cycle refers to the ratio of the amount of time current is flowing (on time) to the amount of time it is not flowing (off time). Used in neuromuscular stimulation, the duty cycle simulates repetitions and rest so as to delay the onset of fatigue. In edema formation, it creates a muscle pump. With neuromuscular stimulation, the recommended duty cycle should be 1:4 or 20% initially (i.e., 10 s on and 40 s off) and should gradually increase as fatigability decreases. To prevent discomfort for the patient, a manual control of the duty cycle is necessary.

DURATION OF TREATMENT

Duration of treatment is the total time the patient is subjected to electrical stimulation. Many units have internal timers. Treatment duration is typically 15 to 30 minutes.

Electrical Stimulating Units

There are several different types of electrical units (see **Box 6.6**). Although it would be much easier to name the units based on the types of current that characterize the stimulation devices, this is not the case. Names are often

---

➤➤ Box 6.6

Application of Neuromuscular Electrical Stimulation

TENS

Indications
- ↓ Posttraumatic pain, acute and chronic
- ↓ Postsurgical pain
- ↑ Analgesia

Contraindications
Patients with pacemakers
Pregnancy (abdominal and/or pelvic area)
Pain of unknown origin

High-Voltage Pulsed

Indications
- ↑ Circulation and joint mobility
- ↑ Muscle re-education and strength
- ↑ Wound and fracture healing
- ↑ Nonunion fracture healing
- ↓ Muscle spasm/spasticity
- ↓ Pain and edema
- ↓ Disuse atrophy
Denervation of peripheral nerve injuries

Contraindications
Pacemakers
Pain of unknown origin
Pregnancy (abdominal and/or pelvic area)
Thrombophlebitis
Superficial skin lesions or infections
Cancerous lesions
Over suspected fracture sites

Interferential

Indications
- ↑ Circulation and wound healing
- ↓ Pain, acute and chronic
- ↓ Reduction of muscle spasm/guarding
- ↓ Posttraumatic and chronic edema
- ↓ Abdominal organ dysfunction

Contraindications
Pacemakers
Pregnancy (abdominal and/or pelvic area)
Thrombophlebitis
Pain of unknown origin
Prolonged use (may increase muscle soreness)

Low-Intensity Stimulation

Indications
- ↑ Nonunion wound healing
- ↑ Fracture healing
Iontophoresis

Contraindications
Malignancy
Hypersensitive skin
Allergies to certain drugs

Parameter	High TENS	Low TENS	Brief-Intense
TABLE 6.2	**PROTOCOL FOR TENS APPLICATION**		
Intensity	Sensory	Motor	Noxious
Pulse frequency	60–100 pps	2–4 pps	Variable
Pulse duration	60–100 μsec	150–250 μsec	300–1000 μsec
Mode	Modulated rate	Modulated burst	Modulated amplitude
Duration	As needed	30 min	15–30 min
Onset of relief	<10 min	20–40 min	<15 min
Duration of relief	Minutes to hours	Hours	<30 min

(Printed with permission from Starkey [1], page 229).

used to show distinction between the characteristics, indications, and parameters of the various units. Unfortunately, many units could fall under the same general title. To complicate matters further, many common names, such as Galvanic, Faradic, and Russian stimulation are still used, and will be discussed later in this section. The more common electrical stimulation units will be discussed.

TRANSCUTANEOUS ELECTRICAL NERVE STIMULATION (TENS)

TENS units are typically portable biphasic generators with parameters that allow pain control via high-frequency, low-frequency, and brief-intense stimulation (**Table 6.2**). The units can produce analgesia and decrease acute and chronic pain, and pain associated with delayed-onset muscle soreness. TENS is often used continuously after surgery in a 30- to 60-minute session, several times a day. It is thought that TENS works to override the body's internal signals of pain (gate theory of pain), or stimulates the re-

lease of endomorphins, a strong, opiate-like substance produced by the body. The unit uses small carbonized silicone electrodes to transmit electrical pulses through the skin (**Figure 6.15**). Most units are small enough to be worn on a belt and are battery powered. The electrodes are taped on the skin over or around the painful site, but may be secured along the peripheral or spinal nerve pathways. For individuals who have allergic reactions to the tape adhesive, or who develop skin abrasions from repeated applications, electrodes with a self-adhering adhesive are available.

HIGH-VOLTAGE PULSED STIMULATION (HVPS)

HVPS units provide a monophasic current with a twin-peak wave form, a relatively short pulse duration and long interpulse interval, and an amplitude range above 150 mV (22). HVPS is often used in muscle re-education and to increase joint mobility, promote wound healing, and decrease pain, edema, and muscle atrophy, but is ineffective in reducing the soreness, loss of range of motion, and loss of strength associated with delayed-onset muscle soreness (DOMS) (23).

NEUROMUSCULAR ELECTRICAL STIMULATION (NMES)

NMES units are designed to elicit a muscle contraction, and are typically biphasic currents with a duty cycle. High-voltage electrical stimulation uses an output of 100 V to 500 V to reduce edema, pain, and muscle spasm during the acute phase. It is also used to exercise muscle and delay atrophy, maintain muscle size and strength during periods of immobilization, re-educate muscles, and increase blood flow to tissues (**Figure 6.16**). Direct current is used primarily to stimulate denervated muscle, and enhance wound healing, and is used during iontophoresis.

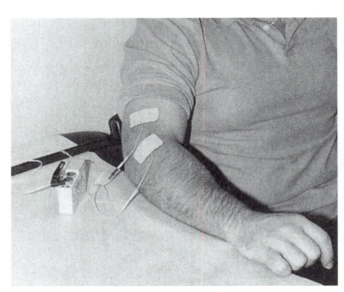

➤ FIGURE 6.15 **Transcutaneous electrical nerve stimulation**. TENS is used to decrease acute and chronic pain to an injured area.

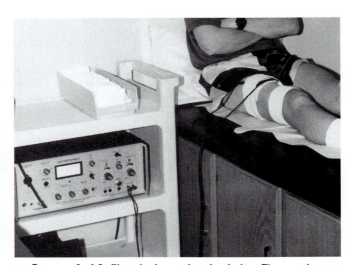

➤ FIGURE 6.16 **Electrical muscle stimulation**. These units are used to stimulate muscle to maintain muscle size and strength during immobilization, re-educate muscles, prevent muscle atrophy, and increase blood flow to tissues to decrease pain and spasm.

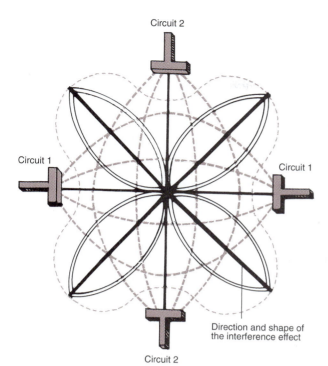

➤ **FIGURE 6.17 Interferential current**. When arranged in a square alignment, the quadripolar electrode setup is actually a bipolar arrangement from two channels. An electric field is created where the currents cross between the lines of electric current flow. The maximum interference effect takes place near the center over the treatment site.

INTERFERENTIAL STIMULATION (IFS)

Interferential current utilizes two separate generators and a quadripolar electrode arrangement to produce two simultaneous AC electrical currents acting on the tissues. The two paired pads are placed perpendicular to each other and the current crosses at the midpoint (**Figure 6.17**). A predictable pattern of interference will occur as the interference effects branch off at 45 angles from the center of the treatment, in the shape of a four-leaf clover. Tissues within this area receive the maximal treatment effect. When the electrodes are properly placed, the stimulation should be felt only between the electrodes, not under the electrodes. Currents range from 1 to 10 Hz (1 to 100 μA) with the paired pads differing from each other by +1 Hz (1). The higher frequencies lower skin resistance, thus eliciting a stronger response with less current intensity. Furthermore, sensory perception is decreased between the pads, allowing for a higher current to be used that increases stimulation. The amplitude and/or beat frequency can be modulated throughout the treatment by selecting the scan or sweep mode, respectively. This modality is used to decrease pain, acute and chronic edema, and muscle spasm; strengthen weakened muscles; improve blood flow to an area; heal chronic wounds; and relieve abdominal organ dysfunction.

LOW-INTENSITY STIMULATION (LIS)

Low-intensity stimulation is the more currently used term to replace the units originally called microcurrent

electrical nerve stimulators (MENS) units. LIS units are available in a variety of waveforms from modified monophasic to biphasic square waves. The units tend to be applied at a subsensory or very low sensory level with a current operating at less than 1000 μA. The devices deliver an electrical current to the body approximately 1/1000 the amperage of TENS, but a pulse duration that may be up to 2500 times longer. The stimulation pathway is not designed to stimulate peripheral nerves to elicit a muscle contraction, but rather is used to reduce acute and chronic pain and inflammation; reduce edema; and facilitate healing in superficial wounds, sprains, strains, fractures, and neuropathies. The efficacy of microcurrent therapy, and subsequently on LIS units, is based primarily on anecdotal evidence rather than valid research. The current is thought to mimic the normal electrical current within the body, which is disrupted with injury, to reduce pain and spasm and improve healing (22). Several studies have shown that microcurrent is ineffective in reducing pain and increasing muscle function associated with delayed-onset muscle soreness (24,25).

GALVANIC STIMULATION

Galvanic stimulation is the common name for any stimulator using direct current.

RUSSIAN CURRENT

Russian current is a type of neuromuscular stimulation that uses an alternating current with frequencies ranging from 2,000 to 10,000 Hz. The current is generated in bursts, with interburst intervals. The number of bps can be manipulated within the therapeutic range. For example, a high-frequency AC current will easily penetrate the skin and provide a high-amplitude, low-frequency (bps) current to the muscle. Russian electrical stimulation is designed to produce an isometric contraction and is useful in muscle re-education. Because it induces an isometric contraction, rather than an isotonic one, strength gains will not transfer across the entire joint, but instead will be restricted to a narrow arc on either side of the joint angle at which the muscle is stimulated. Russian current, however, does permit the athlete to contract actively along with the stimulation, provides an adequate work-to-rest interval, and is usually comfortable for the athlete.

FARADIC CURRENT

Faradic current is a specialized, asymmetrical biphasic wave. Although popular in the past, it is now thought to be of little benefit over symmetrical waves (22).

IONTOPHORESIS

Iontophoresis uses direct current to drive charged molecules from certain medications, such as anti-inflammatories (hydrocortisone), anesthetics (lidocaine), or analgesics (aspirin or acetaminophen), into damaged tissue. It is used as a local anesthetic to treat inflammatory conditions and skin conditions to reduce edema. Contraindications include allergy to the ion being used, decreased sensation, and placing electrodes directly over unhealed or partially healed skin wounds or new scar tissue. No contact should exist between metal or carbon-rubber electrode components and the skin, and electrodes should never be removed or rearranged until the unit has been turned off. The corticosteroid dexamethasone has been very successful in treating overuse conditions, myofascial syndromes, and plantar fasciitis (26).

Iontophoresis is noninvasive and painless, uses a sterile application, and is excellent for those patients who fear injections. It also yields tissue concentrations that are lower than those achieved with injections but greater than those with oral administration, because it avoids enzymatic breakdown in the gastrointestinal tract. A major disadvantage of this treatment is the electrolysis of NaCl in the body by direct current. Electrolysis produces an increased pH (acidic) condition at the cathode (positive electrode), and decreased pH (alkaline) condition at the anode (negative electrode). These pH changes can lead to tissue burns, especially with high intensities or prolonged application. Therefore, the negative electrode should be large, perhaps twice the size of the positive electrode, to reduce current density. With the newer controlled generators and buffered electrodes, athletic trainers can selectively decrease the current density under the anode to decrease the incidence of burns.

Prior to treatment, the skin must be thoroughly cleansed. Next, well-saturated electrodes are applied over the most focal point of tissue inflammation or pain, unless skin irritation is visible. The polarity of the medication determines which electrode is used to drive the molecules into the skin. The medication is placed under the electrode with the same polarity. When the current is applied, the molecules are pushed away from the electrode and driven into the skin toward the injured site. This localized treatment is often preferred over more disruptive systemic treatments.

The athletic trainer can combine ultrasound and a high-voltage pulsed stimulator or interferential stimulation to increase blood flow in the biceps femoris muscle. The electrical current can stimulate a muscle contraction to produce muscle pumping, retard atrophy, and strengthen the muscle.

OTHER TREATMENT MODALITIES

In some clinical settings, an athletic trainer may not have access to expensive electrical modalities. What other treatment modalities might be used to promote healing of the sprinter's biceps femoris strain?

Many of the electrotherapy modalities are costly and may not be readily available in all clinical settings. In addition, state licensure laws may prohibit an athletic trainer from using certain modalities in a nontraditional setting. As such, it becomes necessary to use other treatment modalities to achieve the same results.

Massage

Massage involves the manipulation of the soft tissues to increase cutaneous circulation, cell metabolism, and venous and lymphatic flow to assist in the removal of edema; stretch superficial scar tissue; alleviate soft tissue adhesions; and decrease neuromuscular excitability (see **Box 6.7**). As a result, relaxation, pain relief, edema reduction, and increased range of motion can be achieved. To reduce friction between the patient's skin and hand, particularly over hairy areas, lubricants are often used, i.e., massage lotion, peanut oil, coconut oil, or powder. These lubricants should have a lanolin base or be alcohol free. Massage involves five basic strokes: effleurage (stroking), pétrissage (kneading), tapotement (percussion), vibration, and friction. **Table 6.3** describes the various techniques used in therapeutic massage.

Effleurage is a superficial, longitudinal stroke to relax the patient. When applied toward the heart, it reduces swelling and aids venous return. It is the most commonly used stroke, and begins and ends each massage. Effleurage permits the athletic trainer to evaluate the condition, distribute the lubricant, warm the skin and superficial tissue, and promote relaxation.

Pétrissage consists of pressing and rolling the muscles under the fingers and hands. This "milking" action over deep tissues and muscle increases venous and lymphatic return, and removes metabolic waste products from the injured area. Furthermore, it breaks up adhesions within the underlying tissues, loosens fibrous tissue, and increases elasticity of the skin.

Tapotement uses sharp, alternating, brisk hand movements such as hacking, slapping, beating, cupping,

---

➤➤ **BOX 6.7**

Application of Therapeutic Massage

Indications
Increase local circulation
Increase venous and lymphatic flow
Reduce pain (analgesia)
Reduce muscle spasm
Stretch superficial scar tissue
Improve systemic relaxation
Chronic myositis, bursitis, tendinitis tenosynovitis, fibrositis

Contraindications
Acute contusions, sprains, and strains
Over fracture sites
Over open lesions or skin conditions
Conditions such as: acute phlebitis, thrombosis, severe varicose veins, cellulitis, synovitis, arteriosclerosis, and cancerous regions

TABLE 6.3 **TECHNIQUES OF MASSAGE**

Technique	Use	Method of Application
Effleurage (stroking)	Relaxes patient Evenly distributes any lubricant Increases surface circulation	Gliding motion over the skin without any attempt to move deep muscles Apply pressure with the flat of the hand; fingers and thumbs spread; stroke toward the heart Massage begins and ends with stroking
Pétrissage (kneading)	Increases circulation Promotes venous & lymphatic return Breaks up adhesions in superficial connective tissue Increases elasticity of skin	Kneading manipulation that grasps and rolls the muscles under the fingers or hands
Tapotement (percussion)	Increases circulation Stimulates subcutaneous structures	Brisk hand blows in rapid succession: hacking—with ulnar border slapping—with flat hand beating—with half-closed fist tapping—with fingertips cupping—with arched hand
Vibration	Relaxes limb	Fine vibrations made with fingers pressed into a specific body part
Friction (rubbing)	Loosens fibrous scar tissue Aids in absorption of edema Reduces inflammation Reduces muscular spasm	Small circular motions with the fingers, thumb, or heel of hand Transverse friction is done perpendicular to the fibers being massaged

and clapping to increase blood flow and stimulate peripheral nerve endings. Because this technique is used for stimulation, not relaxation, it is not used in most massage treatments.

Vibration consists of finite, gentle, and rhythmical movement of the fingers to vibrate the underlying tissues. It is used for relaxation or stimulation.

Friction is the deepest form of massage, and consists of deep circular motions performed by the thumb, knuckles, or ends of the fingers at right angles to the involved tissue. These deep circular movements can loosen adherent fibrous tissue (scar), aid in absorption of edema, and reduce localized muscular spasm. Transverse friction massage is a deep friction massage performed across the grain of the

muscle, tendon sheath, or ligament. Cross-friction massage is the most effective technique, and is used to break up adhesions and promote healing of muscle and ligament tears.

One recent study found that blood flow did not significantly increase with effleurage, pétrissage, and tapotement on either a small or large muscle mass (27). Another study found that manual massage did not have a significant impact on the recovery of muscle function following exercise, or on any of the physiological factors associated with the recovery process (28). In both studies, the researchers concluded that light exercise of the affected muscles is probably more effective than massage in improving muscle blood flow (thereby enhancing healing) and temporarily reducing muscle soreness. Because the types and duration of massage are typically based on the athlete's and athletic trainer's preference, its use in athletic settings for these purposes should be questioned.

Traction

Traction is the process of drawing or pulling tension on a body segment. The most common forms involve lumbar and cervical traction. Spinal traction is more commonly used to treat small herniated disc protrusions that may result in spinal nerve impingement, although it may also be used to treat a variety of other conditions (see **Box 6.8**). The effects of spinal traction include distraction of the vertebral bodies, widening of the vertebral foramen, a combination of distraction and gliding of vertebral facets, and stretching and relaxation of the paraspinal muscles and ligamentous structures of the spinal segment.

A distractive force is commonly applied either with a mechanical device or manually by an athletic trainer. Traction may be applied continuously through a low, distracting force for up to several hours; statically with a sustained distracting force applied for the entire treatment time, usually 30 minutes; or intermittently with a distracting force applied and released for several seconds repeatedly over the course of the treatment time. For example, in lumbar traction a split table is used to eliminate friction. A special nonslip harness lined with vinyl is used

➤➤ **BOX 6.8**

Application of Traction

Indications
Herniated disc protrusions
Spinal nerve impingement
Spinal nerve inflammation
Joint hypomobility
Narrowing of intervertebral foramen
Degenerative joint disease
Spondylolisthesis
Muscle spasm and guarding
Joint pain

Contraindications
Unstable vertebrae
Acute lumbago
Gross emphysema
S4 nerve root signs
Temporomandibular dysfunction
Patient discomfort

to transfer the distractive force comfortably to the patient and to stabilize the trunk and thoracic area while the lumbar spine is placed under traction. A distractive force, usually up to one-half of the patient's body weight, is applied for 30 minutes daily for 2 to 4 weeks. Although intermittent traction tends to be more comfortable for the patient, sustained traction is more effective in treating lumbar disc problems. In cervical traction, the patient may be either supine or seated. Again, a nonslip cervical harness is secured under the chin and back of the head to transfer the distractive force comfortably to the patient. Recommended force ranges from 10 to 30 pounds.

With manual traction, the athletic trainer applies the distractive force for a few seconds or sometimes with a quick, sudden thrust. This method has been effective in reducing joint pain when the traction in applied within the normal range of joint movement. Because the athletic trainer can feel the relaxation or resistance, he or she can instantaneously change the patient's position, direction of the force, magnitude of the force, or duration of the treatment.

Continuous Passive Motion (CPM)

Continuous passive motion is a modality that applies an external force to move the joint through a pre-set arc of motion (**Figure 6.18**). It is used primarily postsurgically at the knee, after knee manipulation, or after stable fixation of intra-articular and extra-articular fractures of most joints. It may also be used to improve wound healing, accelerate clearance of a **hemarthrosis** (blood in a joint), and prevent cartilage degeneration in septic arthritis (see **Box 6.9**). The application is relatively pain-free and has been shown to stimulate the intrinsic healing process,

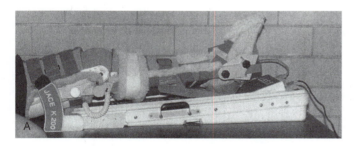

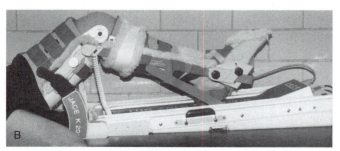

➤ FIGURE 6.18 **Continuous passive motion**. These machines are often used postsurgically to apply an external force to move the joint through a limited range of motion. A, Starting position. B, Ending position.

> ➤➤ BOX 6.9
>
> ## Application of Continuous Passive Motion (CPM)
>
> | Indications | Contraindications |
> |---|---|
> | Postoperative rehabilitation to:
Reduce pain
Improve general circulation
Enhance joint nutrition
Prevent joint contractures
Benefit collagen remodeling
Following knee manipulation
Following joint debridement
Following meniscal or osteochondral repair
Tendon lacerations | Noncompliant patient
If use would disrupt surgical repair, fracture fixation, or lead to hemorrhage in postoperative period
Malfunction of device |

maintain articular cartilage nutrition, reduce disuse effects, retard joint stiffness and the pain-spasm cycle, and benefit collagen remodeling, joint dynamics, and pain reduction (1,29).

 Massage may be used after the acute phase has ended. Stroking and kneading toward the heart may provide some beneficial effects; however, mild exercise may be just as beneficial.

MEDICATIONS

 What medications might be helpful in promoting healing of this injury? Which medications can be recommended and dispensed by an athletic trainer?

Therapeutic drugs are either prescription or over-the-counter medications used to treat an injury or illness. Common drugs used to control pain, inflammation, and muscle spasm include anesthetics, analgesics, nonsteroidal anti-inflammatory drugs (NSAIDs), adrenocorticosteroids, and muscle relaxants. A more detailed presentation of therapeutic drugs can be found in Chapter 26 on Pharmacology.

Local anesthetics eliminate short-term pain sensation in a specific body part or region by blocking afferent (sensory) neural transmissions along peripheral nerves. Many of these drugs can be identified by their "-caine" suffixes (e.g., lidocaine, procaine, and benzocaine). The drugs may be topically applied to skin for minor irritations (burns, abrasions, mild inflammation), introduced into subcutaneous tissues via phonophoresis or iontophoresis (bursitis, tendinitis, contusions), injected by a physician into soft tissue around a laceration for surgical repair (suturing), or injected by a physician near a peripheral nerve to interrupt nerve transmission (nerve block).

Aspirin is the most commonly used drug to relieve pain and inflammation. Because of its anticlotting properties, it is not used during the acute phase. Aspirin is associated with a number of adverse side effects, including gastrointestinal irritation. Stomach distress can be limited by using coated aspirin to delay release of the drug until it reaches the small intestine, or by taking a buffered aspirin to blunt the acidic effects of aspirin in the stomach. With chronic use or high doses (10 to 30 grams), renal problems, liver toxicity, congestive heart failure, hypertension, aspirin intoxication, or poisoning may occur. Normal dosage is 325 to 650 mg every 4 hours.

Acetaminophen (Tylenol) is an analgesic and an **antipyretic** (reduces fever), but does not have any appreciable anti-inflammatory or anticlotting effects. Unlike aspirin, acetaminophen is not associated with gastrointestinal irritation. However, high doses can be toxic to the liver and may be fatal.

Nonsteroidal anti-inflammatory drugs (NSAIDs) are commonly used to dilate blood vessels and inhibit production of prostaglandins. Certain prostaglandins increase local blood flow, capillary permeability, erythema, and edema associated with inflammation, and are believed to decrease the sensitivity of pain receptors to the effects of other pain producing substances, such as bradykinin (1,16). Therefore, these drugs decrease inflammation, relieve mild to moderate pain (analgesia), decrease body temperature associated with fever, increase collagen strength, and inhibit coagulation and blood clotting. The most important time to administer NSAIDs is in the early stages of healing when prostaglandins produce the most detrimental effects of pain and edema. Prolonged use (2 or more weeks) may actually retard the healing process. Examples of NSAIDs include ibuprofen (Advil, Nuprin, Motrin, Rufen), naproxen sodium (Aleve), indomethacin (Indocin), and piroxicam (Feldene). **Table 6.4** lists the more common NSAIDS and suggested dosages.

Ibuprofen and the other NSAIDs are administered primarily for pain relief and anti-inflammatory effects.

TABLE 6.4 NONSTEROIDAL ANTI-INFLAMMATORY DRUGS (NSAIDS)

Generic Name	Brand Name	Single Dose	Maximum Daily Dose	Duration
Over the Counter				
Ibuprofen	Advil, Nuprin, Motrin IB	2 × 200 mg every 4–6 hr	1200 mg	Short
Ketoprofen	Actron, Orudis KT	1 × 12.5 mg every 4–6 hr	75 mg	Short
Naproxen Sodium	Aleve	1 × 220 mg every 8–12 hr	660 mg	Intermediate
Prescription				
Bromfenac	Duract	25 mg	150 mg	Short
Diclofenac Potassium	Cataflam	50 mg	200 mg	Short
Diclofenac Sodium	Voltaren	25, 50, 75 mg XR–100 mg	200 mg	Short
Etodolac	Lodine	200, 300, 400, 500 mg XL–400, 600 mg	1200 mg	Intermediate
Fenoprofen Calcium	Nalfon	200, 300, 600 mg	3200 mg	Short
Flurbiprofen	Ansaid	50, 100 mg	300 mg	Short
Ibuprofen	Motrin, Rufen	300, 400, 600, 800 mg	3200 mg	Short
Indomethacin	Indocin	25, 50 mg SR–75 mg	200 mg	Short/Intermediate
Ketoprofen	Orudis, Oruvail	50, 75 mg SR–100, 150, 200 mg	300 mg	Short
Ketorolac	Toradol	10 mg	40 mg	Short
Meclofenamate	Meclomen	50, 100 mg	400 mg	Short
Mefanamic Acid	Ponstel	250 mg	1000 mg	Short
Nabumetone	Relafen	500, 750 mg	2000 mg	Long
Naproxen Sodium	Anaprox	275, 550 mg	1375 mg	Intermediate
Naproxen	Naprosyn	250, 375, 500 mg	1500 mg	Intermediate
Naproxen	EC-Naprosyn, Naprelen	375, 500 mg	1500 mg	Intermediate
Oxaprozin	Daypro	600 mg	1800 mg	Very long
Piroxicam	Feldene	10, 20 mg	20 mg	Very long
Sulindac	Clinoril	150, 200 mg	400 mg	Intermediate
Tolmetin Sodium	Tolectin	200, 400, 600 mg	2000 mg	Short

However, they are more expensive than aspirin. Although many are still associated with some stomach discomfort, they provide better effects in many patients. Taking the medication after a meal, or with a glass of milk or water will greatly reduce stomach discomfort.

Adrenocorticosteroids are steroid hormones produced by the adrenal cortex. Higher doses, referred to as a pharmacological dose, are typically used to treat endocrine disorders, but can be used to decrease edema, inflammation, **erythema** (inflammatory redness of the skin), and tenderness in a region. These drugs may be topically applied, given orally, or injected by a physician into a specific area, such as a tendon or joint. Examples of these drugs include cortisone, prednisone, and hydrocortisone. Because many of these drugs can lead to breakdown and rupture of structures, long-term use can depress the adrenal glands, and increase the risk of osteoporosis.

Skeletal muscle relaxants are used to relieve muscle spasms. Muscle spasms can result from certain musculoskeletal injuries or inflammation. When involuntary tension in the muscle cannot be relaxed, it leads to intense pain and a buildup of pain-mediating metabolites (e.g., lactate). A vicious cycle is created with the increased pain leading to more spasm, more pain, more spasm, and so on. Skeletal muscle relaxants break the pain-spasm cycle by depressing neural activity causing the continuous muscle contractions, thus reducing muscle excitability. Muscle relaxants do not prevent muscle contraction, but rather attempt to normalize muscle excitability to decrease pain and improve motor function. Examples of muscle relaxants include Flexeril, Soma, and Dantrium.

 Because of legal liability, athletic trainers cannot recommend, prescribe, or dispense medications. The athlete can be seen by the team physician, who may prescribe certain NSAIDs to promote healing, or the athlete may voluntarily take over-the-counter medications as needed. The athletic trainer, however, should monitor the athlete to ensure compliance with manufacturer's suggested guidelines.

Summary

1. Rehabilitation begins immediately after injury assessment with the use of therapeutic modalities to limit pain, inflammation, and loss of range of motion.
2. Therapeutic modalities, with the exception of ultrasound, fall under the electromagnetic spectrum based on their wavelength or frequency. All electromagnetic energy is pure energy that travels in a straight line at the speed of light (300 million meters per second) in a vacuum.
3. Depending on the medium, energy can be reflected, refracted, absorbed, or transmitted.

4. Common therapeutic modalities include cryotherapy, thermotherapy, ultrasound, diathermy, electrical stimulation, massage, traction, continuous passive motion, and medications to promote healing. Although many are used every day in treating athletic injuries, many must be used under the direction of a physician or an individual properly licensed to do so within the individual state. Being a technician and merely applying a modality is not an acceptable athletic training practice.
5. Cryotherapy is used to decrease pain, inflammation, muscle guarding and spasm, and to facilitate mobilization.
6. Thermotherapy is used to treat subacute or chronic injuries to reduce swelling, edema, ecchymosis, and muscle spasm; to increase blood flow and range of motion; to facilitate tissue healing; to relieve joint contractures; and to fight infection.
7. Ultrasound produces thermal and nonthermal effects.
   • Thermal effects include increased blood flow, extensibility of collagen tissue, sensory and motor nerve conduction velocity, and enzymatic activity; and decreased muscle spasm, joint stiffness, inflammation, and pain.
   • Nonthermal effects include decreased edema, and increased blood flow, cell membrane and vascular wall permeability, protein synthesis, tissue regeneration, and the promotion of healing.
8. Diathermy is used to treat joint inflammation (bursitis, tendinitis, synovitis), joint capsule contractures, subacute and chronic inflammatory conditions in deep-tissue layers, osteoarthritis, ankylosing spondylitis, and chronic pelvic inflammatory disease.
9. Electrotherapy is used to decrease pain, re-educate peripheral nerves, delay denervation and disuse atrophy by stimulating muscle contractions, reduce post-traumatic edema, and maintain range of motion by reducing muscle spasm, inhibiting spasticity, re-educating partially denervated muscle, and facilitating voluntary motor function.
10. Iontophoresis is used to introduce ions into the body tissues by means of a direct electrical current. This treatment is beneficial in reducing inflammation, muscle spasm, ischemia, and edema.
11. Massage involves the manipulation of the soft tissues to increase cutaneous circulation, cell metabolism, and venous and lymphatic flow to assist in the removal of edema; stretch superficial scar tissue; alleviate soft tissue adhesions; and decrease neuromuscular excitability. Strokes include effleurage, pétrissage, tapotement, vibration, and friction massage.
12. Traction is the process of drawing or pulling tension on a body segment, and is commonly used on the spine to treat herniated disc protrusion, spinal nerve inflammation or impingement, narrowing of intervertebral foramen, and muscle spasm and pain.

13. Continuous passive motion (CPM) applies an external force to move the joint through a pre-set arc of motion, and is primarily used postsurgically at the knee, after knee manipulation, or after stable fixation of intra-articular and extra-articular fractures of most joints.

14. NSAIDs are commonly used to dilate blood vessels and inhibit production of prostaglandins to decrease inflammation, relieve mild to moderate pain, decrease body temperature associated with fever, increase collagen strength, and inhibit coagulation and blood clotting.

15. Because of the complexity of each of the therapeutic modalities, students should enroll in a separate therapeutic modalities class where they can practice and demonstrate proper clinical skills associated with the application of therapeutic modalities.

16. While using any modality, if the athlete begins to show signs of pain, swelling, discomfort, tingling, or loss of sensation, the treatment should be stopped and the individual should be re-evaluated to determine if the selected modality is appropriate for the current phase of healing.

References

1. Starkey C. Therapeutic Modalities for Athletic Trainers. Philadelphia: FA Davis, 1999.
2. von Nieda K, Michlovitz SL. Cryotherapy. In: Thermal Agents in Rehabilitation. Edited by Michlovitz SL. Philadelphia: FA Davis, 1996.
3. Kimura IF, Gulick DT, Thompson GT. The effect of cryotherapy on eccentric plantar flexion peak torque and endurance. J Ath Train 1997;32(2):124-126.
4. Ho SS, et al. Comparison of various icing times in decreasing bone metabolism and blood flow in the knee. Am J Sports Med 1995;23(1):74-76.
5. Knight KL, Bryan KS, Halvorsen JM. Circulatory changes in the forearm in 1, 5, 10, and 15°C water. Int J Sports Med 1981;4:281.
6. Tsang KK, et al. The effects of cryotherapy applied through various barriers. J Sport Rehab 1997;(4):343-354.
7. Knight KL. Cryotherapy in Sport Injury Management. Champaign, IL: Human Kinetics, 1995.
8. Lessard LA, et al. The efficacy of cryotherapy following arthroscopic knee surgery. JOSPT 1997;26(1):14-22.
9. Edwards DJ, Rimmer M, Keene GC. The use of cold therapy in the postoperative management of patients undergoing arthroscopic anterior cruciate ligament reconstruction. Am J Sports Med 1996;24(2):193-195.
10. Konrath GA, et al. The use of cold therapy after anterior cruciate ligament reconstruction. Am J Sports Med 1996;24(5):629-633.
11. Walsh MT. Hydrotherapy: The use of water as a therapeutic agent. In: Thermal Agents in Rehabilitation. Edited by Michlovitz SL. Philadelphia: FA Davis, 1996.
12. Myer JW, Draper DO, Durrant E. Contrast therapy and intramuscular temperature in the human leg. J Ath Train 1994;29(4):318-322.
13. Myer JW, et al. Cold- and hot-pack contrast therapy: Subcutaneous and intramuscular temperature change. J Ath Train 1997;32(3):238-241.
14. Rennie FA, Michlovitz SL. Biophysical principles of heating and superficial heating agents. In: Thermal Agents in Rehabilitation. Edited by Michlovitz SL. Philadelphia: FA Davis, 1996.
15. Ramirez A, et al. The effect of ultrasound on collagen synthesis and fibroblast proliferation in vitro. Med Sci Sports Exerc 1997;29(3):326-332.
16. Houglum PA. Soft tissue healing and its impact on rehabilitation. J Sport Rehab 1992;1(1):19-39.
17. McDiarmid T, Ziskin MC, Michlovitz SL. Therapeutic ultrasound. In: Thermal Agents in Rehabilitation. Edited by Michlovitz SL. Philadelphia: FA Davis, 1996.
18. Draper DO, Castel JC, Castel D. Rate of temperature increase in human muscle during 1 MHZ and 3 MHZ continuous ultrasound. JOSPT 1995;22(4):142-149.
19. Forest G, Rosen K. Ultrasound treatments in degassed water. J Sport Rehab 1992;1(4):284-289.
20. Klucinec B. Effectiveness of the aquaflex gel pad in transmission of acoustic energy. J Ath Train 1996;31(4):313-317.
21. Draper DO, et al. A comparison of temperature rise in human calf muscles following application of underwater and topical gel ultrasound. JOSPT 1993;17(5):247-251.
22. Holcomb WR. A practical guide to electrical therapy. J Sport Rehab 1997;6(3):272-282.
23. Butterfield DL, et al. The effects of high-volt pulsed current electrical stimulation on delayed-onset muscle soreness. J Ath Train 1997;32(1):15-20.
24. Bonacci JA, Higbie EJ. Effects of microcurrent treatment on perceived pain and muscle strength following eccentric exercise. J Ath Train 1997;32(2):119-123.
25. Denegar CR, et al. The effects of low-volt, microamperage stimulation on delayed onset muscle soreness. J Sport Rehab 1992;1(2):95-102.
26. Guerman SD, et al. Treatment of plantar fasciitis by iontophoresis of 0.4% dexamethasone: A randomized, double-blind, placebo-controlled study. Am J Sports Med 1997;25(3):312-316.
27. Shoemaker JK, Tiidus PM, Mader R. Failure of manual massage to alter limb blood flow: Measures by Doppler ultrasound. Med Sci Sports Exerc 1997;29(5):610-614.
28. Tiidus PM. Manual massage and recovery of muscle function following exercise: A literature review. JOSPT 1997;25(2):107-112.
29. Chiarello CM, Gundersen L, O'Halloran R. The effect of continuous passive motion duration and increment on range of motion in total knee arthroplasty patients. JOSPT 1997;25(2):119-127.

7

Therapeutic Exercise

OBJECTIVES

1. Explain the principles associated with the cognitive model that describes an athlete's adjustment to injury.

2. Identify various psychological influences that can affect an injured athlete, and describe strategies or intervention techniques used to overcome these influences.

3. Explain the athletic trainer's role in dealing with the athlete's psychological concerns that may arise during the therapeutic exercise program, and identify the referral process if warranted.

4. Describe key factors in the development of a therapeutic exercise program.

5. Explain the four phases of a therapeutic exercise program, including the goals of these phases and methodology of implementation.

6. List the criteria used to clear an individual to return to full participation in sport.

T he ultimate goal of therapeutic exercise is to return the injured sport participant to pain-free and fully functional activity. For this to be accomplished, attention must focus on modulating pain and restoring normal joint range of motion, kinematics, flexibility, muscular strength, endurance, coordination, and power. Furthermore, cardiovascular endurance and strength must be maintained in the unaffected limbs.

Psychological influences can inhibit or enhance the progress of the therapeutic exercise program. The athletic trainer must be aware of all physical, psychological, emotional, social, and performance factors that may affect the athlete during rehabilitation. Only then can each component be addressed within a well-organized, individualized exercise program.

In this chapter, several emotional and psychological factors that may affect the injured athlete will be presented. These factors may either inhibit or enhance progress through the rehabilitation program. Next, a therapeutic exercise program following the SOAP note format will be explained. Phases of a therapeutic exercise program will be presented, including criteria used to determine when an individual is ready to progress in the program, and ultimately to return to sport activity. Practical application of the material for the various body segments will be included in Chapters 9 to 16. Due to the extensive nature of the material and the inability to provide in-depth information in a single chapter, students should enroll in a separate therapeutic exercise class to gain a more thorough understanding of the subject area, and to learn the clinical skills necessary to develop a total rehabilitation program.

PSYCHOLOGICAL ASPECTS OF THE INJURED PARTICIPANT

 A high school senior soccer player developed acute Achilles tendinitis 2 days before the post-season tournament, and just learned that he will be unable to participate for the remainder of the season. How might this athlete react to the inability to participate in sport? What impact will this reaction have on his motivation to improve? How can the athletic trainer help this person overcome the physical, psychological, and emotional effects that may hinder progress in the therapeutic exercise program?

To an individual who enjoys sport participation, an injury can be devastating. For many, the development and maintenance of a physically fit body provides a focal point for social and economic success that are important for self-esteem. A therapeutic exercise program must address not only the physical needs in returning the individual to activity, but also the emotional and psychological needs.

In general, there are two models of categorizing an athlete's adjustment to injury: stage and cognitive models.

The **stage model** is often linked to the Kubler-Ross emotional stages that an individual progresses through when confronted with grief. The stages include denial and isolation, anger, bargaining, depression, and acceptance. Although the model has some intuitive appeal, the stereotypical linear pattern of distinct emotional responses has not stood up to empirical scrutiny (1). Furthermore, if individuals react to injury in a linear manner, then the athletic trainer should be able to predict the athlete's progress during rehabilitation. This is rarely the case.

Each person reacts differently to an injury, based on individual coping mechanisms that stem from the interaction of personal and situational factors **(Figure 7.1)**. As such, **cognitive models** were developed to account for the differences. Personal factors, such as performance anxiety, self-esteem/motivation, extroversion/introversion, psychological investment in the sport, coping resources, a history of past stressors (e.g., previous injuries, academics, family life events), and previous intervention strategies influence how an athlete approaches the rehabilitation process. Situational factors may involve the type of sport, relationship with the coach and team members, characteristics of the injury (severity, history, and type), timing of the injury (preseason, in-season, play-offs), level and intensity of the player, point in the athlete's career, and role on the team. All of these factors interact with the cognitive, emotional, and behavioral responses of the athlete to influence the success or failure of a therapeutic exercise program. The cognitive appraisal asks: "What are you thinking

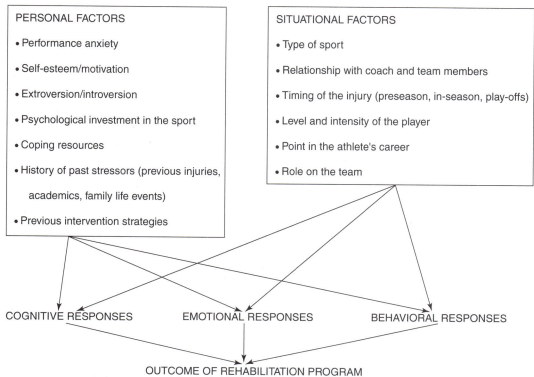

➤ **FIGURE 7.1 Cognitive model of an athletic injury.** Personal factors and situational factors interact with the cognitive, emotional, and behavioral responses of the athlete to influence the success or failure of a therapeutic exercise program.

in regard to this injury?" The emotional response refers to what one is feeling, and the behavioral response focuses on what the athlete is going to do: what are the behavioral rehabilitation consequences (1)?

Goal Setting

Goal setting is one of the most common practices used by athletic trainers to motivate athletes in the recovery program. This practice directs the individual's effort, provides a sense of control that may enhance motivation, persistence, and commitment, and facilitates the development of new strategies to improve performance. It has been found that athletes who set specific personal goals in each training session exhibit an increase in self-efficacy, or the sense of having the power to produce intended outcomes, and have greater satisfaction with their performance (2,3).

The process begins by establishing a strong and supportive rapport between the athletic trainer and athlete, who work in partnership to assist the athlete back to pre-injury status. For success, the athletic trainer must form a genuine relationship with the athlete and listen intently for clues that indicate what the athlete is feeling or not feeling. Goals should be realistic, objective, measurable, and attainable. Guidelines for goal setting for therapeutic exercise can be seen in **Box 7.1.** Long-term goals can reduce the athlete's fears of the unknown, but will do little to motivate the athlete on a day-to-day basis. Therefore, short-term goals should be established to serve as daily motivators. Goals should be personalized and challenging, yet realistic. A timetable for completion should be established, and measured to monitor progress.

Plateaus and setbacks usually occur because something is blocking the athlete's progress. These barriers fall under four general categories: lack of knowledge, lack of skill, lack of risk-taking ability, and lack of social support.

LACK OF KNOWLEDGE

It is imperative to inform the athlete about the injury and recovery process. The athletic trainer should explain why a specific treatment is used, the intended goal, and any side effects or sensations that may be experienced. This helps the athlete understand the process, avoids any surprises, and hopefully, reduces any anxiety the athlete may be experiencing (4).

LACK OF SKILL

When working with an athlete, it is advantageous to explain and demonstrate various techniques to the individual. Although an athlete may respond by telling you that he or she already knows how to complete a specific exercise, he or she may not. For example, lateral step-ups may be indicated for a knee injury. The athlete may report that he or she is capable of performing the skill correctly and

➤➤ **Box 7.1**

Guide to Goal Setting for Therapeutic Exercise
Goals should be:

Specific and Measurable. The athlete must know exactly what to do, and be able to determine if gains are made.

Stated in Positive versus Negative Language. Knowing what to do guides behavior, whereas knowing what to avoid creates a focus on errors without providing a constructive alternative.

Challenging but Realistic. Overly difficult goals set up failure and pose a threat to the athlete. The lower the athlete's self-confidence, the more important success becomes, and the greater the importance of setting attainable goals.

Established on a Time Table for Completion. This allows for a check on progress, and evaluation of whether realistic goals have been set.

Integration of Short-, Intermediate-, and Long-term Goals. A comprehensive program links daily activities with expectations for specific competitions, and for season and career goals.

Personalized and Internalized. The athlete must embrace goals as his or her own, not as something from the outside.

Monitored and Evaluated. Feedback must be provided to assess goals, and the goals should be modified based on progress.

Linked to Life Goals. This identifies sport and rehabilitation as learning experiences in life, and helps the athlete put sport in a broader perspective. This is especially important for athletes whose return to sport is doubtful.

Printed with permission from Heil (7), page 143.

does not need a demonstration. However, while observing the exercise, you notice that the individual is pushing off with the plantar flexors to raise the body, rather than allowing only the heel to touch the floor, which requires the quadriceps to raise the body. The exercise is ineffective if done improperly. Therefore, the athletic trainer should always demonstrate the skill and watch the athlete complete the exercise. Positive reinforcement and suggestions can be added to correct any errors in technique.

LACK OF RISK-TAKING ABILITY

Most individuals experience some level of fear and anxiety of the unknown. These emotions can block the athlete's ability to push themselves to meet the challenges of the exercise program. For example, fear of increased pain, discomfort, or reinjury during an exercise may limit the athlete's motivation to really push himself or herself. Constant positive feedback from the athletic trainer can help overcome many of these obstacles.

SOCIAL SUPPORT

When injured, every athlete needs to feel that he or she is not alone, and is just as important as noninjured athletes. Friends, colleagues, coaches, and the athletic trainer can provide emotional, challenging, material, and informational support to help the athlete feel good about his or her progress and value to the team. It is important to stress the athlete's value as a person, and to maintain connection to the team, friends, family, and any other supportive entities.

Psychological Influences

Five major factors can significantly influence the rehabilitation process: confidence, motivation, anxiety, focus, and the management of pain.

CONFIDENCE

Confidence is perhaps the most critical factor to a complete and timely recovery. Low confidence can lead to a host of negative thinking and talk, which in turn can lead to increasing anxiety, negative emotions, and low motivation, and interfere with the athlete's focus. Four main types of confidence can affect the athlete's recovery: program, adherence, physical, and return-to-sport. *Program confidence* refers to how strongly the athlete believes the rehabilitation program will enable him or her to recover, and is significantly influenced by the athletic trainer's own confidence in the effectiveness of the program. *Adherence confidence* refers to how strongly athletes believe they can complete the prescribed exercise program. This factor can be enhanced by showing the athlete that skills learned in sports, such as goal-setting and understanding the process of rehabilitation, can heighten success in the rehabilitation program. *Physical confidence* is knowing that the athlete's body is capable of handling the demands placed on it during rehabilitation and subsequent competition. Responding well to the rigors of the exercise program, maintaining a positive attitude about the ups and downs of rehabilitation, and using imagery can enhance this factor. *Return-to-sport confidence* relates to the athlete believing that he or she is returning to competition at, or better, than the preinjury status (5).

MOTIVATION

Motivation has the greatest influence on adherence in rehabilitation. Low motivation can result in poor attendance, incomplete exercises, low effort and intensity, lack of attentiveness to instructions, undefined goals, using unspecified pain to avoid exercise, and insupportable excuses. The athletic trainer can enhance motivation through goal setting, reminding the athlete that rehabilitation is a type of athletic performance, improving commitment, providing clear direction and the means to achieve full recovery, and offering deliberate steps to recovery. High motivation will build confidence, reduce anxiety and the perception of pain, and refocus the athlete's attention on the positive aspects of rehabilitation rather than on the negative aspects (5).

ANXIETY

Anxiety is the negative and threatening psychological and physical reaction to the injury, and produces a wide range of physical, cognitive, emotional, social, and performance problems. Many of these signs and symptoms can be seen in **Box 7.2**. Anxiety is often caused by a number of factors, such as pain, slow healing, low confidence, pressure from others, and a lack of familiarity, predictability, and control. Anxiety can restrict oxygen intake and blood flow, increase muscle tension and pain, reduce confidence and motivation, and lead the athlete to focus on the negative, rather than the positive, aspects of rehabilitation. Athletes can control anxiety by using deep breathing, passive and active relaxation, soothing music, smiling, and therapeutic massage. A rehabilitation routine can benefit the athlete's recovery by encompassing all the activities necessary for total preparation, including a review of the goals for that day, mental preparation to ensure prime confidence, motivation, intensity, and focus, and physical preparation such as stretching and warm-up (5).

➤ ➤ **BOX 7.2**

Signs and Symptoms of Anxiety in Rehabilitation

Physical	Muscle tension and bracing; short, choppy breathing; decreased coordination; fatigue; rushed speech; minor secondary injuries or nagging illness with recurrent physical complaints; and sleeping problems.
Cognitive	Excessive negativity and overly self-critical, statements of low confidence in rehabilitation, extreme thinking and unrealistic expectations, and very narrow focus.
Emotional	Anger, depression, irritability, moodiness, and impatience.
Social	Decreased communication, social withdrawal, intolerance and abruptness with others.
Performance	Overall decline in motivation and enjoyment in rehabilitation, loss of interest in sports and other activities, nervousness and physical tension during therapy, trying too hard in therapy or "giving up" in response to obstacles and setbacks, and decrease in school or work performance.

FOCUS

Often misunderstood and ignored, focus is critical in the rehabilitation process. In essence, **focus** is the ability to perceive and address various internal (thoughts, emotions, physical responses) and external (sights, sounds) cues and, when needed, to shift focus to other cues in a natural, effortless manner. Focus differs from concentration in that concentration is usually linked to the ability to attend to one thing for a long period of time. In contrast, focus is the ability to attend to various cues occurring simultaneously, and shift focus when the need arises. For example, an athlete may be executing an exercise and have to shift her focus externally to listen to your instructions for an exercise. Then she will shift her focus internally as she consciously monitors the intensity and any pain she may be experiencing. The ability to focus is often compared to the beam of a Mag-Lite flashlight in that the beam can be adjusted to illuminate a wide area or focused to brighten a narrow area (5).

Cues that interfere with rehabilitation include negative thoughts, anxiety, pain (as an inhibitor), preoccupation with the injury after returning to sport participation, peer pressure to recover quickly, any distraction during physical therapy, and comparisons to others upon return to sport. Facilitating cues may include pain (as information), proprioceptive responses, physical dimensions such as range of motion and strength, information that the athletic trainer provides, support from others, and feedback from the therapeutic exercise equipment. In order to maintain one's prime focus, the athlete must balance the focus on short- and long-term goals, and pay attention to the four principles (Ps) of focus. In general, the athlete should focus on the:

- *Positive* attributes of the rehabilitation rather than the negative.
- *Present* time rather than the past.
- *Process* and what needs to be done on a day-to-day basis to enhance recovery.
- *Progress* as the athlete moves through the rehabilitation program.

The athlete must also avoid being distracted during the exercise session. Too often, distractions in the room (noise, talking, music) can result in the athlete redirecting his or her eyes and attention toward something else rather than internally focusing on the exercise. It is important to learn to control the eyes and only process information that will be of benefit, such as instructions on how to complete the exercise. The use of keywords and rehabilitation imagery may also be helpful. For example, if muscle tension is present, a keyword for this exercise might be relax, or the individual might imagine the muscle relaxing and elongating. Each of these cues help focus the athlete on the task at hand.

PAIN MANAGEMENT

Pain is the most debilitating obstacle to overcome in rehabilitation. It can have significant physical, psychological, and emotional effects on the individual. Athletes must be able to differentiate between benign and harmful pain. **Benign pain** is usually characterized as dull, generalized, not lasting long after exertion, and not associated with swelling, localized tenderness, or long-term soreness. In contrast, **harmful pain** is sharp, localized to the injury site, experienced during and persisting after exertion, and usually is associated with swelling, localized tenderness, and prolonged soreness.

Although pain can be controlled with medication, athletes can use nonpharmacological means to control pain in two manners, namely pain reduction and pain focusing (see **Box 7.3**). Pain reduction techniques (muscle relaxation training, deep breathing, meditation, therapeutic massage) directly affect the physiological aspects of pain by decreasing the actual amount of pain that is present. Pain focusing directs attention onto (association) or away from (dissocia-

---

➤➤ Box 7.3

Pain Management Techniques

PAIN REDUCTION

Deep breathing	Emphasize slow, deep, rhythmical breathing
Muscle relaxation	Passive or progressive relaxation
Meditation	Repetitive focusing on mantra or breathing
Therapeutic massage	Manual manipulation of muscles, tendons, and ligaments (See Chapter 6)

PAIN FOCUSING

External focus	Listening to relaxing or inspiring music; watching a movie; playing chess
Soothing imagery	Generating calming images (lying on a beach, floating in space)
Neutral imaginings	Imagining playing chess or building a model airplane
Rhythmic cognitive activity	Saying the alphabet backwards; meditation
Pain acknowledgment	Giving pain a "hot" color, such as red, then changing it to a less painful "cool" color, such as blue
Dramatic coping	Seeing pain as part of an epic challenge to overcome insurmountable odds
Situational assessment	Evaluating the causes of pain to take steps to reduce it

Reprinted with permission from Taylor and Taylor (5), page 229.

tion) the pain by reducing or altering the perception of pain. Strategies for focusing pain include external focus, such as emotionally powerful or intellectually absorbing activities, pleasant or neutral imaging, rhythmic cognitive activity, dramatic coping, and situational assessment (5).

Interventions

Knowing that an athlete may be very concerned about the physical, psychological, social, and performance ramifications of his or her injury, the athletic trainer can help the athlete confront and overcome the concerns by using a variety of techniques. The more common techniques are discussed below.

COGNITIVE RESTRUCTURING

The athletic trainer should recognize when negative thinking creeps into the rehabilitation process. By restructuring how the athlete views the process, the negative effects can be limited. For example, if the athlete is distressed over the anticipated length of time the exercise program will continue, the athletic trainer might point out how the injury can allow the athlete time to rest and catch up with his or her studies, complete other projects that have been neglected, or simply reevaluate priorities and enjoy the absence of pressure from constant training and competition.

CONCENTRATION SKILLS

Success upon return to sport can be enhanced by teaching the athlete how to focus on skills that will help overcome negative progress. Eating correctly, getting plenty of rest, effectively managing time, and avoiding situations that may lead to reinjury can all help accomplish certain goals during the rehabilitation program.

CONFIDENCE TRAINING

The athlete should be encouraged to direct his or her own course of action and "choose" to succeed. The athlete is made aware of the internal and external factors that affect confidence, and is taught to use those factors to his or her benefit.

COPING REHEARSAL

Use of a performance-enhancing audiotape or videotape can prepare the athlete for challenges ahead. The information allows the athlete to think about several issues that may confront the athlete when he or she returns to sport participation. This allows the athlete to focus on the issues and develop strategies to overcome them prior to actually returning to sport participation.

IMAGERY

Imagery has long been used in the training process to help athletes mentally execute a skill prior to actually performing the skill. In the rehabilitation process, imagery can be used to mentally practice the skills or processes that will hasten a safe return to activity, such as envisioning healing, soothing (pain management), or performance (proper technique of an exercise). Imagery can also be enhanced by preceding it with relaxation exercises, such as passive or progressive relaxation. Relaxation can reduce anxiety and the physical manifestations of pain, and increase the vividness and control in imagery. Mental imagery can serve to motivate the athlete in realizing that this technique can facilitate the athlete's performance upon return to sport activity.

POSITIVE SELF-TALK

When injured, athletes often express negative feelings about the injury, themselves, and occasionally their coaches and teammates. These negative feelings inhibit the athlete and produce a self-defeating attitude. The athletic trainer can redirect these thoughts and feelings into positive, task-oriented thoughts that direct and motivate the athlete to succeed in the rehabilitation process.

The Athletic Trainer's Role

The cognitive, or knowledge, appraisal and response to injury is influenced by the athlete's recognition of the injury, understanding of the goal adjustments, and the athlete's belief that he or she directly influences the success of the exercise program. However, the athletic trainer must not negate the emotional responses that will be exhibited throughout the exercise program. Seriously injured individuals may fear social isolation and loss of income or potential scholarships. This fear of the unknown may lead to increased tension, anger, and depression during the exercise period. If the athlete does not perceive a gradual rate of recovery, frustration and boredom may deter a successful outcome. The athletic trainer should encourage the injured athlete to develop a positive attitude by using social support networks and psychological skills to manage pain, thus directing the athlete's energies into compliance with the treatment protocols. Positive encouragement may allow the athlete to feel better about pushing himself or herself to a higher intensity despite discomfort, fatigue, or pain.

It is critical that the sports medicine team include the athlete as an integral part of the rehabilitation process. This is especially important when goals are established that direct the exercise program. The goals must be realistic and provide some means to measure progress so the athlete can perceive a gradual rate of recovery. Whenever possible, the rehabilitation program should mirror the individual's regular training program, including the level of intensity, frequency, and duration. In some cases, activity modification and creativity may enable the competitive athlete to do limited exercise with the team. This may reduce the feeling of isolation and being left out of daily interaction with the coach and other players. Using graphs or charts to document progress can also help the individual see improvement. The athletic trainer must develop a positive professional relationship with the athlete to assist the athlete in recovering physically and psychologically from the injury.

Referral for Psychological Problems

Athletic trainers seldom have the extensive understanding or clinical training to handle psychological problems. In a recent survey of athletic trainers, 90% indicated that it was important to address the psychological aspects of an injury, but less than 25% had ever referred an athlete for counseling due to the injury, and only 8% had a standard procedure for referral (6). A clearly defined and well-organized procedural plan should be developed to guide the athletic trainer's actions and ensure confidentiality (see **Box 7.4**). Initially, criteria should be developed that establish when psychological distress or clinical issues are evident. During

> ### ▶▶ BOX 7.4
>
> ## Psychological Distress Checklist for Possible Referral
>
> Directions. Place a √ next to each behavior that you observe on a consistent basis in an athlete. The persistent presence of any of these behaviors may warrant a referral. The more items that are checked, the greater the need for a referral.
>
> 1. ___ Not accepting injury
> 2. ___ Denying seriousness or extent of injury
> 3. ___ Displaying depression
> 4. ___ Displaying anger
> 5. ___ Displaying apprehension or anxiety
> 6. ___ Failing to take responsibility for own rehabilitation
> 7. ___ Not adhering to rehabilitation program
> 8. ___ Missing appointments
> 9. ___ Overdoing rehabilitation
> 10. ___ Not cooperating with rehabilitation professional
> 11. ___ Bargaining with rehabilitation professional over treatment or time out of competition
> 12. ___ Frequent negative statements about injury and rehabilitation
> 13. ___ Reduced effort in physical therapy
> 14. ___ Poor focus and intensity in physical therapy
> 15. ___ Unconfirmable reports of pain
> 16. ___ Interfering behaviors outside of rehabilitation, e.g., using injured area
> 17. ___ Inappropriate emotions
> 18. ___ Emotional swings
>
> Reprinted with permission from Taylor (5), page 70.

rehabilitation, several psychological factors can arise, including anxiety, depression, anger, pain, and treatment noncompliance.

As a general rule, any psychological difficulty that persists for more than a few days and interferes with the progress of rehabilitation should be referred to a licensed clinical psychologist or an appropriate counseling center. Failure to address the issues can lead to an escalation in the distress and frustration of the athlete. When a concern arises, the athletic trainer can telephone the clinical psychologist to discuss the symptoms and determine if the athlete should be referred. If a decision is made to refer the athlete, it should be discussed with the athlete to facilitate the process. It should be pointed out that the referral is a positive step in helping the athlete recover and return to sport participation. If possible, it may be advantageous to mention the previous use of a psychologist who had helped other athletes recover. In this manner, the athlete is likely to view the referral as a normal and positive aspect of the rehabilitation process (6,7).

Once referral has been made, it is important for the athletic trainer to follow up with the clinical psychologist and provide any additional information about the athlete's progress. Remember that ethical considerations prohibit mental health professionals from discussing cases with third parties unless the patient gives explicit written permission. In cases involving athletes, it would be beneficial to get this permission in advance, to allow the psychologist and athletic trainer to discuss the athlete's condition and develop strategies to facilitate the rehabilitation process.

Locating an individual with the qualifications and clinical experience of working in a sports rehabilitation setting can be difficult. It may be helpful to investigate the availability of personnel in college and university settings. Many schools may have a clinical psychologist on staff experienced in sports injury rehabilitation. Area hospitals may also be contacted, since many have a psychiatric or psychology department with a clinical psychologist who works with various rehabilitation issues.

 The soccer player is unable to participate for the remainder of the season. Clearly, his emotional and psychological state will have a direct impact on the success or failure of the therapeutic exercise program. Goal setting and intervention strategies can address many psychological influences that may inhibit the program. If progress is inhibited for several days because of suspected psychological issues, the athletic trainer should contact a more highly trained clinical professional for referral.

DEVELOPING A THERAPEUTIC EXERCISE PROGRAM

 The high school soccer player has Achilles tendinitis. Pain increased with active plantar flexion, and

there was an accompanying muscle weakness in plantar flexion. What short- and long-term goals might the athletic trainer and the athlete establish for the therapeutic exercise program? How will progress be measured?

In designing an individualized therapeutic exercise program, several sequential steps help identify the needs of the patient (see **Box 7.5**). First, the individual's level of function is assessed, including range of motion, muscle strength, neurologic integrity, joint stability, and quality of functional activities. Second, the assessment is interpreted, to identify primary and secondary structural or functional deficits. Based on these deficits, lists of short- and long-term goals are established to return the athlete safely to participation. An exercise program is then developed to address each problem. This process is ongoing. As continued assessment of the exercise program occurs, alterations in short-term goals may result in changes in treatment or exercise progression. The process is dependent on the patient's progress and adaptation to the therapeutic exercise program.

Assess the Patient

The subjection evaluation (history of the injury) is recorded in the **Subjective**, or **S**, portion of the SOAP note. This information should include the primary complaint, mechanism of injury, characteristics of the symptoms, functional impairments, previous injuries to the area, and family history. The objective evaluation (observation and inspection, palpation, physical examination tests) establishes a baseline of measurable information, and is recorded in the **Objective**, or **O**, portion of the SOAP note. This information documents the visual analysis of the injury site, symmetry and appearance, determines the presence of a possible fracture, identifies abnormal clinical findings in the bony and soft tissue structures at the injury site, and measures functional testing (active, passive, and resisted range of motion), ligamentous and capsular integrity, neurologic testing, and sport-specific functional testing. In paired body segments, the dysfunction of the injured body part is always compared to the noninjured body part to establish standards for bilateral functional status.

Interpret the Assessment

When assessment is completed, the data is interpreted to identify factors outside normal limits for an individual of the same age and fitness level. Primary deficits or weaknesses are identified. These deficits, along with secondary problems resulting from prolonged immobilization, extended inactivity, or lack of intervention, are organized into a priority list of concerns. Examples of major concerns may include decreased range of motion, muscle weakness or stiffness, joint contractures, sensory changes, inability to walk without a limp, or increased pain with activity. Physical assets are then identified to determine the individual's present functional status. For example, normal gait and bilateral, equal range of motion should be documented. From the two lists, specific problems are then recorded in a section called the *Problem List*, which is a part of the **Assessment**, or **A**, portion of the SOAP note.

Establish Goals

Long-term goals are then established for the individual's expected level of performance at the conclusion of the exercise program and typically focus on functional deficits in performing activities of daily living (ADLs). These goals might include bilateral, equal range of motion, flexibility, muscular strength, endurance, and power; relaxation training; and restoration of coordination and cardiovascular endurance. Next, short-term goals are developed to address the specific component skills needed to reach the long-term goals. The athletic trainer and patient should discuss and develop the goals. The athlete must feel a part of the process, as this may educate and motivate the individual to work harder to attain the stated goals. Many sport-specific factors, such as the demands of the sport; position played; time remaining in the season; regular-season versus postseason or tournament play; game rules and regulations regarding prosthetic braces or safety equipment; the location, nature, and severity of injury; and the mental state of the athlete, may affect goal development.

The short-term goals are developed in a graduated sequence to address the list of problems identified during the assessment. For example, a high-priority short-term goal is the control of pain, inflammation, and spasm. Each short-term goal should be moderately difficult, yet realistic. Specific subgoals should include an estimated time table needed to attain that goal. These subgoals are time dependent, but not fixed, as it is important to take into consideration individual differences in preinjury fitness and functional status, severity of injury, motivation to complete the goals, and subsequent improvement. Constant reinforcement from the athletic trainer to achieve the subgoals can be an incentive to continually progress toward the long-

---

➤➤ **BOX 7.5**

The Rehabilitation Process

1. Assess the present level of function and dysfunction from girth measurements, goniometric assessment, strength tests, neurologic assessment, stress tests, and functional activities.
2. Organize and interpret the assessment to identify factors outside normal limits.
3. Establish short- and long-term goals.
4. Develop and supervise the treatment plan, incorporating therapeutic exercise, therapeutic modalities, and medication.
5. Reassess the progress of the plan, and adjust as needed.

term goals. Long- and short-term goals may be recorded in the Assessment, or A, portion of the note; however, many athletic trainers choose to begin the treatment plan, or P, portion of the note with the objectives. Possible short-term goals for the injured soccer player can be seen in **Box 7.6**.

Develop and Supervise the Treatment Plan

Any therapeutic exercise and therapeutic modality used to achieve the goals is recorded in the **Plan**, or **P**, section of the note, along with any medications prescribed by the physician. In order to return the individual safely to participation, the therapeutic exercise program is divided into four phases. The termination of one phase and initiation of the next may overlap. However, each phase has a specific role. In phase one, the inflammatory response, pain, swell-

ing, and ecchymosis are controlled. Phase two regains any deficits in range of motion at the affected joint and begins to restore proprioception. Phase three regains muscle strength, endurance, and power in the affected limb. Phase four prepares the individual to return to activity and includes sport-specific skill training, regaining coordination, and improving cardiovascular conditioning. These phases and their expected outcomes are discussed in more detail later in the chapter. **Box 7.7** lists the various phases of a therapeutic exercise program.

➤➤ **B o x 7.6**

Short-Term Goals

Week	Goals
1	Control inflammation, pain, and swelling in the right Achilles tendon region
	Restore bilateral active range of motion (ROM) and passive range of motion (PROM), as tolerated
	Protect the involved area, and decrease activity level
	Maintain strength at the knee, ankle, and foot
	Maintain cardiovascular endurance with weight-bearing exercise
2	Restore full bilateral AROM and PROM at the ankle
	Initiate strengthening exercises for the affected lower leg
	Restore bilateral strength at the knee, ankle, and foot
	Maintain cardiovascular endurance and general body strength
2-3	Improve strength of plantar flexors from fair to good
	Maintain full ROM at the knee, ankle, and foot
	Improve cardiovascular endurance
	Begin sport-specific functional patterns with no resistance
3-4	Increase muscle strength, endurance, and power in the lower leg
	Improve cardiovascular endurance
	Restore sport-specific functional patterns with moderate resistance
	Begin functional return to activity with necessary modification
4-5	Improve general body strength, endurance, and power
	Improve cardiovascular endurance
	Increase speed and resistance on sport-specific skills
	Return to full functional activity as tolerated

➤➤ **B o x 7.7**

The Therapeutic Exercise Program

Phase One: Control Inflammation

- Control inflammatory stage and minimize scar tissue with cryotherapy using **PRICE** principles (**P**rotect, **R**estrict activity, **I**ce, **C**ompression, and **E**levation)
- Instruct patient on relaxation and coping techniques
- Maintain range of motion, joint flexibility, strength, endurance, and power in the unaffected body parts
- Maintain cardiovascular endurance

Phase Two: Restore Motion

- Restore ROM to within 80% of normal in the unaffected limb
- Restore joint flexibility as observed in the unaffected limb
- Begin proprioceptive stimulation through closed isotonic chain exercises
- Begin pain-free, isometric strengthening exercises on the affected limb
- Begin unresisted, pain-free functional patterns of sport-specific motion
- Maintain muscular strength, endurance, and power in unaffected muscles
- Maintain cardiovascular endurance

Phase Three: Develop Muscular Strength, Power, and Endurance

- Restore full ROM and proprioception in the affected limb
- Restore muscular strength, endurance, and power using progressive resisted exercise
- Maintain cardiovascular endurance
- Initiate minimal-to-moderate resistance in sport-specific functional patterns

Phase Four: Return to Sport Activity

- Analyze skill performance, and correct biomechanical inefficiencies in motion
- Improve muscular strength, endurance, and power
- Restore coordination and balance
- Improve cardiovascular endurance
- Increase sport-specific functional patterns, and return to protected activity as tolerated

Each phase of the exercise program is supervised and documented. In addition, progress notes are completed on a weekly or biweekly basis. In many health care settings, these records are also used for third party reimbursement of services rendered. They also provide documentation of services provided to an individual should litigation occur.

Reassess the Progress of the Program

Short-term goals should be flexible enough to accommodate the progress of the individual. For example, if therapeutic modalities or medications are used, and the individual attains a short-term goal sooner than expected, a new short-term goal should be written. It is possible that some conditions, such as edema, hemorrhage, muscle spasm, atrophy, or infection, may impede the healing process and delay attaining a short-term goal. Periodic measurement of girth, range of motion, muscle strength, endurance, power, and cardiovascular fitness will determine whether progress occurs. If progress is not seen, the individual should be re-evaluated. The athletic trainer must determine if the delay is due to physical problems, noncompliance, or to psychological influences, necessitating referral to the appropriate specialist (e.g., physician or clinical psychologist). The individual can then continue to progress through the short-term goals until the long-term goals are attained, and the athlete is cleared for full activity.

 Long-term goals for the soccer player might include: pain-free bilateral range of motion, muscle strength, endurance, and power; maintenance of cardiovascular endurance; restoration of normal joint biomechanics; increased proprioception and coordination; restoration of bilateral function of ADLs; and pain-free, unlimited motion in sport-specific skills. Short-term goals were listed in Box 7.6.

PHASE ONE: CONTROLLING INFLAMMATION

 The soccer player has pain and tenderness over the distal portion of the Achilles tendon, and weakness in active plantar flexion. In following acute care protocol, a crushed ice pack was applied to the area. Would it be appropriate to begin any rehabilitation exercises during this initial phase of injury management?

Phase one of the exercise program begins immediately after injury assessment. The primary goal is to control inflammation by limiting hemorrhage, edema, effusion, muscle spasm, and pain. The individual can move into phase two when the following criteria have been attained:

- Control of inflammation with minimal edema, swelling, muscle spasm, and pain

- Range of motion, joint flexibility, muscular strength, endurance, and power are maintained in the general body
- Cardiovascular fitness is maintained at the preinjury level

Collagenous scar formation, a natural component of the repair and regeneration of injured soft tissue, is less efficient and tolerant of tensile forces than the original mature tissue. The length of the inflammatory response is a key factor that influences the ultimate stability and function of scar tissue. The longer the inflammatory process progresses, the more likely the resulting scar tissue will be less dense and weaker in yielding to applied stress. Furthermore, immobilization for more than 2 or 3 weeks may lead to joint adhesions that inhibit muscle fiber regeneration. Therefore, all inflammatory symptoms need to be controlled as soon as possible. **PRICE**, a well-known acronym for protect, restrict activity, ice, compression, and elevation, is used to reduce acute symptoms at an injury site.

Control of Inflammation

Following trauma, hemorrhage and edema at the injury site lead to a pooling of tissue fluids and blood products that increases pain and muscle spasm. The increased pressure decreases blood flow to the injury site, leading to hypoxia (deficiency of oxygen). As pain continues, the threshold of pain is lowered. These events lead to the cyclical pattern of pain-spasm-hypoxia-pain. For this reason, cryotherapy (ice, compression, and elevation) is preferred during the acute inflammation to decrease circulation, cellular metabolism, the need for oxygen, and the conduction velocity of nerve impulses to break the pain-spasm cycle. An elastic compression wrap can decrease hemorrhage and hematoma formation, yet still expand in cases of extreme swelling. Elevation uses gravity to reduce pooling of fluids and pressure inside the venous and lymphatic vessels, to prevent fluid from filtering into surrounding tissue spaces. The result is less tissue necrosis and local waste, leading to a shorter inflammatory phase. **Field Strategy 7.1** explains acute care of soft tissue injuries using the PRICE principle.

Cryotherapy, intermittent compression, and electrical muscle stimulation (EMS) may be used to control hemorrhage and eliminate edema. Electrical therapy has also been shown to decrease pain and muscle spasm, strengthen weakened muscles, improve blood flow to an area, and enhance the healing rate of injured tendons. Transcutaneous electrical nerve stimulation (TENS) might also be used to limit pain (see Chapter 6). The modality of choice is determined by the size and location of the injured area, availability of the modality, and preference of the supervising health care provider. A decision to discontinue treatment and move to another modality should be based on the cessation of inflammation. Placing the back of the hand

---

FIELD STRATEGY 7.1   **ACUTE CARE OF SOFT TISSUE INJURIES**

<u>ICE APPLICATION</u>

- Apply crushed ice for 30 minutes directly to the skin (40 minutes for a large muscle mass such as the quadriceps).
- Ice applications should be repeated every 2 hours when awake (every hour if the athlete is active), and may extend to 72+ hours postinjury.
- Skin temperature can indicate when acute swelling has subsided. For example, if the area (compared bilaterally) feels warm to the touch, swelling continues. If in doubt, it is better to extend the time of a cold application.

<u>COMPRESSION</u>

- On an extremity, apply the wrap in a distal-to-proximal direction to avoid forcing extracellular fluid into the distal digits.
- Take a distal pulse after applying the wrap to ensure the wrap is not overly tight.
- Felt horseshoe-pads placed around the malleolus may be combined with an elastic wrap or tape to limit ankle swelling.
- Maintain compression continuously on the injury for the first 24 hours.

<u>ELEVATION</u>

- Elevate the body part 6 to 10 inches above the level of the heart.
- While sleeping, place a hard suitcase between the mattress and boxspring, or place the extremity on a series of pillows.

<u>RESTRICT ACTIVITY AND PROTECT THE AREA</u>

- If the individual is unable to walk without a limp, fit the person for crutches and apply an appropriate protective device to limit unnecessary movement of the injured joint.
- If the individual has an upper extremity injury and is unable to move the limb without pain, fit the person with an appropriate sling or brace.

---

over the injured site will show any temperature change as compared to an uninjured area. Increased heat may indicate inflammation and edema are still present. A cooler area may indicate diminished circulation in an area.

Effects of Immobilization

The effects of immobilization on the various tissues of the body have been extensively covered in the literature. It is well accepted that muscle tension, muscle and ligament atrophy, decreased circulation, and loss of motion prolong the repair and regeneration of damaged tissues.

MUSCLE

Immobilization can lead to a loss of muscle strength within 24 hours. This is manifested with decreases in muscle fiber size, total muscle weight, mitochondria (energy source of the cell) size and number, muscle tension produced, and resting levels of glycogen and ATP, which reduces muscle endurance. Motor nerves become less efficient in recruiting and stimulating muscle fibers. Immobilization also increases muscle fatigability as a result of decreased oxidative capacity. The rate of loss appears to be more rapid during the initial days of immobilization; however, after 5 to 7 days, the loss of muscle mass dimin-

ishes (8). Although both slow-twitch (type I) and fast-twitch (type II) muscle fibers atrophy, it is generally accepted that with immobilization, there is a greater degeneration of slow-twitch fibers. Muscles immobilized in a lengthened or neutral position maintain muscle weight and fiber cross-sectional area better than muscles immobilized in a shortened position. When shortened, the length of the fibers decreases, leading to increased connective tissue and reduced muscle extensibility. Muscles immobilized in a shortened position atrophy faster and have a greater loss of contractile function.

ARTICULAR CARTILAGE

The greatest impact of immobilization occurs to the articular cartilage, with adverse changes appearing within 1 week of immobilization. The effects depend on the length of immobilization, position of the joint, and joint loading. Intermittent loading and unloading of synovial joints is necessary to ensure proper metabolic exchange necessary for normal function. Constant contact with opposing bone ends can lead to pressure necrosis and cartilage cell (chondrocyte) death. In contrast, noncontact between two surfaces promotes growth of connective tissue into the joint. Diminished weight bearing, and loading and unloading, can also increase bone resorption. In general, articular cartilage will soften and decrease in thickness. Immobilization longer than 30 days can lead to progressive osteoarthritis.

LIGAMENTS

Similar to bone, ligaments adapt to normal stress by remodeling in response to the mechanical demands placed on them. Stress leads to a stiffer, stronger ligament, whereas immobilization leads to a weaker, more compliant structure. This causes a decrease in the tensile strength, thus reducing the ability of ligaments to provide joint stability.

BONE

Mechanical strain on a bone affects the osteoblastic (bone cell formation) and osteoclastic (bone cell resorption) activity on the bone surface. The effects of immobilization on bone, accordingly, are similar to other connective tissues. Limited weight bearing and muscle activity lead to bone loss, and can be detected as early as 2 weeks after immobilization (8). As immobilization time increases, bone resorption occurs, resulting in the bones becoming more brittle and highly susceptible to fracture. Disuse atrophy appears to increase bone loss at a rate 5 to 20 times greater than that resulting from metabolic disorders affecting bone (9). Therefore, non-weight-bearing immobilization should be limited to as short a time as possible.

Effects of Remobilization

Early controlled mobilization can speed the healing process. Bone and soft tissue will respond to the physical demands placed on them, causing the formation of collagen to remodel or realign along the lines of stress, thus promoting healthy joint biomechanics (**Wolff's law**). Continuous passive motion (CPM) can prevent joint adhesions and stiffness, and decrease joint hemarthrosis (blood in the joint) and pain. Early motion, and loading and unloading of joints, through partial weight-bearing exercise maintains joint lubrication to nourish articular cartilage, menisci, and ligaments. This leads to an optimal environment for proper collagen fibril formation. Tissues recover at different rates with mobilization; muscle recovers faster, and articular cartilage and bone respond least favorably.

MUSCLE

Within 3 to 5 days after mobilization, muscle regeneration begins. After 6 weeks, both fast-twitch and slow-twitch muscle fibers can completely recover. Muscle contractile activity rapidly increases protein synthesis. However, maximal isometric tension may not return to normal until 4 months after mobilized activity. The use of electrotherapy (EMS) may be helpful in reeducating muscles, limiting pain and spasm, and decreasing effusion through the pumping action of the contracting muscle. Unfortu-

nately, neither EMS or isometric exercise has been shown to prevent disuse atrophy.

ARTICULAR CARTILAGE

The effects of immobilization, whether there is contact or loss of contact between joint surfaces, can adversely interfere with cartilage nutrition. Articular cartilage generally responds favorably to mechanical stimuli, with structural modifications noted after exercise. Soft tissue changes are reversible if immobilization does not exceed 30 days. These structural changes may not be reversible if immobilization exceeds 30 days.

LIGAMENTS

The bone-ligament junction recovers slower than the mechanical properties in the midportion of the ligament. In addition, other nontraumatized ligaments weaken with disuse. Recovery depends on the duration of immobilization. Studies have shown that, following 12 weeks of immobilization, there was a recovery of 50% of normal strength in a healing ligament after 6 months, 80% after 1 year, and 100% after 1 to 3 years, depending on the type of stresses placed on the ligament and on the prevention of repeated injury (10). Although the properties of ligaments return to normal with remobilization, the bone-ligament junction will take longer to return to normal. This factor must be considered when planning a rehabilitation program.

BONE

Although bone lost during immobilization may be regained, the period of recovery can be several times greater than the period of immobilization. In disuse osteoporosis, a condition involving reduced quantity of bone tissue, bone loss may not be reversible upon remobilization of the limb. Isotonic and isometric exercises during the immobilization period can decrease some bone loss and can hasten recovery after returning to a normal loading environment.

Protection After Injury

The type of protection selected and length of activity modification depend on injury severity, structures damaged, and the philosophy of the supervising health care provider. Several materials can be used to protect the area, including elastic wraps, tape, pads, slings, hinged braces, splints, casts, and crutches. Many of these items were discussed and illustrated in Chapter 3. If an individual cannot walk without pain or walks with a limp, crutches should be recommended. Proper crutch fitting and use are summarized in **Field Strategy 7.2**.

Restricted activity does not imply cessation of activity but simply means "relative rest," decreasing activity to a level below that required in sport, but tolerated by the

FIELD STRATEGY 7.2   FITTING AND USING CRUTCHES AND CANES

FITTING CRUTCHES

1. Have the individual stand erect in flat shoes with the feet close together.
2. Place the crutch tip 2 inches in front, and 6 inches from the outer sole, of the shoe.
3. Adjust crutch height to allow a space of about 2 finger widths between the crutch pad and the axillary skin fold, to avoid undue pressure on neurovascular structures.
4. Adjust the hand grip so the elbow is flexed 25 to 30°, and is at the level of the hip joint (greater trochanter).

FITTING FOR A CANE

1. Place the individual in the same position as above. Adjust the hand grip so the elbow is flexed at 25 to 30°, and is at the level of the hip joint (greater trochanter).

SWING THROUGH GAIT (NON-WEIGHT-BEARING)

1. Stand on the uninvolved leg. Lean forward and place both crutches and the involved leg approximately 12 to 24 inches in front of the body.
2. Body weight should rest on the hands, not the axillary pads.
3. With the good leg, step through the crutches as if taking a normal step. Repeat process.
4. If possible, the involved leg should be extended while swinging forward to prevent atrophy of the quadriceps muscles.

THREE POINT GAIT (PARTIAL WEIGHT-BEARING)

1. Indicated when one extremity can support the body weight, and the injured extremity is to be touched down, or to bear weight partially.
2. As tolerated, place as much body weight as possible onto the involved leg, taking the rest of the weight on the hands.
3. Make sure a good heel-toe technique is used, whereby the heel strikes first, then the weight is shifted to the ball of the foot.
4. Increase the amount of weight bearing by decreasing the force transferred through the arms; mimic a normal gait.

GOING UP AND DOWN STAIRS

1. Place both crutches under the arm opposite the handrail.
2. To go **up** the stairs, step **up with the good leg** while leaning on the rail.
3. To go **down** the stairs, place the crutches down on the next step and step **down with the involved leg.**

USING ONE CRUTCH OR CANE

1. Place one crutch or cane on the uninvolved side and move it forward with the involved leg.
2. Do not lean heavily on the crutch or cane.

recently injured tissue or joint. **Detraining**, or loss of the benefits gained in physical training, can occur after only 1 to 2 weeks of nonactivity, with significant decreases measured in both metabolic and working capacity (11). Strengthening exercises in a weight-lifting program can be alternated with cardiovascular exercises such as jogging or swimming, or use of a stationary bike, or upper body ergometer (UBE). These exercises can prevent the individual from experiencing depression as a result of inactivity, and can be done simultaneously with phase one exercises as long as the injured area is not irritated or inflamed.

After following acute care protocol in treating the Achilles tendon injury, early controlled mobilization, pain-free range-of-motion exercises at the ankle, and general load-bearing, strengthening,

and cardiovascular exercises may be completed as long as the injured area is not irritated.

PHASE TWO: RESTORATION OF MOTION

It is now 4 days postinjury. The acute inflammatory symptoms have subsided. What exercises can now be used to increase flexibility and strength in the Achilles tendon? Are there any modalities that could be used to supplement the exercise program?

After inflammation is controlled, phase two begins immediately. This phase focuses on restoring range of motion and flexibility at the injured site as well as continuing to maintain general body strength and cardiovascular endurance. The phase may begin as early as 4 days after the injury, when swelling has stopped, or may have to wait for several weeks. The injured site may still be tender to touch, but it is not as painful as in the earlier phase. Also, pain is much less evident on passive and active range of motion. If the athlete is in an immobilizer or splint, remove the splint for treatment and exercise. The splint can then be replaced to support and protect the injured site. The individual can move into phase three when the following criteria have been completed:

- Inflammation and pain are under control
- Range of motion is within 80% of normal in the unaffected limb
- Bilateral joint flexibility is restored and proprioception is regained
- Cardiovascular endurance and general body strength is maintained at the preinjury level

Assessment of normal range of motion should be done with a goniometer on the paired, uninjured joint (see Chapter 4). Cryotherapy may be used prior to exercise, to decrease perceived pain, or EMS or thermotherapy may be used to warm the tissues and increase circulation to the region. When the tissue is warmed, friction massage or joint mobilization may be helpful to break up scar tissue to regain normal motion.

Progression in this phase begins gradually with restoration of range of motion, proprioception, and total joint flexibility (see **Box 7.8**). Prolonged immobilization can lead to muscles losing their flexibility and assuming a shortened position, referred to as a **contracture**. Connective tissue around joints has no contractile properties. Connective tissue is supple and will elongate slowly with a sustained stretch; like muscle tissue though, it will adaptively shorten if immobilized. Connective tissue and muscles may be lengthened through passive and active stretching, and proprioceptive neuromuscular facilitation (PNF) exercises.

Passive Range of Motion (PROM)

Two types of movement must be present for normal motion to occur about a joint. Physiological motion, measured by a goniometer, occurs in the cardinal movement planes of flexion-extension, abduction-adduction, and rotation. Ac-

---

> ➤➤ **Box 7.8**

Factors that Limit Joint Motion
- Bony block
- Joint adhesions
- Muscle tightness
- Tight skin or an inelastic dense scar tissue
- Swelling
- Pain
- Fat or other soft tissues that block normal motion

> ➤➤ **Box 7.9**

Contraindications to Joint Mobilization

Acute inflammation	Malignancy
Advanced osteoarthritis	Neurologic signs
Congenital bone deformities	Osteoporosis
Fractures	Premature stressing of surgical structures
Hypermobility	Rheumatoid arthritis
Infections	Vascular disease

Reprinted with permission from Harrelson and Leaver-Dunn (18), page 159.

---

cessory motion, also referred to as **arthrokinematics**, is involuntary joint motion that occurs simultaneously with physiological motion, but cannot be measured precisely. Accessory movements involve the spinning, rolling, or gliding of one articular surface relative to another. Normal accessory movement must be present for full physiological range of motion to occur. If any accessory motion component is limited, normal physiological motion will not occur.

Limited passive range of motion is called **hypomobility**. These discrete limitations of motion prevent pain-free return to competition and predispose an individual to microtraumatic injuries that reinflame the old injury. Restoring passive range of motion prevents degenerative joint changes and promotes healing.

JOINT MOBILIZATION

Joint mobilization utilizes various oscillating forces applied in the open packed position to "free up" stiff joints. The oscillations produce several key benefits in the healing process. They:

- Break up adhesions and relieve capsular restrictions.
- Distract impacted tissues.
- Increase lubrication for normal articular cartilage.
- Reduce pain and muscle tension.
- Restore full range of motion and facilitate healing.

Joint mobilization, however, is contraindicated in several instances (see **Box 7.9**). Maitland described five grades of mobilization (12):

- *Grade I.* A small-amplitude movement at the beginning of the ROM. Used when pain and spasm limit movement early in the ROM.
- *Grade II.* Large-amplitude movement within the mid-range of motion. Used when spasm limits movement sooner with a quick oscillation than with a slow one, or when slowly increasing pain restricts movement halfway into the range.
- *Grade III.* A large-amplitude movement up to the pathologic limit in the range of motion. Used when

pain and resistance from spasm, inert tissue tension, or tissue compression limit movement near the end of the range.

- *Grade IV*. A small-amplitude movement at the very end of the range of motion. Used when resistance limits movement in the absence of pain and spasm.
- *Grade V*. A small-amplitude, quick thrust delivered at the end of the ROM, usually accompanied by a popping sound called a manipulation. Used when minimal resistance limits the end of the range. Manipulation is most effectively accomplished by the velocity of the thrust rather than the force of the thrust.

In performing joint mobilization, the individual is placed in a comfortable position with the joint placed in an open packed position. This allows the surrounding tissues to be as lax as possible and the intracapsular space to be at its greatest. The direction of force is dependent on the contour of the joint surface of the structure being mobilized. The concave-convex rule states that, when the concave surface is stationary and the convex surface is mobilized, a glide of the convex segment should be in the direction opposite to the restriction of joint movement. If the convex articular surface is stationary and the concave surface is mobilized, gliding of the concave segment should be in the same direction as the restriction of joint movement **(Figure 7.2)**. Typical treatment involves a series of three to six mobilizations lasting up to 30 seconds, with one to three oscillations per second (12). **Figure 7.3** demonstrates joint mobilization technique.

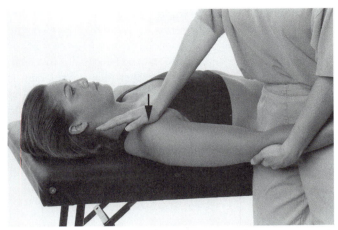

➤ **FIGURE 7.3 Joint mobilization technique**. Posterior humeral glide uses one hand to stabilize the humerus at the elbow while the other hand glides the humeral head in a posterior direction (indicated by the arrow) to increase flexion and medial rotation at the joint.

FLEXIBILITY

Flexibility is the total range of motion at a joint that occurs pain-free in each of the planes of motion. Joint flexibility is a combination of normal joint mechanics, mobility of soft tissues, and muscle extensibility. For example, the hip joint may have full passive range of motion, but when doing active hip flexion from a seated position, as in touching one's toes, resistance from tight hamstrings may limit full hip flexion. Resistance such as this may be generated from tension in muscle fibers or connective tissue.

Muscles contain two primary proprioceptors that can be stimulated during stretching: muscle spindles and Golgi tendon organs. Because muscle spindles lie parallel to muscle fibers, they stretch with the muscle **(Figure 7.4)**. When stimulated, the spindle sensory fibers discharge and through reflex action in the spinal cord initiate impulses to cause the muscle to contract reflexively, thus inhibiting the stretch. Muscles that perform the desired movement are called **agonists**. Unlike muscle spindles, Golgi tendon organs are connected in a series of fibers located in tendons and joint ligaments, and respond to muscle tension rather than length. If the stretch continues for an extended time (over 6 to 8 seconds), the Golgi tendons are stimulated. This stimulus, unlike the stimulus from muscle spindles, causes a reflex inhibition in the **antagonist** muscles. This sensory mechanism protects the musculotendinous unit from excessive tensile forces that could damage muscle fibers.

Flexibility can be increased through ballistic or static stretching techniques. **Ballistic stretching** uses repetitive bouncing motions at the end of the available range of motion. Muscle spindles are repetitively stretched, but because the bouncing motions are of short duration, the Golgi tendon organs do not fire. As such, the muscles resist relaxation. Because generated momentum may carry

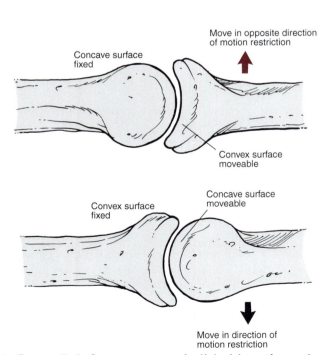

Move in opposite direction of motion restriction

Concave surface fixed

Convex surface moveable

Convex surface fixed

Concave surface moveable

Move in direction of motion restriction

➤ **FIGURE 7.2 Concave-convex rule**. If the joint surface to be moved is convex, mobilize it opposite the direction of motion restriction. If the joint surface of the body segment being moved is concave, move it in the direction of motion restriction.

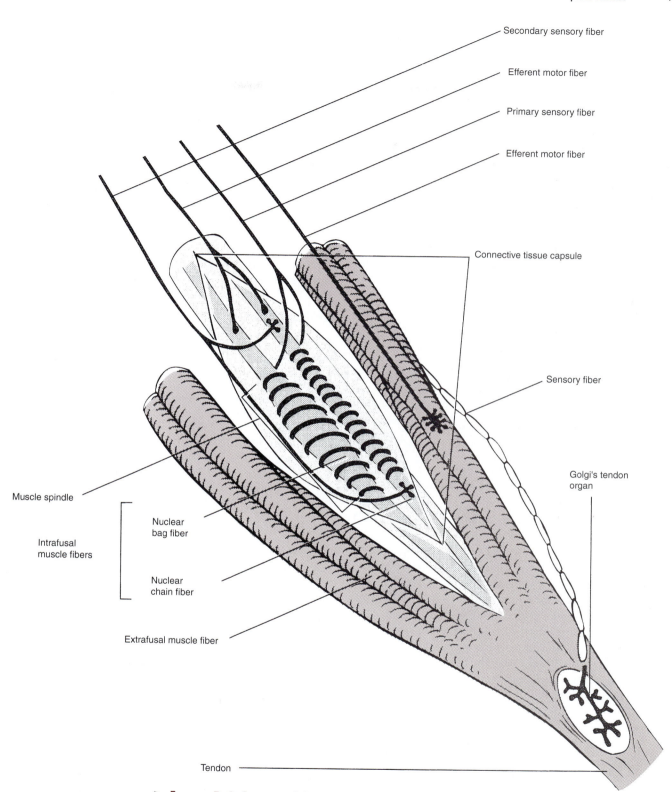

Secondary sensory fiber

Efferent motor fiber

Primary sensory fiber

Efferent motor fiber

Connective tissue capsule

Sensory fiber

Golgi's tendon organ

Muscle spindle

Intrafusal muscle fibers

Nuclear bag fiber

Nuclear chain fiber

Extrafusal muscle fiber

Tendon

➤ **FIGURE 7.4** **Anatomy of the muscle spindle and Golgi tendon organ**.

the body part beyond normal range of motion, the muscles being stretched often remain contracted to prevent overstretching, leading to microscopic tears in the musculotendinous unit. In a **static stretch**, movement is slow and deliberate (see **Box 7.10**). Golgi tendon organs are able to override impulses from the muscle spindles, leading to a safer, more effective muscle stretch. When the muscle is stretched to the point where a mild burn is felt, joint position is maintained statically for about 15 seconds and repeated several times. This technique is often used with vapocoolant sprays to desensitize myofascial trigger points.

Guidelines for Static Stretching to Improve Flexibility

1. Stretching is facilitated by warm body tissues. Therefore, a brief warm-up period is recommended. If it is not possible to jog lightly, stretching could be performed after a superficial heat treatment.
2. In the designated stretch position, position yourself so a sensation of tension is felt.
3. Do not bounce; hold the stretch for 10 to 30 seconds until a sense of relaxation occurs. Be aware of the feeling of relaxation, or "letting go." Repeat the stretch 6 to 8 times.
4. Breathe rhythmically and slowly. Exhale during the stretch.
5. Do not be overly aggressive in stretching. Increased flexibility may not be noticed for 4 to 6 weeks.
6. If an area is particularly resistant to stretching, partner stretching or proprioceptive neuromuscular facilitation (PNF) may be used.
7. Avoid vigorous stretching of tissues in the following conditions:
   - After a recent fracture
   - After prolonged immobilization
   - With acute inflammation or infection in or around the joint
   - With a bony block that limits motion
   - With muscle contractures or when joint adhesions limit motion
   - With acute pain during stretching

Proprioceptive neuromuscular facilitation (PNF) promotes and hastens the response of the neuromuscular system through stimulation of the proprioceptors. The athlete is taught how to perform the exercise through cutaneous and auditory input. The athlete often looks at the moving limb while the athletic trainer moves the limb from the starting to terminal position. Verbal cues are used to coordinate voluntary effort with reflex responses. Words such as "push" or "pull" are commonly used to ask for an isotonic contraction. "Hold" may be used for an isometric or stabilizing contraction, followed by "relax." Manual (cutaneous contact) helps to influence the direction of motion and facilitate a maximal response, because reflex responses are greatly affected by pressure receptors.

These exercises increase flexibility in one muscle group (agonist), and simultaneously improve strength in another muscle group (antagonist). Furthermore, if instituted early in the exercise program, PNF stretches can aid in elongating scar tissue. As scar tissue matures and increases in density, it becomes less receptive to short-term stretches and may require prolonged stretching to achieve deformation changes in the tissue.

PNF technique recruits muscle contractions in a coordinated pattern as agonists and antagonists move through a range of motion. One technique utilizes **active inhibition** whereby the muscle group reflexively relaxes prior to the stretching maneuver. Common methods include contract-relax, hold-relax, and slow reversal-hold-relax (see **Box 7.11**). The athletic trainer stabilizes the limb to be exercised. Alternating contractions and passive stretching of a group of muscles are then performed **(Figure 7.5)**. Contractions may be held for 3, 6, or 10 seconds, with similar results obtained (13).

A second technique, known as **reciprocal inhibition**, uses active agonist contractions to relax a tight antagonist muscle. In this technique, the individual contracts the muscle opposite the tight muscle, against resistance. This causes a reciprocal inhibition of the tight muscle, leading to muscle lengthening. An advantage to PNF exercise is the ability to stretch a tight muscle that may be painful or in the early stages of healing. In addition, movement can occur in a single plane or diagonal pattern that mimics actual skill performance.

Active Assisted Range of Motion (AAROM)

Frequently, passive range of motion at the injured joint may be greater than active motion, perhaps due to muscle

Active Inhibition Techniques

To stretch the hamstring group on a single leg using the three separate PNF techniques, do the following:

CONTRACT-RELAX

1. Stabilize the thigh and passively flex the hip into the agonist pattern until limitation is felt in the hamstrings.
2. The individual then performs an isotonic contraction with the hamstrings through the antagonist pattern.
3. Apply a passive stretch into the agonist pattern until limitation is felt; repeat the sequence.

HOLD-RELAX

1. Passively move the leg into the agonist pattern until resistance is felt in the hamstrings.
2. The individual then performs an isometric contraction to "hold" the position for about 10 seconds.
3. Allow the individual to relax for about 5 seconds.
4. Then apply a passive stretch into the agonist pattern until limitation is felt; repeat the sequence.

SLOW REVERSAL-HOLD-RELAX

1. The individual consciously relaxes the hamstring muscles while doing a concentric contraction of the quadriceps muscles into the agonist pattern.
2. The individual then performs an isometric contraction, against resistance, into the antagonist pattern for 10 seconds.
3. Allow the individual to relax for 10 seconds.
4. The individual then actively moves the body part further into the agonist pattern; repeat the sequence.

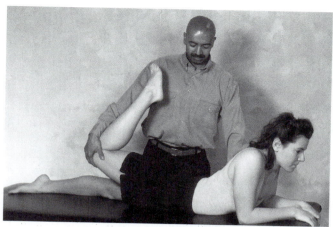

> **FIGURE 7.5 Proprioceptive neuromuscular facilitation.** In performing PNF stretching techniques, the athletic trainer passively stretches a muscle group. In this photo, the hip flexors are being stretched. When slight tension is felt, the athlete isometrically contracts the muscle group against resistance for 3, 6, or 10 seconds. The muscle is then passively stretched again. This process is repeated four to five times.

weakness. A person may be able to sit on top of a table and slide the leg across the tabletop away from the body to fully extend the knee. However, if the individual sits at the edge of the table with his or her legs hanging over the edge then attempts to straighten the knee, the individual may be unable to move the limb voluntarily into full extension. In this situation, normal joint mechanics exist and full PROM is present. However, in order to attain full active range of motion the individual may require some assistance from an athletic trainer, a mechanical device, or the opposite limb to attain full range of motion. Working the limb through available pain-free motion with assistance will more quickly restore normal active range of motion than working the limb within limited voluntary motion.

Active Range of Motion (AROM)

Active range of motion exercises performed by the individual enhance circulation through a pumping action during muscular contraction and relaxation. Full, pain-free, active range of motion need not be achieved before strength exercises are initiated, but certain skills and drills requiring full functional motion, such as throwing, full squats, or certain agility drills, must wait until proper joint mechanics are restored. Active range of motion exercises should be relatively painless, and may be facilitated during certain stages of the program by completing the exercises in a whirlpool to provide an analgesic effect and relieve the stress of gravity on sensitive structures. Examples of active range of motion exercises include spelling out the letters of the alphabet with the ankle, and using a wand or cane with the upper extremity to improve joint mobility. **Field Strategy 7.3** illustrates selected range of motion exercises.

Resisted Range of Motion (RROM)

Resisted range of motion may be either static or dynamic. Static movement is measured with an isometric muscle contraction, and can be used during phases 1 and 2 of the exercise program in a pain-free arc of motion. Dynamic resisted motion (dynamic strengthening) will be discussed in the next section.

Isometric training measures a muscle's maximum potential to produce static force. The muscle is at a constant tension while muscle length and joint angle remain the same. For example, standing in a doorway and pushing outward against the door frame produces a maximal muscle contraction, but joints of the upper extremity do not appear to move. Isometric exercise is useful when motion: (a) is contraindicated by pathology or bracing; (b) is limited because of muscle weakness at a particular angle, called a **sticking point**; or (c) when a painful arc is present. Isometric strength exercises are the least effective training method because, although circumference and strength increase, strength gains are limited to a range of 10° on either side of the joint angle. An adverse, rapid increase in blood pressure occurs when the breath is held against a closed glottis, and is referred to as the **Valsalva effect**. This can be avoided with proper breathing. To perform an isometric contraction, a maximal force is generated against an object, such as the athletic trainer's hand, for about 10 seconds and repeated 10 times per set. Contractions, performed every 20° throughout the available range of motion, are called multiangle isometric exercises.

Proprioception

Proprioception is a specialized variation of the sensory modality of touch that encompasses the sensation of joint movement (**kinesthesia**) and joint position. Sensory receptors located in the skin, muscles, tendons, ligaments, and joints all provide input into the central nervous system (CNS) relative to tissue deformation. Visual and vestibular centers also contribute afferent information to the CNS regarding body position and balance. The ability to sense body position is mediated by cutaneous, muscle, and joint mechanoreceptors.

JOINT MECHANORECEPTORS

Joint mechanoreceptors are found in the joint capsule, ligaments, menisci, labra, and fat pads, and include four types of nerve endings: Ruffini's corpuscles, Golgi receptors, Pacinian corpuscles, and free nerve endings. Ruffini's corpuscles are sensitive to intra-articular pressure and stretching of the joint capsule. Golgi receptors are intraligamentous and become active when the ligaments are stressed at the end ranges of joint movement. Pacinian corpuscles are sensitive to high-frequency vibration and pressure, and the free nerve endings are sensitive to mechanical stress and the deformation and loading of soft tissues that comprise the joint.

FIELD STRATEGY 7.3   RANGE OF MOTION EXERCISES FOR THE LOWER AND UPPER EXTREMITY

A. **Ankle**. Write out the letters of the alphabet using sweeping capital letters. Do all letters three times.

B. **Achilles tendon**. In a seated position, wrap a towel around the forefoot and slowly stretch the Achilles tendon.

C. **Knee**. In a seated position with the knee slightly flexed, wrap a towel around the lower leg and slowly bring the ankle and foot toward the buttocks.

D. **Hip**. Lying down, bring one knee toward the chest. Repeat with the other knee.

E. **Wrist or elbow**. Using the unaffected hand, slowly stretch the affected hand or forearm in flexion and extension.

F. **Shoulder flexion**. With a wand or cane, use the unaffected arm to slowly raise the wand high above the head.

G. **Shoulder lateral (external) rotation**. With a wand or cane, use the unaffected arm to slowly do lateral (external) rotation of the glenohumeral joint.

H. **Shoulder medial (internal) rotation**. With a wand or cane, use the unaffected arm to slowly do medial (internal) rotation of the glenohumeral joint.

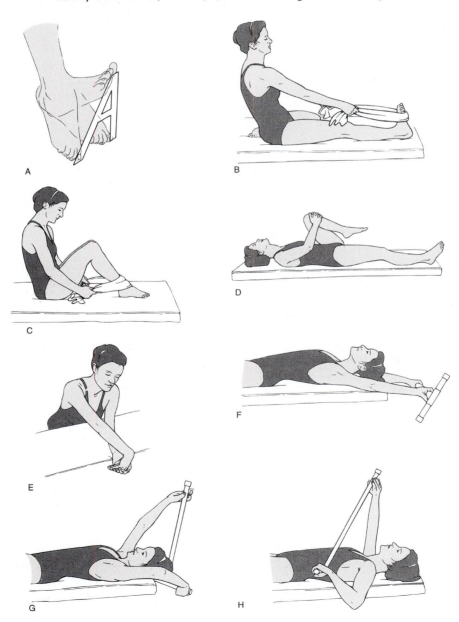

MUSCLE MECHANORECEPTORS

As mentioned earlier, the receptors found in muscle and tendons are the muscle spindles and Golgi tendon organs. Muscle spindles are innervated by both afferent and efferent fibers, and can detect not only muscle length, but more importantly, the rate of change in muscle length. Golgi tendon organs respond to both contraction and stretch of the musculotendinous junction. If the stretch continues for an extended time (over 6 to 8 seconds), the Golgi tendons are stimulated causing a reflex inhibition in the antagonist muscles. This sensory mechanism protects the musculotendinous unit from excessive tensile forces that could damage muscle fibers.

REGAINING PROPRIOCEPTION

Balance involves positioning the body's center of gravity over a base of support through the integration of information received from the various proprioceptors within the body. Even when the body appears motionless, a constant postural sway is caused by a series of muscle contractions that correct and maintain dynamic equilibrium in an upright position. When balance is disrupted, as in falling forward or stumbling, the response is primarily automatic and reflexive. An injury or illness can interrupt the neuromuscular feedback mechanisms. Restoration of the proprioceptive feedback is necessary to promote dynamic joint and functional stability to prevent reinjury.

Like all exercises, proprioceptive exercises must be specific to the type of activity that the athlete will encounter in sport participation. In general, the progression of activities to develop dynamic, reactive neuromuscular control is from slow-speed to high-speed, low-force to high-force, and controlled to uncontrolled activities. An athlete might begin with Romberg's test, which requires the individual to stand with the feet together, arms at the sides, and eyes closed. The athletic trainer looks for any tendency to sway or fall to one side. A single-leg stance test (stork stand) requires the individual to maintain balance while standing on one leg for a specified time with the eyes closed. Then, with the eyes open the athlete can progress to playing catch with a ball. This exercise can be made more difficult by having the athlete balance on a trampoline and playing catch with a ball. Use of a biomechanical ankle platform system (BAPS) board might begin with bilateral balancing and progress to one-legged balancing, dribbling a basketball, or playing catch with a ball. Many of these exercises can be adapted to the upper extremity. An individual can begin in a push-up position and shift his or her weight from one hand to another, or perform isometric or isotonic press-ups, balance on one hand, balance on a BAPS board or ball, or walk on the hands over material of different densities or heights.

Open versus Closed Kinetic Chain Exercises

A common error in developing an exercise program is neglecting to assess the proximal and distal segments of the entire extremity (kinetic chain). A **kinematic chain** is a series of interrelated joints that constitute a complex motor unit, constructed so that motion at one joint will produce motion at the other joints in a predictable manner. Whereas kinematics describes the appearance of motion, **kinetics** involves the forces, whether internal (e.g., muscle contractions or connective tissue restraints) or external (e.g., gravity, inertia, or segmental masses) that affect motion. Initially, a closed kinetic chain (CKC) was characterized when the distal segment of the extremity was in an erect, weight-bearing position, such as the lower extremity when a person is weight bearing. When the distal segment of the extremity is free to move without causing motion at another joint, such as when non–weight bearing, the system was referred to as an open kinetic chain (OKC). When force is applied, the distal segment may function independently or in unison with the other joints. Movements of the more proximal joints are affected by OKC and CKC positions. For example, the rotational components of the ankle, knee, and hip reverse direction when moving from an OKC to CKC position.

Because of incongruities between the lower and upper extremity, particularly in the shoulder region, several authors have challenged the traditional definition of OKC and CKC positions (14-16). Stabilizing muscles in the scapulothoracic region produces a joint compression force that stabilizes the glenohumeral joint much in the same manner as a CKC in the lower extremity. Although debate continues on defining CKC and OKC relative to the upper extremity, there remains general agreement that both CKC and OKC exercises should be incorporated into an upper and lower extremity rehabilitation program.

Injury and subsequent immobilization can affect the proprioceptors in the skeletal muscles, tendons, and joints. In rehabilitation, it is critical that CKC activities be used to retrain joints and muscle proprioceptors to respond to sensory input. CKC exercises are recommended for several reasons (**Box 7.12**). As a result, CKC exercise stimulates the proprioceptors, increases joint stability, increases muscle coactivation, allows better utilization of the SAID principle (Specific Adaptations to Imposed Demands), and permits

---

➤➤ **Box 7.12**

Advantages of Closed Kinetic Chain Exercises

- Provides greater joint compressive forces
- Multiple joints are exercised through weight bearing and muscular contractions
- Velocity and torque are more controlled
- Shear forces are reduced
- Joint congruity is enhanced
- Proprioceptors are re-educated
- Postural and dynamic stabilization mechanics are facilitated
- Exercises can work in spiral or diagonal movement patterns

more functional patterns of movement and greater specificity for athletic activities.

In contrast, OKC exercises can isolate a specific muscle group for intense strength and endurance exercises. In addition, they can develop strength in very weak muscles that may not function properly in a CKC system because of muscle substitution. Although OKC exercises may produce great gains in peak force production, the exercises are usually limited to one joint in a single plane (uniplanar), have greater potential for joint shear, have limited functional application, and have limited eccentric and proprioceptive retraining. However, OKC exercises can assist in developing an athlete-athletic trainer rapport through uniplanar and multiplanar manual therapeutic techniques. **Figure 7.6** illustrates open and closed kinetic chain exercises for the lower extremity.

When range of motion has been achieved, repetition of motion through actual skill movements can improve coordination and joint mechanics as the individual progresses into phase three of the program. For example, a pitcher may begin throwing without resistance or force application in front of a mirror to visualize the action. This can also motivate the individual to continue to progress in the therapeutic exercise program.

 In phase two, passive stretching and active range of motion exercises should be conducted at the ankle. In particular, Achilles tendon stretching and strengthening of the plantar flexors should be a major part of the rehabilitation plan. Cryotherapy, thermotherapy, EMS, or massage can complement the exercise program, as needed. The soccer player should be able to continue many of the exercises at home to supplement the exercise program performed in the athletic training room.

PHASE THREE: DEVELOPING MUSCULAR STRENGTH, ENDURANCE, AND POWER

 The soccer player has regained normal range of motion at the ankle and wants to start playing on an indoor soccer team. Is this a good idea? Will reinjury occur?

Phase three focuses on developing muscular strength, endurance, and power in the injured extremity as compared to the uninjured extremity. The individual can move into phase four when the following criteria have been completed:

- Bilateral range of motion and joint flexibility are restored
- Muscular strength, endurance, and power in the affected limb are equal or near equal to the unaffected limb
- Cardiovascular endurance and general body strength are at or better than the preinjury level
- Sport-specific functional patterns are completed using mild-to-moderate resistance
- Athlete is psychologically ready to return to protected activity

Muscular Strength

Strength is the ability of a muscle or group of muscles to produce force in one maximal effort. Although static strength (isometric strengthening) is used during phases 1 and 2 in a pain-free arc of motion, dynamic strengthening is preferred in phase 3 of the program. Two types of contractions occur in dynamic strength: concentric, in which a shortening of muscle fibers decreases the angle of the associated joint, and eccentric, in which the muscle resists its own lengthening so that the joint angle increases during

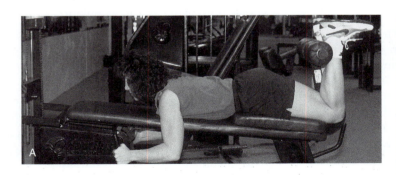

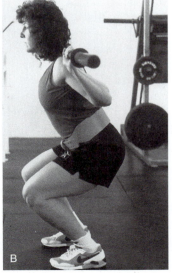

➤ **FIGURE 7.6 Open and closed chain exercises for the lower extremity**. A, Open chain exercise for the hamstrings. B, Closed chain exercise for the hip and knee extensors.

the contraction. Concentric and eccentric may also be referred to as positive and negative work, respectively. Concentric contractions work to accelerate a limb. For example, the gluteus maximus and quadriceps muscles concentrically contract to accelerate the body upward from a crouched position. In contrast, eccentric contractions work to decelerate a limb and provide shock absorption, especially during high-velocity dynamic activities. For example, the shoulder external rotators decelerate the shoulder during the follow-through phase of the overhead throw.

Eccentric contractions generate greater force than isometric contractions, and isometric contractions generate greater force than concentric contractions. In addition, less tension is required in an eccentric contraction. However, one major disadvantage of eccentric training is delayed onset muscle soreness (DOMS). DOMS is defined as muscular pain or discomfort 1 to 5 days following unusual muscular exertion. DOMS is associated with joint swelling and weakness, which may last after the cessation of pain. This differs from acute-onset muscle soreness, where pain during exercise ceases after the exercise bout is completed. To prevent the onset of DOMS, eccentric exercises should progress gradually. Dynamic muscle strength is gained through isotonic or isokinetic exercise **(Figure 7.7)**.

ISOTONIC TRAINING (VARIABLE SPEED/FIXED RESISTANCE)

A more common method of strength training is isotonic exercise, or **progressive resistive exercise** (PRE) as it is sometimes called. In this technique, a maximal muscle contraction generates a force to move a constant load throughout the range of motion at a variable speed. Both concentric and eccentric contractions are possible with free weights, elastic or rubber tubing, and weight machines. Free weights are inexpensive and can be used in diagonal patterns for sport-specific skills, but adding or removing weights from the bars can be troublesome. In addition, a spotter may be required for safety purposes to avoid dropping heavy weights. Theraband, or surgical tubing, is inexpensive and easy to set up, can be used in diagonal patterns for sport-specific skills, and can be adjusted to the patient's strength level by using bands of different tension. Weights on commercial machines can be changed quickly and easily. With several stations utilizing free weights and commercial machines, an individual can do circuit training to strengthen multiple muscle groups in a single exercise session. The machines, however, are typically large and expensive, work only in a single plane of motion, and may not match the biomechanical makeup or body size of the individual.

Isotonic training permits exercise of multiple joints simultaneously, allows for both eccentric and concentric contractions, and permits weight-bearing, closed kinetic chain exercises. A disadvantage is that when a load is applied, the muscle can only move that load through the

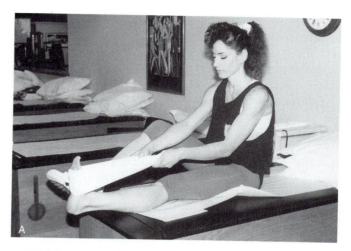

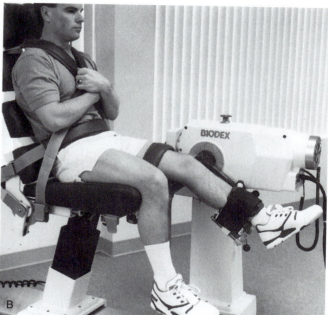

➤ **FIGURE 7.7 Dynamic muscle strengthening.** Dynamic strength may be gained through (A) isotonic exercise, or (B) isokinetic exercise.

range of motion with as much force as the muscle provides at its weakest point. Nautilus and Eagle equipment are examples of variable resistance machines with an elliptical cam. The cam system provides minimal resistance where the ability to produce force is comparatively lower (early and late in the range of motion) and greatest resistance where the muscle is at its optimal length-tension and mechanical advantage (usually the midrange). The axis of rotation generates an isokinetic-like effect, but angular velocity cannot be controlled.

ISOKINETIC TRAINING (FIXED SPEED/VARIABLE RESISTANCE)

Isokinetic training, or accommodating resistance, allows an individual to provide muscular overload and angular movement to rotate a lever arm at a controlled velocity or fixed speed. Theoretically, isokinetic training should activate the maximum number of motor units, which consistently overloads muscles and achieves maximum tension-developing or force output capacity at every point in the range of motion, even at the relatively "weaker" joint angles. Cybex, Biodex, and KinCom are examples of equipment that used this strength training method. Coupled with a computer and appropriate software, torque-motion curves, total work, average power, and torque-to-body weight measurements can be instantaneously calculated to provide immediate, objective measurement to the individual and athletic trainer.

Two advantages of isokinetic training are that a muscle group can be exercised to its maximum potential throughout the full range of motion, and, unlike isotonic training, the dynamometer's resistance mechanism essentially disengages if pain is experienced by the patient. Two disadvantages are the cost of the machine, computer, and software package (ranging from $25,000 to $60,000), and the fact that nearly all available machines do only open chain exercises. For this reason, isokinetic training should be used in conjunction with other modes of resistance training.

Muscular Endurance

Muscular endurance is the ability of muscle tissue to exert repetitive tension over an extended period. The rate of muscle fatigue is related to the endurance level of the muscle (i.e., the more rapidly the muscle fatigues, the less endurance it has). A direct relationship exists between muscle strength and muscle endurance. As muscle endurance is developed, density in the capillary beds increases, providing a greater blood supply, and thus a greater oxygen supply, to the working muscle. Increases in muscle endurance may influence strength gains; however, strength development has not been shown to increase muscle endurance. Muscular endurance is gained by lifting low weights at a faster contractile velocity with more repetitions in the exercise session, or with use of stationary bikes or aquatic therapy, or Stair Master, Nordic Track, or a Slide Board.

Muscular Power

Muscular power is the ability of muscle to produce force in a given time. Power training is started after the injured limb has regained at least 80% of the muscle strength in the unaffected limb. Regaining power involves weight training at higher contractile velocities, or using plyometric exercises.

Plyometric training employs the inherent stretch-recoil characteristics of skeletal muscle through an initial rapid eccentric (loading) prestretching of a muscle, thereby activating the stretch reflex to produce tension prior to initiating an explosive concentric contraction of the muscle. This stretch produces a strong stimulus at the spinal cord level that causes an explosive reflex concentric contraction. The greater the stretch from the muscle's resting length

immediately before the concentric contraction, the greater the load the muscle can lift or overcome. Injury can result if the individual does not have full range of motion, flexibility, and near-normal strength before beginning these exercises. Examples of plyometric exercises include a standing jump, multiple jumps, box jumps or drop jumping from a height, single- or double-leg hops, bounding, leaps, and skips. In the upper extremity, a medicine ball, surgical tubing, plyoback, and boxes can be used. Performing jumping and skipping exercises on grass will reduce impact on the lower extremity during landing. These exercises should be performed every 3 days to allow the muscles to recover from fatigue.

Functional Application of Exercise

Strength, endurance, and power can only be increased by using the **overload principle**: physiological improvements occur only when an individual physically demands more of the muscles than is normally required. This philosophy is based on the **s**pecific **a**daptations to **i**mposed **d**emands (SAID) principle, which states that the body responds to a given demand with a specific and predictable adaptation. Overload is achieved by manipulating intensity, duration, frequency, specificity, speed, and progression in the exercise program.

INTENSITY

Intensity reflects both the caloric cost of the work and the specific energy systems activated. Strength gains depend primarily on the intensity of the overload and not the specific training method used to improve strength. Knight's daily adjusted progressive resistance exercise (DAPRE) is an objective method of increasing resistance as the individual's strength increases or decreases (17). A fixed percentage of the maximum weight for a single repetition is lifted during the first and second sets. Maximum repetitions of the resistance maximum (RM) are lifted in the third set. Adaptations to the amount of weight lifted are then increased or decreased accordingly in the fourth set and in the first set of the next session. The DAPRE guidelines, listed in **Table 7.1**, are based on the concept that if the working weight is ideal, the athlete can perform six repetitions when told to perform as many as possible. If the athlete can perform more than six repetitions, the weight is too light. Conversely, if the athlete cannot lift six repetitions, the weight is too heavy.

For individuals with chronic injuries or early postoperative rehabilitation, the DAPRE method may not be appropriate. Instead, a high-repetition, low-weight exercise may be more productive, particularly in the early phases. High weights can potentially cause a breakdown of the supporting soft tissue structures and exacerbate the condition. Use of smaller weights and submaximal intensities can stimulate blood flow and limit tissue damage. To gain strength and endurance, higher repetitions are required. The athlete

TABLE 7.1 DAILY ADJUSTED PROGRESSIVE RESISTANCE EXERCISE (DAPRE) PROGRAM

Set	Weight	Repetitions
1	50% of RM	10
2	75% of RM	6
3	100% of RM	Maximum
4	Adjusted*	Maximum

# of Repetitions During Set 3	Adjusted Working Weight During Set 4	Weight During Next Day's Exercise Session
0–2	Decrease by 5–10 lb and repeat set	Keep the same
3–4	Decrease by 0–5 lb	Keep the same
5–7	Keep the same	Increase by 5–10 lb
8–12	Increase by 5–10 lb	Increase by 5–15 lb

* Adjusted work weight is gauged on individual differences completed in Set 3.
Adjusted work weight for the next day is gauged on individual differences completed in Set 4.

begins with two or three sets of 10 repetitions, progressing to five sets of 10 repetitions, as tolerated. When the athlete can perform 50 repetitions, 1 pound may be added, and the repetitions reduced to three sets of 10 repetitions. All exercises should be performed slowly, concentrating on proper technique. As strength increases, the DAPRE method or other type of progressive resistance exercise schedule may be used.

DURATION

Duration refers to the estimated time it will take to return the athlete to full (100%) activity, or more commonly to the length of a single exercise session. This time can shorten if pain, swelling, or muscle soreness occur. In general, the individual must participate in at least 20 minutes of continuous activity with the heart elevated to at least 70% of maximal heart rate. This is particularly important when increasing cardiovascular endurance, which will be explained later in the chapter.

FREQUENCY

Frequency refers to the number of exercise sessions per day or week. Although exercise performed twice daily yields greater improvement than exercise done once, the exercise program should be conducted three to four times per week, in most cases. It is critical not to work the same muscle groups on successive days, in order to allow recovery from fatigue and muscle soreness. If daily bouts are planned, strength and power exercises may be alternated with cardiovascular conditioning, or exercises for the lower extremity may alternate with exercises for the upper extremity.

SPECIFICITY

An exercise program must address the specific needs of the athlete. For example, exercises that mimic the throwing action will benefit a baseball pitcher, but are not applicable to a football lineman. If exercises simulate actual skills in the athlete's sport, the more the athlete will tend to be motivated and compliant with the exercise program. The type of exercise (i.e., isometric, isotonic, isokinetic) is also important. Athletes who rely upon eccentric loading must also include eccentric training in their rehabilitation program. Rhythm, or velocity, has also been shown to be specific to that required for the sport skill, with greatest strength gains consistently occurring at training speeds (18).

SPEED

Speed refers to the rate at which the exercise is performed. Initially, exercises should be performed in a slow, deliberate manner at a rate of about 60° per second, with emphasis placed on concentric and eccentric contractions. The athlete should exercise throughout the full range of motion, pausing at the end of the exercise. Large muscle groups should be exercised first, followed by the smaller groups. In addition, the exercise speed should be varied. As strength, endurance, and power increase, functional movements should increase in speed. Surgical tubing can be used to develop a high-speed regimen to produce concentric and eccentric synergist patterns, and isokinetic units may also be used at the highest speeds.

PROGRESSION

To maintain motivation and compliance, an objective improvement should occur each day, whether this is an increase in repetitions or intensity. Muscular strength is improved with a minimum 3 days per week of training that includes 12 to 15 repetitions per bout of 8 to 10 exercises for the major muscle groups (11). If the athlete complains of pain, swelling, or residual muscle soreness, the program may need to be decreased or varied in intensity. An orderly progression, however, should move from range of motion exercises to isometric, isotonic, isokinetic, and functional activities progressing from low-intensity to high-intensity with ever-increasing demands on the athlete as the healing process allows. **Field Strategy 7.4** lists exercises for developing muscular power and strength.

 The soccer player asked to play on an indoor soccer team after full range of motion was achieved at the ankle. However, muscle strength, endurance, and power need to be developed in the affected limb at or near the level of the unaffected limb to prevent reinjury.

PHASE FOUR: RETURN TO SPORT ACTIVITY

 The soccer player has regained near normal strength in the affected limb as compared to the unaffected limb, and maintained cardiovascular

FIELD STRATEGY 7.4   POWER AND STRENGTH EXERCISES

STAIRS

- Use a "low" walking stance and vigorously swing the arms.
- Triple stairs: walk only. One repetition is a round trip from the bottom of the stair-well to the top and back down. Use the walk down as recovery.
- Double stairs: Emphasize technique.
- Single stairs: Emphasize speed.

BOUNDING

- Involves one-foot takeoff and landing for 30 to 40 yards. Swing the arms vigorously to provide a strong movement.
- Run-Run-Bound: Establish the number of bounds (repetitions) and the number of sets.
- Distance: Establish the number of bounds in a given distance.

HOPS (CAN BE PERFORMED ONE-LEGGED OR TWO-LEGGED)

- Single goal: 40-50 yards.
- Double goal: Sequence of 10 hops in each of 3 sets.

UPHILL RUNNING

- Decrease the stride length and make sure foot strike is underneath the body rather than in front.
- Land on the forefoot/toes, not on the heels.

BENCH STEPS WITH BARBELLS

- Step up, up, down, down. Begin with a light weight and add 1 minute daily until consecutive step-ups can be done for a preset period of time.

---

endurance by riding a stationary bike. What additional factors need to be considered to prepare this individual for return to full activity?

The individual can return to his or her sport activity as soon as muscle strength, endurance, and power are restored.

During phase four, the individual should correct any biomechanical inefficiencies in motion; restore coordination and muscle strength, endurance, and power in sport-specific skills; and improve cardiovascular endurance. The individual may be returned to activity if the following goals are attained:

- Coordination and balance are normal
- Sport-specific functional patterns are restored in the injured extremity
- Muscle strength, endurance, and power in the affected limb are equal to that of the unaffected limb
- Cardiovascular endurance is equal to, or greater than, the preinjury level
- The individual receives clearance to return to participation by the supervising physician

Coordination

Coordination refers to the body's ability to execute smooth, fluid, accurate, and controlled movements. Simple movement, such as combing hair, involves a complex muscular interaction using the appropriate speed, distance, direction, rhythm, and muscle tension to execute the task.

Coordination may be divided into two categories: gross motor movements involving large muscle groups, and fine motor movements using small groups. Gross motor movements involve activities such as standing, walking, skipping, and running. Fine motor movements are seen in precise actions, particularly with fingers, such as picking up a coin off a table, clutching an opponent's jersey, or picking up a ground ball with a glove. Coordination and proprioception are directly linked. When an injury occurs and the limb is immobilized, sensory input from proprioceptors and motor commands are disrupted, resulting in an alteration of coordination.

Performing closed kinetic chain activities in phase two of the exercise program can help restore proprioceptive input and improve coordination. Constant repetition of motor activities, using sensory cues (tactile, visual, or proprioceptive) or increasing the speed of the activity over time, can continue to develop coordination in phases three and four. A wobble board, teeter board, ProFitter, or BAPS board is often used to improve sensory cues and balance in the lower extremity. PNF patterns and the Pro-Fitter may also be used to improve sensory cues in the upper and lower extremities. **Field Strategy 7.5** lists several lower extremity exercises used to improve coordination and balance.

Sport-Specific Skill Conditioning

Because sports require different skills, therapeutic exercise should progress to the load and speed expected for the

FIELD STRATEGY 7.5 LOWER EXTREMITY EXERCISES TO IMPROVE BALANCE AND PROPRIOCEPTION

FLAT FOOT BALANCE EXERCISES

1. Stand on one foot (stork stand) and maintain balance for 3 to 5 minutes.
2. Stand on one foot with the toes off the floor and maintain balance for 3 to 5 minutes.
3. Stand on one foot while dribbling a basketball.

BALANCING ON THE TOES

1. Balance on the toes/forefoot using both feet for 3 to 5 minutes, then use only one foot.
2. Balance on the toes while dribbling a basketball.

PROFITTER EXERCISES

1. In a location with a sturdy hand rail, stand on the ProFitter with the feet perpendicular to the long axis of the rails. Gently slide side-to-side, placing pressure first on the toes, then on the heels.
2. Progress to more rapid movement. When you feel comfortable, do the sliding motion without hand support. Document repetitions and sets.

BAPS BOARD EXERCISES

1. Begin in a seated position by rotating the foot clockwise and counterclockwise.
2. Stand with both feet on board (bilateral balancing) with support, and move the platform clockwise and counterclockwise; progress to one foot with support.
3. Do bilateral balancing with no support; progress to one foot with no support.
4. Add dribbling a basketball or catching a basketball to any of these activities.

---

individual's sport. For example, a baseball player performs skills at different speeds and intensities than a football lineman. Therefore, exercises must be coupled with functional training, or specificity of training related to the physical demands of the sport.

As range of motion, muscular strength, and coordination are restored, the individual should work the affected extremity through functional diagonal and sport-specific patterns. For example, in phase three, a baseball pitcher may have been moving the injured arm through the throwing pattern with mild-to-moderate resistance. In phase four, the individual should increase resistance and speed of motion. Working with a ball attached to surgical tubing, the individual can develop a kinesthetic awareness in a functional pattern. When controlled motion is done pain-free, actual throwing can begin. Initially, short throws with low intensity can be used, progressing to longer throws and low intensity. As the player feels more comfortable and is pain-free with the action, the number of throws and their intensity are increased. Similar programs can be developed for other sports.

Cardiovascular Endurance

Cardiovascular endurance, commonly called aerobic capacity, is the body's ability to sustain submaximal exercise over an extended period, and depends on the efficiency of the pulmonary and cardiovascular systems. When an injured individual is unable to continue, or chooses to stop aerobic training, detraining occurs within 1 to 2 weeks (11). If the individual returns to activity without a high cardiovascular endurance level, fatigue sets in quickly and places the individual at risk for reinjury.

Like strength training, maintaining and improving cardiovascular endurance is influenced by an interaction of frequency, duration, and intensity. The American College of Sports Medicine recommends that aerobic training include activity 3 to 5 days per week lasting more than 20 minutes at an intensity of 60 to 90% of maximal heart rate (HRmax) (37). Targeted heart rate can be calculated in two manners:

1. An estimated HRmax for both men and women is about 220 beats/minute. Heart rate is related to age, with maximal heart rate decreasing as an individual ages. A relatively simple calculation is:

$$HRmax = 220 - Age$$

[With a 20 year old athlete working at 80% maximum, the calculation would be: $.8 \times (220 - 20)$ or 160 beats per minute]

2. Another commonly used formula (Karvonen formula) assumes that the targeted heart rate range is between 60 and 90%. The calculation is:

$$Target\ HR\ range = [(HRmax - HRrest) \times 0.60\ and\ 0.90] + HRrest$$

[If an athlete's HRmax is 180 beats/minute and the HRrest is 60 beats/minute, this method yields a target HR range of between 132 and 168 beats/minute.]

Non-weight-bearing exercises, such as swimming, rowing, biking, or use of the UBE can be helpful early in the

FIELD STRATEGY 7.6   CARDIOVASCULAR CONDITIONING EXERCISES

Jumping rope. The rope should pass from one armpit, under the feet, to the other armpit. Jump with the forearms near the ribs at a 45° angle. Rotation occurs at the hand and wrist. Jump with minimal ground clearance.

Two-footed jumps
  Bounce on the balls of the feet.
  Tap heel of one foot to toe of other foot on one jump. Variation: tap toe of same foot to heel of other foot.
  Pepper.
  Arm crossovers and foot crossovers.
One-footed jumps
  One foot hop.
  Rocker step. Rock forward/ backward with feet in a forward straddle.
  Heel strikes and toe taps.
  Jogging steps.

Stair Master. 20 minutes of exercise is recommended 3 to 4 times a week.
Beginner level
  Manual or Pike's Peak mode at Level 2 or 3 for 5 minutes.
  Increase time to 8, 10, 15, and 20 minutes.
Advanced level
  When 20 minutes is comfortable, decrease time to 5 to 8 minutes and increase level intensity, then increase time again. As intensity increases, include a warm-up and cool-down period.

Treadmill
Beginner level
  Begin with a manual mode with a ground level (0° incline) for 5 minutes at approximately 2.5 mph.
  Increase time to 8, 10, 15, and 20 minutes.
Intermediate level
  When 20 minutes is comfortable, increase speed to 3-5.0 mph, and progress to 8, 10, 15, and 20 minutes.
  Allow for warm-up and cool-down periods.
  For example: warm-up at 2.5 mph for 5 minutes
    increase speed to 4.0 to 5.0 mph for 10 minutes
    cool down at 2.5 mph for 5 minutes
    total workout = 20 minutes
Advanced level
  Increase incline during warm-up and decrease incline during cool-down.

Upper Body Ergometer (UBE)
Beginner level
  Start at 120 rpm for 4 minutes, alternating directions: 2 minutes forward, 2 minutes backward.
Intermediate level
  Progress to 90 rpm and increase time to 6, 8, and 10 minutes.
Advanced level
  Alternate directions as tolerated. Duration should not exceed 12 minutes.
  For example: warm-up at 90 rpm for 2.5 minutes
    workout at 60 rpm for 5 minutes
    cool down at 120 rpm for 2.5 minutes

therapeutic program, particularly if the individual has a lower extremity injury. Walking, cross-country skiing, jumping rope, or running can be performed as the condition improves. **Field Strategy 7.6** lists cardiovascular conditioning exercises.

The documentation needed to clear the soccer player for return to full activity includes success-

ful completion of the goals listed in phase 4 and a doctor's medical clearance. The individual should also agree to wear any appropriate taping or protective device to ensure safe return. Remember that all written documentation of the exercise program and written medical clearance should be placed in the individual's file and stored in a safe, secure location for a minimum of 3 to 5 years.

Summary

1. A therapeutic exercise program must address not only the physical needs of the athlete, but also the emotional and psychological needs.
2. Several factors can affect how an athlete reacts to the rehabilitation process, including:
   - Performance anxiety
   - Self-esteem/motivation
   - Extroversion/introversion
   - Psychological investment in the sport
   - Coping resources
   - History of past stressors (previous injuries, academic, family, life events)
   - Previous intervention strategies
3. Goal setting is one of the most common practices used by athletic trainers to motivate athletes in the recovery program.
4. Psychological influences that may affect an athlete's success in the rehabilitation process include confidence, motivation, anxiety, focus, and management of pain.
5. As a general rule, any psychological difficulty that persists for more than a few days and interferes with the progress of rehabilitation should be referred to a licensed clinical psychologist or an appropriate counseling center.
6. Rehabilitation begins immediately after injury assessment:
   - The level of function and dysfunction is assessed.
   - Results are organized and interpreted.
   - A list of patient problems is formulated.
   - Long- and short-term goals are established.
   - A treatment plan is developed, including therapeutic exercises, modalities, and medications.
   - The program is then supervised and periodically reassessed with appropriate changes made.
7. Phase one of the therapeutic exercise program should focus on patient education and control of inflammation, muscle spasm, and pain.
8. Phase two should regain any deficits in range of motion and proprioception at the affected joint as compared to the unaffected joint.
9. Phase three should regain muscular strength, endurance, and power in the affected limb.
10. Phase four prepares the individual to return to activity and includes analysis of motion, sport-specific skill training, regaining coordination, and cardiovascular conditioning.
11. At the conclusion of the exercise program, the supervising physician will determine if the individual is ready to return to full activity. This decision should be based on review of the individual's:
    - Range of motion and flexibility
    - Muscular strength, endurance, and power
    - Biomechanical skill analysis
    - Proprioception and coordination
    - Cardiovascular endurance
12. If additional protective bracing, padding, or taping is necessary to enable the individual to return safely to activity, this should be documented in the individual's file. In addition, it should be stressed that use of any protective device should not replace a maintenance program of conditioning exercises.
13. The athletic trainer should keep a watchful eye on the individual as the person returns to activity. If the individual begins to show signs of pain, swelling, discomfort, or skill performance deteriorates, the individual should be reevaluated to determine if activity should continue or the therapeutic exercise program needs to be reinstituted.

References

1. Wagman D, Khelifa M. Psychological issues in sport injury rehabilitation: Current knowledge and practice. J Ath Train 1996;31(3):257-261.
2. Theodorakis Y, et al. The effect of personal goals, self-efficacy, and self-satisfaction on injury rehabilitation. J Sports Rehab 1996;5(3):214-223.
3. Theodorakis Y, et al. Examining psychological factors during injury rehabilitation. J Sports Rehab 1997;6(4):355-363.
4. Petitpas AJ. Going for the goal. Ath Ther Today 1997;2(4):30-31.
5. Taylor J, Taylor S. Psychological Approaches to Sports Injury Rehabilitation. Gaithersburg, MD: Aspen Publishers, 1997.
6. Larson GA, Starkey C, Zaichknowsky LD. Psychological aspects of athletic injuries as perceived by athletic trainers. Sport Psychologist 1996;10(1):37-47.
7. Heil J. Psychology of Sport Injury. Champaign, IL: Human Kinetics, 1993.
8. Harrelson GL. Physiologic factors of rehabilitation. In: Physical Rehabilitation of the Injured Athlete. Edited by Andrews JR, Harrelson GL, Wilk, KE. Philadelphia: WB Saunders, 1998.
9. Mazess RB, Whedon GD. Immobilization and bone. Calcif Tissue Int 1983;35:265-267.
10. Harrelson GL, Leaver-Dunn D. Range of motion and flexibility. In: Physical Rehabilitation of the Injured Athlete. Edited by Andrews JR, Harrelson GL, Wilk KE. Philadelphia: WB Saunders, 1998.
11. McArdle WD, Katch FI, Katch VL. Exercise Physiology: Energy, nutrition, and Human Performance. Baltimore: Williams & Wilkins, 1996.
12. Maitland GD. Extremity Manipulation. London: Butterworth Publishers, 1977.
13. Nelson KC, Cornelius WL. The relationship between isometric contraction durations and improvement in shoulder joint range of motion. J Sports Med Phys Fitness 1991;31(3):385-388.
14. Wilk KE, Arrigo CA, Andrews JR. Closed and open kinetic chain exercise for the upper extremity. J Sports Rehab 1996;5(1):88-102.
15. Lephart SM, Henry TJ. Functional rehabilitation for the upper and lower extremities. Orthop Clin North Am 1995;26(3):579-592.
16. Dillman CH, Murray TA, Hintermeister RA. Biomechanical differences of open and closed chain exercises with respect to the shoulder. J Sports Rehab 1994;3(3):228-238.
17. Knight KL. Rehabilitating chondromalacia patellae. Phys Sportsmed 1979;7(10):147-148.
18. Harrelson GL, Leaver-Dunn D. Introduction to rehabilitation. In: Physical Rehabilitation of the Injured Athlete. Edited by Andrews JR, Harrelson GL, Wilk, KE. Philadelphia: WB Saunders, 1998.

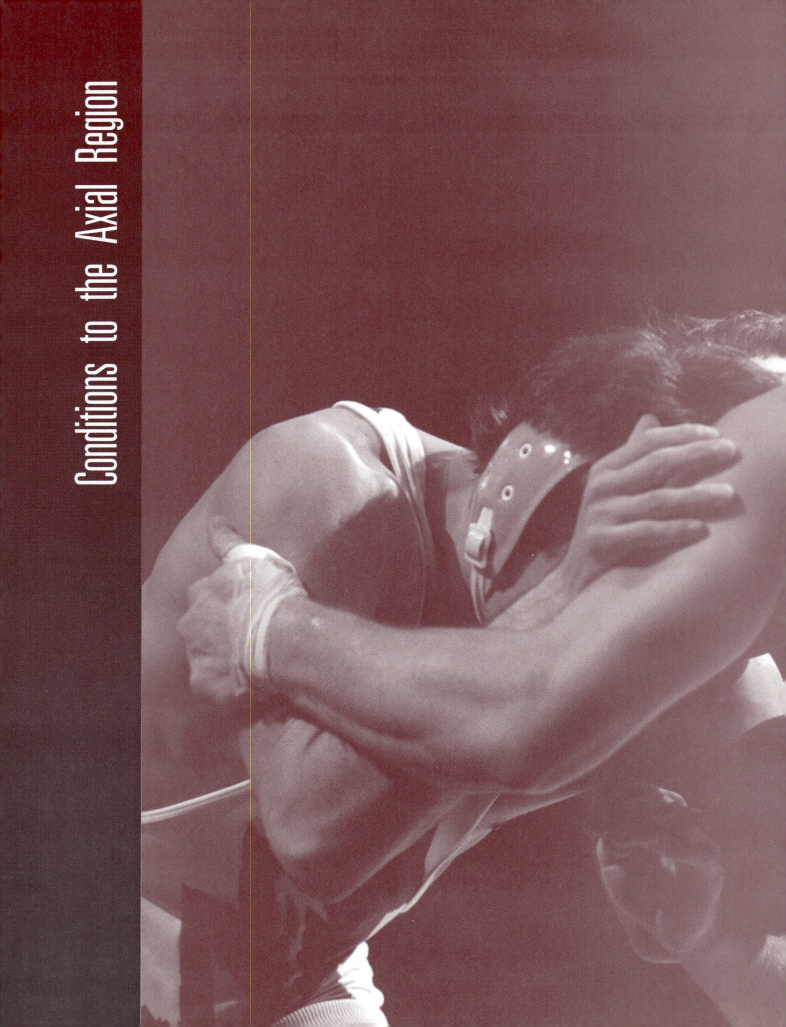

SECTION III

CHAPTER **8**

Head and Facial Conditions

OBJECTIVES

1. Locate the important bony and soft tissue structures of the head and facial region.

2. Recognize the importance of wearing protective equipment to prevent injury to the head and facial region.

3. Identify forces responsible for cranial injuries.

4. Describe signs and symptoms associated with a possible skull fracture.

5. Recognize the critical signs and symptoms that indicate a focal or diffuse cranial injury.

6. Explain the evaluation and management of a cranial injury.

7. Identify the signs and symptoms indicating a facial fracture.

8. Differentiate between an epistaxis and fractured nose.

9. Describe the differences in managing a loose tooth versus a fractured or dislocated tooth.

10. Recognize common external and internal ear conditions and explain their management.

11. Recognize the signs and symptoms indicating a serious eye injury.

12. Describe how to evaluate an eye injury.

The head and facial areas are frequent sites for minor injuries, including lacerations, contusions, and mild concussions. Although intracranial injuries have been associated with sport-related fatalities, measures such as increased standards in protective equipment, rule changes that prohibit leading with the head for contact, and the development and use of the face mask, have significantly decreased the incidence of the injuries since the mid-1970s. A significant decrease has also been seen in eye, ear, and dental injuries when protective equipment is worn.

This chapter begins with a general anatomical review of the head and facial region. Discussion on preventive measures is followed by information on the mechanisms of injury most commonly linked to cranial injuries. The signs, symptoms, and management of the more common focal and diffuse cranial injuries are discussed, followed by steps to include in a thorough assessment of a head injury. The final section discusses the more common facial, nasal, ear, and eye injuries and their management.

ANATOMICAL REVIEW OF THE HEAD AND FACIAL REGION

 A basketball player has fallen backwards, striking his head on the floor. There is a superficial cut on the back of the head that is bleeding profusely. What anatomical structure(s) are likely to have been damaged? How serious is this injury?

The review of anatomy will focus on bony structure, the brain and its coverings, the eye, and the nerve and blood supply to the region. Although the numerous muscles of the face and jaw enable speaking, chewing, and facial expression, these muscles are not commonly involved in sport injuries, and therefore will not be discussed.

Bones of the Skull

The skull is primarily composed of flat bones that interlock at immovable joints called sutures **(Figure 8.1)**. The bones that form the portion of the skull referred to as the cranium protect the brain. The thin bones of the cranium include the frontal, occipital, sphenoid, and ethmoid bones, as well as two parietal bones and two temporal bones. Material properties and thickness of the cranial bones vary, but the strongest is the occipital bone, and the weakest are the temporal bones. The facial bones provide the structure of the face and form the sinuses, orbits of the eyes, nasal cavity, and the mouth. These bones include the paired maxilla, zygomatic, palatine, nasal, lacrimal, vomer, and inferior nasal concha bones, along with the bridge and mandible. The large opening at the base of the skull that sits atop the spinal column is called the foramen magnum.

The Scalp

The scalp is composed of three layers: the skin, subcutaneous connective tissue, and the pericranium. The protective function of these tissues is enhanced by the hair and the looseness of the scalp, which enables some dissipation of force when the head sustains a glancing blow. The scalp and face have an extensive blood supply, which is why superficial lacerations tend to bleed profusely.

The Brain

The four major regions of the brain are the cerebral hemispheres, diencephalon, brain stem, and cerebellum. The entire brain and spinal cord are enclosed in three layers of protective tissue known collectively as the meninges **(Figure 8.2)**. The outermost membrane is the dura mater, a thick, fibrous tissue containing dural sinuses that act as veins to transport blood from the brain to the jugular veins

of the neck. The arachnoid mater is a thin membrane internal to the dura mater, separated from the dura mater by the subdural space. Beneath the arachnoid mater is the subarachnoid space, which is filled with cerebrospinal fluid (CSF) and contains the largest of the blood vessels supplying the brain. The arachnoid mater is connected to the inner pia mater by web-like strands of connective tissue. Whereas the dura mater and arachnoid mater are rather loose membranes, the pia mater is in direct contact with the cerebral cortex. The pia mater contains numerous small blood vessels.

The Eyes

The eye is a hollow sphere, approximately 2.5 cm (1 in) in diameter in adults **(Figure 8.3)**. The anterior eye surface receives protection from the eyelids, eyelashes, and the attached conjunctiva. The conjunctiva lines the eyelids and the external surface of the eye, and secretes mucus to lubricate the external eye. The lacrimal glands, located above the lateral ends of the eyes, continually release tears across the eye surface through several small ducts. The lacrimal ducts, located at the medial corners of the eyes, serve as drains for the moisture. These ducts funnel the moisture into the lacrimal sac and eventually into the nasal cavity.

Like the brain, the eye is surrounded by three protective tissue layers, called tunics. The outer tunic is a thick white connective tissue called the sclera and forms the "white of the eye." The cornea, found in the central anterior part of the sclera, is clear to permit passage of light into the eye. The choroid, the middle covering, is a highly vascularized tissue, which on the anterior eye usually appears blue or brown and contains the pupil. The inner protective layer is the retina, which contains light-sensitive photoreceptor cells that stimulate nerve endings to provide sight.

Nerves of the Head and Face

Twelve pairs of cranial nerves emerge from the brain. These nerves have motor functions, sensory functions, or both. The cranial nerves are numbered and named in accordance with their functions, and are listed in **Table 8.1**.

Blood Vessels of the Head and Face

The major vessels supplying the head and face are the common carotid and vertebral arteries **(Figure 8.4)**. The common carotid artery ascends through the neck on either side to divide into the external and internal carotid artery just below the level of the jaw. The external carotid arteries and their branches supply most regions of the head external to the brain. The middle meningeal artery supplies the skull and dura mater; if it is damaged, serious epidural bleeding can result. The internal carotid arteries send branches to the eyes and supply portions of the cerebral hemispheres and the parietal and temporal lobes of the

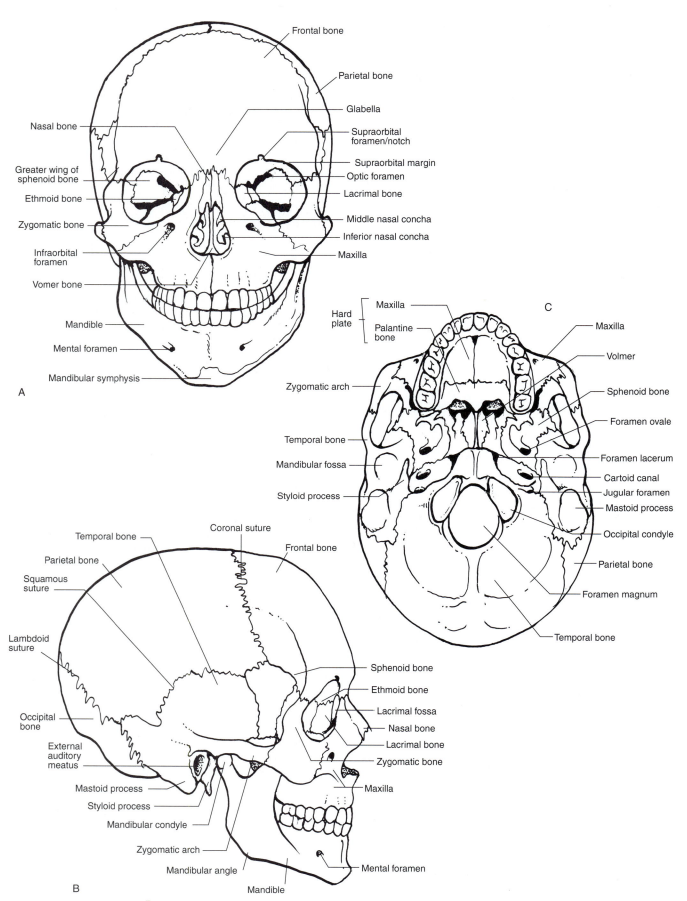

Frontal bone

Parietal bone

Glabella

Supraorbital foramen/notch

Supraorbital margin

Optic foramen

Lacrimal bone

Middle nasal concha

Inferior nasal concha

Maxilla

Nasal bone

Greater wing of sphenoid bone

Ethmoid bone

Zygomatic bone

Infraorbital foramen

Vomer bone

Mandible

Mental foramen

Mandibular symphysis

A

Hard plate

Maxilla

Palantine bone

Maxilla

Volmer

Sphenoid bone

Foramen ovale

Foramen lacerum

Cartoid canal

Jugular foramen

Mastoid process

Occipital condyle

Parietal bone

Foramen magnum

Temporal bone

C

Zygomatic arch

Temporal bone

Mandibular fossa

Styloid process

Temporal bone

Parietal bone

Squamous suture

Lambdoid suture

Occipital bone

External auditory meatus

Mastoid process

Styloid process

Mandibular condyle

Zygomatic arch

Mandibular angle

Mandible

Coronal suture

Frontal bone

Sphenoid bone

Ethmoid bone

Lacrimal fossa

Nasal bone

Lacrimal bone

Zygomatic bone

Maxilla

Mental foramen

B

➤ FIGURE 8.1 Bones of the skull. A, Frontal view. B, Lateral view. C, Inferior view.

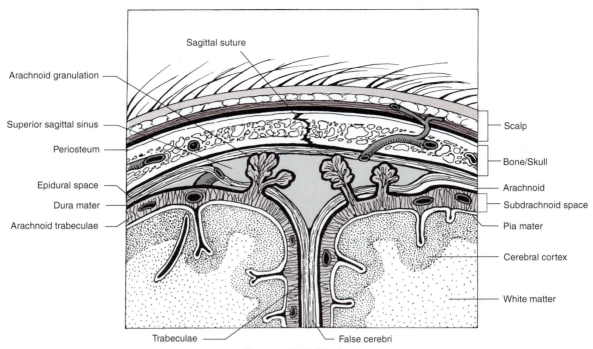

Arachnoid granulation

Superior sagittal sinus

Periosteum

Epidural space

Dura mater

Arachnoid trabeculae

Sagittal suture

Scalp

Bone/Skull

Arachnoid

Subdrachnoid space

Pia mater

Cerebral cortex

White matter

Trabeculae

False cerebri

➤ FIGURE 8.2 Meninges.

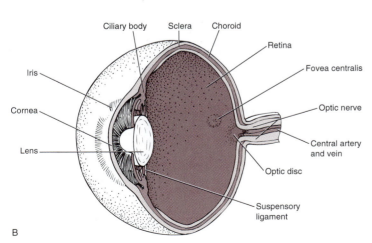

Lacrimal gland

Lacrimal gland ducts

Opening of inferior lacrimal duct

Nasolacrimal duct

Opening of superior lacrimal duct

Superior lacrimal canaliculus

Lacrimal sac

Inferior lacrimal canaliculus

A

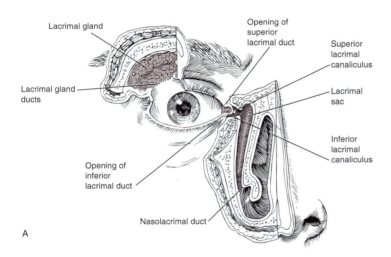

Ciliary body   Sclera   Choroid

Iris

Cornea

Lens

Retina

Fovea centralis

Optic nerve

Central artery and vein

Optic disc

Suspensory ligament

B

➤ FIGURE 8.3 Eye. A, The lacrimal structures of the eye. B, Internal structures of the eye globe.

TABLE 8.1   THE CRANIAL NERVES

Number	Name	Sensory	Motor	Function
I	Olfactory	X		Sense of smell
II	Optic	X		Vision
III	Oculomotor		X	Control of some of the extrinsic eye muscles
IV	Trochlear		X	Control of the remaining extrinsic eye muscles
V	Trigeminal	X	X	Sensation of the facial region and movement of the jaw muscles
VI	Abducens		X	Control of lateral eye movement
VII	Facial	X	X	Control of facial movement, taste, and secretion of tears and saliva
VIII	Vestibulocochlear (acoustic)	X		Hearing and equilibrium
IX	Glossopharyngeal	X	X	Taste, control of the tongue and pharynx, secretion of saliva
X	Vagus	X		Taste, sensation to the pharynx, larynx, trachea, and bronchioles
XI	Accessory		X	Control of movements of the pharynx, larynx, head, and shoulders
XII	Hypoglossal		X	Control of tongue movements

cerebrum. The left and right vertebral arteries and their branches supply blood to the posterior region of the brain.

 Because the scalp and face have an extensive blood supply, superficial lacerations of the head tend to bleed profusely. If there are no signs of a concussion (discussed later in this chapter), the injury is probably a superficial cut of the scalp. This is not serious once bleeding is controlled.

PREVENTION OF HEAD AND FACIAL INJURIES

The most important preventative measure for the head and facial area is use of protective equipment. Many sports, such as baseball/softball, competitive bicycling, fencing, field hockey, football, ice hockey, lacrosse, and wrestling, require some type of head or facial protective equipment for participation. Protective equipment, when properly used, can protect the head and facial area from accidental or routine injuries. It is important to recognize that protective equipment cannot prevent all injuries. To be effective,

equipment must be properly fitted, clean, in good condition, used regularly, and used in the manner for which it was designed.

Protective equipment may include a helmet, face guard, mouth guard, eye wear, ear wear, and throat protector. Helmets protect the cranial portion of the skull by absorbing and dispersing impact forces, thereby reducing cerebral trauma. Face guards protect and shield the facial region from flying projectiles. Mouth guards have been shown to reduce dental and oral soft tissue injuries, as well as cerebral concussions, jaw fractures, and temporomandibular joint injuries. Eye wear, ear wear, and throat protectors reduce injuries to their respective regions. Refer to Chapter 3 to review head and facial protection.

CRANIAL INJURY MECHANISMS

The occurrence of a skull fracture or intracranial injury is dependent on the material properties of the skull, thickness of the skull in the specific area, magnitude and direction of impact, and size of the impact area. In Chapter 5, you learned that direct impact causes two phenomena to occur—deformation and acceleration. When a blow impacts the skull, the bone deforms and bends inward, placing the inner border of the skull under tensile strain, while the outer border is compressed **(Figure 8.5A)**. If the impact is of sufficient magnitude and the skull is thin in the region of impact, a skull fracture will occur at the site where tensile loading occurs. In contrast, if the skull is thick and dense enough at the area of impact, it may sustain inward bending

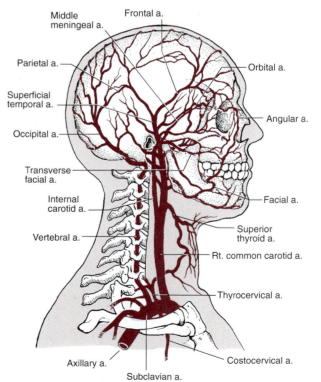

➤ **FIGURE 8.4 Blood supply to the head.** Right lateral view.

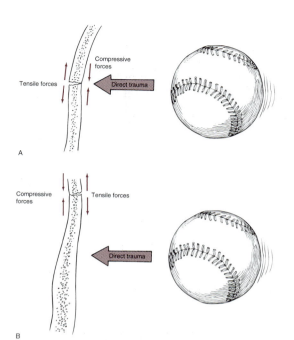

➤ FIGURE 8.5 **Mechanical failure in bone.** When a blow impacts the skull, the bone deforms and bends inward, placing tensile stress on the inner border of the skull. A, If impact is of sufficient magnitude and the skull is thin in the region of impact, a skull fracture occurs at the impact site. B, If the skull is thick and dense enough at the area of impact, it may sustain bending without fracture. However, the fracture may occur some distance from the impact zone in a region where the skull is thinner.

without fracture. A fracture may then occur some distance from the impact zone in a region where the skull is thinner **(Figure 8.5B)**.

On impact, shock waves pass through the skull to the brain, causing it to accelerate. This acceleration can lead to shear, tensile, and compression strains within the brain substance, with shear being the most serious. Axial rotation coupled with acceleration can lead to **contrecoup injuries (Figure 8.6)**, or injuries away from the actual impact site.

Cerebral trauma can lead to **focal injuries**, involving only localized damage (i.e., epidural, subdural, or intracerebral hematomas), or **diffuse injuries** that involve widespread disruption and damage to the function and/or structure of the brain. Although diffuse injuries account for only one-quarter of the fatalities caused by head trauma, they tend to be a more prevalent cause of long-term neurological deficits in individuals. If cerebral injuries are recognized and treated immediately, the severity is limited to the initial structural damage. However, if other factors such as ischemia, hypoxia, cerebral swelling, and hemorrhaging around the brain occur, additional damage and possible neurological dysfunction result. Therefore, it is important for the athletic trainer to work collaboratively with the team physician to accurately assess head injuries, and initiate prompt medical attention to rule out serious underlying problems that may complicate the original injury. A conscious, ambulatory individual should not be considered to have only a minor injury, but rather should be continually assessed to

determine if posttraumatic signs or symptoms indicate a more serious underlying condition.

SKULL FRACTURES

 During hitting practice, a foul tip strikes the head of a baseball player standing near the dugout. The skin is not broken, but the individual is complaining of an intense headache, disorientation, and blurred vision, and cannot recall what happened. Do these signs indicate that a skull fracture may be present?

Skull fractures may be linear (in a line), comminuted (in multiple pieces), depressed (fragments driven internally toward the brain), or basilar (involving the base of the skull) **(Figure 8.7)**. If there is a break in the skin adjacent to the fracture site and a tear in the underlying dura mater, there is a high risk of bacterial infection into the intracranial cavity, which can result in **septic meningitis**. Whenever a severe blow to the head occurs, a skull fracture should always be suspected. However, it is often difficult to detect when a deep scalp hematoma is present.

➤ SIGNS AND SYMPTOMS

Depending on the fracture site, different signs may appear (see **Box 8.1**). For example, a fracture at the eyebrow level may travel into the anterior cranial fossa and sinuses, leading to discoloration around the eyes (**raccoon eyes**). Bony fragments may damage the optic or olfactory cranial nerves, leading to blindness or loss of smell. A basilar fracture above and behind the ear may lead to **Battle's sign**, a discoloration that can appear within minutes behind the ear **(Figure 8.8)**. Blood or CSF may leak from the nose or ear canal. To determine if cerebrospinal fluid is present,

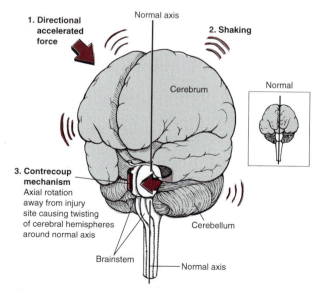

➤ FIGURE 8.6 **Contrecoup injury.** Axial rotation coupled with acceleration is called a contrecoup injury and can lead to injuries away from the actual impact site.

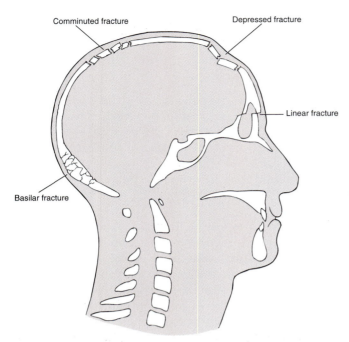

➤ FIGURE 8.7 **Skull fractures.** Fractures of the skull are categorized as linear, comminuted, depressed, or basilar.

gently absorb some of the fluid onto a gauze pad and watch to see if clear fluid separates from the blood. This is called "targeting" or the "halo test," but may not always be reliable. A hearing loss or facial paralysis may also be present. A fracture to the temple region may damage the meningeal arteries, causing epidural bleeding between the dura mater and skull (epidural hematoma). This can be life-threatening and will be discussed in more detail in the section on focal cerebral injuries.

➤ MANAGEMENT

 *A skull fracture can be a life-threatening condition. If any of the signs and symptoms mentioned in Box 8.1 become apparent, activate EMS. **Field Strategy 8.1** summarizes management of a suspected skull fracture.*

➤➤ **BOX 8.1**

Possible Signs of Skull Fractures

- Visible deformity—do not be misled by a "goose egg"; a fracture may be under the site
- Deep laceration or severe bruise to the scalp
- Palpable depression or crepitus
- Unequal pupils
- Discoloration under both eyes (raccoon eyes) or behind the ear (Battle's sign)
- Bleeding or clear fluid (CSF) from the nose and/or ear
- Loss of smell
- Loss of sight or major vision disturbances
- Unconsciousness for more than 2 minutes after direct trauma to the head

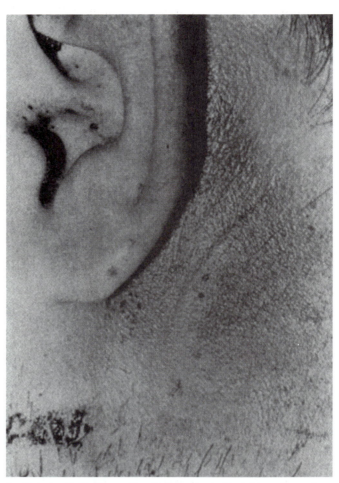

➤ FIGURE 8.8 **Signs of a skull fracture.** Mastoid ecchymosis (Battle's sign), is a discoloration that appears within minutes behind the ear, indicating a basilar skull fracture.

 Signs that indicate a possible skull fracture include deformity, unequal pupils, discoloration around both eyes or behind the ears, bleeding or CSF leaking from the nose and/or ear, and any loss of sight or smell. This athlete did not exhibit any of these "red flags." The athlete should, however, be thoroughly evaluated for head trauma. If any of the signs appear during the assessment, activate EMS.

FOCAL CEREBRAL INJURIES

 A softball player collided with the shortstop, accidentally taking an elbow to the side of the head. The athlete was dazed and removed from the game. After 15 minutes of icing the region, the athlete is complaining of an increasing headache and is experiencing nausea. She is lethargic, disoriented, and sensitive to sunlight. What do these symptoms indicate? How will you manage this injury?

Focal cerebral injuries usually result in a localized collection of blood or hematoma. Within the skull there

FIELD STRATEGY 8.1   EVALUATION AND MANAGEMENT OF A SUSPECTED SKULL FRACTURE

1. Stabilize the head and neck.
2. Activate EMS.
3. Check the ABCs.
4. Take vital signs (pulse, respiration, blood pressure).
5. Observe for:
   Swelling or discoloration around the eyes or behind the ears
   Blood or CSF leaking from the nose or ears
   Pupil size, pupillary response to light, and eye movement.
6. Palpate for depressions, blood, and crepitus. Palpate cervical vertebrae for associated neck injury.
7. Cover any open wounds with a sterile dressing but do not apply pressure.
8. Elevate the upper body and head if there is no evidence of shock, or neck or spinal injury. If present, keep the individual lying flat.
9. Treat for shock and monitor ABCs.
10. Recheck vital signs and symptoms every five minutes until EMS arrives.

is no room for additional accumulation of blood or fluid. Any additional foreign matter within the cranial cavity increases pressure on the brain, leading to significant alterations in neurological function. Depending on the location of the accumulated blood relative to the dura mater, these hematomas are classified as epidural (outside the dura mater), or subdural (deep to the dura mater). A cerebral contusion is also classified as a focal injury; however, there is no mass, occupying lesion associated with this condition.

Epidural Hematoma

An epidural hematoma is very rare in sports. The condition is typically caused by a direct blow to the side of the head and is almost always associated with a skull fracture (**Figure 8.9A**). If the middle meningeal artery or its branches are severed, the subsequent arterial bleeding will lead to a "high-pressure" epidural hematoma.

➤ SIGNS AND SYMPTOMS

The individual will have an initial loss of consciousness at the time of the injury, followed by a lucid interval in which the athlete feels relatively normal, but within 10 to 20 minutes, a decline in mental status occurs. Other signs and symptoms may include increased headache, drowsiness, nausea, vomiting, a decreased level of consciousness, a dilated pupil on the side of the hematoma, and subsequently contralateral weakness and decerebrate posture.

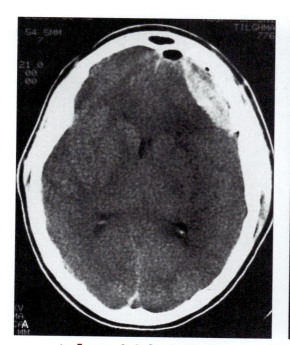
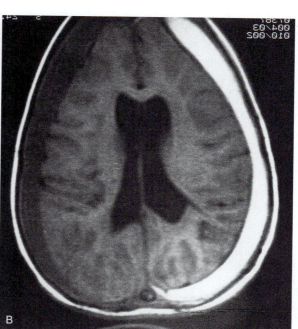

➤ **FIGURE 8.9 Cerebral hematomas**. A, This epidural hematoma resulted from a fracture that extended into the orbital roof and sinus area, leading to rapid hemorrhage in the right frontal lobe of the brain. B, The subdural hematoma on the right side of the brain is fairly evident.

➤ MANAGEMENT

 *Activate EMS. Maintain the ABCs, assess vital signs, and treat for shock. Immediate surgery is needed to **decompress** the hematoma and control arterial bleeding.*

Subdural Hematoma

A subdural hematoma is approximately three times more frequent than an epidural hematoma. Hemorrhaging occurs beneath the dura mater. It is caused by acceleration forces of the head, rather than the impact of the force. Subdural hematomas may be classified as either acute or chronic, and simple or complicated.

➤ SIGNS AND SYMPTOMS

In an acute subdural, bleeding is usually associated with cortical arterial bleeding and tends to be rapid with early loss of consciousness. The condition may become life-threatening in an hour or two. In contrast, a chronic subdural hematoma is associated with bleeding from a cerebral vein, causing low-pressure venous bleeding that clots very slowly **(Figure 8.9B)**. Signs and symptoms may not become apparent for hours, days, or even weeks after injury, when the clot absorbs fluid and expands **(Box 8.2)**.

In a simple subdural hematoma, blood collects in the subdural space but no underlying cerebral injury occurs. Athletes are thus less likely to be rendered unconscious. These individuals seldom demonstrate a deterioration in level of consciousness, and only 13% have a lucid interval. This type of injury accounts for 45% of all acute subdural hematomas and has a 21% mortality rate (1).

In a complicated subdural hematoma, the blood clot generally accompanies simultaneous brain injury. Because of the shear force related to head acceleration, the cerebral cortex is damaged, leading to a rapid accumulation of blood and intracerebral swelling that rapidly increases intracranial pressure. The damage is not due to the mass of the lesion, but rather the increase in intracranial pressure. The mortality rate can be as high as 53%. The individual is

typically knocked out and remains unconscious. Pupillary dilation and retinal changes on the affected side are common. Other signs include a reduced pulse, gradual increase in blood pressure, vomiting, and dyspnea (shortness of breath).

➤ MANAGEMENT

 Activate EMS. Maintain the ABCs, assess vital signs, and treat for shock.

Early diagnosis of a subdural hematoma is essential for a successful recovery. Surgical drainage of the hematoma less than 4 hours after the injury has been shown to result in a mortality rate of less than 40%. The mortality rate increases to 80% if surgery is delayed beyond 4 hours (4).

Cerebral Contusion

A cerebral contusion is a focal injury, but a mass-occupying lesion is not present. Instead, microhemorrhaging of the brain occurs, which is bleeding that is visible on a CT scan as an area of high-density blood interspersed with brain tissue. The common mechanism of injury is striking the occiput as a result of a fall or impact to the frontal lobe. The contusion can occur in any portion of the cortex, brainstem, or cerebellum, but because of the close anatomic relationship between bony ridges and the frontal lobes, these lobes are particularly susceptible to this type of injury.

➤ SIGNS AND SYMPTOMS

Most individuals who sustain a cerebral contusion will experience a loss of consciousness. Subsequently, they may become very alert or become comatose. The danger flag is an individual who has a normal neurologic examination but has symptoms such as headaches, dizziness, or nausea that persist.

➤ MANAGEMENT

 Activate EMS. Maintain the ABCs, assess vital signs, and treat for shock. These individuals should be immediately referred to a physician for further examination, including a CT scan.

➤➤ **BOX 8.2**

Signs and Symptoms of Increasing Intracranial Pressure

- Severe headache
- Nausea or vomiting
- Pupil irregularity
- Confusion, or progressive or sudden impairment of consciousness
- Rising blood pressure
- Falling pulse rate
- Irregular respirations
- Irregular eye tracking or eye movement
- Increased body temperature
- Drastic changes in emotional control

 The softball player is experiencing an increase in intracranial pressure. Activate EMS. Maintain the ABCs, assess vital signs, and treat for shock. Disorientation, headache, and nausea are "red flags" indicating serious intracranial hemorrhage. Activate EMS to transport this individual to the nearest medical facility.

DIFFUSE CEREBRAL INJURIES

 A swimmer misjudged the distance to the wall and collided head-first into the wall. The individual was momentarily stunned, "saw stars," and had blurred vision for about 30 seconds. After 3 or 4 minutes, the individual reports feeling much better except for a slight headache. Can this individual return to activity?

Diffuse injuries are often associated with a **concussion**, characterized by immediate and transient impairment of neural function, such as alteration of consciousness, disturbance of vision, equilibrium, etc., due to mechanical forces. Under normal conditions, the brain balances a series of electrochemical events in billions of brain cells. When shaken or jarred, brain function can be disrupted temporarily without causing injury or damage to brain tissue. For example, mild trauma can result in interruption of cerebral function. Signs and symptoms range from mild to moderate, and are transient and reversible. This can be attributed to the minimal damage to soft tissue structures. As impact magnitude increases with an acceleration injury, both cerebral function and structural damage occur, resulting in more serious signs and symptoms. These include varying degrees of loss of consciousness, headache, confusion, memory loss, nausea, **tinnitus** (ringing in the ears), pupillary changes, dizziness, and loss of coordination. Other related cerebral conditions that may occur as a result of head trauma include posttraumatic headaches, postconcussion syndrome, and second-impact syndrome, all discussed.

Concussions

Concussions may be caused by acceleration or deceleration forces. In football, an acceleration force is generated when an opponent or the ball hits an athlete's head; the site of maximal injury is usually at the point of impact (coup injury). Deceleration forces are generated when an athlete's head strikes the ground; the site of maximal injury is opposite the point of impact (contrecoup injury). Confusion and amnesia are hallmark signs of concussion, but loss of consciousness may or may not occur.

CLASSIFICATIONS OF CONCUSSIONS

To date, there are several different classification schemes that attempt to define the various degrees of brain dysfunction in cerebral concussions **(Table 8.2)**. Dr. Robert C. Cantu, a neurosurgeon, developed a classification that became very popular with a large number of sports medicine clinicians (3). The grading scale used the duration of loss of consciousness (LOC) and posttraumatic amnesia (PTA) to differentiate mild, moderate, and severe concussive injury.

Dr. Joseph S. Torg, an orthopedic surgeon, developed another classification that included six separate grades of concussion (4). Assessment involved evaluating facial ex-

TABLE 8.2	GRADING SCALES FOR ATHLETIC MILD HEAD INJURY		
	Grade I/Mild	Grade II/Moderate	Grade III/Severe
Cantu	No LOC or PTA <1 hour PTA 1–24 hours	LOC <5 minutes PTA >24 hours	LOC >5 minutes
Torg	(Grade I–II) No LOC or amnesia (except PTA)	(Grade III–IV) LOC <few minutes PTA or retrograde amnesia	(Grade V–VI) LOC/coma, confusion, amnesia
CMS	No LOC Confusion with no amnesia	No LOC Confusion with amnesia	LOC
AAN	No LOC Sxs <15 minutes	No LOC Sxs >15 minutes	Any LOC

Adapted from Warren (2), page 16.
CMS = Colorado Medical Society; AAN = American Academy of Neurology; LOC = loss of consciousness; PTA = posttraumatic amnesia; Sxs = symptoms (i.e., confusion, amnesia, etc.).

pression; determining orientation of time, place, and person; testing for any posttraumatic and retrograde amnesia; and evaluating gait.

A single head injury death from second impact syndrome in a high school football player in Colorado more than 6 years ago served as a catalyst for Dr. James Kelly and the Colorado Medical Society to study head injuries and their management. This study culminated in a new classification scale in 1991 entitled *Guidelines for the Management of Concussion in Sports* (5). The guidelines established stricter requirements for assessing the severity of concussions and mandated emergency transport to the nearest hospital for all athletes who were unconscious for any length of time, even if only for a few seconds.

The Quality Standards Subcommittee of the American Academy of Neurology (AAN), in an effort to impose a tighter definition of concussion, developed *The Practice Parameter: The Management of Concussion in Sports* (summary statement) in 1997 (6). The statement made several important modifications to the Colorado Guidelines. These modifications included nine features of concussions frequently observed **(Box 8.3)**, and early and late symptoms of concussions **(Box 8.4)**. While confusion and amnesia remain the most frequently cited symptoms, any disturbance of neural function resulting from mechanical head trauma is sufficient to confirm the presence of cerebral concussion.

One need only look at the various classification systems to see problems with each one. Loss of consciousness may be difficult to detect if it is momentary. By the time the athletic trainer or physician reaches a concussed player on the field, he or she may only be dazed, and it may be impossible to ascertain if LOC has occurred. In using Cantu's classification scale, an athlete with a momentary LOC with an asymptomatic recovery would be considered to have a grade 2 (moderate) injury, and the athlete would miss 1 week of play. Whereas under the Colorado guidelines, this same injury would be seen as a grade 3 (severe) injury and the player would be transported to a hospital and miss up to a month of activity. With Torg's classification, grades 1–3 have normal consciousness with varying levels of posttraumatic and retrograde amnesia. Grade 4 (moderate) is characterized by a loss of consciousness of less than 5 minutes involving a paralytic coma. Both the Cantu and Torg scales focus on mental status testing (confusion and amnesia) and neglect any physical exertional tests. This would lead one to believe that if the individual recovers from the symptoms at rest, the symptoms will not be exacerbated during an exertional competition.

The Colorado Medical Society guidelines state that all individuals who lose consciousness (for even a few seconds) should be transported to the nearest hospital for an immediate neurological evaluation, which may include a CT or MRI scanning. This is not what is practiced in the field routinely by physicians or athletic trainers, as it is just not practical.

A problem that has followed the AAN parameters is that the statement was issued as a practice option, not a standard or guideline. Standards reflect a high degree of certainty based on well-designed research trials or overwhelming evidence from clinical studies. Guidelines identify a particular strategy or strategies that reflect moderate clinical certainty. An option, on the other hand, reflects other strategies for patient management for which there is unclear clinical certainty based on inconclusive or conflicting evidence or opinion. Despite efforts to impose a tighter definition of concussion, more valid in-the-field research is necessary to establish a well-defined standard for classification of concussion. It is no wonder that confusion exists over the classification of concussions.

The usefulness of a grading scale is well established in athletic training to determine the severity of a concussion. The discussion below is a combination of the existing scales, including the recommendations in the Colorado Medical Society guidelines and the American Academy of Neurology. These guidelines define the level of injury and describe the actions that should be taken if such injuries are suspected.

GRADE 1 CONCUSSION

➤ SIGNS AND SYMPTOMS

Although the most common concussion, it is the most difficult to recognize. The athlete is not rendered unconscious and suffers only momentary confusion (e.g., inattentiveness, poor concentration, inability to process information or sequence tasks) without amnesia. The individual may simply report "I had my bell rung." Usually the concussion symptoms or mental status abnormalities on examination resolve in less than 15 minutes.

➤ MANAGEMENT

The individual should be removed from competition and examined immediately and at 5-minute intervals to detect amnesia or postconcussion symptoms at rest or with exertion (see Assessment of Cranial Injuries). If activity provokes early postconcussion symptoms (e.g., unsteady balance [vertigo], headache, nausea, sensitivity to light [photophobia]), the athlete should be disqualified from reentering the game. Players who remain free of symptoms for at least 15 minutes may return to competition. A second mild concussion during the same game eliminates the player from competition that day, with the player returning only if asymptomatic for at least 1 week at rest and with exercise.

GRADE 2 CONCUSSION

➤ SIGNS AND SYMPTOMS

With a grade 2 concussion, transient confusion and no loss of consciousness is present. Concussion symptoms or mental status abnormalities on examination last more than 15 minutes. These abnormalities may include poor concentration, loss of memory of events immediately preceding the injury (**retrograde amnesia**), or loss of memory of events following the injury (**anterograde amnesia**). This memory loss may diminish somewhat, but the player will always have some degree of permanent, though short, memory loss about the injury. Other signs that may be present include moderate dizziness and unsteady gait, blurred vision, tinnitus, and headache.

➤ MANAGEMENT

An athlete with a grade II concussion should be removed from activity and should not be allowed to return that day. The individual may develop "postconcussion syndrome," which can last for several weeks. Frequent on-site examinations should look for signs of evolving intracranial pathology. A physician or neurologist should reexamine the athlete the following day. Return to practice may be allowed only after being asymptomatic for 1 full week at rest and with exertion. A CT or MRI scanning is recommended in all instances where headache or other associated symptoms worsen or persist longer than 1 week. Following a second grade 2 concussion, return to play is delayed until the athlete has had at least 2 weeks symptom-free at rest and with exertion. The season should be terminated if any abnormality on the CT or MRI scan is consistent with brain swelling, contusion, or other intracranial pathology.

GRADE 3 CONCUSSION

➤ SIGNS AND SYMPTOMS

Grade 3 concussions involve any loss of consciousness, either brief (seconds) or prolonged (minutes). With severe concussions, decortication (extension of the legs with flexion of the elbows, wrists, and fingers) or decerebration (extension of all four extremities) are often present (see Figure 4.15). The concussion may also trigger convulsions or collapse of the cardiorespiratory system.

➤ MANAGEMENT

Activate EMS. The individual should be transported from the field to the nearest hospital if still unconscious or if worrisome signs are detected (with cervical spine immobilization, if indicated).

A thorough neurologic examination must be conducted. After a brief (seconds) grade 3 concussion, the athlete should be withheld from play until asymptomatic for 1 week at rest and with exertion. After a prolonged (minutes) grade 3 concussion, the athlete should be with-

TABLE 8.3	WHEN TO RETURN TO PLAY AFTER BEING REMOVED FROM COMPETITION
Grade of concussion	**Time until return to play***
Multiple Grade 1 concussion	1 week
Grade 2 concussion	1 week
Multiple Grade 2 concussion	2 weeks
Grade 3—brief loss of consciousness (seconds)	1 week
Grade 3—prolonged loss of consciousness (minutes)	2 weeks
Multiple Grade 3 concussions	1 month or longer, based on clinical decision of evaluating physician

*Only after being asymptomatic with normal neurologic assessment at rest and with exercise.

Printed with permission from the Quality Standards Subcommittee of the American Academy of Neurology (6), p 584.

held from play for 2 weeks at rest and with exertion. Following a second grade 3 concussion, the athlete should be withheld from play for a minimum of 1 asymptomatic month. The supervising physician may elect to extend the return to play beyond 1 month. As with the grade 2 concussion, a CT or MRI scan is recommended in all instances where headache or other associated symptoms worsen or persist longer than 1 week. Any abnormalities in the scan consistent with brain swelling, contusion, or other intracranial pathology should result in terminating activity for the season, and return to play next season should be highly discouraged. **Table 8.3** summarizes when an athlete may return to play after being removed from competition from either grade of concussion.

Posttraumatic Headaches

Posttraumatic vascular headaches may be confused with a mild concussion or postconcussive headache. A vascular headache is a result of vasospasm, and does not usually occur with impact, but develops shortly afterward.

➤ SIGNS AND SYMPTOMS

Symptoms, such as a localized area of blindness that may follow the appearance of brilliantly colored shimmering lights (scintillating scotoma), are often noted. Posttraumatic migraine headaches, also referred to as footballer's migraine, have been reported in soccer players after repetitive heading of the ball. Also, migraines are characterized by recurrent attacks of severe headache with sudden onset, with or without visual or gastrointestinal problems.

➤ MANAGEMENT

This individual should be immediately referred to a physician for further evaluation and care.

Postconcussion Syndrome

➤ SIGNS AND SYMPTOMS

Postconcussion syndrome may develop after a concussion, and is characterized by persistent headaches, blurred vision, vertigo, memory loss, irritability, and inability to concentrate on even the simplest task. The condition can start from the time of injury to 48 hours after the trauma, and last for several weeks to months after injury (1).

➤ MANAGEMENT

The individual can undergo a CT scan, but the scan is generally normal. There is no definitive treatment other than symptomatic measures to control the headaches. The physician should supervise the level of activity, and prohibit the athlete from returning to activity until the symptoms resolve.

Second Impact Syndrome

Second impact syndrome (SIS) occurs when an athlete who has sustained an initial head injury, usually a concussion, sustains a second head injury before the symptoms associated with the previous one have totally resolved. Most cases have occurred in children and adolescents, although the condition has been linked to ice-hockey, football, and boxing (7).

➤ SIGNS AND SYMPTOMS

In the initial injury, visual, motor, or sensory changes occur, and the individual may have difficulty with thought and memory. Before these symptoms resolve, which may take days or weeks, the individual returns to competition and receives a second blow to the head. This second blow may be relatively minor. The athlete may appear stunned, but often completes the play and sometimes walks off the field unassisted. As the vascular engorgement within the cranium increases intracranial pressure, the brain stem becomes compromised. The athlete collapses with rapidly dilating pupils, progressing to loss of eye movement, coma, and respiratory failure.

➤ MANAGEMENT

The usual interval from second impact to brain stem failure is short, usually 2 to 5 minutes (8).

 Management involves immediate activation of EMS and maintenance of basic life support.

To prevent this problem, it is imperative that any athlete who complains of a headache, light-headedness, visual disturbances, or other neurologic symptoms not be allowed to participate in any athletic event in which head trauma may occur until totally asymptomatic.

 The individual was momentarily stunned, "saw stars," and had blurred vision. This is not uncommon in a grade 1 concussion. However, a lingering headache should signal caution. This individual should be carefully watched for increases in headache, an unsteady gait, nausea, photophobia, or mood swings, dictating immediate evaluation by a physician.

SCALP INJURIES

The scalp is the outermost anatomical structure of the cranium, the first area of contact in trauma. The scalp is highly vascular and bleeds freely, making it a frequent site for abrasions, lacerations, contusions, or hematomas between the layers of tissue. The primary concerns with any scalp laceration are to control bleeding, prevent contamination, and assess for a possible skull fracture. As with any open wound, latex gloves should be worn as part of universal precautions.

Mild direct pressure should be applied to the area with sterile gauze until bleeding has stopped. The wound should be inspected for any foreign bodies or signs of a skull fracture. If a skull fracture is ruled out, the wound should be cleansed with surgical soap or saline solution, covered with a sterile dressing, and the individual referred to a physician for possible suturing.

Abrasions and contusions can be treated with gentle cleansing, topical antiseptics, and ice to control hemorrhage. Hematomas, or "goose eggs," involve a collection of blood between the layers of the scalp and skull. Crushed ice and a pressure bandage are used to control hemorrhage and edema. If the condition does not improve in 24 hours, the individual should be referred to a physician.

ASSESSMENT OF CRANIAL INJURIES

 A skater fell on the ice, landed flat on the back, and bumped his head on the ice. The individual is somewhat disoriented, dizzy, and has a slight headache, but vision appears to be normal. What danger signs indicate that the condition is deteriorating and immediate medical care is warranted?

Any athlete who receives a blow, or any significant acceleration-deceleration-type force, to the head should be thoroughly evaluated for life-threatening conditions. In head injuries, this encompasses gathering a history, observing and inspecting the head and facial area for signs of trauma, and assessing mental status, neurologic integrity, and external provocative tests. These components are not separate and distinct, but rather occur simultaneously. For matters of clarity, these components are presented in separate parts of this section.

Because significant head trauma may also cause neck injury, it should always be assumed that a cervical injury is present. In approaching the individual, the athletic trainer should gather a brief history of the mechanism of injury, duration of unconsciousness, and any other pertinent information from individuals at the scene. Ammonia capsules should never be placed under the nose to arouse the athlete, as he or she may jerk the head and neck, leading to serious complications if a spinal injury is present. An open airway should be established and maintained. If the individual is face down, the head and neck should be stabilized, and the individual log rolled into a supine position while continuing to stabilize the cervical spine. Any mouth guard, dentures, or partial plates should be removed to prevent occluding the airway. On a football player, a pocket mask can be slid between the chin and the lowest portion of the face mask or through the eye hole of the face mask, then positioned over the mouth and nose. Research has shown that this method allows faster activation of rescue breathing or CPR and limits extraneous cervical spine motion that may occur with other face mask removal techniques (9). Rescue breathing and CPR should be initiated as needed.

Vital Signs

Vital signs should be taken early in the assessment to establish a baseline of information that can be periodically rechecked to determine if the individual's status is improving or deteriorating. Vital signs include pulse, respiration, blood pressure, and body temperature. However, with head trauma, body temperature is not as critical as the others. Any abnormal variations, such as falling pulse rate, rising blood pressure, or irregular breathing, indicate increasing intracranial pressure (see **Box 8.2**).

 If present, activate EMS.

1. **Pulse.** A slow, bounding pulse may indicate increasing intracranial pressure. A rapid, weak pulse indicates shock.
2. **Respiration**. Irregular breathing indicates increasing intracranial pressure. Rapid, shallow breathing indicates shock. If the individual shows signs of respiratory difficulty, or collapses into respiratory arrest, immediate action is necessary to initiate and maintain respiratory function.
3. **Blood pressure.** An increase in the systolic blood pressure or a decrease in the diastolic blood pressure indicates rising intracranial pressure. Low blood pressure rarely occurs in a head injury. It may, however, indicate a possible cervical injury or serious blood loss from an injury elsewhere in the body.

History and Mental Status Testing

Confusion and amnesia are the hallmark signs of a concussion. Although disorientation may be present, the cardinal features of confusion include 1) disturbance of vigilance with heightened distractibility, 2) inability to maintain a coherent stream of thought, and 3) inability to carry out a sequence of goal-directed movements (10). The confusion and memory dysfunction may be immediate after injury or may be a delayed process taking several minutes to fully evolve. Because of this, close observation and assessment repeated over a period of time is necessary to see if the evolving neuropathologic change associated with concussion leads to physical signs and symptoms or to the development of memory dysfunction. Initially, the athletic

trainer should call the person's name and gently tap him or her on the cheek or arm to get a response. Slurred speech, difficulty in constructing sentences, or inability to understand commands must be noted. The head and neck should continue to be stabilized throughout the assessment. The following examples may be used to gather the history of the injury and test the mental status of the athlete:

1. **Orientation.** Ask the individual about the time, place, person, and situation (e.g., circumstances surrounding the mechanism of injury).
2. **Concentration**. Recite three digits to the athlete, and ask the individual to recite them backwards. Move to four digits, and then five digits (e.g., 3-1-7, 4-6-8-2, 5-3-0-7-4). Ask the individual to list the months of the year in reverse order.
3. **Memory.** Ask the individual to list the names of competitive teams in prior contests. Name three words or identify three objects for the individual, and ask the athlete to recall the words and objects at 0 and every 5 minutes. Ask the athlete to recall recent newsworthy events or provide details of the contest (plays, moves, strategies, etc.).
4. **Symptoms.** Does the individual have a headache or ringing in the ears? Progressive headaches indicate increasing intracranial pressure and signal danger. Does the individual feel nauseous? Intracranial pressure can stimulate the reflex onset of nausea and vomiting. If this symptom is present, it indicates a fairly serious intracranial injury.
5. **Loss of consciousness.** The Glascow Coma Scale can be used to determine level of consciousness (**Table 8.4**). This information provides a baseline of data that can be periodically rechecked to determine if the athlete's status is improving or deteriorating. Is the individual totally unresponsive, confused, or disoriented? Did he or she lose consciousness? If so, did it occur immediately on direct impact, or did the person progress to unconsciousness? How long was the athlete unconscious? Did the athlete respond to painful stimuli (e.g., squeezing the trapezius, pinching soft tissue between the thumb and index finger in the axilla, knuckle to the sternum, or squeezing the Achilles tendon)? Was there a seizure? Look at the tongue, as it is often bitten during a seizure. Has the individual ever had a head injury before?

Observation and Inspection

Observation of facial expression and function should be performed throughout the evaluation (see Cranial Nerve Assessment below). The following areas and conditions should be assessed in the observation component of the evaluation:

1. **Leakage of cerebrospinal fluid.** Cerebrospinal fluid (CSF) is a clear, colorless fluid that protects and cushions the brain and spinal cord. A basilar skull fracture

TABLE 8.4   GLASGOW COMA SCALE*

Eyes	Open	Spontaneously	4
		To verbal command	3
		To pain	2
		No response	1
Best motor response	To verbal commands To painful stimulus+	Obeys	6
		Localizes pain	5
		Flexion-withdrawal	4
		Flexion-abnormal (decorticate rigidity)	3
		Extension (decerebrate rigidity)	2
		No response	1
Best verbal response++		Oriented and converses	5
		Disoriented and converses	4
		Inappropriate words	3
		Incomprehensible sounds	2
		No response	1
Total			3–15

*The Glasgow Coma Scale is based on eye opening, motor, and verbal response, and is used to monitor changes in level of consciousness. If response on the scale is given a number, then responsiveness of the injured party can be expressed by totaling the figures. Lowest score is 3; highest is 15. A score of 12 or greater is considered to be a mild injury, 9 to 11 is a moderate injury, and 8 or less is a severe head injury.
+Squeeze trapezius, pinch soft tissue between thumb and forefinger or in the axilla, knuckle to sternum; observe arms.
++Arouse injured party with painful stimulus if necessary.

may result in blood and CSF leaking from the ear. A fracture to the cribriform plate in the anterior cranial area may result in blood and CSF leaking from the nose.

2. **Signs of trauma.** Discoloration around the eyes (raccoon's eyes) and behind the ears (Battle's sign) may indicate a skull fracture. A depression, elevation, or bleeding may indicate a skull fracture, laceration, or hematoma. Snoring, which may occur as a result of a fracture to the anterior cranial floor, should be noted.

3. **Skin color.** Skin color and presence of moisture or sweat should be assessed. If shock is setting in, the skin may appear ashen or pale, and may be moist and cool.

4. **Loss of emotional control.** Irritability, aggressive behavior, or uncontrolled crying for no apparent reason indicates cerebral dysfunction.

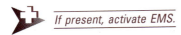

If present, activate EMS.

Palpation

Palpation can help determine possible skull or facial fractures. The athletic trainer should palpate for point tenderness, crepitus, depressions, elevations, swelling, blood, or changes in skin temperature. The following sites can be palpated:

1. Scalp and hair
2. Cervical spinous processes
3. Base of the skull and around the external ear
4. Frontal bone, eye orbit, and bridge of the nose

5. Zygomatic arch (cheek)
6. Upper and lower jaw

Neurologic Examination

Use of myotomes and dermatomes are not an effective technique in assessing cranial injuries because they assess lower motor neuron function associated with the spinal column and spinal nerves. Tests listed in this section directly assess upper motor neuron function of the brain through coordination, sensation, and agility.

1. **Cranial nerve assessment.** Integrity of the cranial nerves can be assessed quickly by sense of smell, vision, eye tracking, smiling, clenching the jaw, hearing, balance, sense of taste, speaking, and strength of shoulder shrugs (see **Table 8.5**).

2. **Pupil abnormalities.** Pupil size and accommodation to light should be equal in both eyes. A dilated pupil on one side may indicate a subdural or epidural hematoma. Dilated pupils on both sides indicate severe cranial injury with death imminent. The athletic trainer should ask the individual to look up, down, and sideways (six cardinal planes of vision). The coordinated and fluid motion of both eyes should be noted. The athlete should be asked about blurred or double vision, or if he or she saw "stars" or flashes of light on impact. Blurred or double vision, abnormal oscillating movements of the eye (nystagmus), or uncoordinated gross movement through the cardinal planes indicate disturbance of the cranial nerves that innervate the eyes and eye muscles.

3. **Babinski's reflex.** The athlete should be lying down with the eyes closed and the leg held in a slightly ele-

TABLE 8.5   CRANIAL NERVE ASSESSMENT

Number	Nerve	Motor Function
I.	Olfactory	Identify familiar odors (chocolate, coffee)
II.	Optic	Test visual fields—Snellen chart (blurring or double vision)
III.	Oculomotor	Test pupillary reaction to light Perform upward and downward gaze
IV.	Trochlear	Perform downward and lateral gaze
V.	Trigeminal	Touch face to note difference in sensation Clench teeth; push down on chin to separate jaws
VI.	Abducens	Perform lateral and medial gaze
VII.	Facial	Close eyes tight Smile and show the teeth
VIII.	Vestibulocochlear (acoustic nerve)	Identify the sound of fingers snapping near the ear Balance and coordination (stand on one foot)
IX.	Glossopharyngeal	Gag reflex; ask the athlete to swallow
X.	Vagus	Gag reflex; ask athlete to swallow or say "Ahhh"
XI.	Accessory	Resisted shoulder shrug
XII.	Hypoglossal	Stick out the tongue

vated and flexed position. Stroke a pointed object along the plantar aspect of the athlete's foot **(Figure 8.10)**. A normal sign is for the toes to curl downward in flexion and adduction. A positive sign suggests an upper motor neuron lesion and is demonstrated by extension of the big toe and abduction (splaying) of the other toes.

4. **Strength**. The athletic trainer should place his or her hands inside the hands of the injured player and ask the athlete to bilaterally squeeze the hands for comparison of grip strength.

5. **Coordination**.

- Finger to nose test. This test can assess balance, depth perception, and ability to focus on an object. With the eyes open and arms out to the side, have the athlete touch the index finger of one hand to the nose, and then alternate with the other hand to the nose. The athletic trainer should observe for any swaying or inability to touch the nose. Then, standing a few feet from the athlete, the athletic trainer should hold a finger in front of the injured individual. The athlete should reach out and touch it while alternating between the right and left hand **(Figure 8.11)**. The athletic trainer can change the

position of his or her finger after two or three touches. A variation is to have the athlete touch his or her nose between each touch of the athletic trainer's finger. The speed of touch between the nose and finger is then progressively increased.

- Gait. The athlete should be asked to walk a straight line, while the athletic trainer notes any swaying or unsteadiness of gait.

6. **Sensation and balance**.

- Finger to nose test. This test can assess sensation and balance, and is performed in a similar manner

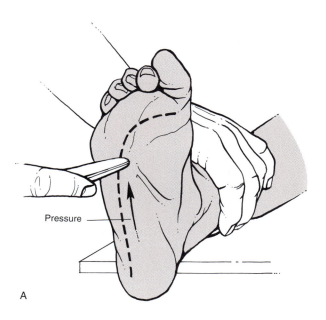

A

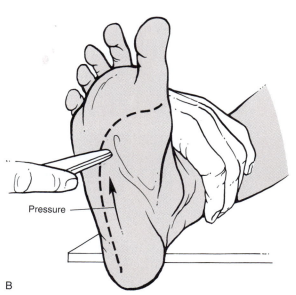

B

➤ **FIGURE 8.10 Babinski's reflex**. Stroke the bottom of the foot along the lateral border moving distally into the middle of the foot over the ball of the foot. A, A normal sign would be the toes curling under (flexing). B, An abnormal sign would show the toes splaying.

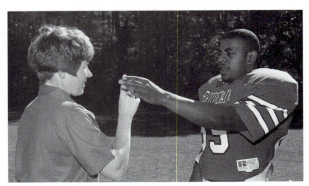

➤ FIGURE 8.11 Finger-to-nose test. With the eyes open and arms out to the side, the athlete should be instructed to touch the index finger of one hand to the nose, and then alternate with the other hand to the nose. The athlete should then alternately touch his or her nose and touch the athletic trainer's finger. The speed of touch is progressively increased while the athletic trainer moves the position of his or her hand. Inability to perform either test indicates physical disorientation and lack of coordination, and should preclude reentry to the game.

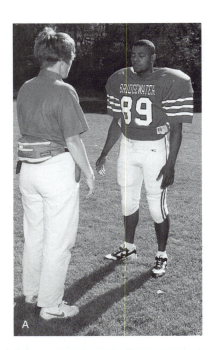

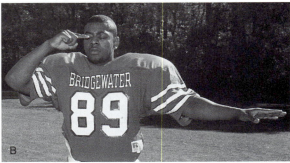

➤ FIGURE 8.12 Romberg test. A, With the eyes closed and the arms at the side, the athlete should be instructed to maintain a standing position. Any sway indicates lack of balance and sensation. B, A variation may include performing the finger-to-nose test with the eyes closed. Again, any sway is a positive sign to preclude the athlete from reentering the contest.

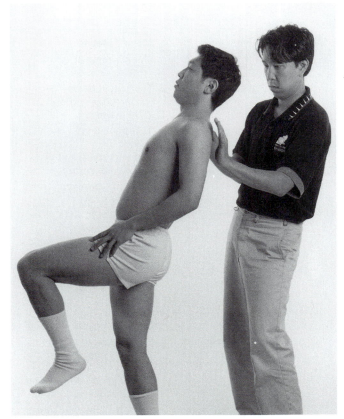

➤ FIGURE 8.13 One-legged (stork) stand. The athlete is instructed to stand and balance on one leg. If this is accomplished, the athlete should then be instructed to lean backwards.

as above, except the eyes are closed. The athletic trainer should observe for any swaying or inability to touch the nose.

- Romberg test. The individual is asked to stand with the feet together, arms at the side, and eyes closed while maintaining balance **(Figure 8.12)**. Variations include raising the arms at 90°, standing on the toes, or touching the nose with the hand while the eyes are closed (finger to nose test). While standing in front of the athlete, the athletic trainer observes for any body sway, indicating a positive test.
- One-legged stand (stork stand). With the eyes closed, have the individual stand on one foot and lean backwards **(Figure 8.13)**.

External Provocative Tests

These tests require the athlete to do exertional activities, such as running or push-ups. Any appearance of associated symptoms is abnormal (e.g., headaches, dizziness, nausea, unsteadiness, photophobia, blurred or double vision, loss of emotional control, or mental status changes). If the assessment has already determined a possible intracranial injury, the athlete should not be subjected to these tests. However, if a possible intracranial injury has not yet been determined, the following tests can be performed:

1. 40-yard sprint
2. 5 sit-ups
3. 5 push-ups
4. 5 knee bends

Determination of Findings

If the individual is not in a crisis situation, vital signs, mental status, and neurologic tests should be completed every 5 to 7 minutes to determine progress of the condition. A standardized assessment of concussion (SAC) developed by McCrea, et al. (11) can be used to evaluate four key mental functions (orientation, immediate memory, concentration, and delayed recall) **(Figure 8.14)**. The form, used to record baseline information and subsequent testing, however, has no definitive guidelines or cutoff scores established for interpreting performance on the examination. The critical part of using the instrument is to collect base-

Orientation

(1 point each)

❏ Month

❏ Date

❏ Day of week

❏ Year

❏ Time (within 1 hour)

Orientation score: 5

Immediate Memory

(1 point for each correct, total over 3 trials)

	Trial 1	Trial 2	Trial 3
Word 1	❏	❏	❏
Word 2	❏	❏	❏
Word 3	❏	❏	❏
Word 4	❏	❏	❏

Immediate memory score: 15

Concentration

Reverse digits

(Go to next string length if correct on first trial. Stop if incorrect on both trials. 1 point each for each string length.)

❏ 3-8-2   5-1-8

❏ 2-7-9-3   2-1-6-8

❏ 5-1-8-6-9   9-4-1-7-5

❏ 6-9-7-3-5-1   4-2-8-9-3-7

Months of the year in reverse order:

(1 point for entire sequence correct.)

Dec-Nov-Oct-Sept-Aug-Jul-Jun-May-Apr-Mar-Feb-Jan

Concentration score: 5

Delayed Recall

(approximately 5 minutes after Immediate Memory: 1 point each)

Word 1   ❏

Word 2   ❏

Word 3   ❏

Word 4   ❏

Word 5   ❏

Delayed recall score: 5

Summary of Total Scores

Orientation	5
Immediate memory	15
Concentration	5
Delayed recall	5
Total score	30

The following may be performed between the Immediate Memory and Delayed Recall portions of this assessment when appropriate:

Neurologic Screening

Recollection of the injury:

Strength:

Sensation:

Coordination

Exertional Maneuvers

1   40-yard sprint

5   sit-ups

5   push-ups

5   knee bends

➤ **FIGURE 8.14 Standardized assessment of concussion (SAC) form.**

line normative data on players during the off-season or preseason camp and then compare each injured player directly with this baseline performance in the event of a concussion to determine the severity of injury and to follow the player's recovery.

If the individual has been evaluated by the team physician on the sideline, and the signs and symptoms linger but appear minor, an individual close to the injured party, such as a parent or roommate, should be informed of the injury and told to look for problematic signs, including changes in behavior, unsteady gait, slurring of speech, a progressive headache or nausea, restlessness, mental confusion, or drowsiness. These danger signs should be fully explained to the observer and provided on an information sheet, such as the one illustrated in **Box 8.5**. **Field Strategy 8.2** summarizes an assessment of a cranial injury.

 The skater was disoriented, dizzy, and had a slight headache, but vision was normal. Although it appears to be a minor head injury, danger signs that indicate a more serious injury include a progressive severe headache, confusion, amnesia, nausea, an unsteady gait, or a falling pulse rate and rising blood pressure. These signs indicate increasing intracranial pressure. If present, activate EMS.

FACIAL CONDITIONS

 A female lacrosse player stepped in front of an opposing player who was taking a shot on goal and was struck on the jaw by the ball. Although she was wearing a mouth guard, bleeding from the mouth is apparent and she is unable to close the jaw with the teeth in their proper alignment. What injury might you expect to find? How will you manage this injury?

Injuries to the cheek, nose, lips, and jaw are very common in sports with moving projectiles (sticks, balls, bats, racquets), in contact sports (football, rugby, or ice hockey), and in sports where collisions with objects occur (diving, skiing, ice hockey, swimming). Many of these injuries can be prevented by wearing properly fitted face masks and mouth guards. Because the facial area has a vast arterial system, lacerations bleed freely and rapid swelling often hides the true extent of injury. **Box 8.6** identifies signs and symptoms of serious facial injuries that necessitate further examination by a physician.

Facial Soft Tissue Injuries

Facial contusions, abrasions, and lacerations are managed the same as elsewhere on the body. Contusions are treated with ice to control swelling and hemorrhage. With abrasions and lacerations, cleanse the wound with a saline solution, apply an antibiotic ointment, and cover with an occlu-

Information Sheet on Follow-up Care for a Head Injury

_____ has recently received a head injury during sport participation, but at this time it does not appear to be serious. Often, many signs and symptoms from a head injury do not become apparent until hours after the initial trauma. As such, we want to alert you to appropriate guidelines to follow for the next 24 hours.

For the rest of the day _____ should:
1. Rest quietly for at least 24 hours.
2. Consume a liquid diet for the next 8 to 24 hours.
3. Apply ice to the head for 15 to 20 minutes every hour to relieve discomfort and swelling.
4. Not use aspirin or other medication for 24 hours without a physician's approval; however, Tylenol may be used.
5. Not consume alcohol or drive a vehicle.

Have someone awaken the individual every 2 hours during the next 24 hours. If any of the following signs or symptoms are observed, seek medical help **immediately:**

- Persistent or increasing headache, particularly if it becomes localized or persists after 48 hours
- Persistent or increasing nausea and/or vomiting
- Mental confusion, disorientation, irritability, or forgetfulness that gets progressively worse
- Loss of appetite
- Drowsiness, lethargy, sleepiness, or difficulty in awakening
- Any visual difficulties, dizziness, or ringing in the ears
- Unequal pupil size; slow or no pupil reaction to light
- Bleeding and/or clear fluid from the nose or ears
- Progressive or sudden impairment of consciousness
- Alterations in breathing pattern or irregular heartbeat
- Difficulty speaking or slurring of speech
- Convulsions or tremors

She/he should not participate or play again without medical clearance by a doctor.

Emergency Phone Numbers:
Ambulance 911
Hospital _____
Remember: If any of the symptoms or signs listed above become apparent, do not delay seeking medical treatment.

sive dressing of gauze or tape. In minor lacerations (less than 1 inch long and an eighth of an inch deep), application of butterfly bandages or Steri-strips can facilitate wound closure. The area requires protection with sterile gauze and tape. The individual can return to participation but, at the conclusion of the event, the individual should see a physician to determine if sutures are needed. Larger and more complicated injuries, such as those with jagged edges

FIELD STRATEGY 8.2 CRANIAL INJURY EVALUATION

1. Stabilize head and neck
2. Check ABCs (if a helmet is worn, remove the face mask but do not remove the helmet or chin strap)
3. Determine initial level of consciousness
4. Activate EMS if necessary
5. Take vital signs (pulse, respiration, blood pressure)
6. History and mental status testing
   - Orientation (time, place, person, situation)
   - Concentration (digits backward, months of the year in reverse order)
   - Memory (names of teams in prior contests, recall of 3 words and 3 objects, recent newsworthy events, details of the contest)
   - Symptoms (headache, nausea, tinnitis)
7. Observation and inspection
   - Leakage of cerebrospinal fluid
   - Signs of trauma (deformity, body posturing, discoloration around the eyes and behind the ears)
   - Loss of emotional control (irritability, aggressiveness, or uncontrolled crying)
8. Palpation
   - Bony and soft tissue structures for point tenderness, crepitus, depressions, elevations, swelling, blood, or changes in skin temperature
9. Neurologic examination
   - Cranial nerve assessment
   - Pupil abnormalities (pupil size, response to light, eye movement, nystagmus, blurred or double vision)
   - Babinski's reflex
   - Strength
   - Coordination (finger to nose test eyes open, gait)
   - Sensation (finger to nose test eyes closed, Romberg test, one-legged stork stand)
10. External provocative test
    - 40-yard sprint
    - 5 sit-ups
    - 5 push-ups
    - 5 knee bends
11. Take vital signs and recheck every 5 to 7 minutes

or damage to nerves, veins, or bony structures, should be referred immediately to a physician.

Temporomandibular Joint Injuries

The temporomandibular joint is a sliding hinge joint stabilized by ligaments, and separated into upper and lower compartments by a fibrocartilage meniscus. Injury occurs when a blow to the mandible transmits the force to the condyles. Injuries may involve intracapsular bleeding (hemarthrosis), inflammation of the capsular ligaments (capsulitis), meniscal displacement, subluxation/dislocation of the condyles, or fracture.

▶ **SIGNS AND SYMPTOMS**

Common signs and symptoms include an inability to open the mouth (normal >40 mm), deviation of the jaw to the side of injury on opening, pain on opening and biting, **malocclusion** (change in bite), joint noise (clicking, popping, crepitus), or an inability to close the mouth (dislocation and meniscus displacement) (11).

▶ **MANAGEMENT**

The athletic trainer should temporarily immobilize the jaw with an elastic bandage wrapped from under the chin over the top of the head, although this is sometimes not needed. Treatment involves refraining from opening the mouth for 7 to 10 days, eating a soft diet, and using ice initially to reduce swelling and pain, then heat. Anti-

---

▶▶ **BOX 8.6**

Facial "Red Flags" Requiring Further Examination by a Physician

- Obvious deformity or crepitus
- Appearance of a long face
- Increased pain on palpation
- Irregular eye movement or failure to accommodate to light
- Malocclusion of the teeth

inflammatories may also assist in reducing pain and inflammation. During the acute period, heavy weightlifting should be restricted.

Facial Fractures

Direct impact can fracture the facial bones, including the mandible (jaw), maxilla (upper jaw), zygomatic (cheek), or nasal bones. The most common fractures occur to the nasal bones (discussed in the next section), followed by the zygomatic and mandible, respectively.

ZYGOMATIC FRACTURES

▶ SIGNS AND SYMPTOMS

With direct impact to the zygomatic bone, the cheek will appear flat or depressed. Swelling and ecchymosis about the eye may occlude vision and hide damage to the orbit. Occasionally the eye on the side of the fracture may appear sunken, or the eye opposite the fracture may appear to be raised. Double vision is common, and paresthesia or anesthesia (numbness) may be present on the affected cheek.

▶ MANAGEMENT

A crushed ice pack may be placed over the area to control swelling; however, avoid pressure or compression over the fracture site. The individual should be referred immediately to a physician. In most cases, the condition can easily be reduced surgically and may not require internal fixation. An exception occurs when the fracture involves the eye orbit, and surgical repair becomes more extensive. Healing usually occurs within 6 to 8 weeks. Special facial protection should be worn for 3 to 4 months. A complication may involve blurred vision over an extended period. As such, individuals in activities requiring eye-hand coordination may not return to their previous level of participation for some time.

MANDIBULAR FRACTURES

▶ SIGNS AND SYMPTOMS

This injury seldom occurs as an isolated single fracture; it is more often a double fracture or fracture-dislocation. The most common fracture sites are the mandibular angle and condyles, both of which lead to malocclusion **(Figure 8.15)**. Because the articulation of words is impossible, changes in speech are apparent. Oral bleeding may occur even though a mouth guard is properly fitted and worn. Pain, discoloration, swelling, and facial distortion may be present.

▶ MANAGEMENT

It is important for the athletic trainer to maintain an open airway with this fracture, as the tongue may occlude the airway. Management involves dressing any open wounds and immobilizing the jaw with an elastic bandage wrapped under the chin and over the top of the head. A

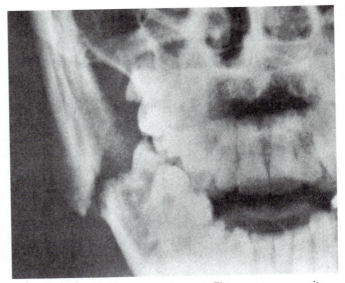

▶ **FIGURE 8.15 Mandibular fracture.** The most common site for a mandibular fracture is near the angle of the jaw, which leads to malocclusion of the teeth.

crushed ice pack may be placed over the area to control swelling; however, avoid pressure or compression over the fracture site. The individual should be referred immediately to a physician. Repair will involve internal fixation (wiring the jaw closed) or using bone plates, which may allow some individuals to return to sport participation. During the healing period, a high-protein, high-carbohydrate liquid diet is required. A weight loss of 5 to 10% is not uncommon. Mild activities, such as stationary bicycling, swimming, and use of light weights, to maintain muscle tone and conditioning are recommended.

MAXILLARY FRACTURES

▶ SIGNS AND SYMPTOMS

If the upper jaw, or midface, is fractured (LeFort fractures), the maxilla may be mobile, giving the appearance of a longer face **(Figure 8.16)**. Nasal bleeding, ecchymosis in the cheek or buccal region, malocclusion, nasal deformity, or a flattening and splaying of the naso-orbital region may be present.

▶ MANAGEMENT

Treatment will involve maintaining the airway. A forward-sitting position will allow for adequate drainage of saliva and blood. A crushed ice pack may be placed over the area to control swelling; however, avoid pressure or compression over the fracture site. The athlete should be referred immediately to a physician. Although reduction and internal fixation are often used to immobilize the region, extensive surgery and possible secondary reconstruction are occasionally necessary to treat the condition.

 As indicated by the apparent malocclusion and inability to close the jaw, the athlete may have a fractured jaw. The athletic trainer should apply

➤ FIGURE 8.16 **Maxillary fractures**. Fractures to the maxilla may involve separation of the palate (A), may extend into the nasal region (B), or may involve complete craniofacial dissociation (C). These midface fractures are commonly referred to as LeFort fractures.

an elastic bandage under the chin and over the top of the head, and refer this person immediately to a physician.

NASAL CONDITIONS

A third baseman covering a hit was struck on the side of the nose when the ball bounced upward unexpectedly. The nose is bleeding and appears to be swollen at the top. What signs and symptoms would indicate that this individual needs to be referred immediately to a physician?

Nasal injuries are common in sports where protective face guards are not worn. Nosebleeds (epistaxis) and nasal fractures are seen frequently. **Box 8.7** identifies signs and symptoms of nasal conditions that necessitate further examination by a physician.

Epistaxis

➤ SIGNS AND SYMPTOMS

Epistaxis, or nosebleed, can be either anterior or posterior. Anterior bleeding originates from superficial blood vessels on the anterior septum and is more common than posterior bleeding from the lateral wall.

➤➤ **BOX 8.7**

Nasal "Red Flags" Requiring Further Examination by a Physician

- Bleeding or CSF from the nose
- Loss of smell
- Nasal deformity or fracture
- Nosebleeds that do not stop within 5 minutes
- Foreign objects that cannot be easily removed

➤ MANAGEMENT

Most nosebleeds will stop spontaneously after applying mild pressure at the nasal bone; however, ice may also be used to stop more persistent bleeding. The head should be tilted slightly forward, reducing the risk of blood traveling down the oropharynx. A nasal plug or pledget may be used, although this is seldom needed. If used, the plug can be coated with topical astringents or soaked with vasoconstrictors, such as tannic acid or a 1% phenylephrine hydrochloride solution, as long as the individual is not allergic to them. The plug should extend externally at least one-half inch. If bleeding continues for more than 5 minutes in spite of manual pressure and ice, refer the individual to a physician. Athletes should be instructed not to blow their noses following significant bouts of epistaxis. Recurrent bouts may need to be treated with nasal cauterization, chemically with silver nitrate sticks, or with electrocautery under local anesthesia.

Nasal Fractures

➤ SIGNS AND SYMPTOMS

Epistaxis is usually present, and the nose may appear flattened and lose its symmetry, particularly with a lateral force. Because of its prominence, the nose is particularly susceptible to lateral displacement (12). Severity can range from a slightly depressed greenstick fracture (seen in adolescents) to total displacement and/or disruption in the bony and cartilaginous parts of the nose. The nasal airway can be obstructed with bony fragments, or the fracture can extend into the cranial region and cause a loss of cerebrospinal fluid. There may be crepitus over the nasal bridge and ecchymosis under the eyes.

➤ MANAGEMENT

The nose should be viewed by standing behind and above the individual, while looking down an imaginary line to determine if the nose is centered. Using a small mirror,

FIELD STRATEGY 8.3   EVALUATION AND MANAGEMENT OF A NASAL INJURY

1. Check ABCs. Bony fragments may occlude the airway
2. Determine responsiveness
3. Check for signs of a concussion and/or skull fracture
4. History
   - Primary complaint (pain, dizziness, disorientation, nausea, vision disturbances, tinnitis)
   - Mechanism of injury
   - Disability from injury (inability to breathe through one side of nose)
5. Observation and inspection
   - Obvious deformity or abnormal deviation
   - Bleeding and/or CSF from the nose
   - Check pupil size, pupillary response to light, eye movement, nystagmus, blurred or double vision that may indicate an associated cranial injury
   - Abnormal breathing rate and pattern
   - Stand behind the individual and look down an imaginary line to see if the nose is deviated
6. Palpation
   - Palpate the two nasal bones with the forefinger and thumb (checking for swelling, depressions, crepitus, mobility, etc.)
   - Check the internal structures of the nasal area for any abnormalities
7. After bleeding is controlled, inspect the internal structures for any abnormalities
8. Apply ice to control hemorrhage, and refer the individual to a physician for further care

the injured individual should look at the nose to determine if it appears normal. Treatment involves controlling bleeding, applying ice to limit swelling and hemorrhage, and referring the individual to a physician for further examination. A nose guard can be worn after a few days to protect the area from additional injury. **Field Strategy 8.3** provides guidelines in the assessment and care of a fractured nose.

 Signs and symptoms that indicate a serious nasal injury include excessive bleeding or CSF from the nose, loss of smell, nasal deformity or fracture, or a nosebleed that does not stop within 5 minutes. If present, the athlete should be referred immediately to a physician.

ORAL AND DENTAL CONDITIONS

 A basketball player was struck in the mouth by an elbow. The inside of the upper lip is bleeding. At least three teeth are loose, and one tooth appears to be broken in half. How should this injury be managed?

The most commonly injured tooth is the maxillary central incisor, which is positioned front and center and receives 80% of all dental trauma (13). During athletic participation, nearly all such injuries are preventable through regular use of mouth protectors. Mouth protectors prevent injury to the lips, teeth, cheek, tongue, mandible, neck, temporomandibular joint (TMJ), and brain by absorbing shock, spreading impact, cushioning the contact

between the upper and lower jaw, and keeping the upper lip away from the incisal edges of teeth. Although certain sports (football, boxing, field hockey, and lacrosse) require mouth guards, few coaches or league officials require the devices in other contact and collision sports. **Box 8.8** identifies signs and symptoms of oral and dental conditions that necessitate further examination by a physician.

Mouth Lacerations

➤ MANAGEMENT

Treatment for minor lacerations is the same as in other lacerations. This includes applying direct pressure to stop bleeding, cleaning the area with a saline solution, applying Steri-strips if needed, and covering the wound with a dry, sterile dressing. Lacerations that extend completely through the lip, or involve the outer lip or large

➤➤ **BOX 8.8**

Oral and Dental "Red Flags" Requiring Further Examination by a Physician

- Lacerations involving the lip, outer border of the lip, or tongue
- Loose teeth either laterally displaced, intruded, or extruded
- Chipped, cracked, fractured, or dislodged teeth
- Any individual complaining of persistent toothache or sensitivity to heat and cold
- Inability to close the jaw
- Malocclusion of the teeth

tongue lacerations, require special suturing. A badly scarred tongue can affect taste and interfere with speech patterns. With tongue lacerations, the wound should be cleansed with water or mouthwash, and referred to a physician for possible suturing. The individual should not be returned to participation until the wound is healed. If sutures are applied, protection is continued for at least 7 days.

Loose Teeth

➤ MANAGEMENT

A loosened tooth may be partially displaced, **intruded, extruded,** or avulsed **(Figure 8.17)**. When the tooth has been displaced outwardly or laterally displaced, the athletic trainer should try to place the tooth back into its normal position, without forcing it. Teeth that are intruded should be left alone; any attempt to move the tooth may result in permanent loss of the tooth or damage to any underlying permanent teeth. The individual should be referred to a dentist immediately. A dental radiograph can rule out damage under the gum line and ensure the tooth is properly replaced. The damaged tooth is then splinted to surrounding teeth for 2 to 3 weeks.

Fractured Tooth

➤ SIGNS AND SYMPTOMS

Fractures may occur through the enamel, dentin, pulp, or root of the tooth. Fractures involving the enamel cause no symptoms and can be smoothed by the dentist to prevent further injury to the lips and inner lining of the oral cavity. Fractures extending into the dentin cause pain and increased sensitivity to cold and heat. Fractures exposing the pulp or root of the tooth lead to severe pain and sensitivity.

➤ MANAGEMENT

The individual should be referred to a dentist who will apply a sedative dressing over the exposed area, and later attach a permanent, composite, resin crown. Fractures exposing the pulp involve more extensive dental work. If

the pulp exposure is small, a pulp-capping procedure placing calcium hydroxide on the area can bridge the exposed area. If successful, it eliminates the need for a root canal. Another treatment involves removing a portion of the pulp in the root canal, leaving uninjured pulp in the root. This has been successful in younger patients whose roots have not yet fully formed. The final method of treatment is a total root canal.

Dislocated Tooth

➤ MANAGEMENT

Teeth that have been totally avulsed from their sockets can often be located in the individual's mouth or on the ground. These teeth can be saved, but time is of the essence. The athletic trainer should hold the tooth by the crown. It is important not to rub the tooth or remove any dirt. If the tooth is rinsed in milk or saline and replaced intraorally within the tooth socket within 30 minutes, the prognosis for successful replanting is 90%. Tap or drinking water will damage the periodontal ligament cells on the root surface and compromise implantation procedures. Implantation that occurs after 2 hours results in a 95% failure rate (14). Semirigid fixation of 7 to 10 days may be followed by root canal therapy. Contact drills and competition are restricted during this period of time, and an appropriate face or mouth guard should be worn to prevent further injury.

With the basketball player, the athletic trainer should: (a) put on latex gloves, (b) stop the bleeding with a sterile gauze pad and compression, (c) cleanse the mouth with a saline solution, and (d) refer the individual immediately to a dentist. The dentist may be able to apply a permanent crown to the tooth.

EAR CONDITIONS

A wrestler was not wearing protective headgear during practice. He is now complaining about a burning, aching sensation on the outer ear. It appears to be somewhat inflamed and sensitive to touch, but no swelling is apparent. How should this injury be managed? What signs might indicate a more serious problem?

Several conditions may affect the ear. Foreign bodies in the ear are usually harmless and easily removed with a speculum. Trauma to the external ear can lead to auricular hematoma or "cauliflower ear," rupture of the eardrum, localized inflammation of the auditory canal, and swimmer's ear. Cauliflower ear is common in wrestlers and completely preventable by wearing proper headgear at all times when on the mat. **Box 8.9** identifies signs and symptoms of ear conditions that necessitate further examination by a physician.

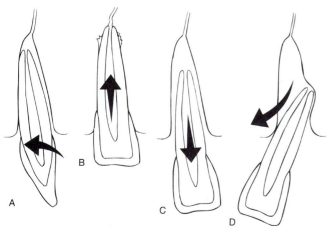

➤ FIGURE 8.17 **Loose teeth.** Loose teeth may involve partial displacement (A), intrusion (B), extrusion (C), or avulsion (D).

Ear "Red Flags" Requiring Further Examination by a Physician

- Bleeding or CSF from the ear canal
- Bleeding or swelling behind the ear (Battle's sign)
- Hematoma or swelling that removes the creases of the outer ear
- Tinnitis or hearing impairment
- Feeling of fullness in the ear; vertigo
- Foreign body in ear that cannot be easily removed
- "Popping" or itching in the ear
- Pain when the ear lobe is pulled

External Ear Injury

➤ SIGNS AND SYMPTOMS

Auricular hematoma, or "cauliflower ear," is a relatively minor injury caused when repeated blunt trauma pulls the cartilage away from the perichondrium. A hematoma forms between the perichondrium and cartilage of the ear, and compromises blood supply to the cartilage. If left untreated, the hematoma forms a fibrosis in the overlying skin, leading to necrosis of the auricular cartilage, resulting is the characteristic "cauliflower ear" appearance **(Figure 8.18)**.

➤ MANAGEMENT

Immediate treatment involves icing the region to reduce pain and swelling. The cold pack can be held in place

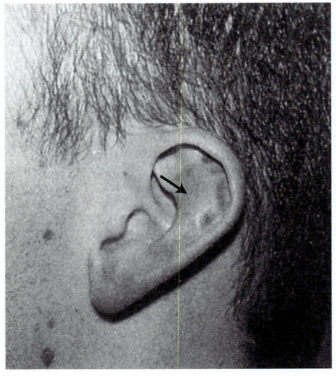

➤ FIGURE 8.18 **Cauliflower ear deformity**. Note how the hematoma has pulled the skin away from the ear cartilage.

by an elastic wrap for at least 20 minutes. If the swelling is still present, the hematoma must be aspirated by a physician to avoid pressure and permanent cartilage damage. Once aspirated, a pressure dressing is applied. The athlete should not take aspirin or nonsteroidal anti-inflammatories (NSAIDs) for several days. It is imperative that the athlete wear protective headgear to prevent reoccurrence.

Internal Ear Injury

A blow to the ear, pressure changes (seen in diving and scuba diving), and infection may injure the eardrum. Although typically seen in water sports, damage to the internal ear may occur in any sport, such as in soccer when a player is hit on the ear by a ball. Any individual with intense pain in the ear, a feeling of fullness, nausea, tinnitis, dizziness, or a hearing loss should be evaluated immediately by a physician. If the eardrum is ruptured, most minor ruptures heal spontaneously. Larger ruptures may necessitate surgical repair.

Localized infections of the middle ear (otitis media) can occur secondary to upper respiratory infections, and are often caused by bacteria, but may also be caused by viruses. Bacterial and viral infections have the same signs and symptoms. When the mastoid area is pressed, the individual will complain of pain and a sense of fullness in the ear. Swelling of the mucous membranes may cause a partial or complete block of the eustachian tube (the connection between the middle ear and pharynx), thus inhibiting hearing. The tympanic membrane may appear red and bulging. Serous otitis is often associated with otitis media and upper respiratory infection. An amber-colored or bloody fluid is seen through the eardrum and is associated with complaints of "ears popping." The supervising physician may prescribe an antibiotic for both conditions for 10 days if there is an infection, or decongestants may be used to shrink the swollen mucous membranes.

If the middle ear of an individual with otitis media is completely filled with fluid, air travel should be discouraged. If the ear is filled with fluid and air, and the eustachian tube is not working properly, the air bubbles will expand on ascent and contract on descent. Both ascent and descent will cause severe pain and may rupture the eardrum. In addition, rupture of the membranes separating the middle ear from the inner ear could also occur with catastrophic results. Therefore, air travel is not recommended until the middle ear has returned to normal appearance and function.

Swimmer's Ear

Swimmer's ear (otitis externa) is a bacterial infection involving the lining of the external auditory canal. It frequently occurs in individuals who fail to dry the canal after being in water, thereby changing the pH of the ear canal's skin.

➤ SIGNS AND SYMPTOMS

In acute conditions, pain is the predominant symptom. In more chronic cases, such as that seen with excessive use of cotton swabs, itching is a more common complaint, with discomfort and pain being secondary. There may or may not be a discharge of pus. Gentle pressure around the external auditory opening and pulling on the pinna will cause increased pain. If left untreated, the infection can spread to the middle ear, causing balance disturbances or hearing loss. Commercial ear plugs may not be helpful in preventing the condition.

➤ MANAGEMENT

Custom ear plugs from an audiologist or otolaryngologist may be necessary. The condition can also be prevented by using ear drops to dry the canal. Virtually all ear drops contain an acidifying agent, either aluminum acetate or vinegar. An effective homemade remedy is equal parts of white vinegar (acetic acid), 70% alcohol, and water. One or two drops after water exposure or after showering is the standard recommendation. If no improvement is seen, the individual should be referred to a physician who may prescribe drops containing broad-spectrum antibiotics.

 The athletic trainer should place ice on the wrestler's ear to control swelling. If any hemorrhage or edema between the perichondrium and cartilage appears to flatten the wrinkles or creases of the ear, the individual should be referred immediately to a physician for follow-up care. Protective ear wear should be worn by all wrestlers at every practice and competition.

EYE CONDITIONS

 A basketball player going up for a rebound was struck in the eye by an opponent's finger. The eye is swollen and closed. Attempts to open the eye produce excessive tearing and discomfort for the individual. What signs and symptoms might indicate a serious underlying condition?

The eyes are exposed daily to potential trauma and injury, yet many eye injuries could be prevented if protective eyewear were worn. This is especially true in racquetball and squash where players are confined to a limited space with swinging racquets and balls traveling at high speeds. Athletes who require corrective lenses should use strong plastic or semirigid rubber frames, and impact-resistant lenses. If glasses are not required, protective eyewear and/or face masks should be worn in sports in which risk of injury is high. Sport participants with only one good eye should consult an ophthalmologist to determine if they should participate in a specific activity, and if so, what protective eyewear can be worn to prevent injury. **Box 8.10** identifies signs and symptoms of ear conditions that necessitate further examination by a physician.

➤➤ **BOX 8.10**

Eye "Red Flags" Requiring Further Examination by a Physician

- Visual disturbances or loss of vision
- Unequal pupils or bilateral, dilated pupils
- Irregular eye movement or failure to accommodate to light
- Severe ecchymosis and swelling (raccoon eyes)
- Suspected corneal abrasion or corneal laceration
- Blood in the anterior chamber
- Embedded foreign body
- Individual complaining of floaters, light flashes, or a "curtain falling over the eye"
- Itching, burning, watery eye that appears pink
- Displaced contact lens that cannot be easily removed

Periorbital Ecchymosis (Black Eye)

➤ SIGNS AND SYMPTOMS

Impact forces can cause significant swelling and hemorrhage into the surrounding eyelids. This discoloration is called **periorbital ecchymosis**.

➤ MANAGEMENT

Trauma to the eye requires inspection for obvious abnormalities, palpation of the orbit for a possible orbital fracture, and assessment of pupillary response to light by shining a concentrated light beam into the eye and noting the bilateral rate of constriction. The ability of an individual to focus clearly on an object must be assessed. The anterior chamber of the eye should be inspected for any obvious bleeding (see Hemorrhage into the Anterior Chamber). Treatment involves controlling the swelling and hemorrhage by using crushed ice or ice water in a latex surgical glove. It is essential that the glove does not have rosin or other powdered substances on it. Due to possible leakage, chemical ice bags should not be used. This condition requires referral to an ophthalmologist for further examination to rule out an underlying fracture or injury to the globe.

Foreign Bodies

➤ SIGNS AND SYMPTOMS

Dust or dirt in the eyes can lead to intense pain and tearing. The individual may resist any attempt to open the eyelids to view the eye.

➤ MANAGEMENT

The foreign body, if not embedded or on the cornea, should be removed and the eye inspected for any scratches, abrasions, or lacerations (see **Field Strategy 8.4**).

 If the foreign object is impaled or embedded, however, do not touch or attempt to remove the object. Activate EMS. Medically trained individuals will stabilize the object and

FIELD STRATEGY 8.4   REMOVING A FOREIGN BODY FROM THE EYE

1. Examine the lower lid by gently pulling the skin down below the eye. Ask the individual to look up, and inspect the lower portion of the globe and eyelid for any foreign object.
2. Examine the upper lid by asking the individual to look downward.
3. Grasp the eyelashes, and pull downward.
4. Place a cotton-tipped applicator on the outside portion of the upper lid.
5. Pull the lid over the applicator, and hold the rolled lid against the upper bony ridge of the orbit.
6. Remove the foreign body with a sterile, moist gauze pad. If you are unable to successfully remove the foreign object, patch both eyes with a sterile, nonpressure oval gauze pad, and refer the individual to a physician for immediate care.

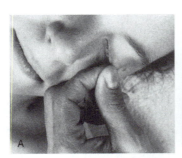
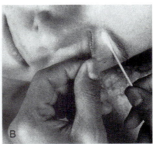
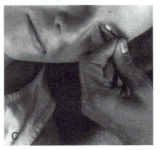

provide rigid protection for the orbit. In the cornea, a fluorescein stain may reveal the object's location, and topical anesthetics may be necessary to facilitate the physician's examination.

Sty

➤ SIGNS AND SYMPTOMS

A sty is an infection of the sebaceous gland of an eyelash or eyelash follicle. The condition starts as a red nodule that progresses into a painful pustule within a few days.

➤ MANAGEMENT

Treatment involves hot, moist compresses. If the pustule does not improve within 2 days, a physician may need to prescribe a topical ointment.

Conjunctivitis (Pinkeye)

➤ SIGNS AND SYMPTOMS

Conjunctivitis is an inflammation, often due to chlorine irritation, or bacterial infection of the conjunctiva,

the membrane between the inner lining of the eyelid and anterior eyeball. The condition leads to itching, burning, and watering of the eye, causing the conjunctiva to become inflamed and red, giving a pinkeye appearance.

➤ MANAGEMENT

The bacterial condition can be highly infectious, so the individual should be referred immediately to a physician for medical treatment.

Corneal Abrasion

➤ SIGNS AND SYMPTOMS

Occasionally a foreign body will scratch the cornea, resulting in a sudden onset of pain, tearing, and photophobia. Blinking and movement of the eye only aggravate the condition. Examination may not reveal a foreign object, but the individual continues to complain that something is in the eye.

➤ MANAGEMENT

Initial management involves covering the eye with a dry sterile dressing. A corneal abrasion is best seen by using a fluorescein dye strip. Soft contacts should be removed prior to applying the dye, as they will absorb the dye and can be ruined. The orange color of the dye is augmented by using a blue light, changing the orange dye to a bright green and illuminating the abrasion. Treatment usually involves a topical ointment, such as 2% homatrophine, to reduce pain, relax cillary muscle spasms, and prevent secondary bacterial infection. An eye patch may be worn for 24 to 48 hours. If used, the patch must be tight enough to ensure that the lids are closed beneath the patch, and firm enough to prevent the lids from opening and closing.

Corneal Laceration

➤ SIGNS AND SYMPTOMS

Lacerations to the cornea are caused by sharp objects, such as a fingernail, darts, skate blades, or broken glass. Signs and symptoms include severe pain, discomfort, decreased visual acuity, distortion or displacement of the pupil.

➤ MANAGEMENT

The pupil should be inspected for symmetry with the opposite eye. Lacerations of the cornea often incarcerate iris tissue, causing distortion and displacement of the pupil. If a laceration is suspected, any pressure on the globe should be avoided to prevent extrusion of the intraocular contents. The eye should be covered immediately with a protective shield with the pressure exerted on the bony orbit, not the soft tissue. The individual should be moved in either the supine or upright position (avoid a prone or head-down position). Therefore, activate EMS for transportation to the nearest medical facility.

Subconjunctival Hemorrhage

➤ SIGNS AND SYMPTOMS

Direct trauma can also lead to **subconjunctival hemorrhage**. Several small capillaries rupture, making the white sclera of the eye appear red, blotchy, and inflamed. The condition looks much worse than it is.

➤ MANAGEMENT

This relatively harmless condition requires no treatment and resolves spontaneously in 1 to 3 weeks. If blurred vision, pain, limited eye movement, or blood in the anterior chamber are present, however, immediate referral to an ophthalmologist is warranted.

Hemorrhage into the Anterior Chamber

Hemorrhage into the anterior chamber **(hyphema)** usually results from blunt trauma from a small ball (squash or racquetball), hockey puck, stick (field hockey or ice hockey), or swinging racquet (squash or racquetball). The small size of the object can fit within the confines of the eye orbit, thereby inflicting direct damage to the eye.

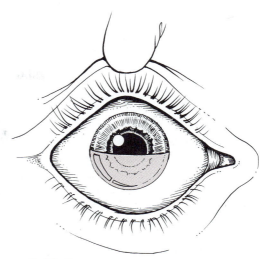

➤ **FIGURE 8.19 Hyphema.** Blood in the anterior chamber of the eye signals a serious eye injury.

➤ SIGNS AND SYMPTOMS

Initially, a red tinge in the anterior chamber may be present, but within a few hours, blood will begin to settle into the anterior chamber, giving a characteristic meniscus appearance **(Figure 8.19)**. Frequently, it occurs in microscopic quantities and can therefore, easily be overlooked. If so, visual acuity may not be affected. Such bleeding, however, indicates that an intraocular injury has occurred that must be identified to prevent recurrent bleeding, which can lead to both massive and destructive results.

➤ MANAGEMENT

 The athletic trainer should activate EMS, as the individual must be transported in a semireclining or seated position. The condition requires hospitalization, bed rest, bilateral patching of the eyes, and sedation. Nonaspirin analgesics are frequently required. The initial hemorrhage usually resolves in a few days with good prognosis for full recovery.

Detached Retina

Damage to the posterior segment of the eye can occur with or without trauma to the anterior segment. A **detached retina** occurs when fluid seeps into the retinal break and separates the neurosensory retina from the retinal epithelium. This can occur days or even weeks after the initial trauma.

➤ SIGNS AND SYMPTOMS

The individual frequently describes the condition with phrases like, "a curtain fell over my eye," or "I keep seeing flashes of light going on and off." Floaters and light flashes are early signs that the retina is damaged.

➤ MANAGEMENT

The athletic trainer should patch both eyes and immediately refer this person to an ophthalmologist, as surgery is often necessary.

Orbital "Blowout" Fracture

A blowout fracture is caused by impact from a blunt object, usually larger than the eye orbit. Upon impact, forces drive the orbital contents posteriorly against the orbital walls. This sudden increase in intraorbital pressure is released in the area of least resistance, typically the orbital floor. The globe descends into the defect in the floor.

➤ SIGNS AND SYMPTOMS

Examination may reveal **diplopia** (double vision), absent eye movement, numbness on the side of the fracture below the eye, and a recessed, downward displacement of the globe. The lack of eye movement becomes evident when the individual is asked to look up, and only one eye is able to move **(Figure 8.20)**.

➤ MANAGEMENT

The athletic trainer should apply ice to the area to limit swelling, being careful not to add additional compression or pressure over the suspected fracture site. The individual should be immediately referred to a physician. Tomograms or radiographs are necessary to confirm a fracture, and surgery is indicated to repair the defect in the orbital floor.

Displaced Contact Lens

Hard contact lenses frequently are involved in corneal abrasions. Foreign objects get underneath the lens and damage the cornea, or the cornea may be injured while putting in or taking out the lens. If irritation is present, the lens should be removed and cleaned. Hard contact lenses can slow the progression of **myopia** (nearsightedness); however, in sports, soft contact lenses are preferred. This is because eye accommodation and adjustment time are less and the lenses can be easily replaced and worn for longer periods of time. In an eye injury, individuals may be able to remove the lens themselves. However, pain or photophobia may preclude them from doing this, and it may become necessary to assist them **(Figure 8.21)**. **Field Strategy 8.5** demonstrates a full assessment of an eye injury.

 The basketball player was struck in the eye by a finger. Attempts to open the swollen, closed eye produced excessive tearing and discomfort for the individual. Signs and symptoms that would

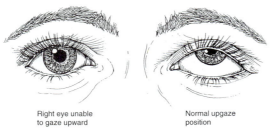

Right eye unable   Normal upgaze
to gaze upward   position

➤ FIGURE 8.20 **Orbital "blowout" fracture.** An orbital fracture can entrap the inferior rectus muscle, leading to an inability to elevate the eye.

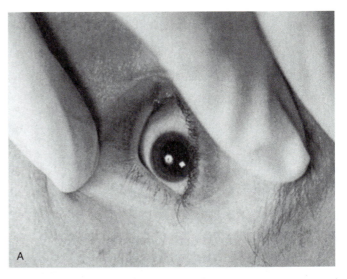

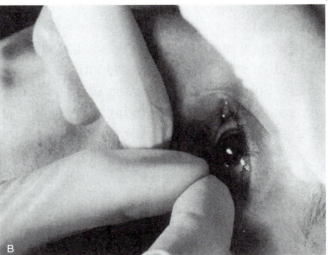

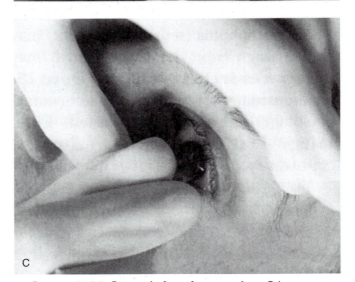

➤ FIGURE 8.21 **Removal of a soft contact lens.** Prior to removing the lens, put on latex gloves that do not have rosin or other powered substances on them. A, Open the upper and lower eyelids to view the contact lens. B, Maneuver the lens below the pupil. C, Remove the lens by pinching it between your thumb and forefinger. Place the lens in a contact lens solution.

FIELD STRATEGY 8.5   EYE EVALUATION

1. Check ABCs
2. Determine responsiveness
3. History
   - Primary complaint. Ask about the level of pain, discomfort, extent of voluntary eyelid movement, and extent of vision.
   - Determine mechanism of injury. Objects larger than the eye orbit may lead to orbital fracture; objects smaller than the eye orbit may lead to direct trauma to the eye globe. Did the trauma result from blunt trauma, a sharp object, or projectile?
4. Observation and inspection
   - Look for obvious deformity or abnormal deviation in the surrounding eye orbit.
   - Observe ecchymosis and extent of swelling in the eyelids and surrounding tissue. If the eyelid is swollen shut and the individual cannot voluntarily open it, do not force it open, as it may cause further damage.
   - Observe any bleeding from deep lacerations of the eyelid.
   - Observe the level of both pupils and the eye globe for anterior or posterior displacement, presence of any corneal lacerations, and bleeding in the anterior chamber.
   - Inspect pupil size, accommodation to light, and sensitivity to light with a penlight.
5. Palpation
   - Carefully palpate the bony rim of the eye orbit, and cheek bone for any swelling, depressions, crepitus, or mobility.
   - Control any bleeding.
6. Special tests
   - Determine eye vision. Compare the vision of the uninjured eye to the injured eye. Is it blurred, sensitive to light, or does the individual have double vision? Can the individual distinguish how many fingers you are holding up in all four quadrants of vision? Can the individual distinguish close objects and objects far away?
   - Determine eye movement. Move your finger through the six cardinal planes of vision. Do the eyes move in a coordinated manner? If one eye moves upward and the other remains in a stationary position, the inferior rectus muscle may be entrapped due to an orbital fracture.
   - Vision disturbances, such as persistent blurred vision, diplopia, sensitivity to light, loss of all or part of a field of vision, dilated pupils, any abnormal eye movement, and throbbing pain or headache, indicate a serious eye injury that warrants immediate referral.

indicate a serious underlying condition include abnormal visual acuity, a corneal abrasion or laceration, and blood in the anterior chamber.

Summary

1. Wearing protective equipment can significantly reduce the incidence and severity of head and facial injuries.
2. Minor injuries, such as nosebleeds, contusions, abrasions, lacerations, and minor concussions, can easily be handled on the field by the athletic trainer. If complications arise or the condition does not improve within a reasonable amount of time, the athletic trainer should immediately consult a physician about the injury.
3. Signs that indicate a possible skull fracture include:
   - Deformity
   - Unequal pupils
   - Discoloration around both eyes or behind the ears
   - Bleeding or CSF leaking from the nose and/or ear
   - Any loss of sight or smell
4. Signs or symptoms of increasing intracranial pressure following head trauma include:
   - Severe headache
   - Pupil irregularity or irregular eye tracking
   - Confusion, or progressive or sudden impairment of consciousness
   - Rising blood pressure and falling pulse rate
   - Drastic changes in emotional control
5. Signs and symptoms of a concussion include:
   - Headache
   - Dizziness or vertigo
   - Lack of awareness of surroundings
   - Nausea and vomiting
   - Deteriorating level of consciousness
   - Disturbance of vigilance with heightened distractibility
   - Inability to maintain coherent thought patterns

- Inability to carry out a sequence of goal-directed movements

6. Injuries that indicate increasing intracranial pressure, memory dysfunction, or gross observable incoordination require immediate referral to a physician.

➤ *Activate EMS.*

7. Fractures to the facial bones often result in malocclusion.

8. The nose is particularly susceptible to lateral displacement from trauma. Simultaneously, the trauma may also lead to a concussion.

9. When a loose tooth has been displaced outwardly or laterally, that athletic trainer should try to place the tooth back into its normal position without forcing it. Teeth that are intruded should be left alone; any attempt to move the tooth may result in permanent loss of the tooth. The individual should be referred to a dentist immediately.

10. A dislocated tooth should be located, rinsed in milk or a saline solution, and replaced intraorally within the tooth socket. The individual should be seen by a dentist within 30 minutes for replacement of the tooth.

11. Cauliflower ear is common in wrestlers and completely preventable by wearing proper headgear at all times when on the mat.

12. A foreign body in the eye, if not embedded or on the cornea, should be removed and the eye inspected for any scratches, abrasions, or lacerations.

13. Direct trauma to the eye can lead to a corneal laceration, rupture of the globe, hemorrhage into the anterior chamber, detached retina, or an orbital fracture. Loss of visual acuity, abnormal eye movement, diplopia, numbness below the eye, or a downward displacement of the globe should signal a serious condition. The individual should be referred immediately to an ophthalmologist.

References

1. Kinderknecht JJ. Head injuries. In: Athletic Injuries and Rehabilitation. Edited by Zachazewski JE, Magee DJ, Quillen WS. Philadelphia: WB Saunders, 1996.
2. Warren WL, Jr, Bailes JE. On the field evaluation of athletic head injuries. Clin Sports Med 1998;17(1):13-26.
3. Cantu RC. Guidelines for return to contact sports after cerebral concussion. Phys Sportsmed 1986;14(10):75-83.
4. Vegso JJ, Torg JS. Field evaluation and management of intracranial injuries. In: Athletic Injuries to the Head, Neck, and Face. Edited by Torg JS. St. Louis: Mosby-Year Book, 1991.
5. Colorado Medical Society. Report of the Sports Medicine Committee: Guidelines for the management of concussion in sports (rev). Denver: Colorado Medical Society, 1991.
6. Quality Standards Subcommittee of the American Academy of Neurology. Practice parameter: The management of concussion in sports. Neurology 1997;48(3):581-585.
7. McCrory PR, Berkovic SF. Second impact syndrome. Neurology 1998;50(3):677-683.
8. Cantu RC, Voy R. Second impact syndrome: A risk in any contact sport. Phys Sportsmed 1995;23(6):27-34.
9. Ray R, Luchies C, Bazuin D, Farrell RN. Airway preparation techniques for the cervical spine-injured player. J Ath Train 1995;30(3):217-221.
10. Kelly JP, Rosenberg JH. Diagnosis and management of concussion in sports. Neurology 1997;48(3):575-580.
11. McCrea M, et al. Standardized assessment of concussion in football players. Neurology 1997;48(3):586-588.
12. Tu HK, Davis LF, Nique TA. Maxillofacial injuries. In: The Team Physician's Handbook. Edited by Mellion MB, Walsh WM, Shelton GL. Philadelphia: Hanley and Belfus, 1997.
13. Woodmansey KF. Athletic mouth guards prevent orofacial injuries. Col Health 1997;45(5):179-182.
14. Kumamoto DP, Jacob M, Nickelsen D. Oral trauma: On-field assessment. Phys Sportsmed 1995;23(5):53-62.

Spinal Conditions

OBJECTIVES

1. Locate and explain the functional significance of the bony and soft tissue structures of the spine.

2. Describe the motion capabilities in the different regions of the spine.

3. Identify the factors that contribute to mechanical loading on the spine.

4. Identify specific strategies in activities of daily living to reduce spinal stress.

5. Identify anatomical variations that may predispose individuals to spine injuries.

6. Explain measures used to prevent injury to the spinal region.

7. Describe common sports injuries and conditions found in the spine and low back area.

8. Describe a thorough assessment of the spine.

9. Identify rehabilitative exercises for the spinal region.

The spine is a complex linkage system that transfers loads between the upper and lower extremities, enables motion of the trunk in all three planes, and protects the delicate spinal cord. Most injuries to the back are relatively minor, consisting of contusions, muscle strains, and ligament sprains. However, acute spinal fractures and dislocations are extremely serious and can lead to paralysis or death. Although sports-related cervical injuries account for only 15% of all spinal cord injuries annually, nearly 92% of these injuries result in quadriplegia (1). Unfortunately, with the increasing prevalence of leisure time in recent years, there has been a concomitant increase in the incidence of spinal injuries and low back pain. Low back problems are especially common in equestrian sports, weightlifting, ice hockey, gymnastics, diving, football, wrestling, and aerobics.

This chapter begins with a review of the intricate anatomical structures that make up the spine, followed by a discussion of the kinematics and kinetics of the spine. Identification of anatomical variations that may predispose individuals to spinal conditions leads into strategies used to prevent injury. Information on common injuries sustained within the various regions of the spinal column during sport participation

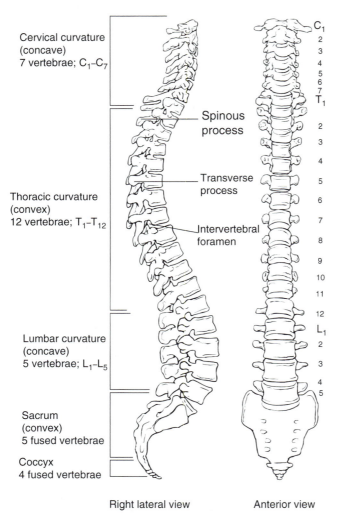

Cervical curvature (concave) 7 vertebrae; C_1–C_7

Spinous process

Transverse process

Intervertebral foramen

Thoracic curvature (convex) 12 vertebrae; T_1–T_{12}

Lumbar curvature (concave) 5 vertebrae; L_1–L_5

Sacrum (convex) 5 fused vertebrae

Coccyx 4 fused vertebrae

Right lateral view   Anterior view

➤ FIGURE 9.1 Vertebral column. Four characteristic curves of the spine can be viewed from the lateral aspect.

is followed by a presentation of techniques used in spinal injury assessment. Finally, examples of general rehabilitation exercises are provided.

ANATOMICAL REVIEW OF THE SPINE

The five regions of the spine—cervical, thoracic, lumbar, sacral, and coccygeal—are all structurally and functionally distinct. There are four normal spinal curves (Figure 9.1). As viewed from the side, the thoracic and sacral curves are convex posteriorly, and the lumbar and cervical curves are concave posteriorly. These curves constitute posture and can be modified by a host of factors, including heredity, disease, and forces, acting on the spine. Abnormal spinal curves are referred to as curvatures and are discussed later in this chapter.

Spinal Column and Vertebrae

The spinal column consists of 33 vertebrae, most of which are separated and cushioned by discs composed of fibrocartilage. There are five regions of the spine based on vertebral structure and function. These include 7 cervical, 12 thoracic, 5 lumbar, 5 fused sacral, and 4 small, fused coccygeal vertebrae. The bony structures of the vertebrae and ribs govern the varying amounts of spinal motion permitted throughout the cervical, thoracic, and lumbar regions. Within these regions, any two adjacent vertebrae and the soft tissues between them are collectively referred to as a motion segment. The motion segment is the functional unit of the spine (Figure 9.2).

A typical vertebra consists of a body, a hollow ring known as the vertebral arch, and several bony processes (Figure 9.3). The superior and inferior articular processes mate with the articular processes of adjacent vertebrae to form the facet joints. The right and left pedicles have

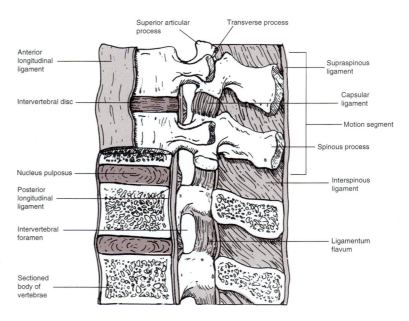

Superior articular process

Transverse process

Anterior longitudinal ligament

Intervertebral disc

Nucleus pulposus

Posterior longitudinal ligament

Intervertebral foramen

Sectioned body of vertebrae

Supraspinous ligament

Capsular ligament

Motion segment

Spinous process

Interspinous ligament

Ligamentum flavum

➤ FIGURE 9.2 Motion segment of the spine. A motion segment includes two adjacent vertebrae and the intervening soft tissues. This is considered to be the functional unit of the spine.

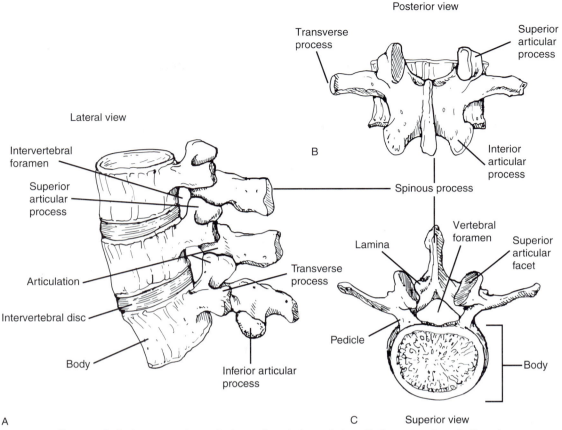

➤ **FIGURE 9.3 Structure of a typical vertebra.** A, Lateral view. B, Posterior view. C, Superior view.

notches on their superior and inferior borders, providing openings between adjacent pedicles, called intervertebral foramina. The spinal nerves pass through these foramina. The spinous and transverse processes serve as handles for muscle attachments. Forming a stacked column, the neural arches, posterior sides of the bodies, and the intervertebral discs form a protective passageway for the spinal cord and associated blood vessels. The thinnest part of the neural arch is called the pars interarticularis (see Figure 9.14). It is the pars region of the vertebrae that is most susceptible to stress fractures.

There is a progressive increase in vertebral size from the cervical region down through the lumbar region. This serves a functional purpose, because when the body is in an upright position, each vertebra must support the weight of all of the trunk positioned above it, in addition to the arms and head. The size and angulation of the vertebral processes also vary throughout the spinal column. This changes the orientation of the facet joints, which limit range of motion in the different spinal regions **(Figure 9.4)**.

Intervertebral Discs

Fibrocartilaginous discs provide cushioning between the articulating vertebral bodies. In the intervertebral disc, a thick ring of fibrous cartilage, the annulus fibrosus, sur-

rounds a gelatinous material known as the nucleus pulposus. The discs serve as shock absorbers and allow the spine to bend. Because the discs receive no blood supply, they must rely upon changes in posture and body position to produce a pumping action that brings in nutrients and flushes out metabolic waste products with an influx and outflux of fluid. Because maintaining a fixed body position curtails this pumping action, sitting in one position for a long period of time can negatively affect disc health.

Ligaments of the Spine

A number of ligaments support the spine (Figure 9.2). Anterior and posterior longitudinal ligaments connect the vertebral bodies of motion segments in the cervical, thoracic, and lumbar regions. The supraspinous ligament attaches to the spinous processes throughout the length of the spine and is enlarged in the cervical region, where it is known as the ligamentum nuchae or "ligament of the neck." Another major ligament, the ligamentum flavum, connects the pedicles of adjacent vertebrae. This ligament contains a high proportion of elastic fibers that keep it constantly in tension, contribution to spinal stability. The interspinous ligaments, intertransverse ligaments, and ligamentum flava, respectively link the spinous processes, transverse processes, and laminae of adjacent vertebrae.

➤ **FIGURE 9.4 Approximate orientations of the facet joints**.
The facet joint orientation in both the sagittal plane (lateral view)
and transverse plane (superior view) shifts progressively throughout the length of the spinal column. A, Cervical vertebrae
(C_3–C_7). B, Thoracic vertebrae. C, Lumbar vertebrae.

**ORIENTATION OF
THE FACETS TO
THE TRANSVERSE PLANE**

**ORIENTATION OF
THE FACETS TO
THE FRONTAL PLANE**

Muscles of the Spine and Trunk

Muscles of the neck and trunk are paired, with one on the
left and one on the right side of the body **(Figure 9.5)**.
These muscles can cause lateral flexion and/or rotation of
the trunk when they act unilaterally, and trunk flexion or
extension when acting bilaterally. Collectively, the primary
movers for back extension are called the erector spinae
muscles. The attachments, actions, and innervations of the
major muscles of the trunk are summarized in **Table 9.1**.

Spinal Cord and Spinal Nerves

The brain and spinal cord make up the central nervous
system. The spinal cord extends from the brain stem to
the level of the first or second lumbar vertebrae. Like the
brain, the spinal cord is encased in the three meninges.
Thirty-one pairs of spinal nerves emanate from the cord,
including 8 cervical, 12 thoracic, 5 lumbar, 5 sacral, and 1
coccygeal. Many of the spinal nerves converge (combine)
and diverge (separate) to form a complex network of in-
terjoining nerves, called a nerve plexus. The more common
ones are the brachial plexus, lumbar plexus, and sacral
plexus. At the distal end of the spinal cord, approximately
at the L_1–L_2 level, a bundle of spinal nerves extends downward through the vertebral canal and is known collectively
as the cauda equina, after its resemblance to a horse's tail.

The spinal cord serves as the major neural pathway
for conducting sensory impulses to the brain and motor
impulses from the brain. It also provides direct connections
between sensory and motor nerves inside the cord, enabling
reflex activity. Deep tendon reflexes are used consistently
in injury assessment to determine possible spinal nerve
damage. Exaggerated, distorted, or absent reflexes indicate
damage to the nervous system, often before other signs
are apparent.

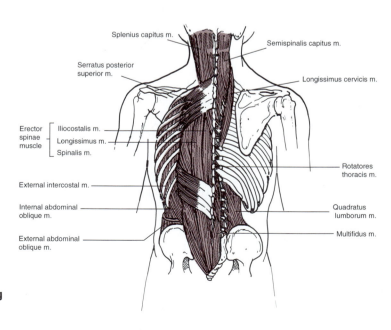

➤ **FIGURE 9.5 Deep posterior back muscles attaching
to the spine.**

TABLE 9.1 **MUSCLES OF THE SPINE**

Muscle	Proximal Attachment	Distal Attachment	Primary Action(s)	Nerve Innervation
Prevertebral muscles (Rectus capitis anterior, rectus capitis lateralis, longus capitis, longus coli)	Anterior aspect of occipital bone and cervical vertebrae	Anterior surfaces of cervical and first three thoracic vertebrae	Flexion, lateral flexion, rotation to opposite side	Cervical nerves (C_1–C_6)
Rectus abdominis	Costal cartilage of ribs 5–7	Pubic crest	Flexion, lateral flexion	Intercostal nerves (T_6–T_{12})
External oblique	External surface of lower eight ribs	Linea alba and anterior iliac crest	Flexion, lateral flexion, rotation to opposite side	Intercostal nerves (T_7–T_{12})
Internal oblique	Linear alba and the lower four ribs	Inguinal ligament, iliac crest, and the lumbodorsal fascia	Flexion, lateral flexion, rotation to same side	Intercostal nerves (T_7–T_{12}, L_1)
Splenius (Capitis and cervicis)	Mastoid process of the temporal bone, transverse processes of C_1–C_3 vertebrae	Lower half of the ligamentum nuchae, spinous processes of C_7–T_6 vertebrae	Extension, lateral flexion, rotation to same side	Middle and lower cervical nerves (C_4–C_8)
The suboccipitals (Obliquus capitus superior and inferior, rectus capitis posterior major and minor)	Occipital bone, transverse process of C_1 vertebra	Posterior surfaces, C_1–C_2 vertebrae	Extension, lateral flexion, rotation to same side	Suboccipital nerve (C_1)
Erector spinae (Spinalis, longissimus, and iliocostalis)	Lower part of the ligamentum nuchae; posterior cervical, thoracic, and lumbar spine; lower nine ribs; iliac crest; posterior sacrum	Mastoid process of the temporal bone, posterior cervical, thoracic, and lumbar spine, 12 ribs	Extension, lateral flexion, rotation to opposite side	Spinal nerves (T_1–T_{12})
Semispinalis (Capitis, cervicis, and thoracis)	Occipital bone, spinous processes of T_2–T_4 vertebrae	Transverse process, C_7–T_{12} vertebrae,	Extension, lateral flexion, rotation to opposite side	Cervical and thoracic spinal nerves (C_1–T_{12})
The deep spinal muscles (Multifidi, rotators, interspinales, intertransversarii, levatores costarum)	Posterior processes of all vertebrae, posterior sacrum	Spinous and transverse processes and laminae of vertebrae below those of the proximal attachment	Extension, lateral flexion, rotation to opposite side	Spinal and intercostal nerves (T_1–T_{12})
Sternocleidomastoid	Mastoid process of the temporal bone	Superior sternum, inner third of the clavicle	Flexion of the neck, extension of the head, lateral flexion, rotation to opposite side	Accessory nerve and C_2 spinal nerve
Levator scapulae	Transverse processes of the first four cervical vertebrae	Vertebral border of the scapula	Lateral flexion	C_3–C_4 spinal nerves, dorsal scapular nerve (C_3–C_5)
The scaleni (Scaleneus anterior, medius, and posterior)	Transverse processes C_1–C_7 vertebrae	Upper two ribs	Flexion, lateral flexion	Cervical nerves (C_3–C_8)
Quadratus lumborum	Last rib, transverse processes of L_1–L_4 vertebrae	Iliolumbar ligament, adjacent lumbar iliac crest	Lateral flexion	T_{12}–L_4 spinal nerves
Psoas major	Sides of 12th thoracic and all lumbar vertebrae	Lesser trochanter of the femur	Flexion	Femoral nerve (L_1–L_3)

THE BRACHIAL PLEXUS

The shoulder region and upper extremity is supplied by the brachial plexus, formed by the C_5 through T_1 nerve roots. The nerve roots converge and diverge to form trunks, division, and cords, and eventually terminate in distal branches that innervate the arm, forearm, and hand **(Figure 9.6)**. The C_5 and C_6 nerve roots form the upper trunk, C_7 forms the middle trunk, and C_8 and T_1 form the lower trunk. Each trunk then divides into anterior and posterior divisions. The posterior divisions

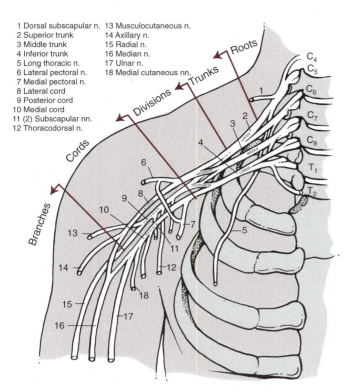

1 Dorsal subscapular n.   13 Musculocutaneous n.
2 Superior trunk   14 Axillary n.
3 Middle trunk   15 Radial n.
4 Inferior trunk   16 Median n.
5 Long thoracic n.   17 Ulnar n.
6 Lateral pectoral n.   18 Medial cutaneous nn.
7 Medial pectoral n.
8 Lateral cord
9 Posterior cord
10 Medial cord
11 (2) Subscapular nn.
12 Thoracodorsal n.

➤ FIGURE 9.6 **Brachial plexus**. The brachial plexus is formed by the segmental nerves C_5 to T_1.

THE SACRAL PLEXUS

A portion of the lumbar plexus (L_4, L_5) forms the lumbosacral trunk and courses downward to form the upper portion of the sacral plexus **(Figure 9.8)**. This plexus supplies the muscles of the buttock region, and through the sciatic nerve, the muscles of the posterior thigh and entire lower leg. The sciatic nerve is composed of two distinct nerves, the tibial nerve and common peroneal nerve. The tibial nerve, formed by the anterior branches of the upper five nerve roots, innervates all of the muscles on the posterior leg with the exception of the short head of the biceps femoris. The common peroneal nerve, formed by the posterior branches of the upper four nerve roots, innervates the short head of the biceps femoris, then divides in the vicinity of the head of the fibula into the deep peroneal nerve and superficial peroneal nerve. These nerves innervate the anterior compartment of the lower leg and lateral compartments of the lower leg, respectively.

KINEMATICS AND MAJOR MUSCLE ACTIONS OF THE SPINE

The vertebral joints enable motion in all planes of movement, as well as circumduction **(Figure 9.9)**. Because the

all converge to form the posterior cord, the anterior division of the upper and middle trunk form the lateral cord, while the anterior division of the lower trunk forms the medial cord.

The posterior cord branches into the axillary and radial nerves, which innervate all shoulder, elbow, wrist, and finger extensors. With the arm in anatomical position, the lateral half of the medial cord joins with the medial half of the lateral cord to form the large median nerve that innervates most of the wrist and finger flexors. The remaining portion of the medial cord terminates as the ulnar nerve, which innervates the flexor carpi ulnaris and the intrinsic muscles of the hand. The remaining portion of the lateral cord terminates as the musculocutaneous nerve, which innervates the main elbow flexors. Minor branches from the medial and lateral cords innervate the pectoral muscles and cutaneous nerves on the medial arm and forearm.

THE LUMBAR PLEXUS

Supplying the anterior and medial muscles of the thigh region is the lumbar plexus, formed by the T_{12} through L_5 nerve roots **(Figure 9.7)**. The posterior branches of the L_2 through L_4 nerve roots form the femoral nerve, innervating the quadriceps, while the anterior branches form the obturator nerve, innervating most of the adductor muscle group.

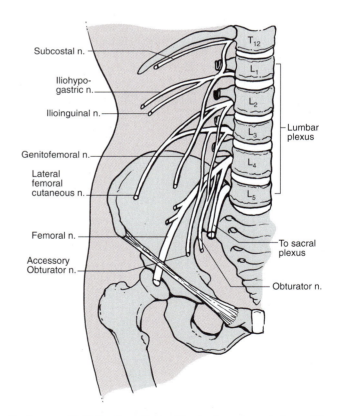

➤ FIGURE 9.7 **Lumbar plexus**. The lumbar plexus is formed by the segmental nerves T_{12} to L_5. Note that the lower portion of the plexus merges with the upper portion of the sacral plexus to form the lumbosacral trunk.

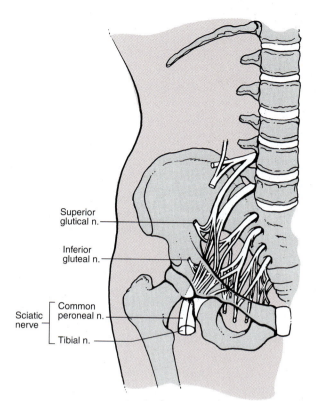

➤ **FIGURE 9.8 Sacral plexus.** The sacral plexus is formed by the segmental nerves L_4 to S_5. This plexus innervates the lower leg, ankle, and foot via the tibial and common peroneal nerves.

(Labels on figure: Superior glutical n., Inferior gluteal n., Sciatic nerve, Common peroneal n., Tibial n.)

motion allowed between any two adjacent vertebrae is small, however, spinal movements always involve a number of motion segments. The range of motion allowed at each motion segment is governed by anatomical constraints that vary through the cervical, thoracic, and lumbar regions of the spine.

Flexion, Extension, and Hyperextension

Spinal flexion is anterior bending of the spine in the sagittal plane, with extension being the return to anatomical position from a position of flexion. The flexion/extension capability of the motion segments at all levels of the spine is relatively small, with a maximum range of 5° at T_1–T_2. The thoracic region permits the largest cumulative range of motion in flexion/extension with 46°, compared to only 16° for both the cervical and lumbar regions (2).

It is important not to confuse spinal flexion with hip flexion or forward pelvic tilt, although all three motions occur during an activity such as touching the toes. Hip flexion consists of anteriorly directed sagittal plane rotation of the femur with respect to the pelvic girdle (or vice versa), and forward pelvic tilt is anteriorly directed movement of the anterior superior iliac spine with respect to the pubic symphysis.

When the spine is extended backward past anatomical position in the sagittal plane, the motion is termed **hyper-**

extension. The range of motion for spinal hyperextension is considerable in the cervical and lumbar regions, ranging as high as 17° at the C_5–C_6 level and 21° at L_5–S_1. The cumulative range of motion for hyperextension is greatest in the cervical region with 64°, followed by the lumbar region with 54°, followed by the thoracic region with 22°. Lumbar hyperextension is required in many sport skills, including several swimming strokes, the high jump and pole vault, wrestling, and numerous gymnastic skills. It has been reported that, during a back handspring, the lumbar curvature may be increased to as much as 20 times that present during relaxed standing (3).

Lateral Flexion and Rotation

Movement of the spine away from anatomical position in a lateral direction in the frontal plane is termed lateral flexion. In the thoracic region, the cumulative range of motion for lateral flexion is approximately 31°, with 23° and 24° permitted in the cervical and lumbar regions, respectively. Spinal rotation capability is greatest in the cervical region, with up to 50° of motion allowed at C_1–C_2. In the thoracic region, approximately 9° of rotation is permitted among the upper six motion segments. From T_7–T_8 downward, however, the range of motion in rotation progressively decreases, with only about 2° of motion allowed in the lumbar spine because of the interlocking of the articular processes there. At the lumbosacral joint, about 5° of rotation is allowed.

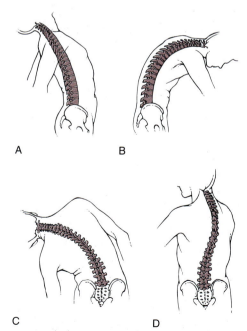

➤ **FIGURE 9.9 Motions of the trunk.** A, Hyperextension in the sagittal plane. B, Flexion. C, Lateral flexion in the frontal plane. D, Rotation in the transverse plane. Extension, the return to anatomical position from a position of flexion, and circumduction, a sequence of movements in which the head traces a circular path, are not shown.

KINETICS OF THE SPINE

 Why is it important to maintain the spine in an erect posture during weight-training exercises?

Forces acting on the spine include body weight, tension in the spinal ligaments and paraspinal muscles, intra-abdominal pressure, and any applied external loads. When the body is in an upright position, the major form of loading on the spine is axial. In this position, body weight, the weight of any load held in the hands, and tension in the surrounding ligaments and muscles all contribute to spinal compression. Intra-abdominal pressure, on the other hand, works like a balloon inside the abdominal cavity to support the adjacent lumbar spine by creating a tensile force that partially offsets the compressive load. Intra-abdominal pressure increases just prior to the lifting of a heavy load, although the mechanism through which this is accomplished is not well understood.

Although most of the axial compression load on the spine is borne by the vertebral bodies and discs, the facet joints also assist with load bearing. When the spine is in hyperextension, the facet joints may bear up to approximately 30% of the load.

Effect of Body Position

One factor that can dramatically affect the load on the spine is body position. When the body is in an upright position, the line of gravity passes anterior to the spinal column **(Figure 9.10)**. As a result, the spine is under a constant, forward bending moment. As the trunk is pro-

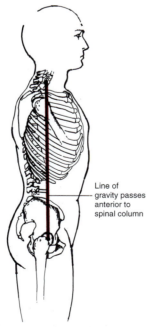

Line of gravity passes anterior to spinal column

➤ **FIGURE 9.10 Line of gravity.** The line of gravity for the head and trunk passes anterior to the spinal column during upright standing. The moment arm for head/trunk weight at any given vertebral joint is the perpendicular distance between the line of gravity and the spinal column.

gressively flexed, the line of gravity shifts farther away from the spine. The farther the line of gravity from the spine, the larger the moment arm for body weight and the greater the bending moment generated. To maintain body position, this moment must be counteracted by tension in the back muscles. The more tension required of these muscles to maintain body position, the greater the compressional load on the spine. In comparison to the load present during upright standing, compression on the lumbar spine increases with sitting, increases more with spinal flexion, and increases still further with a slouched sitting position. During lifting and carrying, holding the load as close to the trunk as possible minimizes the load on the back. **Box 9.1** lists guidelines to reduce spinal stress in daily activities.

Effect of Movement Speed and Impact

Another factor affecting spinal loading is body movement speed. It has been shown that executing a lift in a very rapid, jerking fashion dramatically increases compression and shear forces on the spine, as well as tension in the paraspinal muscles (4). This is one of the reasons that isotonic resistance training exercises should always be performed in a slow, controlled fashion.

For individuals participating in high-speed collision and contact sports, impact forces are an inherent risk for potential spinal injuries. Because the range of motion in the cervical spine is greatest in flexion, a head position of extreme flexion generates the largest bending moment. When combined with axial compression loading, this generates the leading mechanism of injury for severe cervical spine injuries. For example, when a football tackle is executed with the head in a flexed position, the cervical spine is aligned in a segmented column and subjected to both large compressional forces, generated by the cervical muscles, and axial impact forces **(Figure 9.11)**. Impact causes loading along the longitudinal axis of the cervical vertebrae, leading to compression deformation. The intervertebral discs can initially absorb some energy; however, as continued force is exerted, further deformation and buckling occurs, leading to failure of the intervertebral discs, cervical vertebrae, or both **(Figure 9.12)**. This results in subluxation, disc herniation, facet dislocation, or fracture-dislocation at one or more spinal levels.

 Lifting with the trunk erect minimizes the tension requirement for the lumbar muscles because the moment arm for body weight is minimized. Exercises involving trunk flexion should be performed in a slow, controlled manner to progressively strengthen the lumbar extensors.

ANATOMICAL VARIATIONS PREDISPOSING INDIVIDUALS TO SPINE INJURIES

Mechanical stress derived from lateral spinal muscle imbalances or from sustaining repeated impact forces can cause

Preventing Low Back Injuries in Activities of Daily Living

Sitting

- Sit on a firm, straight-backed chair
- Place the buttocks as far back into the chair as possible to avoid slouching
- Sit with the feet flat on the floor
- Avoid sitting for long periods of time, particularly with the knees fully extended

Driving

- Place the seat forward so the knees are level with the hips and you do not have to reach for the pedals
- If the left foot is not working the pedals, place it flat on the floor
- Keep the back of the seat in a nearly upright position to avoid slouching

Standing

- If you must stand in one area for an extended time:
  - ◆ Shift body weight from one foot to the other
  - ◆ Elevate one foot on a piece of furniture to keep the knees flexed
  - ◆ Do toe flexion and extension inside the shoes
- Hold the chin up, keep the shoulders back, and relax the knees

Lifting and carrying

- Use a lumbosacral belt or have assistance when lifting heavy objects. To lift an object:
  - ◆ Place the object close the body
  - ◆ Bend at the knees, not the waist, and keep the back erect
  - ◆ Tighten the abdominal muscles and inhale prior to lifting the object
  - ◆ Exhale during the lift
  - ◆ Do not twist while lifting
- To carry a heavy object:
  - ◆ Hold the object close to the body at waist level
  - ◆ Carry the object in the middle of the body, not to one side

Sleeping

- Sleep on a firm mattress. If needed, place a sheet of ¾-inch plywood under the mattress
- Sleep on your side, and place pillows between the legs
- If you sleep supine, place pillows under the knees. Avoid sleeping in the prone position
- Because waterbeds support the body curves evenly, they may relieve low back pain

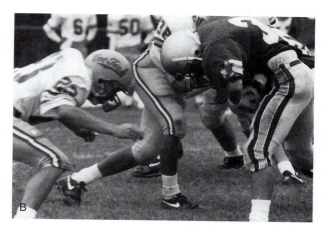

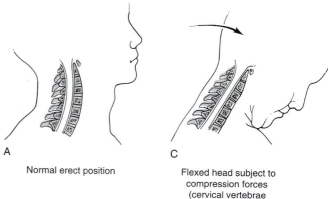

A Normal erect position

C Flexed head subject to compression forces (cervical vertebrae straightened)

➤ FIGURE 9.11 Axial loading. In a normally erect position, the cervical spine is slightly extended (A). When a football tackle is executed with the head flexed at about 30° (B), the cervical vertebrae are aligned in a column and subjected to compressional forces, generated by the cervical muscles, and to axial loading (C).

back pain and/or injury. Excessive spinal curvatures can be congenital or acquired through weight training or sport participation. Defects in the pars interarticularis of the neural arch can be caused by mechanical stress, also placing an individual at risk for serious spinal injury.

Kyphosis

Accentuation of the thoracic curve is called **kyphosis** (**Figure 9.13**). The cause of kyphosis can be congenital, idiopathic (unknown), or secondary to osteoporosis. Congenital kyphosis arises from deficits in the formation of either the vertebral bodies or the anterior and posterior vertebral elements. Idiopathic kyphosis, also known as **Scheuermann's disease**, or osteochondritis of the spine, is common among adolescents, and involves the development of one or more wedge-shaped vertebrae in the thoracic or lumbar regions through abnormal epiphyseal plate behavior (see Figure 9.18B). The individual typically has a round-shouldered appearance, with or without back pain. It may be caused by overtraining with the butterfly stroke, hence the nickname "swimmer's back." However, weight lifters, gymnasts, and football linemen, who overdevelop the pectoral muscles, are also prone to this condition.

Scoliosis

Lateral curvature of the spine is known as **scoliosis**. The lateral deformity, coupled with rotational deformity of the involved vertebrae, may range from mild to severe. Scoliosis may appear as either a "C" or an "S" curve involving the thoracic spine, the lumbar spine, or both. Scoliosis can be structural or nonstructural. Structural scoliosis involves

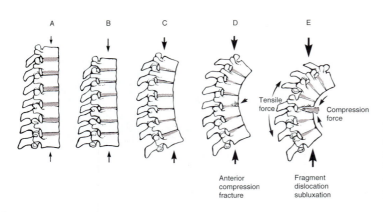

➤ **FIGURE 9.12 Axial loading on the vertebral column causes compressive deformation of the intervertebral discs** (A,B). As load continues and maximum compression deformation is reached, angular deformation and buckling occurs (C). Continued force results in an anterior compression fracture, subluxation, or dislocation (D,E).

an inflexible curvature that persists with lateral bending of the spine. Nonstructural scoliosis curves are flexible and are corrected with lateral bending. Although congenital abnormalities, certain cancers, and leg length discrepancy may lead to scoliosis, approximately 70 to 90% of all cases are idiopathic. Idiopathic scoliosis is most commonly diagnosed between the ages of 10 and 13 years, but can be seen at any age, and is more common in females.

Symptoms associated with scoliosis vary with the severity of the condition. Mild cases (curvature is <20°) are usually asymptomatic and self-limiting. Reassessment should occur every 3 to 4 months until the adolescent has skeletally matured. Active treatment is not necessary as long as the curve is nonprogressive. If skeletally immature and the curve is moderate (20 to 45°) and progressive, bracing is necessary. In many instances, the treatment will allow enough time out of the brace for daily sport participation. In general, relatively unrestricted physical activity is recommended for almost all adolescents with scoliosis. Mild to moderate cases can be treated with strength, flexibility, and overall fitness activities. Severe scoliosis, characterized by extreme lateral deviation and localized rotation of the spine, can be painful and deforming and may require surgery (fusion with spinal instrumentation).

Lordosis

Abnormal exaggeration of the lumbar curve, or **lordosis**, is often associated with weakened abdominal muscles and

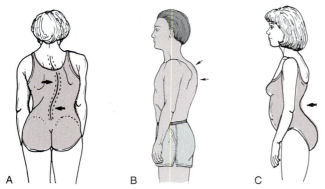

➤ **FIGURE 9.13 Spinal anomalies**. A, Scoliosis. B, Thoracic kyphosis. C, Lordosis.

forward pelvic tilt. Causes include congenital spinal deformity, weakness of the abdominal muscles, poor postural habits, and overtraining in sports requiring repeated lumbar hyperextension such as gymnastics, figure skating, football (linemen), javelin throwing, or swimming the butterfly stroke. Because lordosis places added compressive stress on the posterior elements of the spine, low back pain is a common symptom predisposing many athletes to low back injuries.

Pars Interarticularis Fractures

The pars interarticularis is the weakest bony portion of the vertebral neural arch, the region between the superior and inferior articular facets. A fracture in this region is termed **spondylolysis (Figure 9.14A)**. Although some pars defects may be congenital, they may also be caused by mechanical stress from axial loading of the lumbar spine during repeated weight-loading in flexion, hyperextension (back-arching), and rotation. These repetitive movements cause a shearing stress to the vertebrae, resulting in a stress fracture.

Fractures of the pars interarticularis may range from hairline to complete separation of the bone. A bony defect in spondylolysis tends to occur at an earlier age, typically before age eight, yet often does not produce symptoms until ages 10 to 15. The fracture may heal with less periosteal callus and tends to form a fibrous union more often than fractures at other sites. The condition also has a strong genetic component with prevalence as high as 33% among those with family members who also have the condition (6,7).

A bilateral separation in the pars interarticularis, called **spondylolisthesis**, results in the anterior displacement of a vertebra with respect to the vertebra below it **(Figures 9.14B, 9.15)**. The most common site for this injury is the lumbosacral joint, with 90% of the slips occurring at this level. Spondylolisthesis is often diagnosed in children between the ages of 10 and 15 years, and is more common in boys (5). Unlike most stress fractures, spondylolysis and spondylolisthesis do not typically heal with time, but tend to persist, particularly when there is no interruption in sport participation. Those particularly susceptible to this condition include female gymnasts, interior football line-

Superior articular process

Pedicle

Transverse process

Pars inter-articularis

Superior articular process

Inferior articular process

Isthmus

Inferior articular process

➤ **FIGURE 9.14 Spondylolysis is a stress fracture of the pars interarticularis** (A). Spondylolisthesis is a bilateral fracture of the pars interarticularis accompanied by anterior slippage of the involved vertebra (B).

men, weight lifters, volleyball players, pole vaulters, wrestlers, and rowers.

Although most spondylitic conditions are asymptomatic, when the underlying cause is repeated mechanical stress, low back pain and associated neurological symptoms are likely to occur. The individual may complain of unilateral dull backache aggravated by activity, usually hyperextension and rotation. Standing on one leg and hyperextending the back aggravate the condition. There is demonstrable muscle spasm in the erector spinae muscles or hamstrings, leading to flattening of the lumbosacral curve, but there are usually no sciatic nerve symptoms. Pain may radiate into the buttock region or down the sciatic nerve if the L5 nerve root is compressed. This individual should be referred to a physician.

Slippage is measured by dividing the distance the superior vertebral body has displaced forward onto the inferior by the anteroposterior dimensions of the inferior vertebral body. In mild cases (slippage of 0 to 25%), modifications in training and technique can permit the individual to continue to participate. However, in moderate cases (slippage from 25 to 50%), most physicians will not begin active rehabilitation until the individual is asymptomatic for 4 weeks. At that time, flexibility in the hamstrings and gluteal muscles is combined with strengthening the abdomen and back extensors. If the slip is greater than 50%, the individual will present with flat buttocks, tight hamstrings, and alterations in gait, and a palpable step-off deformity may be present at the level of the defect. This individual will be excluded from participation in contact sports unless the person is asymptomatic and absence of continued slippage has been documented.

PREVENTION OF SPINAL INJURIES

Although most of the load on the spine is borne by the vertebral bodies and discs, the facet joints do assist with some load bearing. Protective equipment can prevent some injuries to the spinal region, particularly over the cervical, sacral, and coccygeal regions. Physical conditioning, however, plays a more important role in preventing injuries to the overall region.

Protective Equipment

Several pieces of equipment can be used to protect the spine. In the cervical region, a neck roll or a posterolateral pad made of a high, thick, and stiff material can be attached to shoulder pads to limit excessive motion of the cervical spine, and has been shown to reduce the incidence of repetitive burners and stingers. Such restraints, however, may also increase the risk of cervical spine injuries by limiting the natural flexibility of the neck. In the upper body, shoulder pads extend over and protect the upper thoracic region. Rib protectors composed of air-inflated, interconnected cylinders can protect a limited region of the thoracic spine. Weight-training belts, abdominal binders, and other similar lumbar/sacral supportive devices support the abdominal contents, stabilize the trunk, and prevent spinal deformity and damage. They place the low back in a more vertical lifting posture, decrease lumbar lordosis, limit pelvic torsion, and lessen axial loading on the spine by increasing intra-abdominal pressure, which, in turn, reduces compressive forces in the vertebral bodies. Many of these protective devices were discussed and demonstrated in Chapter 3.

Physical Conditioning

Flexibility and strengthening of the back muscles is imperative to stabilize the spinal column. Stretching exercises

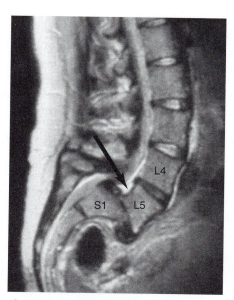

➤ **FIGURE 9.15 Spondylolisthesis**. In this MRI scan of spondylolisthesis, note the anterior shift of the L5 vertebra.

should increase range of motion in the cervical, thoracic, lumbar, and hip regions. In the cervical region, the hands can provide a slow, prolonged stretch in the various motions. Strengthening exercises for the cervical region may involve isometric contractions, manual resistance, use of surgical tubing, or weight training with free weights or specialized machines. Exercises should include neck flexion, extension, lateral flexion, and rotation, as well as scapular elevation. Stabilization of the cervical spine is particularly important for wrestlers and football lineman, who are consistently subjected to extremes of motion at the neck. Exercises to strengthen the thoracic and low back area should involve back extension, lateral flexion, and rotation; abdominal strengthening; and exercises for the lower trapezius and latissimus dorsi. Several of these exercises are shown in **Field Strategy 9.1.**

 FIELD STRATEGY 9.1   EXERCISES TO PREVENT SPINAL INJURIES

FLEXIBILITY EXERCISES

A. **Single-knee-to-chest stretch.** In a supine position, pull one knee toward the chest with the hands. Keep the back flat. Switch to the opposite leg and repeat.

B. **Double-knee-to-chest stretch.** In a supine position, pull both knees to the chest with the hands. Keep the back flat.

C. **Hamstring stretch, seated position.** Place the leg to be stretched straight out, with the opposite foot tucked toward the groin. Reach toward the toes until a stretch is felt.

D. **Hip flexor stretch (lunge).** Extend the leg to be stretched behind you. Place the contralateral leg in front of you. While keeping the back straight, shift your body weight forward.

E. **Lateral rotator stretch, seated position.** Cross one leg over the thigh and place the elbow on the outside of the knee. Gently stretch the buttock muscles by pushing the bent knee across the body while keeping the pelvis on the floor.

F. **Lower trunk rotation stretch.** In a supine position, rotate the flexed knees to one side, keeping the back flat and the feet together.

G. **Angry cat stretch (posterior pelvic tilt).** Kneel on all fours with knees hip-width apart. Tighten the buttocks and arch the back upward while lowering the chin and tilting the pelvis backwards. Relax the buttocks and allow the pelvis to drop downward and forward.

STRENGTHENING EXERCISES

H. **Crunch curl-up.** In a supine position with the knees flexed, flatten the back and curl up to elevate the head and shoulders from the floor. Alternate exercises include diagonal crunch curl-ups and hip crunches.

I. **Prone extension.** In a prone position, raise up on the elbows. Progress to raising up onto the hands.

J. **Alternate arm and leg lift.** In a fully extended prone position, lift one arm and the opposite leg off the surface at least 3 inches. Repeat with the opposite arm and leg.

K. **Double arm and leg lift.** In a fully extended prone position, lift both arms and legs off the surface at least 3 inches. Hold and return to starting position.

L. **Alternate arm and leg extension on all fours;** Kneel on all fours; raise one leg behind the body while raising the opposite arm in front of the body. Ankle and wrist weights may be added for additional resistance.

M. **Back extension.** Use a back extension machine or have another individual stabilize the feet and legs; raise the trunk into a slightly hyperextended position.

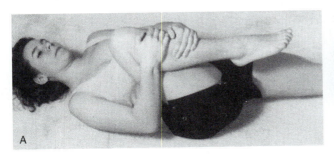

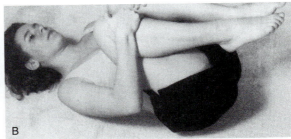

A   B

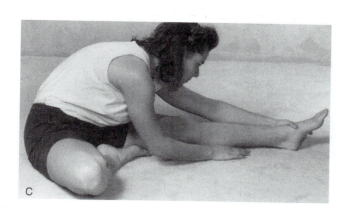

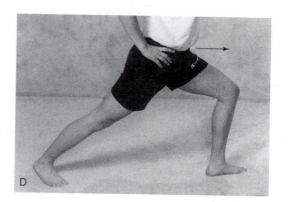

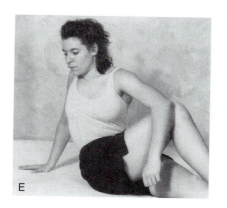

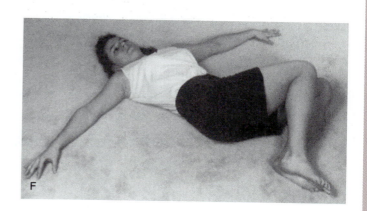

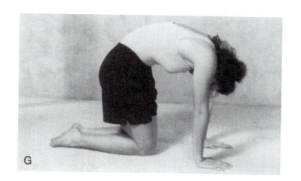

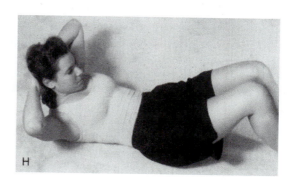

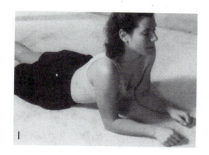

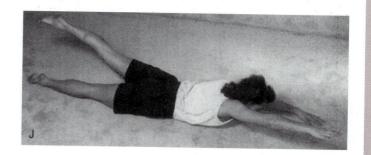

Continued

continued from page 221

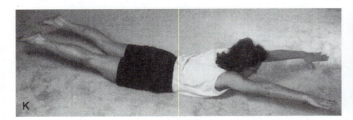

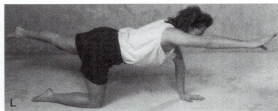

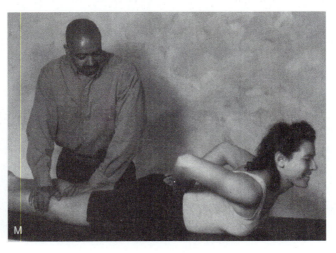

Proper Skill Technique

Proper skill technique is vital in preventing spinal injuries. Helmets are designed to protect the cranial region from injury, but do not prevent axial loading on the cervical spine. Since the 1976 rule change banning spearing in high school football, there has been a large reduction in the incidence of catastrophic spinal injuries, although incidence of spearing continues to occur (8).

Proper lifting technique can also affect spinal loading. It has been shown that executing a lift in a very rapid, jerking fashion dramatically increases compression and shear forces on the spine, as well as tension in the paraspinal muscles. For this reason, isotonic resistance exercises should always be performed in a slow, controlled fashion, inhaling deeply as the lift is initiated and exhaling forcefully and smoothly at the end of the lift. Use of a supportive weight-training belt and a spotter can also prevent injury to the lumbar region during heavy weightlifting.

Poor posture during walking, sitting, standing, lying down, and running may lead to chronic low back strain or ligamentous sprains. All postural deformity cases should be assessed to determine the cause, and an appropriate exercise program should be developed to address the deficits.

CERVICAL SPINE INJURIES

After practice, a wrestler is complaining of a sore neck. There is full range of motion, but he is more comfortable with the head slightly rotated to the right. Point tenderness is present in the muscle mass on the left anterolateral neck. Resisted neck lateral flexion to the left and rotation to the right increase the pain. No change in sensation or grip strength is evident. What injury might you suspect, and how would you manage this injury?

The relatively small size of the cervical vertebrae, combined with the nearly horizontal orientation of the cervical facet joints, makes the cervical spine the most mobile region of the spinal column. As such, this area is especially vulnerable to injury.

Cervical Sprains

Cervical sprains typically occur at the extremes of motion or in association with a violent muscle contraction or external force. Injury can occur to any of the major ligaments traversing the cervical spine, as well as to the capsular ligaments surrounding the facet joints. Minor activity, such as maintaining the head in an uncomfortable posture or sleeping position, can also produce sprains of the neck.

➤ SIGNS AND SYMPTOMS

Symptoms include pain, stiffness, and restricted range of motion, but no neurologic or osseous injury exists. Unlike cervical strains, the symptoms of a severe sprain can persist for several days.

➤ MANAGEMENT

Initial treatment includes rest, cryotherapy, prescribed nonsteroidal anti-inflammatory drugs (NSAIDs), and use of a cervical collar for support. Follow-up treatment may involve continued cryotherapy or superficial heat, gentle stretching, and isometric exercises. Return to competition should not occur until the individual is free of neck pain with and without axial compression, and when range of motion and neck strength are normal. This decision should be made collaboratively with the team physician.

Cervical Strains

Cervical strains usually involve the sternocleidomastoid or upper trapezius, although the scalenes, levator scapulae, and splenius muscles may also be involved. The same mechanisms that cause cervical sprains also cause cervical strains, and in many instances, both injuries occur simultaneously.

➤ SIGNS AND SYMPTOMS

Symptoms include pain, stiffness, and restricted range of motion. Palpation will reveal muscle spasm and increased pain during active contraction or passive stretching of the involved muscle.

➤ MANAGEMENT

Cryotherapy, prescribed NSAIDs, gentle stretching and isometric exercises of the involved muscle, and use of a cervical collar for support will facilitate symptoms subsiding within 3 to 7 days. Follow-up treatment may involve continued cryotherapy or superficial heat, and strengthening the neck muscles through appropriate resistance exercise. Return to competition should not occur until the individual is free of neck pain with and without axial compression, and when range of motion and neck strength are normal. This decision should be made collaboratively with the team physician.

Cervical Spinal Stenosis

Structural spinal stenosis is defined as a narrowing of the sagittal diameter of the cervical spinal canal as compared to the diameter of the corresponding vertebral body (Torg ratio) (9) **(Figure 9.16)**. Recently, the ratio method has been shown to be of low predictive value. Functional spinal stenosis, a more accurate measure of stenosis, is defined as a loss of cerebrospinal fluid (CSF) around the cord, or in more extreme cases as a deformation of the spinal cord. This is documented by magnetic resonance (MR) imaging, contrast-enhanced computed tomography (CT) scans, or myelography (10). As a result of the reduced CSF, the spinal cord's ability to decompress itself is limited, potentially leading to more acute and severe symptoms.

Individuals may remain asymptomatic until a direct blow to the forehead (forced hyperextension) or occiput (hyperflexion) produces neurologic signs. Lateral blows causing rapid lateral flexion with or without rotation can also lead to acute symptoms. The cervical segments most commonly affected are C_5 and C_6.

➤ SIGNS AND SYMPTOMS

Upon impact, the athlete may develop immediate quadriplegia with sensory changes or motor deficits in both arms, both legs, or all four extremities. Sensory changes

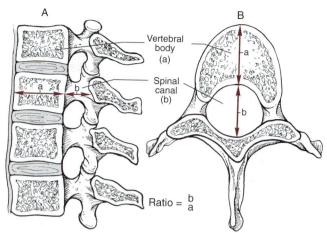

➤ **FIGURE 9.16 Torg's ratio**. The spinal canal/vertebral body ratio is the distance from the midpoint of the posterior aspect of the vertebral body to the nearest point on the corresponding spinolaminar line (a) divided by the anteroposterior width of the vertebral body (b). Torg's ratio is a/b. A, Transverse view. B, Superior view.

may include burning pain, numbness, tingling, or total loss of sensation. Motor changes may include weakness or complete paralysis, with arm weakness greater than leg weakness, secondary to contusion (bruising) of the central portion of the spinal cord (central cord syndrome). The changes are always bilateral, differentiating this condition from a nerve root injury, which is always unilateral. The episode may be transient with full recovery in 10 to 15 minutes, although in some cases, complete recovery does not occur for 36 to 38 hours (11,12). This condition is often called a neurapraxia, since neural changes are only temporary. Stenosis may also occur in the lumbar region, impinging segments of the cauda equina.

➤ MANAGEMENT

Because of the serious nature of this injury, EMS should be activated, and the athlete placed on a spine board.

Structural spinal stenosis may be discovered during routine radiographs, but often an MRI is needed to determine the presence of functional stenosis. An individual who has had an episode of structurally related cervical spinal neurapraxia, with or without transient quadriplegia, is not necessarily predisposed to permanent neurological injury. Individuals with developing spinal stenosis or spinal stenosis associated with congenital abnormalities have returned safely to participation. However, a growing number of physicians have concluded that individuals with functional stenosis of the cervical spine with associated cervical spine instability, or acute or chronic intervertebral disc disease, should be advised to discontinue participation in contact sports (13).

Spear Tackler's Spine

This condition was originally described in 1993 after data was reviewed from the National Football Head and Neck

Injury Registry (14). Four athletes suffered permanent neurologic injury and were found to have the following common characteristics: developmental narrowing of the cervical spinal canal, straightening or reversal of the normal cervical lordotic curve, pre-existing minor posttraumatic radiographic evidence of bony or ligamentous injury, and a past history of using spear-tackling techniques. With flexion of the neck, as is seen in spear tackling, the straightened cervical spine acts like a segmental column, predisposing the spine to permanent neurologic injury with further axial loading.

➤ SIGNS AND SYMPTOMS

As with any catastrophic neck injury, the athlete may develop immediate pain with sensory changes and motor deficits distal to the injury site. Sensory changes may include burning pain, numbness, tingling, or total loss of sensation. Motor changes may include weakness or complete paralysis.

➤ MANAGEMENT

Because of the serious nature of this injury, EMS should be activated, and the athlete placed on a spine board.

Controversy still exists over the return of the athlete to competition. Some neurosurgeons believe that, if the normal cervical lordosis is restored by treatment and the athlete refrains from any further spear-tackling techniques, there is not a high degree of risk for reinjury (15). The majority of neurosurgeons, however, believe that the condition is an absolute contraindication to further participation in contact/collision sports (14,16).

Cervical Fractures and Dislocations

Unsafe practices, such as diving into shallow water, spearing in football, or landing on the posterior neck during gymnastic or trampoline activities, can lead to cervical fractures and dislocations from the axial loading and violent neck flexion. Some fractures, such as those to the spinous process or unilateral laminar fractures, may require only immobilization in a cervical collar. Others, such as a bilateral pars interarticularis fracture of C_2 ("hangman's fracture"), may be treated with a cervical collar or Halo vest immobilization.

➤ SIGNS AND SYMPTOMS

In sports, serious injuries commonly occur at the fourth, fifth, and sixth cervical vertebrae. Because neural damage can range from none to complete severance of the spinal cord, there is a range of accompanying symptoms **(Box 9.2)**. Painful palpation over the spinous processes, muscle spasm, or a palpable defect indicates a possible fracture or dislocation. Radiating pain, numbness, weakness in a myotome, paralysis, and loss of bladder or bowel control are all critical signs of neural damage. If a unilateral cervical dislocation is present, the neck will be visibly tilted

toward the dislocated side, with muscle tightness due to stretch on the convex side and muscle slack on the concave side.

➤ MANAGEMENT

Because spinal cord damage can lead to paralysis or death, a suspected unstable neck injury should be treated as a medical emergency. An unstable neck injury should be suspected in an unconscious athlete, an athlete who is awake but has numbness and/or paralysis, and in a neurologically intact athlete who has neck pain or pain with neck movement. Without moving the head or neck out of alignment, apply light cervical traction while the neck is being stabilized, and assess the ABCs to determine the existence of any life-threatening situation.

Activate EMS and assist the technicians in immobilizing the injured athlete on a spine board.

The wrestler complained of a sore neck and pain over the muscle mass on the left anterolateral neck. Resisted neck lateral flexion to the left and rotation to the right increased the pain. This individual probably has strained the left sternocleidomastoid muscle. Cryotherapy and support from a cervical collar will alleviate some of the discomfort. A mild stretching program and isometric strengthening should be initiated immediately.

BRACHIAL PLEXUS INJURIES

A defensive lineman charged the quarterback preparing to throw a pass, and struck the throwing arm, forcing it into excessive external rotation, abduction, and extension. An immediate burning sensation traveled down the length of the quarterback's arm, and now his thumb is tingling. What might have happened here? Is this a serious injury?

➤ FIGURE 9.17 **Common mechanisms of a brachial plexus stretch**. A blow to the head causing lateral flexion and shoulder depression may lead to a traction injury to the upper trunk of the brachial plexus (A). An injury can also occur when a blow to the supraclavicular region causes lateral flexion with rotation and extension of the cervical spine away from the blow (B). Compression over Erb's point, representing the most superficial passage of the brachial plexus, can also lead to pain and paresthesia radiating into the upper extremity (C).

The brachial plexus is a complex neural structure that innervates the upper extremity and is typically damaged in two manners **(Figure 9.17)**. A stretch injury may be caused when a tensile force leads to forceful downward traction of the clavicle while the head is distracted in the opposite direction, such as when an individual is tackled and subsequently rolls onto the shoulder with the head turned to the opposite side. A stretch injury may also occur when the arm is forced into excessive external rotation, abduction, and extension. The injury usually affects the upper trunk (C_5, C_6) of the brachial plexus, which will lead to a sensory loss or paresthesia in the thumb and index finger. The other mechanism of injury may involve compression of the fixed plexus between the football shoulder pad and the superior medial scapula, where the brachial plexus is most superficial. This site, called Erb's point, is located 2 to 3 cm above the clavicle at the level of the transverse process of the C_6 vertebra.

Burners are graded in three levels **(Table 9.2)**. Grade I burners represent neurapraxia, the mildest lesion. A neuropraxia is a localized conduction block that causes temporary loss of sensation and/or loss of motor function from

selective demyelination of the axon sheath without true axonal disruption. Recovery usually occurs within days to a few weeks. Grade II burners are axonotmesis injuries that produce significant motor and mild sensory deficits that last at least 2 weeks. Axonotmesis disrupts the axon and myelin sheath but leaves the epineurium intact. Axonal regrowth occurs at a rate of 1 to 2 mm per day; full or normal function is usually restored. Grade III burners are neurotmesis injuries, which disrupt the endoneurium. These severe injuries have a poor prognosis, with motor and sensory deficit persisting for up to 1 year. Surgical intervention is often necessary to avoid poor or imperfect regeneration (17).

Acute Burners

➤ SIGNS AND SYMPTOMS

The athlete notices an immediate, severe, burning pain and prickly paresthesia that radiates from the supraclavicular area down the arm into the hand, hence the nickname "burner" or "stinger." Pain is usually transient and subsides in 5 to 10 minutes, but tenderness over the supra-

Grade	Injury	Signs	Prognosis
I	Neurapraxia injury	Temporary loss of sensation and/or loss of motor function	Recovery within days to a few weeks
II	Axonotmesis injury	Significant motor and mild sensory deficits	Deficits last at least 2 weeks. Regrowth is slow, but full or normal function is usually restored
III	Neurotmesis injury	Motor and sensory deficits persist for up to 1 year	Poor prognosis. Surgical intervention is often necessary

TABLE 9.2 CLASSIFICATION OF "BURNERS"

clavicular area and shoulder weakness may persist for hours or days after the injury. Often the individual will try to shake the arm to "get the feeling back." Muscle weakness is evident in actions involving shoulder abduction and external rotation.

➤ MANAGEMENT

When weakness is present, the individual should be removed from competition. A brief nerve root screening can be performed without removing the football uniform. The myotomes are tested bilaterally: shoulder abduction for the C_5 nerve root, elbow flexion for C_6, elbow extension for C_7, thumb extension for C_8, and finger abduction and adduction for T_1. The brachial plexus traction test may also be performed (see Assessment). The test is performed by passively flexing the athlete's head to one side while applying a downward pressure on the opposite shoulder. If pain increases or radiates into the upper arm being depressed, it indicates stretching of the brachial plexus.

If strength and function return completely within 5 minutes, the athlete can return to play (Box 9.3). If any neurologic symptoms persist after this time, the athlete should not be allowed to return to play until full strength, range of motion, and sensation are restored in the cervical spine and extremity. It is also imperative to follow the athlete closely with a postgame examination and successive examinations for several days, to detect any recurrence of weakness.

Treatment may involve ice massage to the upper trapezius and shoulder to decrease pain and inflammation of a secondary muscle strain. A sling may be necessary, particularly with weakness in the rotator cuff muscles. With a grade II or grade III burner, strength training is contraindicated in early rehabilitation, because immature motor end plates may be damaged during resistance training. Range-of-motion exercises for the cervical spine should begin in the supine position and progress to a seated position. Isometric strengthening exercises can progress to diagonal flexion and extension, then to exercise using machines or free weights. After shoulder range of motion is near normal in all planes, closed chain strengthening should be initiated, with progression into isotonic and isodynamic exercise. Scapulothoracic motion should be smooth and isolated, avoiding any muscle substitution. Concentric and eccentric strengthening exercises should be conducted in

---

> ➤➤ **BOX 9.3**

Criteria for Return to Play After a Burner
- No neck pain, arm pain, or dysesthesia (impairment of sensation)
- Full pain-free range of motion in the neck and upper extremity
- Normal strength on manual muscle testing as compared to preseason measurements
- Normal deep tendon reflexes
- Negative brachial plexus traction test

---

external and internal rotation (at 45° abduction), adduction, and extension (17).

Chronic Burners

➤ SIGNS AND SYMPTOMS

In contrast, chronic burners are characterized by more frequent acute episodes that may not produce areas of numbness. Muscle weakness in the shoulder muscles may develop hours or days after the initial injury, and may result in a dropped shoulder or visible atrophy in the shoulder muscles.

➤ MANAGEMENT

These individuals should be examined after the game, during the week, and again the following week, because weakness may not become apparent until days after the initial injury. Initial treatment follows the same parameters of acute burners. The use of lifters, a supplemental pad at the base of the neck, or a modified A-frame shoulder pad supplemented by a cervical collar attached to the posterior aspect of the shoulder pads may limit excessive lateral neck flexion and extension to prevent reoccurrence (see Figure 3.7).

Suprascapular Nerve Injury

The suprascapular nerve may also be damaged with the same mechanisms. This nerve innervates the supraspinatus, infraspinatus, and glenohumeral joint capsule. During motions such as in pitching, spiking, or overhead serving, extreme velocity and torque forces generated during the cocking, acceleration, and release phases subject this nerve and its adjoining artery to rapid stretching.

➤ SIGNS AND SYMPTOMS

Both muscles may appear weak and atrophied, but infraspinatus wasting is usually more apparent because it is not hidden under the trapezius muscle. Because the supraspinatus and infraspinatus are not functioning properly, other problems, such as rotator cuff tendinitis, impingement syndrome, bicipital tenosynovitis, or bursitis of the shoulder, may be present and overshadow this condition.

➤ MANAGEMENT

If an athlete with chronic shoulder problems does not respond well to standard treatment, the individual should be referred to a physician for further evaluation. Once identified, the condition responds well to a flexibility and strengthening program.

 The quarterback experienced a brachial plexus stretch injury. The pain and tingling in the thumb should resolve in a few minutes. If it lingers, or if muscular weakness occurs in shoulder abduction or external rotation, this person should be referred to a physician.

THORACIC SPINE INJURIES

 A 15-year-old butterfly-stroke swimmer is complaining of localized pain and tenderness in the midback region over the thoracic spine. The pain came on gradually and only hurts during the execution of the stroke. Fracture tests are negative. What other condition(s) might be suspected?

The protective rib cage serves to limit movement in the thoracic motion segments. The thoracolumbar junction, however, is a region of potentially high stress during flexion-extension movements of the trunk. Injuries here may involve contusions, strains, sprains, fractures, and apophysitis.

Thoracic Contusions, Strains, and Sprains

Direct blows to the back during contact sports frequently yield contusions to the muscles in the thoracic region. Such injuries range in severity but are generally characterized by pain, ecchymosis, spasm, and limited swelling.

➤ SIGNS AND SYMPTOMS

Thoracic sprains and strains result from either overloading or overstretching muscles in the region through violent or sustained muscle contractions. Painful spasms of the back muscles serve as a protective mechanism to immobilize the injured area, and may develop as a sympathetic response to sprains. The presence of such spasms, however, makes it difficult to determine whether the injury is actually a sprain or strain. Dramatic improvement in a thoracic sprain can be seen in 24 to 48 hours. In contrast, severe strains may require 3 to 4 weeks to heal.

➤ MANAGEMENT

Initial treatment for soft tissue injuries consists of cryotherapy, NSAIDs, and activity modification. Follow-up management may include application of superficial heat, ultrasound, massage, and appropriate stretching and resistance exercise, as needed to recondition the individual.

Thoracic Spinal Fractures and Apophysitis

The rib cage stabilizes and limits motion in the thoracic spine, thereby lessening the likelihood of injury to this area. Thoracic fractures tend to be concentrated at the lower end of the thoracic spine in the transition region between the thoracic and lumbar curvatures.

Large compressive loads, such as those sustained during heavy weight lifting, head-on contact in football or rugby, or landing on the buttock area during tobogganing or snowmobiling, can fracture the vertebral end plates or lead to a **wedge fracture**, named after the shape of the deformed vertebral body (**Figure 9.18A**). Females with **osteopenia**, a condition of reduced bone mineralization, are particularly susceptible to these fractures. More commonly, compressive stress during small, repetitive loads in an activity such as running leads to a progressive compression fracture of a weakened vertebral body. As with any fracture, pain and muscle guarding will be present in the region of the fracture site. Referral to a physician is warranted.

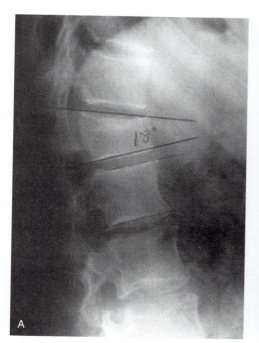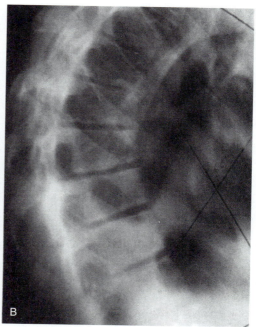

➤ **FIGURE 9.18 Thoracic fracture and apophysitis**. A, Radiograph of a compression wedge fracture in the thoracic region as a result of several compressed motion segments. B, Scheuermann's disease occurs when end plate changes lead to erosion in the anterior vertebral body, which drives a herniated disc forward into the body. In this radiograph, several end plate changes can be seen leading to erosion of the vertebral bodies.

Another leading cause of thoracic fractures among adolescents is **Scheuermann's disease**. This condition, which appears to be related to mechanical stress, involves degeneration of the epiphyseal end plates of the vertebral bodies and typically includes at least three adjacent motion segments. Once the end plate is sufficiently compromised, additional compression from axial and flexion overload forces cause prolapse of the intervertebral disc into the vertebral body **(Figure 9.18B)**. The result is a decrease in spinal height and an accentuation of the thoracic curve, leading to kyphosis. Onset typically occurs at 12 or 13 years of age, with the condition twice as common in girls as in boys. A high incidence of Scheuermann's disease has been documented among gymnasts, trampolinists, wrestlers, and rowers. After referral to a physician, treatment involves modification of activity proportional to the pain. Stretching exercises for the shoulder, neck, and back muscles should be coupled with strengthening the abdominal and spinal extensor muscles. If the kyphosis continues to progress, bracing may be included with the exercise program.

Repeated flexion-extension of the thoracic spine can cause inflammation of the apophyses, the growth centers of the vertebral bodies. Like Scheuermann's disease, apophysitis is a progressive condition characterized by local pain and tenderness. After referral to a physician, treatment for apophysitis includes elimination of the flexion-extension stress, and strengthening abdominal and other trunk muscles.

 The swimmer may have developed apophysitis because of the repeated flexion-extension motions executed during the butterfly stroke. This individual should be referred to a physician for follow-up examination.

LUMBAR SPINE INJURIES

 A weight lifter is experiencing chronic low back pain during the dead lift. What advice would you provide the individual concerning proper lifting technique?

The lumbar spine must support the weight of the head, trunk, and arms, plus any load held in the hands. In addition, the two lower lumbar motion segments (L_4–L_5, L_5–S_1) provide a large range of motion in flexion-extension. It is not surprising, then, that mechanical abuse often results in episodes of low back pain, or that the lower lumbar discs are injured more frequently than any others in the spine.

Lumbar Contusions, Strains, and Sprains

An estimated 80% of the population experiences low back pain (LBP) at some time. Of those, nearly 97% of the pain

stems from mechanical injury to muscles, ligaments, or connective tissue (18) (see **Box 9.4**). Although LBP typically strikes individuals between the ages of 25 and 60 years, with frequency peaking at about age 40, it also occurs in as many as 25% of adolescents and children, ranging down to age 10 (19). Males and females appear to be equally susceptible.

Although several known pathologies may cause LBP, reduced spinal flexibility, repeated stress, and activities that require maximal extension of the lumbar spine are most associated with chronic LBP. During adolescence, the occurrence of LBP increases with age, particularly in sports such as in gymnastics, ballet, figure skating, and football.

➤ SIGNS AND SYMPTOMS

Pain and discomfort can range from diffuse to localized over one area. Pain does not radiate into the buttocks or posterior thigh, nor are there any other signs of neural involvement such as muscle weakness, sensory changes, or reflex inhibition. If a muscle strain is present, pain will increase with passive flexion and active or resisted extension.

➤ MANAGEMENT

Acute protocol is followed to control pain and hemorrhage. After each ice treatment, passive stretching of the low back can help relieve muscle spasm. A corset-type brace can be worn to compress the area (see Figure 3.11). Following the acute stage, a graduated stretching and strengthening program can be initiated. In moderate to severe cases, refer the individual to a physician. Prescription muscle relaxants or NSAIDs may need to be used.

Low Back Pain in Runners

Many runners have muscle tightness in the hip flexors and hamstrings. Tight hip flexors tend to produce a forward body lean, leading to anterior pelvic tilt and hyperlordosis of the lumbar spine. Because the lumbar muscles develop tension to counteract the forward bending moment of the entire trunk when the trunk is in flexion, these muscles are particularly susceptible to strain. This, coupled with tight hamstrings, can lead to a shorter stride.

➤ SIGNS AND SYMPTOMS

Symptoms include localized pain that increases with active and resisted back extension, but radiating pain and neurologic deficits will not be present. Anterior pelvic tilt and hyperlordosis of the lumbar spine may also be present.

➤ MANAGEMENT

Treatment centers on avoiding excessive flexion activities and a sedentary posture (see **Box 9.5**). Flexion causes the mobile nucleus pulposus to shift posteriorly and press against the annulus fibrosus at its thinnest, least-buttressed place. In most cases, this just leads to pain, but in other cases, it may lead to a herniated disc. In addition, physical activity is necessary to pump fluid through the spinal discs to keep them properly hydrated; by interfering with that process, immobility can prolong pain. Ice, NSAIDs, muscle relaxants, TENS, and EMS may be used to reduce pain and inflammation. Lumbar stabilization exercises can be combined with extension exercises, progressive activity, and early mobilization. Aerobic exercise such as walking, swimming, or biking should be included in all programs. If symptoms do not improve within a week, the individual should be referred to a physician to rule out a more serious underlying condition. To decrease the incidence of LBP, training techniques should allow for adequate progression of distance, speed, and hill work, and include extensive flexibility exercises for the hip and thigh region.

Sciatica

Sciatica is an inflammatory condition of the sciatic nerve and is classified in four levels of severity **(Box 9.6)**. The

> ➤➤ **Box 9.5**

Reducing Low Back Pain in Runners

- Wear properly fitted shoes that control heel motion and provide maximum shock-absorption
- Increase flexibility at the hip, knee, ankle plantar flexors, and trunk extensors
- Increase strength in the abdominal and trunk extensor muscles
- Avoid excessive body weight
- Warm up and stretch thoroughly before and after running
- Run with an upright stance rather than a forward lean
- Avoid excessive side-to-side sway
- Run on even terrain and limit hill work. Avoid running on concrete
- Avoid overstriding to increase speed, as this increases leg shock
- Gradually increase distance, intensity, and duration. Do not increase any parameter more than 10% in 1 week
- If orthotics are worn and pain persists, check for wear and rigidity
- Consider alternatives to running, such as cycling, rowing, or swimming

> ➤➤ **Box 9.6**

Classification and Management of Sciatica

- Sciatica only: no sensory or muscle weakness. Modify activity appropriately, and develop rehabilitation and prevention program. Any increased pain requires immediate reevaluation.
- Sciatica with soft signs: some sensory changes, mild or no reflex change, normal muscle strength, normal bowel and bladder function. Remove from sport participation for 6 to 12 weeks.
- Sciatica with hard signs: sensory and reflex changes, and muscle weakness due to repeated, chronic, or acute condition. Normal bowel and bladder function. Remove from participation 12 to 24 weeks.
- Sciatica with severe signs: sensory and reflex changes, muscle weakness, and altered bladder function. Consider immediate surgical decompression.

condition may be caused by a herniated disc, annular tear, myogenic or muscle-related disease, spinal stenosis, facet joint arthropathy, or compression of the nerve between the piriformis muscle.

➤ SIGNS AND SYMPTOMS

If related to a herniated disc, radiating leg pain is greater than back pain, and increases with sitting and leaning forward, coughing, sneezing, and straining. Pain is reproduced during an ipsilateral straight leg raising test, that is, pain is produced on the same side of the elevated leg (see Figure 9.30). With annular tears, back pain is more prevalent and is exacerbated with straight leg raising. Morning pain and muscular stiffness that worsens if chilled or when weather changes (arthritic-like symptoms) are characteristic of myogenic or muscle-related disease. Pain typically radiates into the buttock and thigh region. If lumbar spinal stenosis is present, back and leg pain develop after the individual walks a limited distance and concomitantly increase as distance increases. Pain is not reproduced with a straight leg raising test, but can be reproduced with prolonged spine extension, which is relieved with spine flexion. If a facet joint is involved, pain will be localized over the joint on spinal extension and is exacerbated with ipsilateral lateral flexion. If the sciatic nerve is compressed by the piriformis muscle, pain increases during internal rotation of the thigh. **Table 9.3** lists the more common signs and symptoms that accompany the various etiologies of sciatica.

➤ MANAGEMENT

Referral to a physician is necessary to check for a serious underlying condition. Under normal circumstances, bed rest is usually not indicated, although side-lying with the knees flexed may relieve symptoms. Lifting, bending, twisting, and prolonged sitting and standing aggravate the condition and, therefore, should be avoided. When asymptomatic, abdominal and extensor muscle

TABLE 9.3	SIGNS AND SYMPTOMS OF SCIATICA
Herniated disc	Radiating leg pain is greater than back pain Pain increases with sitting and leaning forward, coughing, sneezing, and straining Neurologic deficits are usually present Positive ipsilateral straight leg raising test
Annular tears	Back pain is more prevalent than leg pain Pain increases with sitting and leaning forward, coughing, sneezing, and straining May have muscle spasm and loss of lordosis Positive ipsilateral straight leg raising test
Myogenic or muscle-related disease	Morning pain and muscle stiffness that worsens if chilled or when weather changes Pain is unilateral or bilateral, not midline Pain extends into the buttock and thigh region only Pain is reproduced with resisted, prolonged muscle contraction and passive stretching of the muscle Contralateral pain with side bending
Spinal stenosis	Back and leg pain develop after walking a limited distance, and increase as distance increases Leg weakness or numbness is present, with or without sciatica Negative straight leg raising test Positive pain on prolonged spine extension, relieved with spine flexion
Facet joint arthropathy	Pain over joint on spinal extension, exacerbated with ipsilateral trunk lateral flexion
Compression from piriformis	Symptoms mimic lumbar disc conditions, except for the absence of true neurologic findings Pain increases with medial rotation of the thigh

strengthening exercises can begin, with gradual return to activity. If symptoms resume, stop activity and refer the individual back to the physician. Occasionally, extended rest is needed for symptoms to resolve totally. If a significant disc protrusion is present, surgery may be indicated.

Lumbar Disc Injuries

Prolonged mechanical loading of the spine can lead to microruptures in the annulus fibrosus, resulting in degeneration of the disc **(Figure 9.19)**. Bulging or protruded discs refer to some eccentric accumulation of the nucleus with slight deformity of the annulus. When the eccentric nucleus produces a definite deformity as it works its way through the fibers of the annulus, it is called a **prolapsed disc**. It is called an **extruded disc** when the material moves into the spinal canal, where it runs the risk of impinging on adjacent nerve roots. Finally, with a **sequestrated disc**, the nuclear material has separated from the disc itself and potentially migrates. The most commonly herniated discs are the lower two lumbar discs at L_4–L_5 and L_5–S_1, followed by the two lower cervical discs. Most ruptures move in a posterior or posterolateral direction as a result of torsion and compression, not just compression.

➤ SIGNS AND SYMPTOMS

Because the intervertebral discs are not innervated, the sensation of pain will not occur until the surrounding soft tissue structures are impinged. When compression is placed on a spinal nerve of the sciatic nerve complex (L_4-S_3), sensory and motor deficits are reflected in the myotome and dermatome patterns associated with the nerve root **(Figure 9.20)**. In addition, alteration in the tendon reflexes will be apparent. A disc need not be completely

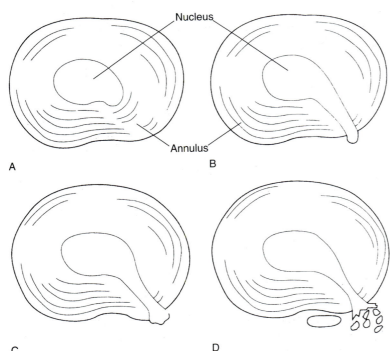

Nucleus

Annulus

A

B

C

D

➤ **FIGURE 9.19 Herniated discs.** Herniated discs are categorized by severity as an eccentrically loaded nucleus progressively moves from **(A)** protruded through, **(B)** prolapsed, and **(C)** extruded, culminating in **(D)** sequestrated when the nuclear material moves into the canal to impinge on the adjacent spinal nerves.

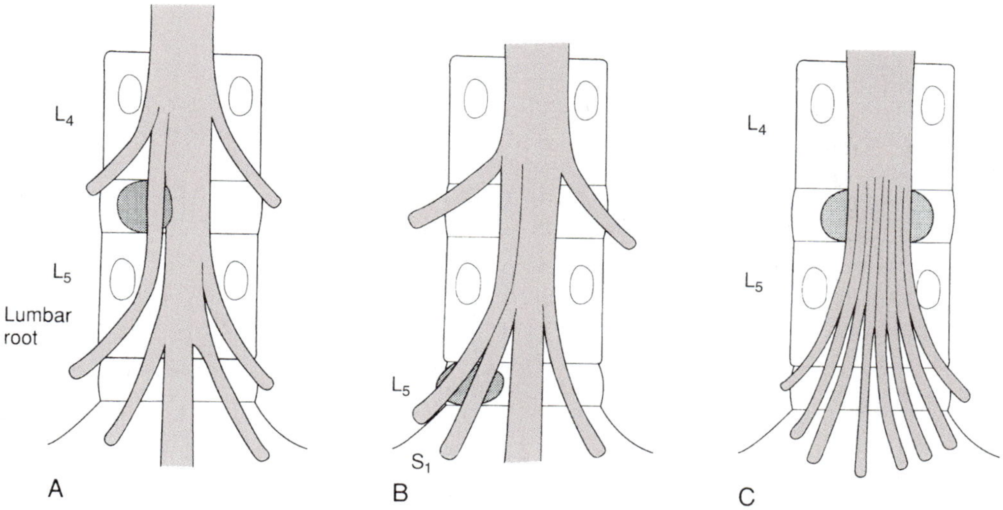

▶ FIGURE 9.20 **Possible effects on the spinal cord and spinal nerves according to the level of herniation.** A, Herniation between L_4 and L_5 compresses the L_5 nerve root. B, Herniation between L_5 and S_1 can compress the nerve root crossing the disc (S_1) and the nerve root emerging through the intervertebral foramina (L_5). C, A posterior herniation at the L_4–L_5 level can compress the dura mater of the entire cauda equina, leading to bowel and bladder paralysis.

herniated to give symptoms. Symptoms include sharp pain and muscle spasms at the site of the herniation that often shoot down the sciatic nerve into the lower extremity. The individual may walk in a slightly crouched position, leaning away from the side of the lesion. Forward trunk flexion or a straight leg raising test (see Figure 9.30) may exacerbate pain and increase distal symptoms. Significant signs indicating the need for immediate referral to a physician include muscle weakness, sensory changes, diminished reflexes in the lower extremity, and abnormal bladder or bowel function. **Table 9.4** outlines physical findings associated with disc herniation in the low back region.

▶ MANAGEMENT

In mild cases, treatment consists of minimizing load on the spine by avoiding activities that involve impact, lifting, bending, twisting, and prolonged sitting and standing. Painful muscle spasms can be eliminated with ice and/or heat, administration of prescribed NSAIDs and/or muscle relaxants, ultrasound, TENS, passive exercise, and gen-

tle stretching. Following resolution of spasm and acute pain, rehabilitation should include spine and hamstring flexibility, spinal strength and stabilization exercises, and functional stabilization control in sports and daily activities.

Lumbar Fractures and Dislocations

Transverse or spinous process fractures result from extreme tension from the attached muscles or from a direct blow to the low back during participation in contact sports, such as football, rugby, soccer, basketball, hockey, and lacrosse. These fractures often lead to additional injury to surrounding soft tissues, but are not as serious as compression fractures. Compression fractures more commonly involve the L_1 vertebra at the thoracolumbar junction. Hyperflexion, or jack-knifing of the trunk, crushes the anterior aspect of the vertebral body. The primary danger with this injury is the possibility of bony fragments moving into the spinal canal and damaging the spinal cord or spinal nerves. Because of the facet joint orientation in the lumbar

TABLE 9.4	PHYSICAL FINDINGS ASSOCIATED WITH A HERNIATED DISC		
Signs and Symptoms	**L_3–L_4 (L_4 root)**	**L_4–L_5 (L_5 root)**	**L_5–S_1 (S_1 root)**
Pain	Lumbar region and buttocks	Lumbar region, groin, and sacroiliac area	Lumbar region, groin, and sacroiliac area
Dermatome and sensory loss	Anterior midthigh over patella, medial lower leg to great toe	Lateral thigh, anterior leg, top of foot, middle three toes	Posterior lateral thigh and lower leg to lateral foot and 5th toe
Myotome weakness	Ankle dorsiflexion	Toe extension (Extensor hallux)	Ankle plantar flexion (Gastrocnemius)
Reduced deep tendon reflex	Quadriceps	Medial hamstrings	Achilles tendon
Straight leg raising test	Normal	Reduced	Reduced

region, dislocations occur only when a fracture is present. Fracture-dislocations resulting from sport participation are rare.

> ▶ SIGNS AND SYMPTOMS

Symptoms will include localized, palpable pain that may radiate down the nerve root if a bony fragment compresses a spinal nerve. Because the spinal cord ends at about L_1 or L_2 level, fractures of the lumbar vertebrae below this point do not pose a serious threat, but should be handled with care to minimize potential nerve damage to the cauda equina. Confirmation of a possible fracture is made with a radiograph or CT scan.

> ▶ MANAGEMENT

 If a fracture or dislocation is suspected, activate EMS for transport to the nearest medical facility.

Conservative treatment consists of initial bed rest, cryotherapy, and minimizing mechanical loads on the low back until symptoms subside, which may take 3 to 6 weeks.

 In supervising the individual doing the dead lift, make sure the individual is using proper technique. The weight may need to be reduced to allow this. Furthermore, make sure the person is wearing a weight belt to help stabilize the low back area.

SACRUM AND COCCYX INJURIES

 An individual is complaining of sharp pain in the sacral region when running on uneven terrain. The pain is becoming so persistent and chronic that it now hurts to sit for an extended time. What injury may be present? What recommendations can made to this person relative to caring for the injury?

Because the sacrum and coccyx are essentially immobile, the potential for mechanical injury to these regions is dramatically reduced. In sport participation, injuries may result from direct blows and stress on the sacroiliac (SI) joint.

Sacroiliac Joint Sprain

Sprains of the sacroiliac joint may result from a single traumatic episode involving bending and/or twisting, repetitive stress from lifting, a fall on the buttocks, excessive side-to-side or up-and-down motion during running and jogging, running on uneven terrain, suddenly slipping or stumbling forward, or wearing new shoes or orthoses. The injury may irritate or stretch the sacrotuberous or sacrospinous ligament, or may lead to an anterior or posterior rotation of one side of the pelvis relative to the other. With rotation of the pelvis, hypomobility results. During healing, the joint on the injured side may become hypermobile,

allowing that joint to subluxate in either an anterior- or posterior-rotated position.

> ▶ SIGNS AND SYMPTOMS

Symptoms may involve unilateral, dull pain in the sacral area that extends into the buttock and posterior thigh. Upon observation, the anterior superior iliac spine (ASIS) or posterior superior iliac spine (PSIS) may appear asymmetrical when compared bilaterally. There may also be a leg-length discrepancy. Muscle spasm is not often seen. Standing on one leg and climbing stairs may also increase the pain. Forward bending reveals a block to normal movement with the PSIS on the injured side moving sooner than on the uninjured side. Lateral flexion toward the injured side increases pain, as do straight leg raises beyond 45°.

> ▶ MANAGEMENT

Treatment for sacroiliac sprains includes cryotherapy, prescribed NSAIDs, and gentle stretching to alleviate stiffness. Flexibility, pelvic stabilization exercises, mobilization of the affected joint, and strengthening exercises for the low back can then begin.

Coccygeal Injuries

Direct blows to the region can produce contusions and fractures of the coccyx. Pain resulting from a fracture may last for several months. Prolonged or chronic pain in the region may also result from irritation of the coccygeal nerve plexus. This condition is termed **coccygodynia**. Treatment for coccygeal pain includes analgesics, use of padding for protection, and a ring seat to alleviate compression during sitting.

 The runner has probably irritated the sacroiliac joint from repeated stress while running on uneven terrain. This individual should ice the region to control inflammation and pain, stretch the low back and buttock region, and run on more even terrain. If conditions do not improve, refer the individual to a physician for further assessment.

ASSESSMENT OF SPINAL INJURIES

 A 17-year-old female high jumper is complaining of pain in the low back and sacroiliac region, aggravated by flexion and hyperextension of the trunk during jumping. How will you progress through the assessment to determine the extent and severity of injury?

Injury assessment of the spine is complex and cannot be rushed. In a traumatic episode, if a fully conscious person is not experiencing severe pain, spasm, or tenderness, it is rare that the individual has sustained a significant spinal injury. It is more likely that the individual has experienced a minor injury, such as a muscular strain or sprain. Even

Red Flags that Warrant Immobilization and Immediate Referral to a Physician

- Severe pain, point tenderness, or deformity along the vertebral column
- Loss or change in sensation anywhere in the body
- Paralysis or inability to move a body part
- Diminished or absent reflexes
- Muscle weakness in a myotome
- Pain radiating into the extremities
- Trunk or abdominal pain that may be referred from the visceral organs
- Any injury in which you are uncertain about the severity or nature

still, it is essential that the injury assessment be performed in a deliberate manner, taking as much time as necessary to perform the examination.

The severity of pain and presence or absence of neurologic symptoms, neck spasm, and tenderness can indicate when a backboard and neck stabilization are needed (20). When in doubt, always assume a severe spinal injury is present and activate the emergency care plan. Do not remove the helmet or move the individual's head, neck, or spine. Once a significant physical finding indicates possible nerve involvement, immobilization and immediate transportation to the nearest medical facility are warranted, regardless of whether a total assessment is completed. **Box 9.7** identifies several signs and symptoms that, if present, necessitate activating EMS.

In cases in which the individual walks into the training room complaining of neck or back pain, it is relatively safe to assume that a serious spinal injury is not present. This section will focus on a spinal assessment in a conscious individual. Specific information related to an acute injury is included where appropriate. **Field Strategy 9.2** summarizes the assessment procedure.

HISTORY

 The high jumper complained of pain in the low back and sacroiliac region, aggravated by flexion and hyperextension of the trunk during jumping. What questions need to be asked to identify the cause and extent of injury?

A history of the injury should include information on the primary complaint, mechanism of injury, characteristics of the symptoms, disability resulting from the injury, previous injuries to the area, and family history that may have some bearing on this specific condition. In a spinal injury, questions should be asked about the location of pain (localized or radiating), type of pain (dull, aching, sharp, burning), presence of sensory changes (numbness, tingling, or absence of sensation), and possible muscle weakness or

paralysis. With a neck injury, questions should be asked to determine both long- and short-term memory loss that may indicate an associated concussion or subdural hematoma. It is important to note the length of time it takes the athlete to respond to the questions. General questions related to a spinal injury are presented in **Field Strategy 9.3.**

 The 17-year-old jumper has been a competitive athlete since seventh grade. The primary complaint is an aching pain when bending over, aggravated with hyperextension and prolonged sitting that produces sharp radiating pain into the low back and sacroiliac region. The condition has been present for 4 weeks and is not getting better. She cannot recall any traumatic episode that led to the condition.

OBSERVATION AND INSPECTION

 Would it be appropriate to do a scan exam to rule out other painful areas? What specific factors should be observed to identify the injury?

Observation should begin as soon as the individual enters the room. Body language can signal pain, disability, and muscle weakness. It is necessary to note the individual's willingness or ability to move, general posture, ease in motion, and general attitude. Clothing and protective equipment may prevent visual observation of abnormalities in the spinal alignment. As such, the individual should be suitably dressed so the back is exposed as much as possible. For girls and women, a bra, halter top, or swimsuit can be worn. Observation should begin with a postural assessment, progress through a scan exam, and gait analysis, and end with an inspection of the injury site.

Posture

Posture assessment can detect congenital or functional problems that may contribute to the injury. Ask the individual to sit down to begin the exam, then stand. The head and neck posture should be observed. Is the head held erect or carried in a forward position? Are any abnormal spinal curvatures present? The individual should have a smooth cervical lordosis with gentle transition into thoracic kyphosis. A "forward" head (ear forward of the acromion) or accentuated cervicothoracic hump creates a constant flexion moment of the head over the spine. The individual should be instructed to lean forward and touch the toes while keeping the knees straight (Adam's position). Observe the vertebrae and contour of the back **(Figure 9.21)**. Look for a hump or raised scapula on one side (convex side of curve) and a hollow (concave side of curve) on the other, indicating scoliosis. The combination of the hump and hollow is due to vertebral rotation.

If a lateral curve is present while standing but disap-

FIELD STRATEGY 9.2   ASSESSMENT FOR A SPINAL INJURY

HISTORY

- ❏ Primary complaint including:
  - ■ Current nature, location, and onset of the condition
- ❏ Mechanism of injury
  - ■ Cause of stress; position of neck, trunk, or low back; direction of force
  - ■ Changes in running surface, shoes, equipment, techniques, or conditioning modes
- ❏ Characteristics of the symptoms
  - ■ Evolution of the onset, nature, location, severity, and duration of pain and weakness
- ❏ Disability resulting from the injury
- ❏ Related medical history
  - ■ Previous injuries to the area, congenital abnormalities, or family history

OBSERVATION AND INSPECTION

- ❏ Observation should analyze:
  - ■ Overall appearance
  - ■ Posture and body symmetry
  - ■ General motor function through a scan exam
  - ■ Gait analysis
- ❏ Inspection at the injury site for:
  - ■ Deformity, swelling, discoloration, hypertrophy or muscle atrophy, visible congenital deformity, or surgical incisions or scars

PALPATION

- ❏ Bony structures to determine a possible fracture
- ❏ Soft tissue structures for skin temperature, swelling, point tenderness, crepitus, deformity, muscle spasm, cutaneous sensation, and pulse

FUNCTIONAL TESTS

- ❏ Active movement
- ❏ Passive movement and end feels
- ❏ Resisted movement

STRESS TESTS

- ❏ Cervical compression and distraction tests
- ❏ Spurling test
- ❏ Brachial plexus traction test
- ❏ Slump test
- ❏ Straight leg raising test
- ❏ Tension or bowstring test
- ❏ Milgram's test
- ❏ Brudzinski-Kernig's test
- ❏ Prone knee bending test
- ❏ Single-leg standing lumbar extension test
- ❏ Hoover test
- ❏ Valsalva's test

NEUROLOGIC TESTS

- ❏ Myotomes
- ❏ Reflexes
- ❏ Dermatomes

SPORT-SPECIFIC FUNCTIONAL TESTS

---

pears on flexion, a nonstructural scoliosis curve is present. With structural scoliosis, the curve remains. Are there any noticeable asymmetries, such as discrepancies in the height of the shoulder or scapula, hip, or patella? A flexed posturing at the hips from tight hip flexors results in a compensatory increase in the lumbar and cervical lordoses. These abnormal postures can lead to tension overload of the posterior cervical muscles, resulting in an inability to maintain the head in an upright position. Obesity with rounded shoulders or a hunched posture, as typically occurs in individuals who overdevelop the anterior chest muscles, can predispose the individual to thoracic outlet syndrome or other chronic strain patterns. Is the trunk rotated so one shoulder is forward? Are the ribs more prominent on one side? Specific postural factors to observe in the head and spinal region are listed in **Field Strategy 9.4.**

Scan Exam

Active movement should not be performed when pain is present over the vertebrae or when motor/sensory deficits are present. If that is not the case, a scan exam can be used

FIELD STRATEGY 9.3 DEVELOPING A HISTORY FOR A SPINAL INJURY

CURRENT INJURY STATUS

1. Were you knocked out or unconscious?
2. How did the injury occur (mechanism)? Did the injury involve twisting of the trunk, a violent stretch, or a jack-knife maneuver?
3. Where is the pain located? Did it come on suddenly or gradually? How severe is the pain? Describe the pain (sharp, aching, burning, radiating, deep or superficial)? Does the severity of symptoms change when you change position?
4. Was there any muscle spasm, numbness, or change in sensation anywhere in the body?
5. Can you move your fingers and toes?
6. Do you have equal muscle strength in the hands?
7. Are there certain activities you cannot perform because of the pain? (Note the gender. Females have a higher incidence of low back pain.)
8. What different activities have you been doing in the last week? (Look for activities such as lifting or carrying heavy objects, or positions involving bending over for long periods of time.)
9. Is there a certain position that alleviates the pain?

PAST INJURY STATUS

1. Have you ever injured your back before? When? How did that occur? What was done for the injury?
2. Have you had any medical problems recently? (Look for possible referred pain from visceral organs, heart, and lungs.)
3. Are you on any medication?
4. Do you have any musculoskeletal problems elsewhere in the body? (These may result in changes in gait or technique that transfer abnormal forces to structures in the spinal region.)
5. Has anyone in your family had a similar problem?

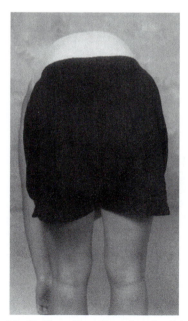

➤ **FIGURE 9.21 Skyline view**. Observing the "skyline" view (Adam's position) of the spine can help assess for the presence of scoliosis. The athletic trainer is looking for an elevated scapula and a curve in the spinal column.

to assess general motor function (**Box 9.8**). It potentially can rule out injury at other joints that may be overlooked due to intense pain or discomfort at the primary injury site. Active movement of the spine may be included in this step and need not be repeated with special tests. It is important to note if there is any hesitation to move a body part, or if the individual prefers to use one side over the other.

Gait Assessment

The individual should be asked to walk several yards while the athletic trainer observes normal body movement. The athletic trainer should stand behind, in front of, and to the side of the individual to observe from all angles. Note subtle posture abnormalities, such as kyphosis, scoliosis, lordosis, or pelvic tilt. A low back injury may produce a forward lean, a lean to one side, or a noticeable limp.

Inspection of the Injury Site

Local inspection at the injury site should include observation for deformity, swelling, discoloration, muscle spasm, atrophy, hypertrophy, scars that might indicate previous surgery, and general skin condition. A step deformity in the lumbar spine may indicate a spondylolisthesis.

FIELD STRATEGY 9.4   POSTURAL ASSESSMENT

<u>ANTERIOR VIEW</u>

- Are the head and neck in the midline of the body? Is the nose centered?
- Does the slope of the shoulder muscles appear bilaterally equal? (The dominant side will usually be lower than the nondominant side.)
- Do both shoulders have a well-rounded musculature with no prominent bony structures?
- Is the space between the arms and body the same on both sides? Are both hands held in the same position?
- Does the rib cage look symmetrical with no rotation?
- Are the folds of the waist at the same height?

<u>SIDE VIEW</u>

- Can you draw an imaginary straight plum line from the ear through the middle of the shoulder, hip, knee, and ankle?
- Does the neck or back have any excessive curves?
- Are the elbows held near full extension?
- Do the chest, back, and abdominal muscles have good tone with no obvious chest deformities?
- Does the pelvis appear to be level?
- Are the knees straight, flexed, or hyperextended? (Normally they should be slightly flexed.)

<u>POSTERIOR VIEW</u>

- Are the head and neck centered? (Note any abnormal prominence of bony structures or muscle atrophy.)
- Does the spine appear to be straight? Have the individual lean over in Adam's position to detect possible scoliosis.
- Are the scapulae at the same height and resting at the same angle? Are both scapulae lying flat against the rib cage?
- Is there any atrophy in the muscle groups of the shoulder and arm?
- Is the olecranon process of each elbow at the same height? Is the space between the body and elbow the same on both sides?
- Do the ribs protrude?
- Are the waist folds level? Are the posterior gluteal folds level?
- Are the skin creases on the posterior knee level?

Gross Neuromuscular Assessment

In an acute injury, a posture and scan exam is not possible. However, it would be beneficial to do a neuromuscular assessment prior to palpation to detect any motor and/or sensory deficits. Without moving the individual, ask the athlete to perform a submaximal, bilateral hand-squeeze test and ankle dorsiflexion. These two actions assess the cervical and lumbar spinal nerves, respectively. Muscle weakness and/or diminished sensation over the hands and feet indicate a serious injury. If any deficits are noted, initiate the emergency care plan and activate EMS. If no deficits are noted, it does not rule out possible neurologic involvement or fracture. Therefore, palpation should be done with the individual maintained in the position found.

 Slight lordosis and anterior pelvic tilt was present in the high jumper. During the scan exam, trunk flexion and extension produced a dull pain in the low back. Lateral flexion to the right caused sharp pain to radiate into the right buttock and poste-

rior leg. A forward straight-leg raise with the right leg was limited and could not be performed without bending the knee. Gait analysis showed a shortened stride on the right side. Visual inspection showed no abnormalities.

PALPATION

 The injury is confined to the low back region. What specific structures need to be palpated to determine if the injury is of bony or soft tissue origin? Can neural involvement be ruled out during palpation?

In injuries that do not involve neural damage, fracture, or dislocation, palpation can proceed in the following manner. Bony and soft tissue structures are palpated to detect temperature, swelling, point tenderness, deformity, crepitus, muscle spasm, and cutaneous sensation. Palpation may be done in a seated, standing, supine, or prone position.

Scan Exam for a Spinal Injury

The athletic trainer should instruct the athlete to perform the skills listed below. During the movements, observe for signs of pain, hesitation to move a body part, or abnormal movement. If present, complete a more thorough evaluation of the affected body part, and if necessary, immobilize the area and refer the athlete to a physician for further care.

- Touch the chin to the chest
- Look up at the ceiling keeping the back straight
- Turn the head sideways in both directions
- Try to touch each ear to the shoulder
- Rotate the trunk sideways keeping the hips stabilized
- Lean forward and touch the toes
- Look up at the ceiling with hyperextension of the trunk
- Lean sideways and do lateral flexion of the trunk
- While placing a hand on a table for support:
  - Do a single straight leg raise forward, backward, and sideways
  - Flex the knee
  - Raise up on the toes
  - Balance on the heels

To relax the neck and spinal muscles, the individual should lie on a table. To palpate posterior neck structures, the individual should be supine. The athletic trainer should reach around the neck with both hands and palpate either side of the spine with the fingertips. Muscle spasms in the erector spinae, sternocleidomastoid muscles, scalene muscles, and/or the upper trapezius may indicate dysfunction of the cervical spine. In the thoracic and low back region, have the individual prone. A pillow or blanket should be placed under the hip region to tilt the pelvis back and relax the lumbar curvature. Muscle spasm in the lower erector spinae, lower trapezius, serratus posterior, quadratus lumborum, latissimus dorsi, or gluteus maximus may indicate dysfunction of the thoracic or lumbar spine. Surface landmarks can facilitate palpation (see **Table 9.5**). Palpate the structures listed below.

TABLE 9.5   SURFACE LANDMARKS ON THE BACK

Vertebra	Bony Landmark
C_2	One finger's breadth inferior to the mastoid process
C_6	Posterior to the cricoid cartilage
C_7 and T_1	Prominent spinous processes in neck
T_2	Top of scapula
T_4	Base of spine of scapula
T_7	Inferior angle of scapula
T_{12}	Lowest floating rib
L_4	Top of iliac crest
L_5	Demarcated by bilateral dimples
S_2	Level of posterior superior iliac spines

Anterior Aspect

1. Hyoid bone, thyroid cartilage, trachea, and carotid arteries.
2. Sternocleidomastoid muscle, manubrium, clavicle, supraclavicular fossa.
3. Sternum, ribs, and costocartilage.
4. Abdomen and inguinal area. Note any abnormal tenderness or masses indicating internal pathology that is referring pain to the spinal region.
5. Iliac crest, anterior superior iliac spine, symphysis pubis.

Posterior Aspect

1. External protuberance of the occiput.
2. Spinous processes. Note any tenderness, crepitus, or deviation from the norm. A noticeable discrepancy can indicate a fracture or vertebral subluxation. Pain and tenderness without positive findings on muscle movement may indicate the problem is not musculoskeletal in origin.
3. Facet joints. The facet articulations are approximately a thumb's breadth to either side of the spinous process. Point tenderness here, especially with extension and rotation to the same side, suggests facet joint pain.
4. Interspinous and supraspinous ligaments, ligamentum flavum, paraspinal muscles, and quadratus lumborum. Trigger points of the paraspinal and shoulder girdle regions will refer pain to a more distal area. Tender points that increase with muscular contraction indicate a localized muscle strain. An area tender to palpation but not painful during muscle contraction may indicate referred pain from another area.
5. Scapula, trapezius, and latissimus dorsi.
6. Iliac crest, posterior superior iliac spine, and sacrum. The interspace between L_4–L_5 lies at the same level as the top of the iliac crest. The S_2 spinous process lies in the middle of a line drawn between the posterior superior iliac spines.
7. Ischial tuberosity, sciatic nerve, and greater trochanter (**Figure 9.22**).

Point tenderness was palpated in the low back region between the L_3 and S_1 vertebrae, with increased pain in the L_4 to L_5 region. Muscle spasm was present on either side of the lumbar region. Pain was also elicited with palpation midway between the ischial tuberosity and greater trochanter.

PHYSICAL EXAMINATION TESTS

The high jumper has concentrated palpable pain in the L_4 to L_5 region, with associated muscle spasm and pain over the sciatic nerve as it

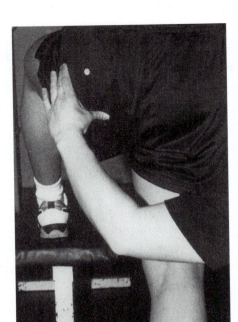

➤ FIGURE 9.22 **Sciatic nerve**. To palpate the sciatic nerve, flex the hip and locate the ischial tuberosity and greater trochanter. The sciatic nerve may be palpated at the midpoint. It is designated here by the white dot.

passes into the posterior thigh. How will you proceed to determine bony versus soft tissue involvement?

Because injuries to the spinal region can be very complex, it is imperative to work slowly through the different tests.

If at anytime, movement leads to increased acute pain or change in sensation, or the individual resists moving the spine, assume that a significant injury is present and activate EMS.

Functional Tests

Goniometry measurements of the spine are not typically taken due to the difficulty of measuring individual regional motions. Completion of gross movement patterns is adequate to determine normal ranges of motion. If motion is limited, further assessment can be conducted.

ACTIVE MOVEMENT

If active movement of the spine was conducted during the scan exam, it need not be repeated here. Look for the individual's willingness to perform the movement. Is the movement fluid and complete? Does pain, spasm, or stiffness block the full range of motion? With movements to the left and right, always compare bilaterally. Cervical, thoracic, and lumbar movement should be tested. The range of motion listed with each trunk movement is lumbar movement and does not include thoracic movement. Spinal movements include:

1. Cervical flexion (80 to 90°)
2. Cervical extension (70°)
3. Lateral cervical flexion (left and right) (20 to 45°)
4. Cervical rotation (left and right) (70 to 90°)
5. Forward trunk flexion (40 to 60°)
6. Trunk extension (20 to 35°)
7. Lateral trunk flexion (left and right) (15 to 20°)
8. Trunk rotation (35 to 50°)

PASSIVE RANGE OF MOTION

Passive movement should not be performed in an acute injury where motor and sensory deficits are present. These deficits indicate a spinal injury, and any movement could be catastrophic. In other injuries where motor and sensory deficits are not present, passive range of motion can be performed if the individual does not have full range of motion. To perform passive motion, place the individual in a supine position. Passively move the cervical region through the various movements. The normal end feel for the cervical spine is tissue stretch in all four movements. Thoracic and lumbar passive movement is seldom performed. End feels can be determined at the extremes of active movement. Like cervical movements, the normal end feels for the thoracic and lumbar movements are tissue stretch.

RESISTED MUSCLE TESTING

Resisted movement is done throughout the full range of motion in the same movements as active muscle testing. It is important to stabilize the hip and trunk during cervical testing to avoid muscle substitution. This can be accomplished by having the individual seated and using one hand to stabilize the shoulder or thorax while the other hand applies manual overpressure. When testing the thoracic and lumbar region, the weight of the trunk will stabilize the hips. Inform the individual not to allow you to move the body part being tested. Maximal force must be applied when testing the major muscle groups to detect early weakness. By repetitively loading the patient's resisting muscle with rapid, consecutive impulses, more subtle weakness can be detected. Cervical movements assessed are demonstrated in **Figure 9.23**. Thoracic and lumbar movements to be tested are demonstrated in **Figure 9.24**.

Stress and Functional Tests

There are several stress tests that can be used in spinal assessment. Only those deemed relevant should be performed.

If any increased pain or change of sensation occurs, the individual should be immobilized and EMS activated.

CERVICAL COMPRESSION TEST

The compression test can detect pressure on a cervical nerve root from degeneration or narrowing of a neural

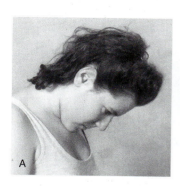
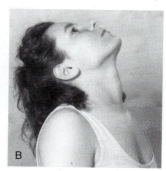
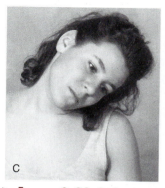
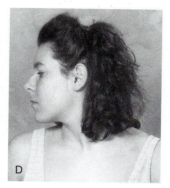

> **FIGURE 9.23 Active movements of the cervical spine**.
A, Flexion. B, Extension. C, Lateral flexion. D, Rotation.

foramen. Carefully compress straight down on the individual's head while the person is sitting on a stable chair or table **(Figure 9.25)**. Increased pain or altered sensation is a positive sign, indicating pressure on a nerve root. The distribution of the pain and altered sensation can indicate which nerve root is involved.

SPURLING TEST (FORAMINAL COMPRESSION TEST)

The Spurling test is a variation of the cervical compression test. The individual extends the neck, then rotates and laterally bends the head to the same side while the examiner applies downward pressure to the top of the head **(Figure 9.26)**. If this position, with or without pressure, reproduces radiating pain into the upper limb, a nerve root impingement due to a narrowing of the neural foramina is suggested. The distribution of the pain and altered sensation can indicate which nerve root is involved.

CERVICAL DISTRACTION TEST

This is performed by placing one hand under the individual's chin and the other around the occiput, and

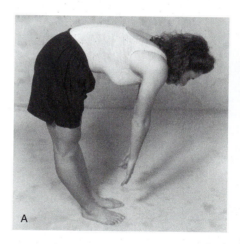
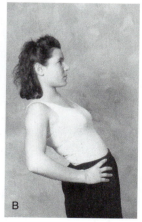
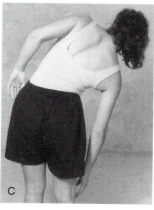
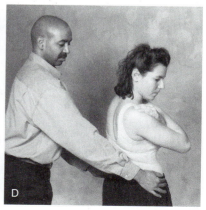

> **FIGURE 9.24 Active movements of the thoracic and lumbar regions**. A, Flexion. B, Extension. C, Lateral flexion. D, Rotation.

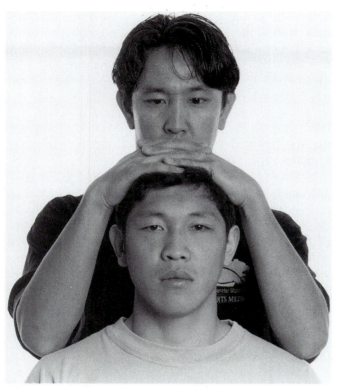

➤ FIGURE 9.25 **Compression test**. With the neck in neutral position, carefully push straight down on the individual's head. Increased pain or altered sensation is a positive sign indicating pressure on a nerve root. The test can also be performed with the neck slightly flexed to one side.

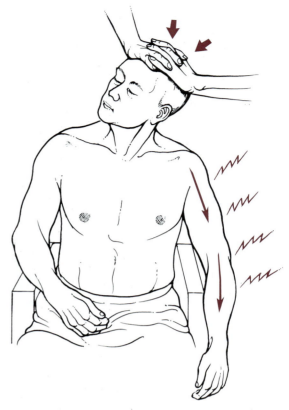

➤ FIGURE 9.26 **Spurling's test**. Have the athlete extend, rotate, and laterally bend the neck. Carefully apply downward pressure on the individual's head. Increased pain indicates cervical nerve root involvement.

then slowly lifting the head **(Figure 9.27)**. The test is positive if pain decreases or is relieved as the head is lifted, indicating that pressure on the nerve root is relieved. If pain increases with distraction, it indicates ligamentous injury.

BRACHIAL PLEXUS TRACTION TEST

This test should not be performed until the possibility of bony trauma has been ruled out. While standing behind the athlete, the athletic trainer passively flexes the athlete's head to one side while applying a downward pressure on the opposite shoulder **(Figure 9.28)**. If pain increases or radiates into the upper arm being depressed, it indicates stretching of the brachial plexus. If pain increases on the side toward the lateral bending, it indicates irritation or compression of the nerve roots between two vertebrae.

SLUMP TEST

With the individual sitting on a table, ask the person to "slump" so that the spine flexes and the shoulders sag forward. With the head erect, ask the individual if any symptoms are produced by the slump **(Figure 9.29A)**. If no symptoms are present, flex the individual's neck and hold the head down with the shoulders slumped forward **(Figure 9.29B)**. If no symptoms are produced, passively extend one of the athlete's knees **(Figure 9.29C)**. If no

symptoms occur, passively dorsiflex the foot of the same leg to see if any symptoms occur **(Figure 9.29D)**. This process is repeated with the opposite leg. A test is positive if symptoms of sciatic pain are reproduced, indicating im-

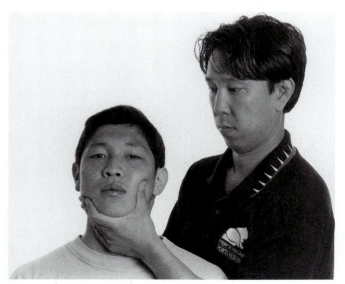

➤ FIGURE 9.27 **Distraction test**. Lift the head slowly. The test is positive if pain is decreased or relieved as the head is lifted, indicating that pressure on the nerve root is relieved. If pain increases with distraction, it indicates ligamentous injury.

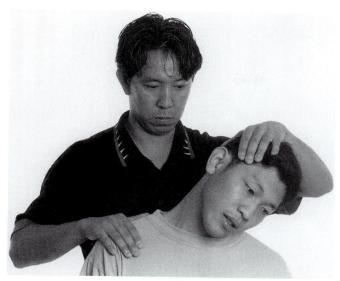

➤ **FIGURE 9.28 Brachial plexus traction test.** Passively apply downward pressure by doing lateral bending away from the involved shoulder and simultaneously depressing the involved shoulder. Radiating pain or a burning sensation indicates injury to the brachial plexus. If pain increases on the side toward the lateral bending, it indicates irritation or compression of the nerve roots between two vertebrae.

pingement of the dura and spinal cord or nerve roots. The pain is usually produced at the site of the lesion.

STRAIGHT LEG RAISING TEST

Also known as Lasègue's test, this test is used to assess sacroiliac joint pain, irritation of the sciatic nerve, or tight hamstrings. The individual is placed in a relaxed supine position with the hip medially rotated and knee extended. The athletic trainer should grasp the individual's heel with one hand and place the other on top of the patella to prevent the knee from flexing. The leg is slowly raised until the individual complains of pain or tightness. The leg is then lowered until the pain is relieved. The individual is then asked to flex the neck onto the chest, or dorsiflex the foot, or to do both actions simultaneously **(Figure 9.30)**.

The neck flexion movement is called Hyndman's sign or Brudzinski's sign. Pain that increases with neck flexion or dorsiflexion indicates stretching of the dura mater of the spinal cord. Pain that does not increase with neck flexion or dorsiflexion indicates tight hamstrings. The sciatic nerve is fully stretched at about 70° of flexion. Hence, pain after 70° usually indicates pain from the lumbar area (facet joints) or sacroiliac joints. Pain that occurs opposite the leg lifted indicates a space-occupying lesion (e.g., herniated disc). The finding of pain when the athletic trainer is testing the opposite (good) leg is sometimes called the well leg raising test of Fajersztajn, a prostrate leg raising test, a sciatic phenomenon, Lhermitt's test, or the crossover sign. Always compare both legs for any difference. Athletes who are very hypermobile (e.g., gymnasts, synchronized swimmers, wrestlers, divers) may not show a positive

straight leg raising test until 110 to 120° of hip flexion, even in the presence of nerve root pathology.

The athletic trainer can then test both legs simultaneously (bilateral straight leg raising). This must be performed carefully, because the athletic trainer is lifting the weight of both lower limbs, thereby placing a large stress on his or her own lumbar spine. If the test causes pain before 70° of hip flexion, the lesion is probably in the sacroiliac joints; if it causes pain after 70°, the lesion is probably in the lumbar spine.

TENSION (BOWSTRING) TEST

A positive straight leg raising test can then be followed by the tension, or bowstring, test. The athletic trainer maintains the leg in the same position, then flexes the knee slightly (20°), reducing the symptoms. Thumb or finger pressure is then exerted over the tibial portion of the sciatic nerve as it passes through the popliteal space to reestablish the painful radiating symptoms. The test indicates tension or pressure on the sciatic nerve and is a modification of the straight leg raising test. An alternative method is to flex both the hip and knee at 90°. The athletic trainer then slowly extends the knee as far as possible while applying pressure in the popliteal space. Replication of tenderness or radiating pain is a positive sign for sciatic nerve irritation.

MILGRAM'S TEST

This test attempts to increase intrathecal pressure, resulting in an increased bulge of the nucleus pulposus. The athlete lies supine and simultaneously lifts both legs off the table 2 to 4 inches, holding this position for 30 seconds. The test is positive if the limbs or affected limb cannot be held for 30 seconds or if symptoms are reproduced in the affected limb. Positive results of this test tend to be limited to the lumbar spine. This test should be performed with caution as it places a high stress load on the lumbar spine.

BRUDZINSKI-KERNIG TEST

This test is similar to the straight leg raising test, but the movements are actively performed by the athlete. In Brudzinki's portion of the test, the athlete is supine with the hands cupped behind the head **(Figure 9.31A)**. The test is positive if the athlete complains of neck and low back discomfort and attempts to relieve the meningeal irritation by involuntarily flexing the knees and hips. In the Kernig position, the athlete lies supine with the hip flexed and knee extended **(Figure 9.31B)**. Pain in the head, neck, or lower back are suggestive of meningeal irritation. If the pain is relieved when the individual flexes the knee, it is considered a positive test indicating meningeal irritation, nerve root involvement or dural irritation. The two parts of the test may be done separately, or together.

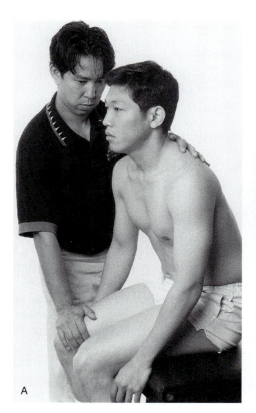

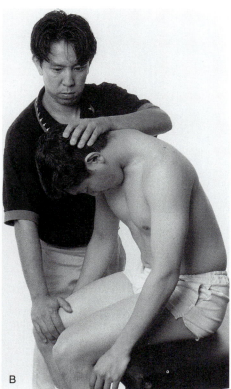

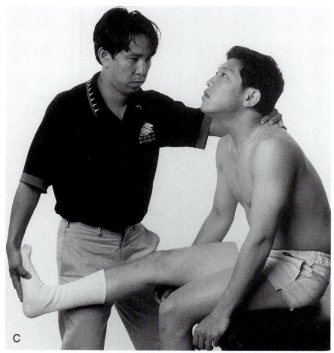

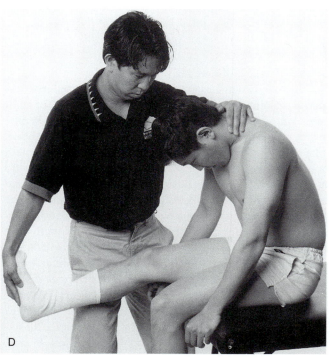

➤ **FIGURE 9.29 Slump test**. The test is performed in several stages. A, With the individual sitting on a table, ask the person to "slump" so that the spine flexes and the shoulders sag forward. B, If no symptoms are present, flex the individual's neck and hold the head down with the shoulders slumped forward. C, If no symptoms are produced, passively extend one of the athlete's knees. D, If no symptoms occur, passively dorsiflex the foot of the same leg to see if any symptoms occur. The test is positive if symptoms of sciatic pain are reproduced, indicating impingement of the dura and spinal cord or nerve roots.

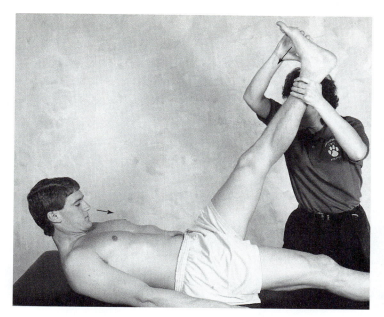

➤ **FIGURE 9.30** **Straight leg raising test**. Passively flex the individual's hip while keeping the knee extended until pain or tension is felt in the hamstrings. Slowly lower the leg until the pain or tension disappears. Then, dorsiflex the foot, have the individual flex the neck, or do both simultaneously. If pain does not increase with dorsiflexion of the ankle or flexion of the neck, it indicates tight hamstrings.

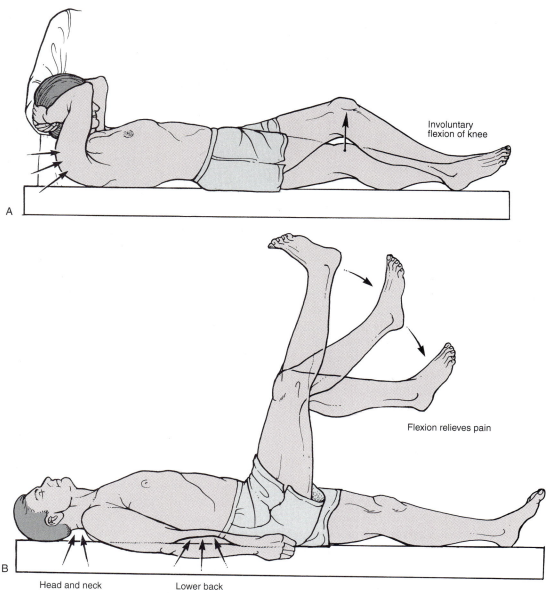

Involuntary flexion of knee

A

Flexion relieves pain

B

Head and neck   Lower back

➤ **FIGURE 9.31** **Brudzinski-Kernig test**. A, In Brudzinki's portion of the test, the athlete lies supine and dorsiflexes the neck. B, In the Kernig portion of the test, the athlete actively flexes the hip with the knee extended. The test is positive if knee extension leads to head, neck, or low back pain that is relieved with knee flexion.

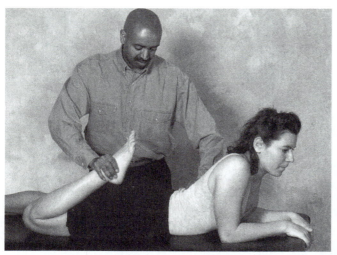

➤ **FIGURE 9.32 Prone knee bending test.** The prone knee bending test is used to indicate an L₂ or L₃ nerve root lesion, and also stretches the femoral nerve.

PRONE KNEE-BENDING TEST

This test is used to indicate an L_2 or L_3 nerve root lesion, and also stretches the femoral nerve. Place the individual prone and passively flex the knee until the foot rests against the buttock. Maintain this position for 45 to 60 seconds **(Figure 9.32)**. Do not allow the hip to rotate during this motion. If the knee cannot be flexed beyond 90° because of a pathological condition, do passive extension of the hip with the knee flexed as much as possible. Unilateral pain in the lumbar region indicates an L_2 or L_3 nerve root lesion. Pain in the anterior thigh indicates tight quadriceps.

SINGLE-LEG STANDING (STORK STANDING) LUMBAR EXTENSION TEST

The athlete stands on one leg and extends the spine while balancing on the single leg **(Figure 9.33)**. The test is repeated with the opposite leg. A positive sign, indicated by pain in the back, is associated with a pars interarticular stress fracture (spondylolisthesis). If the stress fracture is unilateral, standing on the ipsilateral leg causes more pain. If rotation is combined with extension and pain results, it indicates possible facet joint pathology on the side to which rotation occurs.

HOOVER TEST

Because the assessment of lumbopelvic disorders is difficult to do objectively, the Hoover test is used to determine if the patient is really trying or may be a malingerer. The athlete is supine. The athletic trainer's hands cup each heel while the legs remain relaxed on the examining table **(Figure 9.34)**. The athlete is then asked to lift one leg off the table, keeping the knees straight, as in an active straight leg raising test. If the athlete does not lift the leg or the athletic trainer does not feel pressure under the opposite heel, the patient is probably not really trying or may be a

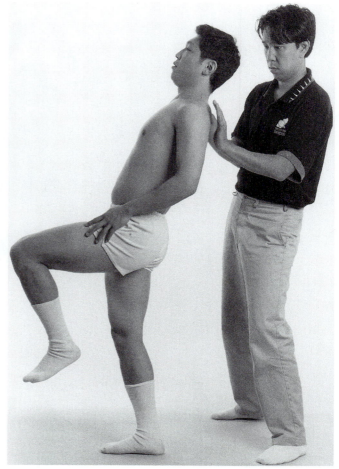

➤ **FIGURE 9.33 One-leg standing (stork standing) lumbar extension test.** While balancing on one leg, the athlete extends the spine. A positive test leads to pain in the back and is associated with a pars interarticularis stress fracture.

malingerer. If the lifted limb is weaker, however, pressure under the normal heel increases, because of the increased effort to lift the weak leg. Bilateral comparison is then made to determine any differences.

VALSALVA'S TEST

Valsalva's maneuver is used to determine the presence of space-occupying lesions (e.g., herniated disc, tumor, or osteophytes). While supine, the athlete is asked to take a deep breath and hold it while bearing down, as if moving the bowels. A positive test is indicated by increased pain, which may be caused by increased intrathecal pressure. Caution should be used with this test. The maneuver increases intrathecal pressure, which can slow the pulse, decrease venous return, and increase venous pressure, all of which may lead to unconsciousness.

Neurologic Tests

Neurologic integrity can be assessed with the use of myotomes, reflexes, and segmental dermatomes and peripheral nerve cutaneous patterns.

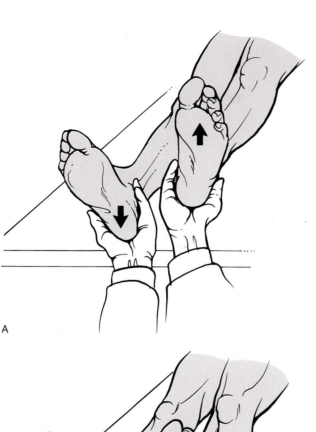

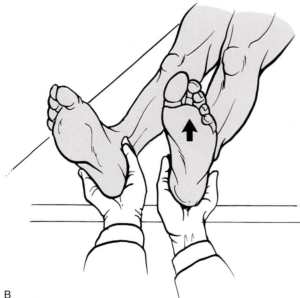

➤ FIGURE 9.34 Hoover test. A, Under normal conditions, when an individual tries to elevate one leg, the action is accompanied by downward pressure by the opposite leg. B, When the athlete attempts to elevate the "weak" leg but the opposite (asymptomatic) leg does not "help", at least some of the weakness is probably feigned.

MYOTOMES

Isometric muscle testing is performed in the upper and lower extremities to test specific myotomes (see **Table 9.6**). These were originally discussed in Chapter 4. Maximal force should be applied when testing the major muscle groups to detect weakness.

REFLEXES

Repetitive tapping of the reflexes may show a gradual decline in the reflex response not otherwise noted in a

TABLE 9.6	MYOTOMES USED TO TEST SELECTED NERVE ROOT SEGMENTS
Nerve Root Segment	**Action Tested**
C_1–C_2	Neck flexion*
C_3	Lateral neck flexion*
C_4	Shoulder elevation
C_5	Shoulder abduction
C_6	Elbow flexion and wrist extension
C_7	Elbow extension and wrist flexion
C_8	Thumb extension and ulnar deviation
T_1	Intrinsic muscles of the hand (finger abduction and adduction)
L_1–L_2	Hip flexion
L_3	Knee extension
L_4	Ankle dorsiflexion
L_5	Toe extension
S_1	Plantar flexion of the ankle, foot eversion, hip extension
S_2	Knee flexion

*These myotomes should not be performed in an individual with a suspected cervical fracture or dislocation, as they may cause serious damage or death.

singe tap. Absent or decreased reflexes are not necessarily pathologic, especially in athletes who have well-developed muscles. Upper-limb reflexes can be increased by having the athlete perform an isometric contraction such as squeezing the knees together during the test. Reflexes in the upper extremity include the biceps (C_5–C_6), brachioradialis (C_6), and triceps (C_7) (see **Table 9.7**). In the lower extremity, the two major reflexes are the patella (L_3–L_4) and Achilles tendon (S_1). Asymmetry between sides should raise suspicion of an abnormality.

CUTANEOUS PATTERNS

The wide variation of dermatomal innervation and the subjectivity of the test make it less useful than motor or reflex testing. If an upper limb peripheral nerve entrapment is suspected, however, then checking for a sensory loss in a peripheral nerve distribution is useful. The segmental nerve dermatome patterns and peripheral nerve cutaneous patterns are demonstrated in **Figure 9.35**. Test bilaterally

TABLE 9.7	DEEP TENDON REFLEXES AND SEGMENTAL LEVELS
Reflex	**Segmental Levels**
Biceps	Cervical 5, 6
Brachioradialis	Cervical 5, 6
Triceps	Cervical 7, 8
Patellar	Lumbar 2, 3, 4
Posterior tibial	Lumbar 4, 5
Medial hamstring	Lumbar 5, Sacral 1
Lateral hamstring	Sacral 1, 2
Achilles	Sacral 1, 2

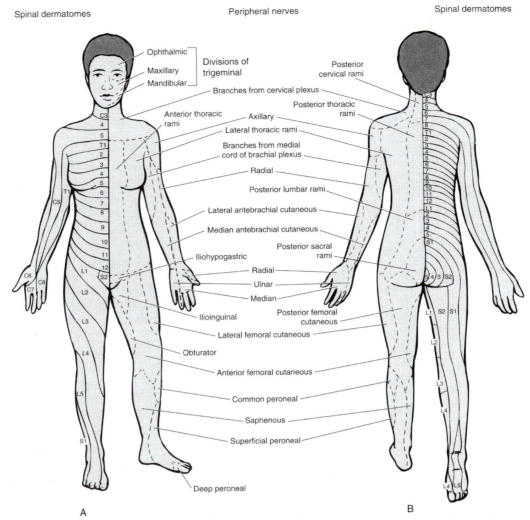

Spinal dermatomes   Peripheral nerves   Spinal dermatomes

Ophthalmic ⎤
Maxillary ⎬ Divisions of
Mandibular ⎦ trigeminal

Posterior
cervical rami

Branches from cervical plexus

Posterior thoracic
rami

Anterior thoracic
rami

Axillary

Lateral thoracic rami

Branches from medial
cord of brachial plexus

Radial

Posterior lumbar rami

Lateral antebrachial cutaneous

Median antebrachial cutaneous

Posterior sacral
rami

Iliohypogastric

Radial

Ulnar

Median

Ilioinguinal

Posterior femoral
cutaneous

Lateral femoral cutaneous

Obturator

Anterior femoral cutaneous

Common peroneal

Saphenous

Superficial peroneal

Deep peroneal

A   B

➤ FIGURE 9.35 **Dermatome patterns for spinal nerve innervations and peripheral nerve distribution patterns**. A, Anterior view. B, Posterior view.

for altered sensation with sharp and dull touch by running the open hand and fingernails over the head, neck, back, thorax, abdomen, and upper and lower extremities (front, back, and sides). Ask if the sensation feels the same on one body segment as compared to the other.

REFERRED PAIN

Pain can be referred to the thoracic spine from various abdominal organs. **Figure 9.36** demonstrates where pain is commonly referred to the torso.

Sport-Specific Functional Testing

Prior to return to play, the individual must have a normal neurologic exam with pain-free range of motion, normal bilateral muscle strength, cutaneous sensation, and reflexes. Axial head compression can be performed on the sideline as an additional safety check. If pain is present, the individual should not return to competition. Sport-specific functional tests that should be performed include walking, bending,

lifting, jogging, running, figure-8 running, karioka running, and sport-specific skills. All must be performed pain-free and with unlimited movement.

 Pain increases in the right lumbar region on resisted trunk extension, lateral flexion, and rotation to the right. The quadriceps reflex is diminished on the right side, and muscle weakness is apparent with knee extension and ankle dorsiflexion. Pain is elicited down the right leg during a straight leg raising test. If you determined a possible sciatica due to an extruded disc at the L4 level, you are correct.

REHABILITATION

 The individual was seen by a physician who prescribed NSAIDs, muscle relaxants, and rest until symptoms subside. When the individual begins rehabilitation, what exercises should be included in the general program?

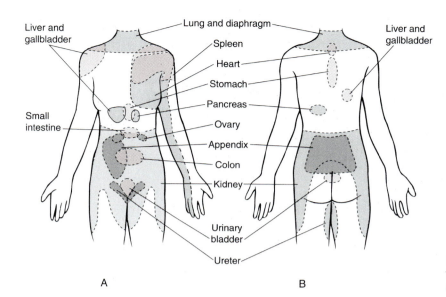

Liver and gallbladder — Lung and diaphragm — Spleen — Heart — Stomach — Pancreas — Ovary — Appendix — Colon — Kidney — Urinary bladder — Ureter

Liver and gallbladder

Small intestine

A   B

➤ **FIGURE 9.36 Referred pain.** Cutaneous patterns to which pain from visceral organs can be referred. A, Anterior view. B, Posterior view.

Rehabilitation programs must be developed on an individual basis and address the specific needs of the patient. Exercises to relieve pain related to postural problems may not address sciatic pain. Therefore, a variety of exercises are listed in this section allowing you to select those appropriate for the patient. The program should relieve pain and muscle tension; restore motion and balance; develop strength, endurance, and power; and maintain cardiovascular fitness. Patient education is also critical in teaching skills and techniques needed to prevent recurrence.

Relief of Pain and Muscle Tension

Maintaining a prolonged posture can lead to discomfort. This can be avoided by doing active range-of-motion exercises to relieve stress on supporting structures, promote circulation, and maintain flexibility. For example, to relieve tension in the cervical and upper thoracic region, neck flexion, extension, lateral flexion, and rotation; shoulder rolls; and glenohumeral circumduction should be performed. In the lower thoracic and lumbar region, exercises such as back extension, side bending in each direction, spinal flexion (avoiding hip flexion), trunk rotation, and walking a short distance can relieve discomfort. However, with nerve root compression injuries, extension exercises may increase discomfort and may be contraindicated. Conscious relaxation training can relax an individual who is generally tense, or release tension in specific muscle groups, such as the upper trapezius. Grade I and II mobilization exercises can be initiated early in the program to relieve pain and stretch tight structures to restore accessory movements to the joints.

Restoration of Motion

Once pain and muscle guarding are relieved, Grade III and IV mobilization exercises can begin. In addition to mobilization exercises, flexibility and range-of-motion exercises can begin. Flexion exercises stretch the lumbar fascia and back extensors, open the intervertebral foramen and facet joints to reduce nerve compression, relieve tension on lumbar vertebrae caused by tight hip flexors, and increase intra-abdominal pressure by strengthening the abdominals. Examples of flexion exercises illustrated in Field Strategy 9.1 included the single- and double-knee to the chest stretches, hamstring stretch, hip flexor stretch, lateral rotator stretch, crunch curl-ups, and diagonal crunch curl-ups. Exercises to stretch the upper thoracic and pectoral region, trunk rotators and lateral flexors, and the hip adductors, abductors, extensors, and medial and lateral rotators should also be added to improve flexibility. Other exercises include bringing both knees to the chest and gently rocking back and forth in a cranial/caudal direction, and in a standing position, shifting the hips from one side to another, lateral trunk flexion and rotation exercises.

Extension exercises improve spinal mobility, reduce load on the intervertebral discs, strengthen the back extensors, and allow for self-mobilization of the motion segments. Back extension exercises in Field Strategy 9.2 included prone extension exercises beginning with raising to the elbows then to the hands, the alternate arm and leg lift, double-arm and leg lift, and alternate arm and leg extension on all fours. Other extension exercises may include prone single-leg hip extension and double-leg hip extension while holding onto a table, beginning with the knee(s) flexed, then with the knee(s) extended.

Pelvic and abdominal stabilizing exercises are used to teach an individual to place the hip in a neutral position to maintain the spine in the most comfortable position and control the forces exerted during repetitive microtrauma. During each exercise, the individual concentrates on maintaining the hip in a neutral position by contracting and relaxing the abdominal muscles. During functional activities, the individual can initiate stabilization contractions before starting any movement. This presets the posture and can reduce stress on the back. Many of these exercises are demonstrated in **Field Strategy 9.5**.

FIELD STRATEGY 9.5   PELVIC STABILIZATION AND ABDOMINAL STRENGTHENING EXERCISES

A. **Stabilization in neutral position.** With the back in a neutral position, slowly shift forward over the arms, adjusting pelvic position as you move. There will be a tendency to "sag" the back, so progressively tighten and relax the abdominal muscles during forward movement and backward movement, respectively.

B. **Stabilization in "two point" position.** Balance on the right leg and left arm. Slowly move forward and back without losing neutral position. Switch to the opposite arm and leg.

C. **Leg exercise.** Without arching the back, lift one leg out behind you. Do not lift the foot more than a few inches from the floor. A variation is to move a flexed knee sideways away from the body, then back to the original position.

D. **Half-knee to stand (lunges).** Move to a standing position while maintaining neutral hip position. Push evenly with both legs. Repeat several times, then switch the forward leg.

E. **Pelvic tilt.** With the hips and knees bent and feet on the floor, do an isometric contraction of the abdominal muscles (posterior pelvic tilt) and hold. Using the phase "tuck the stomach in" may convey the correct motion. Then, arch the back doing an anterior pelvic tilt. Alternate between the two motions until the individual can control pelvic motion.

F. **Bridging.** Keeping the back in neutral position, raise the hips and back off the floor (contract the abdominal muscles to hold the position). Hold for 5 to 10 seconds, drop down, and relax. Repeat. Variations include (a) adding pelvic tilt exercises, (b) lifting one leg off the floor (keeping the back in neutral position), and (c) combining pelvic tilts and one leg lift with bridging.

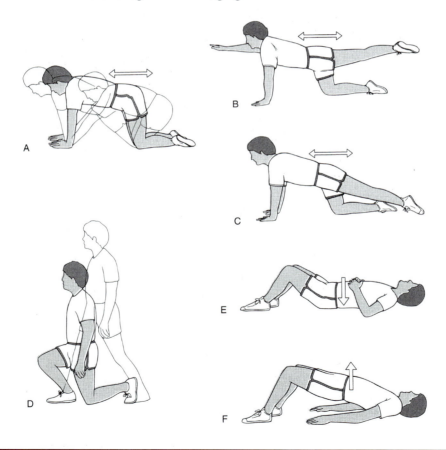

Restoration of Proprioception and Balance

Proprioception and balance are regained through upper and lower extremity closed chain exercises. For example, the upper thoracic region can benefit from push-ups, press-ups, and balancing on a wobble board, ball, ProFitter, or slide board while weight bearing on the hands. Squats, the leg press, lunges, or exercises on a Stair Master, Pro-Fitter, or slide board can restore proprioception and balance in the hip and lower extremity. Stabilization exercises on all fours and use of surgical tubing through functional patterns can also restore proprioception and balance. These exercises should be performed in front of a mirror or videotaped, if available, so the individual can observe proper posture and mechanics. Constant verbal reinforcement from the supervising therapist can also maximize feedback.

Muscular Strength, Endurance, and Power

Isometric contractions to strengthen the neck musculature can progress to manual resistance, surgical tubing, and commercial machines, as available and tolerated. Neck strength is particularly important for wrestlers and football linemen, who need added stability and strength in the cervical region. Abdominal strengthening exercises, such as those listed in Field Strategy 9.5, should begin with pelvic tilts, and progress to crunch curl-ups and diagonal crunch curl-ups to reduce functional lordosis. Progressive prone extension exercises and resisted back extension exercises can increase strength in the erector spinae.

Cardiovascular Fitness

Aquatic exercises are very beneficial because buoyancy can relieve load on sensitive structures. Deep water allows the individual to exercise all muscle groups through a full range of motion without the pain associated with gravity. Performing sport-specific skills against water resistance can apply an equal and uniform force to the muscles, similar to isokinetic strengthening. With low back pain, an upper body ergometer, stationary bicycle, Stair Master, or slide board may be incorporated as tolerated. Jogging can begin when all symptoms have subsided.

After acute symptoms subside, pain and muscle tension should be relieved. Stretching the piriformis, gluteals, and hamstrings should be combined with extension exercises to strengthen the back extensors, to stretch the abdominals, and to reduce pressure on the intervertebral disks. Stabilization exercises, abdominal strengthening, and strengthening the medial rotators of the hip through proprioceptive neuromuscular facilitation (PNF) and Theraband exercises should be major components of the program. As strength is regained, functional activities can be incorporated, with gradual return to full activity.

Summary

1. The spine is a linkage system that transfers loads between the upper and lower extremities, enables motion in all three planes, and serves to protect the delicate spinal cord. Although most injuries to the back are relatively minor and can be successfully managed using the PRICE principles, spinal fractures and nerve conditions do occur.

2. Two adjacent vertebrae and the soft tissues between them are collectively referred to as a motion segment. The motion segment is the functional unit of the spine. The intervertebral disc is a fibrocartilaginous disc that provides cushioning between the articulating vertebral bodies.

3. The interspinous ligaments, intertransverse ligaments, and ligamentum flava, respectively link the spinous processes, transverse process, and laminae of adjacent vertebrae. Collectively, the primary movers for back extension are called the erector spinae muscles.

4. The spinal cord extends from the brain stem to the level of the first or second lumbar vertebrae. Thirty-one pairs of spinal nerves emanate from the cord, with the distal bundle of spinal nerves known as the cauda equina.

5. Anatomical variations that can predispose an individual to spinal injuries include kyphosis, scoliosis, lordosis, and par interarticularis fractures, which can lead to spondylolysis or spondylolisthesis.

6. Functional spinal stenosis is defined as a loss of CSF around the cord, or in more extreme cases as a deformation of the spinal cord. The cervical segments most commonly affected are C_5 and C_6.

7. Signs and symptoms that indicate a serious cervical spine injury include:
   - Pain over the spinous process, with or without deformity
   - Unrelenting neck pain or muscle spasm
   - Abnormal sensations in the head, neck, trunk, or extremities
   - Muscular weakness in the extremities
   - Paralysis or inability to move a body part
   - Absence of weak reflexes

8. Because spinal cord damage can lead to paralysis or death, a suspected unstable neck injury should be treated as a medical emergency. Activate EMS and assist the technicians in immobilizing the injured athlete on a spine board.

9. Brachial plexus injuries are graded in three levels:
   - Neurapraxia injuries—temporary loss of sensation and/or loss of motor function that recovers within 2 weeks
   - Axonotmesis injuries—significant motor and mild sensory deficits that last at least 2 weeks
   - Neurotmesis injuries—severe motor and sensory deficits that persist for up to 1 year with poor prognosis

10. Thoracic fractures tend to be concentrated at the lower end of the thoracic spine. Large compressive loads can lead to a wedge fracture, or Scheuermann's disease can lead to degeneration of the epiphyseal end plates of the vertebral bodies, causing a prolapse of the intervertebral disc into the vertebral body.

11. Runners are particularly prone to low back pain due to tight hip flexors and hamstrings. Symptoms include localized pain that increases with active and resisted back extension, but radiating pain and neurologic deficits will not be present. Anterior pelvic tilt and hyperlordosis of the lumbar spine may also be present.

12. Sciatica may be caused by a herniated disc, annular tear, myogenic or muscle-related disease, spinal stenosis, facet joint arthropathy, or compression of the nerve between the piriformis muscle.

13. The most commonly herniated discs are the lower two lumbar discs at L_4–L_5 and L_5–S_1, followed by the two lower cervical discs. Most ruptures move in a posterior or posterolateral direction as a result of torsion and compression.

14. In assessing a spinal injury, always begin with a thorough history of the injury, and include neurologic tests to determine possible nerve involvement. The severity of pain and presence or absence of neurologic symptoms, neck spasm, and tenderness can indicate when a backboard and neck stabilization are needed.

15. If at anytime, an individual complains of acute pain in the spine, change in sensation anywhere on the body, or the individual resists moving the spine, assume that a significant injury is present, and activate EMS.

References

1. Zachazewski JE, Geissler G, Hangen D. Traumatic injuries to the cervical spine. In: Athletic Injuries and Rehabilitation. Edited by Zachazewski JE, Magee DJ, and Quillen WS. Philadelphia: WB Saunders, 1996.

2. Schultz AB. Mechanics of the human spine. App Mech Rev 1974; 27:1487-1497.

3. Hall SJ. Mechanical contribution to lumbar stress injuries in female gymnasts. Med Sci Sports Exerc 1986;18(6):599-602.

4. Hall SJ. Effect of attempted lifting speed on forces and torque exerted on the lumbar spine. Med Sci Sport Exerc 1985;17(4):440-444.

5. Wilhite JM. Thoracic and lumbosacral spine. In: The Team Physician's Handbook. Edited by Mellion MB, Walsh WM, and Shelton GL. Philadelphia: Hanley & Belfus, 1997.

6. Moeller JL. Contraindications to athletic participation: Spinal, systemic, dermatologic, paired-organ, and other issues. Phys Sportsmed 1996;24(9):57-70.

7. Johnson RJ. Low-back pain in sports: Managing spondylolysis in young patients. Phys Sportsmed 1993;21(4):53-59.

8. Heck JF. The incidence of spearing during a high school's 1975 and 1990 football seasons. J Ath Training 1996;31(1):31-37.

9. Torg JS, et al. Neurapraxia of the cervical spinal cord with transient quadriplegia. J Bone Joint Surg [Am] 1986;68A:1354-1370.

10. Cantu RC. Functional cervical spinal stenosis: A contraindication to participation in contact sports. Med Sci Sports Exerc 1993; 25(3):316-317.

11. Moore J, Rice EL. Neck injuries. In: The Team Physician's Handbook. Edited by Mellion MB, Walsh WM, and Shelton GL. Philadelphia: Hanley & Belfus, 1997.

12. Torg JS. Cervical spine stenosis with cord neurapraxia and transient quadriplegia. Ath Train 1990;25(2):138-146.

13. Cantu RC. The cervical spinal stenosis controversy. Clin Sport Med 1998;17(1):121-126.

14. Torg JS, et al. Spear tackler's spine: An entity precluding participation in tackle football and collision activities that expose the cervical spine to axial injury inputs. Am J Sports Med 1993;21(5):640-649.

15. Wilberger JE. Athletic spinal cord and spine injuries: Guidelines for initial management. Clin Sport Med 1998;17(1):111-120.

16. Torg JS, Ramsey-Emrheim JA. Cervical spine and brachial plexus injuries: Return-to-play recommendation. Phys Sportsmed 1997; 25(7):61-88.

17. Nissen SJ, Laskowski ER, Rizzo RD, Jr. Burner syndrome: Recognition and rehabilitation. Phys Sportsmed 1996;24(6):57-64.

18. Kuritzky L, White J. Low-back pain: Consider extension education. Phys Sportsmed 1997;25(1):57-64.

19. Kujala UM, et al. Lumbar mobility and low back pain during adolescence: A longitudinal three-year follow-up study in athletes and controls. Am J Sports Med 1997;25(3):363-368.

20. Wiesenfarth J, Briner W. Neck injuries: Urgent decisions and actions. Phys Sportsmed 1996;24(1):35-41.

CHAPTER 10

Throat, Thorax, and Visceral Conditions

OBJECTIVES

1. Identify the important bony and soft tissue structures of the throat, thorax, and viscera.

2. List the primary and accessory organs in the female and male reproductive systems.

3. Explain how hormones affect the human body.

4. Identify measures to prevent injuries to the throat, thorax, and viscera.

5. Describe the signs and symptoms, and appropriate management of superficial injuries of the throat, chest wall, and abdominal wall.

6. Describe internal complications of the thoracic area that may occur spontaneously or as a result of direct trauma, and can lead to a life-threatening situation.

7. Describe the signs and symptoms of sternal and rib fractures and their management.

8. Describe the signs and symptoms of intra-abdominal injuries and their management.

9. Identify injuries and conditions of the genitalia related to sport participation.

10. Describe how to assess the throat, thorax, and visceral regions.

Torso injuries occur in nearly every sport, particularly those involving sudden deceleration and impact. Injuries to the reproductive organs, however, are rare, particularly in the female. Although protective equipment and padding is available to protect the anterior throat, thorax, and viscera, only football, men's lacrosse, ice hockey, fencing, catchers in baseball and softball, and goalies in lacrosse and field hockey require specific safety equipment for this vital region. It is estimated that 7 to 10% of all athletic injuries affect the abdomen, the most commonly injured abdominal organs being the spleen, liver, and kidney (1). Most injuries are superficial and easily recognized and managed. Some injuries, however, may involve the respiratory and circulatory system, leading to a life-threatening situation.

This chapter begins with a review of the anatomy of the anterior throat, thorax, and viscera, followed by a brief discussion on prevention of injuries. Common injuries are then presented, followed by internal complications that may occur as a result of trauma or spontaneous rupture. Finally, a step-by-step injury assessment is presented to help determine the extent and seriousness of injury. Because rehabilitation of the region is usually included with other body regions, specific exercises for the thorax and visceral region will not be discussed.

ANATOMICAL REVIEW OF THE THROAT

The throat includes the pharynx, larynx, trachea, esophagus, a number of glands, and several major blood vessels **(Figure 10.1)**. Injuries to the throat are of particular concern because of the life-sustaining functions of the trachea and carotid arteries.

Pharynx, Larynx, and Esophagus

The pharynx, commonly known as the throat, connects the nasal cavity and mouth to the larynx and esophagus below. The pharynx lies between the base of the skull and the sixth cervical vertebra. The laryngeal prominence on the thyroid cartilage that shields the front of the larynx is known as the "Adam's apple." A specialized spoon-shaped cartilage, the epiglottis, covers the superior opening of the larynx during swallowing to prevent food and liquids from entering. If a foreign body does slip past the epiglottis, the

cough reflex is initiated, and the foreign body is normally ejected back into the pharynx. The larynx also contains the vocal cords, two bands of elastic connective tissue surrounded by mucosal folds. When expired air from the lungs passes over the vocal cords, they are capable of producing sound. The hyoid bone, the only bone of the body that does not articulate directly with any other bone, lies just inferior to the mandible in the anterior neck. It is anchored by the narrow stylohyoid ligaments to the styloid processes of the temporal bones, and serves as an attachment point for neck muscles that raise and lower the larynx during swallowing and speech. The esophagus carries food and liquids from the throat to the stomach. It is a muscle-walled tube that originates from the pharynx in the mid-neck and follows the anterior side of the spine. The body of the esophagus is divided into cervical, thoracic, and abdominal regions with upper and lower esophageal sphincters at each end. The coordinated action of the esophagus walls propels food into the stomach. The esophageal sphincters maintain a barrier against reverse movement of the esophageal contents into the pharynx and gastric fluids into the esophagus. When the esophagus is empty, the tube is collapsed.

Trachea

The trachea extends inferiorly from the larynx through the neck down into the midthorax, where it divides into the two right and left bronchial tubes. The tracheal tube is formed by C-shaped rings of hyaline cartilage joined by fibroelastic connective tissue. Smooth muscle fibers of the trachealis muscle form the open side of the C and allow for expansion of the posteriorly adjacent esophagus as swallowed food passes through. Contraction of the trachealis muscle during coughing can dramatically reduce the size of the airway, thus increasing pressure inside the trachea to promote expulsion of mucus.

Blood Vessels of the Throat

The largest blood vessels coursing through the neck are the common carotid arteries **(Figure 10.2)**. At the level of the "Adam's apple," the common carotid arteries divide into external and internal carotid arteries, which provide the major blood supply to the brain, head, and face. Branches from the carotid arteries include the superior thyroid arteries, which supply the thyroid and larynx, facial artery to the face and sinuses, and lingual artery to the mouth and tongue. Several arteries also branch from the left and right subclavian arteries and course upward through the posterior side of the neck. Included are the costocervical trunk, thyrocervical trunk, and vertebral artery.

ANATOMICAL REVIEW OF THE THORAX

The thoracic cavity, or chest cavity, lies anterior to the spinal column and extends from the level of the clavicle

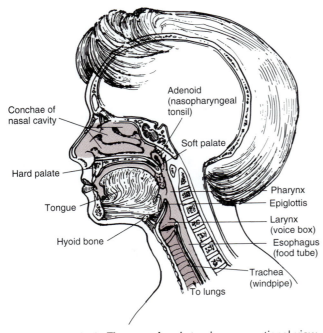

Conchae of nasal cavity

Hard palate

Tongue

Hyoid bone

Adenoid (nasopharyngeal tonsil)

Soft palate

Pharynx

Epiglottis

Larynx (voice box)

Esophagus (food tube)

Trachea (windpipe)

To lungs

➤ FIGURE 10.1 **Throat region**. Lateral cross-sectional view.

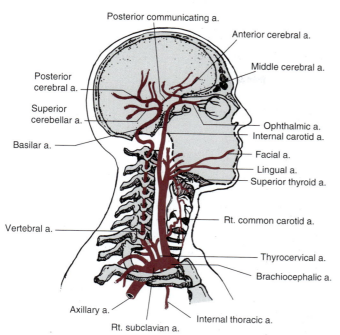

➤ FIGURE 10.2 **Arterial supply to the neck and throat region.**

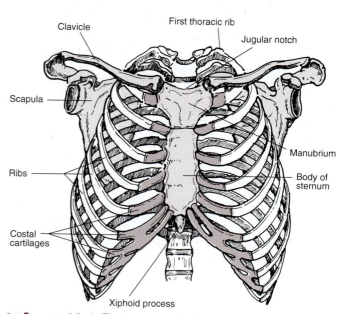

➤ FIGURE 10.3 **Thoracic cage**. Note that only the first seven pairs of ribs articulate anteriorly with the sternum through the costal cartilages.

down to the diaphragm. The major organs of the thorax are the heart and lungs. Although these organs are not commonly injured, internal complications due to direct trauma or spontaneous damage can necessitate emergency action during sport participation.

Thoracic Cage and Pleura

The thorax includes the sternum, ribs, costal cartilages, and thoracic vertebrae. These structures form a protective cage around the heart and lungs **(Figure 10.3)**. The sternum consists of the manubrium, which articulates with the first and second ribs; the body, which articulates with the second through seventh ribs; and the xiphoid process, a trapezoidal projection composed of hyaline cartilage that ossifies around age 40. The costal cartilages of the first seven pairs of ribs attach directly to the sternum, and the costal cartilages of ribs 8 to 10 attach to the costal cartilages of the immediately superior ribs. The last two rib pairs are known as floating ribs because they do not attach anteriorly to any other structure.

The thoracic cavity is lined with a thin, double-layered membrane called the pleura. The pleural cavity is a narrow space between the pleural membranes that is filled with pleural fluid secreted by the membranes, which enables the lungs to move against the thoracic wall with minimal friction during breathing.

Bronchial Tree and Lungs

The primary bronchial tubes branch obliquely downward from the trachea, then branch into approximately 23 levels until the terminal bronchioles are reached **(Figure 10.4)**. These tiny air sacs, called alveoli, serve as diffusion cham-

bers where oxygen from the lungs enters adjacent capillaries, and carbon dioxide from the blood is returned to the lungs. Healthy lungs consist of an elastic network of air passageways and spaces bound together by connective tissue. Although the lungs occupy the majority of the thoracic cavity, each lung weighs only about 0.6 kg (1.25 lb). The left lung is smaller than the right lung, containing a concavity known as the cardiac notch in which the heart is nestled. The lungs extend distally down to the level of, or slightly below, the twelfth rib in 80% of people, and extend down to about the L1 spinal level in about 18%.

Heart

The heart and lungs have an intimate relationship both physically and functionally. The right side of the heart pumps blood to the lungs, where carbon dioxide and oxygen are exchanged. The left side of the heart receives the freshly oxygenated blood from the lungs and pumps it out to the systemic circulation. The vessels interconnecting the heart and lungs are known as the pulmonary circuit, and the vessels that supply the body are known as the systemic circuit **(Figure 10.5)**.

The heart is positioned obliquely to the left of the midline of the body. It is divided into four chambers: the right and left atria superiorly, and the right and left ventricles inferiorly **(Figure 10.6)**. The heartbeat consists of a simultaneous contraction of the two atria followed immediately by a simultaneous contraction of the two ventricles. The contraction phase is known as systole. The phase in which the chambers relax and fill with blood is known as diastole. Two pairs of valves within the heart ensure that blood flow is unidirectional. The atrioventricular valves seal off the atria during contraction of the ventricles to prevent the backflow of blood. The aortic and pulmonary

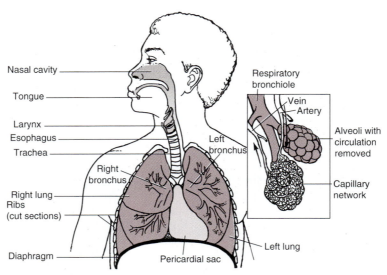

▶ **FIGURE 10.4** **Respiratory system**. A, The trachea, bronchi, and lungs. B, The terminal ends of the bronchial tree are alveolar sacs where oxygen and carbon dioxide are exchanged.

semilunar valves prevent flow of blood from the aorta and pulmonary artery back into the ventricles.

Muscles of the Thorax

The locations, primary functions, and innervations of the muscles of the thoracic region and the muscles of respiration are summarized in **Table 10.1** (also see **Figures 10.7**

and **10.8**). The major respiratory muscle is the diaphragm, a powerful sheet of muscle that completely separates the thoracic and abdominal cavities. During relaxation, the diaphragm is dome-shaped. During contraction, it flattens, increasing the size of the thoracic cavity. This increase in cavity volume causes a decrease in intrathoracic pressure, resulting in inhalation of air into the lungs.

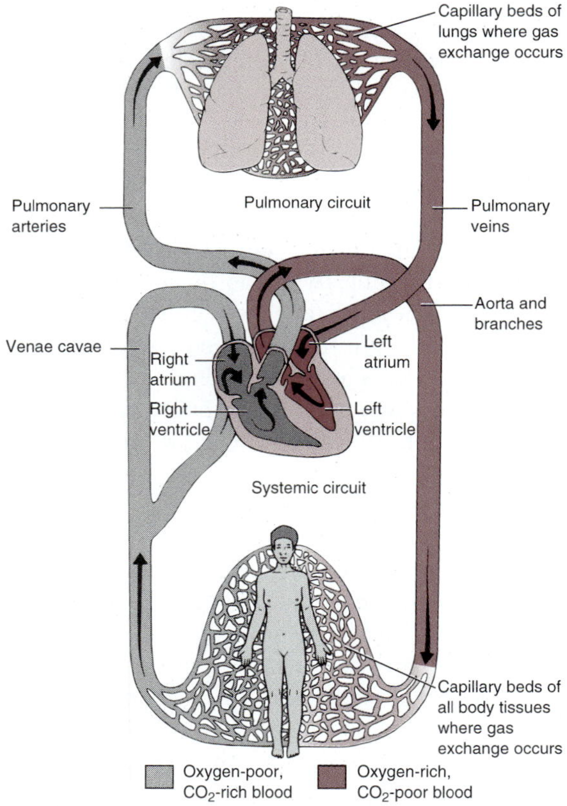

ANATOMICAL REVIEW OF THE VISCERAL REGION

The visceral region includes all organs and structures between the diaphragm and pelvic floor **(Figure 10.9)**. The

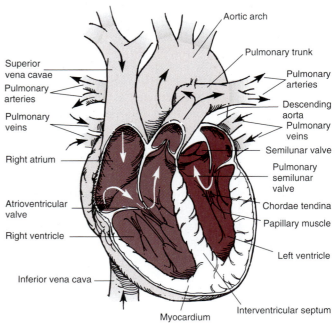

▶ **FIGURE 10.6** **Heart**. Note the arrows that indicate the direction of blood flow through the chambers.

▶ **FIGURE 10.5** **Pulmonary and systemic circuits**.

TABLE 10.1   MUSCLES OF THE THORAX

Muscle	Proximal Attachment	Distal Attachment	Primary Action(s)	Nerve Innervation
Pectoralis minor	Coracoid process of the scapula	Anterior surfaces of ribs 3–5	With ribs fixed, pulls scapula forward and downward, with scapula fixed, pulls upward	Medial pectoral (C_7, C_8, T_1)
Serratus anterior	Vertebral border of scapula	Ribs 1–8 or 9	Protraction and rotation of the scapula	Long thoracic (C_5–C_7)
Subclavius	Groove on inferior surface of clavicle	Costal cartilage of rib 1	Assist to stabilize and depress shoulder girdle	Nerve to subclavius (C_5, C_6)
Levator scapulae	Transverse process of the first four cervical vertebrae	Vertebral border of the scapula	Lateral flexion of the neck	C_3–C_4 nerve roots, Dorsal scapular (C5)
Trapezius	Occipital bone, ligamentum nuchae, C7 and T_1–T_{12}	Acromion, and spine of scapula and lateral clavicle	Stabilizes, elevates, retracts, and rotates scapula; lateral extension of neck	Accessory (cranial nerve XI)
Rhomboids	C7, T_1–T_5	Medial border of scapula	Retracts, rotates, and stabilizes scapula	Dorsal scapular (C_4, C_5)
External intercostals (11 pairs between ribs)	Inferior border of rib above	Superior border of rib below	Elevation of rib cage; assists the diaphragm with inspiration	Intercostal nerves (T_1–T_{11})
Internal intercostals (11 pairs between ribs)	Inferior border of rib above	Superior border of rib below	Depress rib cage; assist with expiration	Intercostal nerves (T_1–T_{11})
Diaphragm	Inferior border of rib cage and sternum; costal cartilages of ribs 6–12; lumbar vertebrae	Central tendon	Inspiration	Phrenic nerve (C_3–C_5)

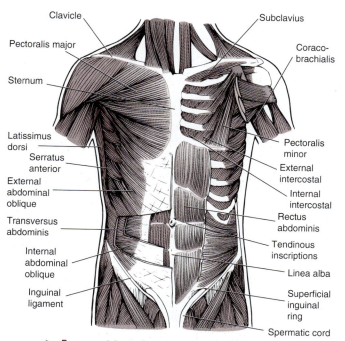

➤ **FIGURE 10.7 Anterior muscles of the trunk.**

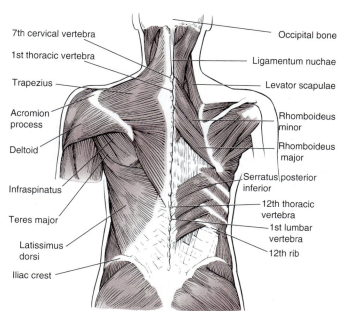

➤ **FIGURE 10.8 Posterior muscles of the trunk.**

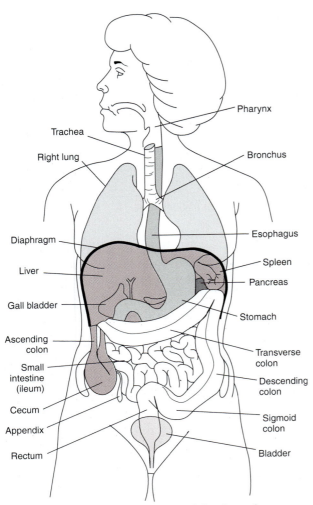

Trachea

Right lung

Pharynx

Bronchus

Diaphragm

Liver

Gall bladder

Esophagus

Spleen

Pancreas

Stomach

Ascending colon

Small intestine (ileum)

Cecum

Appendix

Rectum

Transverse colon

Descending colon

Sigmoid colon

Bladder

➤ **FIGURE 10.9** **Anterior view of the visceral organs.**

solid organs include the spleen, liver, pancreas, kidneys, and adrenal glands. The hollow organs include the stomach, gall bladder, small and large intestines, bladder, and ureters. The pelvic girdle protects the lower abdominal organs.

Pelvic Girdle and Abdominal Cavity

The pelvic girdle, or pelvis, consists of the sacrum, ilium, ischium, and pubis. The joints between these bones are fused in adults, with no movement allowed. The pelvis forms a protective basin around the internal organs of the abdomen and transfers loads between the spine and the lower extremity through the hip joint. The pelvis also provides a mechanical link between the upper and lower extremities. Its primary role is to stabilize the lower trunk while motion occurs in the extremities.

Visceral Organs

The stomach is a J-shaped bag positioned between the esophagus and small intestine. Food is stored in the stomach for approximately 4 hours, during which time it is broken down by hydrochloric acid secreted in the stomach

into a paste-like substance known as **chyme**. A few substances, including water, electrolytes, aspirin, and alcohol are absorbed into the blood stream across the stomach lining without full digestion. The chyme then moves into the small intestine where it is progressively absorbed. The small intestine, about 2 m (6 ft) in length, is responsible for most of the digestion and absorption of food as it is propelled through the small intestine in about 3 to 6 hours by waves of alternate circular contraction and relaxation by a process called **peristalsis**. Water and electrolytes are further absorbed from the stored material in the large intestine, or colon, during the next 12 to 24 hours. Mass peristaltic movements pass through the intestines several times per day to move the feces to the rectum. The vermiform appendix protrudes from the large intestine in the right lower quadrant of the abdomen, and can become a protected environment for the accumulation of bacteria, leading to inflammation of the appendix, or appendicitis.

The liver, located in the upper right quadrant under the diaphragm, produces bile, a greenish liquid that helps break down fat in the small intestine. The liver also absorbs excess glucose from the blood stream and stores it in the form of glycogen for later use. Among its other functions are processing fats and amino acids, manufacturing blood proteins, and detoxifying certain poisons and drugs. These functions can be severely impaired by alcohol abuse, which can result in cirrhosis of the liver. **Hepatitis** is inflammation of the liver caused by a viral infection that can also reduce the liver's efficiency. The gallbladder functions as an accessory to the liver to store concentrated bile on its way to the small intestine.

The spleen, the largest of the lymphoid organs, performs four vital functions: (1) cleansing the blood of foreign matter, bacteria, viruses, and toxins; (2) storing excess red blood cells for later reuse and releasing others into the blood for processing by the liver; (3) producing red blood cells, in the fetus; and (4) storing blood platelets. The pancreas secretes most of the digestive enzymes that break down food in the small intestine and secretes the hormones insulin and glucagon, which lower and elevate blood sugar levels, respectively.

The kidneys filter and cleanse the blood. They are vital for filtering out toxins, metabolic wastes, drugs, and excess ions and excreting them from the body in urine. The kidneys also return needed substances, such as water and electrolytes, to the blood. The ureters connect the kidneys to the urinary bladder, which is an expandable sac that stores urine.

Blood Vessels of the Trunk

The major blood vessel of the trunk is the aorta, with its numerous branches **(Figure 10.10)**. The left and right coronary arteries branch from the ascending aorta to supply the heart muscle. The first arterial branch from the aortic arch is the brachiocephalic artery, which splits into the right common carotid artery and right subclavian artery. The second and third branches from the aortic arch are

The distal portion of the descending aorta becomes the abdominal aorta. The first branch of the abdominal aorta is the celiac trunk that forms the left gastric artery to the stomach, the splenic artery to the spleen, and the common hepatic artery to the liver. Other branches of the abdominal aorta include the superior and inferior mesenteric arteries to the small intestine and the first half of the large intestine, the renal arteries to the kidneys, the ovarian arteries (in females), and the testicular arteries (in males). The distal portion of the abdominal aorta then divides into the common iliac arteries, that further divide into an internal iliac artery to supply the organs of the pelvis, and an external iliac artery, which enters the thigh to become the femoral artery.

Muscles of the Pelvic Girdle

As is the case throughout the neck and trunk, muscles in the pelvic region are named in pairs, with one located on the left and the other on the right side of the body. These muscles cause lateral flexion or rotation when they contract unilaterally, but contribute to spinal flexion or extension when bilateral contractions occur. The locations, primary functions, and innervations of the major muscles of the pelvic girdle are summarized in **Table 10.2**.

ANATOMY OF THE GENITALIA

The reproductive organs of the female and male include the primary and accessory sex organs. The primary sex organs, the ovaries and testes, produce gametes (specifically ovum and sperm, respectively) that, when joined together, develop into a fetus. Important sex hormones influence sexual differentiation and development of secondary sex characteristics, and in the female regulate the reproductive cycle. All sex hormones are predominantly produced by the primary sex organs and belong to the general family known as **steroids**. In the female, estrogen and progester-

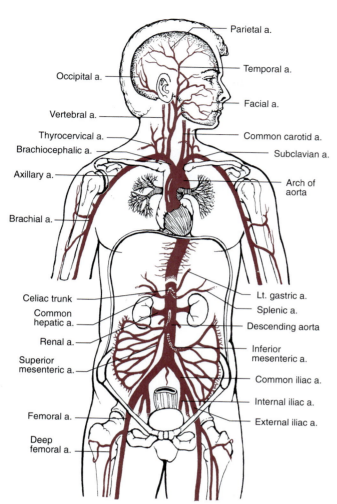

➤ FIGURE 10.10 **Arterial system of the trunk.**

the left common carotid artery and left subclavian artery, respectively. From the thoracic aorta come 10 pairs of intercostal arteries to supply the muscles of the thorax, the bronchial arteries to the lungs, the esophageal artery to the esophagus, and the phrenic arteries to the diaphragm.

TABLE 10.2   MUSCLES OF THE PELVIC GIRDLE

Muscle	Proximal Attachment	Distal Attachment	Primary Action(s)	Nerve Innervation
Rectus abdominus	Costal cartilage of ribs 5–7	Pubic crest	Flexion, lateral flexion	Intercostal nerves (T_6–T_{12})
External oblique	External surface of lower eight ribs	Linea alba and anterior iliac crest	Flexion, lateral flexion, rotation to opposite side	Intercostal nerves (T_7–T_{12})
Internal oblique	Linea alba and the lower four ribs	Inguinal ligament, iliac crest, and the lumbodorsal fascia	Flexion, lateral flexion, rotation to same side	Intercostal nerves (T_7–T_{12}, L_1)
Transverse abdominis	Inguinal ligament, lumbodorsal fascia, cartilages of ribs 6–12, iliac crest	Linea alba and pubic crest	Compression of the abdomen	Intercostal nerves (T_7–T_{12}, L_1)
Quadratus lumborum	Last rib, transverse processes of the first four lumbar vertebrae	Iliolumbar ligament, adjacent iliac crest	Lateral flexion	Spinal nerves (T_{12}, L_1–L_4)

one are produced by the ovaries. In the male, the adrenal cortex and testes produce hormones collectively known as **androgens**, the most active being testosterone. The accessory sex organs transport, protect, and nourish the gametes after they leave the ovaries and testes. In females, the accessory sex organs include the fallopian tubes, uterus, vagina, and vulva. In males, the accessory sex organs include the epididymis, ductus deferens, seminal vesicles, prostate gland, bulbourethral glands, scrotum, and penis.

Female Reproductive System

The female reproductive system includes the ovaries, which produce ova (female eggs); the fallopian tubes, which transport, protect, and nourish the ova; the uterus, which provides an environment for the development of the fertilized embryo; and the vagina, which serves as the receptacle for the sperm **(Figure 10.11)**. These structures are protected by the pelvic girdle and are seldom injured during sport participation.

The ovarian cycle begins at puberty with a release of an ovum, or egg, from the ovary. The ovum, released at ovulation, travels through a fallopian tube to the uterus, where it embeds itself in the uterine wall. The menstrual cycle, lasting anywhere from 28 to 40 days, involves a repeated series of changes within the lining of the uterus, and is controlled by the ovarian cycle. Menses, or the menstrual flow, is a phase in the menstrual cycle lasting 3 to 6 days, when the thickened vascular walls of the uterus, the unfertilized ovum, and blood from the damaged vessels of the endometrium are lost.

The hormones estrogen and progesterone are produced by the ovaries. **Estrogens** help regulate the men-

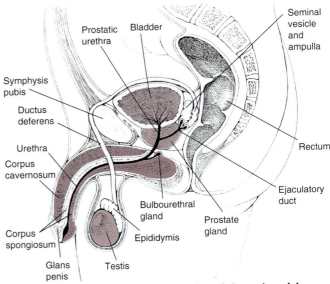

➤ **FIGURE 10.12** **Median section of the male pelvis.**

strual cycle and influence the development of female physical sex characteristics, such as the appearance of breasts, pubic and axillary hair, increased subcutaneous fat—especially in the hips and breasts—and widening and lightening of the pelvis. Estrogens are also responsible for the rapid growth spurt seen in girls between the ages of 10 and 13 years. This growth is short-lived, however, as increased levels of estrogen cause early closure of the epiphyses of long bones, causing females to reach their full height between the ages of 15 to 18 years. In contrast, males may continue to grow until the age of 19 to 21 years. **Progesterones** are responsible for regulating the menstrual cycle and stimulating the development of the uterine lining in preparation for pregnancy.

The external genital organs of the female are known as the vulva, or pudendum. The outer rounded folds, the labia majora, protect the vestibule into which the vagina and urethra open.

Male Reproductive System

The male reproductive system includes the testes, which produce spermatozoa; a number of ducts that store, transport, and nourish the spermatozoa; several accessory glands that contribute to the formation of semen; and the penis, through which urine and semen pass **(Figure 10.12)**. **Testosterone**, the primary androgen produced by the testes, stimulates the growth and maturation of the internal and external genitalia at puberty, and is responsible for sexual motivation. Secondary sex characteristics that are testosterone-dependent include the appearance of pubic, axillary, and facial hair; enhanced hair growth on the chest or back; and a deepening of the voice as the larynx enlarges. Androgens also increase bone growth, bone density, and skeletal muscle size and mass.

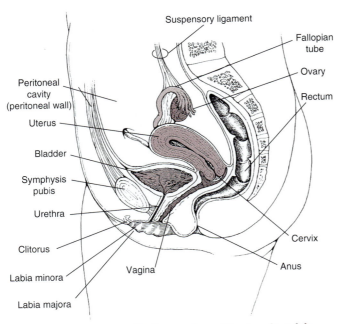

➤ **FIGURE 10.11** **Median section of the female pelvis.**

PREVENTION OF INJURIES TO THE THROAT, THORAX, AND VISCERA

 The throat, thorax, and viscera are vulnerable to direct impact injuries. This is such a critical area, where injuries can be life-threatening. What measures can be taken to prevent injuries to this region?

Injuries to the throat, thorax, and abdomen occur in nearly every sport, yet few sports require protective equipment for all players. In sports where high-velocity projectiles are present, throat and chest protectors are required only for specific players' positions, i.e., a catcher or goalie. As with other body regions, protective equipment, together with a well-rounded physical conditioning program, can reduce the risk of injury. Although proper skill technique can prevent some injuries, this is not a major factor in this body region.

Protective Equipment

Face masks with throat protectors are required only for fencing, baseball/softball catchers, and for goalies in field hockey, ice hockey, and lacrosse. Nearly all lacrosse and ice hockey players wear an optional extended pad attached to the mask to protect the throat region. Many sport participants in collision and contact sports also wear full chest and abdominal protection, such as in fencing, ice hockey, baseball/softball catchers, and goalies in field hockey and lacrosse. In young baseball and softball players (younger than 12 years), it has been suggested that all infield players should wear chest protectors.

Adolescent rib cages are less rigid, placing the heart at a greater risk from direct impact. In this age group, more baseball and softball deaths occur from impacts to the chest than to the head. Shoulder pads can protect the upper thoracic region, and rib protectors can provide protection from rib, upper abdominal, or low back contusions. Body suits made of mesh with pockets can hold rib and hip pads to protect the sides and back. For women, sport bras provide added support to reduce excessive vertical and horizontal breast motion during exercise. Abdominal binders may also be used to reduce the discomfort from hernias. The male genitalia are more susceptible to injury than female genitalia. Protective cups can protect the penis and scrotum from injury and are required for baseball catchers and ice hockey goalies. Much of this protective equipment was illustrated and discussed in Chapter 3.

Physical Conditioning

Flexibility and strengthening of the torso muscles should not be an isolated program, but should include a well-rounded conditioning program for the back, shoulder, abdomen, and hip regions. Range-of-motion and strengthening exercises should include both open and closed kinetic chain activities. Exercises for the thorax and abdominal region are included in the chapters on the hip, shoulder, and spine, and will not be repeated here. The reader should review the appropriate Field Strategies in those chapters to develop a conditioning program for the torso.

 Injuries to the throat, thorax, and viscera can be prevented by wearing appropriate protective equipment. Physical conditioning should include a well-rounded flexibility and strengthening program for the shoulder, back, abdominal, and hip region.

THROAT INJURIES

 An ice hockey player was checked into the sideboard. The opponent's elbow inadvertently struck the player's anterior neck. The player remains on the ice in a supine position coughing, and has difficulty swallowing and speaking. How should this situation be managed?

Although uncommon, lacerations to the neck caused by a skate blade can occur. Bleeding is profuse and, if sufficiently deep, can damage the jugular vein or carotid artery as they pass deep on the lateral side of the neck. Immediate control of hemorrhage is imperative. In addition to blood loss, air may be sucked into the vein and carried to the heart as an air embolism, which may be fatal. Management involves providing firm, direct pressure over the wound followed by an airway assessment. Continuous manual pressure should be applied while the individual is in rapid transit to the nearest medical facility.

Contusions and fractures to the trachea, larynx, and hyoid bone frequently occur during hyperextension of the neck when the thyroid cartilage (Adam's apple) becomes prominent and vulnerable to direct impact forces. A hockey cross-check or slash, a clothesline tackle in football, or a hit or blow to the neck can injure the cartilage.

➤ SIGNS AND SYMPTOMS

Immediate symptoms include hoarseness, dyspnea (difficulty breathing), coughing, difficulty swallowing, and laryngeal tenderness. Significant trauma to the region may result in severe pain, **laryngospasm**, and acute respiratory distress **(Box 10.1)**. Laryngospasm occurs when the adductor muscles of the vocal cords pull together in a shutter-like fashion, and the upper surface of the vocal cords closes over the top, causing complete obstruction. The individual may recover on-site and leave the area to return home, only to have increasing respiratory problems en route. As the internal hemorrhage and swelling increases, the occlusion becomes more complete, and breathing becomes more difficult. Panic and anxiety increase respiration, thereby compounding the problem. Swelling is usually maximal within 6 hours, but may occur as late as 24 to 48 hours after injury. Cyanosis and loss of consciousness may occur with complete occlusion.

➤➤ Box 10.1

Signs and Symptoms of Tracheal and Laryngeal Injuries

- Mild bruising and redness
- Shortness of breath
- Pain and point tenderness
- Subcutaneous crepitation
- Difficulty when swallowing or coughing
- Spasmodic coughing
- Hoarseness or loss of voice*
- Laryngospasm*
- Presence of hemorrhage with blood-tinged sputum*
- Loss of contour of the Adam's apple (thyroid cartilage)*
- Cyanosis or respiratory distress

 Indicates "Red Flags" that necessitate the activation of EMS.

➤ MANAGEMENT

The athletic trainer should immediately reassure the individual to diminish panic and anxiety due to the sudden inability to breathe. An open airway should be maintained and the athlete asked to focus on the breathing rate. Blows to the anterior throat should be reported to another individual, such as a parent or roommate, so observation continues should delayed respiratory problems occur. In cases involving severe anterior neck trauma or spasm, it is important to consider an associated injury to the cervical spine.

 Activate EMS. The individual's neck should be carefully maintained in a neutral position while a cervical collar is applied. As the spasm relaxes, usually in a minute, a loud inspiratory crowing sound is often heard. The individual should be immediately transported to a medical facility. **Field Strategy 10.1** *explains the management of tracheal and laryngeal injuries.*

 Your response to the injured ice hockey player should be to reassure the individual and attempt to maintain an open airway. It may help to have the athlete focus on inhaling and exhaling in a normal breathing pattern to reduce anxiety. If breathing does not return to normal within a few minutes, activate EMS.

THORACIC CONDITIONS

During a collision in a bike race, a rider fell forward onto the handlebars and is now complaining of sharp pain on the lower right side of the rib cage, aggravated by deep breathing, coughing, and palpation over the injured site. During the evaluation, you notice that he is coughing up bright red blood. What possible injuries might be involved in this accident?

Thoracic injuries are frequently caused by sudden deceleration and impact, which can lead to compression and subsequent deformation of the rib cage. The extent of damage depends on the direction, magnitude of force, and point of impact. For example, a glancing blow may contuse

---

 FIELD STRATEGY 10.1   MANAGEMENT ALGORITHM FOR TRACHEAL AND LARYNGEAL INJURIES

If severe anterior throat trauma has occurred:
assume a possible spinal injury and treat accordingly
↓
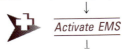 *Activate EMS*
↓
Ensure an open airway:
- If needed, use the jaw-thrust maneuver to achieve a chin-up position
- Apply ice to control swelling, if appropriate
↓
If an obvious deformity is present in the pharynx:
Manually straighten the airway
↓
If a major laceration is present:
- Control hemorrhage with firm manual pressure
- Maintain pressure during assessment
↓
Loosen any restrictive clothing
↓
To reduce panic or anxiety, talk calmly to the individual, assuring him or her that you are there to help
↓
Treat for shock and monitor vital signs until the ambulance arrives

the chest wall, whereas a baseball that directly strikes the ribs may fracture a rib, driving the bony fragments internally and causing subsequent lung or cardiac damage. **Box 10.2** identifies signs and symptoms that indicate a serious thoracic condition.

Stitch in the Side

A "stitch in the side" refers to a sharp pain or spasm in the chest wall, usually on the lower right side, during exertion. Potential causes include trapped colonic gas bubbles, localized diaphragmatic hypoxia with spasm, liver congestion with stretching of the liver capsule, and poor conditioning. Although the frequency of a stitch usually diminishes as the individual becomes more fit, most individuals can run through the sharp pain by:

- Forcibly exhaling through pursed lips
- Breathing deeply and regularly
- Leaning away from the affected side
- Stretching the arm on the affected side over the head as high as possible

Breast Conditions

Excessive breast motion during activity can lead to soreness, contusions, and nipple irritation. Although breast conditions are usually associated with females, men may also have conditions associated with the breast or nipples.

CONTUSIONS

Contusions to the breast may produce fat necrosis or hematoma formation, both of which are painful and may result in the formation of a localized breast mass. Appearance of these lesions on a mammogram may be indistinguishable from a malignant tumor. Although immediate management will involve ice and support, direct trauma should always be recorded on a woman's permanent medical record to avoid any erroneous conclusions when reading a future mammogram.

NIPPLE IRRITATION

Nipple irritation is commonly seen in distance runners when the shirt rubs over the nipples. The resulting friction can lead to abrasions, blisters, or bleeding (**runner's nipples**). This condition can be prevented by applying petroleum based products and band-aids over the nipples to reduce irritation. Initial treatment involves cleansing the wound, applying an antibiotic ointment, and covering the wound with a nonadhering sterile gauze pad. Infection secondary to the injury may involve the entire nipple region or extend into the breast tissue, and may necessitate referral to a physician. **Cyclist's nipples** is a condition not caused by friction, but rather from the combined effects of perspiration and wind-chill that produce cold, painful nipples that may last for several days. Wearing a wind-proof jacket and rewarming the nipples after completion of the event can prevent the irritation.

GYNECOMASTIA

Gynecomastia is an excessive development of the mammary glands, seen particularly in the adolescent male, and is usually bilateral. The nipple is sore and tender to pressure, and more prone to irritation through friction from a shirt. Often it is physiologic and will resolve spontaneously in 6 to 12 months. The condition is increasingly being seen in weight lifters and football players known to be taking anabolic steroids. Other causes include testicular, pituitary, and adrenal pathology. Occasionally, surgical removal of extra breast tissue may be indicated for cosmetic reasons, or a biopsy may be performed to rule out malignancy.

Strain of the Pectoralis Major Muscle

Pectoralis major muscle strains may occur in power lifting particularly while bench pressing, water skiing, football, boxing, wrestling, and basketball, or in sudden deceleration maneuvers, such as when punching in boxing or blocking with an extended arm in football. If the muscle ruptures, the usual mechanism involves an actively contracting muscle overburdened by a load or extrinsic force that exceeds tissue tolerance. A higher incidence of this injury is seen with anabolic steroid abuse (6,7). Steroid use causes muscle hypertrophy and an increase in power secondary to rapid strength gain not accompanied by a concomitant increase in tendon size.

➤ SIGNS AND SYMPTOMS

An audible pop, snap, or tearing sensation is usually accompanied by immediate, marked pain and weakness.

The pain is often described as an aching or fatigue-like pain rather than a sharp pain. With a rupture of the proximal attachment, the muscle will retract toward the axillary fold, causing it to appear enlarged. Swelling and ecchymosis will be limited to the anterior chest wall. If the distal attachment is ruptured, the muscle will bulge medially into the chest region, causing the axillary fold to appear thin **(Figure 10.13)**. Swelling and ecchymosis will occur on the anterior chest wall and upper arm. Shoulder motion will be limited by pain. Horizontal adduction and internal rotation of the shoulder will be weak and accentuate the deformity.

➤ MANAGEMENT

Treatment depends on the extent of damage and follows standard protocol for other muscle strains. Mild and moderate strains (Grades I and II) begin with control of inflammation, protected range-of-motion exercises, and gradual strengthening. Once range of motion has been achieved, strength, endurance, and power are restored. Although surgical treatment of complete pectoralis major ruptures has been successfully performed following delays of up to 5 years after injury, the best results are achieved with prompt recognition and surgery (2).

Costochondral Injury

Costochondral sprains may occur during a collision with another object or as a result of a severe twisting motion of the thorax. This action can sprain or separate the costal cartilage where it attaches to the rib or sternum **(Figure 10.14)**.

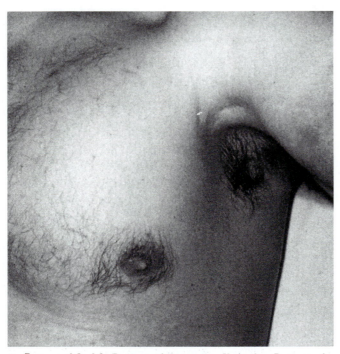

➤ **FIGURE 10.13 Rupture of the pectoralis major.** Rupture of the distal attachment of the pectoralis major can lead to swelling over the muscle belly, and a thin anterior axillary fold.

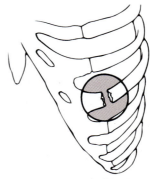

➤ **FIGURE 10.14** **Undisplaced costochondral separation**.

➤ SIGNS AND SYMPTOMS

The individual may hear or feel a pop, but the initial localized sharp pain may be followed by intermittent stabbing pain as the displaced cartilage overrides the bone. A visible deformity and localized pain can be palpated at the involved joint. More severe sprains produce pain during deep inhalation.

➤ MANAGEMENT

Standard acute protocol should be followed to reduce pain and inflammation, and the individual should be referred to a physician. The discomfort usually resolves itself with 3 or 4 weeks of rest and anti-inflammatory medication, but may persist for more than 6 weeks. Occasionally, a physician may choose to inject the site with steroid medication to relieve chronic pain.

Sternal and Rib Fractures

The sternum is rarely fractured in sports, but may occur as a result of rapid deceleration and high impact into an object. The injury causes an immediate loss of breath. Severe pain is aggravated by deep inspiration if the fracture is incomplete, but pain occurs during normal respiration if the fracture is complete. Because of the anatomical location, any suspected fracture should be assessed for underlying cardiac injury, such as a cardiac contusion.

 If the individual shows signs of shock, is pale, or has a rapid, weak pulse, activate EMS.

Stress fractures may be caused by an indirect force, such as a violent muscle contraction in a golf swing, baseball pitch, or crew stroke. Direct blows or compression of the chest can lead to rib fractures, and rarely involve more than one or two ribs. Most rib fractures are minor and undisplaced. The fourth through ninth ribs are the most commonly fractured.

➤ SIGNS AND SYMPTOMS

Intense localized pain over the fracture site is aggravated by deep inspiration, coughing, or chest movement **(Figure 10.15)**. Often, the individual will take shallow breaths and lean toward the fracture site, stabilizing the

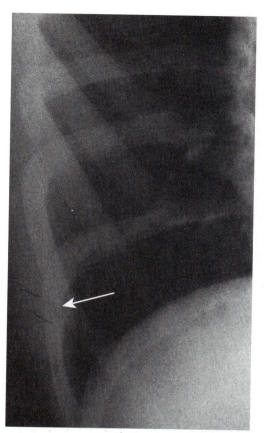

➤ FIGURE 10.15 **Undisplaced fractured rib**. The arrow is pointing to the fracture site.

area with a hand to prevent excessive movement of the chest to ease the pain. A visible contusion and palpable crepitus may be present at the impact site. The athletic trainer should look for any coughing up of blood, especially a bright red or frothy blood. A stethoscope should be used to listen for abnormal or absent breath sounds in the lungs, and the rate and depth of respirations should be recorded. Manual compression of the rib cage in an anteroposterior direction and lateral compression will produce pain over the fracture site (see Figure 10.22). Should any signs of respiratory distress, cyanosis, or shock appear, a thorough assessment for an underlying visceral injury should be conducted. **Box 10.3** identifies other signs and symptoms indicating a possible sternal or rib fracture.

➤ MANAGEMENT

Treatment involves standard acute protocol. A 6-inch elastic bandage can be wrapped around the thorax with circular motions distal to the injury site, or if pain is intense or multiple fractures are suspected, a sling and swathe may be used to immobilize the chest. If one or two ribs are fractured, the individual should be referred immediately to a physician.

However, if three or more ribs are fractured or other serious signs such as those indicating a pneumothorax are present, activate EMS.

➤➤ **Box 10.3**

Signs and Symptoms Indicating a Possible Sternal or Rib Fracture

- History of direct blow, compression of the chest, or violent muscle contraction
- Individual may lean toward the fractured side, stabilizing the area with a hand to prevent movement of the chest
- Localized discoloration or swelling over the fracture site
- Slight step deformity may be visible
- Palpable pain and crepitus at fracture site
- Increased pain on deep inspiration
- Increased pain on trunk rotation and lateral flexion away from the fracture site
- Increased pain on manual compression of the rib cage in an anteroposterior direction or with lateral compression
- Shallow breathing and cyanosis may be present
- Rapid, weak pulse and low blood pressure will be present with multiple fractures, in a fracture that has damaged intercostal vessels and nerves, or if the lung or pleural sac has been penetrated

Pain tends to be most severe during the first 3 to 5 days following injury, at which time it gradually subsides, and ultimately disappears after 3 to 6 weeks. Depending on the sport, the fracture site, the presence of a displaced or nondisplaced fracture, and the number of ribs involved, this individual may be excluded from sport participation during the full healing process. Strapping or taping to reduce chest movement is not recommended since it may aggravate the condition. With a simple fracture, a flak jacket or rib vest can be worn to protect the area from reinjury.

 The bicyclist had sharp pain on the lower right side of the rib cage, aggravated by deep breathing, coughing, and palpation, and had coughed up bright red blood. This individual may have fractured a rib.

 Because deep breathing and coughing aggravate the injury site, and blood was coughed up, bony fragments from the fractured rib may have pierced the lung. This is a serious injury. Activate EMS.

INTERNAL COMPLICATIONS

 The second baseman fielded a line drive and threw the ball to first base. By accident, the ball struck a runner going to second base directly on the sternum. The runner immediately collapsed on the base path. You arrived at the scene to find the player in obvious pain and gasping for air. How will you manage this situation? What underlying serious problems can occur as a result of direct impact to the sternum or ribs?

Several conditions can alter breathing and cardiac function. Hyperventilation is associated with an inability to catch one's breath, and in most instances, is not a serious problem. Direct trauma to the thorax can lead to serious underlying problems, although these conditions are rare in sport participation. Among the more serious complications are pulmonary contusion, pneumothorax, tension pneumothorax, hemothorax, and heart contusions.

Hyperventilation

Hyperventilation is often linked to pain, stress, or trauma in sport participation. During activity, the respiratory rate increases. Rapid, deep inhalations draw more oxygen into the lungs. Conversely, long exhalations result in too much carbon dioxide being exhaled.

➤ SIGNS AND SYMPTOMS

Signs and symptoms include an inability to catch one's breath, numbness in the lips and hands, spasm of the hands, chest pain, dry mouth, dizziness, and occasionally, fainting.

➤ MANAGEMENT

Immediately calm the individual, as panic and anxiety can complicate the condition. Although breathing into a paper bag has proven to be quite successful in restoring the oxygen-carbon dioxide balance, many individuals find it embarrassing. An alternative treatment involves concentrating on slow inhalations through the nose and exhaling through the mouth until symptoms have stopped. The use of breathing into a paper bag is not needed except in severe cases.

Pulmonary Contusion

Pulmonary contusion usually results from nonpenetrating chest trauma, but is rare in sport participation. Force transmitted through the thorax, as in landing on a football or a body slam onto the hard ground, causes bleeding in the alveolar spaces. Breathing may be compromised, and hypoxia may appear 2 to 4 hours after trauma (4). The condition may go undetected until the individual coughs up blood or has other problems, such as pneumothorax, rib fractures, or **subcutaneous emphysema**. Mild contusions heal within days, with the individual returning to full participation in as little as 10 days. In more severe cases, the individual is usually hospitalized and monitored with ventilatory support.

Pneumothorax

Pneumothorax is a condition whereby air is trapped in the pleural space, causing a portion of a lung to collapse. Although the etiology of a pneumothorax can vary, the two most common types are traumatic and spontaneous. A traumatic injury may be caused by a penetrating wound to the chest, such as a stab wound, a fractured rib, or severe chest trauma, that results in a laceration of lung tissue. Air is allowed to escape into the pleural cavity with each inhalation, preventing the lung from expanding fully (**Figure 10.16A**).

A spontaneous pneumothorax occurs unexpectedly, with or without underlying disease. Individuals with spontaneous pneumothorax are commonly tall, lean males, with the condition usually occurring after heavy exertion or running. Other pulmonary conditions that may lead to a spontaneous pneumothorax include asthma, cystic fibrosis, emphysema, and pneumonia (5,6).

➤ SIGNS AND SYMPTOMS

Shortness of breath, cyanosis, severe chest pain on the affected side, deviation of the trachea, and progressive respiratory collapse are the most common symptoms of a traumatic pneumothorax (**Box 10.4**). Other symptoms may

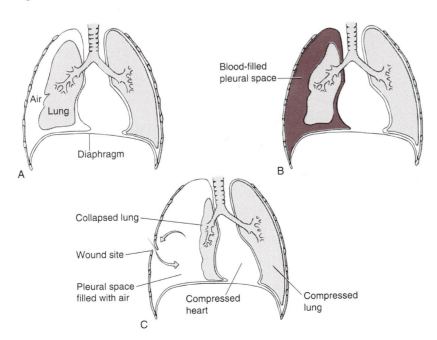

➤ **FIGURE 10.16 Internal complication to the lungs.** A, Pneumothorax. B, Hemothorax. C, Tension pneumothorax. Each condition can become life-threatening if the lung collapses.

➤➤ **BOX 10.4**

Signs and Symptoms that Indicate Possible Pneumothorax

- Sudden onset of sharp chest pain
- Shortness of breath
- Difficulty breathing
- Referred pain to the tip of the shoulder, across the chest, or over the abdomen
- Lightheadedness
- Tightness in chest
- Decreased or absent breath sounds over the collapsed lung
- Asymmetric chest movements on the affected side
- Decrease in blood pressure
- Tachycardia

include asymmetric chest expansion, confusion, fatigue, anxiety, restlessness, and a decrease in blood pressure. Pain may be referred to the shoulder tip, across the chest, or over the abdomen. If not recognized and treated promptly, the condition can develop into tension pneumothorax (discussed below).

With a spontaneous pneumothorax, pain can stop abruptly after onset, leading to a delay in treatment. Shortness of breath and chest discomfort will gradually increase until the individual finally seeks medical care. On the other hand, the symptoms may flare up suddenly, producing acute pain and difficulty in breathing.

➤ MANAGEMENT

Management involves prompt recognition and immediate care. Activate EMS.

Keep the athlete calm and quiet. Have the athlete sit and focus on controlled breathing. If diminished or absent breath sounds are present over the affected lung, do not give the athlete any fluids, and immediately transport the athlete to the nearest medical facility. Because of the risk of recurrence of spontaneous pneumothorax, individuals treated with conservative measures should be counseled to participate only in nonstrenuous activities. For those who want to return to contact and collision sports, and were treated with thoracotomy or other invasive procedures, activity can usually resume after 2 to 4 weeks (7). These individuals, however, should also be counseled about the increased risk of recurrence, especially on the contralateral side. If pneumothorax recurs, the athlete should be advised to discontinue collision and contact sports.

Hemothorax

Hemothorax involves the loss of blood, rather than air, into the pleural cavity **(Figure 10.16B)**. Fractured ribs may tear lung tissue and blood vessels in the chest or chest cavity.

➤ SIGNS AND SYMPTOMS

Severe pain, hypoxia, difficulty breathing, cyanosis, and coughing up frothy blood are the classic signs and symptoms of a hemothorax. As the condition deteriorates, the signs and symptoms of shock appear.

➤ MANAGEMENT

This is a medical emergency. Activate EMS. Treat for shock, and immediately transport this individual to the nearest medical facility.

Tension Pneumothorax

Tension pneumothorax occurs when air progressively accumulates in the pleural space during inspiration and cannot escape on expiration. The pleural space expands with each breath, resulting in the mediastinum being displaced to the opposite side, compressing the heart, uninjured lung, and thoracic aorta **(Figure 10.16C)**.

➤ SIGNS AND SYMPTOMS

Signs and symptoms include tracheal deviation away from the tension pneumothorax, severe difficulty in breathing, absence of breath sounds on the affected side, distention of neck veins, hypotension, and circulatory compromise leading to cyanosis and possible death.

➤ MANAGEMENT

Activate EMS. This is a medical emergency with immediate referral to the nearest medical facility necessary to prevent total collapse of the lung.

Traumatic Asphyxia

Traumatic asphyxia results from direct, massive trauma to the thorax. Classic symptoms include a bluish tinge over the neck and facial regions, subconjunctival hemorrhage, ecchymosis, and minute hemorrhagic spots on the face. Loss of vision has also been reported as a result of retinal edema, but vision may improve within hours or days. Again, immediate recognition and referral to the nearest medical facility is necessary for prompt care.

Heart Injuries

Blunt chest trauma can compress the heart between the sternum and spine, leading to myocardial contusion. The right ventricle is often injured because it lies directly posterior to the sternum. Red blood cells and fluid leak into the surrounding tissues, thereby decreasing circulation to the heart muscle. This action subsequently leads to localized cellular damage and necrosis of the heart tissue. Decreased cardiac output secondary to arrhythmias, or irregular heart beats, are of major concern.

Blunt trauma may also lead to **pericardial tamponade**, the leading cause of traumatic death in youth baseball, but has also occurred in softball, ice hockey, and lacrosse. Massive blunt trauma ruptures the myocardium or lacerates a coronary artery that leads to an increased volume of fluid in the pericardium, and subsequently compresses venous return to the heart. Internal damage can lead to rupture of the ventricles, interventricular septum, chordae tendineae, or the cardiac valves.

➤ SIGNS AND SYMPTOMS

In nearly all cases, the individual collapses within seconds and goes into respiratory arrest.

➤ MANAGEMENT

In many cases, resuscitation is unsuccessful even though it is given immediately after injury. This may be due to structural cardiac disruption caused by the trauma.

Activate EMS. Treatment is the same as for any other chest trauma: maintain an open airway, initiate breathing and chest compressions if necessary, and immediately transport the individual to the nearest medical facility.

Sudden Death in Athletes

Sudden death is defined as an event that is nontraumatic, unexpected, and occurs instantaneously or within minutes of an abrupt change in an individual's previous clinical state. For individuals under 35 years of age, the most common cause is **hypertrophic cardiomyopathy**, with a higher frequency seen in male athletes as compared to females (8). Other causes include abnormalities in the coronary arteries, aortic rupture associated with Marfan's syndrome, and mitral valve prolapse. In individuals over the age of 35, the most common cause is ischemic coronary artery disease. Because of the complexity of sudden death, it is covered in its own chapter (see Chapter 24).

Athletic Heart Syndrome

Athletic heart syndrome is a benign condition associated with physiologic alterations in the heart muscle brought on by repetitive, intensive physical training. These changes may produce abnormalities on electrocardiograms (ECGs) but do not in themselves represent a contraindication to exercise. Individuals with athletic heart syndrome must be fully evaluated by a physician to rule out serious underlying cardiovascular disorders that may place them at risk.

The baseball runner is in obvious respiratory distress. The impact of the ball may have caused hyperventilation or a traumatic pneumothorax. Maintain an open airway, talk and calm the individual, and assess breathing and circulation.

If respirations do not return to normal within minutes, or if respiratory or cardiac irregularities are present, activate EMS.

ABDOMINAL WALL CONDITIONS

A gymnast did a sudden back hyperextension movement after landing on a vault, and felt a sharp pain in the abdominal region. There is marked tenderness and muscle guarding slightly below and to the right of the umbilicus. No swelling or discoloration is visible, but it hurts to do a modified sit-up. What condition may be present? How should the injury be managed?

The muscles of the abdominal wall are strong and powerful, yet flexible enough to absorb impact. Consequently, injuries to the abdominal wall are usually minor. Other conditions, however, such as a contusion to the solar plexus and hernias, can affect sport participation.

Skin Wounds and Contusions

With a skin abrasion, cleanse the wound to prevent contamination, cover the area with a sterile nonstick dressing, and secure the dressing to prevent friction directly over the abrasion.

Lacerations that penetrate the abdominal wall muscles or deeper can be very serious due to possible contamination of the abdominal organs. Activate EMS for immediate transportation to the nearest medical facility.

Because further examination is necessary to rule out intra-abdominal injuries, ointments or creams should not be placed on the wound. Instead, irrigate the wound with sterile water, and cover the area with an absorbent pad to control hemorrhage. Simple contusions to the abdominal wall are evident by tenderness over the area of impact, pain during active contraction of the abdominal muscles, and the absence of referred pain. Treatment involves ice and compression to limit hemorrhage. A pressure dressing may be applied if a large hematoma forms.

Muscle Strains

Muscle strains are caused by direct trauma, sudden twisting, or sudden hyperextension of the spine. The rectus abdominis is the most commonly injured muscle. Complications arise when the epigastric artery or intramuscular vessels are damaged, leading to hematoma formation. Nearly 80% of the hematomas occur below the umbilicus.

➤ SIGNS AND SYMPTOMS

Severe abdominal pain, nausea, vomiting, marked tenderness, and muscle guarding may be present. Straight leg raising or hyperextension of the back increases the pain. A palpable mass may or may not be present. If a mass is present, it will become fixed with contraction of the muscle.

➤ MANAGEMENT

Treatment consists of ice, rest, and early use of nonsteroidal anti-inflammatory drugs (NSAIDs) for the first 36 to 48 hours. Hydrocollator packs and whirlpools can be used with activity modification until the hematoma and soreness ends. Activities such as twisting, turning, or sudden stretching should be avoided until painful symptoms subside.

Solar Plexus Contusion ("Wind Knocked Out")

A blow to the abdomen with the muscles relaxed is referred to as a "solar plexus punch," and results in an immediate inability to catch one's breath (dyspnea). Fear and anxiety complicate the condition. Although the true cause of the breathing difficulty is unknown, it is thought to be caused by diaphragmatic spasm and transient contusion to the sympathetic **celiac plexus**.

➤ MANAGEMENT

Assessment should include a thorough airway analysis. Remove any mouthguard or partial plates. Loosen any restrictive equipment and clothing around the abdomen, and have the individual flex the knees toward the chest. Paradoxical as it may seem, asking the athlete to take a deep breath and hold it, and to repeat this several times, often restores the athlete's breath more quickly. Another method is to have the athlete whistle, as it forces the diaphragm to relax. Because a severe blow may lead to an intra-abdominal injury, reassess the individual at the end of the practice session to rule out any injury that may have been overlooked.

Hernias

A **hernia**, a protrusion of abdominal viscera through a weakened portion of the abdominal wall, can be congenital or acquired. Congenital hernias are present at birth and may be related to family history. Acquired hernias occur after birth and may be aggravated by a direct blow, strain, or abnormal intra-abdominal pressure, such as that exerted during heavy weight lifting or shot-putting. The three most common hernias are the indirect, direct, and femoral hernia **(Figure 10.17)**.

An indirect inguinal hernia is the most common type of hernia in young athletes. A weakness in the peritoneum around the deep inguinal ring allows the abdominal viscera to protrude through the ring into the inguinal canal and occasionally extend into the scrotum. This weakness in the peritoneum is not typically present in women, thus decreasing their risk of acquiring this type of hernia. Large indirect hernias may reduce spontaneously because they cannot extend easily into the inguinal canal. Direct hernias, common in men over 40, result from a weakness in an area of fascia bounded by the rectus abdominis muscle, the inguinal ligament, and the epigastric vessels. Femoral hernias, more commonly seen in women, allow the abdominal viscera to protrude through the femoral ring into the femoral canal, compressing the lymph vessels, connective tissue,

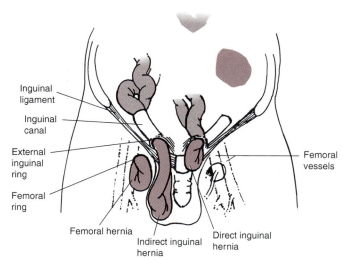

➤ FIGURE 10.17 **Hernias**. A hernia may be classified as (A) indirect, where the small intestine extends into the scrotum, (B) direct, where the small intestine extends through a weakening in the internal inguinal ring, or (C) femoral, where the small intestine protrudes posterior to the inguinal ligament and medial to the femoral artery.

and the femoral artery and vein. The herniation presents as a mass inferolateral to the pubic tubercle and medial to the femoral artery and vein.

➤ SIGNS AND SYMPTOMS

Symptoms vary, but for most hernias the first sign is a visible, tender swelling and an aching feeling in the groin. Many hernias are asymptomatic until the preparticipation exam, when the physician palpates the protrusion by invaginating the scrotum with a finger. Protrusion of the hernia increases with coughing.

➤ MANAGEMENT

The danger of a hernia lies in continued trauma to the weakened area during falls, blows, or increased intra-abdominal pressure exerted during activity. The hernia can twist on itself and produce a strangulated hernia, which can become gangrenous. As a result, most hernias are surgically repaired. Individuals with an indirect hernia repair can begin walking, mild upper extremity exercises, and bicycling within 6 weeks of surgery. Return to noncontact sport participation can occur in 7 weeks and contact sports within 8 to 10 weeks (1).

Repair of direct inguinal and femoral hernias is more extensive. All strenuous activities are prohibited for 3 weeks postsurgery. Return to noncontact sports can occur after 8 weeks and contact sports in 12 weeks. Activities that stretch or pull the abdominal muscles should be avoided. Recommended activities include swimming, biking, and weight training for the upper extremities. Individuals with an unrepaired hernia can participate in noncontact sports; however, surgical repair is recommended to prevent recurrent, irreducible hernias that can lead to small bowel obstruction.

The individual experienced sharp abdominal pain after sudden hyperextension of the back. No swelling or discoloration was present, but pain increased with active contraction of the abdominal muscles. This athlete has a possible strain of the rectus abdominus. Application of ice, compression, and rest will reduce the acute swelling and pain. If a palpable tender hematoma is present, refer the athlete to a physician to rule out damage to the epigastic artery.

INTRA-ABDOMINAL INJURIES

 A 22-year-old football player was struck in the abdomen with a helmet and experienced a sudden onset of abdominal pain in the upper left quadrant that seemed to radiate into the upper chest and left shoulder. Weakness and a light-headed feeling are present. Blood pressure is 96/72, and pulse is weak at 96 beats per minute. What injury might be present?

Trauma to the abdomen can lead to severe internal hemorrhage if organs or major blood vessels are lacerated or ruptured. Injuries can be open or closed, with closed injuries typically caused by blunt trauma. The solid organs are more commonly injured in sport participation. Hollow viscera, if damaged, can leak the contents into the abdominal cavity, causing severe hemorrhage, **peritonitis** (inflammation of the peritoneum), and shock. Many signs and symptoms indicating an intra-abdominal injury are similar in nature, regardless of the organ involved **(Box 10.5)**.

➤➤ **Box 10.5**

Red Flags Indicating a Serious Intra-abdominal Condition

- Abdominal pain, often starting as mild then rapidly increasing in severity
- Nausea, weakness, and thirst
- Individual may lean forward and bring the knees to the chest to reduce tension in the abdominal muscles
- Localized tenderness and rigidity over the injured organ
- Cramps or muscle guarding (splinting)
- Rebound pain with release of deep palpation
- Referred pain to the shoulder tip, back, or groin
- Absence of bowel sounds
- Shallow breathing. Abdominal respiratory motion may be absent
- Coughing up or vomiting blood that looks like used coffee grounds
- Diffuse hemorrhage or distention of the abdomen
- Blood in the urine or stool
- Rapid, weak pulse and decreased blood pressure
- Cyanosis

Variations arise in the area of palpable pain and the site of referred pain.

Acute management of suspected intra-abdominal injuries is also very similar, regardless of the injured organ. Initially, the athletic trainer should keep the individual relaxed while assessing the ABCs. If necessary, activate EMS. The individual should be placed in a supine position with the knees flexed to relax the low back and abdominal muscles. The vital signs should be monitored regularly, and the athlete should be treated for shock. **Field Strategy 10.2** summarizes the acute management of intra-abdominal injuries.

Splenic Rupture

Although rarely injured in sport participation, certain systemic disorders such as infectious mononucleosis can enlarge the spleen, making it vulnerable to injury. The spleen is the most commonly injured abdominal organ and is the most frequent cause of death from abdominal blunt trauma in sport (1). The reason is that the spleen can splint itself and stop hemorrhaging, only to produce delayed hemorrhage days, weeks, or months later, after a seemingly minor jarring motion, such as a cough. Athletes who have infectious mononucleosis should be disqualified from contact and strenuous noncontact sports for at least 3 weeks. After 3 weeks, the individual may return to strenuous noncontact sports if they feel up to activity, the spleen is nonpalpable, and liver function tests are normal. Contact sports are contraindicated for an additional week or longer if the spleen remains palpable or liver function tests are abnormal (9).

➤ SIGNS AND SYMPTOMS

Indications of a splenic rupture include a history of blunt trauma to the left upper quadrant, and a persistent dull pain in the upper left quadrant, left lower chest, and left shoulder, referred to as **Kehr's sign**. This referred pain is caused by irritation of the diaphragm innervated by the phrenic nerves, which arise from the ventral rami of segments C3 to C5. The free blood can also irritate the right side of the diaphragm, in which case pain will be referred to the dermatome patterns in the right shoulder. The individual is often nauseated, cold, and clammy, and will show signs of shock at the time of injury.

 Activate EMS. Maintain an open airway and treat for shock. Refer to Field Strategy 10.2 for further management procedures.

➤ MANAGEMENT

Treatment usually involves nonoperative intravenous therapy, strict bed rest, and intensive monitoring of vital signs. Following a week of hospitalization, the individual should restrict activities for at least 2 weeks. Return to vigorous physical activity is not recommended until 3 to 2 months after injury. If surgical repair is indicated, a mini-

FIELD STRATEGY 10.2 MANAGEMENT ALGORITHM FOR SUSPECTED INTRA-ABDOMINAL INJURIES

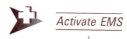 *Activate EMS*
↓

In case of vomiting:
- Roll the person on the side to allow for drainage
- Make certain the airway remains open

↓

Control any external hemorrhage with pressure and a sterile dressing

↓

Lay the individual supine:
- Keep the knees flexed to relax the abdominal muscles
- *Do not* extend the legs or elevate the feet

↓

Record vital signs:
- Respiratory rate and depth (rapid, shallow breathing indicates shock)
- Pulse rate and strength (rapid, weak pulse indicates shock)
- Blood pressure (a marked drop in both readings indicates shock)
- Pupillary response to light (lackluster, dilated pupils indicates shock)

↓

Give nothing by mouth

↓

Treat for shock and monitor vital signs until the ambulance arrives

---

mum 3-month period is needed for the abdominal musculature to heal and regain adequate strength before return to vigorous activity. Most physicians recommend a 6-month interval after a splenectomy before return to contact sports (10).

Liver Contusion and Rupture

A direct blow to the upper right quadrant can contuse the liver, causing significant palpable pain, point tenderness, hypotension, and shock. Pain may be referred to the inferior angle of the right scapula. As with the spleen, systemic diseases, such as hepatitis, can enlarge the liver, making it more susceptible to injury. Those who have an enlarged liver (hepatomegaly) should avoid contact sports until the liver has returned to its normal size or is nonpalpable. If lacerated, the liver is capable of massive bleeding, but often is stopped by the time the wound is exposed in surgery. For this reason, there has been an increasing trend toward nonoperative management (11).

Appendicitis

The vermiform appendix is a pouch extending from the cecum (see Figure 10.9). If it becomes obstructed (for example, with hardened fecal material), venous circulation may be impaired, leading to an increase in bacterial growth and the formation of pus. The resulting inflamed appendix, called **appendicitis**, can lead to ischemia and gangrene. If the appendix ruptures, feces and bacteria are sprayed over the abdominal contents, causing peritonitis.

➤ SIGNS AND SYMPTOMS

Signs and symptoms include acute abdominal pain in the lower right quadrant, loss of appetite, nausea and vomiting, and a low-grade fever. Rebound pain can be elicited at **McBurney's point**, which is one-third the distance between the anterior superior iliac spine (ASIS) and the umbilicus.

➤ MANAGEMENT

Activate EMS. Maintain an open airway and treat for shock. Refer to Field Strategy 10.2 for further management procedures.

Kidney Injuries

Serious injury to the kidney often occurs when the body is extended and the abdominal muscles are relaxed, such as when a receiver leaps to catch a pass. Suspicion should be high if impact is to the midback region, especially if persistent back or significant flank pain is present.

➤ SIGNS AND SYMPTOMS

Pain can be referred posteriorly to the low back region, sides of the buttocks, and anteriorly to the lower abdomen. Individuals may complain of blood in the urine (hematuria), although this is not always indicative of the magnitude of injury.

➤ MANAGEMENT

Treatment involves ice application to control inflammation and pain, treating for shock, and if needed, transporting the individual to the nearest medical facility.

A radiograph or computed tomography (CT) scan may be used to determine the extent of injury. Most injuries are managed conservatively with rest and fluid management. Spontaneous healing and return of good renal function can be expected. Individuals who have a solitary kidney, especially when the kidney is pelvic, iliac, polycystic, or anatomically abnormal, should be counseled about the increased risk of injury. Although contact sports place the remaining kidney at very little risk, participation in contact/collision sports should be individually assessed. Use of a flak jacket or other customized padding may make limited contact/impact sports very safe.

Bladder Injuries

Damage to the bladder is rare, although hematuria may occur. **Hematuria** is characterized by microscopic blood or red blood cells in the urine. Most sport participants void prior to running and competition. Running with an empty bladder increases the risk of gross hematuria (visible blood in the urine), because no fluid cushion exists between the posterior wall and base of the bladder. This condition is commonly seen in long distance runners, hence the name "runner's bladder." Hematuria caused by running rapidly resolves within 24 to 48 hours of rest.

➤ SIGNS AND SYMPTOMS

Massive external trauma associated with pelvic fractures can seriously damage the bladder, leading to lower abdominal pain and tenderness. Bruising in the lower abdominal region may be visible. Palpation may reveal abdominal tenderness, muscle guarding, or rigidity. With a bladder contusion, the individual will be able to void and hematuria is present, either gross or microscopically. With a bladder rupture, the individual is usually unable to void, and a specimen obtained by catheter reveals blood in the pelvic cavity.

➤ MANAGEMENT

Treatment involves using ice to control inflammation and pain, treating for shock, and transporting the individual to the nearest medical facility. A radiograph or CT scan may be used to determine the extent of injury. Most injuries are managed conservatively with rest and fluid management. Spontaneous healing and return of good renal function can be expected.

 The football player had a history of direct trauma to the abdomen, pain in the upper left quadrant, referred pain to the left shoulder, and showed signs of shock. This indicates a possible splenic rupture. Activate EMS.

INJURIES AND CONDITIONS OF THE GENITALIA

 A soccer player was struck in the groin by an opponent's foot. He was not wearing a protective cup at the time. He immediately fell to the ground and drew the knees to the chest while grasping the genital region. What possible conditions can occur as a result of direct trauma to the genitalia? How should this injury be managed? What signs and symptoms would indicate that immediate referral to a physician is warranted?

The male genitalia are more susceptible to injury than female genitalia because several structures are external to the body, and thus exposed to direct trauma. Protective cups can protect the penis and scrotum from injury, and are required for baseball catchers and ice hockey goalies (see Figure 3.12). Direct trauma can damage the penis, urethra, and scrotum, which holds the testes. In addition, congenital variations in testicular suspension make certain individuals susceptible to torsion of the testicle.

Male Genital Injuries

Direct trauma to the groin from a knee, implement, or straddle-like injury, such as falling on a bar, can cause severe pain and dysfunction to the testes and penis. Lacerations are rare, but swelling and hemorrhage inside the scrotal sac can occur. To assist in assessment and follow-up management of an injury to the male genital organs, the individual should be instructed to do periodic self-assessment for pain and swelling, and should be given guidelines on seeking further medical care if necessary.

PENILE INJURIES

Superficial wounds to the penis may involve a contusion, abrasion, laceration, avulsion, or penetrating wound. In addition, the urethra can be damaged. Most injuries resolve without specific treatment. Superficial bleeding may be controlled with a sterile dressing and a cold compress with mild compression to control swelling. Referral to a physician is only necessary if hemorrhage persists or swelling impairs the function of the urethra, leading to an inability to void.

Cyclists may develop transient paresthesia of the penis as a result of pressure on the pudendal nerve. Adjusting the saddle height, tilt, and number of cycling bouts usually resolves the condition. Rising up on the pedals occasionally will also relieve pressure temporarily.

SCROTAL INJURIES

Blunt scrotal trauma can cause a contusion, hematoma, torsion, dislocation, or rupture of the testicle. If the tunica vaginalis ruptures, the vascular and tubercle components of the testes can be seriously damaged. Commonly a knee, foot, or elbow to the groin compresses the testicle against the pelvis, leading to a nauseating, painful condition. Immediate internal hemorrhage, effusion, and muscle spasm

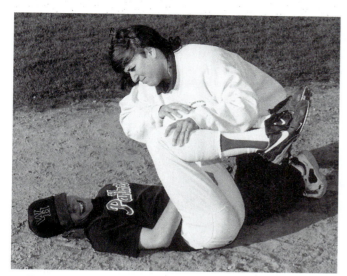

➤ FIGURE 10.18 **Relieving testicular spasm**. To relieve testicular spasm, place the individual on his back and flex the knees toward the chest. After pain has diminished, apply ice to control swelling and hemorrhage.

occur. Testicular spasm can be relieved by placing the individual on his back and flexing the knees toward the chest to relax the muscle spasm **(Figure 10.18)**. After pain subsides, a cold compress should be placed on the scrotum to reduce swelling and hemorrhage.

Occasionally, blunt trauma leads to swelling in the tunica vaginalis, resulting in a traumatic **hydrocele (Figure 10.19A)**. In 9 to 19% of men, the plexus of veins on the posterior testicle can become engorged, constituting a **varicocele**. These lesions may be described as "a bag of worms" adjacent to the testicle and cord **(Figure 10.19B)**. If the plexus ruptures in response to blunt trauma, a rapid accumulation of blood occurs in the scrotum, leading to

a **hematocele**. In nearly 50% of patients with traumatic hematocele, testicular rupture is also present (1).

Pain is not a good indicator of which structure is damaged. Swelling and hemorrhage inside the scrotal sac can enlarge the sac to the size of a tennis ball or grapefruit. Each condition can lead to irreparable testicular damage if evaluation and treatment by a physician is delayed. Treatment for swelling inside the scrotal sac involves aspiration of fluid and injection of a solution to toughen the involved tissues. Symptoms disappear in 85 to 90% of the cases with this treatment (1).

Torsion of the testicle may or may not have a history of trauma. Congenital variations in the testicular suspension can cause rotational twisting of the vascular pedicle and spermatic cord, producing varying degrees of circulatory compromise **(Figure 10.19C)**. It is typically seen at or around puberty, manifesting itself after physical activity. Groin pain may develop gradually or rapidly, sometimes with associated nausea and vomiting. Immediate referral to a physician is necessary if correction of the condition is to be successful. High-resolution ultrasound is used to discover if the blood supply is absent to the testicle and will determine the extent and severity of injury. If corrected within 6 to 8 hours, recovery is nearly 100%.

A scrotal mass may also be indicative of testicular cancer, the most common malignancy in 16- to 35-year-old males. Men who have an undescended or partially descended testicle are at a higher risk of developing testicular cancer than others. The first sign is a slightly enlarged testicle and a change in its consistency. The mass is separate from the cord and epididymis. Often a dull ache or sensation of dragging and heaviness is present in the lower abdomen or groin. Diagnosis is made with ultrasound or transillumination with a bright light. Early detection and surgical treatment yields an excellent survival rate.

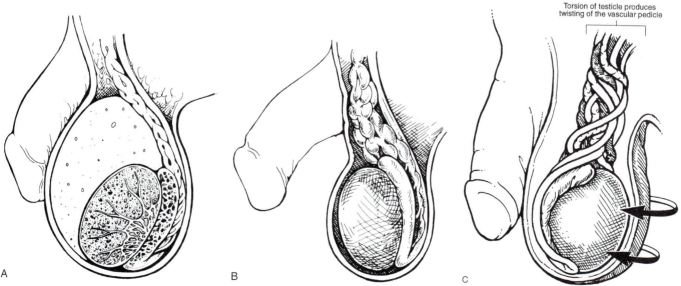

➤ FIGURE 10.19 **Testicular injury**. A, Hydrocele. B, Varicocele. C, Spermatic cord torsion around the tunica vaginalis.

Female Genital Injuries

Injuries to the vulva usually involve straddling or penetration trauma, or can be sustained by falls, resulting in tears from forced perineal stretching during sudden leg abduction. These injuries have occurred in gymnastics, water-skiing, snowmobiling, motorcycling, bicycling, sledding, cross-country skiing, and horseback riding. Nearly all injuries are easily treated by ice application, mild compression, and bed rest. Occasionally, high-speed water-skiing injuries result in water being forced under high pressure into the vulva and vagina, leading to rupture of the vaginal walls. The water may also be forced through the uterus and fallopian tubes, leading to localized pelvic peritonitis. These injuries are easily preventable by wearing a neoprene wetsuit or nylon-reinforced suit.

 Direct trauma to the groin can lead to a laceration, scrotal contusion, hematoma, torsion, dislocation, or rupture of the testicle. The current position of the player will relieve testicular spasm. After the spasm has eased, remove the player from the field, apply cold compresses to reduce swelling and hemorrhage, and encourage the individual to do periodic self-assessment. If persistent pain or swelling of the testicle occurs, the individual should seek immediate medical attention.

ASSESSMENT OF THROAT, THORAX, AND VISCERAL INJURIES

 A 21-year-old female gymnast finished practice an hour ago but is now complaining of vague chest discomfort and shortness of breath. She is also experiencing pain on the top of the right shoulder. How will you progress through this assessment to determine the extent and seriousness of injury?

Injury assessment for thoracic and visceral injuries should focus on the vital signs and history of the injury. Chest or abdominal trauma, although initially appearing superficial and minor, can mask internal hemorrhage and swelling that can seriously compromise function of the vital organs. In addition, the individual's condition can slowly deteriorate, leading to a life-threatening condition. Although general observation and palpation can confirm the possibility of a serious underlying condition, a good understanding of the history of the injury and constant monitoring of vital signs will strengthen the assessment.

While approaching the individual, the athletic trainer should assess consciousness, respirations, and circulation. If the individual is having difficulty breathing, anxiety and panic may make the task more difficult. After ruling out possible spinal injury, the individual should be placed in a supine position with the knees flexed to facilitate breathing. The airway should be open and clear of any blood or

vomitus. The trachea should be in the middle of the throat and should not move during respirations. The athletic trainer should speak in a slow, calm, confident manner and tell the athlete what will transpire, and why. The individual should be assured that any test that causes pain or discomfort will be discontinued. If the difficulty in breathing does not return to normal within a minute or two, the athletic trainer should activate EMS and take vital signs so a baseline of information is established. It is always better to have EMS en route during the assessment than to wait and see if the condition gets any better. Several conditions intensify in severity with time, thereby seriously compromising the health of the injured party. Blood pressure, pulse, respirations, and pupillary response to light should be documented, so comparisons can be made later in the assessment. A decrease in blood pressure may indicate loss of blood volume. Remember, that with an acute abdominal injury, you should never give any water or food to the individual. Not only can the condition be aggravated, but if surgery is needed, any food or fluid in the gastrointestinal tract will make the surgery more dangerous. When the assessment is complete, the vital signs should be monitored frequently, and the athlete should be treated for shock until the ambulance arrives. **Field Strategy 10.3** summarizes assessment of the thorax and visceral regions.

HISTORY

 You have completed the primary survey on the gymnast. She is obviously conscious but does have some shortness of breath. Her pulse is somewhat elevated but you are not sure if that is due to anxiety or an injury. What questions should be asked to determine the cause of this condition?

Since few special tests are available for the region, the athletic trainer must rely heavily on information provided in the history. Musculoskeletal injuries to the ribs, costal cartilage, or abdominal muscles are usually tender at the site of injury. Abdominal pain may indicate a serious abdominal injury, but is also a symptom in conditions as minor as precompetition anxiety. The issue is not to draw a distinction between acute and nonacute pain, but rather between possible surgical and nonsurgical conditions. Athletes tend to tolerate pain better than nonathletes. Consequently, every complaint of thoracic or abdominal pain must be taken seriously.

The athletic trainer should gather information on the primary complaint, mechanism of injury, and the characteristics of the symptoms. Pain that is sudden in onset, severe or explosive, progressive, continuous, and lasts more than 6 hours generally indicates a serious internal problem that necessitates surgical intervention. Persistent pain that awakens the person or occurs during relative inactivity is also a red flag. Pain that is gradual, mild to moderate, intermittent, recurrent, occurs after exercise or after eating,

FIELD STRATEGY 10.3   ASSESSMENT OF THE THORAX AND VISCERAL REGION

HISTORY

☐ Primary complaint including:
- ■ Current nature, location, and onset of the condition

☐ Mechanism of injury
- ■ Position of trunk or abdomen; direction of force

☐ Characteristics of the symptoms
- ■ Evolution of the onset, nature, location, severity, and duration of pain or weakness

☐ Disability resulting from the injury

☐ Related medical history
- ■ Previous injuries to the area, congenital abnormalities, childhood diseases, or allergies, or cardiac, respiratory, vascular, or neurological problems
- ■ Family history

OBSERVATION AND INSPECTION

☐ Observe the general body for:
- • Body position that indicates injury site
- • Difficulty in breathing, shortness of breath, or diminished chest movement
- • Facial expressions that indicate severity of pain
- • Signs of shock

☐ Inspect the injured area for:
- • Muscle symmetry
- • Swelling
- • Discoloration
- • Hypertrophy or muscle atrophy
- • Visible congenital deformity
- • Surgical incisions or scars

PALPATION

☐ Bony structures to determine a possible fracture:
- • Compression in an anteroposterior direction for a rib fracture
- • Lateral compression for costochondral separation

☐ Soft tissue structures to determine temperature, point tenderness, rigidity, and muscle spasm or guarding. Note:
- • Any swelling or loss of continuity in the muscle
- • Rebound tenderness on deep palpation
- • Superficial protrusion or palpable mass

PPHYSICAL EXAMINATION TESTS

☐ Active and resistive movements for muscular strains
☐ Auscultation and percussion for abnormal or absent sounds. Complete this step *prior* to palpation
☐ Neurologic testing for dermatome patterns and referred or radiating pain

---

or resolves partially or completely in less than 6 hours indicates a less serious condition that favors a nonsurgical diagnosis (13). **Table 10.3** identifies some common non-musculoskeletal sources of abdominal pain and the typical signs and symptoms associated with each condition.

The athletic trainer should ask questions about previous injuries to the area, and family history that may have some bearing on this specific condition. Remember that some conditions, such as a ruptured spleen, can delay hemorrhage for hours, days, or weeks after the initial trauma. Other injuries with an acute onset may have signs and symptoms that subside, only to recur later. Inquire about what activities aggravate the pain. Coughing, sneezing,

rapid movements, and walking, especially down stairs, can cause peritoneal irritation. Musculoskeletal pain is often relieved by changing position. In younger athletes who are sexually active, women experience abdominal pain twice as often as men of the same age. However, men tend to have a higher incidence of conditions necessitating surgical intervention. Pain that is sudden in onset and follows an abnormal menstrual period might stem from an ectopic pregnancy, which would constitute a medical emergency. Pain that occurs shortly after a normal menstrual period, is bilateral, and is accompanied by a fever and abdominal pain, but not nausea and vomiting, suggests pelvic inflammatory disease. In addition to the general questions dis-

TABLE 10.3   COMMON NONMUSCULOSKELETAL SOURCES OF ABDOMINAL PAIN

Condition	Signs and Symptoms
Appendicitis (acute)	Inflammation of the appendix resulting in constant pain, progressing in severity; begins in the outer umbilical region, moves to right lower quadrant; nausea, vomiting, and loss of appetite; low-grade fever.
Cholecystitis (acute)	Inflammation of the gall bladder resulting in constant pain in right upper quadrant, onset often follows a meal; nausea and vomiting; tenderness in right upper quadrant and right shoulder; splinting on the right side.
Perforated peptic ulcer	Perforated stomach ulcer resulting in a sudden onset of pain in midepigastric region that spreads and is aggravated by movement; individual is reluntant to move and appears acutely ill; rigid abdomen; grunting respiration; absent bowel sounds.
Ectopic pregnancy	Pregnancy in the fallopian tube, which results in a tubal rupture causing a sudden, severe, and persistent pain, generally following a missed or abnormal period, typically epigastric; often associated with hypotension and tachycardia.
Ovarian cyst	An abnormal cystic tumor of the ovary that is usually benign. Constant pain with sharp, sudden onset; usually in ipsilateral lower area of the abdomen below the umbilicus; may have nausea and vomiting following the pain.
Pelvic inflammatory disease	Chronic inflammation of the pelvis caused by multiple infections including chlamydia and gonorrhea resulting in pain at the end of, or shortly after, a normal menstrual period; bilateral lower quadrant pain aggravated by manipulation of cervix; nausea and vomiting rare; possible cervical discharge; fever.
Urinary calculus	Pain location changes with the movement of the urinary stone, may radiate to the testicle, or groin of the involved side; pain is very severe; individual cannot get comfortable.

Adapted from Berman (13), page 76.

cussed in Chapter 4, specific questions that can be asked for chest and abdominal injuries can be seen in **Field Strategy 10.4**.

 The gymnast has vague, mild chest discomfort on the right side that began about a half hour after practice. Since then, the discomfort has intensified and now she feels pain on the top of the right shoulder. She reports being short of breath and unable to take a deep inhalation without pain. She does not recall any previous chest trauma or injury that might have accounted for her present state, nor does she recall any member of her family having a similar problem.

OBSERVATION AND INSPECTION

 You suspect a pulmonary complication because of the pain on deep inspiration. However, you are not sure if it is superficial or internal. What factors can you observe that might provide clues to help determine if there is an injury to the chest wall or an internal complication?

Observation of body position can give an indication of the site, nature, and severity of injury. For example, in an acute thoracic injury, the individual may lean toward the injured side, using an arm or hand to stabilize the region. In an acute abdominal injury, the individual will lie on the injured side and bring the knees toward the chest to relax the abdominal muscles. Facial expressions can confirm the individual's hesitation to perform any

movement due to severe pain. Chest expansion can reveal the rate and depth of respirations.

Inspection

The individual should be sufficiently undressed to observe the injury site. Inspect the neck, back, chest, abdomen, and groin. Look for deformity, edema, bruising, ecchymosis, and skin color. Deformity may indicate a sternal or rib fracture, costochondral separation, or muscle rupture. An abrasion or localized bruising on the chest wall could suggest a possible rib fracture or internal complication. Diffuse bruising in the axilla and chest wall may indicate a ruptured pectoralis major. A bruise or ecchymosis in the umbilical area (Cullen's sign) indicates intraperitoneal bleeding. Distention in the abdomen may indicate internal hemorrhage. Pale, cold, and clammy skin is associated with shock. Cyanosis, or a bluish skin tinge, indicates a lack of oxygen due to internal pulmonary or cardiac problems. Coughing up bright red or frothy blood indicates a severe lung injury. Vomitus that contains blood that looks like used coffee grounds indicates that blood has been swallowed and partially digested.

The rate and depth of respirations should be noted, particularly if there is any difficulty in catching the breath. If the condition is only transitory, that is, the wind has been knocked out, breathing and color should quickly return to normal. Individuals with an internal injury tend to use rapid and shallow breaths because deep breathing increases pain. The athletic trainer should observe the symmetrical rise and fall of the chest; any abnormal motion may indicate a fractured rib or pneumothorax. If breathing does not return

FIELD STRATEGY 10.4   DEVELOPING A HISTORY FOR A THORACIC OR ABDOMINAL INURY

CURRENT INJURY STATUS

1. How did the injury occur? What position were you in, and from what direction was the force (glancing, direct, or violent muscle contraction)? Does it hurt to take a deep breath?
2. Where is the pain located? How severe is it? When did it begin (sudden or gradual)? Can you describe the pain (sharp, aching, burning, radiating)? Did the pain disappear, then gradually increase (spontaneous pneumothorax, ruptured spleen)? Are you nauseous, lightheaded, or weak?
3. Did you hear any sounds during the incident (rib fracture, costochondral separation, cutaneous emphysema)? Have you had any muscle spasms or cramps with the injury?
4. What motions aggravate the symptoms? In what position are you most comfortable in? How old are you?
5. Have you noticed blood in the urine? Does it occur after long distance running? Is it painful when you urinate? Have you had any recent problems with diarrhea or constipation (bowel obstruction)?

PAST INJURY STATUS

1. Have you ever been injured in this area before? When? What was done for the injury?
2. Do you have a history of diabetes mellitis, rheumatic fever, Marfan's syndrome, low or high blood pressure, or high cholesterol?
3. Do you have a history of cardiovascular disease, congenital coronary artery anomalies, heart murmurs, heart palpitations, chest pains, or shortness of breath? Have you ever fainted before? Have any of these previous conditions occurred after strenuous exercise? Has anyone in your family had a history of any of these conditions?
4. Have you had any medical problems recently? (Look for problems that may be related to referred pain from the visceral organs, heart, and lungs. Remember that some injuries, such as a ruptured spleen, can splint themselves and produce delayed hemorrhage). Do you have any allergies? Are you on any medication?

---

to normal quickly, or if the individual's condition rapidly deteriorates, the injury is significant and EMS should be activated. **Field Strategy 10.5** provides specific observations that can help determine the extent and severity of thoracic or abdominal injuries.

Auscultation and Percussion

If auscultation or percussion is used in the assessment, both should be completed prior to palpation. Because the visceral organs are interconnected by connective tissue, any palpation in the abdomen will move the internal organs, thus giving inaccurate or false sounds.

Auscultation is used to listen very carefully for the presence or absence of sounds in the body, and should precede any physical contact with the individual to prevent alteration of peristalsis by physical stimulation. The stethoscope usually has two heads: the bell and the diaphragm. The bell is used to detect low-pitched sounds, whereas the diaphragm is better at detecting higher-pitched sounds. When using the bell of the stethoscope, light pressure is applied to maintain contact with the skin surface. Firm pressure is applied when using the diaphragm to keep it pressed tightly to the skin. Because the bell or diaphragm must always be in contact with the skin, it is never acceptable to listen through clothing. Be patient. It may take 2

to 3 minutes in each area to adequately evaluate the nature and character of the underlying conditions, particularly bowel sounds.

In the thorax, the flow of air should be heard throughout the various regions of each lung **(Figure 10.20)**. Because most breath sounds are high pitched, the diaphragm is used to evaluate lung sounds. Abnormal sounds include gurgling, popping, snoring, or a high-pitched whistling sound. Absence of air flow indicates pneumothorax, tension pneumothorax, hemothorax, or traumatic asphyxia.

The athletic trainer should also auscultate the heart. Four classic sites are used to determine cardiac sounds: (1) aortic (second intercostal space, right sternal border), (2) pulmonic (second intercostal space, left sternal border), (3) tricuspid (left lower sternal border), and (4) mitral (cardiac apex) (see Figure 10.20). The athletic trainer should be on the right side of the athlete while the athlete is supine. Normally, only the closing of the heart valves can be heard. Murmurs are produced when there is turbulent energy in the walls of the heart and blood vessels. Obstruction to flow or flowing from a narrow to a larger diameter vessel produces the turbulence, which sets up eddies that strike the walls and produce vibrations that can be heard with a stethoscope. Murmurs can also be produced when there is a large volume of blood flowing through a normal opening. Murmurs may be described as "blowing," "rumbling," or

FIELD STRATEGY 10.5   OBSERVATION AND INSPECTION OF THE THORAX AND VISCERA

1. In what position is the individual (standing, leaning to one side, knees drawn to the chest, hands stabilizing an area)? Do the facial expressions indicate pain, anxiety, or panic? Is cyanosis present?
2. Is the trachea centered or deviated to one side (tension pneumothorax)? Does the trachea move during breathing? Are the neck veins distended (traumatic asphyxia)?
3. Does the symmetry of both shoulders appear well rounded with no prominent bony structures? The pectoralis major, anterior axillary fold, and abdominal muscles should look symmetrical.
4. Is there any bruising, ecchymosis, deformity, or muscular atrophy?
5. Does the rib cage look symmetrical and move symmetrically with each breath? Is shallow breathing present? Is the individual coughing up a bright red or frothy blood?
6. Are abrasions, blisters, or bleeding present at the nipples? Are the nipples and breasts bilaterally the same size (gynecomastia)?
7. Is there any bruising or ecchymosis present in the abdomen? (Bruising in the umbilical area indicates intraperitoneal bleeding.) Is the discoloration localized or diffuse? Are there any soft tissue protrusions in the lower abdomen or groin (hernia)?
8. Is the individual grasping an area with the hand? (This may indicate where the pain is, or where the pain is being referred to.)
9. Is the individual pale, cold, clammy, lethargic (shock)?

"harsh." If abnormal sounds are present, such as a click, snap, or a murmur, the individual should be referred to a physician.

In the abdomen, the athletic trainer should auscultate in all four quadrants. Normal bowel sounds in the abdomen make a gurgling sound. Hyperperistalsis with rushes, cramps, and diarrhea suggests gastroenteritis.

 Hypoperistalsis, or a silent abdomen, could indicate a serious underlying problem such as an obstruction or internal hemorrhage. Immediate referral to the nearest medical facility is warranted. Activate EMS.

Percussion is typically used over a bony structure to determine a possible fracture, but it can also be used in the abdominal region to indicate internal complications. The nondominant hand is placed on the individual's abdomen over the various internal organs. The second and third finger of the dominant hand tap on the distal interphalangeal (DIP) joint of the middle finger with a quick rapid motion **(Figure 10.21)**. The tone indicates if the organ is hollow (tympanic) or solid (full). The four quadrants are tested, with facial expressions noted, to indicate any discomfort.

 The gymnast is thin but otherwise healthy, with no sign of trauma on the chest wall or shoulder region. While sitting, she leans to the right side using her right arm to stabilize the chest. Breathing is rapid and shallow. Skin color is pale, and some anxiety is evident in the facial expression. During auscultation, decreased airflow sounds were heard in the lower right lung. Activate EMS, and continue the assessment.

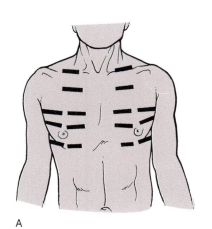
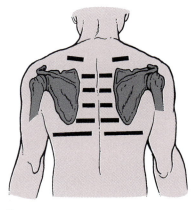
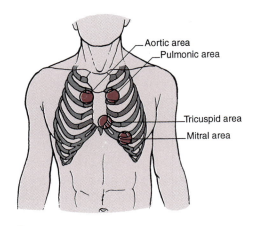

➤ **FIGURE 10.20 Auscultation.** Auscultation is done with a stethoscope to listen at various sites for air exchange in the lobes of the lungs. A, Anterior view. B, Posterior view. C, Cardiac sounds can also be auscultated over four specific sites.

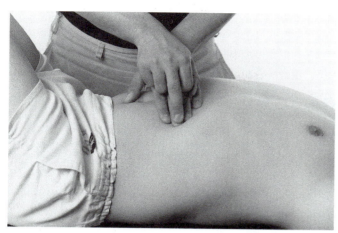

➤ FIGURE 10.21 **Percussion**. Percussion is used in the abdominal region to indicate internal complications, and should be performed prior to palpation.

PALPATION

 You suspect a possible pulmonary injury to the right lung, but cannot totally rule out a visceral injury because of the possibility of referred pain. What anatomical structures in the region can be palpated?

It is important to begin palpation away from the painful area so pain will not be carried over into other areas. Begin with gentle circular motions and feel for deformity, crepitus, swelling, rigidity, muscle guarding, or tenderness. Place the individual in a supine position with the knees flexed for more comfort.

The trachea should be palpated during breathing to ensure that it does not move, as movement may indicate tension pneumothorax. The athletic trainer should palpate the clavicle, sternum, costochondral cartilage, and ribs moving in an anterior-to-posterior direction, noting any

pain, deformity, or crepitus. Possible fractures and costochondral separations are assessed with gentle pressure applied to the sternum and vertebrae in an anteroposterior direction **(Figure 10.22A)**. This action causes the rib cage to bow out laterally. Lateral compression on the sides of the rib cage causes strain on the costochondral junctions **(Figure 10.22B)**. Begin compression superiorly and move down in an inferior direction until the entire area is covered. Pain at a specific site indicates a positive sign.

For the abdomen, begin by gently stroking the abdomen. Underlying peritoneal irritation causes light touch to be perceived as **dysesthesia**, or a disagreeable sensation, and suggests a serious underlying condition. To palpate, use the flat part of several fingers with both hands moving in small circular motions **(Figure 10.23)**. Do not poke or make sudden moves as this may cause the individual to jerk and tighten the muscles. Always begin away from the injured site and move across the abdomen in a straight line. Note any muscle guarding or rigidity. Muscle guarding that cannot be voluntarily relaxed may indicate internal peritoneal hemorrhage. Palpate for tenderness, muscle resistance, and superficial masses or deficits in the continuity of the abdominal wall. Deeper palpation can detect rigidity, swelling, or masses. Rebound tenderness at McBurney's point is indicative of appendicitis. The rebounding pain is caused when the inflamed appendix is impacted by the viscera returning to their normal position. This phenomenon, however, can also occur with peritonitis.

 The rib cage, intercostal muscles, and the abdomen can be palpated for deformity, crepitus, swelling, rigidity, muscle guarding, or tenderness. You completed palpation and found no irregularities or pain in the abdominal region. In the thorax, pain could not be elicited with palpation, but you did notice that the right side of the rib cage is not expanding at the same level as the left side.

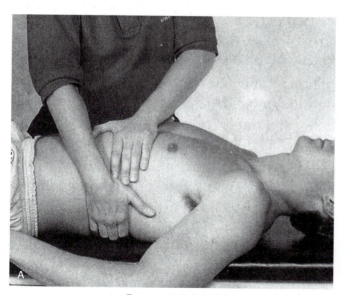
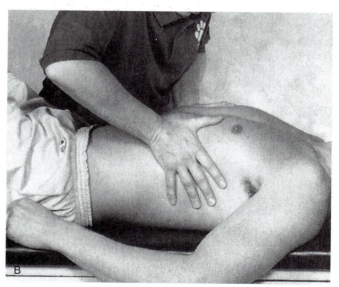

➤ FIGURE 10.22 **Compression of the rib cage in a supine position**. A, Anteroposterior compression for rib fracture. B, Lateral compression for costochondral separation.

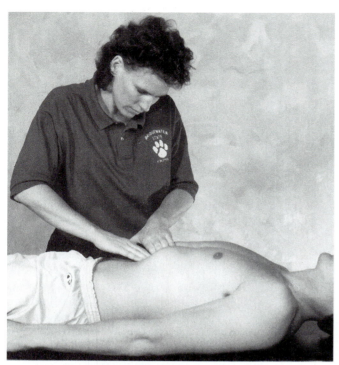

➤ FIGURE 10.23 **Palpation of the abdomen**. Use the flat part of several fingers with both hands moving in small circular motions.

The gymnast is beginning to have more difficulty breathing, and pain is increasing.

PHYSICAL EXAMINATION TESTS

 The condition of the gymnast is slowly deteriorating. Although she remains conscious and fully able to speak, you still have not determined the cause of the problem. You activate EMS. What is your next course of action?

There are very few special tests for the thorax and visceral area. Most of the information must be gathered during the history, observation, and palpation phase of the assessment. If the condition is not serious and a muscular strain is suspected, active, passive, and resisted muscle testing can be performed. Neck and trunk motion, described in Chapters 8 and 9, include flexion, extension, lateral flexion, and rotation. The athletic trainer should note the individual's willingness to perform the motion, ease of motion, and bilateral comparison of motions where applicable.

Vital Signs

The pulse rate and rhythm, blood pressure, temperature, respiratory rate, and characteristics of the breathing pattern should be noted. Any sputum should be checked for the presence of blood. Pink or bloody sputum indicates internal bleeding and should be treated as a serious condition. Painful abdominal conditions are frequently reflected in the vital signs as tachycardia, tachypnea, and elevated temperature. In conditions that involve the upper abdomen (in-

flammatory diseases) or lower lobes of the lung, respirations may be rapid, shallow, painful (grunting), or splinted. Hypotension may result from gastrointestinal bleeding, dehydration, or vagal stimulation.

Neurologic Testing

Neurologic testing in the thorax and abdomen is somewhat limited. Dermatomes vary and often overlap. Although the dermatomes tend to follow the ribs, the absence of only one dermatome may lead to no loss in sensation. Sites for referred pain can indicate the origin of injury and were illustrated in Figure 9.36. Myotome testing includes finger abduction and adduction (T1) and hip flexion (L1–L2). No other myotome testing exists for the axial region. In addition, there are no deep tendon reflexes for the region, though it is always wise to test the deep tendon lumbar and sacral reflexes (patellar reflex and Achilles reflex).

 You determined that muscle testing was not necessary in this assessment, since a more serious, internal pulmonary problem exists. Because of the decreased airflow sounds in the lower right lung, you suspect the gymnast may be experiencing spontaneous pneumothorax. You have already activated EMS. Maintain an open airway, treat for shock, and continue to monitor the vital signs until the ambulance arrives.

Summary

1. Severe blunt trauma to the anterior neck region, thorax, and viscera can have devastating effects leading to serious ventilatory and circulatory compromise.
2. Blows to the throat may result in severe pain, laryngospasm, and acute respiratory distress.
3. A "stitch in the side" is a sharp pain or spasm in the chest wall, usually on the lower right side. Most individuals, however, can run through the pain.
4. Severe blunt trauma to the breast should be documented on a woman's permanent medical record to avoid misreading a mammogram.
5. A pectoralis major muscle strain involves an actively contracting muscle overburdened by a load or extrinsic force that exceeds tissue tolerance. Resisted horizontal adduction and internal rotation of the shoulder will be weak and accentuate the deformity if muscle fibers have been ruptured.
6. Signs and symptoms indicating a possible internal thoracic condition include:
   • Shortness of breath or difficulty in breathing
   • Severe chest pain aggravated by deep inspiration
   • Abnormal chest movement
   • Abnormal or absent breath sounds
7. A hernia is a protrusion of abdominal viscera through a weakened portion of the abdominal wall, and can be congenital or acquired. An indirect ingui-

nal hernia is the most common hernia in young athletes.

8. Signs and symptoms indicating a possible intra-abdominal condition include:
   - Severe abdominal pain
   - Nausea or vomiting
   - Distended abdomen
   - Tenderness, rigidity, or muscle spasm
   - Rebound pain
   - Absence of bowel sounds
   - Blood in the urine or stool

9. Certain injuries may not develop until hours, days, or weeks later. As such, the presumption of possible intrathoracic or intra-abdominal injuries with any blunt trauma necessitates a complete assessment.

10. Injury assessment for the thorax and visceral region should focus on the vital signs and history of the injury.

11. Observation, palpation, and sites of referred pain can confirm suspicions of an existing internal injury.

12. If at anytime, signs and symptoms indicate an intra-thoracic or intra-abdominal injury, EMS should be activated immediately. The vital signs should be monitored every 5 to 7 minutes to determine if the individual is improving or deteriorating.

13. If the individual recovers on site, he or she should be informed of any signs and symptoms that might develop later, indicating that the condition is getting worse. If this occurs, the athlete should then seek immediate medical care.

References

1. Nichols AW. Abdominal and thoracic injuries. In: Athletic injuries and rehabilitation. Edited by Zachazewski JE, Magee DJ, and Quillen WS. Philadelphia: WB Saunders, 1996.

2. Butcher JD, Siekanowicz A, Pettrone F. Pectoralis major rupture: Ensuring accurate diagnosis and effective rehabilitation. Phys Sportsmed 1996;24(3):37-44.

3. Griffiths, and Selesnick. Rupture of the pectoralis major muscle: Diagnosis and treatment. Phys Sportsmed 1997;25(8):119-125.

4. Erickson SM, Rich BSE. Pulmonary and chest wall emergencies: On-site treatment of potentially fatal conditions. Phys Sportsmed 1995;23(11):95-104.

5. Volk, CP, McFarland EG, Horsmon G. Pneumothorax: On-field recognition. Phys Sportsmed 1995;23(10):43-46.

6. Cvengros RD, Lazor JA. Pneumothorax—a medical emergency. J Ath Train 1996;31(2):167-168.

7. Moeller JL. Contraindications to athletic participation: Cardiac, respiratory, and central nervous system conditions. Phys Sportsmed 1996;24(8):47-58.

8. Van Camp SP, et al. Nontraumatic sports death in high school and college athletes. Med Sci Sports Exerc 1995;27(5):641-647.

9. Moeller JL. Contraindications to athletic participation. Spinal, systemic, dermatologic, paired-organ, and other issues. Phys Sportsmed 1996;24(9):57-70.

10. Morden RS, Berman BM, Nagle CE, Jafri SZH. Spleen injury in sports, Part II: Avoiding splenectomy. Phys Sportsmed 1992;20(4):126-139.

11. Ray T, Lemire JE. Liver laceration in an intercollegiate football player. J Ath Train 1995;30(4):324-326.

12. Melekos MD, Asbach HW, Markow SA. Etiology of acute scrotum in 100 boys with regard to age distribution. J Urol 1988;139(5):1023-1025.

13. Bergman RT. Assessing acute abdominal pain: A team physician's challenge. Phys Sportsmed 1996;24(4):72-82.

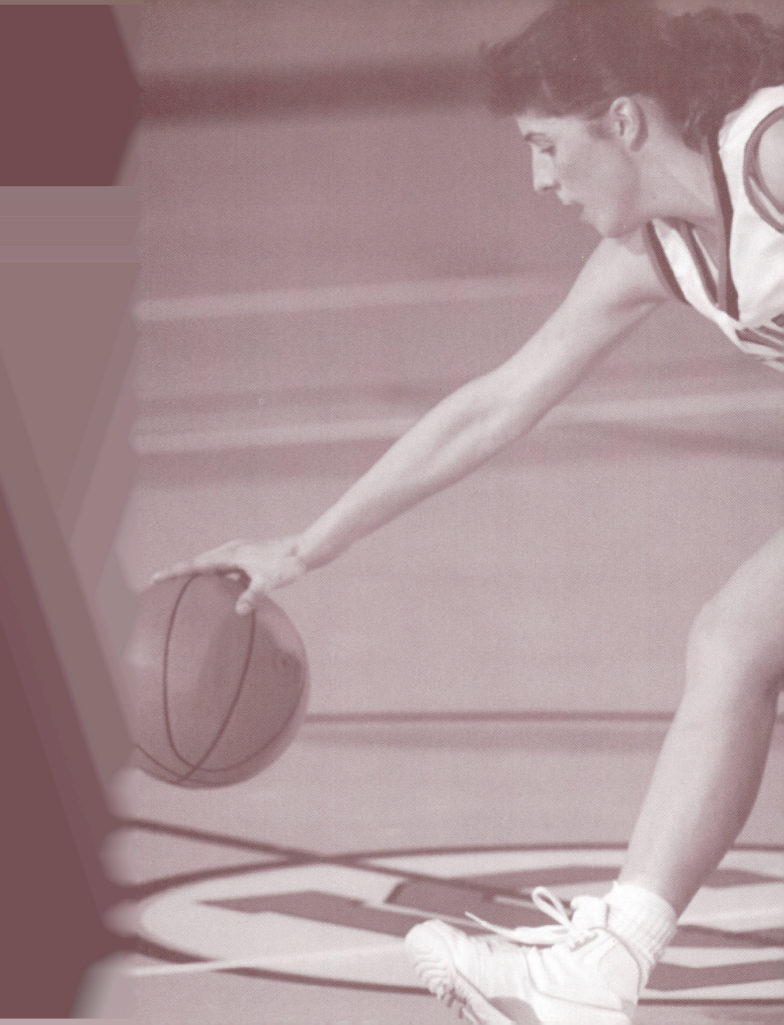

SECTION IV

CHAPTER 11

Shoulder Conditions

OBJECTIVES

1. Identify the important bony and soft tissue structures of the shoulder.

2. Describe the major motions at the shoulder, and identify the muscles that produce them.

3. Describe the phases of the throwing motion, and list common injuries sustained during each phase.

4. Explain general principles and exercises used to prevent injuries to the shoulder.

5. List common mechanisms of injury that may lead to instability in the sternoclavicular (SC) joint, acromioclavicular (AC) joint, and glenohumeral (GH) joint.

6. Explain the criteria for classifying AC joint sprains.

7. Describe the primary anatomical restraints that prevent glenohumeral instabilities; explain the implications of injury to these structures relative to a possible dislocation or subluxation.

8. Define the various cartilaginous lesions that may occur as a result of a glenohumeral dislocation, and identify the typical locations of these lesions.

9. Describe soft tissue pathology in the shoulder region due to overuse; explain management strategies for common soft tissue injuries.

10. Describe a thorough assessment of the shoulder region.

11. Explain general principles and techniques used in developing a rehabilitation exercise program for the shoulder complex.

The loose structure of the shoulder complex enables extreme mobility, but provides little stability. As a result, the shoulder is much more prone to injury than the hip. Shoulder injuries commonly occur in activities involving an overhead motion, such as in baseball, swimming, tennis, volleyball, and weightlifting. In fact, shoulder pain is the most common musculoskeletal complaint among competitive swimmers, with 50 to 80% reporting a history of shoulder pain (1,2). Activities involving overhead motions place significant demands on the shoulder and other joints of the upper extremity, leading to many acute and chronic conditions. Common injuries include bursitis, sprains, rotator cuff and impingement injuries, and bicipital tendinitis. Dislocations of the shoulder articulations are not uncommon in contact sports such as wrestling and football.

This chapter begins with a review of the anatomy of the shoulder region, followed by a synopsis of the kinematics and kinetics of the shoulder joints. Discussion on prevention of injuries is followed by an overview of common injuries to the shoulder complex. Management of specific injuries, the assessment process, and examples of rehabilitation exercises then conclude the chapter.

ANATOMICAL REVIEW OF THE SHOULDER

The shoulder region encompasses five separate articulations: the sternoclavicular (SC) joint, acromioclavicular (AC) joint, coracoclavicular joint, glenohumeral joint (GH), and the scapulothoracic joint. The articulation referred to specifically as the shoulder joint is the glenohumeral joint, whereas the other articulations are joints of the shoulder girdle. The SC and AC joints enhance motion of the clavicle and scapula, enabling the glenohumeral joint to provide a greater range of motion.

Sternoclavicular Joint

As the name suggests, the SC joint consists of the articulation of the superior sternum, or manubrium, with the proximal clavicle (**Figure 11.1**). The SC joint is surrounded by a joint capsule that is thickened anteriorly and posteriorly by four ligaments, including the interclavicular, costoclavicular, and anterior and posterior sternoclavicular ligaments. The anterior sternoclavicular ligament is a broad band supporting the anterior capsule, while the posterior sternoclavicular ligament is smaller and weaker, providing support to the posterior capsule. The costoclavicular ligament runs from the clavicle to the first rib and its adjacent cartilage. The interclavicular ligament provides minimal support to the joint; it runs between the two sternoclavicu-

lar joints, and also attaches to the manubrium. There is a substantial fibrocartilaginous disc between the manubrium and clavicle, which divides the joint almost completely in half. Because of its attachments, the disc adds significant strength to the joint, thereby preventing medial displacement of the clavicle.

The SC joint enables rotation of the clavicle with respect to the sternum. The joint allows motion of the distal clavicle in superior, inferior, anterior, and posterior directions, along with some forward and backward rotation of the clavicle. Thus, rotation occurs at the SC joint during motions such as shrugging the shoulders, reaching above the head, and in most throwing-type activities. Because the first rib is joined by its cartilage to the manubrium just inferior to the joint, motion of the clavicle in the inferior direction is restricted. The close packed position for the SC joint occurs with maximal shoulder elevation.

Acromioclavicular Joint

The AC joint consists of the articulation of the medial facet of the acromion process of the scapula with the distal clavicle (Figure 11.1). As an irregular, diarthrodial joint, limited motion is permitted in all three planes. The joint is enclosed by a capsule, though the capsule is thinner than that of the SC joint. The strong superior and inferior acromioclavicular ligaments cross the joint, providing stability. The coracoacromial ligament, sometimes referred to as the "arch" ligament, also attaches to the inferior lip of the AC joint to serve as a buffer between the rotator cuff muscles and the bony acromion process. The close packed position of the AC joint occurs when the humerus is abducted at 90°.

Coracoclavicular Joint

The coracoclavicular joint is a syndesmosis in which the coracoid process of the scapula and the inferior surface of the clavicle are joined by the coracoclavicular ligament (Figure 11.1). The coracoclavicular ligament, with its conoid and trapezoid branches, resists independent upward movement of the clavicle, downward movement

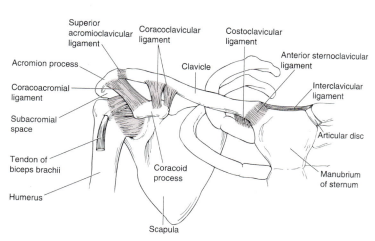

➤ FIGURE 11.1 **Bony and ligamentous structure of the shoulder girdle**.

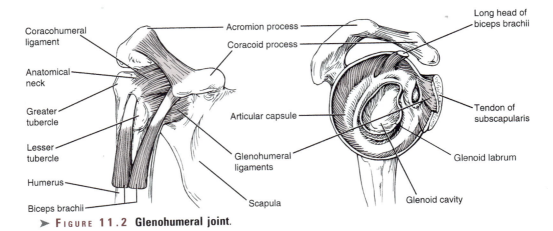

➤ **FIGURE 11.2 Glenohumeral joint.**

of the scapula, and anteroposterior movement of the clavicle or scapula. Very little movement is permitted at this joint.

Glenohumeral Joint

The GH joint is the articulation between the glenoid fossa of the scapula and the head of the humerus. Although the joint enables a greater total range of motion than any other joint in the human body, it is lacking in bony stability **(Figure 11.2)**. This is due partially to the hemispheric head of the humerus, which has three to four times the amount of surface area as compared to the shallow glenoid fossa. Because the glenoid fossa is also less curved than the humeral head, the humerus not only rotates, but also moves linearly across the surface of the glenoid fossa when humeral motion occurs. Humeral head translation is limited by muscle tension (which also limits rotation) during active

positioning of the arm. The largest translations take place during passive movement of the arm at the extremes of the range of motion.

The glenoid fossa is somewhat deepened around its perimeter by the glenoid labrum, a narrow rim of fibrocartilage around the edge of the fossa. The glenohumeral joint capsule is joined by the superior, middle, and inferior glenohumeral ligaments on the anterior side, and the coracohumeral ligament on the superior side. Although joint displacements can occur in anterior, posterior, and inferior directions, the strong coracohumeral ligament protects against superior dislocations. The inferior glenohumeral ligament is the thickest of the ligaments and reinforces the inferior capsule. It is the main static stabilizer in the abducted arm.

The tendons of four muscles, including the supraspinatus, infraspinatus, teres minor, and subscapularis also join the joint capsule **(Figures 11.3, 11.4)**. These muscles,

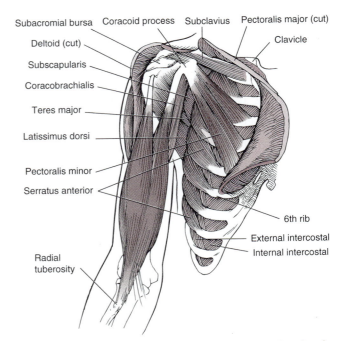

➤ **FIGURE 11.3 Deep posterior muscles that move the glenohumeral joint.**

➤ **FIGURE 11.4 Deep anterior muscles that move the glenohumeral joint.**

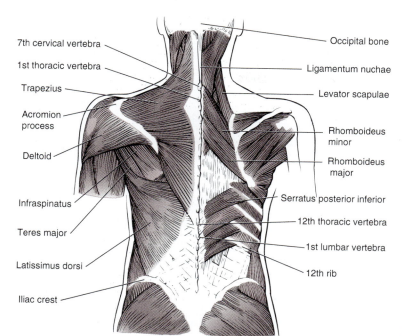

7th cervical vertebra

1st thoracic vertebra

Trapezius

Acromion process

Deltoid

Infraspinatus

Teres major

Latissimus dorsi

Iliac crest

Occipital bone

Ligamentum nuchae

Levator scapulae

Rhomboideus minor

Rhomboideus major

Serratus posterior inferior

12th thoracic vertebra

1st lumbar vertebra

12th rib

➤ **FIGURE 11.5 Superficial and deep posterior muscles of the back.**

referred to as the SITS muscles after the first letter of the muscles' names, are also known as the rotator cuff muscles because they all act to rotate the humerus, and their tendons merge to form a collaginous cuff around the joint. Tension in the rotator cuff muscles helps to hold the head of the humerus against the glenoid fossa, further contributing to joint stability. The joint is most stable in its close packed position when the humerus is abducted and laterally rotated.

Scapulothoracic Joint

Because muscles attaching to the scapula permit its motion with respect to the trunk or thorax, this region is sometimes described as the scapulothoracic joint. Muscles attaching to the scapula include the levator scapula, rhomboids, serratus anterior, pectoralis minor, subclavius, deltoid, subscapularis, supraspinatus, infraspinatus, teres major, teres minor, coracobrachialis, the short head of the biceps brachii, long head of the triceps brachii, and the trapezius (**Figures 11.3, 11.5,** and **11.6**).

The scapular muscles perform two functions. The first is stabilization of the shoulder region. For example, when a barbell is lifted from the floor, the levator scapula, trapezius, and rhomboids develop tension to support the scapula, and in turn, the entire shoulder through the AC joint. The second function is to facilitate movement of the upper extremity through appropriate positioning of the glenohumeral joint. During an overhand throw, for example, the rhomboids contract to move the entire shoulder posteriorly as the arm and hand move backward during the preparatory phase. As the arm and hand then move forward to execute the throw, tension in the rhomboids is released to permit forward movement of the shoulder, enabling medial rotation of the humerus.

Muscles of the Shoulder

A large number of muscles cross the glenohumeral joint, as shown in **Table 11.1.** Identifying the actions of these muscles is complicated by the fact that, due to the large range of motion at the shoulder, the action produced by contraction of a given muscle may change with the orientation of the humerus.

Bursae

The shoulder is surrounded by several bursae, including the subcoracoid, subscapularis, and the most important, the

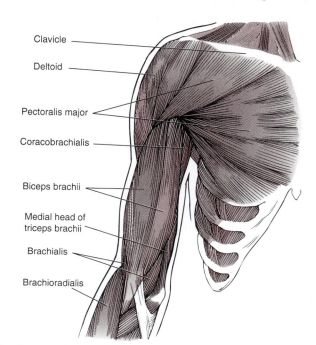

Clavicle

Deltoid

Pectoralis major

Coracobrachialis

Biceps brachii

Medial head of triceps brachii

Brachialis

Brachioradialis

➤ **FIGURE 11.6 Superficial anterior muscles of the shoulder.**

TABLE 11.1   MUSCLES OF THE SHOULDER

Muscle	Proximal Attachment	Distal Attachment	Primary Action(s)	Nerve Innervation
Deltoid	Outer third of the clavicle, top of the acromion, and scapula spine	Deltoid tuberosity of the humerus		Axillary (C_5, C_6)
(Anterior)			Flexion, horizontal adduction	
(Middle)			Abduction, horizontal abduction	
(Posterior)			Extension, horizontal abduction	
Pectoralis major		Lateral aspect of the humerus just below the head		
(Clavicular)	Medial two-thirds of the clavicle		Flexion, horizontal adduction	Lateral pectoral (C_5–T_1)
(Sternal)	Anterior sternum and cartilage of 1st six ribs		Extension, adduction, horizontal adduction	Medial pectoral (C_5–T_1)
Supraspinatus	Supraspinous fossa	Greater tuberosity of the humerus	Abduction, stabilizes shoulder joint	Suprascapular (C_5, C_6)
Coracobrachialis	Coracoid process of the scapula	Medial anterior humerus	Horizontal adduction	Musculocutaneous (C_5–C_7)
Latissimus dorsi	Lower six thoracic and all lumbar vertebrae, posterior sacrum, iliac crest, lower three ribs	Anterior humerus	Extension, adduction	Thoracodorsal (C_6–C_8)
Teres major	Lower, lateral, dorsal scapula	Anterior humerus	Extension, adduction, medial rotation	Subscapular (C_5, C_6)
Infraspinatus	Infraspinous fossa	Greater tubercle of the humerus	Lateral rotation, horizontal abduction	Subscapular (C_5, C_6)
Teres minor	Posterior, lateral border of scapula	Greater tubercle and adjacent shaft of humerus	Lateral rotation, horizontal abduction	Axillary (C_5, C_6)
Subscapularis	Entire anterior surface of scapula	Lesser tubercle of the humerus	Medial rotation	Subscapular (C_5, C_6)
Biceps brachii		Radial tuberosity		Musculocutaneous (C_5–C_7)
(Long head)	Upper rim of the glenoid fossa		Assists with abduction	
(Short head)	Coracoid process of the scapular		Assists with flexion, adduction, medial rotation and horizontal adduction	
Triceps brachii (Long head)	Just inferior to the glenoid fossa	Olecranon process of the ulna	Assist with extension and adduction	Radial (C_5–T_1)

subacromial. The subacromial bursa lies in the subacromial space where it is surrounded by the acromion process of the scapula and the coracoacromial ligament above and the glenohumeral joint below (Figure 11.4). The bursa cushions the rotator cuff muscles, particularly the supraspinatus, from the overlying bony acromion and provides the major component of the subacromial gliding mechanism. This bursa is supplied with free nerve endings, Ruffini endings, and Pacinian corpuscles, and can become irritated when repeatedly compressed during overhead arm action.

Nerves of the Shoulder

Innervation of the upper extremity arises from the brachial plexus, branching primarily from the lower four cervical (C_5–C_8) and first thoracic (T1) spinal nerves **(Figure 11.7)**. The brachial plexus is positioned between the anterior scalene (AS) and middle scalene (MS) muscles in about 60% of individuals, with the C_5 and/or C_6 nerves coursing through or lying anterior to the AS in others. The ventral rami of these nerves divide into upper, middle, and lower trunks, which separate into anterior and posterior divisions, then divide into lateral, medial, and posterior cords (see Chapter 9). This network of nerves passes between the clavicle and first rib at a distance approximately one-third of the length of the clavicle proximal to the glenohumeral joint. Injuries to the clavicle in this region can damage the brachial plexus. Major nerves arising from the brachial plexus that supply the shoulder region are the axillary (C_5, C_6), musculocutaneous (C_5–C_7), dorsal scapular (C_5), subscapular (C_5, C_6), suprascapular (C_5, C_6), and

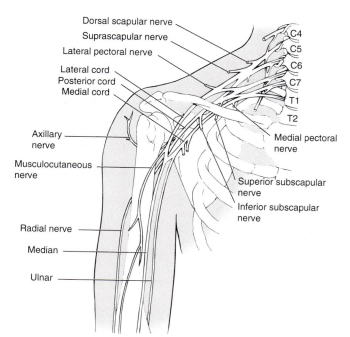

➤ FIGURE 11.7 **Brachial plexus nerve supply to the shoulder region**.

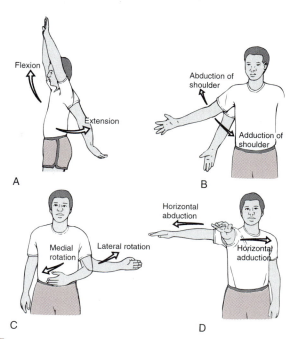

➤ FIGURE 11.9 **Movements of the arm at the shoulder**. A, Flexion and extension. B, Abduction and adduction. C, Medial and lateral rotation. D, Horizontal abduction and adduction. Combined movements are called circumduction.

pectoral nerves (C_5–T_1). The nerve-muscle associations are presented in Table 11.1.

Blood Vessels of the Shoulder

The subclavian artery passes beneath the clavicle to become the axillary artery, providing the major blood supply to the shoulder **(Figure 11.8)**. Branches of the axillary artery include the thoracoacromial trunk, lateral thoracic artery, subscapular artery, and thoracodorsal artery, as well as the anterior and posterior humeral circumflex arteries that supply the head of the humerus.

KINEMATICS AND MAJOR MUSCLE ACTIONS OF THE SHOULDER COMPLEX

The shoulder is the most freely moveable joint in the body, with motion capability in all three planes **(Figure 11.9)**. Sagittal plane movements at the shoulder include flexion (elevation of the arm in an anterior direction), extension (return of the arm from a position of flexion to the side of the body, and hyperextension (elevation of the arm in a posterior direction). Frontal plane movements include ab-

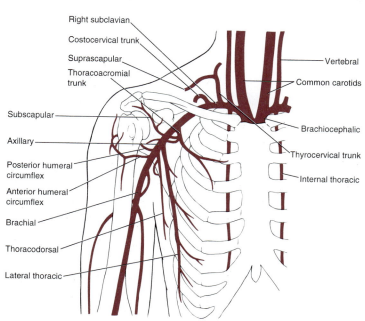

➤ FIGURE 11.8 **Blood supply to the shoulder**.

▶▶ Box 11.1

Phases of the Throwing Motion

- **Wind-up Phase** — From first movement until hands separate. Arms begin with downward swing, then are raised overhead (gathered position). Shoulders and hips rotate as arms go overhead; body shifts from facing target to being perpendicular to the line of throw. Balance is maintained on "stance leg" (right leg) as the lead leg or "stride leg" (left leg) lifts up; hip and knee flex at about chest-high level.
- **Stride Phase** — From hand separation until the lead foot contacts the ground.
- **Cocking Phase** — From foot contact until maximum shoulder external rotation.
- **Acceleration Phase** — From maximum shoulder external rotation until ball release.
- **Deceleration and Follow-through Phase** — From ball release until maximum shoulder internal rotation and balanced position is achieved.

duction (elevation of the arm in a lateral direction) and adduction (return of the arm from a position of abduction to the side of the body). Transverse plane movements include horizontal adduction (horizontally extended arm is moved medially) and horizontal abduction (horizontally extended arm is moved laterally). The humerus can also rotate medially (anterior face of humerus is moved medially) and laterally (anterior face of humerus is moved laterally).

Throwing

Throwing and related motions can produce a variety of both acute and chronic injuries to the shoulder. Throwing styles vary from individual to individual, even across overarm, sidearm, and underarm styles of the throw. To further complicate matters, some sport skills, casually referred to as throwing, actually involve more of a pushing motion than a throwing motion. An example is putting the shot. Nevertheless, overarm throwing can be described in distinct phases **(Box 11.1)**.

Although skillful throwing involves the coordinated action of the entire body, this description focuses on the phases where potential for injury to the shoulder girdle and glenohumeral joint may occur. In the preparatory or cocking phase, the arm and hand are drawn behind the body through horizontal abduction, hyperextension, and maximal external rotation of the humerus **(Figure 11.10)**. Eccentric loading of the horizontal adductors and internal rotators of the shoulder is very high during this action. The subscapularis, in particular, has its peak eccentric activity in the late cocking phase, and serves to protect the anterior joint, which is under extreme tension. The pectoralis major and latissimus dorsi work eccentrically with the subscapularis to further protect the joint. To facilitate this arm motion, the rhomboids must contract concentrically to pull the scapula and the glenohumeral joint posteriorly, while the serratus anterior provides additional scapular stabilization. As the shoulder proceeds into horizontal abduction and sternal rotation, the humeral head tends to sublux, first posteriorly and then anteriorly, against the anterior capsule; consequently, tendinitis of the anterior muscle tendons is quite common (3). Just prior to maximal shoulder external rotation, elbow extension begins. This is immediately followed by the onset of shoulder internal rotation.

During the acceleration or delivery phase, the ball is brought forward and released. Humeral horizontal adduction, elbow extension, and rapid internal rotation of the humerus by the pectoralis major, latissimus dorsi, and subscapularis are coupled with relaxation of the rhomboids to enable anterior movement of the glenohumeral joint. If

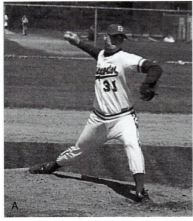
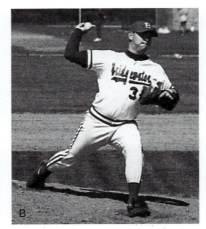
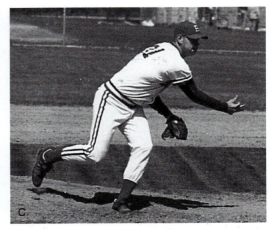

▶ **FIGURE 11.10** The overarm throwing motion. A, Cocking phase. B, Acceleration phase. C, Deceleration and follow-through phase.

> ➤ **Box 11.2**

Common Injuries Sustained During the Throwing Motion

Cocking Phase
- Anterior glenohumeral instability or subluxation
- Anteroinferior glenoid labral tears
- AC joint pathology
- Subacromial bursitis
- Strain to the medial rotators (pectoralis major, latissimus dorsi), biceps brachii, triceps brachii
- Thoracic outlet syndrome

Acceleration Phase
- Anterior subluxation
- Rotator cuff tendinitis/partial tears
- Subacromial bursitis
- Proximal humeral apophysitis
- Glenoid labral pathology
- Strain to the anterior deltoid, pectoralis major, subscapularis, latissimus dorsi
- Bicipital tendinitis or biceps tendon subluxation

Deceleration and Follow-through Phase
- Rotator cuff tendinitis/partial tears
- Triceps tendinitis or biceps tendinitis/rupture
- Teres minor strain
- Posterior glenohumeral subluxation
- Posterior capsulitis
- Glenoid labral pathology
- AC joint pathology

the internal rotators are weak, however, the reduced ability to provide forceful arm depression can lead to increased external rotation, superior humeral migration, and impaired scapular rotation, which can cause or aggravate an impingement syndrome. At ball release, the elbow is almost fully extended and positioned slightly anterior to the trunk. Because throwing can involve a whip-like action of the arm, large stresses can be placed on the tendons, ligaments, and epiphyses of the throwing arm during delivery (3).

Arm deceleration occurs after ball release, until maximal shoulder internal rotation occurs, and consists primarily of a snap-like flexion of the wrist and pronation of the forearm. Large eccentric loads at the elbow and shoulder

decelerate the arm. The infraspinatus, supraspinatus, teres major and minor, latissimus dorsi, and posterior deltoid play major roles in resisting shoulder distraction and anterior subluxation forces. If the rotator cuff muscles are weak, fatigued, or injured, the humeral head will distract and translate in an anterior direction, leading to stress on the posterior capsule. The serratus anterior contracts either concentrically or isometrically to decelerate scapular protraction, and is assisted by the middle trapezius and rhomboids. Injuries common to the specific phases of throwing can be seen in **Box 11.2**.

Coordination of Shoulder Movements

The extensive range of motion afforded by the shoulder is due partially to the loose structure of the glenohumeral joint, and partially to the proximity of the other shoulder articulations and the movement capabilities they provide. Movement at the shoulder typically involves some rotation at the SC, AC, and GH joints. For example, as the arm is elevated past 30° of abduction, or the first 45 to 60° of flexion, the scapula also rotates, contributing approximately one-third of the total rotational movement of the humerus. This important coordination of scapular and humeral movements, known as **scapulohumeral rhythm**, enables a much greater range of motion at the shoulder than if the scapula were fixed **(Figure 11.11)**. Also contributing to the first 90° of humeral elevation is the elevation of the clavicle through approximately 35 to 45° of motion at the SC joint. The AC joint contributes to overall movement capability as well, with rotation occurring during the first 30° of humeral elevation, and then again as the arm is moved past 135° (4).

Glenohumeral Flexion

The muscles that cross the glenohumeral joint anteriorly are positioned to contribute to flexion (Figures 11.4, 11.6). The anterior deltoid and the clavicular pectoralis major are the primary shoulder flexors, with assistance provided by the coracobrachialis and the short head of the biceps

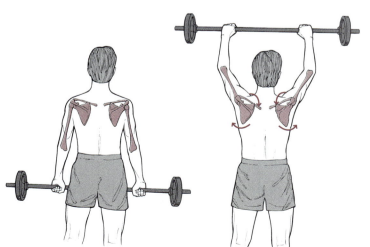

> ➤ **FIGURE 11.11** Scapulohumeral rhythm. The coordinated movement of the scapula needed to facilitate motion of the humerus is known as scapulohumeral rhythm. The arrows indicate the direction the scapulae must rotate to raise the arms.

brachii. Since the biceps brachii also crosses the elbow joint, it is capable of exerting more force at the shoulder when the elbow is in full extension.

Glenohumeral Extension

When extension is unresisted, the action is caused by gravity. Eccentric contraction of the flexor muscles serves as a controlling or braking mechanism. When resistance to extension is offered, the posterior glenohumeral muscles act, including the sternocostal pectoralis, latissimus dorsi, and teres major, with assistance provided by the posterior deltoid and the long head of the triceps brachii (Figures 11.3, 11.5).

Glenohumeral Abduction

The muscles superior to the glenohumeral joint produce abduction and include the middle deltoid and the supraspinatus (Figure 11.3). During the contribution of the middle deltoid, from approximately 90° through 180° of abduction, the infraspinatus, subscapularis, and teres minor produce inferiorly directed force to neutralize the superiorly directed dislocating force produced by the middle deltoid. This action serves an important function in preventing impingement of the supraspinatus and subacromial bursa. The long head of the biceps brachii provides glenohumeral stability during abduction.

Glenohumeral Adduction

As with extension, adduction in the absence of resistance results from gravitational force, with the abductors controlling the speed of motion. When resistance is present, adduction is accomplished through the action of the muscles positioned on the inferior side of the glenohumeral joint, including the latissimus dorsi, teres major, and sternocostal pectoralis (Figure 11.5). The short head of the biceps and long head of the triceps contribute minor assistance. When the arm is elevated above 90°, the coracobrachialis and subscapularis also assist.

Lateral and Medial Rotation of the Humerus

Lateral rotators of the humerus lie on the posterior aspect of the humerus, including the infraspinatus and teres minor, with assistance provided by the posterior deltoid. Muscles on the anterior side of the humerus contribute to medial rotation. These include the subscapularis and teres major, with assistance from the pectoralis major, anterior deltoid, latissimus dorsi, and short head of the biceps (Figure 11.3). **Table 11.2** provides a summary of the primary muscles that act on the arm.

KINETICS OF THE SHOULDER

Although the articulations of the shoulder girdle are interconnected, the glenohumeral joint sustains much greater loads than the other shoulder joints. This is primarily because the glenohumeral joint provides mechanical support for the entire arm. Although the weight of the arm is only approximately 9% of body weight, the length of the horizontally extended arm creates large torques that must be countered by the shoulder muscles. When these muscles contract to support the extended arm, large compressive forces are generated inside the joint. The compressive force acting on the articulating surfaces of the glenohumeral joint when the arm is abducted to 90° has been estimated to reach 90% of body weight (5). Although this load is reduced by about half when the elbow is maximally flexed, due to the shortened moment arm, the shoulder is considered to be a major load-bearing joint.

During the throwing motion, there are two critical instances that increase the potential for shoulder injury. The first is during the cocking phase when the arm has not quite reached maximum lateral rotation and a large internal rotation torque develops at the shoulder, heightening the possibility for a glenoid labral tear. The second occurs just after ball release when both a large compression force and a large horizontal abduction torque are generated at the shoulder, creating potential for rotator cuff tension failure and subacromial impingement (3).

Muscles that attach to the humerus at small angles with respect to the glenoid fossa contribute more to shear than to compression at the joint. These muscles serve the important role of stabilizing the humerus in the fossa when the contractions of the powerful muscles that move the humerus might otherwise dislocate the joint. Maximum shear force has been found to be present at the glenohumeral joint when the arm is elevated approximately 60° (5).

PREVENTION OF SHOULDER INJURIES

Acute and chronic injuries to the shoulder complex are common in sport participation. Many contact and collision

| TABLE 11.2 | PRIMARY MUSCLES PRODUCING MOVEMENT AT THE GLENOHUMERAL JOINT |

Flexion	Extension	Abduction	Adduction	Medial Rotation	Lateral Rotation
Anterior deltoid	Latissimus dorsi	Middle deltoid	Latissimus dorsi	Subscapularis	Infraspinatus
Pectoralis major (clavicular)	Pectoralis major (sternal)	Supraspinatus	Pectoralis major (sternal)	Teres major	Teres major
	Teres major		Teres major		

FIELD STRATEGY 11.1   FLEXIBILITY EXERCISES FOR THE SHOULDER REGION

A. Posterior capsular stretch. Horizontally adduct the arm across the chest while the opposite hand assists the stretch.

B. Inferior capsular stretch. Hold the involved arm over the head with the elbow flexed. Use the opposite hand to assist in the stretching. Add a side stretch.

C. Anterior and posterior capsular stretch. Hold onto both sides of a doorway with your hands behind you. Let the arms straighten as you lean forward. Repeat with your hands in front of you as you lean backward.

D. Medial and lateral rotators. Using a towel, bat, or racquet, pull the arm to be stretched into lateral rotation. Repeat in medial rotation.

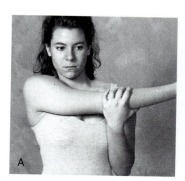
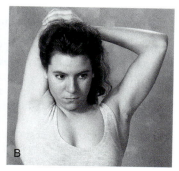
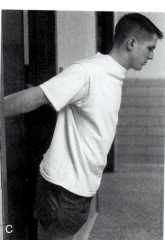
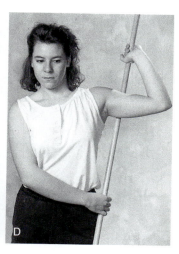

sports do require some protective equipment, but in most cases, flexibility, physical conditioning, and proper technique are the primary factors that can reduce the risk of injury to this vulnerable area.

Protective Equipment

Contact and collision sports such as football, lacrosse, and ice hockey require shoulder pads to protect exposed bony protuberances from impact. Field Strategy 3.3 outlined guidelines for fitting football shoulder pads. Although shoulder pads do prevent some soft tissue injuries in this region, they do not protect the glenohumeral joint from excessive motion. Several other commercial pads and braces used to protect the region were also illustrated in Chapter 3.

Physical Conditioning

Lack of flexibility can predispose an individual to joint sprains and muscular strains. Warm-up exercises should focus on general joint flexibility, and may be performed alone or with a partner using proprioceptive neuromuscular facilitation (PNF) stretching techniques. Individuals using the throwing motion in their sport should increase range of motion in external rotation, as this has been shown to increase the velocity of the throwing arm and decrease shearing forces on the glenohumeral joint (6). Several flexibility exercises for the shoulder complex are demonstrated in **Field Strategy 11.1**.

Strengthening programs should focus on muscles acting on both the glenohumeral and scapulothoracic region. Strength in the infraspinatus, teres minor, and posterior shoulder musculature is necessary to:

- Begin the cocking phase of throwing
- Fix the shoulder girdle during the acceleration phase
- Provide adequate muscle tension, with eccentric contractions, for smooth deceleration through the follow-through phase

In many chronic shoulder problems, particularly among throwers, a weakened supraspinatus is present. Concentric and eccentric contractions with light resistance in the first 30° of abduction can strengthen this muscle. To strengthen the scapular stabilizers, do push-ups or move the arm through a resisted diagonal pattern of external rotation and horizontal abduction. Other strengthening exercises are demonstrated in **Field Strategy 11.2**.

Proper Skill Technique

Coordinated muscle contractions are necessary for the smooth execution of the throwing motion. Any disruption in the sequencing of integrated movements can lead to additional stress on the glenohumeral joint and surrounding soft tissue structures. High-speed photography,

---

 FIELD STRATEGY 11.2   STRENGTHENING EXERCISES FOR THE SHOULDER COMPLEX

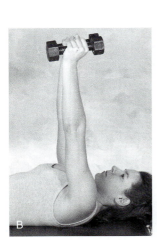

A. Shoulder shrugs. Elevate the shoulders toward the ears and hold. Pull the shoulders back, pinch the shoulder blades together, and hold. Relax and repeat.
B. Scapular abduction (protraction). Thrust the weight directly upward, lifting the posterior shoulder from the table. Relax and repeat.
C. Scapular adduction (retraction). Do bent-over rowing while flexing the elbows. At the end of the motion, pinch the shoulder blades together and hold.
D. Bench press or incline press. Use a weight belt and spotter. Place the hands shoulder-width apart and push the barbell directly above the shoulder joint.
E. Bent arm lateral flies, supine position. With the elbows slightly flexed, bring the dumbbells directly over the shoulders. Lower the dumbbells until they are parallel to the floor, then repeat. An alternative method is to move the dumbbells in a diagonal pattern. In the prone position, the exercise strengthens the trapezius (trap flies).
F. Lat pull-downs. In a seated position, grasp the handle and pull the bar behind the head. An alternative method is to pull the bar in front of the body.
G. Surgical tubing. With the tubing secured, work in diagonal functional patterns similar to those skills experienced in the specific sport.

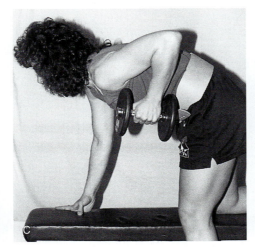

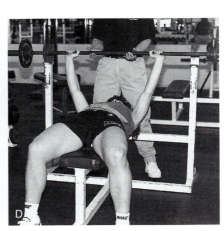

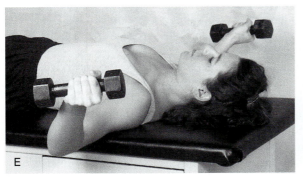

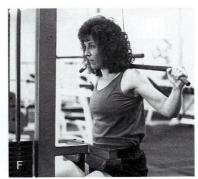

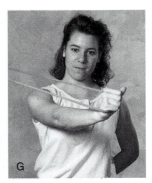

often used to record the mechanics of the throwing motion, can lead to early detection of improper technique. In addition to proper throwing technique, participants in contact and collision sports should be taught the shoulder-roll method of falling, rather than falling on an outstretched arm. This technique reduces direct compression of the articular joints and disperses the force over a wider area.

SPRAINS TO THE SHOULDER COMPLEX

 A soccer player fell on an outstretched arm, and is now complaining of pain on the top of the shoulder. It appears that the distal clavicle is somewhat elevated. There is increased pain over the AC joint with horizontal adduction of the arm across the chest, and with shoulder flexion. What structures may be involved in this injury? How will you manage this condition?

Ligamentous injuries to the SC joint, AC joint, and glenohumeral joint can result from compression, tension, and shearing forces occurring in a single episode, or from repetitive overload **(Figure 11.12)**. A common method of injury is a fall or direct hit on the lateral aspect of the acromion. The force is first transmitted to the site of impact, then to the AC joint and the clavicle, and finally to the SC joint. Failure can occur at any one of these sites. Acute sprains are common in hockey, rugby, football, soccer, equestrian sports, and the martial arts.

Sternoclavicular Joint Sprain

The SC joint is the main axis of rotation for movements of the clavicle and scapula. Nearly all injuries result from compression related to a direct blow, as when a supine athlete is landed on by another participant, or more commonly, by indirect forces transmitted from a blow to the shoulder or a fall on an outstretched arm. The disruption typically drives the proximal clavicle superior, medial, and anterior, disrupting the costoclavicular and sternoclavicular ligaments and leading to anterior displacement.

➤ SIGNS AND SYMPTOMS

First-degree injuries are characterized by point tenderness and mild pain over the SC joint, with no visible deformity. Second-degree injuries cause bruising, swelling, and pain, and the individual will be unable to horizontally adduct the arm without considerable pain. The athlete may

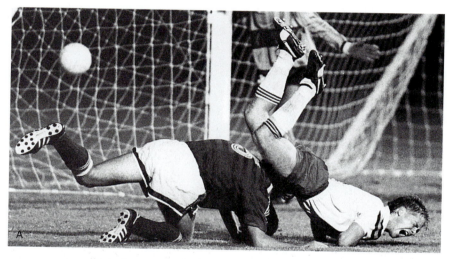
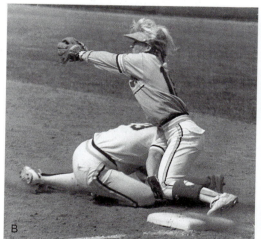
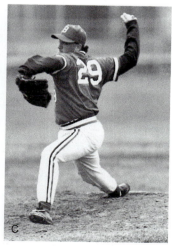

➤ FIGURE 11.12 Common mechanisms of injury to the shoulder. A, Indirect forces. B, Direct forces. C, Microtraumatic repetitive forces.

TABLE 11.3   MANAGEMENT OF A STERNOCLAVICULAR SPRAIN

Signs and Symptoms	First Degree	Second Degree	Third Degree
Deformity	None	Slight prominence of medial end of the clavicle	Gross prominence of medial end of the clavicle
Swelling	Slight	Moderate	Severe
Palpable pain	Mild	Moderate	Severe
Movement	Usually unlimited, but may have discomfort with movement	Unable to abduct the arm or horizontally adduct the arm across the chest without noticeable pain	Limited as in 2°, but pain will be more severe
Treatment	Ice, rest, immobilize with sling/swathe	Ice; rest; immobilize with figure-8, or clavicular strap with sling, for 3 to 4 weeks. Initiate strengthening program after 3 to 4 weeks	⚕ Figure-8 immobilizer with scapulas retracted. Immediately refer to physician. Check radial pulse, swallowing or breathing difficulty. If present, activate EMS.

hold the arm forward and close to the body, supporting it across the chest, indicating disruption of the stabilizing ligaments. In addition, scapular protraction and retraction can reproduce pain associated with ligamentous or disc damage. Third-degree sprains involve a prominent displacement of the sternal end of the clavicle and may involve a fracture. There is a complete rupture of the sternoclavicular and costoclavicular ligaments. Pain is severe when the shoulders are brought together by a lateral force.

Posterior (retrosternal) displacement, although rare, is more serious because of the potential injury to the esophagus, trachea, and subclavian artery. The individual will have a palpable depression between the sternal end of the clavicle and manubrium, is unable to do shoulder protraction, and may have difficulty swallowing and breathing (dyspnea). If the cranial vessels are impinged, dizziness, nausea, and a diminished radial pulse at the wrist may also be present.

➤ MANAGEMENT

First- and second-degree sprains of the SC joint are treated immediately with rest, ice, and anti-inflammatory medication. The arm may be immobilized with a sling and swathe, a figure-eight elastic wrap, or clavicular strap with a sling. Third-degree sprains require immediate reduction of the dislocation by a physician. Immobilization is usually maintained for 3 to 5 weeks; however, a formation of scar tissue may occur. Typically, there is no loss of function, but there remains a high incidence of recurrent sternoclavicular sprains. **Table 11.3** summarizes the signs and symptoms, and management of anterior sternoclavicular sprains.

 Posterior displacement can become life-threatening, and EMS should be activated.

Acromioclavicular Joint Sprain

The AC joint is weak and easily injured by a direct blow, a fall on the point of the shoulder (called a shoulder pointer), or a force transmitted up the long axis of the

humerus during a fall on an outstretched arm. In either case, the acromion is driven away from the clavicle or vice versa. Although often referred to as a "separated shoulder," ruptures of the AC and/or coracoclavicular ligaments can result in an AC dislocation, and therefore, are more correctly referred to as a sprain.

➤ CLASSIFICATION OF INJURY

Like other joint injuries, AC sprains may be classified as a first-degree (mild), second-degree (moderate), or third-degree (severe) sprain. However, because of the complexity of the joint, AC sprains are often classified as Types I–VI based on the extent of ligamentous damage, degree of instability, and where applicable, the direction in which the clavicle displaces relative to the acromion and coracoid process **(Table 11.4)**.

➤ SIGNS AND SYMPTOMS

Type I injuries have no disruption of the AC or coracoclavicular ligaments. Minimal swelling and pain are present over the joint line, and these increase with abduction past 90°. Type II injuries result from a more severe blow to the shoulder. The AC ligaments are torn, but the coracoclavicular ligament, only minimally sprained, is intact. The clavicle rides above the level of the acromion, and a minor step or gap is present at the joint line **(Figure 11.13)**. Pain increases when the distal clavicle is depressed or moved in

TABLE 11.4   CLASSIFICATION OF ACROMIOCLAVICULAR JOINT SPRAINS

Grade	Degree	Injured Structures
Type I	First	Stretch or partial damage of the AC ligament and capsule
Type II	Second	Rupture of AC ligament and partial strain of coracoclavicular ligament
Type III	Second	Rupture of AC ligament and coracoclavicular ligament
Type IV–VI	Third	Rupture of AC ligament and coracoclavicular ligament, and tearing of deltoid and trapezius fascia

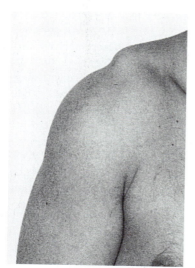

➤ **FIGURE 11.13** Acromioclavicular sprain. With a Type II acromioclavicular sprain, the distal clavicle is elevated by injury to the acromioclavicular and coracoclavicular ligaments.

an anterior-posterior direction, and during passive horizontal adduction. Type III injuries have complete disruption of the AC and coracoclavicular ligaments, resulting in visible dislocation of the AC joint. There will be obvious swelling and bruising, mild elevation of the distal clavicle and, more significantly, depression or drooping of the shoulder girdle. Higher grade injuries (IV–VI) are caused by more violent forces. Extensive mobility and pain in the area may signify tearing of the deltoid and trapezius muscle attachments at the distal clavicle. These rare injuries must be carefully evaluated for associated neurologic injuries.

➤ **MANAGEMENT**

Type I and II injuries are treated with rest, ice, and nonsteroidal anti-inflammatory drugs (NSAIDs), followed by range-of-motion exercises, as tolerated. Immobilization is necessary only if pain is present. The individual may return to sport when pain and strength permit normal use of the extremity, but the area should be padded to protect it from further insult. The majority of Type I and II injuries heal without complications; however, persistent limiting pain occasionally may necessitate a cortisone injection to diminish inflammation. Rehabilitation involves regaining range of motion, and beginning a progressive resistance exercise (PRE) program after active range of motion is bilaterally equal.

The management of Type III injuries is controversial; they are managed both operatively and nonoperatively. Most Type III injuries are treated conservatively, with 90 to 100% having satisfactory results (7,8). Immobilization in a sling for 2 to 4 weeks is followed by pendulum exercises, elbow range-of-motion exercises, isometrics in all planes, and rope-and-pulley exercises for shoulder flexion and abduction as tolerated. If surgery is indicated, pendulum and isometric exercises in all planes are encouraged in the initial stages of rehabilitation, though abduction and flexion to 90° are limited for approximately 3 to 4 weeks (9). Rehabilitation should focus on strengthening the rotator cuff and scapula stabilizers, and on restoring neuromuscular control and arthrokinematics. Return to sports may take as long as 10 to 12 weeks, depending on the return of full, pain-free range of motion and the stability of the joint. Participation in contact sports is usually permitted 3 to 5 months after the injury, depending on functional recovery. **Table 11.5** summarizes the signs and symptoms, and management of acromioclavicular sprains.

In severe cases (Types IV–VI) where total disruption of the supporting ligaments has occurred, the intra-articular disk is damaged, or an intra-articular fracture is in-

TABLE 11.5	**MANAGEMENT OF AN ACROMIOCLAVICULAR SPRAIN**		
Signs & Symptoms	**Type I**	**Type II**	**Type III**
Deformity	None, ligaments are still intact	Slight elevation of lateral clavicle; AC ligaments are disrupted, but coracoclavicular is still intact	Prominent elevation of clavicle; AC ligaments and coracoclavicular ligaments are disrupted
Swelling	Slight	Moderate	Severe
Palpable pain	Mild over joint line	Moderate with downward pressure on distal clavicle; palpable gap or minor step present; snapping may be felt on horizontal adduction	Severe on palpation and depression of acromion process; definite palpable step deformity present
Movement	Usually unlimited, but may have some discomfort on abduction greater than 90°	Unable to abduct the arm or horizontally adduct the arm across the chest without noticeable pain	Limited as in Type II, but pain will be more severe
Stability	No instability	Some instability	Demonstrable instability
Treatment	Ice, NSAIDs, regain full ROM and strength; return to activity as tolerated, with protection	Ice, NSAIDs, immobilize with sling; TENS, interferential EMS for pain relief; ultrasound; strengthening and stability exercises; return to activity with protection	Ice, immobilize, and immediately refer to physician; if treated conservatively, deformity will remain, but function should be within normal limits

volved, open or arthroscopic intervention may be necessary. Immobilization may extend to 4 to 6 weeks. The athlete is permitted to use the arm for activities of daily living, but is restricted from active forward elevation or abduction. Pushing, pulling, or carrying more than 5 pounds is also prohibited. At 6 weeks, a progressive range-of-motion and strengthening regimen begins. Complete sport participation is usually not permitted until isokinetic testing is equal to the contralateral side, which occurs approximately 6 months after surgery.

Glenohumeral Joint Sprain

Damage to the glenohumeral joint can occur when the arm is forcefully abducted (i.e., when making an arm tackle in football), but more commonly is caused by excessive shoulder external rotation and extension (i.e., arm in the overhead position). With the arm externally rotated, the anterior capsule and glenohumeral ligaments are stretched or torn, causing the humeral head to slip out of the glenoid fossa in an anterior-inferior direction **(Figure 11.14)**. A direct blow or forceful movement that pushes the humerus posteriorly can also result in damage to the joint capsule.

➤ **SIGNS AND SYMPTOMS**

In a first-degree injury, the anterior shoulder is particularly painful to palpation and movement, especially when

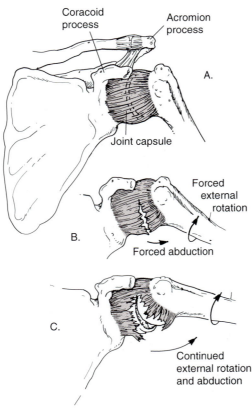

➤ **FIGURE 11.14** Glenohumeral sprains. A, Normal abduction with some stretching of the fibers. B, Forced external rotation and abduction with minimal tears to the joint capsule, leading to a moderate or second-degree sprain. C, Continuation of the forced movement causes a third-degree sprain or shoulder dislocation.

the mechanism of injury is reproduced. Active range of motion may be slightly limited, but pain will not occur on adduction or internal rotation, such as will occur with a muscular strain. A second-degree sprain will produce some joint laxity. Pain, swelling, and bruising are usually severe, and range of motion, particularly abduction, is limited. Treatment includes cryotherapy, rest, NSAIDs, and immobilization with a sling during the initial 12 to 24 hours. Early emphasis is placed on pain-free range-of-motion exercises, elastic-band strengthening, and PNF exercises. Exercises to regain full external rotation and abduction should be delayed at least 3 weeks to allow adequate time for capsular healing. A more extensive resistance program can be started as tolerated.

Glenohumeral Instability

Glenohumeral instability is based on joint play movements, or the relative displacement of the humeral head in the glenoid fossa, and may be classified as anterior, posterior, inferior, or multidirectional instability. Instability can range from a vague sense of shoulder dysfunction (atraumatic instability) to traumatic dislocation. Although glenohumeral instability can occur in any direction, most acute dislocations are anterior, with posterior being the second most frequent (10).

ANTERIOR INSTABILITY

Anterior instability may result from a blow to the posterolateral aspect of the shoulder, but more commonly is caused by excessive indirect forces that push the arm into abduction, external rotation, and extension. Failure of the capsule ligamentous complex, particularly the middle and inferior glenohumeral ligaments, causes the head of the humerus to lodge under the anterior-inferior portion of the glenoid fossa adjacent to the coracoid process. The inferior glenohumeral ligament may be avulsed from the anterior lip of the labrum or in combination with a portion of the labrum, as the humerus slides forward **(Bankart lesion)**.

POSTERIOR INSTABILITY

Posterior instability most often occurs when the humerus is flexed and internally rotated, and a posterior force is directed along the long axis of the humerus, as can occur when blocking in football. Although a single traumatic episode may lead to posterior instability, the condition more commonly results from a series of accumulated microtraumatic episodes.

INFERIOR INSTABILITY

Inferior instability is rare. The primary restraint against inferior translation is the superior glenohumeral ligament. With the arm abducted 45° in neutral rotation, the anterior portion of the inferior glenohumeral ligament is the primary restraint; at 90° of abduction, the entire glenohumeral ligament, particularly the posterior band, is responsible for restricting inferior displacement. Superior translation is limited by the coracoacromial arch and the acromion process (11).

MULTIDIRECTIONAL INSTABILITY

Multidirectional instability (MDI) of the shoulder occurs when damage is done in more than one plane. Acutely, most if not all anterior and posterior dislocations are associated with some preexisting inferior laxity, or laxity in the opposite direction. Pain and/or clicking can occur during simple tasks, such as picking up a box or suitcase. It is essential that the evaluation differentiate between unidirectional and multidirectional instability. Failure to identify the MDI, and subsequent treatment only of a unidirectional instability, can significantly alter joint mechanics, thus predisposing the athlete to continued instability in one or more planes. Treatment is initially conservative, with 50 to 70% responding favorably to rehabilitation and activity modification (11). Surgical repair is indicated for individuals who do not respond to conservative measures.

Glenohumeral Dislocations and Subluxations

The glenohumeral joint is the most frequently dislocated major joint in the body, with the majority of those dislocating in an anterior direction. Dislocations can be acute or chronic.

ACUTE DISLOCATIONS

Many acute dislocations have an associated fracture or nerve damage. Therefore, this injury is considered serious, and necessitates immediate transportation to the nearest medical facility for reduction.

➤ SIGNS AND SYMPTOMS

With an initial dislocation, there is intense pain. Recurrent dislocations may be less painful. Tingling and numbness may extend down the arm into the hand. With a first-time anterior dislocation, the injured arm is often held in slight abduction (20 to 30°) and external rotation, and is stabilized against the body by the opposite hand. Visually, a sharp contour on the affected shoulder, with a prominent acromion process, can be seen when compared to the smooth deltoid outline on the unaffected shoulder **(Figure 11.15)**. The humeral head may be palpated in the axilla anterior to the acromion resting adjacent to the coracoid process. The individual will not allow the arm to be brought across the chest. Assess both the axillary nerve and artery, since both structures can be damaged in a dislocation. A pulse may be taken on the medial proximal humerus over the brachial artery, and the axillary nerve can be assessed by stroking the skin on the upper lateral arm. Ask the individual if it feels the same on both arms. Because the deltoid is not only a key shoulder abductor, but also

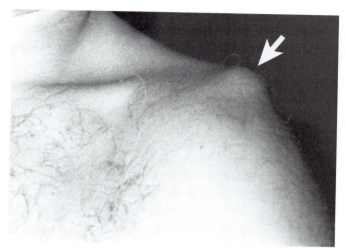

➤ **FIGURE 11.15** Glenohumeral dislocation. In a typical anterior dislocation, the head of the humerus is forced out of the glenoid fossa and comes to rest adjacent to the coracoid process. As a result, the acromion process becomes very prominent (indicated by the arrow), the deltoid musculature appears flat, and the athlete may hold the arm away from the side.

contributes to shoulder flexion and extension, damage to this nerve can be devastating.

Occasionally, a posterior dislocation occurs from a fall on, or blow to, the anterior surface of the shoulder, driving the head of the humerus posterior. If dislocated, the arm will be carried tightly against the chest and across the front of the trunk in rigid adduction and internal rotation. The anterior shoulder will appear flat, the coracoid process is prominent, and a corresponding bulge may be seen posteriorly, if not masked by a heavy deltoid musculature. Any attempt to move the arm into external rotation and abduction produces severe pain. Because the biceps brachii is unable to function in this position, the individual will be unable to supinate the forearm with the shoulder flexed.

➤ MANAGEMENT

Management of a first-time dislocation requires immediate referral to a physician. The athletic trainer should activate EMS to transport the individual to the nearest medical facility.

The injury should be treated as a fracture, with the arm immobilized in a comfortable position. To prevent unnecessary movement of the humerus, a rolled towel or thin pillow can be placed between the thoracic wall and humerus prior to applying a sling. Apply ice to control hemorrhage and muscle spasm as the individual is transported to the nearest medical facility.

A common finding following an anterior dislocation is a **Hill-Sachs lesion**. The lesion is a small defect in the articular cartilage of the humeral head caused by the impact of the humeral head on the glenoid fossa as the humerus dislocates. The lesion is usually located on the posterior aspect of the humeral head, but may be found on the anterior portion of the humeral head following a posterior dislocation, and is then called a reverse Hill-Sachs lesion. The lesion itself is used as a diagnostic tool in determining the severity of the dislocation. In athletes who report that the shoulder dislocated but spontaneously reduced, the lesion may be visible on x-ray. Although the lesion is rarely symptomatic, the condition may lead to early degeneration of the glenohumeral joint.

After reduction, the shoulder is immobilized in a sling. Traditionally, immobilization for 3 to 6 weeks has been advocated, but this has not been proven to diminish the risk of recurrent dislocations (12). When the athlete is able to tolerate movement, range-of-motion exercises can begin, but it is important to avoid an aggressive flexibility program in extension, abduction, and external rotation. Resisted isometric and stretching exercises can begin immediately after the acute phase has ended. Theraband exercises below 90° of abduction can be incorporated early in the program to maintain and improve strength. Interferential current stimulation is used to reduce inflammation, stimulate muscle reeducation, promote deep tissue circulation, and minimize fibrotic infiltration. Strength development of the lateral rotators can reduce strain on the anterior structures of the joint by pulling the humeral head posteriorly during lateral rotation of the shoulder, thus reducing anterior instability. Strong scapula stabilizers (e.g., trapezius, rhomboids, serratus anterior) are also believed to improve anterior stability by placing the glenoid in the optimal position to perform the skill techniques required. Isokinetic internal rotation and adduction can begin within 3 to 4 weeks and advance as tolerated. Complete shoulder rehabilitation exercises are not started until 5 to 6 weeks after removal of the shoulder brace.

CHRONIC DISLOCATIONS

Recurrent dislocations, or "trick shoulders," tend to be anterior dislocations that are intracapsular. The mechanism of injury is the same as acute dislocations; however, as the number of occurrences increase, the forces needed to produce the injury decrease, as do the associated muscle spasm, pain, and swelling. In individuals under the age of 20, the recurrence rate may be as high as 80%, with the majority of these dislocations occurring within 2 years of the initial injury (10). The individual is aware of the shoulder displacing because the arm will give the sensation of "going dead," referred to as the **dead arm syndrome**. Activities in which recurrent posterior subluxations are common include the follow-through of a throwing motion or a racquet swing, the ascent phase of a push-up or a bench press, a linebacker recoil, certain swimming strokes, or during a crew sweep stroke.

► SIGNS AND SYMPTOMS

Pain is the major complaint, with crepitation and/or clicking after the arm shifts back into the appropriate position. Many individuals voluntarily reduce the injury by positioning the arm in flexion, adduction, and internal rotation.

► MANAGEMENT

If the injury does not reduce, the athlete should be placed in a sling and swathe, or the arm may be stabilized next to the body with an elastic wrap. Apply ice to control pain and inflammation, and immediately refer the athlete to a physician for reduction of the injury and further care. After reduction, conservative treatment involves rest and immobilization, restoring shoulder motion, and strengthening the rotator cuff muscles. If persistent instability occurs, surgery may be indicated.

Glenoid Labrum Tears

The glenoid labrum is a fibrocartilaginous rim that lines the glenoid fossa to better receive the humeral head. The capsule and inferior glenohumeral ligament are contiguous with the labrum at their attachment to the glenoid. Tearing of the labrum and inferior glenohumeral ligament (**Bankart lesion**) is associated with recurrent anterior shoulder instability. Tears of the labrum may also occur due to degeneration and aging or trauma. In many instances, the tears are asymptomatic and incidental. Longitudinal or flap tears may occur in the anterior or posterior labrum, with or without associated glenohumeral instability. An injury to the superior labrum may begin posteriorly and extend anteriorly, disrupting the attachment of the long head of the biceps tendon to the superior glenoid tubercle (**SLAP lesion**).

► SIGNS AND SYMPTOMS

The athlete may complain of pain, catching, or weakness, usually when the arm is overhead in an abducted and externally rotated position. The pain is often associated with clicking or popping within the joint. If the tear is a result of a dislocation or subluxation, symptoms of instability may also be present. Superior tears may be symptomatic and can be reproduced with range-of-motion and translation testing, particularly with use of the clunk test and compression rotation test (see Assessment later in this chapter). Speed's test and Yergason's test may also be positive. Axial loading of the joint with forced internal and external rotation and the arm elevated 160° in the scapular plane with the elbow flexed may also reproduce symptoms (anterior impingement "crank" test) (13).

► MANAGEMENT

Treatment is based on the tear pattern and presence or absence of glenohumeral instability. Initial conservative treatment may involve rest, anti-inflammatory medication, and if applicable, rehabilitation exercises. For those individuals who do not respond well to conservative measures, arthroscopic debridement may be necessary.

 The soccer player had pain over the top of the shoulder and an elevated distal clavicle. The AC ligament and coracoclavicular ligament have been injured. Standard acute care protocol should be followed. If pain is present, immobilize the arm in a sling. The individual may return to activity when range of motion and strength have returned to normal, and functional exercise can be performed without pain.

OVERUSE INJURIES

 A swimmer is complaining of a snapping sensation accompanied by pain during the pull phase of the freestyle swimming stroke. The condition has been present for several days, but now it feels as though the humeral head is "popping out" of the joint. What structures may be injured?

Athletes who perform repetitive overhead activities often develop anterior shoulder pain. The glenohumeral capsular ligaments are the prime stabilizers of the shoulder, especially the anteroinferior glenohumeral ligament. As muscles contract to move the arm, they create compressive and shear forces within the joint. The compressive force produced by muscles acting perpendicular to the glenoid fossa will stabilize the humeral head, and muscles acting more parallel to the glenoid will produce a translational shear force. The resultant force derived from the sum of the compressive and shear forces will determine the vector direction of the total joint force. A larger superior shear force will produce impingement, and a larger compressive force will center the humeral head in the glenoid, reducing rotator cuff impingement under the acromion.

During abduction, the strong deltoid and supraspinatus muscles pull the humeral head superiorly, relative to the glenoid fossa. The remaining rotator cuff muscles must counteract (force couple action) this migration by producing an inferior shear force to resist the pull from the supraspinatus and deltoid muscles. If the rotator cuff tendons are weak or fatigued, they are incapable of depressing the humeral head in the glenoid fossa during overhead motions. In addition, fatigue of the infraspinatus and teres minor that resist anterior joint translation may also lead to intracapsular impingement and glenohumeral instability. The resulting compression can lead to impingement of the supraspinatus tendon and subacromial bursa between the acromion, the coracoacromial ligament, and the greater tubercle of the humerus, resulting in a rotator cuff strain, impingement syndrome, bursitis, or bicipital tendinitis.

Rotator Cuff/Impingement Injuries

Chronic rotator cuff tears to the SITS muscles result from repetitive microtraumatic episodes that primarily impinge on the supraspinatus tendon just proximal to the greater tubercle of the humerus **(Figure 11.16)**. Partial tears are usually seen in young individuals, with total tears typically seen in adults over 30 years of age (18). In older age groups, chronic tears can lead to cuff thinning, degeneration, and finally, total rupture of the supraspinatus tendon.

Impingement syndrome implies an actual mechanical abutment of the rotator cuff and the subacromial bursa against the coracoacromial ligament and acromion. This injury is caused from the force overload to the rotator cuff and bursa that occurs during the abduction, forward flexion, and medial rotation cycle of shoulder movements.

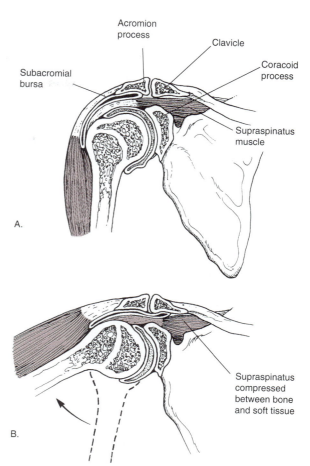

➤ **FIGURE 11.16** Supraspinatus tendon during abduction. A, Normal position. B, Abducted position. Repetitive overhead motions can impinge the muscle or tendon between the acromion process and coracoacromial ligament, resulting in a chronic rotator cuff injury.

In addition to injury to the supraspinatus tendon and subacromial bursa, the glenoid labrum and long head of the biceps brachii may also be injured. The condition is also sometimes called "painful arc" syndrome, or among competitive swimmers, "swimmer's shoulder." **Box 11.3** lists several factors that may increase the risk for an impingement syndrome.

➤ **SIGNS AND SYMPTOMS**

Initially, pain is described as deep in the shoulder and present at night. Activity will increase the pain, but only in the impingement position. As repetitive trauma continues, however, pain becomes progressively worse, particularly between 70 and 120° (hence the name painful arc) of active and resisted abduction. Because forced scapular protraction leads to further impingement and pain in the structures, the individual may be unable to sleep on the involved side. Pain can be palpated in the subacromial space. Atrophy may be apparent in the supraspinatus or infraspinatus fossa in individuals with full-thickness tears. Depending on the severity **(Box 11.4)**, positive results may be elicited in the drop arm test, empty can test, Neer shoulder impingement test, and the anterior impingement test (Hawkins-Kennedy test).

Factors Contributing to an Impingement Syndrome

- Excessive amount of overhead movement (overuse)
- Limited subacromial space under coracoacromial arch, and limited flexibility of coracoacromial ligament
- Thickness of the supraspinatus and biceps brachii tendon
- Lack of flexibility and strength of the supraspinatus and biceps brachii
- Weakness of the posterior cuff muscles (e.g., infraspinatus, teres minor)
- Tightness of the posterior cuff muscles
- Hypermobility of the shoulder joints
- Imbalance in muscle strength, coordination, and endurance of the scapular muscles (e.g., serratus anterior, rhomboids)
- Shape of the acromion
- Training devices (e.g., use of hand paddles, tubing)

➤ MANAGEMENT

Treatment will involve restricting motion below 90° abduction, cryotherapy, NSAIDs, pain-relieving medication, rest, and activity modification. Ultrasound, EMS, interferential therapy, and heat can supplement treatment. Mobility should be maintained with mild stretching exercises, particularly in external rotation at 90°, 135°, and 180° of abduction. Examples of several range-of-motion exercises for the shoulder can be seen later in the chapter in Field Strategy 11.7. Pendulum exercises with abduction and forward flexion up to 90° are initiated early in the rehabilitation process along with rope-and-pulley exercises in flexion, and T-bar exercises in flexion and external rotation, to facilitate clearance of the greater tuberosity under the coracoacromial ligament. In addition, muscles of the rotator cuff should be strengthened, as well as the muscles that perform scapular retraction, depression, and rotation. In terms of strength about the shoulder, adduction should be the strongest, followed by extension, flexion, abduction, internal, and external rotation (10). Exercises such as pull-ups or push-ups should be avoided in the early stages of rehabilitation, as they can impinge on the rotator cuff, thus complicating the condition. **Field Strategy 11.3** discusses the management of an impingement syndrome.

Swimmers present a special problem because many strokes use adduction and internal rotation with excessive propulsion forces. Because of fatigue and lack of coordination in the scapular muscles, this motion may allow subclinical anterior subluxations to occur, thus damaging the glenoid labrum. This anterior lesion may be frayed but not detached, resulting in a roughened leading edge that may mechanically catch during overhead motions. As such, swimmers may feel a snapping sensation or clicking when moving through the pull phase of the stroke, or sense that the shoulder is "going out." Occasionally, a defect or crepitus in the supraspinatus tendon may be palpated just anterior to the acromion process when the arm is extended at the glenohumeral joint. Pain can also be palpated anteriorly over the coracoacromial ligament, laterally at the insertion of the supraspinatus, posteriorly at the insertion of the infraspinatus and teres minor, or over the long head of the biceps tendon. Atrophy of the shoulder muscles with subsequent weakness in the supraspinatus and biceps brachii may also be present. Because rest translates into detraining, other steps may need to be taken to allow continued activity. The intensity and quantity of training need to be reduced, and paddle work eliminated. Stroke mechanics should be assessed to determine if changes are needed to reduce shoulder stress.

Bursitis

Bursitis is not generally an isolated condition, but rather is associated with other injuries, such as an impingement syndrome, or in older individuals with preexisting degenerative changes in the rotator cuff. The large subacromial bursa is commonly injured in swimmers, baseball, softball,

Stages of Impingement Syndrome

Stage 1
- Condition is typically seen in individuals under 25 years old and is reversible
- Localized hemorrhage and edema is present in the supraspinatus tendon
- Minimal pain (like a toothache) with activity, but no restriction or weakness of motion
- Be aware that atrophy of the rotator cuff muscles may be present

Stage 2
- Condition is typically seen in individuals between 25 and 40 years old
- Marked reactive tendinitis with significant pain between 70 and 120° abduction
- Inflammation may affect the biceps brachii tendon and subacromial bursa, leading to thickening and fibrotic changes in the structures
- Limited range of motion in external rotation and abduction
- Possible clicking sounds on resisted adduction and internal rotation

Stage 3
- History of chronic, long-term shoulder pain with significant weakness
- Rotator cuff tear is usually less than 1 centimeter
- May have prominent capsular laxity with multidirectional instability
- Noticeable atrophy of the supraspinatus and infraspinatus muscles
- Arthroscopy may show a damaged labrum

Stage 4
- Rotator cuff tear is greater than 1 centimeter

FIELD STRATEGY 11.3   MANAGEMENT OF AN IMPINGEMENT INJURY

- Use cryotherapy initially; later contrast with moist heat therapy twice a day.
- EMS, interferential current, and TENS may be helpful for pain management.
- Use ultrasound and NSAIDs to reduce inflammation.
- Use selective rest. Concentrate on motions that do not cause pain for 4 to 6 weeks. Avoid abduction above 90°.
- Study skill technique and correct movements that produce shoulder stress.
- Eliminate partner stretching, overhead training, and for swimmers, use of hand paddles.
- Wand and T-bar exercises can improve sport-specific mobility, but should not encourage hypermobility.
- Perform pain-free isometric and Theraband exercises to maintain muscle tone at least two to three times daily. Use low weights and high repetitions.
- Strengthen the lateral rotators (infraspinatus, teres minor) to control superior displacement of the humeral head.
- After 4 to 6 weeks, incorporate isokinetics at high speeds, and Theraband exercises in diagonal patterns.
- Begin a gradual return to activity, as long as the symptoms do not recur.

---

and tennis players. Located between the coracoacromial ligament and the underlying supraspinatus muscle, this bursa provides the shoulder with some inherent gliding ability (Figure 11.4). During an overhead throwing motion, this bursa can become impinged in the subacromial space.

➤ **SIGNS AND SYMPTOMS**

Frequently, sudden shoulder pain is reported during the initiation and acceleration of the throwing motion. Point tenderness can be elicited on the anterior and lateral edges of the acromion process. A painful arc will exist between 70 and 120° of passive abduction. Inability to sleep, especially on the affected side, occurs because of forced scapular protraction that leads to further impingement of the bursa. Pain is often referred to the distal deltoid attachment.

➤ **MANAGEMENT**

Standard acute protocol is followed by referral to a physician. A physician may inject a corticosteroid solution into the subacromial space to relieve the symptoms. In addition, other underlying conditions such as a rotator cuff tear, impingement syndrome, or bicipital tendinitis must be ruled out. Treatment is symptomatic and is the same as for a rotator cuff strain or impingement syndrome.

Bicipital Tendinitis

Injury to the biceps brachii tendon often occurs from repetitive overuse during rapid overhead movements involving excessive elbow flexion and supination activities, such as those performed by racquet sport players, shot-putters, baseball/softball pitchers, football quarterbacks, swimmers, and javelin throwers. Irritation of the tendon occurs as it passes back and forth in the intertubercular (bicipital) groove of the humerus, or it may partially sublux due to laxity of the traverse humeral ligament, a poorly developed

lesser tubercle, or both. A direct blow to the tendon or tendon sheath can lead to bicipital tenosynovitis. Anterior impingement syndrome associated with overhead rotational activity may also damage the tendon.

➤ **SIGNS AND SYMPTOMS**

Pain and tenderness is present over the bicipital groove when the shoulder is internally and externally rotated. In internal rotation, the pain stays medial; in external rotation, the pain is located in the midline or just lateral to the groove. Pain may also be elicited when the tendon is passively stretched in extreme shoulder extension with the elbow extended and forearm pronated. Resisted supination of a flexed elbow while externally rotating the shoulder (Yergason's test) will increase pain, as will forward shoulder flexion of the extended, supinated elbow (Speed's test).

➤ **MANAGEMENT**

Treatment involves restriction of rotational activities that exacerbate symptoms. Because of potential vascular impingement of the biceps tendon when the shoulder is at the side, the arm should be propped or wedged into slight abduction if immobilized in a sling. In early stages, cryotherapy, NSAIDs, ultrasound, EMS, or interferential therapy can control inflammation. Icing before and after activity is combined with a gradual program of stretching and strengthening as soon as pain subsides.

Biceps Tendon Rupture

Prolonged tendinitis can make the tendon vulnerable to forceful rupture during repetitive overhead motions, commonly seen in swimmers, or in forceful flexion activities against excessive resistance, as in weight lifters or gymnasts. The rupture occurs as a result of the avascular portion of the proximal tendon constantly passing over the head of the humerus during arm motion. This condition is often seen in degenerative tendons in older individuals, and in those who have had previous corticosteroid injections into the tendon.

➤ SIGNS AND SYMPTOMS

The individual will often hear and feel a snapping sensation, and experience intense pain. Ecchymosis and a visible, palpable defect can be seen in the muscle belly when the individual flexes the biceps **(Figure 11.17)**. If the muscle mass moves distally as a result of a proximal long-head rupture, a "Popeye" appearance is clearly visible. Partial ruptures may produce only slight muscular deformity but will still be associated with pain and weakness in elbow flexion and supination.

➤ MANAGEMENT

Standard acute care protocol is followed by immediate referral to a physician. Surgical repair is not usually suggested for the noncompetitive athlete or older participant, as return to normal sport activity can occur after completing an appropriate rehabilitation program. Surgical repair and fixation is, however, indicated for competitive athletes in order to restore elbow flexion and forearm supination strength needed for competitive sports participation.

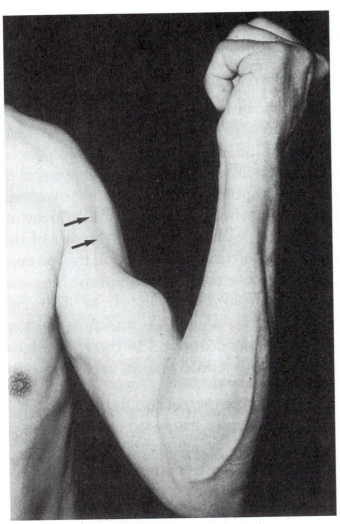

➤ **FIGURE 11.17** Biceps tendon rupture.

> ➤➤ **Box 11.5**
>
> ## Conditions Associated with Thoracic Outlet Syndrome
>
> - Compression of the medial cord of the brachial plexus
> - Compression of the subclavian artery and vein
> - Cervical rib syndrome
> - Scalenus-anterior syndrome
> - Hyperabduction syndrome
> - Costoclavicular space syndrome
> - Poor posture with drooping shoulders

Thoracic Outlet Compression Syndrome

Thoracic outlet compression syndrome is a condition in which nerves and/or vessels become compressed in the proximal neck or the axilla **(Figure 11.18)**. There are two clearly defined forms of this condition. One is a neurologic syndrome that involves the lower trunk of the brachial plexus and is caused by abnormal nerve stretch or compression. Another is a vascular form that involves the subclavian artery and vein, and is more common in men than in women. These and other disorders associated with thoracic outlet syndrome are listed in **Box 11.5**. The condition is often aggravated in activities that require overhead rotational stresses while muscles are loaded, such as weight lifting and swimming.

➤ SIGNS AND SYMPTOMS

If a nerve is compressed, an aching pain, pins-and-needles sensation, or numbness in the side or back of the neck extends across the shoulder down the medial arm to the ulnar aspect of the hand (ulnar nerve distribution). Weakness in grasp and atrophy of the hand muscles may also be present. If arterial or venous vessels are compressed, signs and symptoms vary depending on the specific structure being obstructed. Blockage of the subclavian vein produces edema, stiffness (especially in the hand), and venous engorgement of the arm with cyanosis. If untreated, this may result in thrombophlebitis. The athlete may present these signs and symptoms several hours after a bout of intense exercise. Occlusion of the subclavian artery results in a rapid onset of coolness, numbness in the entire arm, and fatigue after exertional overhead activity. The radial pulse may be obliterated while performing the Adson test, Allen test, or the costoclavicular syndrome (military brace) test. A detailed history is needed, and it is essential to evaluate the cervical spine, shoulder, elbow, and hand for evidence of neural compression. Instability of the shoulder should also be ruled out, and a postural assessment should be conducted.

➤ MANAGEMENT

Immediate referral to a physician is necessary for more extensive assessment to rule out serious vascular involvement. Conservative treatment involves assessing muscle strength and posture. Noted deficits should lead to an

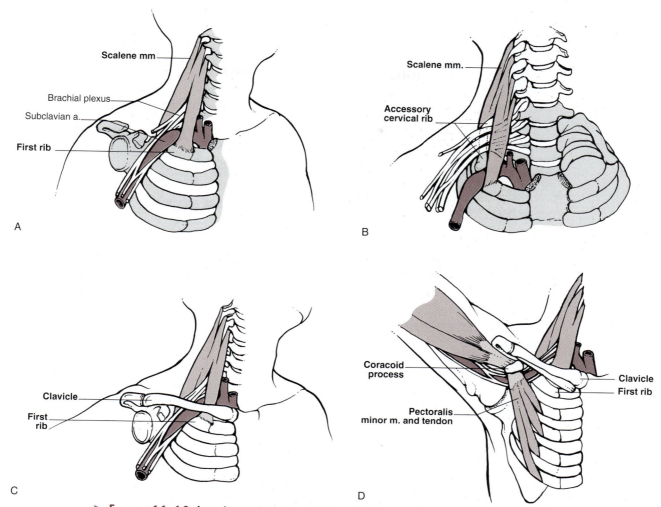

➤ FIGURE 11.18 **Location and etiology of thoracic outlet syndrome**. A, Scalenus anterior syndrome. B, Cervical rib syndrome. C, Costoclavicular space syndrome. D, Hyperabduction syndrome.

appropriate retraining program to develop strength and muscle balance in the shoulder girdle and facilitate the maintenance of a corrected posture. If the condition was precipitated by a sudden increase in activity, treatment involves anti-inflammatory medication, activity modification, and a reassessment of the training program. Return to full activity may occur after range of motion and strength in the shoulder musculature have been regained.

 The swimmer felt that the humeral head was "going out" of the socket and was accompanied by a snapping or catching sensation during the pull phase of the freestyle stroke. An anterior subluxation of the joint may be present due to chronic damage of the anteroinferior lip of the glenoid labrum. The supraspinatus tendon may also be injured. This individual should be referred to the team physician for further care.

FRACTURES

 A young gymnast lost her balance on a dismount and fell on an outstretched arm. She immediately felt intense pain in the shoulder region and is now unable to move the arm. The shoulder appears to sag down and forward, and there is a noticeable bump in the midclavicular region. What possible condition might you suspect? How should the injury be managed?

Most fractures to the shoulder region result from a fall on the point of the shoulder, rolling over onto the top of the shoulder, or indirectly, by falling on an outstretched arm. Clavicular fractures are more common than fractures to the scapula and proximal humerus, with nearly 80% occurring in the midclavicular region (10).

Clavicular Fractures

Because of the S-shaped configuration of the clavicle, it is highly susceptible to compressive forces caused by a blow or fall on the point of the shoulder, a direct blow to the bone by an opponent or object, or falling on an outstretched arm. Activities that have a high incidence of clavicular injury include ice hockey, football, martial arts, lacrosse, gymnas-

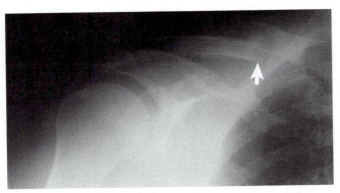

➤ FIGURE 11.19 Midclavicular fracture. The arrow indicates the fracture site.

tics, weight lifting, wrestling, racquetball, squash, and bicycling.

➤ SIGNS AND SYMPTOMS

The sternocleidomastoid muscle pulls the proximal bone fragment upward, allowing the distal shoulder to collapse downward and medially from the force of gravity and the pull of the pectoralis major muscle **(Figure 11.19)**. Swelling, ecchymosis, and a deformity may be visible and palpable at the fracture site. Greenstick fractures, typically seen in adolescents, will also produce a noticeable deformity. Pain occurs with any shoulder motion, and may radiate into the trapezius area. In older adults, fractures of the distal clavicle may involve tears of the coracoclavicular ligament, resulting in an increased deformity. Complications, although rare, may arise if bony fragments penetrate local arteries or nerves.

➤ MANAGEMENT

Immediate treatment involves immobilization in a sling and swathe. After assessment by the physician, a figure-eight brace or strapping is used to pull the shoulder backward and upward for 4 to 6 weeks in young adults and 6 or more weeks in older adults **(Figure 11.20)**. Although this immobilization prevents movement in nearly all planes,

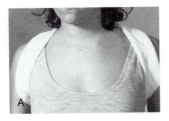

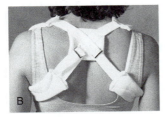

➤ FIGURE 11.20 Figure-eight clavicular straps. A, Anterior view. B, Posterior view.

it will not prevent scapular elevation. As a result, healing may be delayed and an excessive callus formation may form at the fracture site. This bump tends to remodel to some degree over a period of years but may never completely disappear. After immobilization, gentle isometric and mobilization exercises should begin with gradual return to sports.

Scapular Fractures

Scapular fractures may involve the body of the scapula, the spine of the scapula, the acromion process, the coracoid process, or the glenohumeral joint. Avulsion fractures to the coracoid process result from direct trauma, or forceful contraction of the pectoralis minor or short head of the biceps brachii. Fractures to the glenoid area are associated with shoulder subluxations and dislocations. In this case, treatment is dictated by the shoulder dislocation rather than the fracture, and often requires open reduction and internal fixation or shoulder reconstruction.

➤ SIGNS AND SYMPTOMS

Most fractures result in minimal displacement and exhibit localized hemorrhage, pain, and tenderness. It is critical, however, to rule out underlying pulmonary injury (e.g., pneumothorax or hemothorax) resulting from a possible accompanying rib fracture. The individual is reluctant to move the injured arm and prefers to maintain it in adduction.

➤ MANAGEMENT

The arm should be immediately immobilized in a sling and swathe and referred to a physician. Cryotherapy is used during the first 48 hours to minimize hematoma formation. Complications may arise from scarring and adhesions in the muscles overlying the scapula. Other muscles in the region must then compensate for this limited scapular motion, leading to overuse injuries. The amount of adhesions in the area can be reduced with an early program of passive and active stretching exercises.

Epiphyseal and Avulsion Fractures

Strength of the epiphyseal plate is only one-fifth that of the joint capsule and supporting ligaments (10). Epiphyseal centers around the shoulder region remain unfused for a longer span of time than is typically seen at other epiphyseal sites. For example, the medial clavicular growth plate does not close until age 25, and is often misdiagnosed as a sternoclavicular subluxation/dislocation. The proximal humeral epiphysis does not close until age 18 to 21 years of age. An epiphyseal fracture at this site, called **little league shoulder**, is often caused by repetitive medial rotation and adduction traction forces placed on the shoulder during pitching **(Figure 11.21)**. Catchers may also get this fracture since they throw the ball as hard and often as pitchers, but with less of a windup. The injury usually occurs during

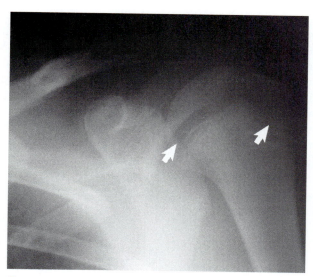

➤ FIGURE 11.21 **Epiphyseal fracture to the proximal humeral growth center**. The arrows indicate the fracture site.

the deceleration and follow-through phases of throwing or pitching.

Avulsion fractures to the coracoid process can be seen in a young individual when forceful, repetitive throwing places too much stress on the growth plate. Fractures of the greater and lesser tubercle are often associated with anterior and posterior glenohumeral dislocations, respectively. When the tubercle cannot be maintained in a stable position, open reduction and internal fixation is often required.

➤ SIGNS AND SYMPTOMS

With an epiphyseal fracture, the athlete will complain of acute shoulder pain when attempting to throw hard, which, if ignored, may result in an acute displacement of the weakened physis. Pain may be elicited with deep palpation in the axilla. With an avulsion fracture, pain can be elicited by deep palpation over the specific bony landmark.

➤ MANAGEMENT

 The arm should be immobilized in a sling and swathe. Apply ice to control pain and swelling, and refer the athlete immediately to a physician for further care.

Radiographs are necessary to see the widened epiphyseal line and demineralization. Treatment is conservative with symptoms disappearing after 3 to 4 weeks of rest. If activity is resumed too quickly, the condition may recur.

Humeral Fractures

Humeral fractures result from violent compressive forces from a direct blow, a fall on the upper arm, or a fall on an outstretched hand with the elbow extended. The surgical neck is the most common site for proximal humeral fractures, and may display an appearance similar to a dislocation (**Figure 11.22**).

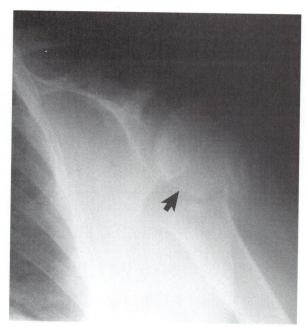

➤ FIGURE 11.22 **Fracture to the surgical neck of the humerus**. The arrow indicates the fracture site.

➤ SIGNS AND SYMPTOMS

Pain, swelling, hemorrhage, discoloration, an inability to move the arm, an inability to supinate the forearm, and possible paralysis may be present. The arm is often held splinted against the body.

➤ MANAGEMENT

 The arm should be immobilized in a sling and swathe. Apply ice to control pain and swelling, and refer the athlete immediately to a physician for further care.

Fortunately, these fractures are often impacted, which facilitates closed reduction and allows early mobilization after 3 to 4 weeks of immobilization. Early complications of fracture to the proximal humerus include brachial plexus injury and/or vascular injury. Late complications include shoulder stiffness, malunion, nonunion, avascular necrosis, and myositis ossificans.

 After falling on an outstretched arm, the gymnast's shoulder appeared to sag down and forward, and had a visible bump in the midclavicular region. Any shoulder movement caused severe pain. These signs indicate a possible clavicular fracture. The arm should be immobilized with a sling and swathe, and the athlete should be transported to the nearest physician for further care.

ASSESSMENT

 A volleyball player is complaining of pain in the right arm every time the arm is abducted above 90°. Pain is localized on the anterior shoulder and aggravated with horizontal adduction. What

biomechanical factors are involved in this injury? How will you assess this individual?

The shoulder complex is a complicated region to assess because of the number of important structures located in such a small area. Furthermore, the biomechanical demands on each structure during overhead motion are not fully understood, so identification of all injured structures is difficult. As a result, each joint must be methodically assessed to determine limitation of function. Improper bio-mechanical skill technique is a leading cause of many acute and overuse injuries at the shoulder. Assessment of the individual's sport-specific techniques may determine if improper technique contributed to the injury. By correcting minor mechanical flaws in technique and identifying flexibility and strength deficits, many shoulder injuries can be prevented. It is also important to remember pain may be referred from the cervical region, heart, spleen, lungs, and other internal organs to the shoulder region. **Field Strategy 11.4** summarizes a shoulder assessment.

 FIELD STRATEGY 11.4   SHOULDER ASSESSMENT HISTORY

HISTORY

- Primary complaint including:
  Current nature, location, and onset of the condition
- Mechanism of injury
  Cause of stress; position of neck, shoulder, and arm; direction of force
  Changes in throwing style, equipment, overhead motion techniques, or conditioning modes
- Characteristics of the symptoms
  Evolution of the onset, nature, location, severity, and duration of pain and weakness
- Disability resulting from the injury
- Related medical history
  Previous injuries to the area, congenital abnormalities, or family history

OBSERVATION AND INSPECTION

- Observation should analyze:
  Overall appearance
  Posture and body symmetry
  Scapulae position on posterior chest wall
- Inspection at the injury site for:
  Deformity, swelling, discoloration, hypertrophy, or muscle atrophy in the supraspinatus and infraspinatus, or visible congenital deformity

PALPATION

- Bony structures to determine a possible fracture
- Soft tissue structures for skin temperature, swelling, point tenderness, crepitus, deformity, muscle spasm, cutaneous sensation, and pulse

FUNCTIONAL TESTS

- Active movement
- Passive movement and end feels
- Resisted movement

STRESS TESTS

- Serratus anterior weakness
- Sternoclavicular joint instability
- Acromioclavicular joint instability
- Glenohumeral joint instability
- Glenoid labrum pathology
- Rotator cuff pathology and impingement syndrome
- Biceps brachii pathology
- Thoracic outlet compression syndrome tests

NEUROLOGIC TESTS

- Myotomes
- Reflexes
- Dermatome

SPORT-SPECIFIC FUNCTIONAL TESTS

HISTORY

 What information should be gathered from the volleyball player complaining of anterior shoulder pain during shoulder abduction and horizontal adduction?

Questions about a shoulder injury should focus on the current primary complaint, past injuries to the region, and other factors that may have contributed to the current problem (referred pain, alterations in posture, change in technique, or overuse). Many conditions may be related to family history, age, improper biomechanical execution of skills, and recent changes in training programs. Questions should be open-ended to allow the individual to fully describe the injury. Because the shoulder and upper arm are common sites for referred pain from orthopedic or visceral origins, a complete examination of the cervical spine, thorax, and abdomen may be indicated, particularly when the athlete presents a vague history of injury to the shoulder girdle. In addition to the general questions discussed in Chapter 4, specific questions related to the shoulder region can be seen in **Field Strategy 11.5**.

 The volleyball player is midway through the competitive season. During the day, he directs the swimming program at a local health club and

swims 3 to 5 miles/day. The pain started gradually 2 months ago, but now it hurts to raise the arm and wakes him up at night when he sleeps on the affected side. Although he has had a sore shoulder numerous times before, he has never seen a physician.

OBSERVATION AND INSPECTION

 After taking a thorough history, what specific factors should be observed in the postural exam and during inspection of the injury site?

On-the-field assessment may be somewhat limited because uniforms and protective equipment may obscure the region from observation and assessment. Initially, you may have to slide your hands under the pads to palpate the region and determine the presence of a possible fracture or major ligament damage. If necessary, the pads could be cut and gently removed to more fully expose the area. After the initial exam, the individual may need to be removed from the field to complete a more comprehensive assessment in the examination room.

In an ideal clinic situation, women should wear a bathing suit or halter top so the entire shoulder and arm can be fully exposed. Complete a postural exam, looking for

---

 FIELD STRATEGY 11.5   DEVELOPING A HISTORY OF THE INJURY

<u>CURRENT INJURY STATUS</u>

1. Where is the pain (or weakness) located? How would you rate the pain (weakness)? What type of pain is it (dull ache, throbbing, sharp, intermittent, red-hot, burning, or radiating)?
2. Did the pain come on suddenly (acute) or gradually (overuse)? Was the pain greatest when the injury first occurred, or did it get worse the second or third day?
3. (If acute, ask:) What were you doing at the time of the injury? Was there a direct blow? Did you fall? How (outstretched arm, rolling over the shoulder or side of the shoulder)? (If chronic, ask:) What different activities have you been doing in the last week? (Look for changes in technique, frequency, duration, intensity, or changes in equipment.)
4. Did you hear any sounds during the incident? Any snaps, pops, or cracks? Did you notice any swelling, discoloration, muscle spasms, or numbness with the injury?
5. What actions or motions bring on the pain? It is worse in the morning, during activity, after activity, or at night? Does it wake you up at night? In what part of the arm motion does it hurt the worst? Does the arm tire easily? When the pain sets in, how long does it last?
6. Are there certain activities you are unable to perform because of the pain? Which ones?
7. What has been done for the condition?
8. How old are you? (Remember that many shoulder problems are age-related.) Which hand is dominant?

<u>PAST INJURY STATUS</u>

1. Have you ever injured your shoulder before? How did that occur? What was done for the injury? Did you have any difficulty returning to your full functional status?
2. Have you had any medical problems recently? (Look for problems that may refer pain to the area.) Are you on any medication?

faulty posture or congenital abnormalities that could place additional strain on the anatomical structures. The individual should be viewed from the anterior, lateral, and posterior views. The position of the head should be noted. A head that is tilted or rotated may suggest a muscle spasm, pressure on a cervical nerve root, or stretching of the cervical nerves. The position of the scapulae on the chest wall should also be noted. The base of the spine of the scapula should be at the T4 level, and the inferior pole of the scapula should be at the T7 level. The medial borders should be an equal distance from the vertebral spinous processes. Is the medial border elevated (winged) off the chest wall? With a chronic or acutely weakened serratus anterior muscle, the affected side will usually be depressed (lower on the chest wall), protracted (further from the vertebral spinous processes), and elevated (winged) off the chest wall, all reflecting a weakened muscle in spasm or one with decreased flexibility. The position of the arm should be noted. Is it splinted alongside the body, or does it simply hang limp at the side? A painful shoulder is often held in an elevated position by the athlete. During movement, assess the athlete's willingness to move the involved arm, and the symmetry and fluid scapular motion. Inspection should be performed at the specific injury site, looking for obvious deformity, swelling, discoloration, symmetry, hypertrophy, muscle atrophy, or previous surgical incisions. The affected limb should always be compared with the unaffected limb. Specific areas to focus on in this region are summarized in **Field Strategy 11.6**.

 No anomalies are observed during the postural exam. Slight swelling is present on the anterior lip of the acromion process and over the bicipital groove.

PALPATION

 Pain and swelling appear to be confined to the anterior shoulder. Where should palpation begin, and what specific factors are you looking for?

Bilateral palpation can determine temperature, swelling, point tenderness, crepitus, deformity, muscle spasm, and cutaneous sensation. Increased skin temperature could indicate inflammation or infection. Decreased skin temperature could indicate a reduction in circulation. Swelling should be differentiated between localized extra-articular swelling and joint effusion. In the shoulder, intra-articular swelling would prevent full adduction of the arm against the body. Crepitus may indicate an inflamed subacromial bursa, bicipital tenosynovitis, or an irregular articular surface. Vascular pulses can be taken at the radial and ulnar arteries in the wrist, brachial artery on the medial arm, or axillary artery in the armpit.

 FIELD STRATEGY 11.6 **POSTURAL ASSESSMENT OF THE SHOULDER REGION**

ANTERIOR VIEW

1. Check that the neck and head are in the midline of the body.
2. Follow the clavicles distally and note any deformity that may indicate a possible fracture.
3. Look to make sure both shoulders have a well-rounded deltoid cap with no prominent acromion process present.
4. Check the level of the shoulders. The dominant side will usually be lower than the nondominant side.
5. Note the color of the hand. This may indicate a vascular problem.

POSTERIOR VIEW

1. Note any abnormal prominence of bony structures or muscle atrophy in the supraspinatus or infraspinatus. Are the scapulae at the same height and resting at the same angle? Are the medial borders an equal distance away from the spinous processes?
2. Are the spines of the two scapula and inferior angles bilaterally even? (The base of the spine should be at the T4 level; the inferior angle at the T7 level.)
3. Note any "winging" of the scapula.
4. Note the presence of any scoliosis, or lateral curvature, of the spine.
5. Note any scars or muscular atrophy, particularly in the supraspinatus or infraspinatus.
6. Is there any swelling or discoloration present?

LATERAL VIEW

1. Note the attitude of the head and neck in relation to the shoulders. Is the head jutting forward or backward?
2. Note any kyphosis (rounded shoulders).

Fractures can be assessed through palpation of pain at the fracture site, compression of the humeral head against the glenoid fossa, compression along the long axis of the humerus, percussion on a specific bony landmark, or by using a tuning fork. If a fracture or dislocation is suspected, circulatory and neural integrity distal to the site should be assessed immediately. This can be performed by taking a pulse at the sites indicated above and stroking the palm and dorsum of both hands to determine the presence of similar findings.

If a fracture is suspected, immobilize the extremity in an appropriate sling or splint, monitor vital signs, and activate EMS, if necessary, to transport the individual to the nearest medical facility.

Stand behind the individual to begin bilateral palpation, moving proximal to distal. The following structures should be palpated, leaving the most painful area for last.

Anterior Palpation

1. Sternocleidomastoid muscle
2. Sternoclavicular joint, interclavicular ligament, sternoclavicular ligament, and sternal end of the clavicle
3. Clavicle and costoclavicular ligament
4. AC joint, acromion process, and acromioclavicular ligament
5. Coracoid process, pectoralis minor, short head of the biceps brachii, and coracoacromial ligament
6. Pectoralis major and anterior deltoid muscle
7. Greater tuberosity and the distal attachments of the supraspinatus, infraspinatus, and teres minor
8. Biceps brachii muscle and tendon. Palpate the bicipital groove with the arm in external rotation. The lesser tubercle is medial to the groove where the subscapularis is attached
9. With the arm extended, the subacromial bursa and supraspinatus tendon

Lateral Palpation

1. Middle deltoid muscle and greater tubercle
2. Glenohumeral capsule

Posterior Palpation

1. Posterior deltoid and trapezius muscles
2. Spine of the scapula, medial and lateral borders, and inferior angle
3. Rhomboid muscles, latissimus dorsi, serratus anterior, levator scapulae, and scaleni

 Crepitus and point tenderness were elicited just anterior to the acromion process when the arm was passively flexed and extended. The bicipital groove was also point tender. The anterior shoul-

der was warm to the touch, and swelling was noted anterior to the acromion process and over the bicipital groove.

PHYSICAL EXAMINATION TESTS

 There are several painful areas. How will you determine what structures have been injured, and how severe this injury is?

The athlete should always be placed in a comfortable position for the physical examination. Depending on the history, some tests are compulsory, while others may be used to confirm or exclude tests. Proceed cautiously through the assessment, and always compare the injured limb with the noninjured limb.

Functional Tests

The athletic trainer must remember that the arm and shoulder may act as an open kinetic chain when the hand is free to move or as a closed kinetic chain when the hand is fixed to a relatively immovable object. Depending on the sport-specific skills performed by the athlete and when the pain occurs, the components of the kinetic chain can have different effects on the shoulder. The first movements to be performed are active movements.

ACTIVE MOVEMENTS

Active movements may be performed in a seated or prone position, with the most painful movements done last. Since pain is frequently referred from the cervical region into the shoulder, active range of motion (AROM) should be performed initially at the neck. Neck flexion, extension, rotation, and lateral flexion should be assessed for fluid motion and presence of pain. If pain is elicited on active motion at the neck, a full neck evaluation should be completed.

 If findings are significant, the neck should be immobilized in a cervical collar and EMS should be activated to transport the athlete to the nearest medical facility.

If no problems are noted during neck movement, continue with the shoulder evaluation. The individual should perform gross movement patterns at the shoulder. The arms should be viewed from an anterior and posterior view. When standing behind the individual, make sure the scapula and humerus move together in a freely coordinated motion. To facilitate active movement, Apley's Scratch Test is used to measure gross movement patterns at the shoulder and arm **(Figure 11.23)**.

The advantage of these simple tests is that they quickly assess bilateral symmetry in gross motor movements. Any deficit can be easily seen and investigated in further detail.

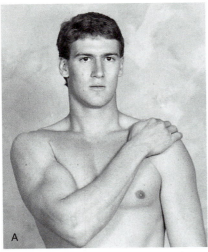
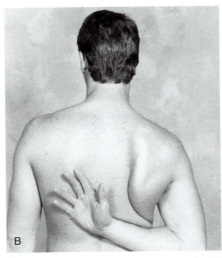
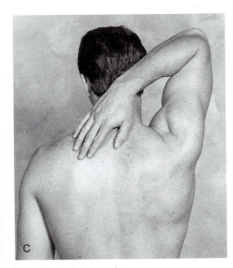

➤ FIGURE 11.23 Apley's scratch test. A, Medial rotation and adduction. The athlete reaches in front of the head to touch the opposite shoulder. B, Medial rotation, extension, and adduction. The athlete reaches behind the back to touch the inferior angle of the opposite scapula. C, Abduction, flexion, and lateral rotation. The athlete reaches behind the head to touch the superior angle of the opposite scapula.

The individual motions listed below can also be assessed at the shoulder. The numbers in parentheses are normal ranges of motion for each movement.

- Shoulder abduction (170 to 180°)
- Shoulder flexion (160 to 180°)
- Shoulder extension (50 to 60°)
- Lateral or external rotation (80 to 90°)
- Medial or internal rotation (60 to 100°)
- Adduction (50 to 70°)
- Horizontal abduction/adduction (130°)
- Upward/downward rotation of the scapula

Goniometry measurements for the glenohumeral joint are illustrated in **Figure 11.24**.

PASSIVE RANGE OF MOTION

If the individual is able to perform full range of motion during active movements, apply gentle pressure at the extremes of motion to determine end feel. Tissue stretch is the normal end feel for shoulder flexion, extension, lateral rotation, medial rotation, abduction, and horizontal abduction; adduction is tissue approximation. Horizontal adduction can be tissue stretch or tissue approximation. Abduction of the shoulder can be bone to bone or tissue stretch.

RESISTED MUSCLE TESTING

The hip and trunk should be stabilized during muscle testing to prevent any muscle substitution. Begin with the muscle on stretch and apply resistance throughout the full range of motion. As the athletic trainer moves through the various motions, he or she should begin with gentle stress, and ask the athlete to perform the motion several times to note any weakness or fatigue. It is common at the shoulder

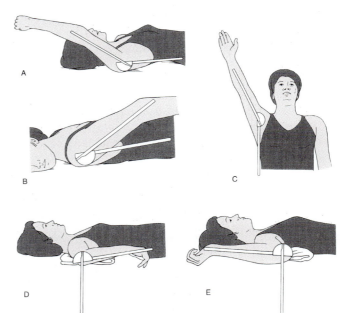

➤ FIGURE 11.24 Goniometry measurements. A, Shoulder flexion. Align the proximal arm with the midaxillary line of the thorax with the fulcrum close to the acromion process. Align the distal arm along the humerus in line with the lateral epicondyle of the humerus. B, Shoulder extension. Use the same landmarks used for shoulder flexion. C, Shoulder abduction. The proximal arm is parallel to the midline of the sternum with the fulcrum close to the acromion process. Align the distal arm with the humerus using the medial epicondyle for reference. D–E, Lateral and medial rotation. Flex the elbow at 90° with the fulcrum centered over the olecranon process. The proximal arm is placed perpendicular to the floor with the distal arm aligned with the olecranon process and ulnar styloid process.

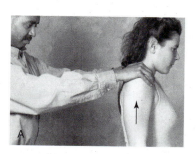
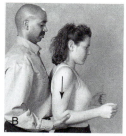
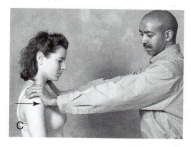
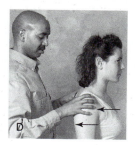

➤ FIGURE 11.25 **Manual muscle testing for the scapula.** Myotomes are listed in parentheses. A, Elevation (C4). B, Depression. C, Protraction. D, Retraction. Arrows indicate the direction the athlete moves the scapula against applied resistance.

to have painful arcs. Therefore, it is important to move the extremity throughout the full range of motion, and note if movement through an isolated range of motion is particularly painful. Avoid any sudden or jarring motions, as this may lead to undue pain. Note any lag, muscle weakness, or painful arc. Delay working those muscles that cause extreme pain until the final phase of muscle testing. **Figure 11.25** demonstrates resisted scapular motions to be tested, and **Figure 11.26** demonstrates glenohumeral and elbow motions to be tested.

Stress Tests

At this point in the assessment, the history, observation, palpation, and functional testing should have established a strong suspicion of what structures may be damaged. In using stress tests, perform only those tests that are absolutely necessary **(Table 11.6)**. As the athletic trainer moves through the various functional tests, he or she should begin with gentle stress, and apply it several times to note any weakness or instability. It is common at the shoulder to

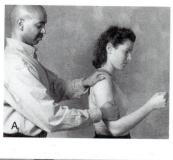
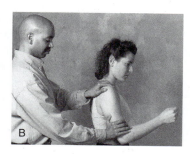
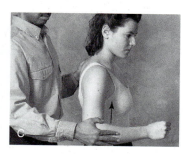
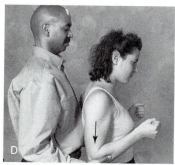
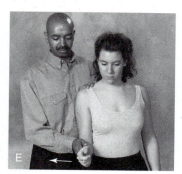
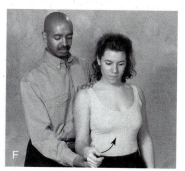
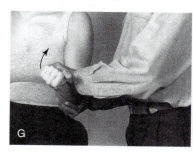
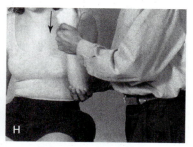

➤ FIGURE 11.26 **Manual muscle testing for the glenohumeral and elbow.** Myotomes are listed in parentheses. A, Flexion. B, Extension. C, Abduction (C5). D, Adduction. E, External or lateral rotation. F, Internal or medial rotation. G, Elbow flexion (C6). H, Elbow extension (C7). Arrows indicate the direction the athlete moves against applied resistance.

TABLE 11.6   COMMON SPECIAL TESTS PERFORMED AT THE SHOULDER

Sternoclavicular joint	Sternoclavicular instability test
Acromioclavicular joint	Acromioclavicular instability test Piano key test Acromioclavicular distraction/compression test
Glenohumeral instability, anterior	Apprehension test ("crank test") Relocation test Anterior load and shift test
Glenohumeral instability, posterior	Posterior load and shift test Posterior apprehension test
Glenohumeral instability, inferior	Sulcus sign
Labral lesions	Clunk test Compression rotation test
Impingement tests	Neer shoulder impingement test Anterior impingement test (Hawkins-Kennedy test)
Muscle tendon pathology	Serratus anterior weakness test Lift-off test for subscapularis Drop arm test Empty can (Centinela) supraspinatus test Transverse humeral ligament test Yergason's test Speed's test
Thoracic outlet syndrome	Adson's test Allen test Costoclavicular syndrome (military brace) test

have painful arcs. Therefore, it is important to move the extremity slowly throughout the full range of motion, and note if movement through an isolated range of motion is particularly painful. Avoid any sudden or jarring motions, as this may lead to undue pain.

STERNOCLAVICULAR INSTABILITY TEST

With the athlete in a seated position, the athletic trainer should apply pressure to the medial clavicular head to force the clavicle downward, upward, anteriorly, and posteriorly to determine any instability or increased pain. Pain present in all movements may stem from a SC sprain, damage to the SC joint disc, or a complete disruption

of the joint capsule, indicating a possible dislocation or subluxation of the joint.

ACROMIOCLAVICULAR INSTABILITY TEST

The athletic trainer should grasp the distal clavicle and apply pressure in all four directions to determine stability and any increase in pain. Pressure is then applied to the tip of the shoulder, which compresses the acromioclavicular joint and may also increase pain.

PIANO KEY SIGN

If a step deformity is noted at the AC joint, the athletic trainer should apply a downward pressure on the distal end of the clavicle. The pressure may produce a bobbing motion, which would indicate damage to the coracoclavicular ligament.

ACROMIOCLAVICULAR (AC) DISTRACTION/COMPRESSION

If the AC joint is unstable, downward traction on the upper extremity will lead to downward movement of the acromion process away from the clavicle. Assessment involves grasping the arm in one hand, and applying steady downward traction while palpating the joint with the other hand **(Figure 11.27A)**. A positive test will produce pain and/or joint movement. Horizontal adduction of the humerus across the chest compresses the AC joint and will also lead to increased pain if the joint is injured **(Figure 11.27B)**.

APPREHENSION TEST ("CRANK TEST") FOR ANTERIOR INSTABILITY

This test involves positioning the individual in a supine position and slowly abducting and externally rotating the individual's humerus **(Figure 11.28A)**. If the individual will not allow passive movement to the extremes of motion, or apprehension or alarm is shown in the facial expression, it is a positive sign for chronic anterior subluxation or dislocation of the glenohumeral joint. This motion should always be done slowly to prevent recurrence of a dislocation.

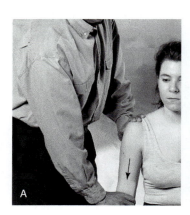
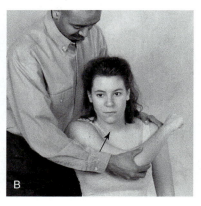

➤ **FIGURE 11.27 Acromioclavicular testing.** A, Acromioclavicular traction. B, Acromioclavicular compression. Arrows indicate the direction the athletic trainer moves the arm.

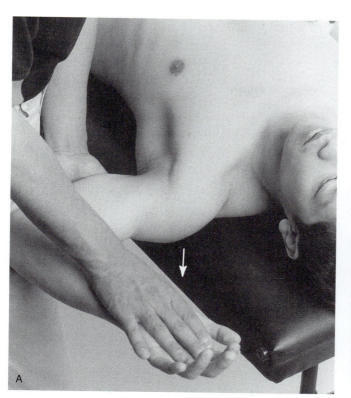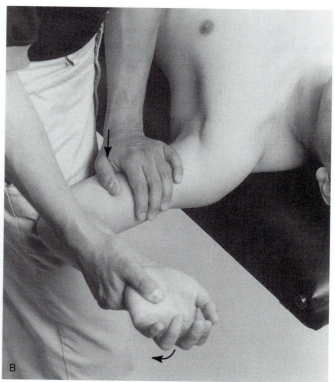

> **FIGURE 11.28 Glenohumeral anterior instability.** A, Apprehension or "crank" test. The athletic trainer applies abduction and lateral rotation to the arm. B, Relocation test. The athletic trainer applies abduction and lateral rotation combined with posterior translation of the humerus.

RELOCATION TEST FOR ANTERIOR INSTABILITY

Position for this test is identical to the apprehension test. If the athlete demonstrates a positive apprehension test, the athletic trainer slowly applies a posterior stress to the arm **(Figure 11.28B)**. The athlete's apprehension and pain should diminish, and further lateral rotation of the glenohumeral joint may be possible before the apprehension returns. This test is positive if pain decreases during the maneuver, even if there was no apprehension. If the arm is released (release test) in the newly acquired range, any pain and forward translation of the head indicates a positive sign. The resulting pain from this release procedure may be caused by anterior shoulder instability, labral lesion (Bankart lesion or SLAP lesion superior labrum, anterior-posterior), or bicipital tendinitis. This release should be done slowly as it may dislocate the joint, leading to distrust on the part of the patient. Therefore, lateral rotation should be released before the posterior stress is released (14).

ANTERIOR LOAD AND SHIFT TEST

With the athlete seated and the hand of the test arm resting on the thigh, the athletic trainer stands or sits slightly behind the athlete and stabilizes the shoulder with one hand over the clavicle and scapula. The head of the

humerus is grasped with the other hand, placing the thumb over the posterior humeral head and the fingers over the anterior humeral head **(Figure 11.29)**. The athletic trainer then gently pushes the humerus into the glenoid to "seat" it properly in the glenoid fossa. This is the "load" portion of the test, and is necessary for true translation to occur. If the load is not applied, movement will be greater and the "feel" will be altered. While pushing the humeral head anteriorly (anterior instability) or posteriorly (posterior instability), the amount of translation should be noted. This is the "shift" portion of the test. Normally the head will translate 0 to 25% of the diameter of the humeral head. The test is positive if translation is between 25% and 50%, and the head feels as if it riding over the glenoid rim, but spontaneously reduces (14).

POSTERIOR LOAD AND SHIFT TEST

In a posterior load and shift test, posterior translation of 50% of the humeral head is considered normal. Differences between the normal and injured sides should be bilaterally compared in terms of the amount of translation and the ease with which it occurs. This comparison, along with the athlete's symptoms, is considered more important than the amount of movement occurring. If MDI is present, both anterior and posterior translation may be excessive

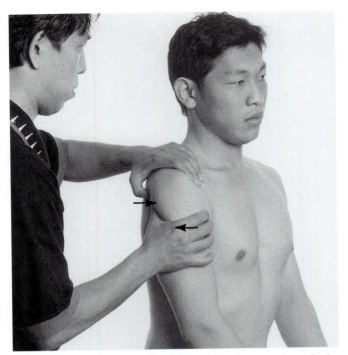

> ▶ FIGURE 11.29 **Load and shift test**. The humerus is pushed into the glenoid to "load" the humeral head. The athletic trainer then pushes the humeral head anteriorly (anterior instability) or posteriorly (posterior instability), noting the amount of "shift" or translation.

on the affected side as compared to the normal side. The test may also be done in a supine position.

POSTERIOR APPREHENSION TEST

With the athlete supine, the arm is moved into forward flexion and internal rotation as a steady downward force is applied on the elbow to drive the humeral head posteriorly on the glenoid fossa **(Figure 11.30)**. While applying the axial load, the athletic trainer horizontally adducts and medially rotates the arm. A positive test is indicated by a look of apprehension or alarm on the individual's face, or the athlete's resistance to further motion or the reproduction of the symptoms. Reproducing pain is more likely to occur than apprehension. A positive sign indicates a possible posterior dislocation.

SULCUS SIGN

Traction is applied to the humerus to determine the integrity of the supportive structures. If the space widens between the acromion process and humeral head, producing an indentation or "sulcus," this indicates a positive test for inferior instability. To differentiate this test from the AC distraction test, note that the humerus and scapula are distracted away from the clavicle in the AC distraction test, whereas in the sulcus test, only the humerus is distracted away from both the clavicle and scapula.

CLUNK TEST

With the athlete supine, one hand is placed on the posterior aspect of the shoulder under the humeral head. The humerus is grasped above the elbow and the arm is fully abducted over the athlete's head. The hand over the humeral head applies a slow push in an anterior direction, while the other hand moves the humerus into lateral rotation **(Figure 11.31A)**. A positive test results in a clunk or grinding sound, indicating a tear of the labrum. This test may also cause apprehension if anterior instability is present.

COMPRESSION ROTATION TEST

With the athlete supine, the arm is positioned at about 20° abduction, and the elbow is flexed. The humerus is slowly compressed into the glenoid fossa by pushing on the elbow with one hand while the other hand rotates the humerus medially and laterally **(Figure 11.31B)**. If a snapping or catching sensation is present when the humeral head is felt, the test is positive for a labral tear (Bankart or SLAP lesion).

NEER SHOULDER IMPINGEMENT TEST

With the athlete seated and the arm placed in anatomical position, the athlete's posterior shoulder is stabilized.

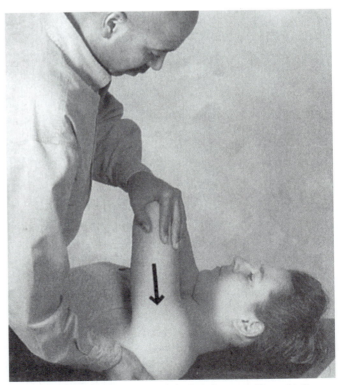

> ▶ FIGURE 11.30 **Posterior apprehension test**. The athletic trainer applies a steady downward force on the elbow to displace the humeral head posteriorly on the glenoid fossa.

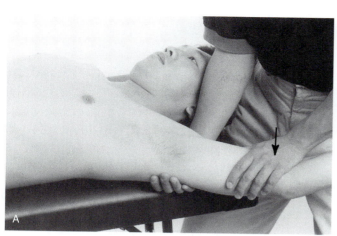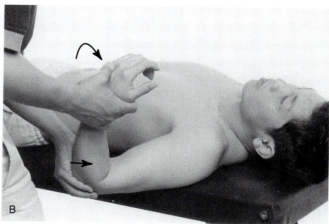

➤ FIGURE 11.31 **Glenoid labral pathology**. A, Clunk test. Using the hand placed under the humeral head, apply an anterior force while the other hand rotates the humerus into lateral rotation. B, Compression rotation test. With the arm slightly abducted and the elbow flexed, apply a compressive force along the long axis of the humerus while the other hand rotates the humerus medially and laterally.

The athlete's arm is grasped at the elbow joint, and the arm is passively moved through forward flexion (**Figure 11.32A**). The test is positive if pain occurs with motion, particularly near the end of the range of motion. A positive test indicates impingement of the supraspinatus or long head of the biceps tendon between the greater tuberosity of the humerus and the acromion process or coracoacromial arch.

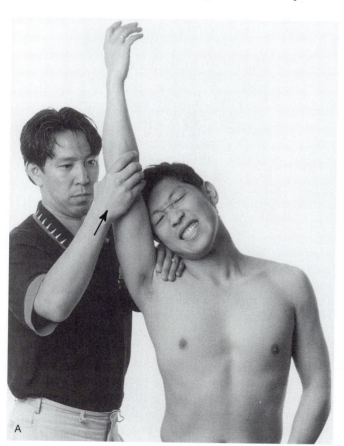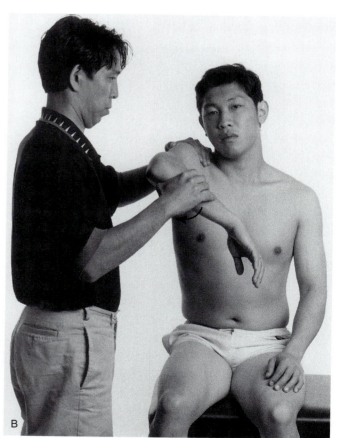

➤ FIGURE 11.32 **Anterior impingement tests**. A, Neer shoulder impingement test. The arm is internally rotated and forcibly flexed forward to jam the greater tuberosity against the anteroinferior surface of the acromion. B, Anterior impingement test. An alternative method is to forcibly medially rotate the proximal humerus when the arm is forward flexed to 90° (Hawkins-Kennedy impingement test).

ANTERIOR IMPINGEMENT TEST

This test involves internally rotating and abducting the humerus through shoulder flexion while depressing the scapula, thus jamming the greater tubercle underneath the anteroinferior border of the acromion process. The arm is returned to 90° of abduction (with the elbow flexed at 90°), and then horizontally adducted across the chest while maintaining internal rotation of the humerus **(Figure 11.32B)**. Pain or apprehension on the individual's face may indicate an overuse injury to the supraspinatus or biceps brachii tendon. This test is also called the Hawkins-Kennedy impingement test.

SERRATUS ANTERIOR WEAKNESS

Weakness of the serratus anterior, often called winging of the scapula, is determined by having the individual perform a push-up against the wall **(Figure 11.33)**. If the muscle is weak, or the long thoracic nerve is involved, the medial border of the scapula will pull away from the chest wall.

LIFT-OFF TEST FOR SUBSCAPULARIS

The athlete stands with the dorsum of the hand on the lumbar region of the back. The hand is then lifted

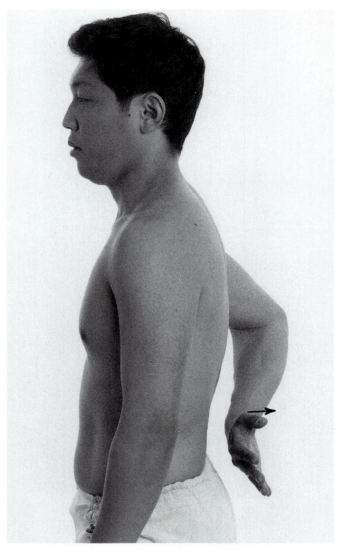

➤ **Figure 11.34 Lift-off test**. Failure to lift the hand away from the small of the back indicates a weakened subscapularis muscle, scapular instability, or weak rhomboids.

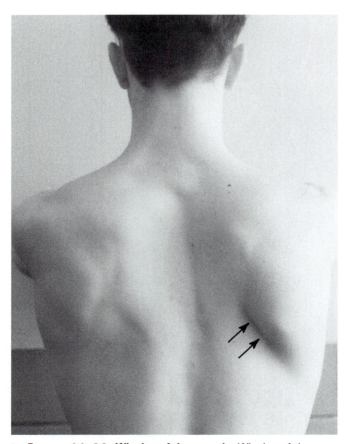

➤ **Figure 11.33 Winging of the scapula**. Winging of the scapula can result from weakness in the serratus anterior or injury to the long thoracic nerve. The arrows indicate the elevated vertebral border of the right scapula.

away from the back **(Figure 11.34)**. An inability to do this indicates a lesion of the subscapularis muscle. Abnormal motion of the scapula during the test indicates scapular instability. If the medial border of the scapula wings during the test, the rhomboids may also be affected.

DROP ARM TEST

To test the integrity of the supraspinatus muscle and tendon, the shoulder is abducted to 90° with no humeral rotation. The athlete is asked to slowly lower the arm to the side. If positive, the arm will not lower smoothly, or increased pain will occur during the motion. An alternative test is to abduct the arm again at 90° with no rotation, and ask the individual to hold that position. Apply downward resistance to the distal end of the humerus **(Figure 11.35A)**. A positive test is indicated if the individual is unable to maintain the arm in the abducted position.

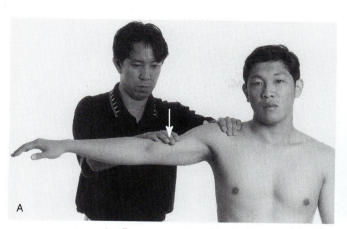
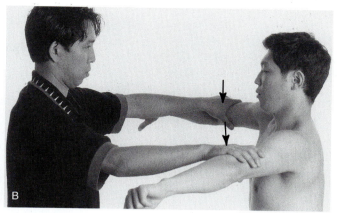

➤ FIGURE 11.35 **Supraspinatus testing.** A, Drop-arm test. Abduct the humerus to 90°. Apply mild downward pressure on the distal humerus. B, Empty can test. Horizontally adduct the arm approximately 30 to 60° with the humerus internally rotated. Apply mild downward pressure on the distal humerus.

EMPTY CAN (CENTINELA) TEST FOR SUPRASPINATUS PATHOLOGY

Both arms are positioned at 90° abduction. The arms are then horizontally adducted approximately 30° to 60°, and the humerus is internally rotated with the thumbs pointing downward ("empty can position") **(Figure 11.35B)**. The athletic trainer applies a downward pressure proximal to the elbow. Pain and/or weakness should be assessed. The arms should rebound to the 90° abducted position. A positive test indicates a tear to the supraspinatus muscle or tendon.

TRANSVERSE HUMERAL LIGAMENT TEST

To test for a torn transverse humeral ligament, place the shoulder in 90° of abduction and external rotation with the elbow flexed at 90°. The athletic trainer places the fingers over the bicipital groove. An audible and/or palpable snap, which may be accompanied by pain, will occur as the arm is moved into internal rotation **(Figure 11.36)**.

YERGASON'S TEST FOR BICIPITAL TENDINITIS

The athlete should be positioned with the elbow flexed at 90°, and the arm should be stabilized against the body with the forearm pronated. The athletic trainer asks the individual to supinate the forearm, flex the elbow, and externally rotate the humerus. Simultaneously, the athletic trainer resists the motion with one hand while applying downward traction on the elbow with the other hand **(Figure 11.37A)**. The test is positive if pain is elicited over the bicipital groove, or the tendon snaps out of the groove.

SPEED'S TEST FOR BICIPITAL TENDINITIS

In this test, the tendon moves over the bone during motion, rather than simply placing tension on it. This provides a more effective, accurate result than Yergason's

test. The arm is supinated with the elbow fully extended. The athletic trainer places one hand over the bicipital groove, and resists forward flexion of the arm with the other hand. A positive test will result in tenderness over the groove **(Figure 11.37B)**.

ADSON'S TEST FOR THORACIC OUTLET SYNDROME

The athletic trainer palpates the radial pulse. The individual turns the head toward the affected shoulder and extends the head while the athletic trainer slowly extends and laterally rotates the humerus **(Figure 11.38A)**. The

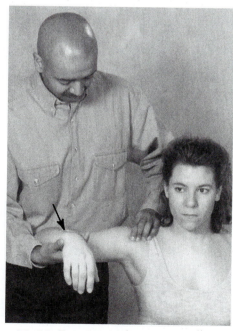

➤ FIGURE 11.36 **Transverse humeral ligament test.** Place the extended arm in 90° of abduction and external rotation. Place your fingers over the bicipital groove and move the arm into internal rotation. If positive, an audible or palpable snap, which may be accompanied by pain, will occur during internal rotation.

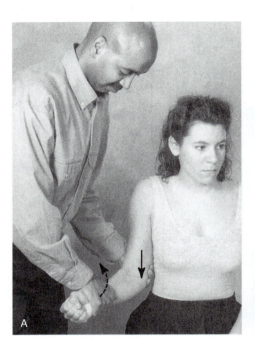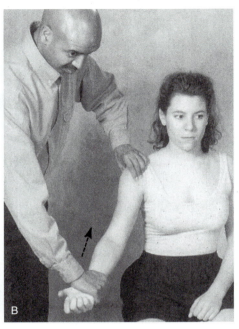

➤ FIGURE 11.37 Bicipital tendinitis. A, Yergason's test. Stabilize the flexed arm against the body with the forearm pronated. Ask the individual to supinate the forearm, flex the elbow, and externally rotate the humerus while you apply resistance. Simultaneously apply downward traction on the elbow with the other hand. B, Speed's test. Supinate the hand with the elbow fully extended. With one hand over the bicipital groove, resist forward flexion of the arm.

athletic trainer then instructs the athlete to take a deep breath and hold it. A diminished or absent pulse indicates a positive test verifying that the subclavian artery is being occluded between the anterior and middle scalene muscles. This is sometimes referred to as the anterior scalene syndrome test.

ALLEN TEST FOR THORACIC OUTLET SYNDROMES

Similar to Adson's test, the athletic trainer palpates the radial pulse while the individual abducts the shoulder, flexes the elbow to 90°, and looks toward the opposite

shoulder **(Figure 11.38B)**. The athletic trainer then instructs the individual to take a deep breath and hold it. A diminished or absent pulse indicates a positive test, suggesting that the pectoralis minor muscle is compressing the neurovascular bundle. Note, however, that this test often produces false-positive results.

An alternative position, called the Halstead maneuver, is done with the arm extended and the athlete's neck hyperextended and rotated to the opposite side. The athletic trainer finds the radial pulse and applies a downward traction to the arm. An absent or diminished pulse indicates a positive test for thoracic outlet syndrome.

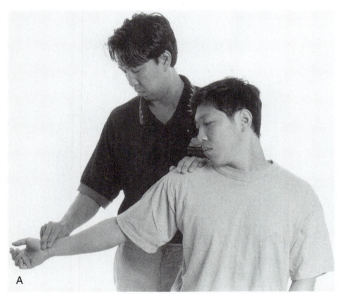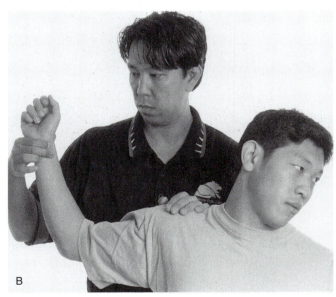

➤ FIGURE 11.38 Thoracic outlet compression syndrome. A, Adson's maneuver. Extend and externally rotate the humerus while the individual extends the head. B, Allen test. Abduct the shoulder and flex the elbow while the individual looks toward the opposite shoulder. An alternative position is to extend the elbow and apply downward traction while the individual hyperextends the neck and rotates the head to the opposite side (Halstead maneuver).

COSTOCLAVICULAR SYNDROME (MILITARY BRACE) TEST FOR THORACIC OUTLET SYNDROME

The athlete stands in a relaxed position while the athletic trainer stands behind the individual and palpates the radial pulse. The athlete then retracts the shoulders as if coming to military attention. The athletic trainer then extends and abducts the arm to 30° while the athlete hyperextends the neck **(Figure 11.39)**. If the radial pulse diminishes or disappears, it indicates that the subclavian artery is being blocked by the costoclavicular structures of the shoulder.

Neurologic Assessment

Neurologic integrity can be assessed with the use of myotomes, reflexes, and cutaneous patterns, which include both the segmental dermatomes and peripheral nerve patterns.

MYOTOMES

Isometric muscle testing should be performed in the following motions to test specific myotomes in the upper extremity: scapular elevation **(C4)**, shoulder abduction **(C5)**, elbow flexion and/or wrist extension **(C6)**, elbow extension and/or wrist flexion **(C7)**, thumb extension and/or ulnar deviation **(C8)**, and abduction and/or adduction of the hand intrinsics **(T1)**. These tests are demonstrated in Figures 11.25 and 13.30.

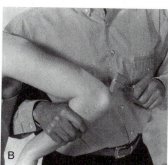
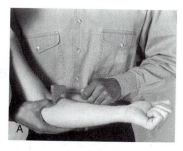

➤ **FIGURE 11.40 Reflex testing.** A, Biceps reflex (C5, C6). B, Triceps reflex (C7).

REFLEXES

Reflexes in the upper extremity include the biceps **(C5–C6)** and triceps **(C7)**. The biceps reflex is tested with the individual's arm flexed and supported by the athletic trainer's forearm. The examiner's thumb is placed over the biceps tendon and the thumb is struck with the reflex hammer using a quick downward thrust **(Figure 11.40A)**. A normal response is slight elbow flexion. The triceps reflex is tested with the individual's arm abducted and extended with the elbow flexed. The triceps tendon is placed on a slight stretch, and the triceps tendon is then tapped with the reflex hammer **(Figure 11.40B)**. A normal response is slight elbow extension.

CUTANEOUS PATTERNS

The segmental nerve dermatome patterns for the shoulder region are illustrated in **Figure 11.41**. The peripheral nerve cutaneous patterns are illustrated in **Figure 11.42**. Bilateral testing should be performed for altered sensation with sharp and dull touch by running the open hand and fingernails over the neck, shoulder, anterior and posterior chest walls, and down both sides of the arms.

Sport-Specific Functional Tests

Occasionally, sport-specific functional movements are the only activities that reproduce the signs and symptoms. Throwing a ball, performing a swimming stroke, doing the arm part of jumping jacks, or doing an overhead serve or spike may replicate the painful pattern. The athletic trainer should look for smooth coupled motion of the scapulothoracic joint and glenohumeral joint. Disharmony constitutes

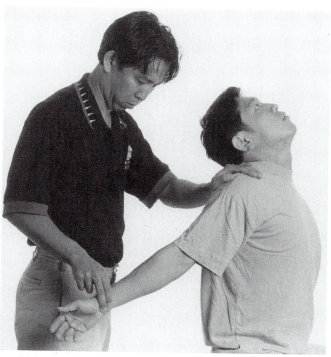

➤ **FIGURE 11.39 Costoclavicular syndrome test.** The athlete retracts the shoulders as if coming to military attention. The arm is extended and abducted about 30° while the head and neck are hyperextended. If the radial pulse disappears, it indicates the subclavian artery is blocked by the costoclavicular structures in the shoulder.

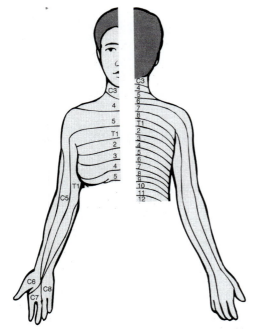

➤ **FIGURE 11.41** Dermatome patterns for the shoulder region.

scapulothoracic dyskinesia, or an inability to perform fluid voluntary movements. Based on your knowledge of the mechanics of the motion, it may be possible to narrow down the few definitive results of the assessment to determine the actual injury. These movements are also commonly used to determine when the individual can return to sport participation. All functional patterns should be fluid and pain-free.

💡 You found a painful arc of motion between 60 and 120° of abduction and flexion of the glenohumeral joint during active, passive, and resisted motion. Pain increased when the arm was horizontally adducted, as the greater tubercle of the humerus slid under the acromion process. Positive results were found with the drop-arm test, empty can (Centinela) supraspinatus test, impingement test, Yergason's test, and Speed's test. Neurologic tests were normal. This individual has an impingement syndrome involving the supraspinatus tendon, subacromial bursa, and long head of the biceps brachii.

REHABILITATION

❓ The volleyball player has a painful shoulder as a result of an impingement syndrome. What will be the priorities in rehabilitating this injury and returning the player to full functional status?

Rehabilitation of the shoulder region must involve range-of-motion and strengthening exercises for the entire shoulder complex in a functional progression. Progress within any program is dictated by the type and severity of injury, amount of immobilization, and the supervising physician's treatment plan. In a general sense, restoration of active range of motion should precede strengthening exercises that focus on specific strength deficits. Strengthening exercises for the scapular stabilizers should not be overlooked, since they play a key role in each phase of the throwing

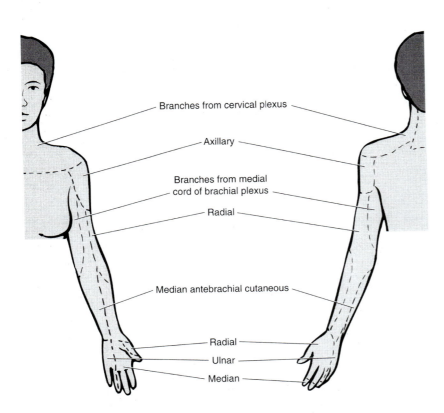

Branches from cervical plexus

Axillary

Branches from medial cord of brachial plexus

Radial

Median antebrachial cutaneous

Radial

Ulnar

Median

➤ **FIGURE 11.42** Cutaneous patterns for the peripheral nerves.

motion. In addition to restoring range of motion and strength, proprioception and cardiovascular fitness levels must be maintained.

Restoration of Motion

Gentle range-of-motion exercises, such as Codmans' circumduction and pendulum swings, are often used immediately after injury. The exercise is performed by making small circles and a pendulum motion in flexion and extension, and in horizontal abduction and adduction. The range of motion increases as pain-free motion is regained. Exercises can progress to active assistive T-bar exercises in the supine position **(Field Strategy 11.7)**. In throwing activities, the range of motion needed to adequately complete the cocking phase exceeds 90° of external rotation when the arm is abducted 90° (6). Special attention should be focused on regaining this additional range of motion,

---

FIELD STRATEGY 11.7   RANGE-OF-MOTION EXERCISES FOR THE GLENOHUMERAL JOINT

Wand and T-bar exercises. Hold the stretch for 5 to 10 seconds and repeat 10 to 20 times per session. Initially, range-of-motion exercises can be performed two to three times daily.

A. **Supine shoulder flexion**. Grasp the wand with both hands palm-down, at waist height. Raise the wand directly overhead, leading with the uninvolved arm until a stretch is felt in the involved shoulder. If an impingement syndrome is present, this exercise can be performed palm-up.

B. **Shoulder abduction**. Hold the wand with the involved arm palm-up, uninvolved arm palm-down. With the uninvolved arm, push the wand sideward and upward toward the involved side until a stretch is felt in the involved shoulder.

C. **Shoulder adduction/horizontal adduction**. Reverse hand positions from exercise B. Pull the wand toward the uninvolved side until a stretch is felt in the involved shoulder.

D. **Shoulder internal/external rotation**. Keeping both palms down, abduct the shoulders and flex the elbows. Move the wand upward toward the head, then return to waist level.

E. **Shoulder horizontal abduction/adduction**. Keeping both palms down, push the wand across the body with the uninvolved arm, then pull back across the body. Do not allow the trunk to twist.

F. **Supine external rotation**. Abduct the shoulder and flex the elbow to 90°. Grip the T-bar in the hand on the involved arm. Use the opposite arm to push the involved arm into external rotation. Perform external rotation with the arm abducted at 135° and 180°.

G. **Supine internal rotation**. With the arms in the same position as in exercise F, use the uninvolved arm to push the involved arm into internal rotation.

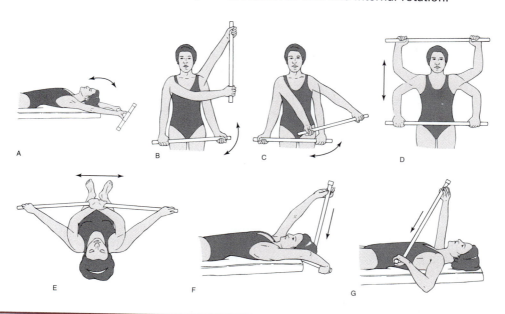

but not to the point of hypermobility. A rope-and-pulley system can augment active, assistive glenohumeral flexion and abduction. Shoulder shrugs performed in three directions (superior, anterior, and posterior) can increase scapular range of motion.

Restoration of Proprioception and Balance

Closed chain exercises may be performed after acute inflammation has been controlled. Shifting body weight from one hand to the other may be performed on a wall, table top, or unstable surface, such as a foam mat or BAPS board. Push-ups and exercises in a frontal and sagittal plane can be performed on a ProFitter or slide board, if available. Step-ups can be completed on a box, stool, or Stair Master. This activity can progress to stepping up and down on boxes of differing heights arranged so the exercise is performed in diagonal patterns, circles, figure eights, or any other pattern.

Use of free weights can develop balance, coordination, and skill in moving through diagonal patterns. It is imperative, however, to include a transference of proprioceptive training to the actual throwing motion. This is accomplished with a slow, deliberate rehearsal of the throwing motion incorporating visual feedback through the use of mirrors or videotape. As the motion is performed, biomechanical errors are corrected. When motion is perfected, speed of movement and distance of throw are gradually increased.

Muscular Strength, Endurance, and Power

Gentle, resisted isometric exercises can begin immediately after injury, or after surgery, while the arm is still immobilized. With the glenohumeral joint in a resting position, a slow, mild overload is applied. A disadvantage of isometric exercise is that strength gains are relatively specific to the joint angle at which the exercise is performed. Therefore, to strengthen the joint, isometric contractions must be performed at multiple positions. As the individual improves, a more moderate isometric overload is applied. Finally, a higher, rapid, unexpected resistance is provided at various positions including the end of the range of motion required for throwing.

Once range-of-motion approximates are normal for the individual, open chain kinetic exercises can be performed in a prone, sidelying, supine, or standing position to add gravity as resistance **(Field Strategy 11.8)**. A sandbag or dumbbell can be used for added resistance. The athlete should complete 50 to 100 repetitions with a 1-pound weight, and should not progress in resistance until 100 repetitions are achieved. Resistance should be limited to 5 pounds, as this decreases the chance of rotator cuff inflammation during the strengthening program. Careful attention should be directed to a potential painful arc of motion during concentric and eccentric contractions, as pain can further aggravate the injury. Therefore, work within a pain-free arc of motion with light resistance to the point of fatigue.

Muscular strength and endurance can be developed through PNF-resisted exercises in diagonal patterns to mimic functional skills, or surgical tubing can be used through a functional pattern. As strength improves, free weights or machine weight exercises for the upper body are incorporated. Many of these exercises were demonstrated in **Field Strategy 11.2**.

Plyometric exercises may involve catching a weighted ball using a quick, eccentric stretch of the muscle to facilitate a concentric contraction in throwing the ball. The exercise can progress through various one- and two-arm

---

 FIELD STRATEGY 11.8   **REHABILITATION EXERCISES FOR THE SHOULDER COMPLEX**

Progressive exercises should begin when pain subsides.

Exercises should be controlled, while focusing on the line of movement.

Begin with gravity as resistance, progress to light dumbbells or sandbags, then incorporate the exercises listed in Field Strategy 11.2.

A. **Sidelying medial and lateral rotation**. With the elbow flexed, perform lateral and medial rotation.

B. **Prone horizontal abduction (90°)**. The arm hangs over the table with the hand rotated outward. Raise the arm and laterally rotate the humerus until it is parallel to the floor.

C. **Prone horizontal abduction (100°)**. With the arm abducted at 100°, raise the arm and laterally rotate the humerus.

D. **Prone flexion and extension**. With the hand rotated outward as far as possible, raise the arm forward into flexion. Repeat, moving the arm into extension.

E. **Prone medial and lateral rotation**. With the shoulder abducted 90° and the elbow flexed, perform lateral and medial rotation. Repeat in the supine position.

F. **Prone rows (scapular adduction)**. With the shoulder abducted 90° and the elbow flexed, raise the arm off the table as if pinching the shoulder blades together. Do not raise the chest off the table.

G. **Wall push-ups and press-ups**.

Continued

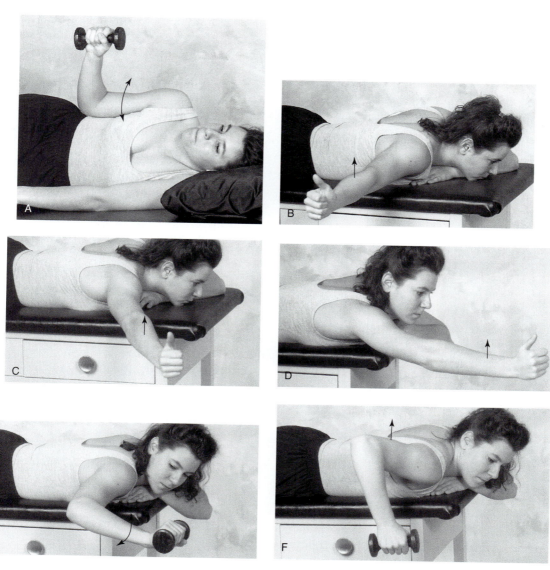

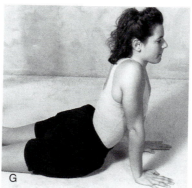

chest passes and overhead passes. A minitramp may also be used to do plyometric bounding push-ups.

Cardiovascular Fitness

General body conditioning should be maintained throughout the rehabilitation program. Several examples of programs were provided in Field Strategy 7.6, and included use of a jump rope, Stair Master, treadmill, and upper body ergometer (UBE).

 The volleyball player should increase range of motion in external rotation, restore strength in the rotator cuff and scapulothoracic musculature, regain proprioception and balance, and restore proper throwing mechanics through a functionally progressive throwing program.

Summary

1. The shoulder complex does not function in an isolated fashion; rather a series of joints work together in a coordinated manner to allow complicated patterns of motion. Because of this, injury to one structure can affect other structures.
2. The throwing motion occurs in several distinct phases: wind-up, stride, cocking, acceleration, deceleration, and follow-through.
3. The scapulohumeral rhythm is the combined scapular and glenohumeral movement that allows coordinated shoulder motion.
4. A moderate sternoclavicular sprain is characterized by pain and swelling over the joint and an inability to horizontally adduct the arm without increased pain. The arm is typically held forward and close to the body.
5. A moderate acromioclavicular sprain is characterized by an elevated distal clavicle, indicating that the coracoclavicular ligament and the AC ligaments have been torn. The individual will typically have a depressed or drooping shoulder.
6. Glenohumeral instability may be classified as anterior, posterior, inferior, or multidirectional. Anterior instability indicates injury to the middle and inferior glenohumeral ligaments, and may have an associated Bankart lesion. Multidirectional instability is often associated with pain and/or clicking during simple tasks.
7. Anterior glenohumeral dislocations are more common than posterior dislocations. The injured arm is often held in slight abduction and external rotation, and is stabilized against the body.
8. A Hill-Sachs lesion may occur with an anterior dislocation; a reverse Hill-Sachs lesion may occur with a posterior dislocation. A SLAP lesion is a superior labral tear that may disrupt the attachment of the

long head of the biceps tendon, and may occur with or without associated glenohumeral instability.
9. Impingement syndromes involve an actual abutment of the supraspinatus tendon and subacromial bursa under the coracoacromial ligament and acromion process. The glenoid labrum and long head of the biceps brachii may also be injured.
10. Thoracic outlet compression syndrome may involve compression of the lower trunk of the brachial plexus or the subclavian artery and vein. If a nerve is compressed, an aching pain or numbness may extend across the shoulder to the ulnar aspect of the hand. If arterial or venous vessels are compressed, coolness, numbness in the entire arm, and fatigue occur after exertional, overhead activity.
11. The surgical neck is the most common site for proximal humeral fractures in adults. Adolescents, however, have a high degree of proximal humeral epiphyseal fractures due to repetitive medial rotation and adduction traction forces placed on the shoulder during pitching motions.
12. Pain may be referred to the shoulder from other areas of the body, particularly the heart, lungs, visceral organs, and cervical spine region.
13. Injuries that should be immediately referred to a physician include:

   - Obvious deformity suggesting a suspected fracture, separation, or dislocation
   - Significant loss of motion or weakness in the myotomes
   - Joint instability
   - Abnormal sensations in either the segmental dermatomes or peripheral cutaneous patterns
   - Absent or weak pulse distal to the injury
   - Any significant, unexplained pain

14. If referred, remove the individual from activity and immobilize the limb in a sling and swathe, or another commercial product that adequately pads and supports the limb. Apply cryotherapy to reduce inflammation and swelling, and transport the individual in an appropriate manner.
15. Pain-free functional tests should be performed before clearing the individual for reentry into sports participation. The individual should also have bilateral strength, flexibility, and muscular endurance, and a high cardiovascular level, before returning to participation. Whenever possible, protective equipment or padding should be used to prevent reinjury.

References

1. Koehler SM, Thorson DC. Swimmer's shoulder: Targeting treatment. Phys Sportsmed 1996;24(11):39-50.
2. McMaster WC, Roberts A, Stoddard T. A correlation between shoulder laxity and interfering pain in competitive swimmers. Am J Sports Med 1998;26(1):83-86.

3. Fleisig GS, Escamilla RF, Andrews JR. Biomechanics of throwing. In: Athletic Injuries and Rehabilitation. Edited by Zachazewski JE, Magee DJ, and Quillen WS. Philadelphia: WB Saunders, 1996.

4. Hamill J, Knutzen KM. Biomechanical Basis of Human Movement. Baltimore: Williams & Wilkins, 1995.

5. Kent BE. Functional anatomy of the shoulder complex: A review. J Am Phys Ther Assoc 1971;51:867-888.

6. Irrgang JJ, Witney SL, Harner CD. Nonoperative treatment of rotator cuff injuries in throwing athletes. J Sport Rehab 1992; 1(3):197-222.

7. Lemos MJ. The evaluation and treatment of the injured acromioclavicular joint in athletes. Am J Sports Med 1998;26(1):137-144.

8. Hutchinson MR, Ahuja FS. Diagnosing and treating clavicle injuries. Phys Sportsmed 1996;24(3):26-36.

9. Wilk KE, Harrelson GL, Arrigo C, Chmielewski T. Shoulder rehabilitation. In: Physical Rehabilitation of the Injured Athlete. Edited by Andrews JR, Harrelson GL, Wilk KE. Philadelphia: WB Saunders, 1998.

10. Magee DJ, Reid DC. Shoulder injuries. In: Athletic Injuries and Rehabilitation. Edited by Zachazewski JE, Magee DJ, Quillen WS. Philadelphia: WB Saunders, 1996.

11. Starkey C, Ryan JL. Evaluation of Orthopedic and Athletic Injuries. Philadelphia: FA Davis, 1996.

12. Hulstyn MJ, Fadale PD. Shoulder injuries in the athlete. Clin Sports Med 1997;16(4):663-679.

13. Wang DH. New exam for glenoid labral tears. Phys Sportsmed 1997;25(2):15.

14. Magee DJ. Orthopedic Physical Assessment. Philadelphia: WB Saunders, 1997.

CHAPTER 12

Upper Arm, Elbow, and Forearm Conditions

OBJECTIVES

1. Identify the important bony and soft tissue structures in the upper arm, elbow, and forearm.

2. Describe the motions at the elbow, and identify the muscles that produce them.

3. Explain what forces produce the loading patterns responsible for common injuries in the upper arm, elbow, and forearm.

4. Describe measures used to prevent injuries to the upper arm, elbow, and forearm.

5. List the signs and symptoms associated with a contusion to the region, and explain what potentially serious conditions might develop if a contusion is improperly managed.

6. List the four types of bursae injuries or conditions, and explain the management of each type.

7. Explain the signs and symptoms associated with the different degrees of a joint sprain.

8. Explain the management of an elbow dislocation.

9. Describe what motions will be painful and weak in a flexor and extensor strain.

10. Contrast medial epicondylitis and common extensor tendinitis.

11. Name the three major peripheral nerves that course through the elbow region, and describe the various differences in muscle weakness and sensory loss seen for each nerve, if it is injured.

12. Describe the various types of fractures found at the elbow, and their management.

13. Demonstrate a thorough assessment of the elbow region.

14. Demonstrate common rehabilitation exercises for the elbow.

The arms perform lifting and carrying tasks, cushion the body during collisions, and lessen body momentum during falls. Performance in many sports is also contingent on the ability of the arms to effectively swing a racquet or club, or to position the hands for throwing and catching a ball. The elbow is second only to the shoulder as the most commonly dislocated joint. In children under 10 years of age, it is the most commonly dislocated joint (1). Furthermore, the elbow is believed to be second only to the knee in overuse injuries; with common extensor tendinitis, also known as lateral **epicondylitis** (inflammation of the epicondyle) as the most frequent overuse injury in athletes (2,3). Medial epicondylitis and "little league elbow" are other overuse injuries commonly seen in adolescents.

This chapter begins with a review of anatomy, and an overview of the kinematics and kinetics of the upper arm, elbow, and forearm. Discussion on measures to prevent injury to the region is followed by information on common injuries and their management. Finally, the injury assessment process is presented, followed by examples of rehabilitation exercises.

ANATOMICAL REVIEW OF THE ELBOW

Although the elbow may be generally thought of as a simple hinge joint, the elbow actually encompasses three articulations: the humeroulnar, humeroradial, and proximal radioulnar joints. The bony structure of the elbow and forearm are displayed in **Figure 12.1**. Several strong ligaments

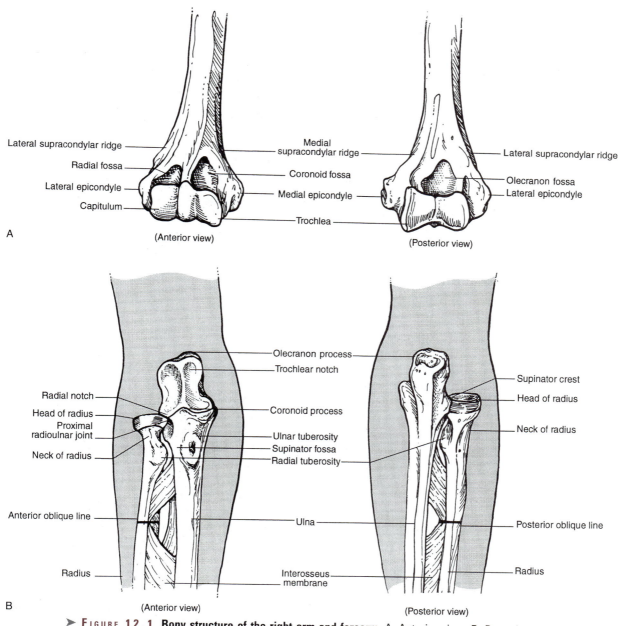

➤ **FIGURE 12.1 Bony structure of the right arm and forearm.** A, Anterior view. B, Posterior view.

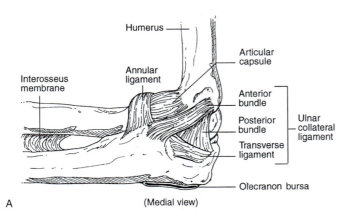

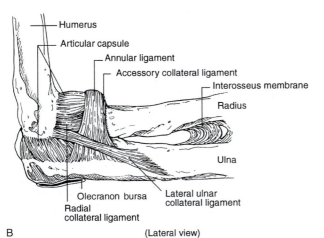

➤ **FIGURE 12.2** Major ligaments (A) and olecranon bursa (B) of the left elbow.

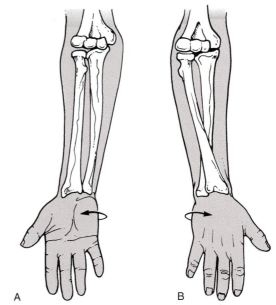

➤ **FIGURE 12.3** Forearm movements. A, Supination occurs when the radius and ulna are parallel to each other. B, Pronation involves the rotation of the radius over the ulna.

bind these articulations together, and a single joint capsule surrounds all three **(Figure 12.2)**. Twenty-three muscles associated with the elbow provide dynamic stability.

Humeroulnar Joint

The hinge joint at the elbow is the humeroulnar joint, where the trochlea of the humerus articulates with the reciprocally shaped trochlear fossa of the ulna. Motion capabilities are primarily flexion and extension, although in some individuals, particularly women, a small amount of overextension (5 to 15°) is allowed. The joint is most stable in the close packed position of extension.

Humeroradial Joint

The humeroradial joint, just lateral to the humeroulnar joint, is formed between the spherical capitellum of the humerus and the proximal radius. This is a gliding joint, with motion restricted to the sagittal plane by the adjacent humeroulnar joint. The close packed position is with the elbow flexed at 90° and the forearm supinated about 5°.

Proximal Radioulnar Joint

The annular ligament binds the head of the radius to the radial notch of the ulna, forming the proximal radioulnar

joint. This is a pivot joint, with forearm pronation and supination occurring as the radius rolls medially and laterally over the ulna **(Figure 12.3)**. The closed packed position is at 5° of forearm supination.

Carrying Angle

The angle between the longitudinal axes of the humerus and the ulna when the arm is in anatomical position is known as the carrying angle. The angle is so-named because it causes the forearm to angle away from the body when a load is carried in the hand. Given that loads are typically carried with the forearm in a neutral rather than a fully supinated position, however, the functional significance of the carrying angle is questionable. Nevertheless, the size of the carrying angle at the elbow is one of the skeletal differences between females and males, and is attributed to differences in the shape of the trochlea. With the elbow fully extended and the forearm fully supinated, the carrying angle ranges from approximately 10 to 15° in adults, and is generally greater in females than in males.

Ligaments of the Elbow

The elbow is reinforced by capsuloligamentous structures that are thickenings of the capsule. These form the medial and lateral ligamentous complexes. The medial (ulnar) collateral ligament, the most important ligament for stability of the elbow joint, is divided into three oblique bands denoted by their anatomical location—anterior, transverse, and posterior. The anterior oblique band is taut throughout the elbow's full range of motion (ROM) and is the primary restraint against valgus forces. The transverse oblique band provides little, if any, support to the medial elbow. The posterior oblique band is a fan-shaped capsular thickening that is generally taut when the elbow is flexed beyond 90°. The lateral (radial) collateral ligament complex consists of four components: the lateral ulnar collateral, radial collateral, annular, and the accessory ligaments. The radial collateral ligament, which runs from the lateral epicondyle of the humerus and terminates at the annular ligament, resists varus forces. A posterior portion of this ligament extends distally to the lateral ulna, and is referred to as the lateral ulnar collateral ligament. The annular ligament fits tightly around the radial head and upper portion of the neck, and permits pronation and supination of the forearm as the radius internally and externally rotates on the ulna. During extreme supination, the anterior fibers of the annular ligament are taut; during extreme pronation, the posterior fibers are taut. The accessory lateral collateral ligament is a superficial layer of fibers that blends with the annular ligament to insert onto the supinator tubercle of the ulna.

Bursae of the Elbow

Although there are several small bursae about the elbow, the most clinically relevant is the subcutaneous olecranon bursa between the olecranon and skin surface. This bursa can become enlarged by a hematoma, chronic irritation, or rheumatoid synovitis, and may require surgical excision to relieve symptoms.

Muscles of the Elbow

A number of muscles cross the elbow, including several that also either cross the shoulder or extend down into the hand and fingers. The tendinous attachments of muscles near the medial and lateral aspects of the elbow are often irritated and inflamed by repetitive stresses associated with poor technique or overtraining in sports such as tennis, golf, and baseball pitching. The muscles considered to be primary movers of the elbow are summarized in **Table 12.1**.

Nerves of the Elbow

The major nerves of the elbow and forearm descend from the brachial plexus and include the musculocutaneous (C_5–C_7), median (C_5–T_1), ulnar (C_8–T_1), and radial nerves (C_5–T_1) **(Figure 12.4)**. The musculocutaneous nerve provides motor supply to the flexor muscles of the anterior arm, and sensory innervation to the skin of the lateral forearm. The median nerve supplies most of

TABLE 12.1	MUSCLES OF THE ELBOW			
Muscle	**Proximal Attachment**	**Distal Attachment**	**Primary Action(s)**	**Nerve Innervation**
Biceps brachii		Tuberosity of the radius	Flexion; assists with supination	Musculocutaneous (C_5, C_6)
(Long head)	Superior rim of the glenoid fossa			
(Short head)	Coracoid process of the scapula			
Brachioradialis	Upper two-thirds of the lateral supracondylar ridge of the humerus	Styloid process of the radius	Flexion	Radial (C_5, C_6)
Brachialis	Anterior, lower half of the humerus	Anterior coronoid process of the ulna	Flexion	Musculocutaneous (C_5, C_6)
Pronator teres		Lateral midpoint of the radius	Assists with flexion and pronation	Median (C_6, C_7)
(Humeral head)	Medial epicondyle of the humerus			
(Ulnar head)	Coronoid process of the ulna			
Pronator quadratus	Lower fourth of the anterior ulna	Lower fourth of the anterior radius	Pronation	Anterior interosseous (C_8, T_1)
Triceps brachii		Olecranon process of the ulna	Extension	Radial (C_6–C_8)
(Long head)	Just inferior to the glenoid fossa			
(Lateral head)	Upper half of the posterior humerus			
(Medial head)	Lower two-thirds of the posterior humerus			
Anconeus	Posterior, lateral epicondyle of the humerus	Lateral olecranon and posterior ulna	Assists with extension	Radial (C_7, C_8)
Supinator	Lateral epicondyle of the humerus and adjacent ulna	Lateral upper third of radius	Supination	Posterior interosseous (C_5, C_6)

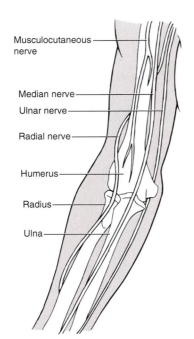

➤ FIGURE 12.4 Nerves of the elbow region.

the flexor muscles of the anterior forearm and the skin on the palmar aspect of the hand, including the thumb, index finger, and middle finger, and the lateral half of the ring finger. The ulnar nerve provides innervation to the flexor carpi ulnaris and the medial half of the flexor digitorum profundus, and to the skin on the medial border of the hand including the little finger and medial half of the ring finger. The radial nerve, the largest branch of the brachial plexus, passes anteriorly to the lateral epicondyle at the elbow, then divides into the superficial and deep branches to continue along the posterolateral aspect of the forearm. The radial nerve supplies all the arm and forearm extensor muscles, and the skin on the posterior aspect of the arm and forearm. Specific nerve-muscle associations are shown in Table 12.1.

Blood Vessels of the Elbow

The major arteries of the elbow and forearm region are the brachial, ulnar, and radial arteries **(Figure 12.5)**. The brachial artery courses down the medial side of the arm, providing blood supply to the flexor muscles of the arm. The deep brachial artery branches off to supply the triceps brachii. At the elbow, the brachial artery forms an **anastomosis**, or a network of communicating blood vessels, to supply the elbow joint. The main branch of the brachial artery crosses the anterior aspect of the elbow where the brachial pulse can be readily palpated. Distal to the elbow, the brachial artery splits into the ulnar and radial arteries. The ulnar artery supplies the medial forearm and via one of its branches, the common interosseous artery, supplies the deep flexors and extensors of the forearm. The radial artery, which courses along the anterior aspect of the radius, supplies the lateral forearm muscles. Pulses can be

taken for both arteries on the anterior aspect of the wrist (see Figure 4.7).

KINEMATICS AND MAJOR MUSCLE ACTIONS OF THE ELBOW

The three associated joints at the elbow allow motion in two planes. Flexion and extension are sagittal plane movements that occur at the humeroulnar and humeroradial joints, and pronation and supination are longitudinal rotational movements that take place at the proximal radioulnar joint.

Flexion and Extension

The elbow flexors include those muscles crossing the anterior side of the joint **(Figure 12.6)**. The primary elbow flexor is the brachialis. Because the distal attachment of the brachialis is the coronoid process of the ulna, the muscle is equally effective when the forearm is in supination and pronation. Another elbow flexor, the biceps brachii, has both long and short heads attached to the radial tuberosity via a single common tendon. The muscle contributes effectively to flexion when the forearm is supinated, because it is slightly stretched. When the forearm is pronated, the muscle is less taut and consequently less effective. The brachioradialis, a third elbow flexor, is most effective when the forearm is in a neutral position (midway between full pronation and full supination). Other flexor muscles that cross the elbow are important dynamic stabilizers of the joint. The flexor carpi ulnaris and flexor digitorum superficialis, in particular, provide significant stability to the medial elbow during activities such as throwing.

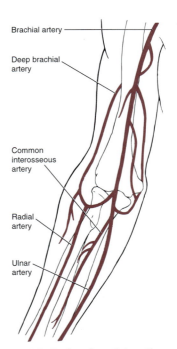

➤ FIGURE 12.5 Arteries of the elbow region.

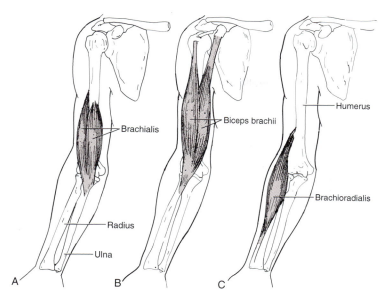

➤ **FIGURE 12.6 Primary flexor muscles of the elbow.** A, Brachialis. B, Biceps brachii. C, Brachioradialis.

The triceps is the major elbow extensor **(Figure 12.7)**. Although the three heads have separate origins, they attach to the olecranon process of the ulna through a common distal tendon. The small anconeus also assists with extension at the elbow.

Pronation and Supination

Pronation and supination of the forearm occur when the radius rotates around the ulna. There are three radioulnar articulations: the proximal, middle, and distal radioulnar joints. The proximal and distal joints are pivot joints. The middle radioulnar joint is a syndesmosis, with an elastic interconnecting membrane permitting supination and pronation, but preventing longitudinal displacement of one bone with respect to the other. The primary pronator muscle is the pronator quadratus, which attaches to the distal ulna and radius **(Figure 12.8)**. The pronator teres, which

crosses the proximal radioulnar joint, assists with pronation. As the name suggests, the supinator is the muscle primarily responsible for supination **(Figure 12.9)**. During resistance or when the elbow is flexed, the biceps also participates in supination.

KINETICS OF THE ELBOW

Although the elbow is not considered to be a weight-bearing joint, it sustains significant loads during daily activities. For example, it has been estimated that the compressive load at the elbow reaches 300 Newtons (N) (67 lb) during activities such as dressing and eating, 1700 N (382 lb) when the body is supported by the arms when rising from a chair, and 1900 N (427 lb) when pulling a table across the floor (3). Large forces are generated by muscles crossing the elbow during forceful pitching and throwing motions, as well as during weight lifting and many resis-

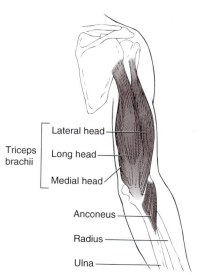

➤ **FIGURE 12.7 Primary extensor muscles of the elbow are the triceps brachii and the anconeus.**

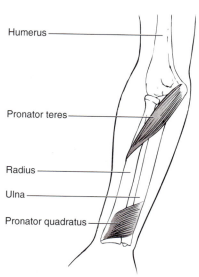

➤ **FIGURE 12.8 Primary pronators of the elbow are the pronator quadratus and pronator teres.**

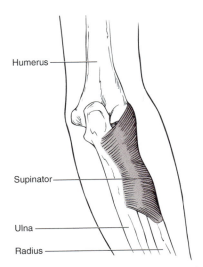

▶ FIGURE 12.9 **Primary supinator of the elbow is the supinator muscle**.

tance training exercises. In fact, during an activity such as pitching, varus torques on the order of 120 Nm must be generated by the elbow muscle to resist valgus stress (4). The triceps, wrist flexor-pronator muscles, and anconeus must develop tension to assist the ulnar collateral ligament in resisting the valgus load. During the execution of many skills in gymnastics and wrestling, the elbow does function as a weight-bearing joint.

Since the attachment of the elbow extensors to the ulna is closer to the joint center than the attachments of the elbow flexors on the radius and ulna, the extensor moment arm is shorter than the flexor moment arm. This means that the elbow extensors must generate more force than the elbow flexors to produce the same amount of joint torque. This translates to greater joint compression forces during extension than during flexion, when movements with comparable speed and force requirements are executed.

PREVENTION OF ELBOW INJURIES

The elbow is often subjected to compressive forces when the arm is placed in a position to cushion a fall or lessen body impact with another object. Microtraumatic forces caused by repetitive valgus and varus stresses can also lead to overuse injuries, many of which are related to poor skill technique. Few sports require protective equipment at the elbow. Therefore, physical conditioning and proper skill technique are major factors in preventing injury to this region.

Protective Equipment

Standard shoulder pads may not extend far enough to protect the upper arm. Many football lineman have an additional biceps pad attached to the shoulder pads to protect this vulnerable area. Hockey and lacrosse players also have special pads to protect the elbow during falls and collisions. Commercially available padded elbow sleeves or neoprene sleeves are worn in many sports to protect the olecranon from direct trauma and abrasions, particularly when playing on artificial turf. Counterforce braces, commonly seen in racquet sports, reduce muscle tensile forces that can lead to medial or lateral epicondylitis. Hinged braces add compression and support to the elbow to reduce excessive varus and valgus forces.

Physical Conditioning

Many of the muscles that move the elbow also move the shoulder or wrist. Therefore, flexibility and strengthening exercises must focus on the entire arm. General flexibility exercises for the shoulder can be used in conjunction with warm-up exercises that mimic specific sport skills. For example, a tennis player may begin the warm-up session with slow, controlled forehand and backhand strokes, gradually increasing intensity. A pitcher or outfielder may begin with short, controlled throws, increasing the distance and intensity as the arm is warmed up. Strengthening exercises for the shoulder can be combined with those listed in **Field Strategy 12.1**. These exercises are designed to improve general strength in elbow flexion and extension, forearm pronation and supination, wrist flexion and extension, and radial and ulnar deviation. Begin with light resistance and progress to a heavier resistance.

FIELD STRATEGY 12.1   EXERCISES TO PREVENT INJURY TO THE ELBOW REGION

Begin all exercises with light resistance using dumbbells or surgical tubing.

A. **Biceps curl.** Support the involved arm on the leg, and fully flex the elbow. This can also be performed bilaterally in a standing position with a barbell.

B. **Triceps curl.** Raise the involved arm over the head. Extend the involved arm at the elbow. This can also be performed bilaterally in a supine or standing position with a barbell.

C. **Wrist flexion.** Support the involved forearm on a table or your leg with the hand off the edge. With the palm facing up, slowly do a full wrist curl and return to the starting position. Repeat.

D. **Wrist extension.** Support the involved forearm on a table or your leg with the hand off the edge. With the palm facing down, slowly do a full reverse wrist curl and return to the starting position. Repeat.

E. **Forearm pronation/supination.** Support the involved forearm on a table or your leg with the hand over the edge. With surgical tubing or a hand dumbbell, roll the forearm into pronation, then return to supination. Adjust the surgical tubing and reverse the exercise, stressing the supinators. Be sure the elbow remains stationary.

F. **Ulnar/radial deviation.** Support the involved forearm on a table or your leg with the hand over the edge. With surgical tubing or a hand dumbbell, perform ulnar deviation. Reverse directions and perform radial deviation. An alternate method is to stand with the arm at the side holding a hammer or weighted bar. Raise the wrist in ulnar deviation. Repeat in radial deviation.

G. **Wrist curl-ups.** To exercise the wrist extensors, grip the bar with both palms facing down. Slowly wind the cord onto the bar until the weight reaches the top, then slowly unwind the cord. Reverse hand position to work the wrist flexors.

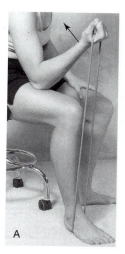
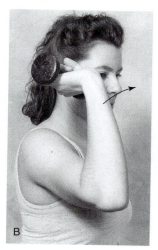
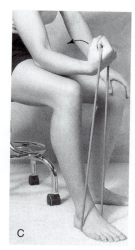
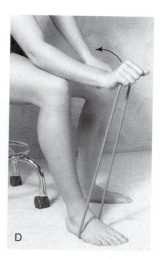

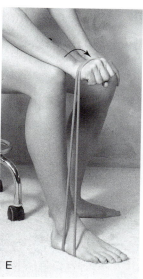
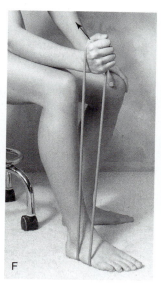
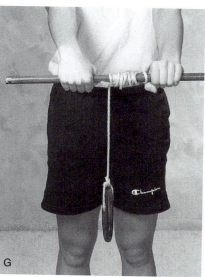

Proper Skill Technique

Nearly all overuse injuries are directly related to repetitive throwing-type motions that produce microtraumatic tensile forces on the surrounding soft tissue structures. Children who pitch sidearm motions are three times more likely to develop problems than those who use a more traditional overhead technique (2). Movement analysis can detect improper technique in the acceleration and follow-through phase that contribute to these excessive tensile forces. High-speed photography may aid in this analysis. Another preventative measure, already discussed in the shoulder chapter, is teaching sport participants the shoulder-roll method of falling. Falling on an extended hand or flexed elbow is the most common mechanism for acute injuries in the upper extremity. Excessive compressive forces can be transmitted along the long axis of the bones, leading to a fracture or dislocation.

CONTUSIONS

 A football player is complaining of pain in his right arm during blocking drills. Palpation reveals a hardened mass of soft tissue over the distal anterior arm that is very tender and sore. There is good bilateral strength but the pain is getting worse. What potentially serious condition might develop? How will you manage this condition?

Direct blows to arm and forearm are frequently associated with contact and collision sports. Contusions occur more frequently over bony prominences. For volleyball players, the very nature of the sport leads to trauma on the radial side of the forearm **(Figure 12.10)**.

➤ SIGNS AND SYMPTOMS

Bruising can lead to internal hemorrhage, rapid swelling, and hematoma formation that can limit ROM. Chronic blows to the anterior arm or near the distal attachment of the deltoid muscle, however, may result in the development of ectopic bone (a proliferation of bone ossification in an abnormal place) in either the belly of the muscle **(myositis ossificans)** or as a bony outgrowth (exostosis) of the underlying bone. Because of the proximity of the brachialis muscle belly to the joint, it is a common site for the development of myositis ossificans (an accumulation of mineral deposits within muscle tissue) after trauma. Another vulnerable site is just proximal to the deltoid's insertion on the lateral aspect of the humerus where the bone is least padded by muscle tissue. Standard shoulder pads do not extend far enough to protect the area, and the edge of the pad itself may contribute to the injury. The developing mass can become painful and disabling if the radial nerve is contused, leading to transitory paralysis of the extensor forearm muscles.

"Tackler's exostosis" (blocker's spur), commonly seen in football linemen, is not a true myositis ossificans, because the ectopic formation is not infiltrated into the muscle, but rather is an irritative exostosis arising from the bone. A painful bony mass, usually in the form of a spur with a sharp edge, can be palpated on the anterolateral aspect of the humerus.

➤ MANAGEMENT

Treatment for contusions will involve ice, compression, elevation, and rest, followed by nonsteroidal anti-inflammatory drugs (NSAIDs) and gentle, pain-free ROM exercises. Aggressive stretching and strengthening exercises should be avoided so as not to further injure muscle tissue. If conservative measures do not alleviate the condition, refer the individual to a physician for further care. A more serious condition has developed. Visible radiograph changes in the muscle can be noted after 2 to 3 weeks. As the condition progresses and becomes chronic, a painful **periostitis** (inflammation of the periosteum) and **fibrositis** (inflammation of fibrous tissue) may develop. Surgical excision of the calcification is seldom necessary because function is not usually impaired. The area should be protected with a special pad during participation. However, if function is adversely affected, surgery should be delayed until the calcification is mature, usually in 12 to 18 months, as it may redevelop.

 The football player may be developing myositis ossificans in the brachialis muscle. Standard acute care should be followed with referral to a physician for further assessment and possible radiographs.

OLECRANON BURSITIS

 A wrestler has acute swelling about an inch in diameter on the proximal posterior ulna. What condition is present, and how will you manage it?

The subcutaneous olecranon bursa is the largest bursa in the elbow region. The lubricating function of the bursa facilitates smooth gliding of the skin over the olecranon process during elbow flexion and extension. The superficial location predisposes the bursa to either direct macrotrauma or cumulative microtrauma by repetitive elbow flexion and

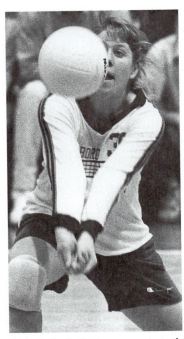

➤ **FIGURE 12.10** Volleyball players contuse the forearms during the early part of the season with repetitive compression of soft tissue structures.

extension **(Box 12.1)**. The bursitis may be acute or chronic, aseptic or septic.

Acute and Chronic Bursitis

A fall on a flexed elbow can lead to an acutely inflamed bursa. Constantly leaning on one's elbow or repetitive pressure and friction can lead to a chronic inflamed bursa.

➤ SIGNS AND SYMPTOMS

The acutely inflamed bursa will present with an immediate tender, swollen area of redness in the posterior elbow. If the bursa ruptures, a discrete, sharply demarcated goose egg is visible directly over the olecranon process **(Figure 12.11)**. Approximately one-half of patients with olecranon bursitis have a history of an abrupt onset of pain and swelling; the other half have a more insidious onset over a few weeks leading to chronic inflammation (5). Motion is limited at the extreme of flexion as tension increases over the bursa.

➤ MANAGEMENT

Acute management involves ice, rest, and a compressive wrap applied for the first 24 hours. Significant distention may necessitate aspiration, for comfort, followed by a compressive dressing for several days. Chronic bursitis is managed with cryotherapy, NSAIDs, and use of elbow cushions to protect the area from further insult. In long-term cases of chronic bursitis, the bursa may be aspirated

or totally excised, although there is a risk of poor wound healing over the olecranon process.

Septic and Nonseptic Bursitis

Occasionally, the bursa can become infected, regardless of acute trauma to the area. Septic bursitis is sometimes related to seeding from an infection at a distant site, such as **paronychia** (infection of the folds of skin surrounding a fingernail), cellulitis of the hand, or forearm infection. Nonseptic bursitis can also be caused by crystalline deposition disease or rheumatoid involvement, and has been associated with atopic dermatitis.

➤ SIGNS AND SYMPTOMS

Individuals with septic bursitis are more likely to show traditional signs of infection, including malaise (lethargy), fever, pain, localized heat, restricted motion, tenderness, and swelling at the elbow. These signs and symptoms usually present within 1 week of developing symptoms. Approximately half will have a skin lesion overlying the bursa, 92 to 100% will have bursal tenderness, and 40 to 100% have peribursal cellulitis (5). In contrast, nonseptic bursitis is associated with an overlying skin lesion in 5% of the cases, bursal tenderness in 45% of cases, and cellulitis in 23 to 25% of cases.

➤ MANAGEMENT

An athlete with an infected bursa should be referred to a physician. The physician will generally aspirate the bursa and take a culture of the fluid to determine the presence of septic bursitis. After aspiration, the elbow is immobilized in a sling, and continuous hot packs and appropriate antibiotics are typically prescribed.

 The wrestler has acute olecranon bursitis. Standard acute care should resolve the condition, though additional padding can help prevent recurrence.

SPRAINS

 After practice, a football lineman is complaining of anterior elbow pain. He reports that the initial acute pain occurred after falling on a hyperextended arm. Palpation reveals deep tenderness over the anterior joint line, and extreme tenderness on the anteromedial side on passive full elbow extension. What condition may have occurred? How can you determine if the collateral ligaments supporting the joint are injured?

At the elbow, acute tears to ligamentous and joint structures are rare, but may occur during a fall on an extended hand, producing a hyperextension injury, or through a valgus/varus tensile force. More commonly, however, repetitive tensile forces irritate and tear the ligaments, particularly the ulnar (medial) collateral ligament. If the ulnar collateral

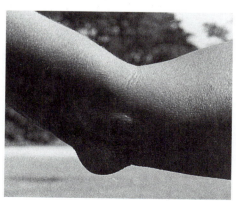

➤ **FIGURE 12.11 Olecranon bursitis.** When the olecranon bursa ruptures, a discrete, sharply demarcated goose egg is visible directly over the olecranon process.

ligament is damaged, the ulnar nerve may also be affected. A history of pain localized on the medial aspect of the elbow during the late cocking and acceleration phases of throwing is common. Examination will reveal point tenderness on the joint line, and increased pain and instability with the valgus stress test applied to the elbow at 15 to 20° flexion (see Assessment later in this chapter). Ice, compression, NSAIDs, and rest are followed by early, protected ROM exercises to stretch the forearm flexor-pronator group and the forearm extensors.

Anterior Capsulitis

Anterior joint pain caused by hyperextension is usually attributed to acute anterior capsulitis, rather than chronic, repetitive throwing. Microtears in the capsule are usually not sufficient to cause dislocation. The individual will have diffuse, anterior elbow pain after a traumatic episode, with deep tenderness on palpation, particularly on the anteromedial side. A strain to the pronator teres should be ruled out, as well as entrapment of the median nerve as it courses through the pronator teres. When this occurs, tingling or numbness of the thumb and index finger are usually noted. The condition is managed with immobilization for 3 to 5 days, after which active ROM exercises can begin as pain allows.

Dislocations

In adolescents, the most common traumatic injury to the elbow is subluxation or dislocation of the proximal radial head, often associated with an immature annular ligament. Sometimes referred to as "nursemaid's elbow" or "pulled-elbow syndrome," the condition results from longitudinal traction of an extended and pronated upper extremity, such as when a young child is swung by the arms. This causes a small tear in the annular ligament that allows the radial head to migrate out from under the annular ligament.

If an athlete is unable to pronate and supinate the forearm without pain, refer the individual immediately to a physician. Immobilization for 3 to 6 weeks in flexion is usually necessary (6).

Most ulnar dislocations occur in individuals younger than 20 years, with a peak incidence in early adolescence (6). The mechanism of injury is usually hyperextension, or a sudden, violent unidirectional valgus force that drives the ulna posterior or posterolateral. Sixty percent have associated fractures of the medial epicondyle, radial head, coronoid process, and olecranon process (7).

➤ SIGNS AND SYMPTOMS

Immediately on impact, a snapping or cracking sensation is followed by severe pain, rapid swelling, total loss of function, and an obvious deformity (**Figure 12.12**). The anterior capsule, brachialis muscle, and flexor and extensor muscle masses may also be disrupted. The arm is frequently held in flexion, with the forearm appearing shortened. The olecranon and radial head are palpable posteriorly, and a

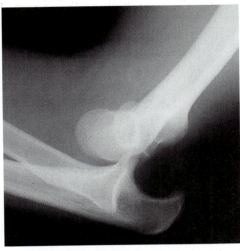

➤ **FIGURE 12.12 Elbow dislocation.** Posterior dislocations produce a snapping or cracking sensation followed by immediate, severe pain, rapid swelling, and total loss of function.

slight indentation in the triceps is visible just proximal to the olecranon (**Box 12.2**).

Nerve palsies are common, making pre- and post-reduction neurovascular examination critical. Ulnar nerve dysfunction is usually transient. If damaged, numbness will extend into the little finger. The median nerve, however, may become trapped within the joint, within a healing medial epicondyle fracture or looped anteriorly into the joint. Persistent unexplained pain and median nerve dysfunction (e.g., finger flexor weakness or numbness in the palm of the hand) necessitate immediate reevaluation by a physician.

➤ MANAGEMENT

*Management involves immediate immobilization in a vacuum splint. Activate EMS to transport the individual to the nearest medical facility, since early reduction minimizes the amount of muscle spasm. Management of an elbow dislocation is discussed in **Field Strategy 12.2**.*

➤➤ **Box 12.2**

Signs and Symptoms of a Posterior Elbow Dislocation

- Snapping or cracking sensation
- Immediate, severe pain with rapid swelling, primarily on the medial aspect of the elbow
- Total loss of function
- Obvious deformity as the olecranon is pushed posteriorly
- The elbow will be slightly flexed and supported, if possible, by the uninjured arm
- Pain is predominantly localized over the medial aspect of the elbow
- If there is an associated fracture, crepitation may be palpated

FIELD STRATEGY 12.2 MANAGEMENT ALGORITHM FOR POSTERIOR ELBOW DISLOCATION

Consider this injury to be an emergency. Activate EMS

↓

Apply ice immediately to reduce swelling and inflammation

↓

To rule out circulatory impairment, assess:
- Radial pulse
- Skin color
- Blanching of the nails

↓

To rule out nerve impairment, assess motor and sensory function:
- Have the patient (if able) flex, extend, abduct, and adduct the fingers with the person looking away:
  Stroke the palm and dorsum of the hand in several different locations with a blunt and sharp object
  Ask him or her to identify where you are touching, and whether the object is sharp or dull

↓

Immobilize the area with a vacuum splint or other appropriate splint

↓

Take vital signs, recheck pulse and sensory functions, and treat for shock

↓

Transport immediately to the nearest medical facility

Closed reduction under general or regional anesthesia is necessary. In cases where the forearm flexors, extensors, and annular ligament have maintained their integrity with no associated fracture, limited immobilization and early ROM and proprioceptive neuromuscular facilitation (PNF) exercises have proven quite successful (8). Recurrent dislocations are rare, and are often related to laxity in the lateral ulnar collateral ligament of the elbow, leading to posterolateral rotary subluxation. Most commonly, a recurrent dislocation in the first 6 months after initial injury is due to a missed osteochondral fracture. Elbow dislocations involving fractures of the radial head and capitellar fracture dislocations are more complex and require internal fixation.

The football lineman has probably injured the anterior capsule of the joint. This is evident by the anterior joint pain. During assessment, a valgus and varus stress test at 15 to 20° of elbow flexion should be performed to rule out injury to the supporting collateral ligaments.

STRAINS

A volleyball player is complaining of vague forearm pain aggravated during overhead spiking drills. Palpation elicits point tenderness on the proximal anterior arm. Pain increases with resisted elbow flexion and wrist ulnar deviation. What muscles may be involved here? How will you manage this injury?

Muscular strains commonly result from inadequate warm-up, excessive training past the point of fatigue, and inadequate rehabilitation of previous muscular injuries. Less commonly, they may occur as a result of a single massive contraction or sudden overstretching. **Field Strategy 12.3** summarizes management of isolated muscular strains.

Flexor Strains

Injury to the elbow flexors (brachialis, biceps brachii, and brachioradialis) is usually self-limiting. Occasionally, however, the distal biceps brachii may rupture following a sudden eccentric load (e.g., during weight lifting or trying to catch oneself during a fall).

➤ SIGNS AND SYMPTOMS

Injury will result in point tenderness on the anterior distal arm. Pain will increase with passive elbow extension and resisted elbow flexion. With a biceps brachii rupture, ecchymosis will be present in the antecubital area, weakness in supination and elbow flexion will be present, and the distal biceps brachii tendon will not be palpable.

➤ MANAGEMENT

Treatment involves standard acute care with ice, compression, elevation, and protected rest. Activity modification, NSAIDs, and a gradual active ROM and strengthening exercise program should be initiated as tolerated. Treatment for a rupture may involve a nonoperative approach or surgical repair. However, recent studies have found a significant loss of elbow flexion (30%) and supina-

Control inflammation, swelling, and pain:
Use ice, compression, elevation, NSAIDs, and rest if necessary

↓

Use ice, ultrasound, EMS, interferential current, or thermotherapy to
precede therapeutic exercise

↓

Restore ROM (Assess flexibility at the shoulder region, since limitations
there may increase stress at the elbow)

↓

Perform isometric exercises throughout a pain-free ROM

↓

Progress to isotonic exercises with light resistance, building from
1 to 5 lb, throughout a pain-free range

↓

Improve neuromuscular control with closed kinetic chain exercises,
such as:
Shifting a weighted ball in the hand, press-ups, or walking on the
hands in a push-up position between boxes of varying heights

↓

Add surgical tubing exercises as tolerated

↓

When pain-free, ensure adequate warm-up and gradual return to
functional exercises

↓

Recommend activity modification, biomechanical analysis of skill
performance, or equipment modifications

↓

If involved in a throwing activity:
- Begin functional throwing with a light toss over a distance of
  20–30 feet for 5 minutes, progressing to 15–20 minutes
- When the individual can throw for 15–20 minutes, gradually
  increase the distance to 150 feet
- When proper throwing mechanics are present, gradually
  increase velocity

↓

Continue a strengthening and stretching program as return to activity is initiated

---

tion (40%) strength with a nonoperative approach (9,10). Although this decreased level of function may suffice for daily activities, the distal biceps tends to scar to the brachialis muscle, illuminating the normal contour of the muscle. Surgical repair to reattach the avulsed distal biceps tendon to the radial tuberosity provides the greatest likelihood of maximal functional results and return to sports.

Extensor Strains

With a triceps strain, the mechanism is generally a decelerating type injury. It has been reported in tennis and baseball players, and in weight lifters with a history of anabolic steroid use or local steroid injections (11).

➤ SIGNS AND SYMPTOMS

Passive flexion and resisted elbow extension will produce discomfort. In more moderate strains, acute pain and swelling, and a palpable defect, will be present. Occasionally, a direct blow to the posterior elbow, or an uncoordinated triceps contraction during a fall, can result in an acute rupture of the tendon. In addition to the tendon rupture, 80% of all injuries involve an olecranon avulsion fracture (7). Spontaneous ruptures of the tendon can occur, but these are rare, usually associated with systemic diseases or steroid use.

➤ MANAGEMENT

Treatment involves standard acute care with ice, compression, elevation, and protected rest.

If a palpable defect is noted or an avulsion fracture is suspected, immobilization in a sling is followed by immediate referral to a physician for possible surgical reattachment.

Compartment Syndrome

The deep fascia of the forearm encloses the wrist and finger flexor and extensor muscle groups in a common sheath. The two groups are separated into compartments by an interosseous membrane between the radius and ulna. The wrist and finger flexors are in the anterior compartment; the wrist and finger extensors are in the posterior compartment. The condition is often secondary to an elbow fracture or dislocation, crushing injury, forearm fracture, post-ischemic edema, or excessive muscular exertion, as in weight lifting. Hemorrhage or edema causes increased pressure within the compartment, leading to excessive pressure on neurovascular structures and tissues within the space.

➤ SIGNS AND SYMPTOMS

Onset is usually rapid and can be recognized by swelling, discoloration, absent or diminished distal pulse, and subsequent onset of sensory changes and paralysis. Severe pain at rest, aggravated by passive stretching of the muscles in the compartment, signals a potential problem.

➤ MANAGEMENT

 Treatment involves immobilization of the forearm and wrist. Apply ice to limit pain and swelling, and elevate the forearm above the heart. No external compression should be applied to the area, as the neurovascular structures are already compressed by the swelling. Immediate referral to a physician is necessary since a fasciotomy may be needed to decompress the area.

 The volleyball player may have a mild strain of the common wrist and finger flexor muscle tendons that has been aggravated during repeated overhead spiking drills. Ice, compression, and protected rest should be accompanied by stretching and strengthening exercises for the elbow flexors. If any vascular or sensory changes are present, the individual should be immediately referred to a physician.

OVERUSE CONDITIONS

 A little league baseball pitcher is complaining of pain on the medial elbow that is aggravated during the acceleration phase of throwing. Palpation reveals point tenderness on the medial epicondyle of the humerus, and pain during active elbow flexion and forearm pronation. What condition(s) might be present? How will you manage the injury?

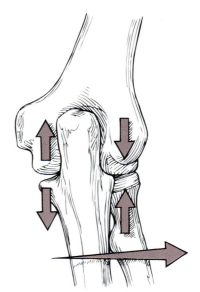

➤ FIGURE 12.13 **An excessive valgus force can lead to both medial tensile stress and lateral compression stress, causing injury to both sides of the joint.**

The throwing mechanism discussed in Chapter 11 can also lead to overuse injuries at the elbow. During the initial acceleration phase, the body is brought rapidly forward, but the elbow and hand lag behind the upper arm. This results in a tremendous tensile valgus stress being placed on the medial aspect of the elbow, particularly the ulnar collateral ligament and adjacent tissues. As acceleration continues, the elbow extensors and wrist flexors contract to add velocity to the throw. This whipping action produces significant valgus stress on the medial elbow and concomitant lateral compressive stress in the radiocapitellar joint **(Figure 12.13)**. At ball release, the elbow is almost fully extended and is positioned slightly anterior to the trunk. At release, the elbow is flexed approximately 20 to 30°. As these forces decrease, however, the extreme pronation of the forearm places the lateral ligaments under tension. During deceleration, eccentric contractions of the long head of the biceps brachii, supinator, and extensor muscles decelerate the forearm in pronation. Additional stress occurs on structures around the olecranon as pronation and extension jam the olecranon into its fossa. Impingement can occur during this jamming.

Epicondylitis is a common, chronic condition seen in activities involving pronation and supination, such as in tennis, javelin throwing, pitching, volleyball, and golf. The condition is sometimes referred to as a **tendinosis** because degeneration, rather than inflammatory conditions, exist. Often the individual will reveal a pattern of poor technique, fatigue, and overuse.

Medial Epicondylitis

Medial epicondylitis is caused by repeated, medial, tension/lateral compression (valgus) forces placed on the arm during the acceleration phase of the throwing motion. Valgus

Signs and Symptoms of Medial Epicondylitis

- Swelling, ecchymosis, and point tenderness over the humeroulnar joint
- Pain over the medial epicondyle, extending distally 1 to 2 cm along the track of the flexor carpi radialis and pronator teres
- Increased pain with resisted wrist flexion and forearm pronation
- Increased pain with valgus stress at 30° flexion
- Negative Tinel's sign, at the cubital tunnel, for ulnar neuritis

forces often produce a combined flexor muscle strain, ulnar collateral ligament sprain, and ulnar neuritis. The two most commonly involved tendons are the pronator teres (humeral head) and the flexor carpi radialis, which originates along the medial supracondylar ridge and a portion of the medial epicondyle (11). If the medial humeral growth plate is affected, it is called "little league elbow," discussed later in the chapter. Simultaneously, lateral compressive and shearing forces generated in the olecranon fossa can damage the lateral condyle of the humerus and radial head, leading to capitellar osteochondral injuries. Posterior stresses may lead to triceps strain, synovial impingement, olecranon fractures, or loose bodies and degenerative joint changes.

➤ SIGNS AND SYMPTOMS

Assessment will reveal swelling, ecchymosis, and point tenderness over the humeroulnar joint, or over the flexor/pronator origin, slightly distal and lateral to the medial epicondyle. Pain is usually severe and aggravated by resisted wrist flexion and pronation, and by a valgus stress applied at 15 to 20° of elbow flexion (Box 12.3). If the ulnar nerve is involved, tingling and numbness may radiate into the forearm and hand, particularly the fourth and fifth fingers.

➤ MANAGEMENT

Most conditions can be managed with ice, NSAIDs, and immobilization in a sling for 2 to 3 weeks with the wrist in slight flexion. Transcutaneous electric nerve stimulation (TENS), high-voltage galvanic stimulation, ultrasound, and interferential current are used to decrease pain and inflammation. Early ROM exercises and gentle, resisted isometric exercises should progress to isotonic strengthening and use of surgical tubing. Activity should not resume until the individual can complete all functional tests pain-free. A functional brace may limit valgus stress and allow early resumption of strenuous activities. In moderate injuries, throwing or overhead motions should be avoided for up to 6 to 12 weeks (7).

*With intra-articular injuries, ulnar nerve problems, or moderate to severe cases of pain or instability, referral to a physician is indicated. **Field Strategy 12.4** describes management of medial epicondylitis.*

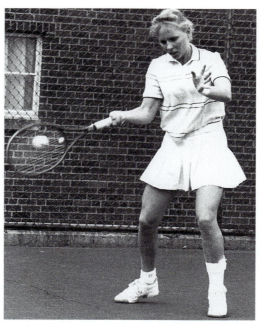

➤ FIGURE 12.14 **Common extensor tendinitis**. Eccentric loading of the elbow extensor muscles occurs with excessive forearm pronation and wrist flexion during the deceleration phase of a tennis stroke or a throwing motion.

Common Extensor Tendinitis (Lateral Epicondylitis)

Pain over the lateral epicondyle denotes extensor tendon overload, and is the most common overuse injury in the adult elbow. The condition is typically caused by eccentric loading of the extensor muscles, predominantly the extensor carpi radialis brevis, during the deceleration phase of the throwing motion or tennis stroke **(Figure 12.14)**. Faulty mechanics ("leading" with the elbow, off-center hits in racquet sports), poorly fitted equipment (handle too small, string too tight), and age (30 to 50 years of age) all contribute to this condition (7).

➤ SIGNS AND SYMPTOMS

Pain will be anterior or just distal to the lateral epicondyle, and may radiate into the forearm extensors during and after activity. With repetition, pain becomes more severe and increases with resisted wrist extension, the "coffee cup" test (pain increases while picking up a full cup of coffee), and the tennis elbow test **(Box 12.4)**.

Signs and Symptoms of Lateral Epicondylitis

- Pain anterior or just distal to the lateral epicondyle that may radiate into the forearm extensors
- Pain initially subsides but becomes more severe with repetition
- Pain increases with resisted wrist extension
- Positive "coffee cup" test and tennis elbow test

FIELD STRATEGY 12.4 **MANAGEMENT ALGORITHM FOR MEDIAL EPICONDYLITIS**

Limit pain and inflammation with ice, compression, NSAIDs, and rest

↓

In the adolescent, if an apophyseal fracture or an avulsion fracture of the medial epicondyle is suspected:

Refer the individual to a physician

↓

Avoid all activities that lead to pain; immobilization may be necessary if simple daily activities cause pain

↓

Other therapies may also supplement the treatment plan:
Ice massage, contrast baths, ultrasound therapy, EMS, interferential current, and friction massage over the flexor tendons

↓

Maintain ROM and strength at the wrist and shoulder

↓

Stretching exercises, within pain-free motions, should include:
Wrist flexion/extension, forearm pronation/supination, and radial and ulnar deviation

↓

Begin with fast contractions using light resistance:
• Perform tennis ball squeezes and other strengthening exercises within pain-free ranges
• Add surgical tubing as tolerated
• Work up to 3–5 sets of 10 repetitions per session before moving on to heavier resistance

↓

Incorporate early, closed chain exercises such as press-ups, wall push-ups, or walking on the hands

↓

Add strengthening exercises for all shoulder, elbow, and wrist motions

↓

Do a biomechanical analysis of the throwing motion to determine proper technique, and make adjustments as necessary

↓

After return to protected activity:
• Continue stretching exercises before and after practice
• Continue ice after practice to control any inflammation
• Return to full activity as tolerated

➤ MANAGEMENT

Initially, ice, compression, NSAIDs, rest, and support will alleviate symptoms. Grasping an object with the forearm pronated is highly discouraged until acute symptoms resolve. Rehabilitation should focus on increasing the strength, endurance, and flexibility of the extensor muscle group. Wrist extension curls or lifts should be performed, and proper equipment and mechanics for the sport should be evaluated. A counterforce strap placed 2 to 3 inches distal to the elbow joint can limit excessive muscular tension placed on the epicondyle, and is usually sufficient to eliminate symptoms. **Field Strategy 12.5** describes management of common extensor tendinitis.

Neural Entrapment Injuries

The ulnar nerve passes behind the medial epicondyle of the humerus through the cubital tunnel to rest against the posterior portion of the ulnar collateral ligament **(Figure 12.15)**. Here the nerve is vulnerable to compression and tensile stress, which may be caused by trauma (acute or chronic), cubital valgus deformity, irregularities within the ulnar groove, or subluxation as a result of a lax ulnar collateral ligament. The individual will complain of a shocking sensation along the medial aspect of the elbow, radiating as if they were "hitting their crazy bone." Palpation or percussion in the ulnar groove will generally reproduce tingling and numbness down the medial aspect of the fore-

1. Ice, compression, elevation, NSAIDs, and rest to limit pain and inflammation.
2. Immobilize wrist in slight extension to allow for functional use of the hand.
3. Cryotherapy, ultrasound, thermotherapy, EMS, interferential current, and friction massage over the extensor tendons may be helpful.
4. Avoid strong gripping activities and activities that aggravate symptoms.
5. Perform stretching exercises within pain-free motion, including wrist flexion/ extension, forearm pronation/supination, and radial and ulnar deviation.
6. Do isotonic strengthening exercises, and add surgical tubing exercises as tolerated. Begin with fast contractions using light resistance.
7. Work up to 3 to 5 sets of 10 repetitions per session before moving on to heavier resistance.
8. Continue active ROM and strengthening exercises for all shoulder, elbow, and wrist motions.
9. Incorporate early, closed chain exercises, such as press-ups, wall push-ups, or walking on the hands.
10. Do a biomechanical analysis of the skills to determine if improper technique may have contributed to the problem, and make appropriate changes.
11. After return to activity, continue stretching exercises before and after practice, and ice after practice to control any inflammation. Return to full activity as tolerated.

arm into the ring and little finger (Tinel's sign). Pain is usually not present, and ROM is not limited. Because the ulnar nerve innervates several intrinsic muscles of the hand, grip strength may be weak.

The median nerve travels across the cubital fossa, passing between the two heads of the pronator teres and the two heads of the flexor digitorum superficialis, to give off its largest branch, the anterior interosseous nerve. Compression may be caused by hypertrophied muscles, particu-

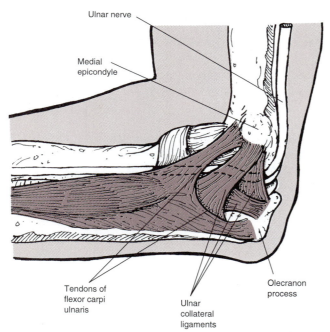

➤ **FIGURE 12.15 Ulnar nerve.** As the ulnar nerve passes through the cubital tunnel between the ulnar collateral ligament and the olecranon fossa, it passes under the two heads of the flexor carpi ulnaris. This tendon is slack during extension, but becomes taut during flexion, contributing to ulnar nerve compression.

larly the pronator teres, or by compression from fibrous arches near the flexor digitorum superficialis muscle, bicipital aponeurosis, or supracondylar process. Often called **"pronator syndrome,"** pain is felt in the anterior proximal forearm, and is aggravated with pronation activities. Numbness may occur in the anterior forearm, or middle and index fingers and thumb.

The radial nerve may be damaged during a midshaft humeral fracture. Less frequently, direct trauma or entrapment occurs at the elbow as the nerve passes anterior to the cubital fossa, pierces the supinator muscle, and runs posterior again into the forearm **(radial tunnel syndrome)**. The terminal branch, the posterior interosseous nerve, supplies all the deeper-lying extensor muscles of the forearm. When injured, symptoms often mimic lateral epicondylitis. An aching lateral elbow pain may radiate down the posterior forearm. Significant point tenderness can be elicited over the supinator muscle, and resisted supination is generally more painful than wrist extension. Extensor weakness of the wrist, called **wrist drop**, is seen in extreme cases, but no sensory loss tends to be present.

➤ MANAGEMENT

The athlete should be immediately referred to a physician. Treatment for neural entrapment depends on the frequency, duration, intensity, magnitude, and cause of the problem. If recognized early, complete rest and NSAIDs can help acute cases. If the injury is secondary to direct blows, a pad can protect the area. Occasionally, chronic nerve damage may require surgery to release any pressure or constriction on the nerve.

 The little league pitcher may have medial epicondylitis caused by excessive valgus forces generated during the throw. Standard acute care is

followed by early ROM exercises to prevent joint stiffness and adhesions. If sensory changes occur on the ulnar aspect of the hand, indicating possible ulnar nerve involvement, or if the condition does not improve in 3 to 4 days, this individual should be referred immediately to a physician.

FRACTURES

 A pole vaulter lost his grip on the pole and fell to the ground on a flexed elbow. Immediate pain and deformity is evident just proximal to the elbow. What is the probable injury? How will you assess possible damage to the neurovascular structures of the arm?

Displaced and undisplaced fractures to the humerus, radius, and ulna usually result from violent compressive forces in direct trauma, such as impact with a helmet or implement, a fall on a flexed elbow or outstretched hand with or without a valgus/varus stress, or tensile forces associated with throwing. Because major nerves and vessels run along the bones, serious neurovascular injury can result from the jagged bone fragments. Fractures to the growth plates are also common in javelin throwers, gymnasts, water polo and tennis players, and adolescent baseball/softball pitchers, whereas stress fractures have been reported in gymnasts, volleyball players, and weight lifters (1,12).

Epiphyseal and Avulsion Fractures

Because the closing growth plate of the medial epicondyle in adolescents is sensitive to tension stress, a repetitive or sudden contraction of the flexor-pronator muscle group may result in a partial or complete avulsion fracture of the medial epicondyle of the humerus. Referred to as "**little league elbow**," the tension stress is related to throwing curve balls and other breaking pitches that require forceful pronation. Use of this term, however, negates the fact that other individuals, such as golfers, gymnasts, javelin throwers, tennis players, bowlers, squash and racquetball players, wrestlers, and weight lifters are also susceptible to the condition. Fracture to the secondary growth center of the lateral epicondyle is similar to a medial epicondyle fracture, and is treated in a similar manner.

➤ SIGNS AND SYMPTOMS

In the initial phase of the injury, the athlete will complain of aching during performance, but no limitations of performance or residual pain will be present. As the condition progresses, an aching pain during activity will limit performance, and a mild postexercise achiness will be present. Some localized tenderness can be elicited directly over the epicondyle. In severe cases, pain can be severe with point tenderness, swelling, and ecchymosis directly on the epicondyle.

➤ MANAGEMENT

Standard acute protocol is followed in the initial stages of injury with activity modification. If performance is lim-

ited because of the pain and postexercise pain is present, the athlete should be referred to a physician. The fracture is managed conservatively with rest and immobilization in a sling for as little as 2 to 3 weeks. However, throwing is usually not allowed for 6 to 12 weeks. Surgery is only necessary if a valgus instability is present, the medial epicondyle is incarcerated within the elbow joint, or ulnar nerve symptoms are present.

Stress Fractures

Stress fractures to the diaphysis of the ulna can occur during intensive weight lifting. Bilateral distal radial and ulnar fractures have been found in young individuals who lift heavy weights or lose control of the barbells, resulting in added shear stress. For this reason, adolescents in a weight-lifting program should be properly instructed and supervised to prevent injury.

Osteochondritis Dessicans

An unusual complication of repetitive stress to the skeletally immature elbow is osteochondritis dessicans. The mechanism is attributed to lateral compressive forces exerted during the throwing motion that can damage the radial head, capitellum, or both. In young athletes with open growth plates (ages 12 to 15 years), a focal lesion can lead to destruction of the overlying articular cartilage with fragmentation and softening of the underlying subchondral bone. A microfracture (loose bodies) and eventual avascular necrosis lead to further joint degeneration.

An associated osteochondrosis condition, called Panner's disease, occurs at a younger age (ages 7 to 10 years), and encompasses the entire capitellum. Pain is present over the lateral and anterior elbow and increases with deep palpation or pronation-supination. Elbow extension may be limited by 20° or more secondary to synovitis and a deformed capitellar congruity (1). Loose body formation is much less likely to occur in Panner's disease.

➤ SIGNS AND SYMPTOMS

Signs and symptoms of osteochondritis dessicans will mirror little league elbow. Pain with be present with activity and improve with rest. There may be occasional clicking or locking of the elbow. Swelling and tenderness is centralized over the radiocapitellar joint. Grating may be present during passive pronation and supination, and the athlete may have limited full extension. A flexion contracture of the dominant elbow, in a sport that requires throwing, necessitates referral to a physician.

➤ MANAGEMENT

Management involves referral to a physician. Treatment is usually conservative, with rest for 6 to 18 months. If no loose body is present, no further treatment may be needed. If a fragment is displaced, then surgery may be necessary to reattach a large articular fragment or to excise a small fragment.

Displaced and Undisplaced Fractures

Supracondylar fractures, caused by falling on an outstretched hand, occur largely in children. A catastrophic complication from this fracture is ischemic necrosis of the forearm muscles known as **Volkmann's contracture**. The brachial artery or median nerve can be damaged by the fractured bone ends, leading to major circulatory or neural impairment to the forearm and hand. As a result, the hand is cold, white, and numb. Severe pain in the forearm is aggravated by passive extension of the fingers. These symptoms indicate a serious problem.

Immobilize the arm in a vacuum splint, and activate EMS to immediately transport the individual to the nearest medical facility. Do not assume that the presence of a radial or ulnar pulse indicates adequate circulation to the forearm muscles.

Fracture of the olecranon process of the ulna results from direct trauma, such as being struck with a field hockey or lacrosse stick, or falling on a flexed elbow. The tension of the triceps pulls the bone fragment superiorly. Because this fracture is intra-articular, it does not respond to conservative treatment and requires surgical intervention.

The head of the radius may be fractured as a result of a valgus stress that tears the ulnar collateral ligament, leading to traumatic compressive and shearing stress on the radial head (see Figure 12.13). The fracture may be nondisplaced (Type I), displaced (Type II), or comminuted (Type III). Tenderness can be elicited on palpation of the radial head, and swelling can be seen lateral to the olecranon. Flexion and extension may or may not be limited. In contrast, passive pronation and supination is painful and restricted. There may be an associated valgus instability of the elbow or axial instability of the forearm. A nondisplaced fracture is treated nonoperatively with early ROM exercises to prevent joint stiffness. If more than one-third of the articular surface is involved, more than 30° of angulation, or more than 3 mm or more of fracture gap, open reduction is recommended (7).

The "**nightstick fracture**," seen in football and hockey players, is caused by a direct blow to the forearm that fractures the ulna. After closed reduction, splinting or casting for 7 to 10 days is needed to allow initial swelling and discomfort to subside. If a radial head dislocation or distal radial ulnar joint subluxation is present, open reduction and internal fixation is necessary.

In gymnastics, a unique forearm fracture occurs as a result of wearing leather grips with enclosed dowels. These dowels help grip the horizontal bar. Instead of allowing the individual to continue around the circle during a giant swing maneuver, the leather grip "catches" or grabs onto the bar and holds the hand in position, causing the forearm to "wrap around" and sustain multiple fractures. Severe pain and disability with this fracture require immediate immobilization in a vacuum splint.

Activate EMS to transport this individual to the nearest medical facility.

Fracture Management

Fractures should be suspected in all elbow and forearm injuries. Palpation, compression, traction, and percussion, which can assist in determining possible fractures, are explained in **Field Strategy 12.6**. In addition, a neurological and circulatory assessment should be conducted. If the radial nerve is damaged, forearm supination and extension at the elbow, wrist, or fingers is weak, and sensory changes may occur on the dorsum of the hand. If the median nerve is damaged, active wrist and finger flexion is weak, and sensory changes may occur on the palm of the hand.

If the ulnar nerve is damaged, ulnar deviation and finger abduction and adduction are weak, and sensory changes may occur on the ulnar border of the hand. The athletic trainer should take a pulse at the wrist, at the ulnar and radial arteries, or blanch the fingernails and note capillary refill. Apply a vacuum splint, and immediately transport the athlete to the nearest medical facility.

The pole vaulter fell on a flexed elbow and now has deformity just proximal to the elbow. This indicates a possible supracondylar fracture. Immobilize the arm in a vacuum splint, and take a pulse at the radial and ulnar artery, check capillary refill at the fingernails, and check bilateral sensation on the palm and dorsum of the hand. Activate EMS to transport this individual to the nearest medical facility.

ASSESSMENT OF THE ELBOW

Two weeks ago on a cold and windy day, a javelin thrower experienced extreme pain on the posteromedial aspect of the right elbow during a series of throws. She iced periodically throughout the night, and practiced the next day with only mild discomfort. She has iced daily for the past week and had the elbow strapped for support. Today she noticed muscle weakness when picking up her book bag, and an inability to extend the elbow fully without sharp pain. How will you conduct the evaluation?

The elbow's primary role is to position the forearm and hand in the most appropriate position to perform efficient motion. Biomechanical errors in throwing technique at the shoulder can place additional stress at the elbow. Because use of equipment is often associated with overuse problems, find out if the individual uses a bat, racquet, field hockey or lacrosse stick, or other implement. Check for proper

FIELD STRATEGY 12.6 **DETERMINING A POSSIBLE FRACTURE IN THE UPPER ARM AND FOREARM**

A. **Compression.** Palpate the region for any pain, deformity, crepitus, or loose bodies. Ask if the individual heard any cracking sounds that might indicate a possible fracture. Apply gentle compression along the long axis of the bone. Then encircle the distal ulna and radius with your hand, and give mild compression. This will produce some distraction at the proximal end of the ulna and radius. Increased pain in either position indicates a possible fracture.

B. **Distraction.** Slowly distract the bones. If pain is eased, this may indicate a possible fracture. If pain increases, it indicates soft tissue damage.

C. **Percussion.** Gently tap the superficial bony landmarks. Vibrations will travel along the bone and cause increased pain at the fracture site. For example, tap the following sites:
 - Humerus—medial and lateral epicondyles
 - Ulna—olecranon process and distal styloid process
 - Radius—distal styloid process

D. **Tuning fork.** Tap a tuning fork, and place the base on the superficial bone sites mentioned above. Increased pain indicates a possible fracture.

Any positive signs indicate a possible fracture. Immobilize the limb in a vacuum splint or other appropriate splint or sling, and transport the individual to the nearest medical facility.

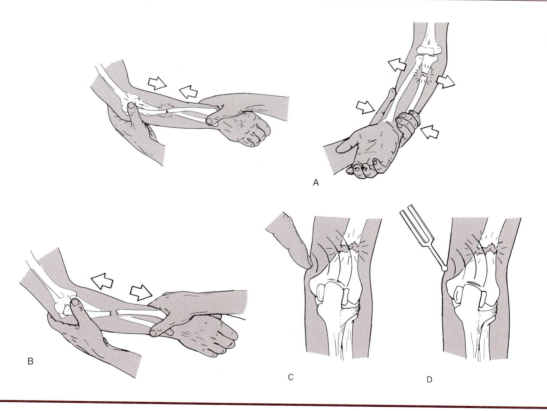

grip size, excessive string tension, and excessive racquet weight or stiffness, and assess skill technique to rule out possible contributing factors. During the evaluation, keep in mind that pain may be referred from the cervical region, shoulder, or wrist. As in any assessment, both elbows should be fully visible to allow for bilateral comparison. **Field Strategy 12.7** summarizes an assessment of the upper arm, elbow, and forearm.

HISTORY

What questions need to be asked to determine the javelin thrower's primary complaint? Could age, gender, or the sport-specific skills be a factor in this injury?

The onset and location of symptoms are two of the most critical facts surrounding elbow trauma. This information

FIELD STRATEGY 12.7   ELBOW EVALUATION

<u>HISTORY</u>

- Primary complaint including:
  - Current nature, location, and onset of the condition
- Mechanism of injury
  - Cause of stress; position of the arm and elbow; direction of force
  - Changes in throwing style, equipment, overhead motion techniques, or conditioning modes
- Characteristics of the symptoms
  - Evolution of the onset, nature, location, severity and duration of pain and weakness
- Disability resulting from the injury
- Related medical history
  - Previous injuries to the area, congenital abnormalities, or family history

<u>OBSERVATION AND INSPECTION</u>

- Observation should analyze the carrying angle and position of function
- Inspect the injury site for deformity, swelling, discoloration, hypertrophy or muscle atrophy, visible congenital deformity, or surgical incisions or scars

<u>PALPATION</u>

- Bony structures to determine a possible fracture
- Soft tissue structures for skin temperature, swelling, point tenderness, crepitus, deformity, muscle spasm, cutaneous sensation, and pulse

<u>FUNCTIONAL TESTS</u>

- Active movement
- Passive movement and end feels
- Resisted movement

<u>STRESS TESTS</u>

- Ligamentous instability tests
- Common extensor tendinitis test
- Medial epicondylitis test
- Tinel's sign for ulnar neuritis
- Elbow flexion test for ulnar neuritis
- Test for pronator teres syndrome
- Pinch grip test

<u>NEUROLOGIC TESTS</u>

- Myotomes
- Reflexes
- Dermatomes

<u>SPORT-SPECIFIC FUNCTIONAL TESTS</u>

forms the basis for determining the cause-and-effect relationship between the mechanism and the onset of injury. To gather information about the primary complaint, ask questions that focus on the individual's perception of pain, weakness, or sensory changes. When was the problem first noticed? Is it acute or has the problem progressively gotten worse? Ask specific questions related to equipment, technique, and recent changes in training intensity, frequency, or duration. Is there any noticeable locking, catching, or general muscle weakness? Are there specific actions that aggravate the condition, such as throwing? In addition to the general questions discussed in Chapter 4, specific questions to ask in an elbow evaluation are listed in **Field Strategy 12.8**.

The 17-year-old javelin thrower has been working on a new throwing style this past month. Two weeks ago, she began to add velocity to the throw and experienced sharp pain on the posteromedial aspect of the elbow. Today she noticed muscle weakness when picking up her book bag, and an inability to fully extend the elbow without sharp pain. In addition, her little finger feels funny.

OBSERVATION AND INSPECTION

What specific factors should be observed during the assessment? Would it be advantageous also to assess the shoulder and wrist?

FIELD STRATEGY 12.8 DEVELOPING A HISTORY OF THE INJURY

CURRENT INJURY STATUS

1. Where is the pain (or weakness) located? How would you rate the pain (weakness)? What type of pain is it (dull ache, throbbing, constant, intermittent, burning, or radiating)?
2. Did the pain come on suddenly (acute) or gradually (overuse)? Was the pain greatest when the injury first occurred or did it get worse the second or third day?
3. (If acute, ask:) What were you doing at the time of the injury? Was there a direct blow? Did you fall? How (outstretched arm, flexed elbow)? (If chronic, ask:) What different activities have you been doing in the last week? (Look for changes in technique, frequency, duration, intensity, or changes in equipment.)
4. Did you hear any sounds during the incident? Any snaps, pops, or cracks? Did you notice any swelling, discoloration, muscle spasms, or numbness with the injury?
5. What actions or motions bring on the pain? It is worse in the morning, during activity, after activity, or at night? Does it wake you up at night? In what part of the arm motion does it hurt the worst? Does the arm tire easily? When the pain sets in, how long does it last?
6. Are there certain activities you are unable to perform because of the pain? Which ones?
7. What has been done for the condition?
8. How old are you? (Remember that common extensor tendinitis (tennis elbow) often occurs in older individuals or in individuals that do a great deal of flexion and extension in their jobs. Dislocation of the radial head is seen in young children who have had the arm jerked in a distractive manner). Which hand is dominant?

PAST INJURY STATUS

1. Have you ever injured the elbow before? How did that occur? What was done for the injury? Did you have any difficulty returning to your full functional status?
2. Have you had any medical problems recently? (Look for problems that may refer pain to the area.) Are you on any medication?

Both arms should be clearly visible for bilateral comparison. With an acute injury, it is critical early in the assessment to recognize possible fractures and dislocations. If the individual is in great pain or is unable or unwilling to move the elbow, complete the assessment in a position most comfortable for the individual. First observe the position of the arm. Is there a noticeable deformity? How is the individual holding the arm? If swelling is present in the joint, the individual may be unable to fully extend the elbow, resulting in a slightly flexed position. This **resting position** allows the joint to have maximal volume to accommodate intra-articular swelling. Note the position of the olecranon relative to the epicondyles of the humerus. In a normal, flexed position, the olecranon process and two epicondyles of the humerus should form an isosceles triangle. In an extended position, the olecranon process and two epicondyles form a straight line.

If the history has indicated an insidious onset of elbow trauma, observe full-body posture, especially the neck and shoulder area, for possible referral of symptoms. Note the carrying angle of the arms. Normally the individual should have a slight valgus angle with the forearm fully supinated and elbow extended. Angles greater than 20° are referred to as **cubital valgus**; angles less than 10° are referred to as **cubital varus**. Baseball pitchers may exhibit cubital valgus in the throwing arm, an adaptation to repeated valgus

loading during the throwing motion. The alignment of the forearm and humerus is normally fully extended, though extension beyond 0° **(cubital recurvatum)** is common, especially in female athletes. The elbow is then placed in the position of function: 90° of flexion with the hand held halfway between supination and pronation. Inspect the cubital fossa for swelling, which may place pressure on the neurovascular structures as they pass through the area. The cubital fossa is a triangular area bounded laterally by the brachioradialis muscle and medially by the pronator teres muscle. The biceps brachii tendon, median nerve, and brachial artery pass through the fossa. Inspect the entire region for symmetry and any abnormal deformity, muscle atrophy, hypertrophy, swelling, discoloration, or previous surgical incisions.

 An abnormal carrying angle does not exist in either arm. Joint effusion and swelling are visible on the medial and posteromedial aspect of the humerus over the medial epicondyle and cubital tunnel. No other visible signs are apparent.

PALPATION

 Weakness occurs during wrist flexion, and swelling is visible on the medial and posteromedial aspect

of the humerus. The individual is unable to fully extend the elbow without sharp pain. Where will you begin palpation so the discomfort is not compounded?

Bilateral palpation should determine temperature, swelling, point tenderness, crepitus, deformity, muscle spasm, and cutaneous sensation. Pulses can be taken at the radial and ulnar arteries at the wrist, and at the brachial artery in the cubital fossa. Begin palpation in a proximal-to-distal direction, leaving the most painful areas for last. Support the injured arm during palpation, and compare bilaterally.

Anterior Palpation

1. Cubital fossa, biceps brachii tendon, median nerve, and brachial artery
2. Coracoid process and head of radius

Lateral Palpation

1. Lateral supracondylar ridge and brachioradialis muscle
2. Lateral epicondyle, common wrist extensors, and supinator muscle
3. Radial collateral ligament
4. Annular ligament and head of the radius. This is facilitated by supination and pronation of the forearm

Posterior Palpation

1. Triceps muscle
2. Olecranon process and olecranon fossa. This is facilitated with the elbow flexed at 45° to relax the triceps
3. Olecranon bursa. Grasp the skin overlying the olecranon process and note any thickening or presence of loose bodies
4. Ulnar nerve in the cubital tunnel
5. Ulnar border distal to the styloid process at the wrist

Medial Palpation

1. Medial supracondylar ridge
2. Medial epicondyle and common wrist flexor-pronator tendons and muscles
3. Ulnar collateral ligament

Swelling and point tenderness were elicited at the medial epicondyle, medial joint line, medial olecranon process, and medial superior ridge of the olecranon fossa. Palpation in the cubital tunnel caused an extremely painful tingling sensation to travel down the ulnar aspect of the forearm into the little finger.

PHYSICAL EXAMINATION TESTS

Swelling and pain appear to be centered on the medial aspect of the humerus and involve the medial border of the olecranon process and ole-cranon fossa. Furthermore, it appears the ulnar nerve may be involved. How will you proceed to confirm your suspicions about the extent of this injury?

If a fracture or dislocation is suspected, do not attempt any special tests. Immobilize the arm in an appropriate splint, and refer the individual to a physician. For other injuries, do only those tests necessary to assess the current injury.

Functional Tests

The athletic trainer should determine the available range of motion in elbow flexion/extension, forearm pronation/supination, and wrist flexion/extension. If trauma is suspected to the ulnar, median, or radial nerves, range-of-motion testing of the thumb and fingers should also be performed.

ACTIVE MOVEMENTS

The athletic trainer should stabilize the upper arm against the body to prevent muscle substitution. As with previous assessments, bilateral comparison with the uninvolved arm should always be completed. In addition, painful active movements should be performed last to prevent painful symptoms from overflowing into the next movement. The individual motions listed below can be assessed. The numbers in parentheses are normal ranges of motion for each movement.

- Flexion at the elbow (140 to 150°)
- Extension at the elbow (0 to 10°)
- Supination of the forearm (90°)
- Pronation of the forearm (90°)
- Flexion of the wrist (80 to 90°)
- Extension of the wrist (70 to 90°)

During elbow extension, remember that some females can extend as much as 5 to 15° below the straight line. Bilateral comparison will verify whether this extra motion is normal for this individual. In performing active pronation and supination, instruct the individual to flex the elbow to 90° and secure the elbow next to the body, to avoid any glenohumeral motion. The individual can hold a pencil in the closed fist and perform both motions in a continuous pattern. Goniometry measurements are demonstrated in **Figure 12.16**.

PASSIVE MOVEMENTS

If the individual is able to perform full ROM during active movements, apply gentle overpressure at the extremes of motion to determine end feel in both arms for bilateral comparison. Flexion at the elbow provides an end feel of tissue approximation. In extension, end feel is bone to bone. Supination and pronation have an end feel of tissue stretch. If the individual is unable to perform full active movement, passive movement can determine the available ROM and end feel.

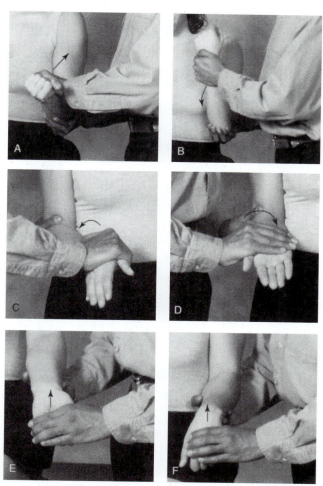

➤ FIGURE 12.16 Goniometry measurement. A, Elbow flexion and extension. Center the fulcrum over the lateral epicondyle of the humerus. Align the proximal arm along the humerus, using the acromion process for reference. The distal arm is aligned along the radius, using the styloid process for reference. B, Forearm supination. The fulcrum is centered medial to the ulnar styloid process. The proximal arm is parallel to the midline of the humerus, and the distal arm is placed across the palmar aspect of the forearm just proximal to the styloid processes of the radius and ulna. C, Forearm pronation. The fulcrum is centered lateral to the ulnar styloid process. The arms are placed in the same position but on the dorsal aspect of the forearm.

➤ FIGURE 12.17 Resisted manual muscle testing for the elbow. The myotomes are listed in parentheses. A, Elbow flexion (C6). B, Elbow extension (C7). C, Forearm supination. D, Forearm pronation. E, Wrist flexion (C7). F, Wrist extension (C6).

RESISTED MUSCLE TESTING

Stabilize the individual's elbow against the body. Begin with the muscle on stretch and apply resistance proximal to the wrist throughout the full ROM. Do bilateral comparison with the uninvolved side. To avoid allowing finger flexors or extensors to assist during movement, instruct the individual to keep the thumb and fingers relaxed. As always, painful motions should be delayed until last. **Figure 12.17** demonstrates motions that should be tested.

Stress Tests

Stress tests are performed when you have a clear indication of what structures may be damaged. Use only those tests deemed relevant, and always compare the results to the uninvolved arm.

LIGAMENTOUS INSTABILITY TESTS

Because of the amount of rotation that occurs at the shoulder, it is difficult to get an accurate valgus or varus stress at the elbow. To compensate for this, the athletic trainer should perform these tests at multiple angles from full extension to 20 to 30° of flexion. When the olecranon is "unlocked" from the olecranon fossa, the ligamentous structures are isolated. With the individual seated, stabilize the arm and apply a valgus or abduction force to the distal forearm to stress the ulnar collateral ligament **(Figure 12.18A)**. A varus or adduction force is then applied at the forearm in the various angles to stress the radial collateral ligament **(Figure 12.18B)**. Apply the force several times with increasing overpressure, and note any pain or joint laxity.

COMMON EXTENSOR TENDINITIS TEST (LATERAL EPICONDYLITIS OR TENNIS ELBOW TEST)

The athletic trainer should stabilize the individual's flexed elbow and palpate the lateral epicondyle. The individual should make a fist and pronate the forearm. The athletic trainer then instructs the athlete to radially deviate and extend the wrist while the athletic trainer resists the motion **(Figure 12.19A)**. A positive sign is indicated if

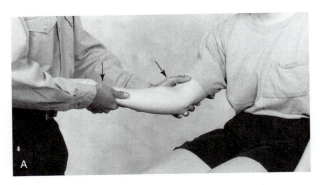
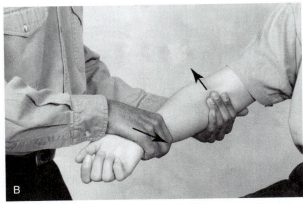

➤ FIGURE 12.18 Ligamentous instability tests. A, To stress the ulnar collateral ligament, apply a valgus force at multiple angles. B, To stress the radial collateral ligament, apply a varus force at multiple angles. Arrows indicate the direction the athletic trainer applies stress.

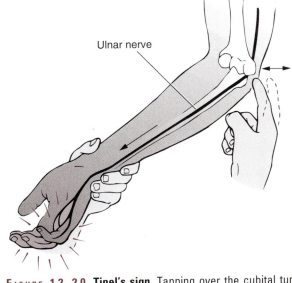

Ulnar nerve

➤ FIGURE 12.20 Tinel's sign. Tapping over the cubital tunnel will produce a tingling sensation down the ulnar nerve into the forearm and hand. A positive Tinel's sign indicates ulnar nerve entrapment.

MEDIAL EPICONDYLITIS TEST

With the flexed elbow stabilized against the body and the forearm supinated, the athletic trainer palpates the medial epicondyle. The athletic trainer extends the wrist and elbow while the athlete resists this movement. A positive sign is indicated by pain over the medial epicondyle of the humerus.

TINEL'S SIGN FOR ULNAR NEURITIS

The cubital tunnel is tapped on the posteromedial side of the elbow. A positive sign is indicated by a tingling sensation that runs down the ulnar aspect of the forearm into the medial half of the fourth finger and all of the fifth **(Figure 12.20)**.

severe pain is present over the lateral epicondyle of the humerus. The same results can be elicited by passively stretching the extensor muscles by simultaneously pronating the forearm, flexing the wrist, and extending the elbow **(Figure 12.19B)**. Additional discomfort can be produced by testing the extensor digitorum communis of the third digit by applying resistance distal to the proximal interphalangeal joint with the wrist extended **(Figure 12.19C)**.

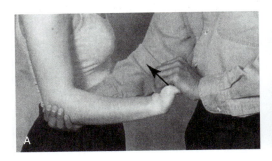
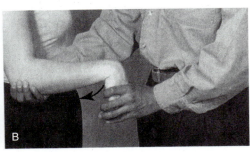
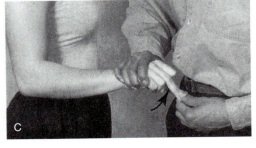
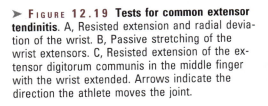

➤ FIGURE 12.19 Tests for common extensor tendinitis. A, Resisted extension and radial deviation of the wrist. B, Passive stretching of the wrist extensors. C, Resisted extension of the extensor digitorum communis in the middle finger with the wrist extended. Arrows indicate the direction the athlete moves the joint.

ELBOW FLEXION TEST FOR ULNAR NEURITIS

This test determines whether the ulnar nerve is entrapped in the cubital tunnel. Ask the athlete to completely flex the elbow and hold it in that position for 5 minutes. A positive test is indicated by tingling or numbness in the ulnar nerve distribution pattern of the forearm and hand.

TEST FOR PRONATOR TERES SYNDROME

The athlete sits with the elbow flexed at 90°. The examiner strongly resists forearm pronation while the elbow is extended. A positive test is indicated by tingling or paresthesia in the median nerve distribution in the forearm and hand.

PINCH GRIP TEST

Ask the individual to pinch the tip of the index finger and thumb together **(Figure 12.21)**. Normally, there should be a tip-to-tip pinch. If an abnormal pulp-to-pulp pinch is performed, the anterior interosseous nerve, an extension of the median nerve, may be entrapped at the elbow as it passes between the two heads of the pronator teres.

Neurologic Testing

Neurologic integrity can be assessed with the use of myotomes, reflexes, and cutaneous patterns, which include both segmental dermatomes and peripheral nerve patterns.

MYOTOMES

Isometric muscle testing of the myotomes should be performed in the loose-packed position and include scapular elevation (C_4), shoulder abduction (C_5), elbow flexion and/or wrist extension (C_6), elbow extension and/or wrist flexion (C_7), thumb extension and/or ulnar deviation (C_8), and abduction and/or adduction of the hand intrinsics (T_1).

REFLEXES

Reflexes in the upper extremity include the biceps (C_5–C_6), brachioradialis (C_6), and triceps (C_7). The individual should be relaxed with the elbow flexed. The biceps and triceps reflex testing was explained in Figure 11.40. The brachioradialis reflex is tested in a similar manner. The elbow is flexed and supported by the examiner's forearm, with the wrist in slight ulnar deviation. Using a reflex hammer, strike the brachioradialis tendon at the distal end of the radius **(Figure 12.22)**. In some individuals, the tap may need to be applied 2 to 3 inches proximal to the wrist. A slight jerk in elbow flexion is a normal sign.

CUTANEOUS PATTERNS

The segmental nerve dermatome patterns for the elbow region are demonstrated in **Figure 12.23**. The peripheral nerve cutaneous patterns are demonstrated in **Figure 12.24**. Test bilaterally for altered sensation with sharp and dull touch by running the open hand and fingernails over the neck, shoulder, and anterior and posterior chest walls, and down both sides of the arms and hands.

Sport-specific Functional Tests

Remember that the elbow is in the middle of the upper extremity kinetic chain. Therefore, it must function properly to position the hand so that daily activities can be performed smoothly and efficiently. Activities such as combing the hair, throwing a ball, lifting an object, or pushing an object should be performed pain-free. Ask the individual to perform those skills needed to complete their daily living activities and sport-specific tasks. Each movement should be pain-free and fluid.

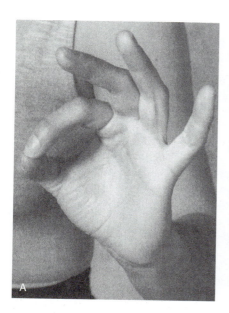
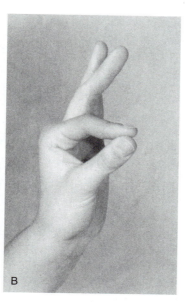

➤ FIGURE 12.21 **Pinch grip test**. Ask the individual to make an O with the thumb and forefinger. A, Normal tip-to-tip. B, Abnormal pulp-to-pulp signifies entrapment of the interior interosseous nerve.

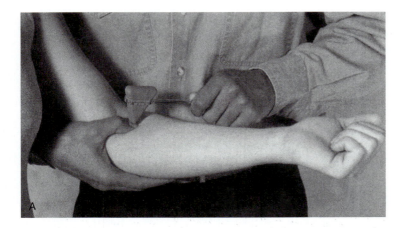

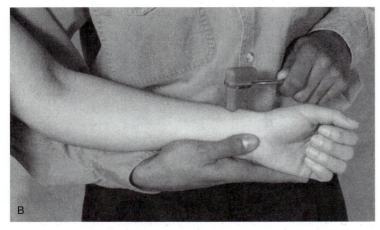

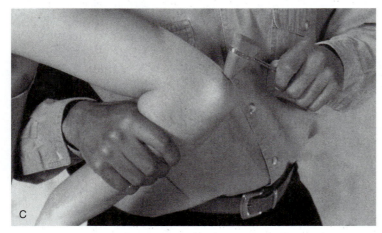

➤ FIGURE 12.22 Reflex testing. A, Biceps reflex. B, Brachioradialis reflex. C, Triceps reflex.

The athlete should be referred to a physician if any of the conditions listed in **Box 12.5** are present.

💡 *Active and passive elbow flexion is limited by about 10°, which may be due to intra-articular swelling. Passive terminal extension is painful, and increased pain and muscle weakness are evident in wrist flexion and pronation. Valgus stress produces only slight pain and no laxity. Tinel's sign is positive. This individual may have an impingement injury involving ulnar neuritis, posterior impingement of the olecranon process in the fossa, and a*

strain of the flexor-pronator group. This individual needs to be referred to a physician.

REHABILITATION

 The javelin thrower has a painful elbow as a result of overuse while learning a new technique. After the physician assesses and treats the individual, what exercises should be included in the general rehabilitation program for this elbow injury?

Rehabilitation of the upper arm, elbow, and forearm must involve exercises for the entire kinetic chain, since

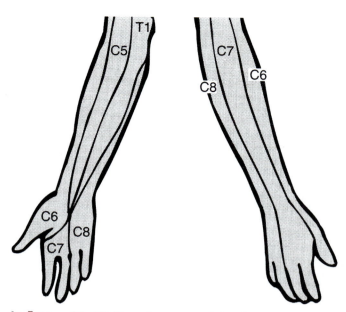

➤ FIGURE 12.23 Dermatomes around the elbow region.

muscles in the upper arm cross the shoulder and elbow, and muscles in the forearm cross the elbow and wrist. Traumatic injuries to the elbow often require immobilization. Although the elbow is immobilized, early ROM and strengthening exercises can be conducted at the wrist, hand, and shoulder. In overuse injuries where immobilization is usually not present, pain may be exacerbated by certain motions. The exercise program should focus on early mobilization in the available pain-free motions, and expand to the other motions once pain has subsided. Individuals who are involved in throwing-type activities should also be sure to include scapular stabilization exercises, along with strengthening exercises for the shoulder. The reader should refer to Chapter 11 for appropriate shoulder exercises. This section will focus on only those exercises specifically for the upper arm, elbow, and forearm. Hand and finger exercises are discussed in Chapter 13.

Restoration of Motion

ROM exercises focus on elbow flexion and extension, forearm pronation and supination, wrist flexion and extension, and wrist radial and ulnar deviation. The individual can use the opposite hand to apply a low-load, prolonged stretch in the various motions to minimize joint trauma and increase flexibility **(Figure 12.25)**. The upper body ergometer (UBE) is also an effective ROM tool.

Restoration of Proprioception and Balance

Closed chain exercises may be performed immediately after the acute phase of injury. Shifting body weight from one hand to the other may be performed on a wall, table top, or unstable surface, such as a foam mat or BAPS board. Push-ups and exercises in a frontal and sagittal plane can be performed on a ProFitter or slide board, if available. Step-ups can be completed on a box, stool, or Stair Master. This activity can progress to stepping up and down on boxes of differing heights, arranged so the exercise is performed in diagonal patterns, circles, or figure 8s.

As with the shoulder injury, the throwing motion should be rehearsed using mirrors or videotape. As the

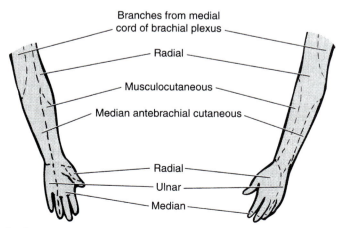

➤ FIGURE 12.24 Cutaneous sensation patterns for the peripheral nerves at the elbow region.

Branches from medial cord of brachial plexus
Radial
Musculocutaneous
Median antebrachial cutaneous
Radial
Ulnar
Median

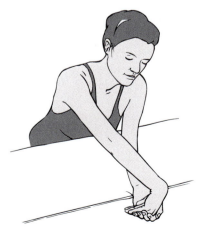

➤ FIGURE 12.25 Range-of-motion exercises can be facilitated by using the opposite hand to apply a sustained stretch.

motion is performed, biomechanical errors at the elbow are corrected. When motion is perfected, speed of movement and distance of throw are gradually increased.

Muscular Strength, Endurance, and Power

Gentle, resisted isometric exercises can begin immediately after injury or after surgery while the arm is still immobilized. As the individual improves, more overload is applied. Once normal ROM is achieved, apply a resistance force in an unanticipated direction to make the individual adjust to the resistance. Open kinetic chain exercises can be performed in the various motions using light-weight dumbbells. Many of these exercises were demonstrated in Field Strategy 12.1. The individual should complete 30 to 50 repetitions with a 1-pound weight, and should not progress in resistance until 50 repetitions are achieved. With the forearm supported on a table, perform wrist curls, reverse wrist curls, pronation, and supination. A weighted bar or hammer can be used for radial and ulnar deviation, and for pronation and supination. Another common exercise is the wrist curl-up, using a broomstick with a light weight suspended on a 3- to 4-foot rope. The individual slowly winds the rope up around the stick, then slowly unwinds the rope. PNF resisted exercises and surgical tubing are used for concentric and eccentric loading.

Plyometric exercises may involve catching a weighted ball and using a quick eccentric stretch of the muscle to facilitate a concentric contraction in throwing the ball. The exercise can progress through various one- and two-arm chest passes and overhead passes. A minitramp may also be used to do plyometric bounding push-ups.

Cardiovascular Fitness

General body conditioning should be maintained throughout the rehabilitation program. Several examples of programs were provided in Field Strategy 7.6 and included use of a jump rope, Stair Master, treadmill, and upper body ergometer (UBE).

 The javelin thrower should focus on restoring ROM in elbow flexion/extension, forearm pronation/supination, wrist flexion/extension, and radial and ulnar deviation. Isometric strengthening exercises should begin immediately in pain-free motions, with active exercises beginning as soon as normal ROM is achieved. The program should also include general body conditioning and strengthening exercises for the shoulder, elbow, and wrist.

Summary

1. The elbow encompasses three articulations: the humeroulnar, humeroradial, and proximal radioulnar joints.

2. The medial collateral ligament is the most important ligament for stability of the elbow joint, and is divided into the anterior, transverse, and posterior oblique bands.

3. The major nerves of the elbow and forearm include the musculocutaneous, median, ulnar, and radial nerves.

4. Chronic blows to the arm can result in the development of ectopic bone, either in the belly of the muscle (myositis ossificans) or as an outgrowth (exostosis) of the underlying bone.

5. The subcutaneous olecranon bursa is the largest bursa in the elbow region. Bursitis may be acute or chronic, aseptic or septic.

6. In adolescents, the most common traumatic injury to the elbow is subluxation or dislocation of the radial head, referred to as "nursemaid's elbow" or "pulled-elbow syndrome."

7. Most ulnar dislocations occur in individuals younger than 20, with a peak incidence in early adolescence. The mechanism is usually hyperextension, or a sudden, violent unidirectional valgus force that drives the ulna posterior or posterolateral. Because 60% of all elbow dislocations have an associated fracture, the limb should be immobilized in a vacuum splint and the athlete transported immediately to the nearest medical facility.

8. Chronic injuries result from inadequate warm-up, excessive training past the point of fatigue, inadequate rehabilitation of previous injuries, or neglect of seemingly minor conditions that progress to major complications.

9. Repetitive throwing motions place a tremendous tensile stress on the medial joint structures (medial collateral ligament, ulnar nerve, and common flexor tendons), and concomitant lateral compressive stress in the radiocapitellar joint.

10. Medial epicondylitis will produce severe pain on resisted wrist flexion and pronation, and with a valgus stress applied at 15 to 20° of elbow flexion.

11. Common extensor tendinitis will produce severe pain on resisted wrist extension and supination, and with a varus stress applied at 15 to 20° of elbow flexion.

12. Lateral compressive forces on the radiocapitellar joint can lead to osteochondritis dessicans in the skeletally immature elbow.

13. During assessment, pain may be referred from other areas of the body, particularly the cervical neck, shoulder, and wrist.

14. Should a decision be made to refer an individual to a physician for care, immobilize the limb by wrapping the arm to the body, or using a sling and swathe, posterior splint, vacuum splint, or a commercial product that can pad and protect the area.

References

1. Sobel J, Nirschl RP. Elbow injuries. In: Athletic Injuries and Rehabilitation. Edited by Zachazewski AE, Magee DJ, Quillen WS. Philadelphia: WB Saunders, 1996.

2. Stanitski CL. Combating overuse injuries: A focus on children and adolescents. Phys Sportsmed 1993;21(1):87-106.

3. Rettig AC, Patel DV. Epidemiology of elbow, forearm, and wrist injuries in the athlete. Clinics Sport Med 1995;14(2):289-297.

4. Werner SL, Fleisig GS, Dillman CJ, Andrews JR. Biomechanics of the elbow during baseball pitching. J Orthop Sports Phys Ther 1993;17(6):274-278.

5. Salzman KL, Lillegard WA, Butcher JD. Upper extremity bursitis. Am Fam Phys 1997;56(7):1797-1806.

6. Ring D, Waters PM. Management of fractures and dislocations of the elbow in children. Acta Ortho Belgica 1996;62(S1):58-65.

7. Mehlhoff TL, Bennett JB. Elbow injuries. In: The Team Physician's Handbook. Edited by Mellion MB, Walsh WM, Shelton GL. Philadelphia: Hanley & Belfus, 1997.

8. Blackard D, Sampson JA. Management of an uncomplicated posterior elbow dislocation. J Ath Train 1997;32(1):63-67.

9. Williams JS Jr, Hang DW, Bach BR Jr. Distal biceps rupture in a snowboarder. Phys Sportsmed 1996;24(12):67-70.

10. Pearl ML, Bessos K, Wong K. Strength deficits related to distal biceps tendon rupture and repair. Am J Sports Med 1998;26(2):295-296.

11. Caldwell GL Jr, Safran MR. Elbow problems in the athlete. Orthop Clin North Am 1995;26(3):465-485.

12. Thein LA. The child and adolescent athlete. In: Athletic Injuries and Rehabilitation. Edited by Zachazewski AE, Magee DJ, Quillen WS. Philadelphia: WB Saunders, 1996.

CHAPTER 13

Wrist and Hand Conditions

OBJECTIVES

1. Identify the important bony and soft tissue structures of the wrist and hand.

2. Describe the pathways of the median, ulnar, and radial nerves, and identify the motor and sensory components of each nerve.

3. Describe the motions of the wrist and hand, and identify the muscles that produce them.

4. Explain what forces produce the loading patterns responsible for common injuries of the wrist and hand.

5. Describe measures that can be taken to prevent injuries to the wrist and hand.

6. Explain how to identify and manage general sprains and dislocations of the wrist and hand.

7. Explain how to identify and manage acute strains and tendinopathies of the wrist and hand.

8. Describe the more common nerve entrapment syndromes associated with the median, ulnar, and radial nerves at the wrist and hand.

9. Explain the various types of fractures that may occur in the wrist and hand, and describe their management.

10. Describe a thorough assessment of the wrist and hand.

11. Describe general rehabilitation exercises for the wrist and hand.

The wrist and hand are used extensively in activities of daily living and in nearly all sport skills. Injuries to the region often result from the natural tendency to sustain the force of a fall on the hyperextended wrist (**Figure 13.1**). Pubescent and adolescent athletes have a higher incidence of hand and wrist injuries than adult athletes (1). Many of these injuries are directly related to specific sports. For example, in wrestling, football, hockey, and skiing, forced abduction of the thumb can damage the ulnar collateral ligament of the thumb, leading to an injury called a gamekeeper's thumb. Receivers in football and catchers in baseball and softball are subject to "mallet" deformity of the finger, caused when a ball hits the end of

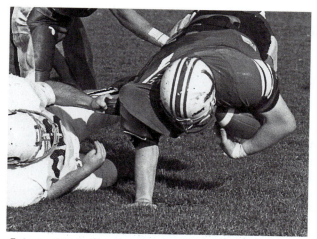

➤ FIGURE 13.1 **Sustaining the force of a fall with a hyperextended wrist can result in serious injuries to the wrist and hand.**

the finger and avulses an extensor tendon from its distal attachment.

This chapter begins with a review of the anatomy, kinematics, and kinetics of the wrist and hand. A discussion of prevention of injury is followed by information on common injuries to the wrist and hand and their management. Finally, assessment techniques and rehabilitation exercises are presented.

ANATOMICAL REVIEW OF THE WRIST AND HAND

The wrist and hand are composed of numerous small bones and articulations. These function effectively to enable the dexterous movements performed by the hands during both daily living and sport activities.

Wrist Articulations

The wrist consists of a series of radiocarpal and intercarpal articulations **(Figure 13.2)**. Most wrist motion occurs at the radiocarpal joint, a condyloid joint where the radius articulates with the scaphoid, lunate, and triquetrum. The joint allows sagittal plane motions (flexion, extension, and hyperextension) and frontal plane motions (radial deviation and ulnar deviation), as well as circumduction.

During wrist motions, the scaphoid and lunate exhibit significant nonplanar motions. Wrist flexion and extension, for example, elicit flexion and extension as well as radial and ulnar deviation of the scaphoid and lunate. When the wrist moves through radial and ulnar deviation, the scaphoid and lunate deviate radially and ulnarly, but also flex and extend (2). The scaphoid and lunate do not, however, move as a unit, having separate axes of rotation. The axes of rotation for the lunate and triquetrum are close, but are oriented differently from the axes of the scaphoid (3).

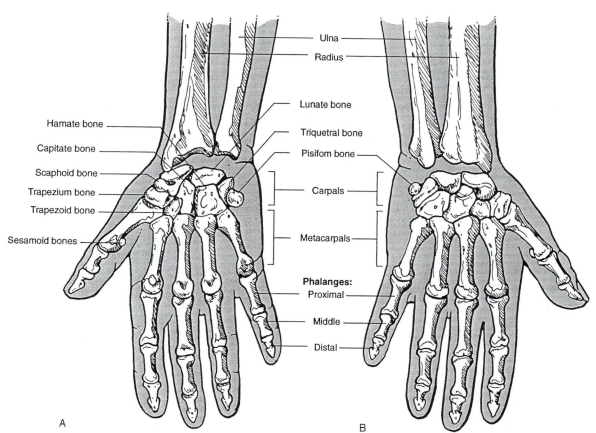

➤ FIGURE 13.2 **Bones of the forearm, wrist, and hand.** A, Anterior view. B, Posterior view.

Alternately, the bones of the distal carpal row function as a single unit and are separated by gliding joints that contribute little to wrist motion. The distal carpal bones are directly linked to the motion of the third metacarpal (4).

The distal radioulnar joint is immediately adjacent to the radiocarpal joint. The triangular fibrocartilage (TFC) is the cartilaginous disc overlying the distal ulnar head, between it and the ulnar carpal column (lunate and triquetral bones). It makes up a portion of the triangular fibrocartilage complex (TFCC), which acts as a stabilizer of the distal radioulnar joint. The TFCC is also the ulnar continuation of the radius, providing an articular surface for the carpal condyle. Although the ulna and radius share the articular disc, they have separate joint capsules. The volar radiocarpal, dorsal radiocarpal, radial collateral, and ulnar collateral ligaments reinforce the radiocarpal joint capsule. Its close packed position is in extension with radial deviation.

Hand Articulations

A large number of joints are required to provide the extensive motion capabilities of the hand. Included are the carpometacarpal (CM), intermetacarpal (IM), metacarpophalangeal (MP), and interphalangeal (IP) joints. The fingers are numbered digits one through five, with the first digit being the thumb.

CARPOMETACARPAL AND INTERMETACARPAL JOINTS

The CM joint of the thumb is a classic saddle joint. A capsule surrounding the joint serves to restrict motion. The flexion-extension axis and abduction-adduction axis at the joint are not perpendicular to each other or to the bones and do not intersect (5). The articulating trapezium and metacarpal bones at the joint appear to have greater congruence, or better fit, in males than in females, which may predispose the female joint to osteoarthritis (6).

The CM joints of the four fingers are essentially gliding joints, although some anatomists have described them as modified saddle joints. The CM and IM joints of the fingers are mutually surrounded by joint capsules that are reinforced by the dorsal, volar, and two interosseous CM ligaments. Among these, the V-shaped interosseous ligaments are the strongest, providing very strong interconnections between the bases of the adjacent metacarpals.

METACARPOPHALANGEAL JOINTS

The knuckles of the hand are formed by the MP joints. These are condyloid joints where the rounded distal heads of the metacarpals articulate with the concave proximal ends of the phalanges. The MP joints are each enclosed in a capsule reinforced by strong collateral ligaments. A dorsal ligament also merges with the MP joint of the thumb. Close packed positions of the MP joints in the

fingers and thumb are full flexion and opposition, respectively.

INTERPHALANGEAL JOINTS

The proximal interphalangeal (PIP) and distal interphalangeal (DIP) joints of the fingers, and the single IP joint of the thumb, are all hinge joints. Subtle differences in the geometry of the articulating bone surfaces, and soft tissue restraints govern the motion capabilities at the PIP joints. An articular capsule joined by volar and collateral ligaments surrounds each IP joint. These joints are most stable in the close packed position of full extension.

Muscles of the Wrist and Hand

Given the numerous, highly controlled, precision movements of which the hand and fingers are capable, it is no surprise that a relatively large number of muscles are responsible. There are nine extrinsic muscles that cross the wrist and 10 intrinsic muscles that have both of their attachments distal to the wrist. The muscles of the wrist and hand are shown in **Figures 13.3** (anterior) and **13.4** (posterior), and their locations and actions are summarized in **Table 13.1**.

RETINACULA OF THE WRIST

The fascial tissue surrounding the wrist is thickened into strong fibrous bands called retinacula that form protective passageways through which tendons, nerves, and blood vessels pass. On the palmar side of the wrist, the flexor retinaculum protects the extrinsic flexor tendons and the median nerve as they pass into the hand through the carpal tunnel. Within the tunnel, the tendons are enclosed in bursal tissue and tenosynovium. On the dorsal side of the wrist, the extensor retinaculum provides a passageway for the extrinsic extensor tendons.

TENDON SHEATHS

At the level of the metacarpal heads, the flexor tendons enter a flexor tendon sheath, a double-walled hollow tube sealed at both ends **(Figure 13.5)**. Filled with synovial fluid, the sheath provides low-friction gliding and nutrition for the flexor tendons. The sheath is supported by a series of retinacular thickenings, called annular pulleys or cruciform pulleys depending on their configuration, that prevent tendon bowstringing with flexion. The second (A2) and fourth (A4) annular pulleys, located at the proximal and middle phalanges respectively, are the most important for preventing tendon bowstringing during active flexion.

Nerves of the Wrist and Hand

The median, ulnar, and radial nerves are major terminal branches of the brachial plexus that provide motor and

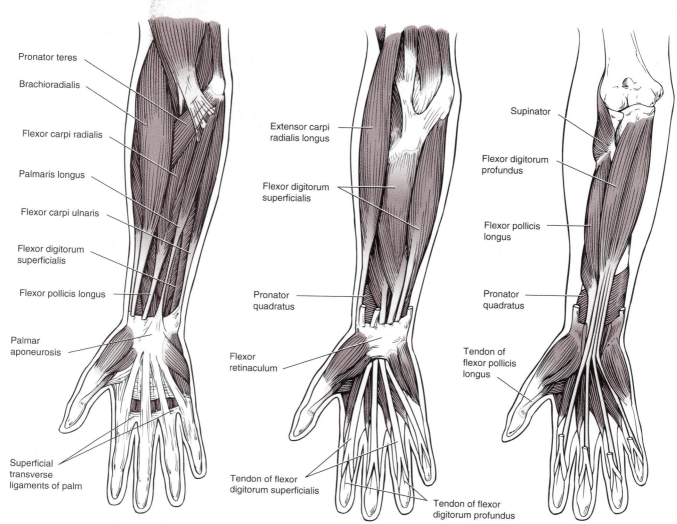

> ▶ FIGURE 13.3 Anterior muscles of the forearm, wrist, and hand.

sensory innervation to the wrist and hand **(Figure 13.6)**. The median nerve supplies the majority of the flexor muscles of the wrist and hand, as well as the intrinsic flexor muscles on the radial side of the palm, and cutaneous sensation to the skin on the lateral two-thirds of the palm and the dorsum of the second and third fingers. The ulnar nerve innervates the flexor carpi ulnaris and the ulnar portion of the flexor digitorum profundus, along with most of the intrinsic muscles of the hand. It also provides cutaneous sensation to the fifth and half of the fourth finger on both dorsal and palmar sides. The radial nerve divides into superficial and deep branches distal to the lateral epicondyle of the elbow. The superficial branch supplies the skin on the dorsum of the hand. The deep branch innervates most of the extensor muscles of the forearm. Specific nerve-muscle associations are presented in Table 13.1.

Blood Vessels of the Wrist and Hand

The major vessels supplying the muscles of the wrist and hand are the radial and ulnar arteries **(Figure 13.7)**. The radial artery supplies the muscles on the radial side of the

forearm, as well as the thumb and index finger. The ulnar artery divides into anterior and posterior interosseous arteries to supply the deep flexor muscles and extensor muscles of the forearm, respectively. In the palm, the radial and ulnar arteries merge to form the superficial and deep palmar arches. Another connecting branch from these arteries forms the carpal arch on the dorsal side of the wrist. Digital arteries branch from the palmar arches to supply the fingers, and branches from the carpal arch run distally along the metacarpal bones. The radial artery is superficial on the anterior aspect of the wrist, where the pulse is readily palpable.

KINEMATICS AND MAJOR MUSCLE ACTIONS OF THE WRIST AND HAND

The wrist is capable of sagittal and frontal plane movements, as well as rotary motion **(Figure 13.8)**. Flexion occurs when the palmar surface of the hand is moved toward the anterior forearm. Extension involves the return of the hand to anatomical position from a position of flexion, and hyperextension occurs when the dorsal surface

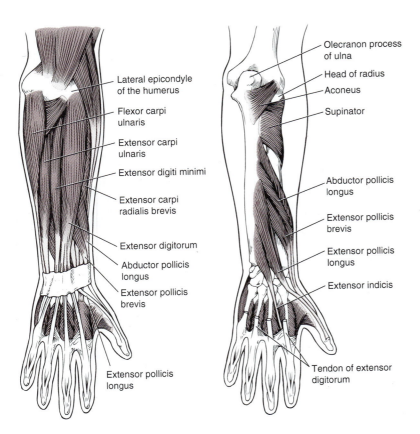

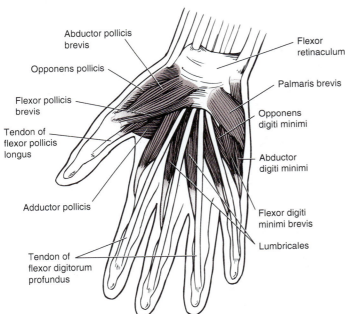

➤ **FIGURE 13.4 Posterior muscles of the forearm, wrist, and hand.**

of the hand is brought toward the posterior forearm. Movement of the hand toward the radial side of the arm is radial deviation, with movement in the opposite direction known as ulnar deviation. Rotational movement of the hand through all four directions is termed circumduction.

Flexion

The major flexor muscles of the wrist are the flexor carpi radialis and flexor carpi ulnaris (Figure 13.3). The palmaris longus, which is often absent in one or both forearms,

contributes to flexion when present. The flexor digitorum superficialis and flexor digitorum profundus assist with flexion at the wrist when the fingers are completely extended, but when the fingers are in flexion these muscles cannot develop sufficient tension to assist.

Extension and Hyperextension

The extensor carpi radialis longus, extensor carpi radialis brevis, and extensor carpi ulnaris produce extension and hyperextension at the wrist. The other posterior wrist

TABLE 13.1 MAJOR MUSCLES OF THE HAND AND FINGERS

Muscle	Proximal Attachment	Distal Attachment	Primary Action(s)	Nerve Innervation
Extrinsic Muscles				
Extensor pollicis longus	Middle dorsal ulna	Dorsal distal phalanx of thumb	Extension of MP and IP joints of thumb	Radial (C_7, C_8)
Extensor pollicis brevis	Middle dorsal radius	Dorsal proximal phalanx of thumb	Extension at MP and CM joints of thumb	Radial (C_7, C_8)
Flexor pollicis longus	Middle palmar radius	Palmar distal phalanx of thumb	Flexion at IP and MP joints of thumb	Median (C_8, T_1)
Abductor pollicis longus	Middle dorsal ulna and radius	Radial base of 1st metacarpal	Abduction at CM joint of thumb	Radial (C_7, C_8)
Extensor indicis	Distal dorsal ulna	Ulnar side of the extensor digitorum tendon	Extension at MP joint of 2nd digit	Radial (C_7, C_8)
Extensor digitorum	Lateral epicondyle of humerus	Base of 2nd and 3rd phalanges, digits 2–5	Extension at MP, proximal and distal IP joints, digits 2–5	Radial (C_7, C_8)
Extensor digiti minimi	Proximal tendon of extensor digitorum	Tendon of extensor digitorum distal to 5th MP joint	Extension at 5th MP joint	Radial (C_7, C_8)
Flexor digitorum profundus	Proximal 3/4 of ulna	Base of distal phalanx, digits 2–5	Flexion at distal and proximal IP joints and MP joints, digits 2–5	Ulnar and median (C_8, T_1)
Flexor digitorum superficialis	Medial epicondyle of humerus	Base of middle phalanx, digits 2–5	Flexion at proximal IP and MP joints, digits 2–5	Median (C_7, C_8, T_1)
Intrinsic Muscles				
Flexor pollicis brevis	Ulnar side, 1st metacarpal	Ulnar, palmar base of proximal phalanx of the thumb	Flexion at MP joint of the thumb	Median (C_8, T_1)
Abductor pollicis brevis	Scaphoid and trapezium bones	Radial base of 1st phalanx of thumb	Abduction at 1st CM joint	Median (C_8, T_1)
Opponens pollicis	Scaphoid bone	Radial side of 1st metacarpal	Opposition at CM joint of the thumb	Median (C_8, T_1)
Adductor pollicis	Capitate, distal 2nd and 3rd metacarpals	Ulnar proximal phalanx of thumb	Adductor and flexion at CM joint of thumb	Ulnar (C_8, T_1)
Abductor digiti minimi	Pisiform bone	Ulnar base of proximal phalanx, 5th digit	Abduction and flexion at 5th MP joint	Ulnar (C_8, T_1)
Flexor digiti minimi brevis	Hamate bone	Ulnar base of proximal phalanx, 5th digit	Flexion at 5th MP joint	Ulnar (C_8, T_1)
Opponens digiti minimi	Hamate bone	Ulnar metacarpal of 5th metacarpal	Opposition at 5th CM joint	Ulnar (C_8, T_1)
Dorsal interossei (four muscles)	Sides of metacarpals, all digits	Base of proximal phalanx, all digits	Abduction at 2nd and 4th MP joints, radial and ulnar deviation of 3rd MP joint, flexion of MP joints 2–4	Ulnar (C_8, T_1)
Palmar interossei (three muscles)	2nd, 4th, and 5th metacarpals	Base of proximal phalanx, digits 2, 4, and 5	Adduction and flexion at MP joints, digits 2, 4, and 5	Ulnar (C_8, T_1)
Lumbricales (four muscles)	Tendons of flexor digitorum profundus, digits 2–5	Tendons of extensor digitorum, digits 2–5	Flexion at MP joints of digits 2–5	Median and ulnar (C_8, T_1)

muscles may also assist with extension movements, particularly when the fingers are in flexion. Included are the extensor pollicis longus, extensor indicis, extensor digiti minimi, and extensor digitorum (Figure 13.4). Research on tennis players indicates that wrist flexion at ball contact during a backhand stroke concomitant with eccentric contraction of the wrist extensor muscles is a leading mechanism for the development of tennis elbow or lateral epicondylitis (7).

Radial and Ulnar Deviation

The flexor and extensor muscles of the wrist cooperatively develop tension to produce radial and ulnar deviation of

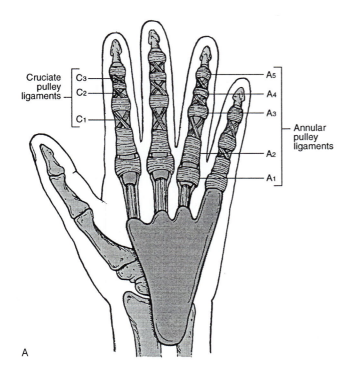

A

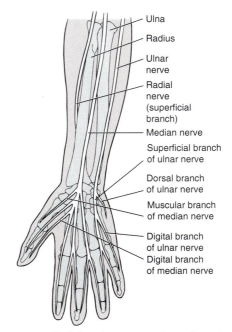

➤ FIGURE 13.6 **Peripheral nerve supply to the wrist and hand**.

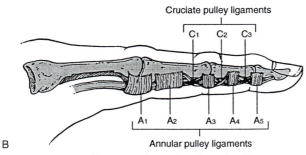

B

➤ FIGURE 13.5 **Flexor tendons, sheath, and pulley system**. The tendons from the finger flexors pass through strong annular pulleys (A1 through A5), which keep the tendons and their encircling sheath closely applied to the phalanges. The thin, pliable cruciate pulleys (C1 through C3) collapse to allow full digital flexion.

the hand at the wrist. The flexor carpi radialis and extensor carpi radialis act to produce radial deviation, and the flexor carpi ulnaris and extensor carpi ulnaris cause ulnar deviation.

Carpometacarpal Joint Motion

The CM joint of the thumb allows a large range of movement, comparable to that of a ball-and-socket joint. The fifth CM joint permits significantly less range of motion, however, and only a very small amount of motion is allowed at the second through fourth carpometacarpal joints, due to the presence of restrictive ligaments.

Metacarpophalangeal Joint Motion

The MP joints of the fingers allow flexion, extension, abduction, adduction, and circumduction **(Figure 13.9)**.

Among the fingers, abduction is defined as movement away from the middle finger and adduction is movement toward the middle finger. The MP joint of the thumb functions more as a hinge joint, with the primary movements being flexion and extension.

Interphalangeal Joint Motion

The IP joints permit flexion and extension, and in some individuals, slight hyperextension. These are classic hinge joints.

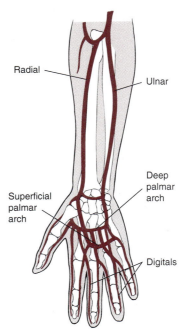

➤ FIGURE 13.7 **Blood supply to the wrist and hand**.

Extension

Flexion

Hyper-
extension

Radial deviation

Ulnar deviation

A

B

➤ **FIGURE 13.8 Directional movement capabilities at the wrist.** A, Sagittal plane movements. B, Frontal plane movements.

KINETICS OF THE WRIST AND HAND

The extrinsic flexor muscles of the hand are more than twice as strong as the strongest extrinsic extensor muscles. This should come as little surprise given that the flexor muscles of the hand are used extensively in everyday activities involving gripping, grasping, or pinching movements, while the extensor muscles rarely exert much force.

Three types of hand grips are predominantly used in sport activities **(Figure 13.10)**. The power grip, typified by the baseball bat grip, is one in which the fingers and thumb are used to clamp the grip of the bat against the palm of the hand. The wrist is held in a position of ulnar deviation and slight hyperextension to increase the tension in the flexor tendons. In contrast to the power grip, the precision grip, exemplified by the baseball grip, involves use of the semiflexed fingers and thumb to pinch the ball against the palm, with the wrist in slight hyperextension. A third grip that is intermediate to the two previously described might be termed a lateral pinch, also referred to as the "fencing grip." Fencing requires both power and

precision. The grip on the foil is essentially a power grip, but with the thumb aligned along the long axis of the foil handle, it enables precise control of the direction of force application.

PREVENTION OF WRIST AND HAND INJURIES

The very nature of many contact and collision sports places the wrist and hands in an extremely vulnerable position for injury. The hands are almost always the first point of contact to cushion the body during collisions, deflect flying objects, or to lessen body impact during a fall. Falling on

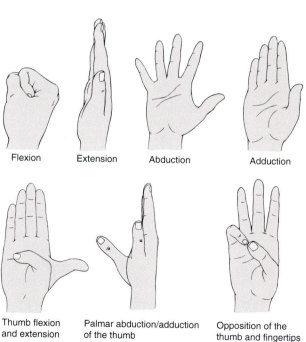

Flexion   Extension   Abduction   Adduction

Thumb flexion
and extension

Palmar abduction/adduction
of the thumb

Opposition of the
thumb and fingertips

➤ **FIGURE 13.9 Directional movement capabilities at the fingers and thumb.**

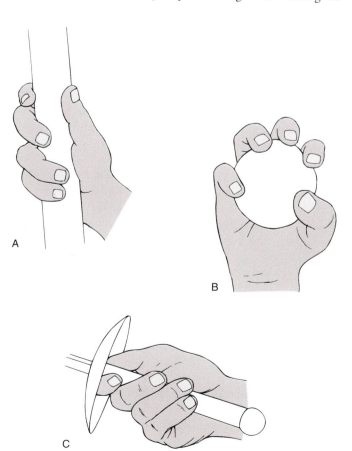

A

B

C

➤ **FIGURE 13.10 Hand grips.** Muscles of the hand contract to provide several grips, including power (A), precision (B), and fencing grips (C).

an outstretched hand is the leading cause of fractures and dislocations at the distal forearm, wrist, and hand. Although several pads and gloves are available, few sports require protective padding for the region.

Protective Equipment

Goalies, baseball and softball catchers, and field players in many sports such as hockey and lacrosse are required to wear wrist and hand protection (see Figure 3.8). The padded gloves prevent direct compression from a stick, puck, or ball. Several other gloves have extra padding placed at high impact areas, aid in gripping, and protect the hand from abrasions, particularly when playing on artificial turf, or on a baseball or softball field. Whenever possible, protective pads and gloves should be worn during sport participation to lessen the risk of injury.

Physical Conditioning

Several muscles that move the wrist and hand cross the elbow. As such, flexibility and strengthening exercises for the wrist and hand must also include exercises for the elbow, which were illustrated in Field Strategy 12.1. These exercises included general strength in elbow flexion and extension, forearm pronation and supination, wrist flexion and extension, and radial and ulnar deviation. Other exercises, such as squeezing a tennis ball or a spring-loaded grip device, can be used to strengthen the finger flexors.

Proper Skill Technique

Unlike the shoulder and elbow, which is subjected to excessive stress during a throwing-type motion, nearly all wrist and hand injuries result from direct trauma. Although analysis of specific movements may detect improper technique, in many cases, the analysis is incidental. An important skill technique, however, that can prevent injury of the wrist and hand is proper instruction on the shoulder-roll method of falling. Here, the force of impact is dispersed over a wider area, lessening the risk for injury from direct axial loading on the extended wrist.

CONTUSIONS AND ABRASIONS

 A softball player dove for a ball on the infield and sustained an abrasion on the palmar side of the throwing hand. What immediate and long-term concerns are there in cleaning this superficial wound?

Direct impact to the back of the hand can produce a soft, painful, bluish discoloration. Although many contusions are minor, always be alert for an underlying fracture. Initial treatment involves ice, compression, elevation, and rest. Symptoms will usually disappear in 2 to 3 days. If not, refer the individual to a physician for follow-up care.

Abrasions must be thoroughly cleansed of all foreign matter. A soap wash for 10 minutes using surgical soap, with a water-soluble iodine solution and brush, can remove imbedded foreign matter. Once cleansed, an antiseptic is applied and the wound is covered with a nonocclusive dressing. The dressing is changed daily, and the wound is inspected for signs of infection.

 If the wound appears red, swollen, or purulent, or is hot and tender, refer the individual immediately to a physician.

 After cleansing the abrasion on the palm of the hand, apply an antiseptic and a nonocclusive dressing. Check the wound daily for signs of infection.

SPRAINS

 A hurdler fell after hitting the hurdle, and landed on an outstretched hand used to cushion the fall. Muscle testing and stress tests were inconclusive. Radiographs were negative, and the physician diagnosed the injury as a wrist sprain. How would you treat this condition? Can the individual return to practice?

Ligamentous sprains in the wrist and hand are the result either of a single episode of trauma, or of repetitive stress. When due to a single episode, the severity of injury is independent on:

- Characteristics of the injury force (its point of application, magnitude, rate, and direction)
- Position of the hand at impact
- Relative strength of the carpal bones and ligaments

Most injuries to the region result from a compressive load applied while the hand is in some degree of extension, although hyperflexion or rotation may also lead to injury. Unfortunately, because of the need to perform simple daily activities, most individuals do not allow ample time for healing. Consequently, many sprains are neglected, leading to chronic instability.

Wrist Sprains

Axial loading on the proximal palm during a fall on an outstretched hand is the leading cause of wrist sprains (8). Gymnasts have a high incidence of dorsal wrist pain when excessive forces are exerted on the wrist, producing combined hyperextension, ulnar deviation, and intercarpal supination. These excessive forces occur during vaulting, floor exercise, or during pommel horse routines. Divers who enter the water with the hands in extension, and skaters and wrestlers who fall on an extended hand, are also prone to this injury.

➤ SIGNS AND SYMPTOMS

Assessment will reveal point tenderness on the dorsum of the radiocarpal joint. Pain increases with active or passive extension.

➤ MANAGEMENT

After immobilization of the joint, and referral to a physician to rule out a fracture or carpal dislocation, treatment involves decreasing intensity of training, cryotherapy before and after practice, nonsteroidal anti-inflammatory drugs (NSAIDs), and the use of an appropriate bandage, taping technique, or splint to prevent excessive hyperextension. As pain decreases, range-of-motion exercises and wrist- and hand-strengthening exercises, such as those listed in Field Strategy 12.1, can begin.

Gamekeeper's Thumb

The thumb is exposed to more force than the fingers by virtue of its position on the hand. Integrity of the ulnar collateral ligament at the MP joint is critical for normal hand function because it stabilizes the joint as the thumb is pushed against the index and middle fingers while performing many pinching, grasping, and gripping motions. **Gamekeeper's thumb** is common in football, baseball/softball, hockey, and in skiing when the individual falls on the ski pole (skier's thumb) **(Figure 13.11)**. When the MP joint is near full extension and the thumb is forcefully abducted away from the hand, tearing of the ulnar collateral ligament at the MP joint occurs.

➤ SIGNS AND SYMPTOMS

The palmar aspect of the joint is painful and swollen, and may have visible bruising. Instability is detected by replicating the mechanism of injury, or by stressing the thumb in flexion. With partial tears, only moderate laxity is present and a definite end feel is present. In more severe cases, laxity greater than 35° and the absence of an end feel indicate total rupture of the ulnar collateral ligament. Bilateral comparison, as well as assessment of laxity at other major joints, will help determine normal joint laxity for the individual.

➤ MANAGEMENT

Initial treatment includes ice, compression, elevation, and referral to a physician for further care. With no instability, treatment involves early mobilization accompanied by cryotherapy, contrast baths, ultrasound, and NSAIDs. Strapping or taping the thumb can prevent reinjury. If there is joint instability, a thumb spica cast may be applied for 3 to 6 weeks, followed by further taping for another 3 to 6 weeks during risk activities. Severe cases require surgical repair.

Interphalangeal Collateral Ligament Sprains

Excessive varus/valgus stress and hyperextension can damage the collateral ligaments of the fingers. Ligament failure usually occurs at its attachment to the proximal phalanx or, less frequently, in the midportion. Hyperextension of the proximal phalanx can stretch or rupture the volar plate on the palmar side of the joint **(Figure 13.12)**.

➤ SIGNS AND SYMPTOMS

An obvious deformity may not be present, unless there is a fracture or total rupture of the supporting tissues that causes a dorsal dislocation. Rapid swelling makes assessment difficult. A radiograph is needed to rule out an associated dislocation or fracture.

➤ MANAGEMENT

After standard acute care, a mild sprain can be treated by taping the injured finger to an adjacent finger (buddy taping). This provides some support and mobility, but should not be used on an acutely swollen, painful finger because of possible constriction to the vascular flow. If more support is needed, the involved joint can be splinted in extension with a molded polypropylene splint to avoid flexion contractures.

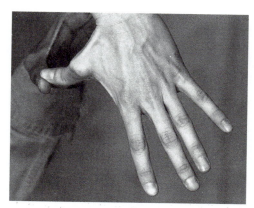

➤ FIGURE 13.11 Clinical appearance of a Gamekeeper's thumb.

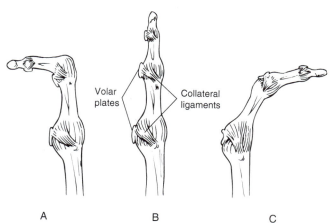

➤ FIGURE 13.12 Collateral ligaments and volar plate of the fingers can be damaged in hyperextension injuries. A, Flexion. B, Extension. C, Hyperextension.

Dislocations

An acute dislocation and subluxation of the distal radioulnar joint (DRUJ) can be an isolated injury, or may occur in conjunction with a fracture of the radius. The mechanism of injury almost always involves hyperextension. If an ulna dorsal dislocation of the joint occurs, hyperpronation is also present, while a ulna volar dislocation occurs in conjunction with hypersupination. Because the triangular fibrocartilage complex functions as a sling to support the ulnar border of the wrist, and connects the distal ulna to the ulnar side of the radius, dislocation of the DRUJ can result in damage to some portion of this complex or to its attachments. The clinical appearance of a DRUJ dislocation can vary significantly depending on the presence or absence of an associated fracture. Generally, when dislocated or subluxated, the joint is deformed, swollen, and very painful. Swelling may be so extensive as to obscure the prominence of the ulnar head. In a dorsal dislocation, the ulnar head is more prominent dorsally. In volar dislocations, the wrist typically appears narrow as a result of an overlap of the distal parts of the radius and ulna; if soft-tissue swelling is not excessive, a depression may be noted near the sigmoid notch of the radius where the ulnar head is normally located. Flexion and extension of the elbow are normal unless there is an associated fracture, but pronation and supination of the forearm is limited.

 Immediate action involves immobilization of the limb in a vacuum splint and immediate transport to a physician.

Because of the shape of the lunate and its position between the large capitate and lower end of the radius, this carpal bone is particularly prone to dislocation during axial loading that causes displacement in a volar direction **(Figure 13.13)**. The dorsum of the hand will be point tender, and a thickened area on the palm can be palpated just distal to the end of the radius, if not obscured by swelling. Passive and active motion may not be painful.

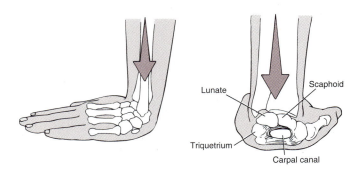

➤ FIGURE 13.13 **Lunate dislocation**. A, The lunate can dislocate during a fall on an outstretched hand when the load from the radius compresses the lunate in a volar direction. B, If the bone moves into the carpal tunnel, the median nerve can become compressed, leading to sensory changes in the first and second fingers.

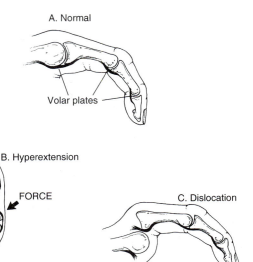

➤ FIGURE 13.14 **Metacarpal phalangeal (MP) dislocation**. A, The volar plates protect the anterior joint capsules of the fingers. B, Hyperextension can tear the anterior capsule and supporting ligaments. C, As the force continues, the capsule ruptures, dislocating the phalanx. The resulting deformity signals a serious dislocation.

If the bone moves into the carpal tunnel, compression of the median nerve leads to pain, numbness, and tingling in the first and second fingers.

MP joint dislocations are rare, but readily recognizable as a serious injury. Hyperextension causes the anterior capsule to tear, allowing the proximal phalanx to move backward over the metacarpal and stand at a 90° angle to the metacarpal **(Figure 13.14)**.

The most common dislocation in the body occurs at the PIP joint **(Figure 13.15)**. Because digital nerves and vessels run along the sides of the fingers and thumb, dislocations here are potentially serious. The mechanism of injury is usually hyperextension and axial compression, such as when a ball hits the end of the finger and forces it into

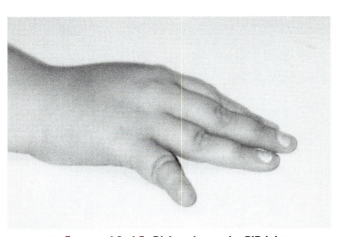

➤ FIGURE 13.15 **Dislocation at the PIP joint**.

hyperextension. A swollen, painful finger is the most frequent initial complaint. Pain will be present at the joint line and will increase when the mechanism of injury is reproduced. If inadequately cared for, dislocations at the PIP joint can result in a painful, stiff finger with a fixed flexion deformity called a "**coach's finger**."

DIP dislocations usually occur dorsally and may be associated with an open wound. The individuals often reduce the injury themselves. As with MP joint dislocations, injuries to the collateral ligaments at the PIP and DIP joints can involve ruptures of the volar plate. Because of the probability of entrapping the volar plate in an IP joint, which can lead to permanent dysfunction of the finger, no attempt should be made to reduce a finger dislocation by an untrained individual.

Immediate treatment for all dislocations involves immobilization in a wrist or finger splint, application of ice to reduce swelling and inflammation, and immediate referral to a physician.

The prognosis and rehabilitation program will depend on the extent of tissue damage and instability. Simple DRUJ dislocations may be stabilized after the internal fixation of associated fractures, and are immobilized in an above-the-elbow cast. Range-of-motion exercises should be started 6 weeks after fixation. Following a dislocation of the lunate, the wrist is immobilized in moderate flexion with a silicone cast for 3 to 4 weeks. The wrist is then placed into neutral position and protected from any wrist extension, particularly during sport participation. This condition is often overlooked until complications, such as flexor tendon contractures and median nerve palsies, arise from chronic dislocations. In a dislocation of the PIP joint, the finger may be splinted in about 30° of flexion with active motion started at 10 to 14 days. Immobilization for a DIP joint dislocation involves splinting the DIP joint with a volar splint for approximately 3 weeks. The PIP joint can be left free so motion can continue at this joint. Protective splinting is continued for at least 3 weeks until the finger is pain-free (9).

The physician diagnosed the hurdler's injury as a mild wrist sprain. Applying tape or a splint to reduce excessive wrist extension can permit the individual to continue performing. Cryotherapy, thermotherapy, EMS, and interferential current may also be used to enhance optimal healing.

STRAINS

While holding a jersey tightly in one hand in an effort to stop the opposing player, a football player felt a sharp pain in the distal phalanx of the ring finger. Upon release of the jersey, the player was unable to flex the DIP joint of the ring finger. What structure(s) are responsible for motion at this joint? How would you assess which structures are damaged?

Muscular strains occur as a result of excessive overload against resistance, or overstretching the tendon beyond its normal range. In mild or moderate strains, pain and restricted motion may not be a major factor. In many injuries, muscular strains occur simultaneously with a joint sprain. The joint sprain takes precedence in priority of care, especially with an associated dislocation. As a result, tendon damage may go unrecognized and untreated.

Jersey Finger (Profundus Tendon Rupture)

This injury typically occurs when an individual grips an opponent's jersey while the opponent simultaneously twists and turns to get away. This jerking motion may force the fingers to rapidly extend, rupturing the flexor digitorum profundus tendon from its attachment on the distal phalanx, hence the name "jersey finger." The ring finger is most commonly involved, because this finger assumes a position of slight extension relative to the other, more flexed, fingers during grip.

➤ SIGNS AND SYMPTOMS

If avulsed, the tendon can be palpated at the proximal aspect of the involved finger; it will typically have a hematoma formation along the entire flexor tendon sheath. If a portion of bone is also avulsed, it may become trapped distal to the A4 pulley over the middle phalanx, or distal to the A2 pulley, or it may retract all the way into the palm. Because of the avulsion, the individual will be unable to flex the DIP joint against resistance.

➤ MANAGEMENT

After standard acute care, the individual should be referred to the physician for further care. In cases where the tendon has retracted into the palm, surgical reattachment of the tendon must be performed within 7 to 10 days, before permanent contracture occurs. More distal retraction can wait up to 3 months, provided no further retraction develops (10).

Mallet Finger

Mallet finger, or baseball finger, occurs when an object hits the end of the finger while the extensor tendon is taut, such as when catching a ball. The resulting forceful flexion can avulse the lateral bands of the extensor mechanism from its distal attachment, or the tendon may remain attached to an avulsed piece of bone or fracture fragment, leaving a characteristic mallet deformity (**Figure 13.16**).

➤ SIGNS AND SYMPTOMS

Unlike the jersey finger, where the flexor tendon retracts into the proximal aspect of the finger, isolated rup-

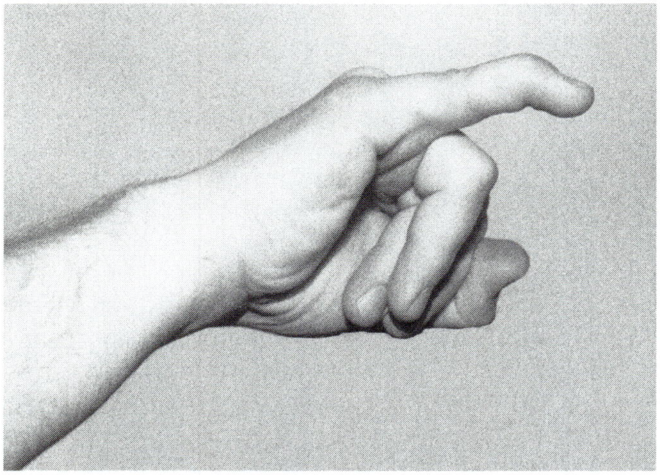

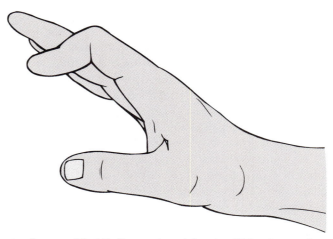

> FIGURE 13.16 **Mallet finger**. Mallet finger is caused when the extensor tendon is avulsed from the attachment on the distal phalanx. The tendon may also avulse a small piece of bone, leading to an avulsion fracture.

ture of the extensor tendon usually does not retract. Examination reveals pain, swelling, and a variable lack of active extension at the DIP joint.

> MANAGEMENT

After standard acute care, the individual should be referred to the physician for further care. Treatment usually involves splinting the DIP joint in complete extension for 6 to 8 weeks. Motion at the PIP and MP joints, however, is highly encouraged. An additional 6 to 8 weeks of splinting should be employed during athletic participation (10). Soft tissue irritation or ulceration on the dorsum of the DIP may occur secondary to splinting. To avoid this, keep the splint dry and alternate its position between the dorsal and palmar aspects of the finger. Extreme hyperextension of the distal phalanx may also impair vascular supply to the tip of the finger, leading to further skin damage.

Boutonniere Deformity

A boutonniere deformity is caused by blunt trauma to the dorsal aspect of the PIP joint, or by rapid, forceful flexion of the joint against resistance. The central slip of the extensor tendon ruptures at the middle phalanx, leaving no active extensor mechanism intact over the PIP joint.

> SIGNS AND SYMPTOMS

The deformity is usually not present immediately, but develops over 2 to 3 weeks as the lateral slips move in a palmar direction and cause hyperextension at the MCP joint, flexion at the PIP joint, and hyperextension at the DIP joint **(Figure 13.17)**. Because the head of the proximal phalanx protrudes through the split in the extensor hood, this condition is sometimes referred to as a "buttonhole rupture." The PIP joint will be swollen and lack full extension.

> FIGURE 13.17 **Boutonniere deformity**. With a boutonniere deformity, the proximal joint flexes while the distal joint hyperextends.

> MANAGEMENT

Any injury that limits PIP extension to 30° or less, and produces dorsal tenderness over the base of the middle phalanx, should be treated as an acute tendon rupture and immediately referred to a physician. Initial treatment involves splinting the PIP joint in complete extension for 5 to 6 weeks with the DIP joint free to move, to avoid adhesions.

Tendinopathies

Individuals involved in strenuous and repetitive training often inflame tendons and tendon sheaths in the wrist and hand. The tendon injury may be macrotraumatic, involving acute tissue destruction, or microtraumatic, from chronic loading. Overuse can lead to derangement of both the mechanic and physiologic components of the normal tendon, and is clinically referred to as tendinitis. Tendons are most at risk for injury when tension is applied rapidly at an oblique angle. Tendons already under tension, and muscles maximally innervated or stretched, are other risk factors for rupture (11).

TRIGGER FINGER

Snapping flexor tendons, or trigger finger, may be present in individuals who have multiple, severe trauma to the palmar aspect of the hand, or who do repeated movement and clenching of the fingers. It most commonly occurs to the middle or ring finger, but may occur at the thumb and other fingers. Repeated trauma and inflammation results in a thickening of the tendon sheath as it passes over the proximal phalanx. A nodule can form and grow within the thickened, synovium-lined tendon sheath that eventually prevents the tendon from sliding within the annular ligaments of the finger. Flexion occurs and the finger becomes locked in flexion when the nodule becomes

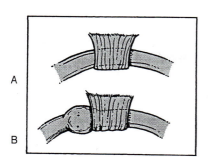

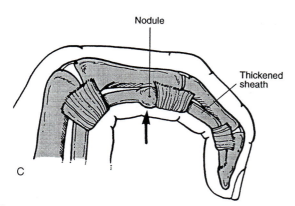

➤ **Figure 13.18** **Trigger finger.** A, Under normal conditions, the flexor tendons slide within the synovial sheaths under the annular ligaments at the proximal and middle phalanx. B, Repeated trauma can cause a nodule to form in the tendon sheath, or the sheath may become thickened. C, Flexion occurs and the finger becomes locked in flexion when the nodule becomes too thick or the sheath too constricted. D, The finger is then unable to reextend.

too thick, or the sheath too constricted to allow the finger to be actively reextended **(Figure 13.18)**.

➤ SIGNS AND SYMPTOMS

This locking usually occurs when the individual first wakens from sleep. A painful popping sensation is often perceived when the flexed PIP joint is passively returned to extension. Additional palpable crepitus may indicate an underlying systemic disease (e.g., systemic sclerosis, rheumatoid arthritis, granulomotous infection) (12).

➤ MANAGEMENT

Treatment includes NSAIDs, resting the finger, splinting when necessary, and possible cortisone injections into the sheath (intralesional injection). Often, however, an incision proximal to the palpable nodule is necessary to cut the annular ligament and allow the tendon to slide freely.

DE QUERVAIN'S TENOSYNOVITIS

Athletes who must use a forceful grasp, combined with repetitive use of the thumb and ulnar deviation are particularly at risk for de Quervain's tenosynovitis. Sports such as racquet sports, golf, fly fishing, and javelin and

discus throwing place a high demand on the abductor pollicis longus (APL) and extensor pollicis brevis (EPB). These two tendons share a single synovial tendon sheath that travels through a bony groove over the radiostyloid process, then turns sharply as much as 105° to enter the thumb when the wrist is in radial deviation. Tenosynovitis results from friction between the tendons, the stenosing sheath, and the bony process **(Figure 13.19)**. The tendons slide within the sheath not only during movements of the thumb, but also in movements of the wrist with the thumb fixed, as in bowling and throwing.

➤ SIGNS AND SYMPTOMS

The individual will complain of pain over the radial styloid process that increases with thumb and wrist motion. Palpation reveals point tenderness over the tendons, at or just proximal to the radial styloid, and occasionally crepitation. Movements of the thumb are painful, and snapping of the tendons during the throwing motion may be present. Pain is reproduced in two manners: (1) abducting the thumb against resistance, and (2) flexing the thumb and cupping it under the fingers, then flexing the wrist in ulnar deviation to stretch the thumb tendons (see Finkelstein's test and Figure 13.32). Swelling and inflammation of the first dorsal compartment are occasionally present.

➤ MANAGEMENT

Treatment is conservative with ice, rest, and NSAIDs as prescribed by a physician. If symptoms are not relieved, steroid injections or immobilization with a thumb spica for three weeks, or both, may be helpful. In severe cases, surgical decompression may be necessary.

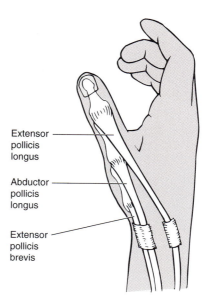

Extensor pollicis longus

Abductor pollicis longus

Extensor pollicis brevis

➤ **Figure 13.19** **Tenosynovitis.** The abductor pollicis longus and extensor pollicis brevis share the same synovial sheath. Excessive friction among the tendons, sheath, and bony process lead to tenosynovitis of the tendons.

INTERSECTION SYNDROME

Intersection syndrome is a tendinitis or friction tendinitis in the first and second dorsal compartments. It has been described in rowers, indoor racket players, canoeists, and weight lifters who overuse the radial extensors of the wrist by excessive curling (13). The muscle and tendons of these two compartments traverse each other at a 60° angle, two to three finger breadths proximal to the wrist joint on the dorsal aspect (4 to 6 cm proximal to Lister's tubercle). The condition has also been described as a stenosing tenosynovitis of the sheath of the second compartment (the radial extensors) where it traverses the muscle bellies of the first compartment (APL and EPB).

➤ SIGNS AND SYMPTOMS

Examination reveals point tenderness on the dorsum of the forearm, two to three finger breadths proximal to the wrist joint, as well as crepitation or squeaking with passive or active motion, and visible swelling along the course of the affected tendons.

➤ MANAGEMENT

Treatment consists of ice massage, rest, NSAIDs, splinting, and avoiding exacerbating activities. A corticosteroid injection may be necessary to relieve acute symptoms. Rehabilitation should consist of range-of-motion exercises and wrist extensor strengthening. If conservative treatment fails, a tenosynovectomy and a fasciotomy of the APL muscle may be necessary.

Ganglion Cysts

Ganglion cysts are benign tumor masses typically seen on the dorsal aspect of the wrist, although they may occur on the volar aspect **(Figure 13.20)**. Associated with tissue sheath degeneration, the cyst itself contains a jelly-like, colorless fluid of mucin, and is freely mobile and palpable. Occurring spontaneously, cysts seldom cause any pain or loss of motion. As the ganglion increases in size, discomfort from the pressure may occur. Treatment is symptomatic; aspiration, injection, and rupture of the cyst have not

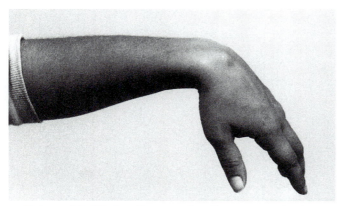

➤ FIGURE 13.20 **Ganglion cyst**. Ganglion cysts are benign tumor masses associated with tissue sheath degeneration.

proven successful, as the condition may recur. Surgical excision remains the treatment of choice (8).

 The football player's flexor digitorum profundus tendon was avulsed from the distal phalanx, preventing flexion of the DIP joint. When rehabilitation begins, range-of-motion and strength in the finger flexors must be restored.

FINGERTIP INJURIES

 A shot putter pinched a finger under the shot, causing blood to accumulate under the fingernail. The fingertip is extremely painful from the increasing pressure. What must you keep in mind in deciding whether or not to relieve the pressure?

Direct trauma to the nail bed, such as that caused when the finger is impacted by a ball, jammed into an object, or crushed when stepped on, can lead to a subungual hematoma. Infections can also occur in the nailfold, leading to a condition called paronychia.

Subungual Hematomas

Direct trauma to the nail bed can result in blood forming under the fingernail, called a subungual hematoma. Increasing pressure can lead to throbbing pain. After ruling out an underlying fracture, soak the finger in ice water for 10 to 15 minutes to numb the area and reduce bleeding under the nail bed. If it is not absolutely necessary to relieve the blood from the nail, do not do so, as this opens an avenue for infection. If discomfort is so great the individual is unable to perform, however, drain the hematoma under the direction of a physician. Cut a hole through the nail with a rotary drill or a number 11 surgical blade, or melt a hole through the nail with the end of a paper clip heated to a bright red color. **Field Strategy 13.1** explains how to properly care for a subungual hematoma. After draining the blood, check the area daily for signs of infection. If present, refer the athlete immediately to a physician for further care.

Paronychia

Paronychia is an infection along the nail fold, commonly seen with a hangnail, or in individuals whose hands are frequently immersed in water. The nail fold becomes red, swollen, and painful, and can produce purulent drainage. The condition is treated with warm water soaks and germicide. In more severe cases, the physician may recommend systemic antibiotics and drainage of localized pus, or may perform a partial-nail resection. The area is then protected with a dry, sterile dressing.

 The shot putter has a subungual hematoma. If it is not absolutely necessary to relieve pressure

FIELD STRATEGY 13.1 MANAGEMENT ALGORITHM FOR SUBUNGUAL HEMATOMA*

To numb the area and reduce hemorrhage:
soak the finger in ice water for 10–15 minutes

↓

Clean your hands thoroughly with antiseptic soap and water;
apply latex gloves

↓

Thoroughly cleanse the finger with:
- Antiseptic soap, or
- An antibacterial solution

↓

Make a hole through the nail. Either:

Cut the hole, using: *OR:*   Melt the hole with the end
- A sterile #11 surgical blade, or   of a paper clip heated to
- A rotary drill, cleaned and   bright red
  disinfected with iodine solution

↓

Have the individual exert mild pressure on the distal pulp
of the finger to drive excess blood through the hole

↓

Watch carefully for signs of shock. Treat accordingly by:
- Placing the individual in a supine position, and
- Elevating the feet above the level of the heart

↓

Soak the finger in an iodine solution for 10 minutes

↓

Cover the phalanx with a sterile dressing;
apply a protective splint

↓

Follow up:
- Do not apply heat for 48 hours
- Check the finger daily for signs of infection;
  if any appear, refer immediately to a physician

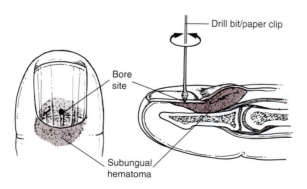

*Due to the nature of opening a wound and the potential for subsequent infection, this procedure should be discussed with the supervising physician and documented as a standing order.

under the nail, do not do so, as this opens an avenue for infection. Any drainage of fluid should be done in accordance with standing orders from the supervising physician, and should follow universal safety precautions.

NERVE ENTRAPMENT SYNDROMES

 A long-distance cyclist is complaining of bilateral numbness in the little finger and medial half of the ring finger, and an inability to adduct the little finger. The individual can not recall an incident that could have caused this condition, but stated that training distance has significantly increased this past week. What possible factors are involved in this condition, and what suggestions can be made to alleviate the symptoms yet allow this cyclist to continue training?

Nerve entrapment syndromes, or compressive neuropathies, can be subtle and are often overlooked. They occur in activities such as bowling, cycling, karate, rowing, baseball/softball, field hockey, lacrosse, rugby, weight lifting, and handball, and in wheelchair athletes. Mechanisms of injuries most commonly involve repetitive compression, contusion, or traction. A compressive neuropathy may also be caused by anatomical structures such as anomalous muscles or vessels, fibrous bands, osteofibrous tunnels, or muscle hypertrophy. Pathologic structures such as ganglia, lipomas, osteophytes, aneurysms, and localized inflammation can also compress a nerve (11). Discussion of compressive neuropathies will be limited to those found in the distal forearm, wrist, and hand **(Box 13.1)**.

Median Nerve Entrapment

The median nerve lies medial to the brachial artery in the cubital fossa, and passes distally between the two heads of the pronator teres. At the distal margin, the nerve divides to form the anterior interosseous nerve to supply the flexor

> ➤ **Box 13.1**

Nerve Entrapment Syndromes

Median Nerve
- Anterior interosseous syndrome
- Carpal tunnel syndrome

Ulnar Nerve
- Ulnar tunnel syndrome
- Cyclist's palsy
- Bowler's thumb

Radial Nerve
- Distal posterior interosseous nerve syndrome
- Superficial radial nerve entrapment

pollicis longus, the flexor digitorum superficialis to the index and middle digits, and the pronator quadratus. The main trunk of the median nerve continues distally beneath the fibrous arch of the flexor digitorum superficialis. The palmar cutaneous branch supplies sensation to the volar wrist, thenar eminence, and palm. The median nerve continues through the carpal tunnel beneath the flexor retinaculum to supply sensation to the palm and the radial three and one-half digits. The deep motor branch supplies the abductor pollicis brevis, opponens pollicis, superficial head of the flexor pollicis brevis, and the two lateral lumbricales.

ANTERIOR INTEROSSEOUS NERVE SYNDROME

Seen sporadically in athletes, anterior interosseous nerve (AIN) syndrome can occur after a set of strenuous or repetitive elbow motion exercises. Structurally, there may be compression of the nerve by fibrous bands from the deep head of the pronator teres or flexor digitorum superficialis, affecting any or all of the muscles innervated by the nerve. There is, however, no sensory cutaneous portion of the nerve, hence no sensory changes. This syndrome has been reported in "junk" baseball pitchers, weight lifters, gymnasts, tennis players, swimmers, and football players (11).

➤ SIGNS AND SYMPTOMS
The athlete will present in one of two ways:

- Acute onset—the individual suddenly loses use of the flexor pollicis longus and index finger profundus tendons
- Slow, insidious onset—gradual weakening of these muscles becomes apparent with weakness during heavy activity

Examination reveals weakness or loss of flexion of the IP joint of the thumb and DIP joint of the index finger. The individual characteristically is unable to make a circle with the index finger and thumb.

➤ MANAGEMENT
Initial treatment involves splinting the extremity and avoiding heavy activity. If no return of function is noted after 6 months, surgical intervention and decompression of the nerve may be necessary.

CARPAL TUNNEL SYNDROME

Carpal tunnel syndrome (CTS) is the most common compression syndrome of the wrist and hand, although it is not commonly seen in the athletic population. CTS may be caused by direct trauma, repetitive overuse, or anatomical anomalies, and is typically seen in the dominant extremity. Sporting activities that predispose athletes to CTS include those that involve repetitive or continuous flexion and extension of the wrist, such as cycling, throwing sports, racquet sports, archery, and gymnastics.

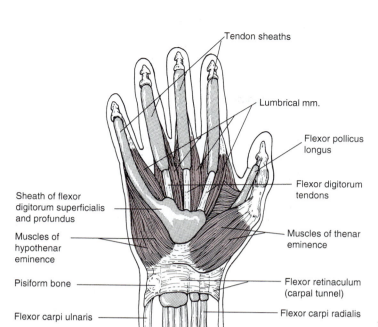

Tendon sheaths

Lumbrical mm.

Flexor pollicus longus

Flexor digitorum tendons

Sheath of flexor digitorum superficialis and profundus

Muscles of thenar eminence

Muscles of hypothenar eminence

Pisiform bone

Flexor retinaculum (carpal tunnel)

Flexor carpi ulnaris

Flexor carpi radialis

Flexor tendons

➤ FIGURE 13.21 **Carpal tunnel**. The flexor tendons of the fingers pass through the carpal tunnel in a single synovial sheath.

The carpal tunnel is formed by the floor of the volar wrist capsule, with the roof formed by the transverse retinacular ligament traveling from the hook of the hamate and pisiform on the lateral side to the volar tubercle of the trapezium and tuberosity of the scaphoid on the medial side. This unyielding tunnel accommodates the median nerve, the finger flexors in a common sheath, and the flexor pollicis longus in an independent sheath **(Figure 13.21)**. Any irritation of the synovial sheath covering these tendons can produce swelling or edema that puts pressure on the median nerve.

➤ SIGNS AND SYMPTOMS

The individual will report that pain wakes them in the middle of the night and is often relieved by shaking the hands. Pain, numbness, tingling, or a burning sensation may be felt only in the fingertips on the palmar aspect of the thumb, index, and middle finger. Grip strength and pinch strength may be limited. Symptoms are reproduced when direct compression is applied over the median nerve in the carpal tunnel for about 30 seconds. A positive Phalen and Tinel's sign indicates a possible CTS (see Figures 13.34 and 13.35).

➤ MANAGEMENT

Individuals with suspected CTS should be referred to a physician for care. Immobilization in slight wrist extension with a dorsal splint is used to rest the wrist for up to 3 to 5 weeks, particularly at night when symptoms occur. An ice cup or ice bag, NSAIDs, or in some situations, diuretics, can initially reduce swelling and pain in the area caused by tenosynovitis. Use of a compression wrap should be avoided, since this adds additional compression on the already impinged structures. More than half of the individuals with this condition respond well to conservative treat-

ment, although symptoms may recur, necessitating a corticosteroid injection into the canal. In cases that do not respond well to conservative treatment, surgical decompression or carpal tunnel release can be performed.

Ulnar Nerve Entrapment

The ulnar nerve passes through the ulnar groove posterior to the medial epicondyle, to enter the cubital tunnel formed by the aponeurosis and two heads of the flexor carpi ulnaris. The nerve continues distally between the flexor digitorum profundus dorsally and the flexor carpi ulnaris palmarly. The palmar cutaneous nerve arises in the midforearm to supply the proximal hypothenar eminence. The dorsal cutaneous nerve arises 5 to 8 cm proximal to the ulnar styloid and supplies the dorsum of the ulnar side of the hand. At the wrist, the nerve courses between the hook of the hamate and pisiform, then passes through Guyon's canal to move distally into the fingers **(Figure 13.22)**. The superficial branch supplies the overlying palmaris brevis, then becomes entirely sensory to supply the hypothenar eminence and ring and small fingers. The deep branch curves around the hook of the hamate to supply the ulnar intrinsics, ending its terminal branch in the first dorsal interossei.

ULNAR TUNNEL SYNDROME

Compression of the ulnar nerve may occur as the nerve enters the ulnar tunnel, or as the deep branch curves around the hook of the hamate and traverses the palm. This condition is frequently seen in cycling, racquet sports, and in baseball/softball catchers, hockey goalies, and handball players that experience repetitive compressive trauma to the palmar aspect of the hand. Distal ulnar nerve palsy may

Transverse carpal ligament
(Flexor retinaculum)

Deep branch of ulnar nerve

Volar carpal ligment

Guyon's canal

Ulnar artery

Ulnar nerve

➤ FIGURE 13.22 Impingement of the ulnar nerve. The ulnar nerve can become impinged in the tunnel of Guyon as it runs under the ligament between the hamate and pisiform.

also be seen as a push-up palsy, following fractures of the hook of the hamate, or caused by a missed golf shot or baseball swing.

➤ SIGNS AND SYMPTOMS

The lesion may present with motor, sensory, or mixed symptoms. Coincident involvement of the median nerve is common. The individual will complain of numbness in the ulnar nerve distribution, particularly in the little finger, and will be unable to grasp a piece of paper between the thumb and index finger (see Froment's sign, Figure 13.37). Slight weakness in grip strength and atrophy of the hypothenar mass may also be present. Tapping just distal to the pisiform bone will produce a tingling sensation that radiates into the little finger and ulnar aspect of the ring finger (positive Tinel's sign).

➤ MANAGEMENT

Treatment involves splinting, NSAIDs, and avoidance of any precipitating activity. If symptoms do not disappear within 6 months of conservative treatment, surgical decompression of Guyon's canal may be necessary.

CYCLIST'S PALSY

Cyclist's palsy, also linked to ulnar nerve entrapment, occurs when a biker leans on the handlebar for an extended period of time, leading to swelling in the hypothenar area. Symptoms mimic the more serious ulnar nerve entrapment syndrome, but in this condition, symptoms usually disappear rapidly after completion of the ride. Properly padding the handlebars, wearing padded gloves, varying hand position, and properly fitting the bike to the rider can greatly reduce the incidence of this condition.

BOWLER'S THUMB

Bowler's thumb involves compression of the ulnar digital sensory nerve, on the medial aspect of the thumb in the web space, while gripping the ball. Constant pressure on this spot can lead to scarring in the area. The radial digital nerve of the index finger is similarly at risk in racquet sports.

➤ SIGNS AND SYMPTOMS

Numbness, tingling, or pain may develop on the medial aspect of the thumb. Athletic trainers develop similar symptoms from excessive use of dull scissors, or added pressure on the thumb as one cuts through thick tape jobs or pads. The individual may have swelling or thickening over the medial palmar aspect at the base of the thumb. Although there is no true motor involvement, grip strength may be decreased secondary to pain.

➤ MANAGEMENT

Treatment depends on the stage of injury. Since the predominant cause is inflammatory in nature, treatment is directed at reducing inflammation. Cryotherapy, immobilization with a molded plastic thumb guard, NSAIDs, and corticosteroid injection, if needed, are usually successful in relieving symptoms.

Radial Nerve Entrapment

The radial nerve bifurcates near the radiocapitellar joint to become the posterior interosseous and superficial radial nerves. The posterior interosseous nerve travels between the two heads of the supinator, around the proximal radius, and under the forearm extensors to supply the terminal articular branches to the wrist. The superficial radial nerve travels underneath the brachioradialis to become subcutaneous in the distal forearm and supply sensation to the dorsoradial portion of the hand, including the first web space and the proximal phalanges of the first three digits. The most common compressive neuropathy of the radial nerve, which occurs at the radial tunnel, was discussed in Chapter 12.

DISTAL POSTERIOR INTEROSSEOUS NERVE SYNDROME

Compression of the distal posterior interosseous nerve occurs as it passes dorsally over the distal radius and enters the wrist capsule. Gymnasts are particularly prone to this injury because of repetitive and forceful wrist dorsiflexion.

➤ SIGNS AND SYMPTOMS

The athlete usually complains of a deep, dull ache in the wrist that is reproduced with forceful wrist extension or deep palpation of the forearm with the wrist in flexion. Because the condition can often be confused with carpal instability, ganglions, and wrist sprains, the examiner should perform several tests for carpal stability.

➤ MANAGEMENT

If the condition does not improve after following standard acute care and activity modification, refer the individual to a physician for further care.

SUPERFICIAL RADIAL NERVE ENTRAPMENT

The superficial branch of the radial nerve can be compressed at the wrist as it pierces the deep fascia to become subcutaneous between the tendons of the extensor carpi radialis longus and brachioradialis. This constriction is made worse by sports that require repeated pronation and supination, such as batting, throwing, and rowing; by gloves that are strapped too tight; or by tight wrist bands, commonly seen in racquet sports.

➤ SIGNS AND SYMPTOMS

The individual will complain of burning pain, sensory changes, and night pain over the dorsoradial aspect of the wrist, hand, dorsal thumb, and index finger. Typically, the Finkelstein test is negative, but Tinel's sign over the wrist is positive. The athlete denies any pain with motion of the wrist, which rules out a tendinitis-, arthritis-, or impingement-type syndrome.

➤ MANAGEMENT

If the condition does not improve after following standard acute care and activity modification, refer the individual to a physician for further care.

 The cyclist may have compressed the ulnar nerve while leaning on the handlebars during the recent increased training. To alleviate symptoms, suggest padding the handlebars, wearing padded gloves, varying hand position, and properly fitting the bike to the rider.

FRACTURES TO THE WRIST AND HAND

 A football player had his hand stepped on by another player. Immediate pain and a cracking sensation were felt in the palm of the hand. Observation reveals noticeable swelling on the dorsum of the hand. Palpation of the third metacarpal and percussion on the distal end of the third finger cause increased pain. What should you suspect? How will you immobilize the hand?

Fractures of the distal ulna and radius, and the carpal bones are usually caused by axial loading when an individual falls on an outstretched hand. The majority are simple and nondisplaced. With the advent of external orthoses, many fractures can be immobilized adequately to allow individuals to continue with regular sport participation. Specific rules governing special protective equipment, however, require that braces, casts, or any unyielding substances on the elbow, forearm, wrist, or hand be padded on all sides so as not to endanger other players. Once the fracture has reached a stage where external support is no longer necessary during daily activities, a splint may be worn during sport participation only.

Distal Radial and Ulnar Fractures

The distal radial epiphyseal plate is the classic location for the stress injury commonly called "gymnast's wrist." In contrast to other growth-plate overuse syndromes in adolescents, this fracture is caused by compression. Repetitive performance on the pommel horse and uneven bars causes excessive wrist loading, leading to pain over the dorsum of the wrists. Pain increases as the wrist is carried into maximum dorsiflexion, as occurs in vaulting, tumbling, and beam work. Diffuse tenderness is typically present over the dorsum of the midcarpal area, but edema, discoloration, and clinical instability are generally not present. Pain increases with the extremes of wrist motion. The distal ulnar physis may also be involved. Treatment involves splinting, NSAIDs, and the avoidance of the offending exercises until asymptomatic. Complete resolution of symptoms may require up to 3 to 6 months or longer. A dorsal block splint may be beneficial for practice and competition to avoid extremes of wrist extension.

Fractures to the distal radius and ulna present a special problem. One or both bones may be fractured, or one bone may be fractured with the other bone dislocated at the elbow or wrist joint **(Table 13.2)**. A Colles's fracture oc-

TABLE 13.2	RADIAL AND ULNAR FRACTURES
Common Name	**Bone and Soft Tissue Damage**
Monteggia's fracture	Fracture of distal ulna with an associated dislocation of the radial head
Galeazzi's fracture	Fracture of distal radius with associated dislocation or subluxation of the distal radioulnar joint
Colles' fracture	Fracture of distal metaphysis of the radius, with displacement of distal fragment dorsally
Smith's fracture	Fracture of distal radius, with displacement of distal fragment toward palmar aspect (reverse Colles')

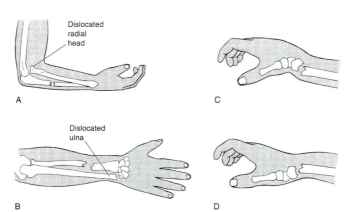

➤ FIGURE 13.23 **Forearm fractures**. A, Monteggia's fracture. B, Galeazzi's fracture. C, Colles's fracture. D, Smith's fracture.

curs within one and a half inches of the wrist joint, and results in a "dinner-fork" deformity when the distal segment displaces in a dorsal and radial direction. A reverse of this fracture is Smith's fracture, which tends to move toward the palmar aspect (volar) **(Figure 13.23)**. Swelling and hemorrhage may lead to circulatory impairment, or the median nerve may be damaged as it passes through the forearm.

 As a result, immediate immobilization in a vacuum splint and referral to a physician is necessary. In many instances, open reduction and internal fixation with rigid plates and screws is necessary to restore function.

Scaphoid Fracture

Scaphoid fractures account for 60 to 70% of all carpal bone injuries in the general population, and are the most common wrist bone fracture in the athlete (14). Often, the individual will fall on the wrist, have normal radiographs, and be discharged with a diagnosis of a wrist sprain without further care. Yet several months later, the individual will continue to experience persistent wrist pain. Radiographs at this time may reveal an established nonunion fracture of the scaphoid **(Figure 13.24)**. Because of a poor blood supply to the area, aseptic necrosis, or death of the tissue, is a common complication with this fracture.

➤ SIGNS AND SYMPTOMS

Assessment will reveal a history of falling on an outstretched hand. If pain is present during palpation of the anatomical snuff box **(Figure 13.25)**, which lies directly over the scaphoid, or with inward pressure along the long axis of the first metacarpal bone, suspect a fracture. Pain will also increase during wrist extension and radial deviation.

➤ MANAGEMENT

 Treatment involves ice, compression, immobilization in an appropriate splint, and immediate referral to a physician.

Nondisplaced scaphoid fractures are usually handled with a long-arm thumb cast, which originates from above

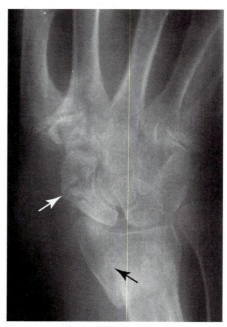

➤ FIGURE 13.24 **Scaphoid fracture**. Nonunion fractures of the scaphoid occur when there is a poor blood supply to the area. Note this individual also has a fractured radius.

the elbow to prevent rotation (but allows some flexion and extension of the elbow), and extends over the DIP joint of the thumb. The cast is changed at 2-week intervals to ensure proper molding around the forearm. At 6 weeks postinjury, the cast is replaced by a short-arm thumb cast originating proximal to the wrist, but leaving the DIP joint free to move. Follow-up radiographs are taken at 3- to 4-week intervals to monitor healing and detect signs of delayed union, nonunion, malunion, or avascular necrosis. Some fractures may take several weeks or months to heal. During this time, the individual may participate with a padded, short-arm thumb cast or silicone cast (14). Displaced scaphoid fractures are secured with internal fixation.

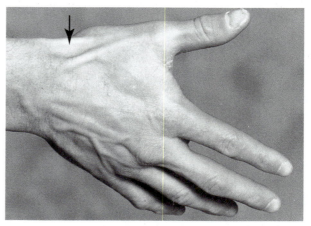

➤ FIGURE 13.25 **Anatomical snuff box**. The scaphoid forms the floor of the anatomical snuff box. It is bounded by the extensor pollicis brevis medially and the extensor pollicis longus laterally. Increased pain during palpation in this region indicates a possible fracture to the scaphoid bone.

Hamate Fracture

Direct impact to the hamate may also lead to a nonunion fracture. This typically occurs when an athlete strikes a stationary object with a racquet or club in full swing. Once fractured, the ligamentous insertions of the transverse carpal ligament, the pisohamate ligament, the short flexor, and the opponens digiti minimi act to displace the fragment and prevent union.

➤ SIGNS AND SYMPTOMS

Physical examination will reveal tenderness over the hypothenar muscle mass. Painful abduction of the small finger against resistance will be present, as well as decreased grip strength.

➤ MANAGEMENT

Treatment involves ice, compression, immobilization in an appropriate splint, and immediate referral to a physician.

Radiographs and tomograms using a carpal tunnel view with the wrist in extension will confirm the diagnosis. Care is usually symptomatic, with a protective orthoses worn for 4 to 6 weeks until tenderness subsides. It may be 2 to 3 months before a racquet or bat will feel comfortable in the hand again.

Triquetrum Fractures

Fractures of the triquetrum are fairly common and caused by impingement of the ulnar styloid into the dorsum of the triquetrum. The ulna tends to shear a portion of bone away from the triquetrum (chip fracture).

➤ SIGNS AND SYMPTOMS

The athlete will usually report a history of an acute wrist dorsiflexion injury (chip fracture) or direct trauma (body fracture) to the wrist area. Pain in the dorsal wrist will be present over the triquetrum.

➤ MANAGEMENT

Treatment involves ice, compression, immobilization in an appropriate splint, and immediate referral to a physician.

Immobilization in a short-arm cast with mild extension of the wrist for 4 to 6 weeks is the treatment of choice; however, some fractures may become nonunion and require surgical excision.

Kienbock's Disease

A true lunate fracture is rare in sports. However, avascular necrosis of the lunate, or Kinebock's disease, can affect young athletes. Its cause has yet to be determined, but it is thought to arise either because of repetitive trauma or an unrecognized lunate fracture. The athlete usually complains of dorsal wrist pain, swelling, and weakness of the wrist associated with use. A history of trauma may or may not be present. Early radiographs are needed to ascertain the correct diagnosis, as the preferred treatment is early surgical intervention.

Metacarpal Fractures

Uncomplicated fractures of the metacarpals result in severe pain, swelling, and deformity **(Figure 13.26)**. A unique fracture involving the neck of the fifth metacarpal is called a Boxer's fracture. It occurs when an individual punches an object with a closed fist leading to rotation of the head of the metacarpal over the neck.

➤ SIGNS AND SYMPTOMS

Increased pain and a palpable deformity will be present in the palm of the hand directly over the involved metacarpal. Gentle percussion and compression along the long axis of the bone will increase pain at the fracture site (see **Field Strategy 13.2**). These same techniques can be used to detect possible fractures in the carpals and phalanges.

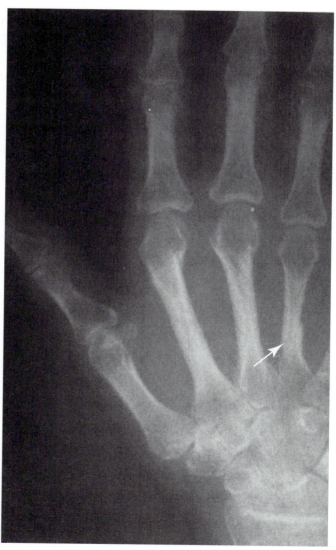

➤ FIGURE 13.26 **Metacarpal fracture**. Uncomplicated fracture of the fourth metacarpal.

FIELD STRATEGY 13.2   DETERMINING A POSSIBLE FRACTURE TO A METACARPAL

1. Palpate for pain along the shaft of the bone.
2. Apply compression along the long axis of the bone (A).
   • Positive sign occurs if pain is felt at the injury site.
3. Apply percussion or vibration at the end of the bone (B).
   • Positive sign occurs if pain is felt at the injury site.
4. Apply distraction at the end of the bone (C).
   • Positive sign occurs if pain is decreased. Increased pain may indicate a ligamentous injury.

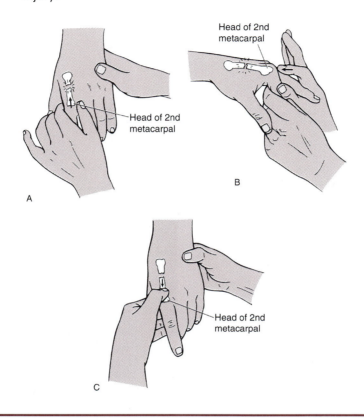

➤ MANAGEMENT

Fractures should be immobilized in the position of function, with the palm face down and fingers slightly flexed. Ice is applied to reduce hemorrhage and swelling; an elastic compression bandage should not be applied to a swollen hand, as it may lead to increased distal swelling in the fingers. The athlete should be referred immediately to a physician for further care.

Bennett's Fracture

A Bennett's fracture is an articular fracture of the proximal end of the first metacarpal. It is typically due to axial compression, as occurs when a punch is thrown with a closed fist or the individual falls on a closed fist. The pull of the abductor pollicis longus tendon at the base of the metacarpal displaces the shaft proximally. A small medial fragment, however, is held in place by the deep volar ligament, leading to a fracture-dislocation **(Figure 13.27)**.

➤ SIGNS AND SYMPTOMS

Pain and swelling are localized over the proximal end of the first metacarpal, but deformity may or may not be present. Inward pressure exerted along the long axis of the first metacarpal will elicit increased pain at the fracture site.

➤ MANAGEMENT

Acute care consists of ice, compression, immobilization in a wrist splint, and immediate referral to a physician for further care.

The preferred treatment for this fracture is closed reduction and percutaneous pinning for less than 3 mm of fracture displacement, and open reduction and fixation for greater displacements (10).

Phalangeal Fractures

Fractures of the phalanges are very common in sport participation, and are difficult to manage. They may be caused due to the strong pull of the flexor and extensor tendons. The four fingers move as a unit. Failure to maintain the longitudinal and rotational alignments of the fingers can lead to long-term disability in grasping or manipulating small objects in the palm of the hand. This deformity often results in a finger overlapping another when a fist is made.

➤ MANAGEMENT

Acute care involves ice to reduce pain and swelling. With the hand immobilized in a full wrist splint, place gauze pads or a gauze roll under the fingers to produce about 30° finger flexion, and reduce the pull of the flexor tendons. Refer the individual immediately to a physician for care. Immobilization will depend upon the type of fracture and its location, and may vary from 2 to 4 weeks.

The football player probably fractured the third metacarpal when the other player stepped on his hand. Immobilize the hand in the position of function with a wrist splint, apply ice to reduce swelling, and transport the individual to the physician.

ASSESSMENT OF THE WRIST AND HAND

A young gymnast has increased pain on the dorsum of the wrist when weight bearing on his hands. Pain increases with hyperextension and ulnar deviation and with passive wrist flexion and extension. How will you assess this injury?

The wrist and hand are difficult to evaluate because of the number of anatomical structures providing motor and sensory function to the region. A thorough examination often takes longer than other joints of the body because of the multiples structures and joints involved, and the importance of the hand to everyday function. In assessing this region, two major objectives must be kept in mind. First, the injury or condition must be evaluated as accurately as possible to ensure adequate treatment. Second, the athletic trainer must ascertain the remaining function to determine whether the athlete will have any incapacity in performing sport-specific skills and activities of daily living.

The athletic trainer must also keep in mind that if the mechanism of injury involves axial loading at the wrist, additional assessment may be necessary at the elbow or shoulder. Albeit uncommon, pain at the wrist and hand may also be referred from the cervical spine, shoulder, and elbow, which may necessitate assessment of these joints prior to assessing the wrist and hand. **Field Strategy 13.3** outlines a full wrist and hand assessment.

HISTORY

What information must be gathered from the gymnast to identify the primary complaint and ascertain if other factors such as sport-specific skills contributed to this injury?

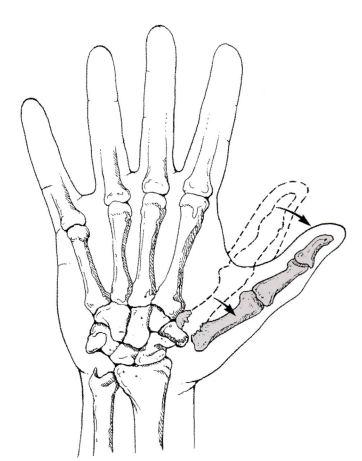

➤ FIGURE 13.27 **Bennett's fracture.** A Bennett's fracture is usually associated with a dislocation of the metacarpophalangeal (MP) joint of the thumb. An avulsion fracture, however, occurs when a segment of the metacarpal is held in place by the deep volar ligament.

by having the fingers stepped on or impinged between two hard objects such as a football helmet and the ground, or by hyperextension that may lead to a fracture-dislocation **(Figure 13.28)**.

➤ SIGNS AND SYMPTOMS

Increased pain will be present with circulative compression around the involved phalanx. Gentle percussion and compression along the long axis of the bone will increase pain at the fracture site. Particular attention should be given to a possible fracture of the middle and proximal phalanges. These fractures tend to have marked deformity

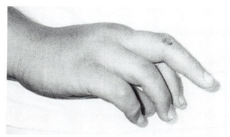

➤ FIGURE 13.28 **Phalangeal fracture.** This finger was crushed between two football helmets during a tackle, fracturing the phalanx.

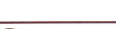

FIELD STRATEGY 13.3   WRIST AND HAND EVALUATION

HISTORY

- Primary complaint including:
  - Current nature, location, and onset of the condition
  - Mechanism of injury
  - Cause of stress; position of arm, wrist, and hand; direction of force
  - Changes in throwing style, equipment, overhead motion techniques, or conditioning modes
  - Characteristics of the symptoms
  - Evolution of the onset, nature, location, severity and duration of pain and weakness
  - Disability resulting from the injury
  - Related medical history
  - Previous injuries to the area, congenital abnormalities, or family history

OBSERVATION AND INSPECTION

- Observation should analyze general shape, contour, and posture of the hand (see Field Strategy 13.4)
- Inspection at the injury site for deformity, swelling, discoloration, hypertrophy or muscle atrophy, visible congenital deformity, or surgical incision or scars

PALPATION

- Bony structures, to determine a possible fracture
- Soft tissue structures, to determine skin temperature, swelling, point tenderness, crepitus, deformity, muscle spasm, cutaneous sensation, and pulse

FUNCTIONAL TESTS

- Active range of motion
- Passive range of motion
- Resisted manual muscle testing

STRESS TESTS

- Wrist and finger ligamentous instability tests
- Finkelstein's test for de Quervain's tenosynovitis
- Carpal tunnel compression test
- Phalen's wrist flexion test
- Tinel's signs for ulnar neuritis
- Pinch-grip test for anterior interosseous nerve entrapment
- Froment's sign for ulnar nerve paralysis

NEUROLOGICAL TESTS

- Myotomes
- Reflexes
- Dermatomes

SPORT-SPECIFIC FUNCTIONAL TESTS

Questions about a wrist injury should focus on the primary complaint, past injuries, and other factors that may have contributed to the current problem (demands of the sport, changes in technique, overuse, occupational requirements, or referred pain). For example, ask how the injury occurred. Is the region subjected to repetitive trauma, such as from constant impact from a ball, racquet, bat, or stick? Determine what symptoms are currently present, and how they progressed. Is the pain localized, general, or does it radiate into the forearm? What activities increase or decrease pain? What recent changes, if any, have occurred in the training program? In addition to general questions discussed in Chapter 4, specific questions for the wrist and hand region are listed in **Field Strategy 13.4**.

 The 16-year-old gymnast has been working quite extensively on pommel horse and floor exercise routines in preparation for an upcoming competition. Pain on the dorsal wrist was first noticed after practice 3 to 4 weeks ago, but the pain has intensified and is now present whenever he is weight bearing on his hands. He has been icing both wrists for the past week after practice and taking over-the-counter anti-inflammatories.

FIELD STRATEGY 13.4 DEVELOPING A HISTORY OF THE INJURY

<u>CURRENT INJURY STATUS</u>

1. How did the injury occur (mechanism)? Was the region subjected to repetitive impact from a ball, bat, racquet, or stick?
2. Where is the pain? How severe is it? Did it come on gradually or suddenly? What type of pain is it (sharp, aching, burning, radiating)? Does it wake you up at night (possible carpal tunnel syndrome)?
3. Did you hear any sounds during the incident, such as snaps, cracks, or pops? Was there any swelling, discoloration, muscle spasms, or numbness with the injury?
4. Are there certain activities you cannot perform because of the pain? What actions or motions replicate the pain? At what angle of wrist or finger motion does it hurt the worst? Does your elbow or shoulder bother you?

<u>PAST INJURY STATUS</u>

1. Have you ever injured your wrist or fingers before? When? How did that occur? What was done to treat the injury?
2. Have you had any medical problems recently? (You are looking for possible referred pain from the cervical neck, shoulder, or elbow.)

OBSERVATION AND INSPECTION

What specific factors should be observed at the injury site? Since pain is present in both wrists, can you still do bilateral comparison?

The entire arm should be exposed for observation and inspection. Although the individual may have a wrist injury, the elbow and shoulder region may also need to be evaluated, depending on the mechanism of injury. First observe the position of the wrist, hand, and fingers. Is there a noticeable deformity? How is the individual holding the wrist and hand? If swelling is present in a specific joint, the individual may be unable to fully extend that joint, supporting it in a slightly flexed position. When a possible fracture or dislocation is not present, observe the individual's willingness and ability to place the hand in the various positions requested. The functional position of the wrist, sometimes called the position of rest, is with the wrist in 20 to 35° of extension and 10 to 15° of ulnar deviation. This position allows for the greatest amount of flexion of the fingers. Inspect the palm of the hand for palmar creases. Swelling in one or more of the hand compartments may obliterate these lines. With bilateral comparison, the dominant hand tends to be slightly larger than the nondominant hand. Inspect the specific injury site for obvious abrasions, deformity, swelling, discoloration, symmetry, hypertrophy, muscle atrophy, or previous surgical incisions. **Field Strategy 13.5** summarizes observations at the wrist and hand, from dorsal and palmar views.

Bilateral comparison reveals slight swelling over the dorsal aspect of the wrist. No bilateral differences are visible in the thenar or hypothenar muscle masses. The fingers appear to be normal, with no discoloration or swelling present.

PALPATION

Pain and swelling are confined over the dorsal aspect of both wrists. Where will you begin palpation? What specific factors are you looking for?

With an acute injury, if the individual is in great pain, unable or unwilling to move the wrist or hand, determine the possibility of a fracture or dislocation before moving the wrist or hand. Perform the fracture tests, including compression, percussion, vibration, and traction. If a fracture is suspected, treat accordingly.

Immobilize the wrist and hand in a vacuum splint or wrist splint, apply ice to control pain and inflammation, and immediately transport the individual to a physician.

Palpate the wrist and hand proximal to distal. Begin on the dorsal aspect, then move to the palmar aspect. Support the individual's hand throughout the palpation. Bilateral palpation can determine temperature, swelling, point tenderness, crepitus, deformity, muscle spasm, and cutaneous sensation. Temperature changes may indicate inflammation, infection, or a reduction in circulation. Crepitus may indicate tenosynovitis, an irregular articular surface, or possible fracture. Circulation can be assessed by blanching the fingernails. Squeeze the nail; initially it should turn white, but color should return immediately upon release of pressure. Pulses can also be taken at the radial and ulnar arteries in the wrist.

Dorsal Aspect

1. Radial styloid process and tubercle of the radius
2. Styloid process of the ulna
3. Finger and thumb extensors and thumb abductor

FIELD STRATEGY 13.5   OBSERVATION AND INSPECTION OF THE WRIST AND HAND

<u>DORSAL VIEW</u>

1. Check bilateral shape and contour of the bony and soft tissue structures of the fore-arm, wrist, and hand. Note how the individual moves the hand into the requested positions.
2. Note skin color, presence of ganglions, or muscular wasting. Do the hands appear healthy? Many vascular problems, such as peripheral vascular disorders, Raynaud's disease, or diabetes mellitus, may be indicated by changes in skin color and temperature.
3. Note any localized swelling, effusion, or synovial thickening at the MP or IP joints.
4. Observe for any angular deformities of the fingers that may indicate a previous fracture or dislocation.
5. With the forearm in pronation, note whether or not the distal phalanx fails to remain in an extended position (possible mallet finger).
6. Observe the fingernails for any abnormality or change in color during blanching.

<u>PALMAR VIEW</u>

1. Check the smooth contours of the bony and soft tissue structures of the forearm, wrist, and hand.
2. Look for muscle wasting in the thenar eminence (median nerve) and hypothenar eminence (ulnar nerve) that may indicate a nerve injury.
3. Have the individual flex the MP and PIP joints, and keep the DIP joint extended. Note any angular deformity of the fingers that may indicate a previous fracture.
4. Note any localized swelling, effusion, or synovial thickening at the MP, PIP, and DIP joints. (This may be more visible on the dorsal view.)
5. Check skin color and presence of any abrasions or scars. Scars may decrease the mobility of a joint because of the formation of scar tissue around the tendons and joint.

4. Palpate the carpal bones on the dorsal and palmar aspect at the same time

Scaphoid. Lies distal to the radial styloid process and forms the floor of the anatomical snuff box. Tenderness is indicative of a possible fracture

Lunate. Lies just distal to the radial tubercle, and is easily palpated during wrist flexion

Triquetrum. Lies one finger's breadth distal to the ulnar styloid process

Pisiform. Slightly flex the wrist, and palpate on the medial palmar side

Trapezium. Lies distal to the anatomical snuff box. Take a radial pulse in the anatomical snuff box

Trapezoid. Lies medial to the trapezium

Capitate. Lies distal to the lunate and a slight indentation before the metacarpal

Hamate. Lies distal to the triquetrum; the hook of the hamate is more easily palpated on the palmar aspect

5. Metacarpal bones and phalanges. Palpate the MP, PIP, and DIP joints for synovial thickening, swelling, and tenderness

Palmar Aspect

1. Flexor tendons
2. Carpal transverse arch that forms the carpal tunnel, and the longitudinal arch comprised of the carpal bones, metacarpals, and phalanges

3. Palmar fascia and intrinsic muscles within the thenar and hypothenar muscle masses

 Swelling and extreme point tenderness were apparent over the dorsum of the radiocarpal joint. Circulation and sensation are normal.

PHYSICAL EXAMINATION TESTS

 Pain appears to be centralized over the radiocarpal joint. What specific tests should be performed to determine the extent and seriousness of this injury?

Perform special tests in a comfortable position, and begin with gentle stress. Note what part of the range of motion is most painful. Do not force the wrist or hand through any sudden motions, nor otherwise cause undue pain. Proceed cautiously through the assessment.

Functional Tests

The athletic trainer should determine the available range of motion in forearm pronation/supination, wrist flexion/extension, radial/ulnar deviation, finger flexion/extension, finger abduction/adduction, thumb flexion/extension, thumb abduction/adduction, and opposition of the thumb and little finger. As always, bilateral comparison is critical to determine normal or abnormal movement.

ACTIVE MOVEMENTS

In determining active movements at the wrist and hand, perform the most painful movements last. Finger active motion is usually done in a continuous pattern of flexion and extension. Ask the individual to: (a) make a tight fist (flexion), (b) straighten the fingers (extension), (c) spread the fingers (abduction), and (d) bring the fingers together (adduction). Note how fluidly each digit moves throughout the range of motion. If one finger does not move through the full ROM, that finger can be evaluated separately. The movements listed below can be assessed. The number in parentheses are normal ranges of motion for each movement.

- Pronation/supination of the forearm (85 to 90°)
- Wrist flexion (80 to 90°)
- Wrist extension (70 to 90°)
- Radial deviation (15°)
- Ulnar deviation (30 to 45°)
- Finger flexion and extension
- Finger abduction and adduction
- Thumb flexion, extension, abduction, and adduction
- Opposition of the thumb and little finger (tip to tip)

Technique for taking goniometry measurements of wrist flexion and extension, and radial and ulnar deviation, are listed in **Figure 13.29**.

PASSIVE MOVEMENTS

If the individual is unable to perform active movements in all ranges, assess passive movements. Slight overpressure at the end of each motion can test the end feel

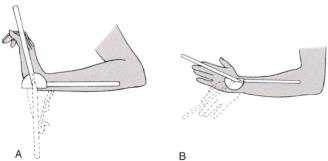

A   B

➤ FIGURE 13.29 **Goniometry measurement.** A, Wrist flexion and extension. The fulcrum is centered over the lateral aspect of the wrist close to the triquetrum. Align the proximal arm along the lateral aspect of the ulna using the olecranon process as reference. Align the distal arm along the midline of the fifth metacarpal. B, Radial and ulnar deviation. Center the fulcrum over the middle of the dorsum of the wrist close to the capitate. Align the proximal arm with the midline of the forearm using the lateral epicondyle as reference. Align the distal arm along the midline of the third metacarpal.

of each joint. Normal end feel for the wrist and finger joints is tissue stretch; however, in thin individuals, end feel for pronation may be bone-to-bone. Passive movements tested are the same as the active movements listed.

RESISTED MUSCLE TESTING

Active movements are tested using resisted movements throughout the full range of motion. The individual can be standing or seated. The proximal joint is stabilized, and a mild resistance is applied to the distal joint. **Figure 13.30** demonstrates motions that should be tested.

Stress Tests

Stress tests are performed when you have a clear indication of what structures may be damaged. Use only those tests deemed relevant, and always compare the results to the uninvolved arm.

LIGAMENTOUS INSTABILITY TEST FOR THE WRIST

With the elbow flexed at 90° and the forearm pronated, grip the distal forearm with one hand. With the other hand grasping across the metacarpals, apply a varus (ulnar deviation) and valgus (radial deviation) stress to the wrist joint. Pain or laxity indicates damage to the ulnar collateral and radial collateral ligaments that support the wrist, and may also elicit signs of trauma to the triangular fibrocartilage.

LIGAMENTOUS INSTABILITY TEST FOR THE FINGERS

Stabilize the thumb or finger with one hand proximal to the joint being tested. Apply valgus and varus stresses to the joint to test the integrity of the collateral ligaments **(Figure 13.31)**. Do bilateral comparison with the uninvolved hand. This test is used for gamekeeper's thumb and joint sprains of the fingers.

FINKELSTEIN'S TEST

Have the individual make a fist with the thumb inside the fingers **(Figure 13.32)**. Stabilize the forearm, and flex the wrist in an ulnar direction. A positive Finkelstein's test, indicating de Quervain's tenosynovitis, produces pain over the abductor pollicis longus and extensor pollicis brevis tendons at the wrist. Because the test may be uncomfortable for even a healthy individual, all positive tests should be compared bilaterally to the uninvolved wrist.

CARPAL TUNNEL COMPRESSION TEST

Exert even pressure with both thumbs directly over the carpal tunnel, and hold for at least 30 seconds **(Figure**

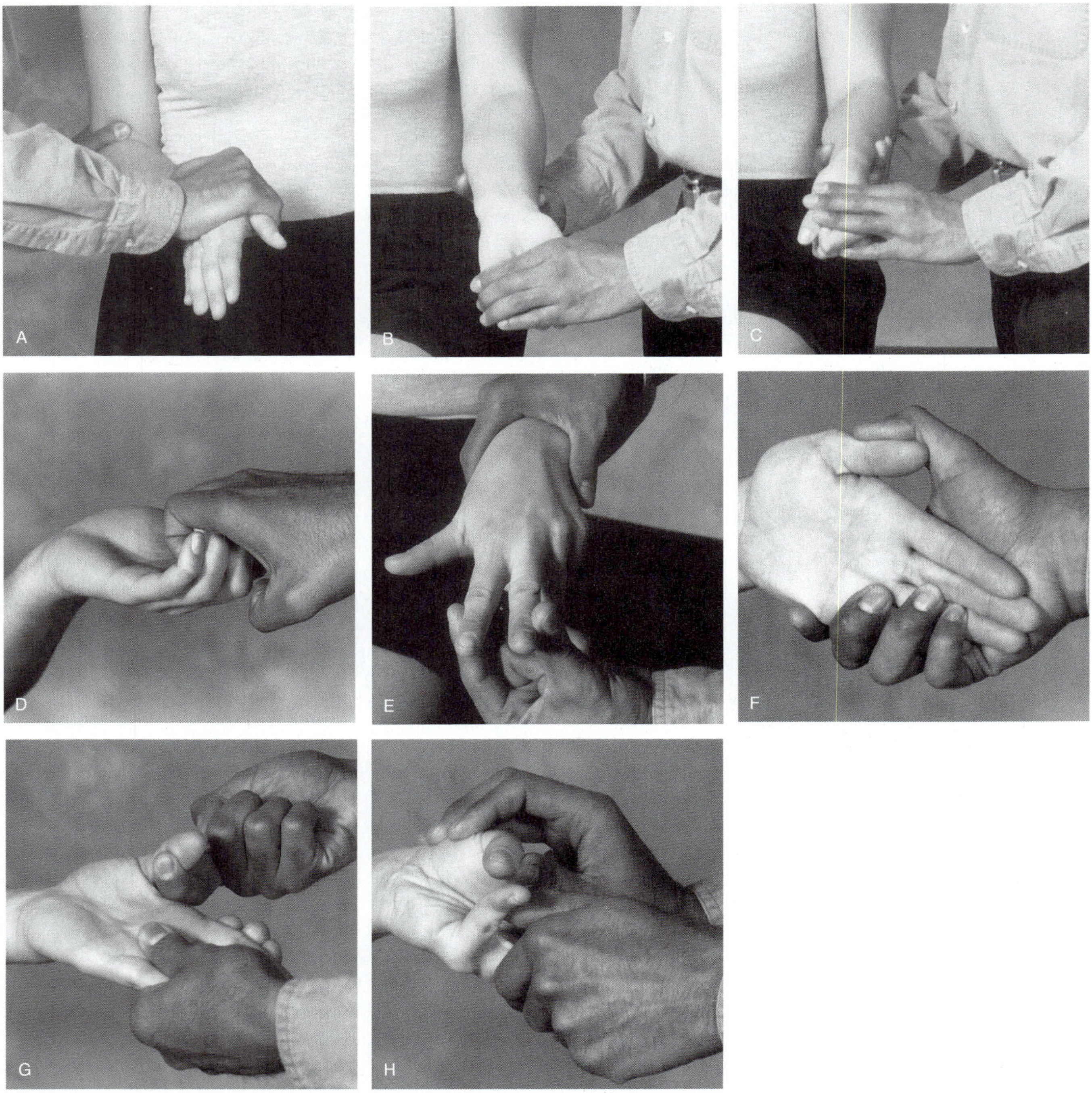

➤ **FIGURE 13.30 Resisted manual muscle testing**. A, Forearm supination and pronation. B, Wrist flexion and extension. C, Ulnar and radial deviation. D, Finger flexion and extension. E, Finger abduction and adduction. F, Thumb flexion and extension. G, Thumb abduction and adduction. H, Opposition.

13.33). A positive test produces numbness or tingling into the palmar aspect of the thumb, index finger, and middle finger.

PHALEN'S (WRIST FLEXION) TEST

Place the dorsum of the hands together to maximally flex the wrists. Hold this position for 1 minute by gently pushing the wrists together **(Figure 13.34)**. Ensure that

the athlete does not shrug the shoulders during the test, as this causes compression of the median branch of the brachial plexus as it passes through the thoracic outlet. An alternative position is to have the examiner apply overpressure during passive wrist flexion and hold the position for 1 minute. A positive test, indicating either median nerve or ulnar nerve compression, produces numbness or tingling into the specific nerve distribution pattern. If the median nerve is compressed, sensory changes will be evident in

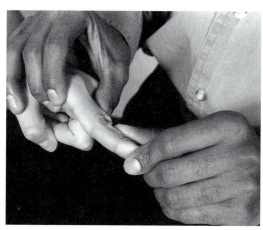

➤ FIGURE 13.31 **Ligament instability test**. To stress the ligamentous structures around the joints, apply varus and valgus forces at the specific joint.

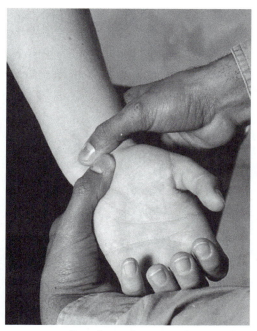

➤ FIGURE 13.33 **Carpal tunnel compression test**. Compression over the carpal tunnel may lead to tingling into the palmar aspect of the thumb, index finger, and middle finger, and indicates a carpal tunnel syndrome.

the thumb, index finger, third finger, and lateral half of the ring finger. If the ulnar nerve is compressed, sensory changes will occur in the fifth finger and medial half of the ring finger.

TINEL'S SIGN

To test for median nerve compression, tap over the carpal tunnel at the wrist **(Figure 13.35)**. A positive test produces numbness or tingling in the median nerve distribution. This test can also be adapted for ulnar nerve com-

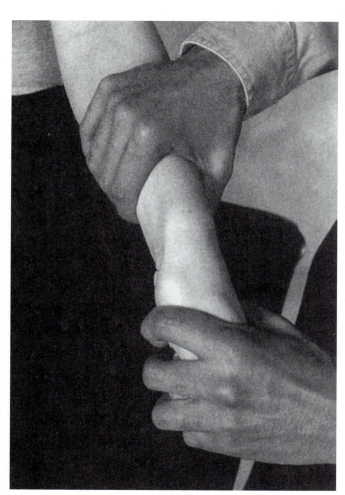

➤ FIGURE 13.32 **Finkelstein's test**. Have the individual make a fist with the thumb inside the fingers. Flex the wrist in an ulnar direction. A positive Finkelstein's test indicates tenosynovitis of the thumb tendons.

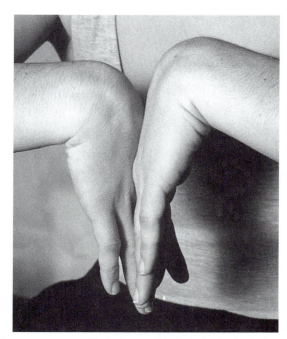

➤ FIGURE 13.34 **Phalen's test**. Phalen's (wrist flexion) test indicates that the median or ulnar nerve is compressed if it produces numbness or tingling into the specific nerve distribution pattern.

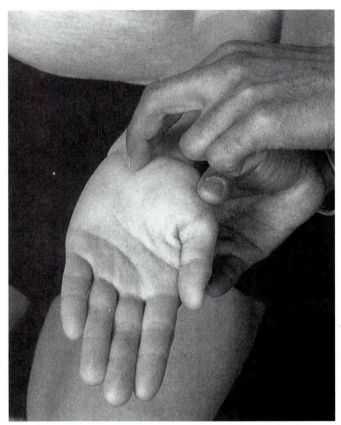

➤ FIGURE 13.35 **Tinel's sign**. Tinel's sign at the wrist is also used to indicate median nerve compression.

pression in the hypothenar mass and radial nerve compression on the dorsoradial aspect of the wrist.

PINCH GRIP TEST FOR ENTRAPMENT OF THE ANTERIOR INTEROSSEOUS NERVE

Ask the individual to pinch the tip of the index finger and thumb together **(Figure 13.36)**. If an abnormal pulp-

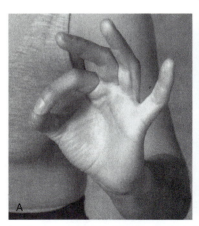

➤ FIGURE 13.36 **Pinch grip test**. Ask the individual to make an O with the thumb and forefinger. A, Normal tip-to-tip. B, Abnormal pulp-to-pulp signifies entrapment of the interior interosseous nerve.

to-pulp pinch is performed, the anterior interosseous nerve, an extension of the median nerve, may be entrapped at the elbow as it passes between the two heads of the pronator teres.

FROMENT'S SIGN FOR ULNAR NERVE PARALYSIS

The patient grasps a piece of paper between the thumb and forefinger **(Figure 13.37)**. The examiner attempts to pull the paper away. If the distal phalanx of the thumb flexes to hold the paper, it indicates paralysis of the adductor pollicis muscle indicative of ulnar nerve damage.

ALLEN TEST FOR CIRCULATION

Ask the athlete to quickly open and close the hand several times and then squeeze the hand tightly. Place your thumb and index finger over the radial and ulnar arteries, compressing them. The athlete then opens the hand while pressure is maintained over the arteries. One artery is tested by releasing the pressure over that artery to see if the hand flushes. The other artery is then tested in a similar fashion. Bilateral comparison can then determine the effectiveness of the two arteries, and which artery provides the major blood supply to the hand.

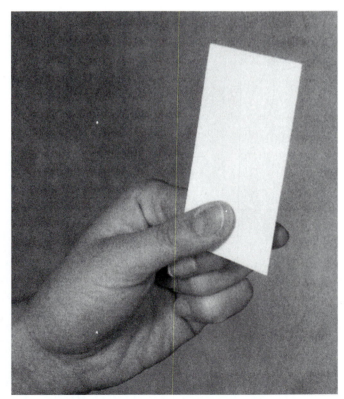

➤ FIGURE 13.37 **Froment's sign**. If the individual flexes the distal phalanx of the thumb to prevent a piece of paper from being pulled away, the positive Froment's test indicates paralysis of the adductor pollicis muscle resulting from possible ulnar nerve damage.

Neurologic Testing

Neurologic integrity can be assessed with the use of myotomes, reflexes, and segmental dermatomes and peripheral nerve cutaneous patterns.

MYOTOMES

Isometric muscle testing to test the myotomes should be performed in the loose-packed position and include: scapular elevation (C_4), shoulder abduction (C_5), elbow flexion and/or wrist extension (C_6), elbow extension and/or wrist flexion (C_7), thumb extension and/or ulnar deviation (C_8), and abduction and/or adduction of the hand intrinsics (T_1).

REFLEXES

Reflexes in the upper extremity include the biceps (C_5–C_6), brachioradialis (C_6), and triceps (C_7). These were discussed and demonstrated in Chapters 11 and 12.

CUTANEOUS PATTERNS

The segmental nerve dermatome patterns for the wrist and hand region are demonstrated in **Figure 13.38**. The peripheral nerve cutaneous patterns are demonstrated in **Figure 13.39**. Test bilaterally for altered sensation with sharp and dull touch by running the open hand and fingernails over the shoulder and down both sides of the arms and hands.

Sport-specific Functional Tests

Because the wrist, hand, and fingers are vital to perform activities of daily living, individuals should be assessed for

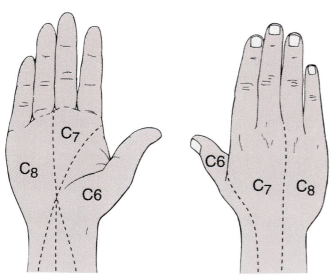

➤ FIGURE 13.38 Segmental dermatomes for the wrist and hand.

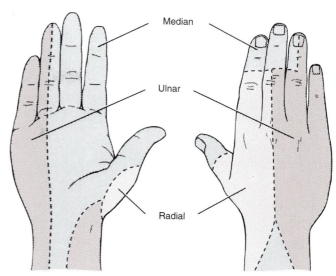

➤ FIGURE 13.39 Cutaneous nerve distribution patterns for the wrist and hand.

manual dexterity and coordination. Can they hook, pinch, and grasp an object? Can they comb their hair, hold a fork, brush their teeth, or pick up a briefcase? Prior to return to sport, the individual should be able to perform these simple functional skills in addition to having bilateral range of motion and strength in the wrist and fingers. Conditions that must be referred to a physician are listed in **Box 13.2**.

➤➤ **Box 13.2**

Conditions that Warrant Immediate Referral to a Physician

- Suspected fracture or dislocation
- Significant pain and/or excessive swelling in soft tissues or around joints
- Joint instability
- Loss or impairment of motion or function
- Presence of any sensory or circulatory changes

 The gymnast had localized pain over the distal radiocarpal joint that increased with active and passive wrist extension, and axial loading of the wrist joint with the wrist in hyperextension and ulnar deviation. A varus stress (ulnar deviation) placed on the wrist joint also increased pain. Although you think the individual may have a wrist sprain, this athlete should be referred to a physician to rule out a stress lesion of the distal radial epiphysis, or a dislocation of the lunate.

REHABILITATION

 Radiographs were negative and the gymnast was diagnosed with a wrist sprain. He was placed in a wrist splint to prevent excessive hyperextension

until the symptoms calmed down. What exercises should be included in the general rehabilitation program to help this athlete maintain his fitness?

Injuries to the wrist and hand often require immobilization; however, early range-of-motion and strengthening exercises should be conducted at the elbow and shoulder. Many of the exercises for the wrist and hand were discussed and demonstrated in Chapter 12, because they are often combined with rehabilitation of the elbow.

Restoration of Motion

Immobilization typically results in joint contractures and stiffness in the fingers; therefore, active range-of-motion exercises should begin as soon as possible. In the acute phase, exercises can be performed using cryokinetic techniques. Ice immersion is alternated with active range-of-motion exercises. The individual can use the opposite hand to apply a low-load, prolonged stretch in the various motions to minimize joint trauma and increase flexibility. As inflammation decreases, a warm whirlpool or paraffin bath may be used to facilitate motion.

Restoration of Proprioception and Balance

Closed chain exercises may involve shifting body weight from one hand to the other on a wall, tabletop, or unstable surface, such as a foam mat or BAPS board. Push-ups and step-ups on a box, stool, or Stair Master can also be used. Precision techniques to restore dexterity can be performed by picking up and manipulating the following objects: (a) coins of different thicknesses; (b) playing cards; (c) small objects of differing shapes; (d) large, light objects; and (e) large, heavy objects. In addition, the individual can tear tape, use scissors to cut paper, or juggle balls of different sizes.

Muscular Strength, Endurance, and Power

Once range-of-motion approximates normal for the individual, open chain kinetic exercises are performed in the various motions using light-weight dumbbells. Many of these exercises were listed and explained in Field Strategy 12.1. The individual should complete 30 to 50 repetitions with a 1-lb weight, and should not progress in resistance until 50 repetitions are achieved. With the forearm supported on a table, perform wrist curls, reverse wrist curls, pronation, and supination. Wrist curl-ups using a light weight suspended from a broomstick on a 3- to 4-foot rope can be used to increase strength in the wrist flexors and extensors. A weighted bar or hammer can be used for radial and ulnar deviation, and pronation and supination. PNF resisted exercises, surgical tubing, or strong rubber bands can be used in all motions for concentric and eccentric loading. Gripping exercises using a tennis ball or putty can be combined with pinching small and large objects.

Plyometric exercises may involve catching a weighted ball in a single hand and throwing it straight up and down, or using a minitramp to do bounding push-ups.

Cardiovascular Fitness

General body conditioning should be maintained throughout the rehabilitation program. Several examples of programs were provided in Field Strategy 7.6, and included use of a jump rope, Stair Master, treadmill, and upper body ergometer (UBE).

 As pain decreases, range-of-motion exercises for the fingers and wrist can begin immediately. Gripping exercises, precision dexterity skills, PNF resisted exercises, and surgical tubing can be incorporated early in the program with other wrist and hand strengthening exercises. General body conditioning and strengthening exercises for the shoulder and elbow can be performed as long as the condition is not aggravated.

Summary

1. Most wrist motion occurs at the radiocarpal joint. The triangular fibrocartilage is the cartilaginous disc that acts as a stabilizer of the distal radioulnar joint, and serves as the ulnar continuation of the radius.

2. The CM joint of the thumb is a classic saddle joint, which allows it to have more motion than the CM joints of the other 4 digits.

3. Retinacular tissue is found throughout the hand, forming protective passageways through which tendons, nerves, and blood vessels pass.

4. Most injuries to the wrist are a result of axial loading on the proximal palm during a fall on an outstretched hand.

5. Excessive varus/valgus stress and hyperextension can damage the collateral ligaments of the fingers. Ligament failure usually occurs at its attachment to the proximal phalanx or, less frequently, in the mid-portion.

6. The most common dislocation in the body occurs at the PIP joint. Because digital nerves and vessels run along the sides of the fingers and thumb, dislocation can be serious if it is reduced by an untrained individual.

7. Muscular strains occur as a result of excessive overload against resistance, or stretching the tendon beyond its normal range. Ruptures of a muscle tendon may cause the tendon to retract, necessitating surgical reattachment of the tendon in its proper position.

8. Chronic overuse of a tendon can lead to a tendinitis or friction tendinitis in one or more of the dorsal tunnels. Treatment usually consists of ice, rest,

NSAIDs, splinting, and avoiding exacerbating activities.

9. Carpal tunnel syndrome is the most common compression syndrome of the wrist and hand. It is characterized by pain and numbness that wakes the individual in the middle of the night, and is often relieved by shaking the hands.

10. Compression of the ulnar nerve will lead to weakness in grip strength, atrophy of the hypothenar mass, and loss of sensation over the little finger.

11. If pain is present during palpation of the anatomical snuff box, or with inward pressure along the long axis of the first metacarpal bone, suspect a fracture of the scaphoid.

12. Any injury that impairs the function of the hand or fingers should be referred to a physician. Immobilize the area in a vacuum, wrist, or finger splint to prevent further damage, apply ice to control hemorrhage and swelling, and transport the individual in an appropriate manner.

References

1. Rettig AC, Patell DV. Epidemiology of elbow, forearm, and wrist injuries in the athlete. Clin Sports Med 1995;14(2):289-297.

2. Short WH, Werner FW, Fortino MD, Mann KA. Analysis of the kinematics of the scaphoid and lunate in the intact wrist joint. Hand Clin 1997;13(1):93-108.

3. Sennwald GR, Zdravkovic V, Kern HP, Jacob HA. Kinematics of the wrist and its ligaments. J Hand Surg [Am] 1993;18(5):805-814.

4. Kobayashi M, Berger RA, Linscheid R, An KN. Intercarpal kinematics during wrist motion. Hand Clin 1997;13(1):143-149.

5. Hollister A, et al. The axes of rotation of the thumb carpometacarpal joint. J Orthop Res 1992;10(3):454-460.

6. Ateshian GA, Rosenwasser MP, Mow VC. Curvature characteristics and congruence of the thumb carpometacarpal joint: Differences between female and male joints. J Biomech 1992;25(6):591-607.

7. Knudson D, Blackwell J. Upper extremity kinematics of the one-handed backhand drive in tennis players with and without tennis elbow. Int J Sports Med 1997;18(2):79-82.

8. Tiedeman JJ, Ferlic TP. Hand and wrist injuries. In: The Team Physician's Handbook. Edited by Mellion MB, Walsh WM, Shelton GL. Philadelphia: Hanley & Belfus, Inc, 1997.

9. Bruckner JD, Alexander CAH, Lichtman DM. Acute dislocations of the distal radioulnar joint. Instruct Course Lec 1996;45:27-36.

10. Mastey RD, Weiss APC, Akelman E. Primary care of hand and wrist athletic injuries. Clin Sports Med 1997;16(4):705-724.

11. Plancher KD, Peterson RK, Steichen JB. Compressive neuropathies and tendinopathies in the athletic elbow and wrist. Clin Sports Med 1996;15(2):331-371.

12. Sheon RP. Repetitive strain injury: Diagnostic and treatment tips on six common problems. Postgrad Med 1997;102(4):72-81.

13. Servi JT. Wrist pain from overuse: Detecting and relieving intersection syndrome. Phys Sports Med 1997;25(12):41-44.

14. Griggs SM, Weiss AC. Bony injuries of the wrist, forearm, and elbow. Clin Sports Med 1997;15(2):373-400.

Lower Extremity

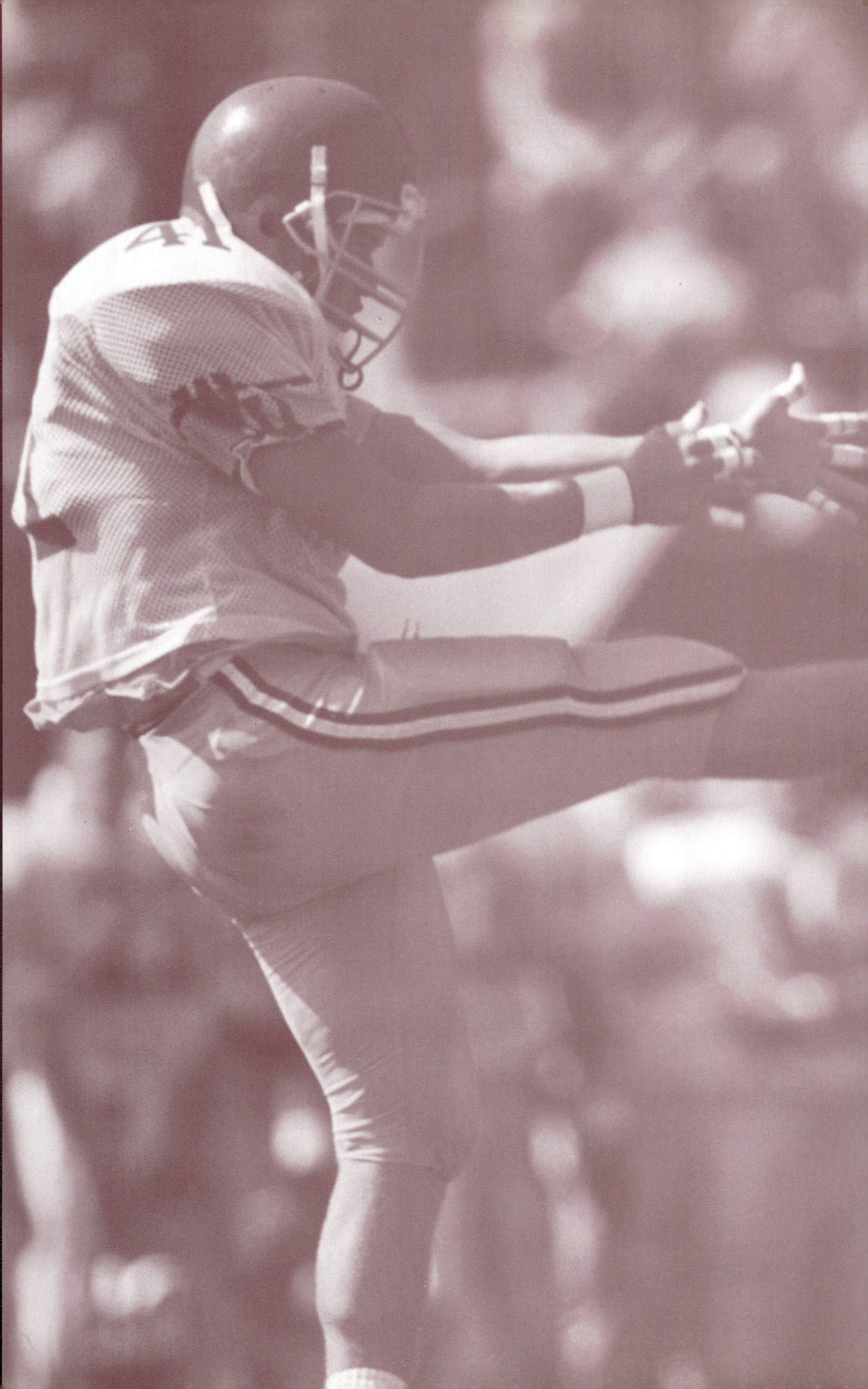

SECTION V

CHAPTER 14

Pelvis, Hip, and Thigh Conditions

OBJECTIVES

1. Identify the important bony and soft tissue structures of the pelvis, hip, and thigh.

2. Describe the functions of the various soft tissue structures that support the sacroiliac joint, sacrococcygeal joint, and hip joint.

3. Identify the major nerves and blood vessels that course through the pelvic and proximal femoral region.

4. Describe the motions of the hip, and identify the muscles that produce them.

5. Explain what forces produce loading patterns responsible for common injuries of the pelvis, hip, and thigh.

6. Identify specific measures that can prevent injury to the region.

7. Describe the signs and symptoms associated with a hip pointer and quadriceps contusion, and explain what adverse conditions may result if the injury receives inadequate management.

8. Describe the three common sites for bursitis, and explain the management of this condition.

9. List the signs and symptoms of a hip joint sprain, and describe the position an individual will likely be found in if the hip is dislocated.

10. List the signs and symptoms seen in first-, second-, and third-degree strains of the muscles that move the hip, and explain the management of each injury.

11. List the characteristic signs and symptoms indicating a possible vascular or neural disorder in the pelvis, hip, or thigh.

12. List and describe the various types of fractures that can occur in the pelvis, hip, and thigh, and explain their management.

13. Describe a thorough assessment of the hip region.

14. Describe general rehabilitation exercises for the hip region.

Although the pelvis, hip, and thigh have a sturdy anatomical composition, this region can be subjected to large, potentially injurious forces when individuals engage in sports or exercise. For example, the soft tissues of the anterior thigh often sustain compressive forces, particularly during contact sports. Although the resulting contusions are not usually serious, mismanagement of these injuries can lead to more serious problems. Daily activities such as sitting, walking, and climbing stairs rarely involve stretching of the hamstrings. This inflexibility, and a strength imbalance between the hamstrings and the more frequently exercised quadriceps, place the sport participant at a higher risk for strains of the hamstrings. Because of their strong bony stability, the hip and pelvis are seldom injured; however, since the hip sustains repetitive forces of four to seven times body weight during walking and running, the joint is subject to stress-related injuries.

This chapter begins with a review of the anatomy, kinematics, and kinetics of the pelvis, hip, and thigh. Next, preventative measures will be discussed, followed by information on basic injuries to the region. A step-by-step injury assessment process is then followed by examples of rehabilitation exercises for the region.

ANATOMY OF THE PELVIS, HIP, AND THIGH

The pelvis, hip, and thigh have an extremely stable bony structure that is further reinforced by a number of large, strong ligaments and muscles. This region is anatomically well-suited for withstanding the large forces to which it is subjected during daily activities.

The Pelvis

The pelvis, or pelvic girdle, consists of a protective bony ring formed by four fused bones—the two innominate bones, the sacrum, and the coccyx **(Figure 14.1)**. The innominate bones articulate with each other anteriorly at the pubic symphysis, and with the sacrum posteriorly at the sacroiliac joints. Each innominate bone consists of three fused bones—the ilium, ischium, and pubis. Among these, the ilium forms the major portion of the innominate bone, including the prominent iliac crests. The anterior superior iliac spine (ASIS) is a readily palpable landmark. The posterior superior iliac spine (PSIS) is typically marked by an indentation in the soft tissues just lateral to the sacrum. The pelvis protects the enclosed inner organs, transmits loads between the trunk and lower extremity, and provides a site for a number of major muscle attachments.

SACROILIAC JOINTS

The sacroiliac (SI) joints form the critical link between the two pelvic bones. Working with the pubic symphysis, they help to transfer the weight of the torso and skull to

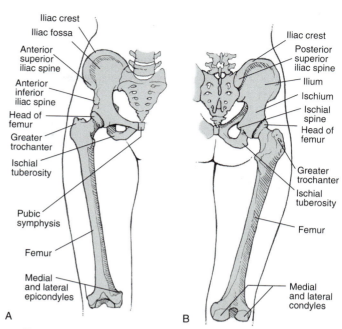

> **FIGURE 14.1 Pelvis and femur**. A, Anterior view. B, Posterior view.

the lower limbs, provide elasticity to the pelvic ring, and conversely, act as a buffer to decrease impact forces from the foot as they are transmitted to the spine and upper body.

The SI joints are both synovial and syndesmosis joints. The synovial portion of the joint is C-shaped, with the convex iliac surface of the C facing an anterior and inferior direction. The articular surface of the ilium is covered with fibrocartilage; the articular surface of the sacrum is covered with hyaline cartilage and is three times thicker than that of the ilium. The size, shape, and texture of the articular surfaces vary across the lifespan. In children, the surfaces are smooth. In adults, irregular depressions and elevations are formed that fit into one another. As a result, the articulation is very strong and has a limited range of motion. In older individuals, portions of the joint surfaces may be obliterated by adhesions.

The strong fibers of the interosseous sacroiliac ligaments bind the anterior portion of the ilium and the posterior portion of the sacrum, filling the void behind the articular surfaces of these bones **(Figure 14.2)**. The joint is also strengthened anteriorly and posteriorly by the dorsal and ventral sacroiliac ligaments **(Figure 14.3)**. The dorsal SI ligament runs transversely to bind the posterior ilium to the upper portion of the sacrum, and vertical fibers connect the lower sacrum to the PSIS. The ventral SI ligament lines the anterior portion of the pelvic cavity attaching onto the anterior portion of the sacrum. Two accessory ligaments also assist in maintaining the stability of the SI joint. The sacrotuberous ligament arises from the ischium to merge with the inferior fibers of the dorsal SI ligaments. The sacrospinous ligament, indirectly supporting the sacrum, runs from the ischial spine and attaches to the coccyx.

Plane of cut

Ileum

Sacrum

Dorsal sacroiliac ligament

Sacral canal

Interosseus sacroiliac ligament

Sacroiliac joint

Ventral sacroiliac ligament

Ischial tuberosity

Coccyx

Sacrospinous ligament

Sacrotuberous ligament

➤ **FIGURE 14.2 Transverse section of the pelvis.** The strong interosseous sacroiliac ligament lies anterior to the dorsal sacroiliac ligament and consists of short fibers that connect the tuberosity of the sacrum to the ilium.

SACROCOCCYGEAL JOINT

The sacrococcygeal joint is usually a fused line (symphysis) united by a fibrocartilaginous disc. Occasionally, the joint is freely movable and synovial, but with advanced age, the joint may fuse and be obliterated.

PUBIC SYMPHYSIS

The pubic symphysis is a cartilaginous joint with a disc of fibrocartilage, called the interpubic disc, located between the two joint surfaces. A small degree of spreading, compression, and rotation occurs between the two halves of the pelvic girdle at this joint.

Bony Structure of the Thigh

The femur, a major weight-bearing bone, is the longest, largest, and strongest bone in the body (Figure 14.1). Its weakest component is the femoral neck, which is smaller in diameter than the rest of the bone, and is weak internally because it is primarily composed of cancellous bone. The head of the femur is angled at approximately 125° in the frontal plane. This relationship, known as the **angle of inclination (Figure 14.4)**, allows the femur to angle medially downward from the hip during the support phase of walking and running, producing single-leg support beneath the body's center of gravity. Because women have a wider pelvis, this angulation tends to be more pronounced in

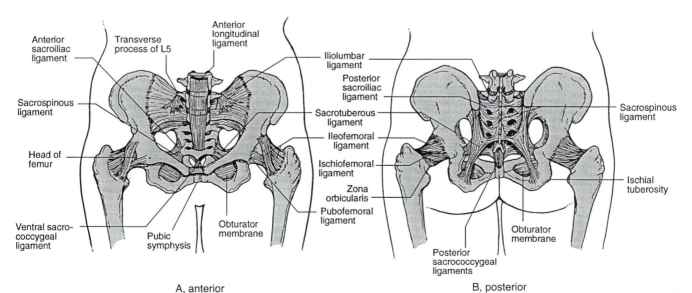

Anterior sacroiliac ligament

Transverse process of L5

Anterior longitudinal ligament

Iliolumbar ligament

Posterior sacroiliac ligament

Sacrotuberous ligament

Ileofemoral ligament

Ischiofemoral ligament

Zona orbicularis

Pubofemoral ligament

Sacrospinous ligament

Sacrospinous ligament

Head of femur

Ischial tuberosity

Ventral sacro-coccygeal ligament

Pubic symphysis

Obturator membrane

Obturator membrane

Posterior sacrococcygeal ligaments

A, anterior

B, posterior

➤ **FIGURE 14.3 Ligaments of the pelvis and hip.** A, Anterior view. B, Posterior view.

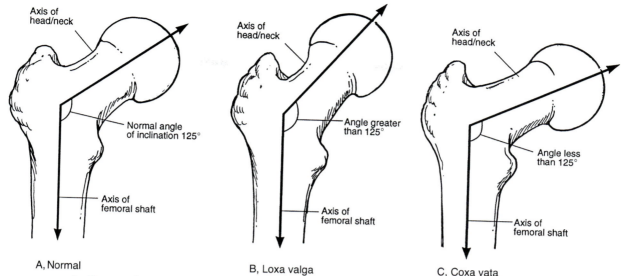

A, Normal   B, Loxa valga   C, Coxa vata

➤ FIGURE 14.4 **Angle of inclination**. In the frontal plane, the femoral head normally assumes a 125° angle with the long axis of the femur (A). This angle allows the femur to angle medially downward from the hip during the support phase of walking and running, producing single-leg support beneath the body's center of gravity. Because women have a wider pelvis, this angulation tends to be slightly increased, called coxa valga (B); a decrease is called coxa vara (C).

women, called **coxa valga**; a decreased angle of inclination is called **coxa vara**.

In the transverse plane, the relationship between the femoral head and femoral shaft is called the angle of **torsion**, which is normally 15° **(Figure 14.5)**. A decreased angle between the femoral condyles and femoral head is called **retroversion**; an increased angle is called **anteversion**.

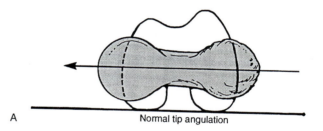

A   Normal tip angulation

The Hip Joint

The hip is the articulation between the concave acetabulum of the pelvis and the head of the femur, and functions as a classic ball-and-socket joint **(Figure 14.6)**. The acetabulum angles obliquely in an inferior, anterior, and lateral direction. Because the socket is deep, it provides considerable bony stability to the joint. Both articulating surfaces are covered with friction-reducing joint cartilage. The cartilage on the acetabulum is thickened around the periphery where it merges with the U-shaped fibrocartilaginous acetabular labrum, which further contributes to stability of the joint.

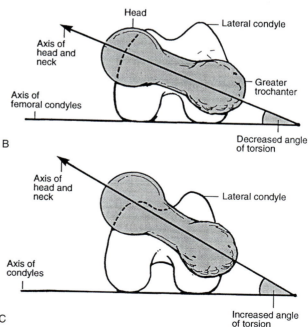

➤ FIGURE 14.5 **Angle of torsion**. A, In the transverse plane, deviations may also occur from the norm. B, A decreased angle between the femoral condyles and femoral head is called retroversion; C, An increased angle is called anteversion.

Hip Joint Capsule

The joint capsule of the hip, the coxofemoral joint, is large and loose. It completely surrounds the joint, attaching to the labrum of the acetabular socket. It also passes over a fat pad internally to join to the distal aspect of the femoral neck. Because the capsular fibers attaching to the femoral neck are arranged in a circular fashion, they are known as the zona orbicularis (see Figure 14.4). The zona orbicularis is an important contributor to hip stability.

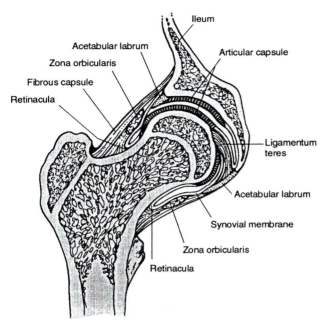

➤ FIGURE 14.6 **Coronal section of the hip joint**. The epiphysis of the head of the femur is entirely within the joint capsule. The ligamentum teres is a synovial tube that is fixed superiorly at the fovea on the head of the femur and opens inferiorly at the acetabular foramen where it is continuous with the synovial membrane covering the fat in the acetabular fossa. The ligament is taut during adduction of the hip joint, as occurs when crossing the legs.

Ligaments of the Hip Joint

Several large, strong ligaments support the hip (Figure 14.3). On the anterior aspect, the extremely strong Y-shaped iliofemoral ligament, sometimes referred to as the Y ligament of Bigelow, extends from the anterior inferior iliac spine (AIIS) to the intertrochanteric line on the femur, enabling it to limit hip hyperextension. The pubofemoral ligament, also located anteriorly, connects the pubic ramus to the intertrochanteric line, limiting abduction and hyperextension of the hip. The ischiofemoral ligament reinforces the hip posteriorly, extending from the posterior acetabular rim of the ischium in a superior, lateral direction, attaching to the inner surface of the greater trochanter of the femur. The spiraling nature of this ligament causes it to limit extension of the hip. Tension in these major ligaments acts to twist the head of the femur into the acetabulum upon hip extension, as occurs when a person rises from a seated position.

Within the joint, the ligamentum teres serves as a conduit for the medial and lateral circumflex arteries but provides little support to the hip joint (see Figure 14.6). The inguinal ligament, which runs from the ASIS and inserts at the pubic symphysis, serves to contain the soft tissues as they course anteriorly from the trunk to the lower extremity. The structure demarcates the superior border of the femoral triangle.

Femoral Triangle

The femoral triangle is formed by the inguinal ligament superiorly, the sartorius laterally, and the adductor longus medially **(Figure 14.7)**. This region is significant in that the femoral nerve, artery, and vein are located within the area. The femoral pulse can be palpated as it crosses the crease between the thigh and abdomen. In addition, if there is an infection or active inflammation in the lower extremity, enlarged lymph nodes may be palpated in this region.

Bursae

Four primary bursae are present in the hip and pelvic region. The iliopsoas bursa is positioned between the iliopsoas and the articular capsule, serving to reduce the friction between these structures. The deep trochanteric bursa provides a cushion between the greater trochanter of the femur and the gluteus maximus at its attachment to the iliotibial tract. The gluteofemoral bursa separates the gluteus maximus from the origin of the vastus lateralis. Finally, the ischial bursa serves as a weight-bearing structure when an individual is seated, cushioning the ischial tuberosity where it passes over the gluteus maximus.

Q-Angle

The **Q-angle** is defined as the angle between the line of resultant force produced by the quadriceps muscles and the line of the patellar tendon (see Figure 15.3). One line

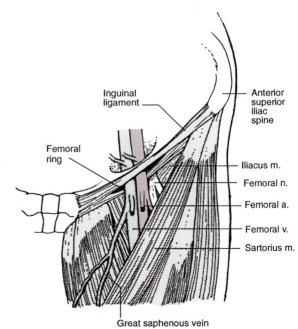

➤ FIGURE 14.7 **Femoral triangle**. The triangle is bounded by the inguinal ligament superiorly, the adductor longus medially, and the sartorius laterally. The femoral artery, vein, and nerve pass through this area to enter the thigh.

is drawn from the middle of the patella to the ASIS of the ilium, and a second line is drawn from the tibial tubercle through the center of the patella. The normal Q-angle ranges from approximately 13° in males to approximately 18° in females when the knee is fully extended. This angle can predispose an athlete to patellar injuries, and is explained in more detail in Chapter 15.

Muscles of the Hip Joint

A number of large, strong muscles cross the hip, enhancing its stability. The muscles of the hip are summarized in

Table 14.1, and the actions of the major muscles are discussed later in the chapter.

Nerves of the Pelvis, Hip, and Thigh

The major nerve supply to the pelvis, hip, and thigh arises from the lumbar and sacral plexi. The **lumbar plexus** is formed from the first four lumbar spinal nerves (**Figure 14.8**). It innervates portions of the abdominal wall and psoas major, with branches into the thigh region. The largest branch is the femoral nerve (L_2–L_4) that supplies muscles and skin of the anterior thigh. Another branch,

TABLE 14.1   MUSCLES OF THE HIP

Muscle	Proximal Attachment	Distal Attachment	Primary Action(s)	Nerve Innervation
Rectus femoris	Anterior inferior iliac spine (AIIS)	Patella	Hip flexion and knee extension	Femoral (L_2–L_4)
Iliopsoas (Iliacus)	Iliac fossa and adjacent sacrum	Lesser trochanter	Hip flexion	L_1 and femoral (L_2–L_4)
(Psoas major)	12th thoracic and lumbar vertebrae, and lumbar discs	Lesser trochanter		(L_1–L_3)
Sartorius	Anterior superior iliac spine (ASIS)	Upper medial tibia	Assists with flexion, abduction, and lateral rotation	Femoral (L_2, L_3)
Pectineus	Pectineal crest of pubic ramus	Medial, proximal femur	Flexion and adduction	Femoral (L_2, L_3)
Tensor fasciae latae	Anterior crest of the ilium and ASIS	Iliotibial band	Assists with flexion, abduction, and medial rotation	Superior gluteal (L_4–S_1)
Gluteus maximus	Posterior ilium, iliac crest, sacrum, and coccyx	Gluteal tuberosity of the femur and iliotibial band	Hip extension and lateral rotation	Inferior gluteal (L_5–S_2)
Gluteus medius	Between posterior and anterior gluteal lines on posterior ilium	Superior, lateral greater trochanter	Abduction	Superior gluteal (L_4–S_1)
Gluteus minimus	Between anterior and inferior gluteal lines on posterior ilium	Anterior surface of the greater trochanter	Medial rotation	Superior gluteal (L_4–S_1)
Gracilis	Anterior, inferior pubic symphysis	Medial, proximal tibia	Adduction	Obturator (L_3, L_4)
Adductor magnus	Inferior ramus of pubis and ischium	Entire linea aspera	Adduction	Obturator (L_3, L_4)
Adductor longus	Anterior pubis	Middle linea aspera	Adduction	Obturator (L_2, L_3)
Adductor brevis	Inferior ramus of the pubis	Upper linea aspera	Adduction	Obturator (L_3, L_4)
Semitendinosus	Medial ischial tuberosity	Proximal, medial tibia	Hip extension and knee flexion	Tibial (L_5, S_1)
Semimembranosus	Lateral ischial tuberosity	Proximal, medial tibia	Hip extension and knee flexion	Tibial (L_5, S_1)
Biceps femoris (long head)	Posterior, lateral ischial tuberosity Lateral ischial tuberosity	Head of fibula and condyle of tibia	Hip extension and knee flexion	Tibial (L_5–S_2)
(short head)	Lateral linea aspera		Knee flexion	Common peroneal (L_5, S_1)
Lateral rotators	Sacrum, ilium, and ischium	Posterior greater trochanter	Lateral rotation	L_5–S_2

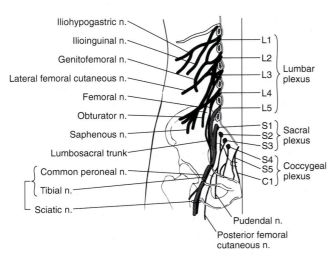

Iliohypogastric n.
Ilioinguinal n.
Genitofemoral n.
Lateral femoral cutaneous n.
Femoral n.
Obturator n.
Saphenous n.
Lumbosacral trunk
Common peroneal n.
Tibial n.
Sciatic n.

L1
L2
L3
L4
L5
} Lumbar plexus

S1
S2
S3
} Sacral plexus

S4
S5
C1
} Coccygeal plexus

Pudendal n.
Posterior femoral cutaneous n.

➤ **FIGURE 14.8 Lumbar plexus and sacral plexus.**

the obturator nerve (L_2–L_4), provides innervation to the hip adductor muscles.

The **sacral plexus** is positioned just anterior to the lumbar plexus, and has some intermingling of fibers with the lumbar plexus. The lower spinal nerves, including L_4 through S_4, spawn the sacral plexus (Figure 14.8). Twelve nerve branches arise from the sacral plexus. The most major is the sciatic nerve (L_4, L_5, S_1–S_3), which is the largest and longest single nerve in the body. The sciatic nerve passes through the greater sciatic notch of the pelvis, courses through the gluteus maximus muscle, and then innervates the hamstrings and adductor magnus. The tibial and common peroneal nerves that branch from the sciatic nerve in the posterior thigh region are discussed in Chapters 15 and 16.

Blood Vessels of the Pelvis, Hip, and Thigh

The external iliac arteries become the femoral arteries at the level of the thighs, providing the major blood supply to the lower extremity **(Figure 14.9)**. The femoral artery gives off several branches in the thigh region, including the deep femoral artery, which serves the posterior and lateral thigh muscles, and the lateral and medial femoral circumflex arteries, which supply the region of the femoral head.

KINEMATICS AND MAJOR MUSCLE ACTIONS OF THE HIP

Since the hip is a ball-and-socket joint, the femur can move in all planes of motion. The massive muscles crossing the hip, however, tend to limit range of motion, particularly in the posterior direction.

Pelvic Positioning

During many sport activities, the positioning of the pelvic girdle facilitates motion of the femur at the hip. For example, abduction of the leg during the preparatory phase of a kick in one of the martial arts is made easier by a lateral tilt of the pelvis toward the side opposite the kicking leg. Likewise, flexion at the hip is assisted by posterior pelvic tilt, and extension at the hip is enhanced by anterior pelvic tilt.

Flexion

The major hip flexors are the iliacus and psoas major, referred to jointly as the iliopsoas because of their common attachment at the femur **(Figure 14.10)**. Four other muscles cross the anterior aspect of the hip to contribute to hip flexion. These include the pectineus, rectus femoris, sartorius, and tensor fascia latae. Because the rectus femoris is a two-joint muscle active during both hip flexion and knee extension, it functions more effectively as a hip flexor when the knee is in flexion, as occurs when a person kicks a ball. The sartorius is also a two-joint muscle. Crossing from the ASIS to the medial surface of the proximal tibia just below the tuberosity, the sartorius is the longest muscle in the body.

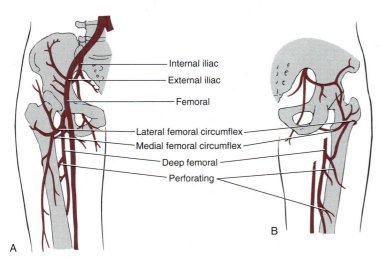

Internal iliac
External iliac
Femoral
Lateral femoral circumflex
Medial femoral circumflex
Deep femoral
Perforating

A

B

➤ **FIGURE 14.9 Arterial supply to the hip and thigh region.** A, Anterior view. B, Posterior view.

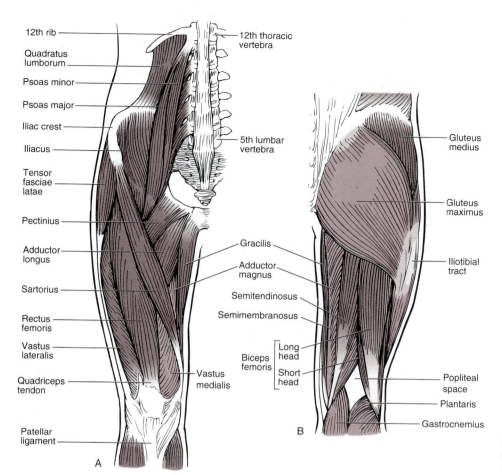

12th rib

Quadratus lumborum

Psoas minor

Psoas major

Iliac crest

Iliacus

Tensor fasciae latae

Pectinius

Adductor longus

Sartorius

Rectus femoris

Vastus lateralis

Quadriceps tendon

Patellar ligament

A

12th thoracic vertebra

5th lumbar vertebra

Gracilis

Adductor magnus

Semitendinosus

Semimembranosus

Biceps femoris — Long head / Short head

Vastus medialis

B

Gluteus medius

Gluteus maximus

Iliotibial tract

Popliteal space

Plantaris

Gastrocnemius

➤ **FIGURE 14.10 The superficial muscles of the hip and thigh.** A, Anterior view. B, Posterior view.

Extension

The hip extensors are the gluteus maximus and the three hamstrings: the biceps femoris, semitendinosus, and semimembranosus. The gluteus maximus is usually active only when the hip is in flexion, as occurs during stair climbing or cycling, or when extension at the hip is resisted. The nickname "hamstrings" derives from the prominent tendons of the three muscles, which are readily palpable on the posterior aspect of the knee. The hamstrings cross both the hip and knee, contributing to hip extension and knee flexion.

Abduction

The gluteus medius is the major abductor at the hip, with assistance from the gluteus minimus. The hip abductors are active in stabilizing the pelvis during single-leg support of the body, and during the support phase of walking and running (see Chapter 16). For example, when body weight is supported by the right foot during walking, the right hip abductors contract isometrically and eccentrically to prevent the left side of the pelvis from being pulled downward by the weight of the swinging left leg. This allows the left leg to move freely through the swing phase without scuffing the toes. If the hip abductors are too weak to perform this function, then lateral pelvic tilt occurs with every step.

Adduction

The hip adductors include the adductor longus, adductor brevis, and adductor magnus. These muscles are active during the swing phase of gait, bringing the foot beneath the body's center of gravity for placement during the support phase. The relatively weak gracilis assists with hip adduction. The hip adductors also contribute to flexion and internal rotation at the hip, especially when the femur is externally rotated.

Medial and Lateral Rotation of the Femur

Although several muscles contribute to lateral rotation of the femur, there are six that function solely as lateral rotators. These are the piriformis, gemellus superior, gemellus inferior, obturator internus, obturator externus, and quadratus femoris (**Figure 14.11**). Lateral rotation of the femur of the swinging leg occurs to accommodate the lateral rotation of the pelvis during the stride.

The major medial rotator of the femur is the gluteus minimus, with assistance from the tensor fascia latae, sem-

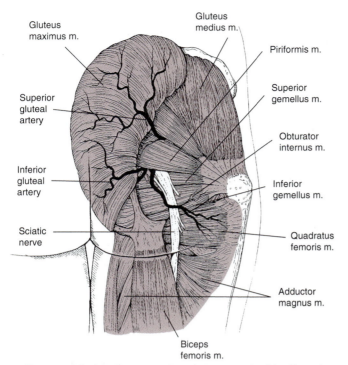

➤ FIGURE 14.11 **Deep muscles of the posterior hip**. Note that the sciatic nerve passes inferior to the piriformis muscle to enter the posterior thigh.

itendinosus, semimembranosus, gluteus medius, and the four adductor muscles. The medial rotators are relatively weak; the estimated strength is approximately one-third that of the lateral rotators. **Table 14.2** summarizes the muscles responsible for the various motions at the hip joint.

KINETICS OF THE HIP

Forces at the Hip During Standing

The hip is a major weight-bearing joint that is subject to extremely high loads during sport participation. During upright standing, with weight evenly distributed on both legs, the weight supported at each hip is one-half the weight of the body segments above the hip. However, the total load on each hip in this situation is greater than the weight supported because tension in the large, strong hip muscles further adds to compression at the joint.

Forces at the Hip During Gait

Compression on the hip is approximately the same as body weight during the swing phase of normal walking gait, but increases to at least six times body weight during the stance phase (1). Body weight, impact forces translated upward through the skeleton from the foot, and muscle tension all contribute to this compressive load. Forces on the hip increase along with walking or running speed. Use of a crutch or cane on the side opposite an injured lower limb is beneficial in that it serves to more evenly distribute the load between the legs throughout the gait cycle.

PREVENTION OF INJURIES TO THE PELVIS, HIP, AND THIGH

The hip joint is well protected within the pelvic girdle and is seldom injured. Several factors, such as wearing protective equipment, wearing shoes with adequate cushion and support, and participating in an extensive physical conditioning program, however, can reduce the incidence of acute and chronic injuries to the region.

Protective Equipment

Several collision and contact sports require special pads composed of hard polyethylene covered with layers of Ensolite to protect vulnerable areas such as the iliac crests, sacrum and coccyx, and genital region. A girdle with special pockets can hold the pads in place. The male genital region is best protected by a protective cup placed in the athletic supporter. Special commercial thigh pads may also be used to prevent contusions to the anterior thigh, and neoprene sleeves can provide uniform compression, therapeutic warmth, and support for a quadriceps or hamstrings strain. Many of these items can be seen in Chapter 3.

Physical Conditioning

Exercises to prevent injury to the pelvis, hip, and thigh are primarily concerned with flexibility and strengthening muscles in the area. **Field Strategy 14.1** demonstrates specific exercises for the hip flexors, extensors, adductors, abductors, and medial and lateral rotators. Exercises for the quadriceps, hamstrings, and tensor fascia latae can be seen in Chapter 15, regarding the knee.

| TABLE 14.2 | HIP MOVEMENTS AND INVOLVED MUSCLES | | | | |

Flexion	Extension	Abduction	Adduction	Medial Rotation	Lateral Rotation
Iliopsoas	Gluteus maximus	Gluteus medius	Pectineus	Gluteus medius	Piriformis
Rectus femoris	Biceps femoris	Gluteus minimus	Adductor brevis	Gluteus minimus	Obturator internus
Pectineus	Biceps femoris	Gluteus minimus	Adductor magnus	Tensor fasciae latae	Obturator externus
Sartorius	Semitendinosus	Tensor fasciae latae	Adductor longus		Superior gemelli
Tensor fasciae latae	Semimembranosus	Sartorius	Adductor magnus		Inferior gemelli
	Adductor magnus	Piriformis	Gracilis		Quadratus femoris
					Gluteus maximus

FIELD STRATEGY 14.1   EXERCISES TO PREVENT INJURY AT THE THIGH, HIP, AND PELVIS

The following exercises can be performed for motions at the hip. Exercises for the hamstrings, quadriceps, and iliotibial band, which also cross the knee joint, can be seen in Chapter 15.

A. **Hip flexor stretch (lunge).** Place the leg to be stretched in front of you. Bend the contralateral knee as you move the hips forward. Keep the back straight. Alternative method: Place the foot on a chair or table and lean forward until a stretch is felt.

B. **Lateral rotator stretch, seated position.** Cross one leg over the thigh and place the elbow on the outside of the knee. Gently stretch the buttock muscles by pushing the bent knee across the body while keeping the pelvis on the floor.

C. **Adductor stretch, standing position.** Place the leg to be stretched out to the side. Slowly bend the contralateral knee. Keep the hips in a neutral or extended position.

D. **Theraband or tubing exercises.** Secure Theraband or surgical tubing to a table. Perform hip flexion, extension, abduction, adduction, and medial and lateral rotation in a single plane or in multidirectional patterns.

E. **Full squats.** A weight belt should be worn during this exercise. Place the feet at shoulder width or wider. Keep the back straight by keeping the chest out and the head up at all times. Flex the knees and hips to no greater than 90°. Begin the upward motion by extending the hips first.

F. **Hip extension.** With the trunk stabilized and the back flat, extend the hip while keeping the knee flexed. Alternate legs.

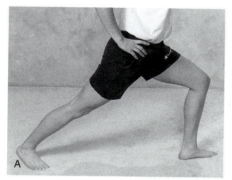

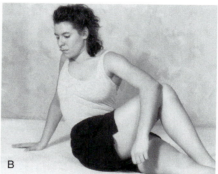

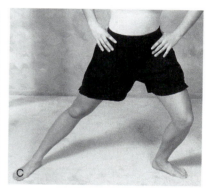

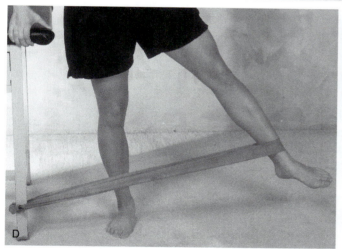

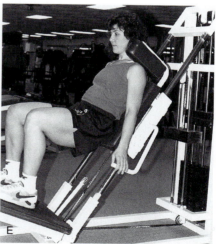

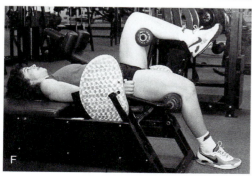

Shoe Selection

Sport activities take place on a variety of terrains and floor surfaces. Shoes should adequately cushion impact forces, and support and guide the foot during the stance and final pushoff phases of running, regardless of the terrain or surface. Inadequate cushioning in the heel region can transmit forces up the leg, leading to inflammation of the hip joint, or stress fractures of the femoral neck or pubis. Therefore, it is important to purchase shoes that provide an adequate heel cushion, and a thermoplastic heel counter, which can maintain its shape and firmness even in adverse weather conditions. The soles should be designed for the specific type of surface the athlete is participating on to avoid slipping or sliding.

CONTUSIONS

A football player took a direct blow to the antero-lateral hip from an opponent's shoulder during a tackle. Immediate severe pain, spasm, and loss of function forced the player to remove himself from the field. How would you differentiate a soft tissue injury from a possible fracture?

Direct impact to soft tissue, such as a kick to the thigh or a fall onto a hard surface, causes a compressive force to crush soft tissue. The condition may be mild and resolve itself in a matter of days, or the bleeding and swelling may be more extensive, resulting in a large, deep hematoma that takes months to resolve. Contusions may occur anywhere in the hip region, but are typically seen on the crest of the ilium, called a hip pointer, or in the quadriceps muscle group, referred to as a charley horse.

Hip Pointer

A **hip pointer** generally refers to a contusion of the iliac crest over the tensor fascia latae muscle belly with an associated hematoma, but the term may also be used to identify tearing of the external oblique muscle from the iliac crest, periostitis of the crest, and trochanteric contusions.

➤ SIGNS AND SYMPTOMS

Because so many trunk and abdominal muscles attach to the iliac crest, any movement of the trunk will be painful, including coughing, laughing, and even breathing. Immediate pain, discoloration, spasm, and loss of function will prevent the individual from rotating the trunk or laterally flexing the trunk toward the injured side. Extreme tenderness is present over the iliac crest, and abdominal muscle spasm may be present. Within 24 to 48 hours, the swelling is more diffuse, and ecchymosis is visibly evident. In severe injury, the individual may be unable to walk or bear weight, even with crutches, because of the intense pain caused by muscular tension at the injury site. **Table 14.3** lists the signs and symptoms of the various grades of hip pointers.

TABLE 14.3	SIGNS AND SYMPTOMS OF HIP POINTERS
Injury Grade	**Signs and Symptoms**
Grade I	Normal gait and normal posture
	Slight pain on palpation
	Little or no swelling present
	Full trunk range of motion (ROM)
	Return to activity may take 3 to 7 days
Grade II	Abnormal gait pattern
	Posture may be slightly flexed toward the side of injury
	Noticeable pain on palpation of iliac crest, with visible swelling
	Active trunk ROM will be painful and limited, especially lateral flexion to the opposite side, and trunk rotation
	Return to activity may take 5 to 14 days
Grade III	Severe pain, swelling, and ecchymosis
	Gait is slow, with short stride length and swing-through
	Posture may have severe tilt to injured side
	Trunk ROM is painful and limited in all directions
	Return to activity may take 14 to 21 days

➤ MANAGEMENT

Treatment will involve ice, compression, and total inactivity during the first 2 to 3 days following injury.

If intense pain was palpated directly over the iliac crest, the individual should be referred to a physician to rule out a fracture of the iliac crest, because the same mechanism of injury may cause both injuries.

With an uncomplicated hip pointer, the athlete can return to activity in 3 to 7 days; however, the area should be protected with a pad to prevent reinjury. In a grade II or III injury, crutches should be used by the athlete. Nonsteroidal anti-inflammatory drugs (NSAIDs) are indicated after 48 hours. Later treatment may include heat therapy, ultrasound, transcutaneous electrical nerve stimulation (TENS), and pain-free range-of-motion (ROM) exercises as tolerated. As soon as pain-free active range-of-motion (AROM) exercise can be accomplished, progress to resistive exercise, including lower extremity and trunk strengthening. Gradual return to activity, possibly wearing a dense foam donut pad fitted into a custom-formed plastic shell, or a compression garment, may be worn to protect the area from further injury.

Quadriceps Contusion

The most common site for a quadriceps contusion is the anterolateral thigh. If the contusion is located adjacent to the intermuscular septum, pain and hemorrhage tend to resolve more rapidly. Contusions within the muscle itself are often associated with greater tearing, hemorrhage, and pain, and a greater tendency toward abnormal pathology.

Severity of the injury is almost always underestimated and undertreated.

➤ SIGNS AND SYMPTOMS

Immediately after impact, pain and swelling may be extensive. In a mild contusion, the individual will have mild pain and swelling, and will be able to walk without a limp. Passive flexion beyond 90° may be painful, but resisted knee extension may cause less discomfort. In a moderate contusion, the individual can flex the knee only between 45° and 90°, and will walk with a noticeable limp. If severe, effusion frequently develops over a 24-hour period. Initially, there is little evidence of bruising, but within 24 hours, progressive bleeding and swelling occur, preventing knee flexion beyond 45°. There may be a palpable, firm hematoma, resulting in an inability to contract the quadriceps or do a straight-leg raise.

➤ MANAGEMENT

Treatment involves ice application and a compressive wrap for the first 24 to 48 hours applied with the knee in maximal flexion **(Figure 14.12)**. This position preserves the needed flexion and limits intramuscular bleeding and spasm. After 48 hours, reevaluation may necessitate continuation of the ice, compression, and flexion for another 12 to 24 hours.

Continued swelling despite proper acute care protocol indicates continued hemorrhage; immediate referral to a physician is necessary to assess the level of bleeding.

The athlete should be placed on crutches if unable to perform a pain-free gait, kept non-weight-bearing for 48 hours, and returned to partial weight-bearing in a pain-free range. If range of motion has not improved after 2 days, continue with acute care protocol and non-weight-bearing. If motion is possible, initiate gentle passive and active pain-free stretching with daily ice treatments and use of NSAIDs. Proprioceptive neuromuscular facilitation

(PNF) exercise patterns may be used to strengthen, relax, or gain range of motion. Isometric quadriceps strengthening and hamstrings resistive exercises can progress to an active stretching and progressive resistance strengthening program. Pulsed ultrasound or high-voltage galvanic stimulation (HGVS) may be helpful in the early stages to reduce edema. Continuous ultrasound, hydrotherapy, and massage should be avoided in the early stages as they may irritate the inflammatory process, but may be used in later stages to aid recovery. When full range of motion has been restored, full weight-bearing gait should be resumed, the progressive strengthening program can be expanded, and cycling, jogging, running, and functional activities specific to the sport can be incorporated. **Field Strategy 14.2** explains the care of a quadriceps contusion.

Myositis Ossificans

Myositis ossificans is an abnormal ossification involving bone deposition within muscle tissue. It may stem from a single traumatic blow, or repeated blows, to the quadriceps. Several risk factors following a quadriceps contusion can predispose an athlete to this condition **(Box 14.1)**. Common sites are the anterior and lateral thigh, but it may also occur on the hip, groin, leg, and lateral aspect of the midhumerus. Although the precise mechanism that triggers the bone formation has yet to be established, it is thought that during resolution of the hematoma, within a week after injury, the existing fibroblasts involved in the repair process begin to differentiate into osteoblasts (2). The evidence of calcification on a radiograph becomes visible after 3 to 4 weeks. As the calcification continues to progress, a palpable, firm mass can be felt in the deep tissues. After 6 to 7 weeks, the mass generally stops growing and resorption occurs. Total resorption may not fully occur, however, leaving a visible cortical-type bony lesion **(Figure 14.13)**.

➤ SIGNS AND SYMPTOMS

Examination reveals a warm, firm, swollen thigh nearly 2 to 4 cm larger than the unaffected side. A palpable, painful mass may limit passive knee flexion to 20 to 30°. Active quadriceps contractions and straight-leg raises may be impossible.

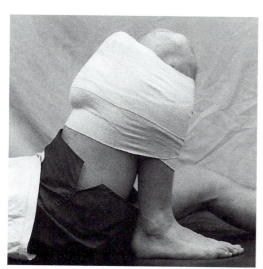

➤ FIGURE 14.12 **Ice a quadriceps contusion with the knee in maximal flexion to place the muscles on stretch**.

➤➤ **Box 14.1**

Risk Factors for Developing Myositis Ossificans

- Innate predisposition to ectopic bone formation
- Continuing to play after injury
- Early massage, hydrotherapy, or thermotherapy during acute stage
- Passive, forceful stretching
- Too rapid a progression in rehabilitation program
- Premature return to play
- Reinjury of same area

FIELD STRATEGY 14.2   MANAGEMENT ALGORITHM FOR A QUADRICEPS CONTUSION

<u>Acute Phase</u> (first 24-48 hours)
- Ice and compression with knee flexed at 120°
- Crutches, with partial- or non-weight-bearing
- Pain-free passive and active ROM
- NSAIDs after 24 hours

<u>Subacute Phase</u> (2-5 days)
- Cryotherapy and passive stretching exercises
- NSAIDs
- Active ROM and pain-free resisted PNF relaxation and strengthening exercises
- Continue partial-weight-bearing until 90° flexion attained
- High-voltage galvanic stimulation (HVGS), hot packs, or hydromassage (when no swelling is present)
- Swimming with gentle kicking exercises

<u>Final Phase</u>
- Discontinue crutches (when no limp is present)
- Cycling, light jogging, or running as tolerated
- HVGS
- Radiograph at 3 weeks to rule out myositis ossificans

<u>Return to Play</u>
- Range of motion within 10° of unaffected leg
- Bilaterally equal strength and endurance
- Work on jumping, starts, stops, changing directions, sprinting
- Must pass all functional tests
- Consider protective padding to prevent reinjury

➤ MANAGEMENT

Refer this individual to a physician.

Treatment will include ice, compression, elevation, crutches, and protected rest. NSAIDs are only indicated after 48 hours because they inhibit platelet function and promote hemorrhage. Periodic radiographs will generally be taken until the abnormal ossification matures. This typically occurs within 6 to 12 months. In cases where the mass fails to reabsorb completely, many individuals return safely to participation, with adequate protection from subsequent blows. Surgery is only indicated in cases where activity is limited by pain, weakness, and decreased range of motion. Excision before the mass matures may result in reformation, sometimes larger than the original mass.

Acute Compartment Syndrome

A serious complication of a quadriceps contusion is the development of an acute compartment syndrome. Compartment syndrome is defined as increased tissue pressure in a closed facial compartment that compromises circulation to the nerves and muscles found within that compartment. The condition often follows severe blunt trauma to the thigh, but may also occur as a result of a crushing injury or fracture of the femur.

➤ SIGNS AND SYMPTOMS

The athlete will complain of a progressive, severe pain that occurs with passive motion and isometric contraction of the quadriceps. As pressure increases within the compartment, decreased femoral sensation and motor weakness may occur, although distal pulse and capillary refill may be normal.

➤ MANAGEMENT

The athletic trainer should apply ice to reduce swelling, and immediately refer the athlete to a physician.

Because motor function of the femoral nerve is difficult to assess in the presence of a large hematoma, diagnosis

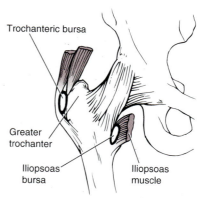

➤ **FIGURE 14.14 Bursa of the hip**. Bursitis at the hip may involve the trochanteric bursa, iliopsoas bursa, or ischial bursa.

➤ **FIGURE 14.13 Myositis ossificans**. With myositis ossificans, full resorption of the calcification may not occur, leaving a visible cortical-type bony lesion.

is based on compartment pressure measurements taken by a physician. Pressure readings greater than 40 mm Hg pressure usually indicate surgical intervention consisting of an anterior or anterolateral skin incision, fasciotomy, and evacuation of the hematoma (2).

 Palpate the anterolateral hip region for a possible fracture. If point tenderness, swelling, and discoloration are found in the soft tissues above or below a bony structure, the athlete may have a hip pointer. If point tenderness is elicited over a bony structure, a fracture may be present.

BURSITIS

A 20-year-old woman is complaining of pain while running on the city streets. Pain is localized on the posterior aspect of the greater trochanter, and occasionally is accompanied by a snapping sensation. What structures are located in this area that might be irritated? What other factors may be contributing to this injury?

Bursitis is common in runners and joggers; it typically affects the greater trochanteric bursa, iliopsoas bursa (iliopectineal), and ischial bursa **(Figure 14.14)**. Development of bursitis is usually a result of two mechanisms. The most common mechanism is inflammation secondary to excessive friction or shear forces due to overuse. The other mechanism is posttraumatic bursitis, which stems from direct blows and contusion that cause bleeding in the bursa, which then leads to inflammation (3).

Greater Trochanteric Bursitis

The greater trochanteric bursa lies between the greater trochanter and the gluteus maximus and tensor fascia latae (iliotibial tract). Seen commonly in female runners because of the wider pelvis and larger Q angle, it is also seen in runners who cross their feet over the midline as they run, thereby functionally increasing the Q angle, and in cross-country skiers and ballet dancers. Because streets are crowned to allow for run-off, the condition usually affects the down leg of runners, referring to the leg closest to the gutter.

➤ **SIGNS AND SYMPTOMS**

Trochanteric bursitis is characterized by a burning or aching pain over or just posterior to the tip of the greater trochanter that intensifies with walking or exercise. The condition is aggravated by contraction of the hip abductors against resistance, or during hip flexion and extension on weight-bearing. Referred pain may also move distally into the lateral aspect of the thigh. If accompanied by sudden sharp pain that occurs during certain movements, it can be secondary to a snapping hip problem (see below).

Iliopsoas Bursitis

The iliopsoas bursa can be irritated when the iliopsoas muscle repeatedly compresses the bursa against either the joint capsule of the hip or the lesser trochanter of the femur. Osteoarthritis of the hip may also lead to the condition.

➤ **SIGNS AND SYMPTOMS**

Pain is felt more medial and anterior to the joint, and cannot be easily palpated. With the knee supported to relax the muscles, point tenderness may be elicited with the hip and knee flexed and the leg externally rotated. Passive rotary motions at the hip, and resisted hip flexion, abduction, and external rotation, may also produce increased pain. Iliopsoas bursitis may also be associated with symptoms of a snapping hip syndrome.

Ischial Bursitis

Direct bruising from a fall can lead to compression of the ischial bursa; however, there is often a history of prolonged sitting, especially with the legs crossed or on a hard surface, hence the nickname, "benchwarmer's bursitis." Although it is relatively uncommon, it must be differentiated from a hamstring tear at the tendinous attachment, or an epiphyseal fracture.

➤ SIGNS AND SYMPTOMS

Pain is aggravated by prolonged sitting, uphill running, and even carrying a wallet in the back pocket. With the hip flexed, point tenderness can be palpated directly over the ischial tuberosity. Pain increases with passive and resisted hip extension.

Management of Bursitis

Treatment for bursitis includes cryotherapy, deep friction massage, protected rest, NSAIDs, and a stretching program for the involved muscle(s). The use of ultrasound or interferential current may also be helpful. A postural examination and biomechanical analysis of the running motion can be done by trained professionals to determine if certain factors contributed to the individual's condition. Different shoes, orthotics, or altering the running technique may correct the problem and avoid recurrence. If the condition does not rapidly improve, a bone scan should be conducted to rule out possible femoral neck stress fractures. Individuals who do not respond to conservative treatment may require local injections with anesthetics and cortisone, or surgery may be necessary.

Snapping Hip Syndrome

Chronic bursitis can lead to **snapping hip syndrome**, a condition very prevalent in dancers, runners, and cheerleaders, which may develop secondary to a variety of both intra- and extra-articular causes **(Box 14.2)**. The most common cause is snapping of the iliotibial tract over the greater trochanter, which can also result in trochanteric bursitis.

➤ SIGNS AND SYMPTOMS

Snapping hip syndrome is characterized by a snapping sensation either heard or felt during certain motions at the hip, rather than pain. It usually occurs when an individual laterally rotates and flexes the hip joint while balancing on one leg. If the iliopsoas bursa is affected, the individual may complain of snapping in the medial groin.

➤ MANAGEMENT

The condition is usually handled with NSAIDs and a rehabilitation program to address specific deficits: muscle tightness, muscle imbalance, poor training techniques, or poor biomechanics of movement. If associated with pain or a sense of hip joint instability, however, the individual should be referred to a physician.

➤ ➤ **Box 14.2**

Causes of Snapping Hip Syndrome

Intra-articular causes:
- Osteocartilaginous nodules occurring in the synovial membrane of the joint (synovial chondromatosis)
- Loose bodies
- Osteocartilaginous exostosis
- Subluxation of the hip
- Negative pressure in the joint capsule

Extra-articular causes:
- Iliotibial band friction syndrome
- Snapping of the iliopsoas over the iliopectineal eminence on the medial aspect of the inferior ilium
- Snapping of the iliofemoral ligaments over the femoral head
- Snapping of the long head of the biceps femoris over the ischial tuberosity

The runner probably has trochanteric bursitis caused by the iliotibial tract snapping over the greater trochanter during the running motion. Because of the characteristic wider pelvis in women, and the fact that she is running on city streets crowned for water runoff, she is at risk for additional stress to the lateral soft tissue structures of the hip region. The individual should increase flexibility in the iliotibial tract and alter her running direction to prevent the same leg from being the down leg when running in the street.

SPRAINS AND DISLOCATIONS

An ice hockey player was checked into the boards by an opponent with his hip and knee flexed at 90°. The impact drove the femur posteriorly. The individual is now lying on the ice in great pain with the hip slightly flexed and internally rotated in a fixed position. From the player's position, you have determined that EMS should be activated immediately. What can you do for the individual while the ambulance is on the way?

Hip joint sprains are rare because of the multitude of movements allowed at the ball-and-socket joint, and the level of protection provided by layers of muscles that add to its stability. Injury can occur in violent twisting actions or in catastrophic trauma when the knee strikes a stationary object, such as in an automobile accident when the knee is driven into the dashboard. Traumatic hip dislocations in children are rare, but are more common than femoral neck fractures. This may be largely due to the pliable cartilage composition of the acetabulum during the early- to midteen years.

➤ SIGNS AND SYMPTOMS

Symptoms of a mild or moderate hip sprain mimic those of synovitis, or stress fractures about the hip, and involve pain on hip rotation. Severe hip sprains and dislocations result in immediate intense pain, and an inability to walk or even move the hip. The hip remains in a characteristic flexed and internally rotated position indicating a posterior, superior dislocation **(Figure 14.15)**.

➤ MANAGEMENT

Treatment for a mild-to-moderate sprain is symptomatic and may include cryotherapy, NSAIDs, rest, and protected weight-bearing on crutches until walking is pain-free. Radiographs or bone scans are usually taken to rule out degenerative joint disease, slipped femoral capital epiphysis, and femoral stress fractures.

With a hip dislocation, activate EMS. Because the sciatic nerve may be damaged, the athletic trainer should assess nerve function. This can be done by running the fingers down both lower legs of the athlete and asking the individual where you are touching the leg, and what it feels like. Is there full or partial sensation? It is imperative not to move the individual until the ambulance arrives, because of a possible fracture to the posterior rim of the acetabulum or head of the femur. Movement may damage the blood supply to the head of the femur and cause avascular necrosis, or cause further damage to surrounding soft tissue structures, complicating joint reduction and thus lengthening the individual's recovery time. The vital signs should be monitored frequently and the individual treated for shock.

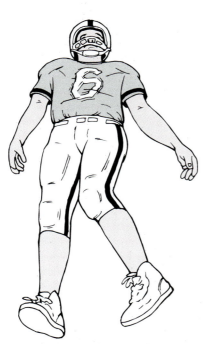

➤ **FIGURE 14.15 Hip dislocation.** Most hip dislocations drive the head of the femur posterior and superior, leaving the leg in a characteristically flexed and internally rotated position.

While the ambulance is en route, talk to the individual in a calm, reassuring voice, assess the ABCs, monitor the vital signs, and check for nerve and circulatory impairment at the lower leg and ankle. If possible, cover the athlete to maintain body heat to prevent the onset of shock. Do not move the individual until medical help arrives.

STRAINS

 A female body builder is complaining of a dull ache in the midbuttock region that increases when she goes up and down stairs. Recently, the pain has extended down the back of her leg, and really hurts when she sits and extends the knee with the tibia and femur internally rotated. What possible injury may be present? Should this individual be referred to a physician?

Muscular strains of the hip and thigh muscles are frequently seen not only in sport, but in many occupations involving repetitive motions. Strains may range from mild to severe, with the severity of symptoms paralleling the amount of disruption to the fibers (see Table 5.2).

Quadriceps Strain

A strain of the quadriceps is less common than hamstring strains. An explosive muscular contraction of the rectus femoris can lead to an avulsion fracture at the proximal attachment on the anterior inferior iliac spine (AIIS), but tears more commonly occur in the midsubstance of the muscle belly. Because the rectus femoris is the most superficial muscle of the quadriceps, any disruption in its continuity is easily visible. The vastus lateralis and vastus medialis are more rarely injured, but when injury does occur, it is usually in the mid- to upper-third of the muscle belly.

➤ SIGNS AND SYMPTOMS

In a grade I injury, the athlete will complain of tightness in the anterior thigh, but gait will be normal. No swelling or pain can be palpated, although passive knee flexion beyond 90° may be painful. In a grade II injury, the individual will report a snapping or tearing sensation during an explosive jumping, kicking, or running motion, followed by immediate pain and loss of function, and if severe, an inability to bear weight. The knee may be kept in extension to protect the injured area. Assessment will reveal tenderness, swelling, a palpable defect if continuity is disrupted, discoloration, pain on passive knee flexion between 45 and 90°, and pain and weakness during resisted knee extension. Grade III strains are extremely painful, and ambulation is not possible. Palpation will reveal an obvious defect in the muscle. Resisted knee extension is not possible, and ROM is severely limited. An isometric contraction may reveal a muscle bulge or defect in the quadriceps

➤➤ Box 14.3

Signs and Symptoms of a Quadriceps Strain

- Snapping or tearing sensation at AIIS or at mid-thigh during an explosive movement
- Increased pain or weakness elicited during:
  - Passive knee flexion
    - Grade I: Beyond 90° will be painful
    - Grade II: Limited to 45 to 90°
    - Grade III: Limited to <45°
  - Active knee extension with a flexed hip
  - Resisted knee extension
- Isolated rectus femoris strain will produce increased pain and weakness during:
  - Passive knee flexion and hip extension
  - Active knee extension and hip flexion
  - Resisted hip flexion with the knee flexed at 45°

muscles, especially the rectus femoris of the thigh. **Box 14.3** lists the signs and symptoms of a quadriceps strain.

Hamstrings Strains

The hamstrings are the most frequently strained muscles in the body and are typically caused by a rapid contraction of the muscle during a ballistic action, or a violent stretch. Several factors can increase the risk of injury **(Box 14.4)**.

A hamstrings strain has a reputation of being both chronic and recurring. Most sport participants are fully aware of limited motion after a strain, and concentrate on regaining flexibility through an aggressive stretching program. However, these individuals fail to restrengthen the hamstrings adequately, setting up a muscle imbalance with the quadriceps. During the initial swing phase of gait, the hamstrings act to flex the knee. In late swing, the hamstrings contract eccentrically to decelerate knee extension and reextend the hip in preparation for the stance phase. The hamstrings are also important dynamic stabilizers at the knee. Atrophy in the medial hamstrings (semitendinosus and semimembranosus) can contribute to anteromedial instability at the knee. Conversely, muscle atrophy of the biceps femoris can contribute to anterolateral instability at the knee. Collectively, hamstrings function antagonistically to resist the quadriceps, and thus may

➤➤ Box 14.4

Risk Factors for Hamstring Strains

- Poor flexibility
- Poor posture
- Muscle imbalance
- Improper warm-up
- Muscle fatigue
- Lack of neuromuscular control
- Previous injury
- Overuse
- Improper technique

protect an injured or surgically repaired anterior cruciate ligament.

➤ SIGNS AND SYMPTOMS

In mild strains, the individual will complain of tightness and tension in the muscle. In second- and third-degree strains, the individual may report a tearing sensation or feeling a "pop," leading to immediate pain and weakness in knee flexion. In more severe cases, a sharp pain will be present in the posterior thigh that may occur during mid-stride. The individual will limp and be unable to do heel-strike or fully extend the knee. Pain and muscle weakness are elicited during active knee flexion. If assessed early enough, a noticeable defect in the muscle belly may be palpated. Frequently, profuse swelling and ecchymosis will become visible in the popliteal fossa 1 to 2 days after injury. Although total rupture of the ischial origin is rare, it can result from a sudden forceful flexion of the hip joint when the knee is extended and the hamstring muscles contract powerfully. **Box 14.5** lists the signs and symptoms of a hamstrings strain.

Adductor (Groin) Strain

Adductor strains are common in activities that require quick changes of direction, and explosive propulsion and acceleration. A strength imbalance between the hip abductors and adductors may be a predisposing factor in many of these injuries. The more severe strains are typically at the muscles' proximal attachment on the hip, particularly the adductor longus. Milder strains may occur more distally at the musculotendinous junction.

➤ SIGNS AND SYMPTOMS

The individual will often experience an initial "twinge" or "pull" of the groin muscles, and be unable to walk because of the intense, sharp pain. As the condition worsens, increased pain, stiffness, and weakness in hip adduction and flexion become apparent. Running straight

➤➤ Box 14.5

Signs and Symptoms of a Hamstrings Strain

- History of poor posture, inflexibility, and muscle imbalance
- Injury often occurs when muscle function suddenly changes from a stabilizing knee flexor to an active hip extensor, as occurs in sprinting, and may occur midstride
- Sharp pain in the posterior thigh
- Increased pain or weakness during:
  - Passive knee extension
  - Passive hip flexion
  - Active knee flexion
  - Active hip extension with an extended knee
- Resisted knee flexion:
  - Medial hamstrings—tibia internally rotated
  - Lateral hamstrings—tibia externally rotated
- Resisted hip extension with an extended knee

➤➤ Box 14.6

Signs and Symptoms of an Adductor Strain

- No pain with running straight ahead or backward, but pain with sliding sideways
- Increased pain or weakness during:
  - Passive hip abduction
  - Active hip adduction
  - Resisted hip adduction

ahead or backwards may be tolerable, but any side-to-side movement will lead to more discomfort and pain. Localized tenderness can be palpated on the ischiopubic ramus, lesser trochanter, or musculotendinous junction. Increased pain will be present during passive stretching with the hip extended, abducted, and externally rotated, and with resisted hip adduction. Occasionally, a palpable defect may be found, indicating a more serious injury. **Box 14.6** lists the signs and symptoms of an adductor strain.

Gluteal Muscles

Because of their size and strength, the gluteal muscles are rarely injured except in activities that require muscle overload, such as power weight lifting and rowing. Symptoms will be similar to those in other muscular strains. Passive stretching and resisted hip extension or abduction will cause discomfort. **Box 14.7** lists the signs and symptoms of gluteal strains.

Piriformis Syndrome

The sciatic nerve passes through the sciatic notch beneath the piriformis muscle to travel into the posterior thigh (Figure 14.11). In about 10 to 15% of the population, the nerve passes through or above the muscle, subjecting the nerve to compression from trauma, hemorrhage, or spasm of the piriformis muscle. The incidence of piriformis syndrome has been reported to be six times more prevalent in women than men (3). A history of prolonged sitting, overuse, a recent increase in activity, or buttock trauma may be reported. Resulting symptoms may mimic a herniated lumbar disc problem with nerve root impingement. In a herniated disc problem, pain is usually increased on coughing, sneezing, or straining on defecation, indicating

epidural involvement, which is not noted in a piriformis syndrome.

➤ SIGNS AND SYMPTOMS

Low back pain is not usual, although the individual may complain of a dull ache in the midbuttock region, pain that worsens at night, difficulty walking up stairs or on an incline, and weakness or numbness down the back of the leg. Assessment will reveal point tenderness in the midbuttock region over the greater sciatic notch, and weakness on active hip external rotation and passive internal rotation. The individual may stand with the leg in slight external rotation. Pain can be elicited with the individual supine and the hip flexed, adducted and internally rotated (reverse Patrick's test), as this stretches the piriformis muscle. Straight leg raising may be limited. **Box 14.8** lists signs and symptoms of piriformis syndrome.

Management of Strains

Treatment for muscle strains involves immediate ice, compression, elevation, and protected rest. NSAIDs are typically used for the first 7 to 10 days. Whenever possible, the injured muscle(s) should be iced in a stretched position and crutches used if the individual walks with a limp. In severe strains, a compression wrap may be indicated from the toe to groin, to prevent venous thrombosis and distal edema.

 If the condition does not improve within 2 to 5 days, refer the individual to a physician to rule out other underlying conditions.

Nontraumatic diagnostic possibilities may include an avulsion fracture, osteitis pubis, myositis ossificans, hip joint disease, nerve entrapment, hernia-related conditions, urologic disorders, and gynecologic problems.

After the acute inflammatory phase has progressed to resolution of the hematoma, pain-free gentle stretching and isometric contractions can begin, with cryotherapy and electrical modalities. Compression shorts can provide symptomatic relief and expedite return to play. If compres-

➤➤ **Box 14.8**

Signs and Symptoms of Piriformis Syndrome

- History of prolonged sitting, overuse, or recent increase in activity
- Dull ache in the midbuttock region that worsens at night
- Numbness or weakness may extend down the back of the leg
- Increased pain or weakness during:
  - Passive hip flexion, adduction, and internal rotation
  - Active hip external rotation
  - Resisted hip external rotation

➤➤ **Box 14.7**

Signs and Symptoms of a Gluteal Strain

- History of muscle overload or repetitive muscular contractions, as occurs in weight lifting or rowing
- Increased pain or weakness during:
  - Passive hip flexion with the knee flexed
  - Active hip extension with the knee flexed
  - Resisted hip extension with the knee flexed

sion shorts are not available, a hip spica wrap or compressive wrap can provide both warmth and support. Active stretching, progressive resistance exercises, soft tissue mobilization, and swimming, cycling, mild jogging, and stair climbing can begin when the region is pain-free and range of motion is within 10° of the uninvolved limb (2,4). Several stretching and strengthening exercises were discussed in Field Strategy 14.1; other exercises for muscles crossing the knee joint can be seen in Field Strategy 15.1. When jogging is comfortable, skipping and rope jumping may begin. Rapid stops, starts, and direction changes are not allowed until the individual can achieve full pain-free motion. The individual should not be returned to sport participation until normal muscle strength and power are achieved.

 The female body builder may have a piriformis syndrome. This individual should be treated with rest, NSAIDs, muscle relaxants, and a strong stretching program for the hip external rotators. If the condition does not improve within a week, the individual should be referred to a physician to rule out a herniated intervertebral disc condition.

VASCULAR AND NEURAL DISORDERS

 A 12-year-old soccer player is seen limping after a game. When asked about a possible injury, he reports that his groin and knee have hurt ever since the start of the season, nearly 10 weeks ago. When the parents were questioned about the pain, they reported that the pain comes and goes. They have been having the child ice the hip and stretch the groin muscles, but have not thought that it was serious enough to see a physician. What would be your recommendation?

Vascular disorders should be suspected in any lower extremity injury caused by a high-velocity, low-mass projectile, and in an injury where no physical findings support the continued discomfort. If an acute circulatory problem exists, the lower leg and foot may appear pale or cyanotic, be cool to the touch, or have diminished or totally absent pulse. Immobilization of the limb and transportation to the nearest medical center are the priorities to restore proper circulation to the involved extremity. Other vascular problems are more insidious, but can be just as serious. Neural entrapment is very rare in the hip region, particularly as a result of sport participation.

Legg-Calvé-Perthes Disease

Legg-Calvé-Perthes disease, or avascular necrosis of the proximal femoral epiphysis, is a noninflammatory, self-limiting disorder of the hip seen in young children, especially males, between the ages of 3 and 12 (5). It is consid-

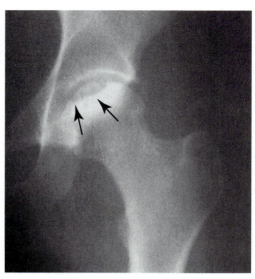

➤ **FIGURE 14.16 Osteochondrosis of the left femoral head (Legg-Calvé-Perthes disease).** Note the destruction of the articular cartilage. In mild cases, no restriction of activity is indicated.

ered to be an osteochondrosis condition of the femoral head, caused by diminished blood supply to the capital region of the femur. This leads to a progressive necrosis of the bone and marrow of the epiphysis of the femoral head **(Figure 14.16)**. The natural history of the condition occurs in the following stages (6):

- Edema develops at the synovial membrane and capsule over 1 to 6 weeks.
- Necrosis of the femoral epiphysis occurs, lasting from several months to 1 year.
- Regeneration/resorption lasts 1 to 3 years. Granulation tissue invades necrotic bone, leaving isolated areas of bone sequestered. Connective tissues invade the area, leading to resorption and replacement by new immature bone that results in a weakened subchondral support system.
- Repair occurs when new, normal bone replaces dead bone. Outcome is related to the percentage of epiphysis involved, patient's age, and promptness of diagnosis.

➤ SIGNS AND SYMPTOMS

The most common complaint is a gradual onset of a limp and mild hip or knee pain of several months' duration. The pain is most often referred to the groin region, but up to 15% of patients report knee pain as the primary symptom (7). Pain is generally activity related, which often contributes to delayed recognition. Examination will reveal a decreased range of motion in hip abduction, extension, and external rotation due to muscle spasm in the hip flexors and adductors.

➤ MANAGEMENT

This condition should be suspected in this age group when pain in the groin, anterior thigh, or knee region cannot be explained.

If pain persists for more than 1 week after initial acute care, or if the individual continues to limp after activity, immediate referral to a physician is needed to rule out nontraumatic causes of the pain that have similar signs and symptoms.

Possibilities include a slipped capital femoral epiphysis (discussed later in the chapter), septic arthritis, transient synovitis, juvenile rheumatoid arthritis, or a bone tumor. Confirmation of the condition is made through radiographs, bone scans, or magnetic resonance images (MRIs).

Treatment depends on the extent of the disease and philosophy of the supervising physician. Nonoperative treatment may involve several different progressive protocols, including:

- Therapy to improve hip range of motion
- Non-weight-bearing in a brace
- Weight-bearing in a brace that limits hip motion
- Weight-bearing in a brace that allows free movement

Treatment can be quite extensive, sometimes taking 1 to 2 years, and may involve immobilization, non-weight-bearing, and possible surgery to prevent any further deformity of the femoral head caused by the avascular necrosis.

Venous Disorders

A direct blow from a baseball, softball, puck, or helmet may damage a vein causing thrombophlebitis or phlebothrombosis. **Thrombophlebitis** is an acute inflammation of a vein; **phlebothrombosis** is a thrombosis, or clotting, in a vein without overt inflammatory signs and symptoms and is discussed in more detail in Chapter 16. Superficial thrombophlebitis (ST) is the preferred term for inflammation of superficial veins; the term deep venous thrombosis (DVT) is preferred for problems with deep veins.

➤ SIGNS AND SYMPTOMS

Superficial thrombophlebitis may present itself as acute, aching or burning pain and superficial tenderness. It is usually more painful than DVT and may be associated with varicose veins.

➤ MANAGEMENT

Treatment may involve anticoagulant therapy, external support with compression stockings or elastic bandages, ambulation and lower extremity exercises particularly with hydrotherapy, periodic elevation of the extremity, and avoidance of long-term sitting or standing in one position. The most reliable signs are chronic swelling and edema in the involved extremity, and a positive Homan's sign (see Figure 16.37).

Toxic Synovitis

An infrequent condition occurring largely in children is **toxic synovitis** of the hip. The transient inflammatory condition is characterized by a painful hip joint accompanied with an antalgic gait and limp.

Early referral to a physician is necessary to rule out septic arthritis of the hip and other more serious conditions that may require surgery to drain the septic joint, relieve pressure, and preserve blood supply to the femoral head.

Rest is the key to treatment, with appropriate medication and traction for prompt resolution.

Obturator Nerve Entrapment

The obturator nerve is derived from the anterior portion of the lumbar plexus (L_2–L_4), and innervates the adductor brevis, long, and magnus; the obturator externus; and the gracilis, as well as providing sensory innervation for the hip joint and distal, medial thigh. A fascial entrapment of the obturator nerve may occur where it enters the thigh as a result of pelvic tumors, obturator hernias, or pelvic and proximal femoral fractures.

➤ SIGNS AND SYMPTOMS

A characteristic clinical pattern of exercise-induced medial thigh pain ranges from the adductor muscle origin distally along the medial thigh. This pain may be described as vague groin or medial knee pain.

➤ MANAGEMENT

An athlete who reports vague groin or medial knee pain should be referred to a physician, especially after no definitive positive signs are reached during special stress tests for the hip and knee regions. Surgical intervention is necessary to release the obturator nerve.

Return to competition usually occurs within several weeks of treatment.

The soccer player's symptoms have been present for more than 10 weeks, and icing and stretching the groin muscles have not improved the injury. Because of the age of the athlete, the vague groin and knee pain, and the length of disability that has now resulted in a noticeable limp, you should recommend that the child see a physician immediately. He may have Legg-Calvé-Perthes disease or another degenerative condition involving the hip joint.

HIP FRACTURES

A tall, thin high school sophomore basketball player is complaining of diffuse knee and groin pain on his left side. It is uncomfortable to run and do shooting drills, and he notes that he cannot balance on his left leg, or walk without a limp. What might you suspect with these symptoms? How will you manage this injury?

Major fractures of the pelvic girdle and hip often result from severe direct trauma, as occurs when an individual is thrown from a horse onto hard ground, when a hockey player collides with the side boards, or in rugby or football when another player falls on top of a downed player. In sports where this is most likely to occur (e.g., football and hockey), the pelvic region is usually adequately protected by padding to prevent such injuries. Traumatic pelvic fractures are therefore seldom seen in sport participation. Fractures that may be seen in this region include avulsion and apophyseal fractures, epiphyseal fractures, and stress fractures.

Avulsion Fractures

Individuals who perform rapid, sudden acceleration and deceleration moves are at risk for avulsion fractures of the ASIS with the displacement of the sartorius, the AIIS with rectus femoris displacement, the ischial tuberosity with hamstrings displacement, and the lesser trochanter with iliopsoas displacement **(Figure 14.17)**. Many of these apophyseal sites do not unite with the bone until ages 18 to 25, and thus continue to be prone to fracture during an individual's competitive interscholastic and intercollegiate years.

➤ SIGNS AND SYMPTOMS

The individual will complain of sudden, acute, localized pain that may radiate down the muscle. Examination will reveal severe pain, swelling, and discoloration directly over the tendinous attachment on the bony landmark. In a completely displaced avulsion fracture, a gap may be palpated between the tendon's attachment and the bone.

Pain increases with passive stretching of the involved muscle, and during active and resisted motion.

➤ MANAGEMENT

Depending on the fracture site, immobilization from an elastic compression spica wrap may limit motion and decrease pain. After fitting the individual with crutches, refer the individual immediately to a physician for radiograph examination.

Ice, rest, modified activity, and protected weight-bearing with crutches for 4 to 6 weeks will provide adequate healing for an undisplaced fracture. Range-of-motion exercises should be discouraged until the fracture has healed, but isometric exercises can be performed if pain-free. Once healed, restoration of range of motion and strength should be initiated, with gradual return to activity. If returned to vigorous activity too soon, a bony prominence may form at the site of the avulsion.

Slipped Capital Femoral Epiphysis

An epiphyseal fracture seen in adolescent boys ages 12 to 15 occurs across the capital femoral epiphysis, the growth plate at the femoral head. The condition is sometimes referred to as adolescent coxa vara. The condition is commonly seen in an obese adolescent with underdeveloped sexual characteristics and, occasionally, in rapidly growing slender boys. In a slipped capital femoral epiphysis, the femoral head slips at the epiphyseal plate and displaces inferiorly and posteriorly relative to the femoral neck **(Figure 14.18)**. As the proximal femoral growth plate deterio-

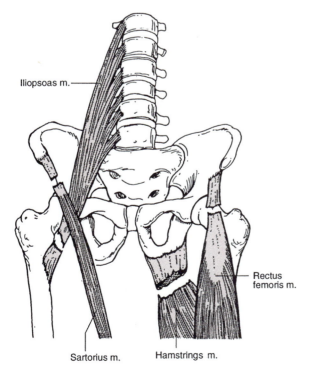

Iliopsoas m.

Rectus femoris m.

Sartorius m.   Hamstrings m.

➤ FIGURE 14.17 **Avulsion fractures.** Several major muscles attach to the pelvis that can be avulsed from their bony attachments during muscular action.

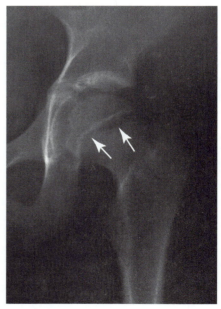

➤ FIGURE 14.18 **Slipped capital femoral epiphysis.** An epiphyseal fracture, seen in adolescents ages 12 to 15, occurs through the growth plate at the femoral head. With this fracture, the patient will be unable to internally rotate the femur.

rates, the individual begins to develop a painful limp with groin pain. Pain may also be referred to the anterior thigh or knee region. The condition may lead to synovitis of the hip and an accompanying psoas major spasm.

➤ SIGNS AND SYMPTOMS

Early signs and symptoms may go undetected. Frequently, the only complaint is diffuse knee pain. In later stages, the individual will feel more comfortable holding the leg in slight flexion. The individual will be unable to touch the abdomen with the thigh because the hip externally rotates with flexion, and will be unable to rotate the femur internally or stand on one leg. If the obturator nerve is damaged during the fracture, an aching pain may be referred to the groin, medial thigh, or knee.

➤ MANAGEMENT

After fitting the individual with crutches, refer the individual immediately to a physician for radiograph examination.

Radiographs of the hip will confirm the condition and rule out other possible conditions, such as tumors, bone cysts, and underlying osteochondromas, that may also lead to hip pain. Prognosis is good with early detection, though those with more severe slips are likely to have residual deformity and progressive disability. In nearly all cases, surgery is indicated.

Stress Fractures

Stress fractures to the pubis, femoral neck (most common), and proximal third of the femur are seen in individuals who do extensive jogging or aerobic dance activities, to the point of muscle fatigue. Several factors can increase the risk of sustaining a stress fracture **(Box 14.9)**.

➤ SIGNS AND SYMPTOMS

Signs and symptoms usually involve a diffuse or localized aching pain in the anterior groin or thigh region during weight-bearing activity that is relieved with rest. Night pain is a frequent complaint, and an antalgic gait may be present. Deep palpation in the inguinal area will produce discomfort. Diffuse or localized swelling may also be present. Increased pain on the extremes of hip rotation, an abduction lurch, and an inability to stand on the involved

leg (positive Trendelenburg sign or "one-legged hop" test) may indicate a femoral neck stress fracture.

➤ MANAGEMENT

Bone scans or MRIs are frequently used for early diagnosis, to prevent delayed treatment. Subsequent radiographs will show periosteal bone formation and a faint fracture line. If diagnosed early enough, rest is indicated for at least 1 to 4 weeks, with no weight-bearing activity until the fracture is completely healed. Stress fractures of the ischium and pubis may require 2 to 3 months of rest. Biking and swimming can maintain cardiovascular fitness; however, the whip kick and scissors kick should be avoided. Displaced stress fractures of the femoral neck require surgical pin fixation to prevent a complete fracture and avascular necrosis of the femoral head.

Osteitis Pubis

Osteitis pubis is an inflammatory process involving continued stress on the pubic symphysis from repeated overload of the adductor muscles, or from repetitive running activities.

➤ SIGNS AND SYMPTOMS

The most common complaint is a gradual onset of pain in the adductor musculature, which is aggravated by kicking, running, and pivoting on one leg. Pain over the pubic symphysis and lower abdominal muscles will increase with sit-ups and abdominal muscle strengthening exercises. Pain may also radiate distally into the groin or medial thigh.

➤ MANAGEMENT

Treatment is symptomatic with ice, protected rest, and NSAIDs until the condition is resolved; however, prolonged rest extending over 2 to 3 months may be required to alleviate symptoms. Hydrotherapy exercises, such as running, cycling, stretching, and strengthening the hip abductors and adductors while in the water, may also help in rehabilitation. Use of a stationary bike and light jogging may be added as tolerated.

Displaced and Nondisplaced Pelvic Fractures

Major fractures of the pelvis seldom occur in sport participation except in activities such as equestrian sports, ice hockey, rugby, skiing, and football. There are three distinct mechanisms involved in traumatic pelvic fractures:

- Avulsion or traction injury of the bony origin or attachment of muscle (see Avulsion Fractures)
- Direct compression, with disruption of the pelvic osseous ring
- Direct blow to the pelvis itself

Because the pelvis is a closed ring, an injury to one location in the pelvis will cause a countercoup fracture or sprain on

---

➤➤ Box 14.9

Risk Factors for Stress Fractures of the Femur
- Sudden increase in training (mileage, intensity, or frequency)
- Change in running surface or terrain
- Improper footwear
- Biomechanical abnormalities
- Nutritional and hormonal factors (anorexia, amenorrhea, osteopenia)

the other side of the pelvic ring. For example, if the superior and inferior pubic rami are fractured on the right side, there often will be sacroiliac disruption on the left side.

➤ SIGNS AND SYMPTOMS

This crushing injury produces severe pain, total loss of function, and in many cases, severe loss of blood leading to hypovolemic shock. The extent of blood loss is unknown because hemorrhage within the pelvic cavity is not visible. In addition, possible internal injuries to the genitourinary system, such as rupture of the bladder or laceration of the urethra, may also occur. In dramatic, severe fractures, this internal damage and subsequent shock can lead to death. A possible pelvic fracture can be determined with slight compression of the sides of the ilium and the ASIS. Fractures of the acetabulum can be detected by gently placing upward pressure on the femur against the acetabulum (see Assessment).

➤ MANAGEMENT

If a fracture is suspected, initiate the emergency procedures plan, and activate EMS. Cover the individual with a blanket to maintain body temperature. Monitor vital signs frequently, and watch for signs of internal hemorrhage and shock. When EMS arrives, place the individual on a long spine board in the position found. Elevate the foot of the board 8 to 12 inches to reduce pooling of blood and fluids in the pelvic region and lower extremities during transportation.

Sacral and Coccygeal Fractures

Fractures of the sacrum and coccyx rarely occur in sports, but are typically caused by a direct blow onto the sacrococcygeal area. This can occur in horseback riding or in other activities involving a fall on the buttock region. When it occurs, it is an extremely painful injury.

The athlete should be referred immediately to a physician. These fractures usually heal without any functional impairment. In rare cases, coccygodynia, or persistent severe pain, can occur, which is very difficult to treat because of the rich complex of pain nociceptors in the area.

The fractures heal within 6 weeks and often show evidence of fibrous union even though clinically healed. Return to competition should be restricted only if pain interferes with the activity.

Femoral Fractures

Fractures of the femoral shaft can be very serious because of potential damage to the neurovascular structures from bony fragments. Femoral shaft fractures are caused by tremendous impact forces, such as shearing or torsion forces when an alpine skier falls, or from direct compressive forces in football, ice hockey, or rugby. Fractures may be open or closed, with significant bleeding at the fracture site in

---

> ➤➤ **Box 14.10**

Signs and Symptoms of Femoral Fractures
Displaced fracture
- Shortened limb deformity
- Severe angulation with the thigh externally rotated
- Swelling into the soft tissues
- Severe pain
- Total loss of function
- Loss of, or change in, distal neurovascular functions
Nondisplaced fractures
- Extreme pain on palpation
- Crepitation
- Muscle weakness
- Muscle spasm
- Swelling into the soft tissues

---

either case. Signs and symptoms indicating a femoral fracture can be seen in **Box 14.10**.

➤ MANAGEMENT

It is not unusual for significant bleeding in the thigh to lead to hypovolemic shock, similar to that seen in pelvic fractures. Be alert to this factor, and treat for shock. Vascular damage may lead to impaired circulation distal to the injury, causing a pale, cold, pulseless foot. Treatment involves initiating the emergency procedures plan and activating EMS. This fracture is best immobilized in a traction splint, which should be applied by trained personnel. Any bleeding should be covered with a dry, sterile dressing to protect the area from further contamination. Distal neurovascular function should be assessed immediately and monitored frequently. Palpate a pulse at the posterior tibial artery and dorsalis pedis artery. Look for pale skin at the foot, and feel for cool skin temperature. Stroke the dorsum and plantar aspect of both feet, and ask the individual if the feeling is the same on the involved leg as on the uninvolved leg. The leg should be totally immobilized and the individual transported immediately to the nearest medical facility.

Table 14.4 summarizes signs and symptoms of the various fractures seen in the pelvis and thigh region.

The high school basketball player could not balance on one leg without severe pain, and had a noticeable limp. These two red flags signal a serious injury of the femur, acetabulum, or hip joint. If pain increases with axial compression along the long axis of the femur, fit the individual with crutches, instruct him to do a non-weight-bearing gait, and immediately refer him to a physician.

ASSESSMENT

A lacrosse player has come into the athletic training room complaining of groin pain in her right

TABLE 14.4   FRACTURES AND ASSOCIATED SIGNS AND SYMPTOMS

Fracture	Common Sites	Signs and Symptoms
Avulsion and apophyseal	ASIS, AIIS, ischial tuberosity, lesser trochanter	Severe pain and tenderness over bony landmark Increased pain with active motion of involved muscle
Epiphyseal	Capital femoral epiphysis	Unable to internally rotate the thigh Possible pain in groin, medial thigh, or knee
Stress	Pubis, femoral neck, proximal third of femur	May have point tenderness over fracture site Pain is worse before and after activity; relieved with rest Possible limp as the fracture progresses
Pelvic girdle	Wing of ilium or acetabulum	Severe pain over fracture site Total loss of function Positive fracture tests Will show signs of shock
Femoral	Shaft of femur or femoral neck	Severe angulation with thigh externally rotated Shortened limb; swelling into soft tissue Severe pain and crepitation at fracture site Total loss of function and signs of shock Positive fracture tests Vascular damage may lead to pale, cold, pulseless foot

leg during running and cutting motions, which is occasionally accompanied with a clicking sensation. Why can't you assume the injury is only related to soft tissue injury?

The lower extremity works as a unit to transmit load from the upper body to the ground through a closed kinetic chain. In the closed chain, the foot, ankle, leg, and hip also absorb force from the ground and dissipate the stress throughout the various structures. When excessive loads and stress exceed the tissues' yield points, injury occurs. Furthermore, the hip is a common site for referred pain from visceral, low back, and knee conditions. Evaluations must therefore be inclusive, particularly with adolescents complaining of groin pain. In the absence of direct trauma to the hip, or in situations where improvement is not seen in 2 to 5 days, always refer the individual to a physician to rule out serious underlying conditions. **Field Strategy 14.3** summarizes a total hip evaluation.

HISTORY

 What information should be gathered from the lacrosse player complaining of vague groin pain and a clicking sensation during running and cutting activities? What questions can identify the four main components of the primary complaint to differentiate soft tissue injury versus a possible fracture or joint disruption?

Many conditions at the hip may be related to family history, age, congenital deformity, improper biomechanical execution of skills, and recent changes in training programs, surfaces, or foot attire. The athletic trainer should gather information on the mechanism of injury, associated symptoms, the progression of symptoms, any disabilities that

may have resulted from the injury, and related medical history. For example, deep groin pain may originate in the hip joint itself, or be referred from the lumbar spine or sacroiliac joint. **Box 14.11** identifies other conditions that may cause groin pain. Sacroiliac pathology almost always manifests itself with pain over the PSIS of the affected side. Trochanteric bursitis usually presents with pain in the posterior aspect of the greater trochanter. In addition to general questions discussed in Chapter 4, specific questions related to the pelvis, hip, and thigh region can be seen in **Field Strategy 14.4**.

 The 20-year-old lacrosse player has had chronic groin pain for the past 2 weeks. The athlete pointed to the right groin and stated that the pain is occasionally accompanied by a sensation

➤➤ **Box 14.11**

Conditions That May Cause Groin Pain

- Referred pain from the bowel, bladder, testicle, kidney, abdomen, rectum, hip joint, sacroiliac joint, pubic symphysis, lymph nodes, or rectus abdominis muscle
- Apophysitis, stress fracture, or avulsion fracture
- Osteitis pubis
- Toxic synovitis of the hip
- Testicular torsion or rupture
- Testicular cancer and other neoplasms
- Ovarian cysts
- Pelvic inflammatory disease
- Urinary tract infections
- Avascular necrosis of the femoral head, or slipped capital femoral epiphysis
- Lymphadenopathy
- Hernia
- Osteoarthritis

FIELD STRATEGY 14.3   HIP EVALUATION

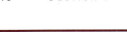

HISTORY

- Primary complaint including:
  - Current nature, location, and onset of the condition
- Mechanism of injury
  - Cause of stress; position of hip, knee, and ankle; direction of force
  - Changes in kicking style, equipment, running technique, or conditioning modes
- Characteristics of the symptoms
  - Evolution of the onset, nature, location, severity, and duration of pain and weakness
- Disability resulting from the injury
- Related medical history
  - Previous injuries in the area, congenital abnormalities, or family history

OBSERVATION AND INSPECTION

- Observation should analyze general posture and gait (see Field Strategy 14.5)
- Inspection at the injury site for deformity, swelling, discoloration, hypertrophy or muscle atrophy, visible congenital deformity, or surgical incision or scars

PALPATION

- Bony structures, to determine a possible fracture
- Soft tissue structures, to determine skin temperature, swelling, point tenderness, crepitus, deformity, muscle spasm, cutaneous sensation, and pulse

FUNCTIONAL TESTS

- Active range of motion
- Passive range of motion
  - Sacroiliac compression and distraction test
  - "Squish" test
  - Sacroiliac rocking (knee-to-shoulder) test
  - Approximation (transverse posterior stress) test
  - Patrick's (Faber) test
- Resisted manual muscle testing

STRESS TESTS

- Leg length measurement
- Contracture tests
  - Thomas test
  - Gaenslen's test
  - Kendall rectus femoris test
  - Patrick's (Faber) test
  - Hamstrings contracture test
  - 90°-90° straight-leg-raising test
- Straight leg raising (Lasègue's) test
- Trendelenburg's test
- Long sitting test
- Ober's test
- Sign of the buttock test

NEUROLOGIC TESTS

- Myotomes
- Reflexes
- Dermatomes

SPORT-SPECIFIC FUNCTIONAL TESTS

FIELD STRATEGY 14.4 DEVELOPING A HISTORY OF THE INJURY

CURRENT INJURY STATUS

1. Where is the pain (or weakness) located? How severe is the pain (weakness)? Does the pain radiate? (Hip pain may be referred pain, so ask additional questions if you suspect a visceral, low back, lumbar, or knee problem.)
2. Did the pain come on suddenly (acute) or gradually (overuse)? Was the pain greatest when the injury first occurred, or did it get worse the second or third day?
3. (If acute, ask:) What were you doing at the time of the injury? What position was the leg in when the injury occurred? (If chronic, ask:) What different activities have you been doing in the last week? (Look for changes in technique, frequency, duration, intensity, or changes in shoes, equipment, or running surface.)
4. Did you hear any sounds during the incident? Any snaps, pops, or cracks? (Snapping may indicate bursitis; tearing may indicate a muscle strain.) Can you bear weight on the leg or balance on the leg? Did you notice any swelling, discoloration, muscle spasms, or numbness with the injury?
5. What actions or motions bring on the pain? It is worse in the morning, during activity, after activity, or at night? Does it wake you up at night? When the pain sets in, how long does it last?
6. Are there certain activities you are unable to perform because of the pain? Which ones?
7. What has been done for the condition?
8. How old are you? (Remember that many problems are age-related.) Which leg is dominant?

PAST INJURY STATUS

1. Have you ever injured your hip or low back before? How did that occur? What was done for the injury? Did you have any difficulty returning to your full functional status?
2. Have you had any medical problems recently? (Look for problems that may refer pain to the area.) Are you on any medication? Do you have any musculoskeletal problems elsewhere in the body? (This may lead to changes in gait or technique that transfer abnormal forces to structures in the lower limb.) What shoes do you wear?

of clicking or snapping deep in that area. It also hurts to turn her right leg outward, and to go up and down stairs. She has been icing the groin and taking over-the-counter NSAIDs, but the condition isn't getting better, and she is concerned that she may have a serious groin strain.

OBSERVATION AND INSPECTION

 Would a posture and gait analysis be indicated with this individual? Why? What specific postural factors might contribute to pain in the hip and pelvic region?

In the examination room, the individual should wear running shorts to allow full view of the lower extremity. On the field, however, this may not be possible as protective equipment or the uniform may obstruct the view. In these cases, determination of the condition may rest more heavily on palpation and stress tests. With individuals who are nonambulatory, complete all observations, inspection, and palpation for possible fractures and dislocations prior to moving the individual.

If time permits, a full postural assessment and gait analysis should be completed. The individual should be viewed from anterior, lateral, and posterior positions. Note the position of the ilium relative to the sacroiliac joint **(Figure 14.19)**. If contranutation occurs at the SI joint, it indicates anterior torsion of the joint, or posterior rotation of the sacrum on the ilium on one side; the limb on that side will probably be medially rotated. Contranutation occurs when the ASIS is lower and the PSIS is higher on one side.

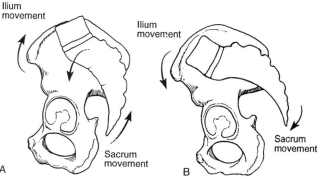

➤ **FIGURE 14.19 Abnormal pelvic tilt.** Movements of nutation (A) and contranutation (B) occurring at the sacroiliac joint.

As a result, the iliac bones move apart and the ischial tuberosities approximate. Contranutation is limited by the posterior sacroiliac ligaments. **Nutation** is the backward rotation of the ilium on the sacrum. If nutation occurs on only one side, the ASIS is higher and the PSIS is lower on that side. The iliac innominate bones move together, and the ischial tuberosities move apart, resulting in an apparent or functional short leg on the same side. Nutation is limited by the anterior sacroiliac ligaments, the sacrospinous ligament, and the sacrotuberous ligament. Nutation occurs when a person assumes a pelvic tilt position; contranutation occurs when a person assumes a lordotic or anterior pelvic tilt position.

Observe for symmetry in the region. Note any visible congenital deformity, such as excessive femoral torsion, abnormal positioning of the patella, toeing in, or toeing out. An increase in the angle of torsion greater than 15° (anteversion) is evidence of external femoral rotation characterized by a toe-out gait. When the angle is decreased (retroversion), the femur internally rotates, causing a toe-in position of the feet. An increase in the angle of inclination (coxa valga), may be visible through either **genu varum**, or laterally positioned patellae. Decreases in this angle (coxa vara), may be visible with **genu valgum** or medially positioned, "squinting" patellae. Also, observe for visible swelling, discoloration, hypertrophy, muscle atrophy, or previous surgical incisions. Specific areas on which to focus in this region are summarized in **Field Strategy 14.5**.

After completing a static exam, observe the individual walking from an anterior, posterior, and lateral view. Note any abnormalities in gait. Ask the person if any actions cause pain or discomfort. In adolescent boys who limp, ask when the limp started. Does the pain or limp come and go? What activities make it worse, better? You are investigating the possibility of a congenital defect in the femoral head with these questions and observations. Inspect the specific injury site for obvious deformities, discoloration, edema, and scars that might indicate previous surgery, and note the general condition of the skin. As always, do bilateral comparison.

 You observed a slight anterior pelvic tilt on the lacrosse player, which may be due to excellent muscle tonus in the legs. No other abnormal postural aspects were present. Gait appeared nor-

---

 FIELD STRATEGY 14.5   POSTURAL ASSESSMENT OF THE HIP REGION

ANTERIOR VIEW

- The iliac crests should be level. Leg length discrepancies may alter the height on one side, leading to lateral pelvic tilt. Ask the person to stand on one leg, and view the level of the iliac crests (Trendelenberg's test).
- The anterior superior iliac spines should be level and an equal distance from the center of the body.
- The greater trochanters should be level.
- Both thighs should look the same. Ask the athlete to contract the quadriceps. Check for hypertrophy or atrophy. Check the patella's relative position and alignment, and note any internal or external rotation of the thigh.
- Check the skin for normal contours, discolored lesions, bruising, ecchymosis, and scars indicating a previous injury or surgery. Note any signs of circulatory impairment or varicose veins.

POSTERIOR VIEW

- The iliac crests should be level.
- The posterior superior iliac spines should be level and an equal distance from the center of the body. Uneven skin depressions may indicate lateral pelvic tilt.
- Are the gluteals bilaterally symmetrical? Any atrophy may indicate an L_5–S_1 nerve root pathology. The gluteal and knee folds should be level.
- The ischial tuberosities should be level. The hamstrings and calf muscles should have equal bulk.
- Check the popliteal fossa for abnormal bruising that may indicate a recent hamstring strain.

LATERAL VIEW

- Check to see if there is excessive lumbar lordosis or flat back caused by anterior or posterior pelvic tilt, respectively. Anterior pelvic tilt may also be indicative of hip flexion contractures.
- Check that one hip is not rotated forward or backward more than the other.
- Is genu recurvatum (hyperextension of the knees) present?
- Check for any skin abnormalities, bruising, discoloration, or scars indicating previous injuries or surgery.

mal, although when asked to slide sideways, she noted some discomfort in the medial groin region.

PALPATION

 With pain centered on the anterior, medial groin region, where you will begin to palpate the various structures? Should you start in the groin, or begin away from the painful area?

Bilateral palpation can determine temperature, swelling, point tenderness, crepitus, deformity, muscle spasm, and cutaneous sensation. Vascular pulses can be taken at the femoral artery in the groin, popliteal artery in the posterior knee, and posterior tibial artery and dorsalis pedis artery in the foot (see Figures 15.5 and 16.14). Proceed proximal to distal, but leave the most painful area to last. Have the individual non-weight-bearing, preferably on a table. When the individual is prone on the table, always place a pillow under the hip and abdominal area to reduce strain on the low back region.

Pain during palpation of bony structures may indicate a displaced avulsion fracture or femoral shaft fracture. Compression, distraction, percussion, or use of a tuning fork on specific bony landmarks may also be used to determine a possible fracture. For example, to determine a possible fracture to the acetabulum, or the femoral neck or head, slowly apply a compressive force to the hip through the longitudinal axis of the femur by pushing through the femoral condyles **(Figure 14.20)**. A possible pelvic fracture can be determined with the sacroiliac compression and distraction test (see Figure 14.22).

 If you suspect a fracture, immediately assess circulatory and neural integrity distal to the fracture site, activate EMS, take vital signs, and treat for shock.

Anterior Palpation

1. Iliac crest, ASIS, tensor fascia latae, and sartorius
2. Inguinal ligament, lymph nodes, pubic symphysis,

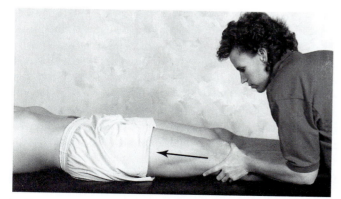

➤ **FIGURE 14.20 Axial compression of the femur.** Increased pain with gentle compression along the long axis of the femur indicates a possible fracture of the femur or acetabulum.

greater trochanter, trochanteric bursa, and abductors (gluteus medius and gluteus minimis)
3. Femoral triangle, femoral artery, iliopsoas bursa, and flexor and adductor muscles (pectineus, adductor brevis, adductor longus, adductor magnus, and gracilis)
4. Quadriceps muscles (vastus lateralis, rectus femoris, vastus medialis, vastus intermedius)

Posterior Palpation

1. Iliac crest and PSIS
2. Ischial tuberosity, ischial bursa, hamstring muscles (biceps femoris is lateral; semitendinosus and semimembranosus are medial), and greater trochanter
3. Sacroiliac, lumbosacral, and sacrococcygeal joints

 Palpable pain was elicited in the anteromedial groin area with the hip and knee flexed, and the leg externally rotated. No other painful sites were palpable.

PHYSICAL EXAMINATION TESTS

 Pain appears to be isolated in the anteromedial groin region. What special tests can be performed to determine if the injury is muscular, capsular, or neurovascular?

Always perform physical examination tests in a comfortable position for the athlete, and begin with gentle stress. Pain and muscle spasm may prevent an accurate assessment of the extent of weakness or instability, so do not force the limb through any sudden motions, or otherwise cause unnecessary pain. Proceed cautiously through the examination.

Functional Tests

The athletic trainer should determine the available range of motion in hip flexion/extension, hip abduction/adduction, hip internal/external rotation, and knee flexion/extension. As always, bilateral comparison is critical to determine normal or abnormal movement.

ACTIVE MOVEMENTS

Active movements can be performed in a seated or prone position, with the most painful movements done last. The movements listed below can be assessed. The number in parentheses are normal ranges of motion for each movement.

- Knee extension (0 to 15°)
- Lateral rotation (40 to 60°)
- Medial rotation (30 to 40°)
- Hip flexion (110 to 120°) with knee flexed
- Abduction (30 to 50°)

- Adduction (30°)
- Knee flexion (0 to 135°)
- Hip extension (10 to 15°)

Measuring range of motion at the hip with a goniometer is demonstrated in **Figure 14.21**.

PASSIVE RANGE OF MOTION

If the individual is able to perform full range of motion during active movements, apply gentle pressure at the extremes of motion to determine end feel. The end feel for hip flexion and adduction is tissue approximation; hip extension, abduction, and medial and lateral rotation are tissue stretch. Passive movements at the pelvic joint also stress the ligamentous structures at these joints, and will be discussed in this section. When testing passive movement, the aim is to reproduce the patient's symptoms, not just pain or discomfort.

Sacroiliac Compression (Transverse Anterior Stress) and Distraction Test

With the individual supine, apply a cross-arm pressure down and outward to the ASIS with your thumbs **(Figure 14.22)**. Repeat with pressure applied down through the

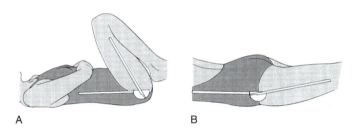

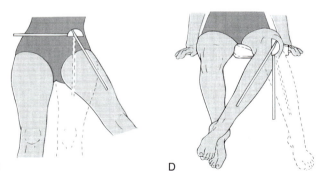

➤ **FIGURE 14.21 Goniometry measurements for the hip. A,** Hip flexion. Center the fulcrum over the greater trochanter of the femur. Align the proximal arm with the lateral margin of the pelvis. Align the distal arm along the lateral midline of the femur, using the lateral epicondyle as reference. **B,** Hip extension. Alignment is the same as for measuring hip flexion, except that the individual is prone. **C,** Hip abduction and adduction. Center the fulcrum over the anterior superior iliac spine (ASIS) of the extremity being measured. Align the proximal arm along an imaginary horizontal line extending to the other ASIS. Align the distal arm along the middle of the femur, using the midline of the patella for reference. **D,** Hip medial and lateral rotation. Center the fulcrum over the anterior aspect of the patella. Align the proximal arm perpendicular to the floor. Align the distal arm, using the crest of the tibia and a point midway between the two malleoli for reference.

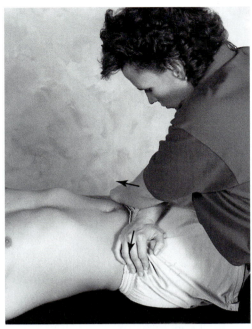

➤ **FIGURE 14.22 Sacroiliac compression and distraction test.** Apply a cross-arm pressure down and outward to the ASIS with your thumbs. Repeat with pressure applied down through the anterior portion of the ilium, spreading the SI joint. Unilateral pain or posterior leg pain may indicate a sprain to the anterior sacroiliac ligaments. Sharp pain elsewhere may indicate a pelvic fracture.

anterior portion of the ilium, spreading the SI joint. Unilateral gluteal or posterior leg pain may indicate a sprain to the anterior sacroiliac ligaments. Sharp pain elsewhere along the pelvic ring with outward pressure, or with bilateral compression of the iliac crests, may indicate a pelvic fracture.

"Squish" Test

With the individual supine, push both ASISs downward and inward at a 45° angle. This action stresses the posterior sacroiliac ligaments, and is positive if pain is present.

Sacroiliac Rocking (Knee-to-Shoulder) Test

This test is also called the sacrotuberous ligament stress test. In a supine position, the athletic trainer fully flexes the individual's knee and hip toward the opposite shoulder and adducts the hip **(Figure 14.23)**. The hip and knee must both demonstrate no pathology, and have full range of motion. The sacroiliac joint is rocked by flexion and adduction of the hip. If bringing a single knee to the chest causes pain in the posterolateral thigh, it may indicate irritation of the sacrotuberous ligament. If pain is produced in the area around the PSIS when pulling the leg toward the opposite shoulder, it indicates sacroiliac ligament irritation.

Approximation (Transverse Posterior Stress) Test

In a side-lying position, a downward force is applied over the iliac crest **(Figure 14.24)**. The movement causes for-

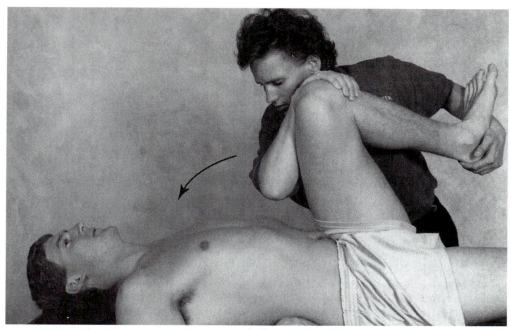

➤ FIGURE 14.23 **Sacroiliac rocking (knee-to-shoulder) test**. The athlete's knee and hip are fully flexed toward the opposite shoulder, and the hip is adducted. The SI joint is rocked by flexion and adduction of the hip. Pain in the posterolateral thigh indicates irritation of the sacrotuberous ligament. Pain in the region of the PSIS when pulling the leg toward the opposite shoulder indicates sacroiliac ligament irritation.

ward pressure on the sacrum. A positive test will produce pain or a feeling of pressure on the sacroiliac joints, indicating a sprain of the posterior sacroiliac ligaments or a sacroiliac lesion, or both. Sharp pain along the pelvic ring may indicate a fracture.

Patrick's (Faber) Test

In a supine position, the foot and ankle of the involved leg are rested on the contralateral knee. The flexed leg is then slowly lowered into abduction **(Figure 14.25)**. The final position of *f*lexion, *ab*duction, and *e*xternal *r*otation (Faber) at the hip should place the involved leg on the table or at least near a horizontal position with the opposite leg. Overpressure on the knee of the involved leg and the contralateral iliac crest may produce pain in the sacroiliac joint on the side of the involved leg, denoting possible pathology.

Resisted Muscle Testing

Stabilize the hip during manual muscle testing to prevent any muscle substitution. Begin with the muscle on stretch, and apply resistance throughout the full range of motion.

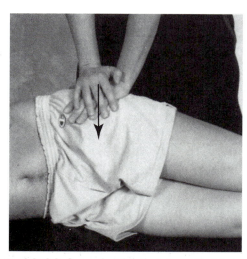

➤ FIGURE 14.24 **Approximation test**. In a side-lying position, apply a downward force over the iliac crest. Increased pain or a feeling of pressure on the sacroiliac joints indicates a possible joint sprain. Pain or pressure in the sacroiliac joints indicates a possible sacroiliac lesion or sprain of the posterior sacroiliac ligaments, or both. Sharp pain may indicate a possible pelvic fracture.

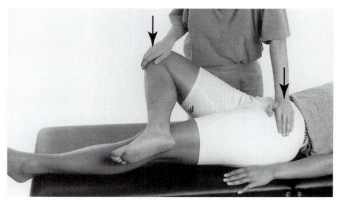

➤ FIGURE 14.25 **Patrick's (Faber) test**. Also called the figure-4 test, the foot and ankle of the involved leg is rested on the contralateral knee. Overpressure on the knee of the involved leg and the contralateral iliac crest may produce pain in the sacroiliac joint on the side of the involved leg, indicating pathology.

Note any muscle weakness when compared to the uninvolved limb. As always, painful motions should be delayed until last. **Figure 14.26** demonstrates motions that should be tested.

Stress Tests

Always be alert to possible congenital defects and epiphyseal injuries when dealing with adolescents. As you progress through the assessment process, perform only those tests you believe to be absolutely necessary.

LEG LENGTH MEASUREMENT

Nutation (backward rotation) of the ilium on the sacrum results in a decrease in leg length, as does contranuta-tion (anterior rotation) on the opposite side. If the iliac bone on one side is lower, the leg on that side is usually longer. Anatomical discrepancy, or true leg length, is measured in a supine position with the ASISs square, level, and balanced. The legs should be parallel to each other, with the heels approximately 6 to 8 inches apart. Using a flexible tape measure, obtain the distance from the distal edge of the ASIS to the distal aspect of the medial malleolus of each ankle **(Figure 14.27A)**. The measurement is repeated on the other side, and the results are compared. A difference of 1.0 to 1.3 cm (0.5 to 1 inch) is considered normal.

Apparent leg length discrepancies as a result of lateral pelvic tilt, or flexion or adduction contractures are measured from the umbilicus to the medial malleolus of each ankle **(Figure 14.27B)**. The test is meaningful only if the test for true leg length discrepancy is negative.

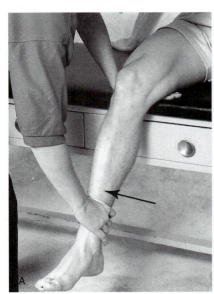
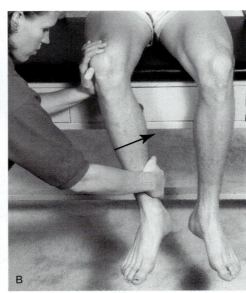
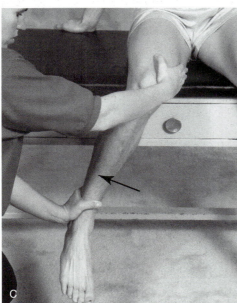
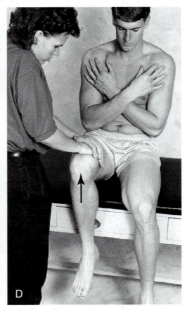

➤ **FIGURE 14.26 Resisted manual muscle testing**. A, Knee extension (L3). B, Lateral hip rotation. C, Medial hip rotation. D, Hip flexion (L2). E, Hip abduction. F, Hip adduction. G, Knee flexion (S2). H, Hip extension (S1). Myotomes are listed in parentheses.

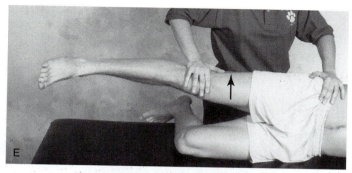

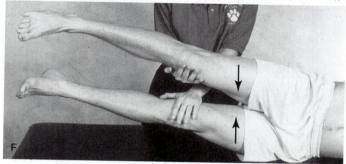

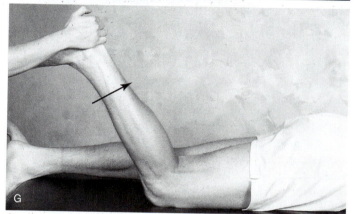

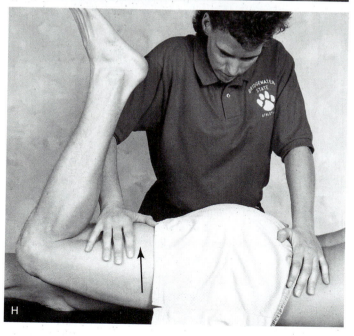

➤ FIGURE 14.26 *Continued.*

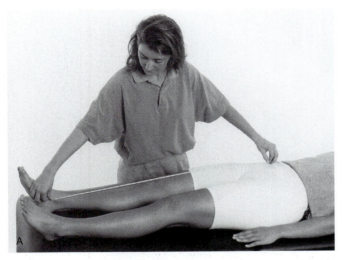

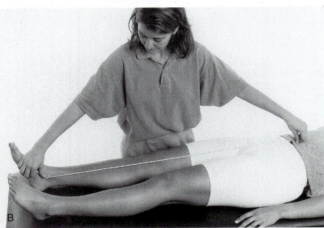

➤ **FIGURE 14.27 Measuring leg length.** A, To measure leg length, make sure the pelvis is square, level, and balanced. For anatomical discrepancy, or true leg length, measure from the ASIS to the distal aspect of the medial malleolus of each ankle. B, For apparent leg length discrepancies, measure from the umbilicus to the medial malleolus of each ankle.

THOMAS TEST FOR FLEXION CONTRACTURES

In a supine fully extended position, observe any noticeable lumbar lordosis. If contractures are present, you may be able to slip your hand under the low back. Ask the individual to flex the uninvolved leg to the chest and hold it in that position. This should flatten the lumbar region. If the test is negative, the straight leg will remain in contact with the table. If the test is positive, however, the straight leg (involved leg) will rise off the table **(Figure 14.28)**. Both legs are tested and compared.

GAENSLEN'S TEST

A modification of the Thomas test, Gaenslen's test is used to place a rotatory stress on the SI joint by forcing one hip into hyperextension. The athlete is positioned so that the test hip extends beyond the edge of the table. Both legs are drawn onto the chest and then one is slowly lowered

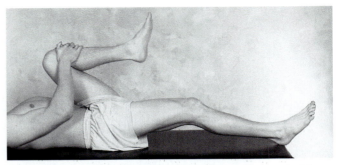

➤ **FIGURE 14.28 Thomas test.** To perform a Thomas test for flexion contractures, ask the individual to flex the uninvolved leg to the chest and hold it. A positive test occurs when the extended leg moves up off the table, indicating hip flexion contractures.

into extension **(Figure 14.29)**. The other leg is tested in a similar fashion for comparison. A positive test is indicated with pain in the sacroiliac joints. An alternative position is with the athlete in a side-lying position with the upper leg (test leg) hyperextended at the hip. The lower leg is flexed against the chest. Stabilize the pelvis while extending the hip of the uppermost leg. Increased pain may be caused by an ipsilateral sacroiliac joint lesion, hip pathology, or an L4 nerve root lesion.

KENDALL TEST FOR RECTUS FEMORIS CONTRACTURE

The individual lies supine on the table with both knees flexed at 90° over the edge of the table. The individual flexes the unaffected knee to the chest and holds it in that position. The other knee should remain flexed at 90°. If the knee slightly extends, a contracture in the rectus femoris may be present on that leg **(Figure 14.30)**. If the results are positive, palpate the muscle for tightness to confirm the contracture. If there is no palpable tightness, the condition may be due to tight joint structures (capsular or ligamentous). If the hip abducts during the test, it may be due to iliotibial band tightness. Ober's test should then be performed bilaterally (see Figure 14.34).

PATRICK'S (FABER OR FIGURE-FOUR) TEST

In a supine position, rest the foot and ankle of the involved leg on the contralateral knee. The flexed leg is then slowly lowered into abduction (see Figure 14.25). The final position should place the involved leg on the table or at least near a horizontal position with the opposite leg. If the leg is unable to relax to this position and remains above the opposite leg, it may indicate a iliopsoas spasm or hip joint contracture.

HAMSTRING CONTRACTURE TEST

In a seated position on a table, flex the hip, bringing one leg against the chest to stabilize the pelvic region. Ask

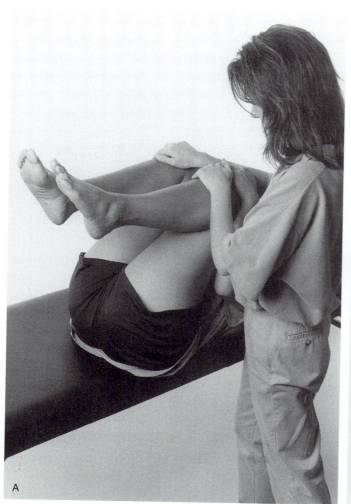
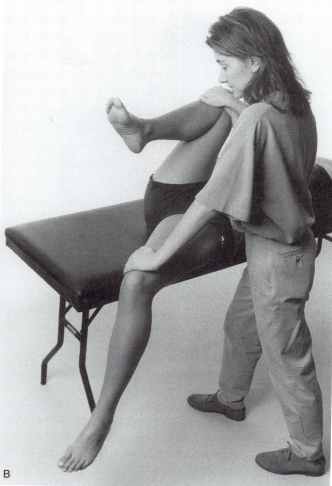

➤ **FIGURE 14.29 Gaenslen's sign.** A, Position the athlete so the involved hip extends beyond the edge of the table. B, Both legs are drawn onto the chest, and then one is slowly lowered into extension. Increased pain signals an ipsilateral sacroiliac joint lesion, hip pathology, or an L4 nerve root lesion.

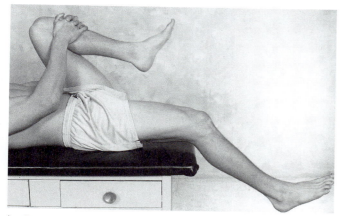

➤ **FIGURE 14.30 Kendall test.** The Kendall test is similar to the Thomas test, except the individual lies supine with both knees flexed over the edge of the table. The uninvolved leg is flexed to the chest and held. A positive test occurs when the leg flexed over the end of the table extends.

the individual to touch the toes of the extended leg **(Figure 14.31)**. Inability to do so indicates tight hamstrings on the extended leg. Test both legs and compare.

90°-90° STRAIGHT LEG RAISING TEST

With the individual supine, flex the hip to 90° with the knees bent. Grasp behind the knee to stabilize the hip at 90°, and extend each knee one at time. For normal flexibility in the hamstrings, knee extension should be within 20° of full extension. Nerve root symptoms may also result, as this position is similar to the slump test done in a supine rather than a sitting position.

STRAIGHT LEG RAISING (LASÈGUE'S) TEST

Although this test is typically used to stretch the dura mater of the spinal cord and assess possible intervertebral disc lesions, it is also used to rule out tight hamstrings. In a supine position, passively flex the individual's hip while

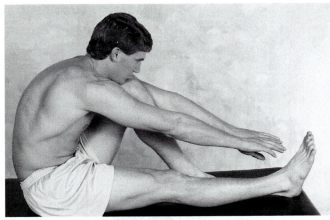

➤ FIGURE 14.31 **Hamstring contractures**. The athlete flexes one hip against the chest to stabilize the pelvic region. The test is positive if the individual cannot touch the toes of the extended leg.

keeping the knee extended, until the individual complains of tightness or pain **(Figure 14.32)**. Slowly lower the leg until the pain or tightness disappears. Then, dorsiflex the foot, have the individual flex the neck, or perform both actions simultaneously. Pain that increases with dorsiflexion and neck flexion, or both, indicates stretching of the dura mater of the spinal cord. Pain that does not increase with dorsiflexion or neck flexion usually indicates tight hamstrings. If both legs are passively raised simultaneously, and pain occurs prior to 70° of flexion, it indicates sacroiliac joint problems.

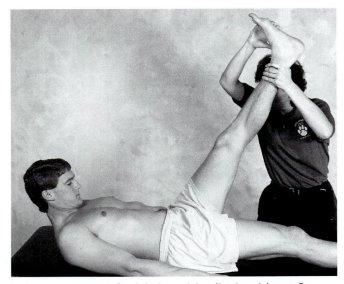

➤ FIGURE 14.32 **Straight leg raising (Lasègue's) test**. Passively flex the individual's hip while keeping the knee extended, until pain or tension is felt in the hamstrings. Slowly lower the leg until the pain or tension disappears. Then, dorsiflex the foot, have the individual flex the neck, or do both simultaneously. If pain does not increase with dorsiflexion of the ankle or flexion of the neck, it indicates tight hamstrings.

TRENDELENBURG'S TEST

The individual is asked to stand, or balance first on one leg and then on the other leg **(Figure 14.33)**. While the individual is balancing, examine the movement of the pelvis. If the pelvis on the side of the nonstance leg rises, the test is considered negative, because the gluteus medius muscle on the opposite (stance) side is lifting it up as it normally does in a one-legged stance. If the pelvis on the side of the nonstance leg falls, however, the test is considered positive, indicating weakness or instability of the hip abductor muscles, primarily the gluteus medius on the stance side. Although the examiner is watching what happens on the nonstance side, it is the stance side that is being tested.

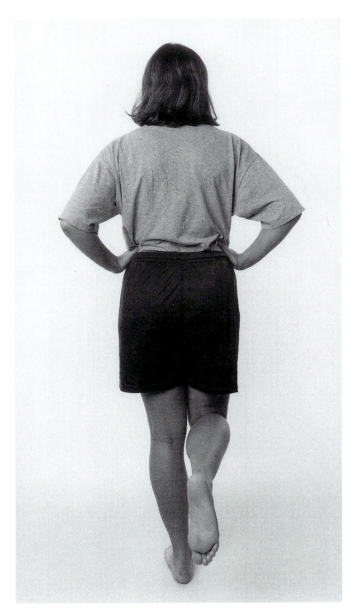

➤ FIGURE 14.33 **Trendelenburg test**. If an individual is unable to stand on the left leg with the hips level, it indicates weakness in the left hip abductors.

LONG SITTING TEST

The athlete is asked to lie supine with the legs straight. The examiner places the thumbs over the medial malleoli, ensuring that the malleoli are level. The athlete is then asked to sit up while the examiner observes whether one leg moves from a long position to a short position (moves proximally). If one leg moves up farther than the other, there is a functional leg length difference resulting from pelvic dysfunction caused by pelvic torsion or rotation. For example, if the right leg moves proximally, it indicates anterior rotation of the right ilium on the sacrum. If the reverse occurs, i.e., the right leg moves from a short position to a longer position, it indicates posterior rotation of the right ilium on the sacrum.

OBER'S TEST

To test the tensor fascia latae (iliotibial band) for contracture, have the individual lie on the side with the lower leg slightly flexed at the hip and knee for stability. Stabilize the pelvis with one hand to prevent the pelvis from shifting posteriorly during the test. Passively abduct and slightly extend the hip so the iliotibial tract passes over the greater trochanter **(Figure 14.34)**. Although the original Ober's test called for the knee to be flexed at 90°, the iliotibial tract has a greater stretch if the knee is extended. Slowly lower the upper leg. If the iliotibial band is tight, the leg will remain in the abducted position. If the knee is flexed during the test, greater stress is placed on the femoral nerve, which may result in neurological signs (i.e., pain, tingling, or paresthesia).

BUTTOCK TEST

This test determines the presence of pathology in the buttock region, such as a bursitis, tumor, or abscess that may restrict hip flexion. The straight-leg-raising test is performed as above. If a restriction is reached in hip flexion,

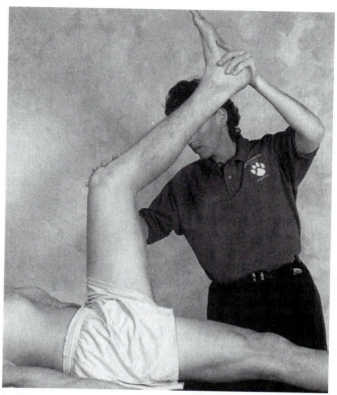

> FIGURE 14.35 **Sign of the buttock test**. Do a unilateral straight-leg-raising test. If a restriction is felt, flex the knee. If hip flexion increases, a problem may exist in the lumbar spine. A positive buttock test occurs when hip flexion does not increase.

flex the individual's knee to see if hip flexion will increase **(Figure 14.35)**. If a problem exists in the lumbar spine, hip flexion will increase, denoting a negative buttock test. A positive buttock test is determined when hip flexion does not increase after the knee is flexed.

Neurologic Assessment

Neurologic integrity can be assessed with the use of myotomes, reflexes, and cutaneous patterns including segmental dermatomes and peripheral nerve patterns.

MYOTOMES

Isometric muscle testing in the loose packed position should be performed in the following motions to test specific segmental myotomes: hip flexion (L_1, L_2); knee extension (L_3); ankle dorsiflexion (L_4); toe extension (L_5); ankle plantar flexion, foot eversion, or hip extension (S_1); and knee flexion (S_2). Testing of these motions are demonstrated in Figure 14.26 and Figure 16.31.

REFLEXES

There are no specific reflexes to test the pelvic or hip area. Other reflexes in the lower extremity, demonstrated

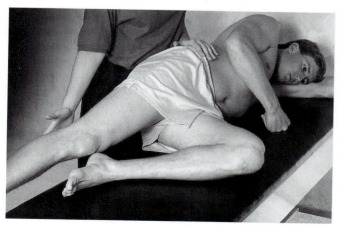

> FIGURE 14.34 **Ober's test**. Passively abduct and slightly extend the hip. Slowly lower the extended leg. If the iliotibial band is tight, the leg will remain in the abducted position.

in Figure 15.27, include the patella (L_3, L_4) and Achilles tendon reflexes (S_1).

CUTANEOUS PATTERNS

In testing cutaneous sensation, the athletic trainer should run a sharp and dull object over the skin, i.e., blunt tip of taping scissors vs. flat edge of taping scissors. With the individual's eyes closed or looking away, he or she should be asked to distinguish sharp and dull, and pinpoint the area being tested. Segmental nerve dermatome patterns for the pelvis, hip, and thigh region are demonstrated in **Figure 14.36**; peripheral nerve distribution patterns are demonstrated in **Figure 14.37**.

Sport-Specific Functional Tests

Functional tests should be performed before clearing any individual for reentry into sports participation. The individual should be able to perform activities pain-free, with no limp or antalgic gait. Examples of functional activities include walking, going up and down stairs, jogging, squatting, jumping, running straight ahead, running sideways, and changing directions while running. Whenever possible, protective equipment or padding should be used to prevent reinjury.

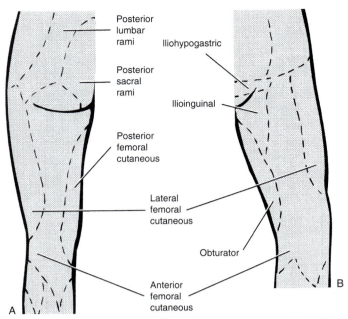

▶ **FIGURE 14.37 Peripheral nerve cutaneous patterns for the pelvis, hip, and thigh region.** A, Anterior view. B, Posterior view.

 You have completed the assessment of the lacrosse player. In addition to the palpable pain anteromedial to the hip joint, you found pain and weakness on passive rotary motions at the hip, especially hip extension, adduction, and internal rotation. Pain was also elicited on resisted hip flexion, abduction, flexion, and external rotation. A snapping sensation occurred when the individual balanced on the right leg and flexed the hip with the femur externally rotated. Bilateral normal results were found in end feels, cutaneous sensation, and other stress tests. This individual has iliopsoas bursitis secondary to snapping hip syndrome.

REHABILITATION OF THE HIP

 After being referred to the team physician, the lacrosse player is doing ice therapy to control inflammation and pain. What exercises should be included in the rehabilitation program to address the deficits in muscle tightness and muscle imbalance?

Rehabilitation for the hip area should restore motion and proprioception; improve muscular strength, endurance, and power; and maintain cardiovascular fitness. In addition to focusing on muscles that move the hip, exercises should also involve the quadriceps and hamstrings muscle groups.

Restoration of Motion

Range-of-motion exercises for the hip region should focus on the hip flexors, extensors, abductors, adductors, and

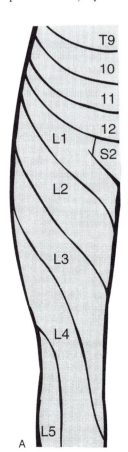
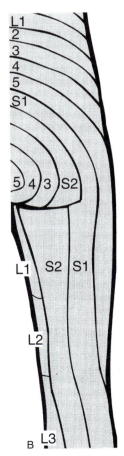

▶ **FIGURE 14.36 Segmental nerve dermatome patterns for the pelvis, hip, and thigh region.** A, Anterior view. B, Posterior view.

medial and lateral rotators, and the quadriceps and hamstrings. Several of the stretching exercises were demonstrated in Field Strategy 14.1; other ROM exercises for muscles crossing the knee joint may appear in Field Strategy 15.1. These exercises can be active or passive, and should include PNF stretching techniques.

Restoration of Proprioception and Balance

Proprioception and balance are regained in the early stages of exercise with activities such as shifting one's weight while on crutches, doing straight leg raises while weight-bearing on one leg, performing bilateral minisquats, and using the BAPS board, slide board, or minitramp. Straight leg raises can be further supplemented with ankle weights and surgical tubing or Theraband. Attaching the tubing to the opposite limb from the one on which you are working can develop balance in one limb while strengthening the other. Movement patterns can work in a single plane or in multidirectional patterns.

Muscular Strength, Endurance, and Power

Isometric exercises may be used early to strengthen the muscle groups. Open chain exercises such as straight leg raises can be completed in a single plane or in multidirectional patterns, and can be supplemented with ankle weights or tubing. Closed chain exercises may include minisquats and modified lunges, and should progress to full squats and lunges. Resistance may be added with handheld weights, a weighted bar, or use of a leg-press machine. A variety of commercial isotonic and isokinetic machines are available to strengthen the individual muscle groups, using open and closed chain technique.

Cardiovascular Fitness

Cardiovascular fitness exercises can include early use of an upper body ergometer (UBE) or hydrotherapeutic exercise. Running in water and performing sport-specific exercises in deeper water can allow the individual to maintain sport-specific functional skills in a non-weight-bearing position. When range of motion is adequate, a stationary bike should be used, beginning with a light-to-moderate load, increasing the load as tolerated. A slide board may also be used. Light jogging can begin with one-quarter speed, and progress to half speed, three-quarter speed, and full sprints. Plyometric exercises including jumping, skipping, and bounding can be combined with running, side-to-side running, or cutting and changing directions. Timed sprints, shuttle runs, karioca runs, hops or vertical jump tests may be used to measure return to full activity. At that time, the individual should have bilaterally equal range of motion, balance, muscular strength, endurance, and power, and an appropriate level of cardiovascular fitness for the specific sport.

The lacrosse player should focus on range-of-motion exercises for the hip flexors and adductors, in addition to general range-of-motion exercises for the entire hip region. Furthermore, exercises for the hip muscles should include closed chain exercises to improve muscular strength, endurance, and power. Proprioception, balance, and cardiovascular fitness should be at or better than the preinjury level.

Summary

1. The sacroiliac joints help to transfer the weight of the torso and skull to the lower limbs, provide elasticity to the pelvic ring, and conversely, act as a buffer to decrease impact forces from the foot as they are transmitted to the spine and upper body.

2. The hip joint is the most stable joint in the body, protected by a deep, bony socket called the acetabulum, and stabilized by several strong ligaments, including the iliofemoral, pubofemoral, and ischiofemoral ligaments.

3. Compression on the hip is approximately the same as body weight during the swing phase of normal walking, but increases to at least six times body weight during the stance phase.

4. Muscle imbalance and dysfunction, congenital abnormalities, and postural deviations can predispose an individual to injury.

5. Contusions are typically seen on the crest of the ilium, called a hip pointer, or in the quadriceps muscle group, referred to as a charley horse. Severe quadriceps contusions can lead to myositis ossificans or an acute compartment syndrome.

6. Bursitis can result from inflammation secondary to excessive friction or shear forces, or can stem from a direct blow that causes bleeding in the bursa. The greater trochanteric bursa is the most commonly injured.

7. The hamstrings are the most frequently strained muscle group in the body. Injuries are typically caused by a rapid contraction of the muscle during a ballistic action, or by a violent stretch.

8. Adductor strains are common in activities that require quick changes of direction, and explosive propulsion and acceleration.

9. Piriformis syndrome is six times more prevalent in women than men, and can mimic signs and symptoms associated with a herniated lumbar disc problem with nerve root impingement.

10. In adolescents, any unexplained groin pain associated with a gradual onset of a limp should be referred to a physician to rule out Legg-Calvé-Perthes disease or a slipped capital femoral epiphysis.

11. Avulsion fractures may occur in individuals who perform rapid, sudden acceleration and deceleration moves, with the following sites being most affected:
    - ASIS—proximal sartorius muscle or tensor fascia latae
    - AIIS—proximal rectus femoris muscles
    - Ischial tuberosity—proximal hamstrings attachment
    - Lesser trochanter—distal iliopsoas attachment
12. Refer an individual to a physician if any of the following conditions are suspected:
    - Obvious deformity suggesting a dislocation or fracture
    - Significant loss of motion or palpable defect in a muscle
    - Severe joint disability that may be evident by a noticeable limp
    - Excessive soft tissue swelling, particularly in the quadriceps
    - Any adolescent with groin pain that does not improve within 5 to 7 days, or is associated with a gradual onset of a limp
    - Any abnormal or absent reflexes, or weakness in a myotome
    - Abnormal sensations in either the segmental dermatomes or peripheral cutaneous patterns
    - Absent or weak pulse
13. Radiographs, bone scans, or MRIs can be used to rule out underlying bone cysts, tumors, osteochondromas, or congenital defects that could lead to permanent disability.

References

1. Nordin M, Frankel VH. Basic Biomechanics of the Musculoskeletal System. Philadelphia: Lea and Febiger, 1992.
2. Sanders B, Nemeth WC. Hip and thigh injuries. In: Athletic Injuries and Rehabilitation. Edited by Zachazewski JE, Magee DJ, Quillen WS. Philadelphia: WB Saunders, 1996.
3. Esposito PW. Pelvis, hip and thigh injuries. In: The Team Physician's Handbook. Edited by Mellion MB, Walsh WM, Shelton GL. Philadelphia: Hanley and Belfus, 1997.
4. Best TM, Garrett WE. Hamstring strains: Expediting return to play. Phys Sportsmed 1996;24(8):37-44.
5. Ruane JJ, Rossi TA. When groin pain is more than 'just a strain.' Navigating a broad differential. Phys Sportsmed 1998;26(4):78-103.
6. Gerberg LF, Micheli LJ. Traumatic hip pain in active children: A critical differential. Phys Sportsmed 1996;24(1):69-74.
7. Paletta GA, Adrish JT. Injuries about the hip and pelvis in the young athlete. Clin Sports Med 1995;14(3):591-628.

CHAPTER 15

Knee Conditions

OBJECTIVES

1. Identify the important bony and soft tissue structures of the knee region.
2. Identify the primary and secondary ligamentous restraints of the knee.
3. Describe the motions of the knee, and identify the muscles that produce them.
4. Explain what forces produce the loading patterns responsible for common injuries at the knee.
5. Explain the basic principles in the prevention of knee injuries.
6. Describe the causes and management of bursitis at the knee.
7. Identify the structures injured in each type of unidirectional and multidirectional instability, and describe their management.
8. List the signs and symptoms associated with a meniscal lesion.
9. List the various factors that can predispose an individual to patellofemoral pain.
10. Describe common patella injuries and their management.
11. Differentiate between an osteochondral fracture and osteochondritis dissecans.
12. Describe a thorough assessment of the knee and patellofemoral joint.
13. Explain the basic principles associated with rehabilitation of the knee.

The knee is a large, complex joint that is frequently injured in sport participation. During walking and running, the knee moves through a considerable range of motion while bearing loads equivalent to three to four times body weight. The knee is also positioned between the two longest bones in the body, the femur and tibia, creating the potential for large, injurious torques at the joint. These factors, coupled with minimal bony stability, make the knee susceptible to injury, particularly during participation in field and/or contact sports. The knee is the predominant site of injury among runners, and is one of the most frequently injured joints in basketball and volleyball players (1,2,3).

This chapter begins with a review of the anatomy of the knee, and discusses its kinematics and kinetics. General principles to prevent injuries will then be followed by discussion of common injuries to the knee complex. Finally, a step-by-step injury assessment of the region is presented, and examples of rehabilitative exercises will be provided.

ANATOMICAL REVIEW OF THE KNEE

The knee is a large synovial joint including three articulations within the joint capsule. The weight-bearing joints are the two condylar articulations of the tibiofemoral joint, with the third articulation being the patellofemoral joint. The soft tissue connections of the proximal tibiofibular joint also exert a minor influence on knee motion.

Bony Structure of the Knee

The proximal bone of the knee joint is the femur, which was discussed in Chapter 14. The prominent posterior ridge of the femur, the linea aspera, serves as an attachment for many of the muscles that move the hip and knee. As it reaches its distal end, the shaft of the femur broadens to form the medial and lateral epicondyles. Running between the epicondyles on the anterior surface of the femur is the femoral trochlea, through which the patella glides as the knee moves into flexion and extension **(Figure 15.1)**.

The lateral epicondyle is wider than the medial epicondyle. Arising from the most superior crest of the medial epicondyle is the palpable adductor tubercle. Inferior to each epicondyle are the medial and lateral condyles, the medial condyle being the longer. Sharing a common anterior surface, they bifurcate posteriorly and are separated by the deep intercondylar notch.

Corresponding to the femoral condyles are the medial and lateral tibial plateaus. The medial tibial plateau (condyle) is 50% larger than the lateral tibial plateau to accommodate for the longer medial femoral condyle. Separating the two tibial plateaus are the intercondylar eminences, which are raised areas that match the femur's intercondylar notch. On the anterior aspect of the tibia is the prominent tibial tubercle, which serves as the distal attachment of the

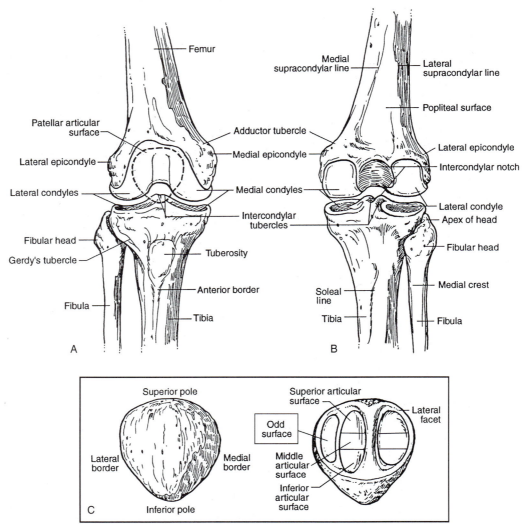

➤ FIGURE 15.1 Bony structures of the knee. A, Anterior view. B, Posterior view. C, Patella.

infrapatellar ligament. The patella, a sesamoid bone located in the quadriceps (patellar) tendon, improves the biomechanical function of the extensor mechanism, and protects the anterior portion of the knee. The head of the fibula, although not directly a part of the knee joint, does serve as a site for several soft tissue attachments that support and stabilize the knee.

Tibiofemoral Joint

The distal femur and proximal tibia articulate to form two side-by-side condyloid joints known collectively as the **tibiofemoral joint (Figure 15.2)**. These joints function together primarily as a modified hinge joint because of the restricting ligaments, with some lateral and rotational motions allowed. Because the medial and lateral condyles of the femur differ somewhat in size, shape, and orientation, the tibia rotates laterally on the femur during the last few degrees of extension to produce "locking" of the knee. This phenomenon, known as the **"screwing-home" mechanism**, brings the knee into the close packed (most stable) position of full extension.

Menisci

The **menisci**, also known as semilunar cartilages because of their half-moon shapes, are discs of fibrocartilage firmly attached to the superior plateaus of the tibia by the coronary ligaments and joint capsule. They serve several functions, such as absorption and dissipation of force, lubrication and

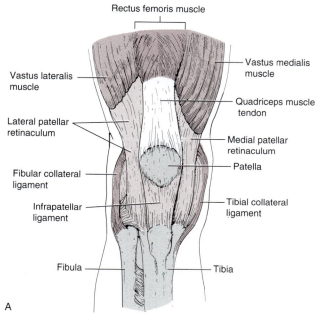

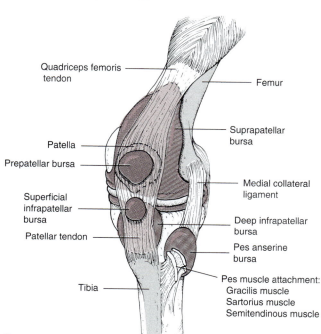

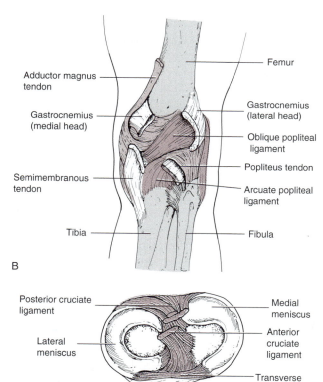

▶ **FIGURE 15.2 Knee**. A, Ligaments of the knee (anterior view). B, Ligaments of the knee (posterior view of superficial and deep structures). C, Bursae of the knee. D, Superior surface of tibia with menisci and associated structures.

➤➤ Box 15.1

Functions of the Menisci

- Deepen the articulation and fill the gaps that occur during knee motion
- Aid in lubrication and nutrition of the joint
- Reduce friction during movement
- Increase area of contact between the condyles, thus improving weight distribution
- Provide shock absorption by dissipating stress over the articular cartilage, thus decreasing cartilage deterioration
- Assist the ligaments and capsule in preventing hyperextension
- Prevent the joint capsule from entering the joint during the locking mechanism, by directing the movement of the femoral articular condyles

nourishment of the joint structures, and congruency of the joint surfaces to improve weight distribution **(Box 15.1)**.

When viewed in cross section, the menisci are thicker along the lateral margin and thinner on the medial margin, serving to deepen the concavities of the tibial plateaus. When viewed from above, the medial meniscus is semicircular, whereas the lateral meniscus is somewhat more circular (Figure 15.2D). The inner edges of both menisci are unattached to the bone, but the two ends of the menisci, known as the anterior and posterior horns, are attached to the intercondylar tubercles. The anterior horns of each meniscus are joined to each other by the transverse ligament, and are connected to the infrapatellar tendon via the patellomeniscal ligaments. The medial meniscus is also attached to the deep medial collateral ligament and fibers from the semimembranosus muscle. It is injured much more frequently than the lateral meniscus. This is partly because the medial meniscus is more securely attached to the tibia, and therefore less mobile. The lateral meniscus is a smaller and more freely moveable structure. In addition to its attachments to the joint capsule, intercondylar tubercles, and transverse ligament, the lateral meniscus is attached to the posterior cruciate ligament through the meniscofemoral ligament (ligament of Wrisberg), and to the popliteus muscle via the joint capsule and coronary ligament. Contraction of the popliteus serves to retract the lateral meniscus. During flexion and extension of the knee, the menisci move posteriorly and anteriorly, respectively.

Joint Capsule and Bursae

The thin articular capsule at the knee is large and lax, encompassing both the tibiofemoral and patellofemoral joints. Anteriorly it extends about 2.5 cm above the patella to attach along the edges of the superior patellar surface. The deep bursa formed by this capsule above the patella, the suprapatellar bursa, is the largest in the body (Figure 15.2C). It lies between the femur and quadriceps femoris tendon, and functions to reduce friction between the two structures.

Posteriorly, two other bursae communicate with the joint capsule, the subpopliteal and semimembranosus bursae. The subpopliteal bursa lies between the lateral condyle of the femur and the popliteal muscle. The semimembranosus bursa lies between the medial head of the gastrocnemius and the semimembranosus tendon.

During flexion and extension, synovial fluid moves throughout the bursal recesses to lubricate the articular surfaces. In extension, the gastrocnemius and subpopliteal bursae are compressed, driving the synovial fluid anteriorly. In flexion, the suprapatellar bursa is compressed, forcing fluid posteriorly. When the knee is in a semiflexed position, or open packed position, the synovial fluid is under the least pressure. This position provides relief of pain caused by swelling in the joint capsule and surrounding bursae.

Three other key bursae associated with the knee, but not contained in the joint capsule, are the prepatellar, superficial infrapatellar, and deep infrapatellar bursae. The prepatellar bursa is located between the skin and anterior surface of the patella, allowing free movement of the skin over the patella during flexion and extension. The superficial infrapatellar bursa is located between the skin and patellar tendon. Inflammation of this bursa due to excessive kneeling is sometimes referred to as "housemaid's knee." The deep infrapatellar bursa is located between the tibial tubercle and the infrapatellar tendon, and is separated from the joint cavity by the infrapatellar fat pad. This bursa reduces friction between the ligament and the bony tubercle.

Ligaments of the Knee

Because the shallow articular surfaces of the tibiofemoral joint contribute little to knee stability, the stabilizing role of the ligaments crossing the knee is of great significance. Two major ligaments of the knee are the anterior and posterior **cruciate ligaments** (Figure 15.2D). The name cruciate is derived from the fact that these ligaments cross each other, with anterior and posterior referring to their respective tibial attachments. These ligaments are termed intracapsular because they are located within the articular capsule, and **extrasynovial** because they lie outside the synovial cavity. The anterior cruciate ligament (ACL) stretches from the anterior aspect of the intercondyloid fossa of the tibia just medial and posterior to the anterior tibial spine in a superior, posterior direction to the posterior medial surface of the lateral condyle of the femur. The ACL is a critical stabilizer that prevents:

- Anterior translation (movement) of the tibia on a fixed femur
- Posterior translation of the femur on a fixed tibia
- Internal and external rotation of the tibia on the femur
- Hyperextension of the tibia

The ACL has two discrete bands: an anteromedial and a posterolateral bundle, with a third, intermediate band occasionally present. When the knee is fully extended, the femoral attachment of the anteromedial bundle is anterior to the attachment of the posterolateral bundle. When the knee is flexed, the positions are reversed, causing the ACL to wind on itself. The result of this action is that varying portions of the ACL are taut as the knee moves through a normal range of motion (ROM). When the knee is fully extended, the posterolateral bundle is taut; when the knee is fully flexed, the anteromedial bundle is taut. The ACL is frequently subject to deceleration injuries; internal tibial torque is the most dangerous loading mechanism, particularly when combined with an anterior tibial force (4).

The shorter and stronger posterior cruciate ligament (PCL) runs from the posterior aspect of the tibial intercondyloid fossa in a superior, anterior direction to the lateral anterior medial condyle of the femur. It consists of a large anterolateral and a smaller posteromedial bundle. The PCL is considered to be the primary stabilizer of the knee and resists posterior displacement of the tibia on a fixed femur. The PCL's posterior fibers are taut when the knee is fully extended, and the anterior fibers are taut when it is fully flexed.

The medial and lateral **collateral ligaments** are referred to respectively as the tibial and fibular collateral ligaments, after their distal attachments. Formed by two layers, the deep fibers of the medial (tibial) collateral ligament (MCL) merge with the joint capsule and medial meniscus to connect the medial epicondyle of the femur to the medial tibia. The superficial layer originates from a broad band just below the adductor tubercle and is separated from the deep layer by a bursa. The two layers insert just below the pes anserinus, the common attachment of the semitendinosus, sartorius, and gracilis, thereby positioning the ligament to resist medially directed shear (valgus) and rotational forces acting on the knee. As a unit, the MCL is taut in complete extension. In midrange, its posterior fibers are most taut; in complete flexion, the anterior fibers are the most taut.

The lateral (fibular) collateral ligament (LCL) connects the lateral epicondyle of the femur to the head of the fibula, contributing to lateral stability of the knee. The ligament is separated from the lateral meniscus by a small fat pad. The LCL is the primary restraint against varus forces when the knee is between full extension and 30° of flexion, and provides secondary restraint against external rotation of the tibia on the femur.

Other Structures Stabilizing the Knee

Several other structures also contribute to knee integrity. Posteriorly, the oblique popliteal ligament forms an extension of the semimembranosus tendon, and the arcuate popliteal ligament connects the lateral condyle of the femur to the head of the fibula. Together these two ligaments are called the **arcuate-popliteal complex**, providing support to the posterior joint capsule. The complex limits anterior displacement of the tibia relative to the femur, as well as hyperextension and hyperflexion of the knee. It becomes taut during internal and external tibial rotation, and during valgus and varus loading of the knee.

Although the knee is only partially surrounded by a joint capsule, the capsule is reinforced by several tendons, including the expanded tendons of the quadriceps, the tendon of the semimembranosus, and the iliotibial (IT) band. Laterally, the IT band is a broad, thickened band of fascia that extends from the tensor fascia latae over the lateral epicondyle of the femur to Gerdy's tubercle on the lateral tibial plateau. This resisting band is well supplied with free nerve endings that transmit signals for pain and proprioception to the brain, enhancing the structure's ability to promote lateral knee stability. The tissue under the IT band is a lateral extension and invagination of the knee joint capsule. **Table 15.1** lists the structures providing stability to the knee.

Patellofemoral Joint

The patella (kneecap) is a triangular bone that rests between the femoral condyles to form the patellofemoral joint (Figure 15.2A). The posterior surface of the patella is composed of three distinct facets, each covered with up to 5-mm thickness of hyaline cartilage (Figure 15.1C). A central vertical ridge separates the medial and lateral regions, each having a superior, middle, and inferior articular surfaces. The odd facet, lying medial to the medial facet, has no articular subdivisions.

In the sagittal plane, the patella serves to increase the angle of pull of the patellar tendon on the tibia, thereby improving the mechanical advantage of the quadriceps muscles to produce knee extension. During knee flexion and extension, the patella tracks within the femoral trochlear groove. When the knee is fully extended, the patella

TABLE 15.1	STRUCTURES CONTRIBUTING TO THE STABILITY OF THE KNEE		
Tibial Motion	**Primary Restraints**	**Secondary Restraints**	
Anterior translation	ACL	MCL, LCL; middle third of mediolateral capsule, IT band	
Posterior translation	PCL	MCL, LCL; posterior third of mediolateral capsule; popliteus tendon; anterior and posterior meniscofemoral ligaments	
Valgus rotation	MCL	ACL, PCL; posterior capsule when knee is fully extended	
Varus rotation	LCL	ACL, PCL; posterior capsule when knee is fully extended	
Lateral rotation	MCL, LCL	Popliteus corner, ACL, PCL	
Medial rotation	ACL, PCL	Anteroposterior meniscofemoral ligaments	

Adapted from Irrgang JJ, Safran MR, and Fu FH (5), page 627.

rests on the distal portion of the femoral shaft, just proximal to the femoral groove. During flexion, the patella makes initial contact with the groove at 10 to 20° of flexion and becomes seated within the groove as the knee approaches 20 to 30°. At this time, the lateral border of the trochlea is prominent, forming a barrier against lateral displacement of the patella. Although the greatest amount of contact with the surface area is reached between 60° and 90° of flexion, the greatest compressive forces are exerted on the patella at 30° of flexion (6).

Patellar positioning is maintained and restrained by the patellar retinaculum. The lateral retinaculum originates from the vastus lateralis and the IT band, and inserts on the patella's lateral border. The medial retinaculum originates from the distal portion of the vastus medialis and adductor magnus, and inserts on the medial border of the patella. The superior portion of the knee's joint capsule thickens and inserts on the patella's superior border, forming the medial and lateral patellofemoral ligaments.

The Q-angle is defined as the angle between the line of resultant force produced by the quadriceps muscles and the line of the patellar tendon **(Figure 15.3A)**. One line is drawn from the middle of the patella to the anterior superior iliac spine (ASIS) of the ilium, and a second line is drawn from the tibial tubercle through the center of the patella. The normal Q-angle ranges from approximately 13° in males to approximately 18° in females, when the knee is fully extended. A Q-angle less than 13° or greater than 18° is considered abnormal, and can predispose the sport participant to patellar injuries or degeneration. There

is controversy in the literature, however, regarding the significance of the Q-angle. Some investigators have suggested that clinical measurements of the Q-angle actually underestimate the lateral force component of the quadriceps pull on the patella (7,8).

Another measurement, similar to the Q-angle, is the **A-angle**, which measures the relationship of the patella to the tibial tubercle **(Figure 15.3B)**. This measurement consists of a vertical line that divides the patella in half. A second line is drawn from the tibial tubercle to the apex of the inferior pole of the patella. An A-angle of 35° or greater has been linked to increased patellofemoral pain, although some have questioned the reliability of this measurement because of the difficulty in consistently finding appropriate landmarks.

Muscles Crossing the Knee

The muscles of the knee develop tension to produce motion at the knee and also contribute to the knee's stability. The attachments and primary actions of the muscles crossing the knee are summarized in **Table 15.2**.

Nerves of the Knee

The tibial nerve (L_4, L_5, S_1–S_3) is the largest and most medial continuation of the sciatic nerve. It innervates all of the muscles in the hamstring group except the short head of the biceps femoris, and also supplies all muscles in the calf of the leg **(Figure 15.4)**.

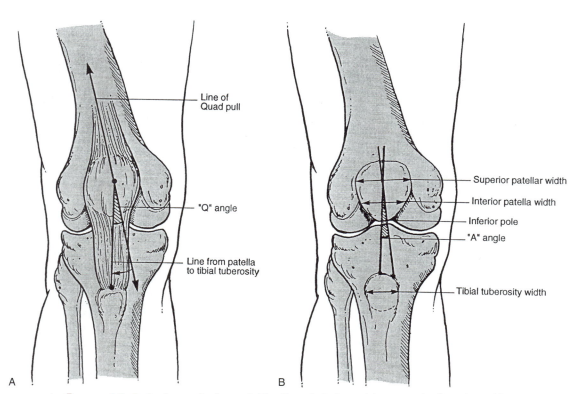

Line of Quad pull

"Q" angle

Line from patella to tibial tuberosity

Superior patellar width

Interior patella width

Inferior pole

"A" angle

Tibial tuberosity width

A   B

▶ **FIGURE 15.3 Angles at the knee.** A, The Q-angle is formed between the line of quadriceps pull and the imaginary line connecting the center of the patella to the center of the tibial tubercle. B, The A-angle measures the relationship of the patella to the tibial tubercle.

TABLE 15.2   MUSCLES ACTING ON THE KNEE

Muscle	Proximal Attachment	Distal Attachment	Primary Action(s)	Nerve Innervation
Rectus femoris	Anterior inferior iliac spine (AIIS)	Patella	Extension	Femoral (L_2, L_3, L_4)
Vastus lateralis	Greater trochanter and lateral linea aspera	Patella	Extension	Femoral (L_2, L_3, L_4)
Vastus intermedius	Anterior femur	Patella	Extension	Femoral (L_2, L_3, L_4)
Vastus medialis	Medial linea aspera	Patella	Extension	Femoral (L_2, L_3, L_4)
Semitendinosus	Ischial tuberosity	Proximal, medial tibia at pes	Knee flexion and medial rotation	Sciatic (L_5, S_1, S_2)
Semimembranosus	Ischial tuberosity	Proximal, medial tibia	Knee flexion and medial rotation	Sciatic (L_5, S_1, S_2)
Biceps femoris	*Long head:* ischial tuberosity. *Short head:* lateral linea aspera	Fibular head and lateral condyle of tibia	Knee flexion and lateral rotation	Sciatic (L_5, S_1, S_2)
Sartorius	Anterior superior iliac spine (ASIS)	Proximal medial tibia at pes	Knee flexion and medial rotation	Femoral (L_2, L_3)
Gracilis	Symphysis pubis and the pubic arch	Proximal medial tibia at pes	Knee flexion and medial rotation	Obturator (L_2, L_3)
Popliteus	Lateral condyle of the femur	Posterior, medial tibia	Knee flexion and medial rotation	Tibial (L_4, L_5)
Gastrocnemius	Posterior medial and lateral femoral condyles	Calcaneus, via the Achilles tendon	Knee flexion	Tibial (S_1, S_2)
Plantaris	Posterior femur above lateral condyle	Calcaneus	Knee flexion	Tibial (S_1, S_2)

The common peroneal nerve (L_4, L_5, S_1, S_2) is the lateral branch of the sciatic nerve. It innervates the short head of the biceps femoris in the thigh, then passes through the popliteal fossa to wind laterally along the subcutaneous surface to just below the proximal head of the fibula, where it can be easily damaged. As it passes between the fibula and the peroneus longus muscle, it subdivides into the superficial and deep peroneal nerves. An articular branch to the knee may arise either from the deep peroneal nerve or from both deep and superficial peroneal nerves as a terminal branch of the common peroneal nerve.

The femoral nerve (L_2–L_4) courses down the anterior aspect of the thigh adjacent to the femoral artery to supply the quadriceps group. The L_2 and L_3 branches of the femoral nerve also innervate the sartorius.

Blood Vessels of the Knee

Just proximal to the knee, the main branch of the femoral artery becomes the popliteal artery. The popliteal artery courses through the popliteal fossa and then branches, forming the medial and lateral superior genicular, the middle genicular, and the medial and lateral inferior genicular arteries that supply the knee (**Figure 15.5**). The superior and inferior genicular arteries intertwine with each other about the knee.

KINEMATICS AND MAJOR MUSCLE ACTIONS OF THE KNEE

The knee functions primarily as a hinge joint. The different shapes of the femoral condyles, however, serve to complicate joint function.

Flexion and Extension

The primary motions permitted at the tibiofemoral joint are flexion and extension. Knee flexion is primarily carried out by the hamstrings, also assisted by the popliteus, gastrocnemius, gracilis, and sartorius. In addition, the flexor musculature has a secondary responsibility of rotating the tibia. The flexors attaching on the tibia's medial side (e.g., semitendinosus, semimembranosus, gracilis, and sartorius) internally rotate the tibia, while those attaching on the lateral side (e.g., biceps femoris) externally rotate the tibia. Knee extension is carried out by the quadriceps femoris muscle group. Although the name implies four muscles, most clinicians describe five: the vastus lateralis, vastus intermedius, vastus medialis, vastus medialis oblique (VMO), and rectus femoris. The VMO is a discrete group of fibers arising from the medial femoral condyle and the fascia of the adductor magnus. Each muscle has a common attachment on the tibial tubercle via the patella and infrapatellar ligament.

In the terminal 20° of knee extension, the tibia externally rotates approximately 15° in what is called the "screw-home" mechanism. In full extension, the joint's close packed position, maximal bony contact occurs between the femur and tibia, resulting in the joint being anatomically "locked." This rotation occurs because the articulating surface of the medial condyle of the femur is longer than that of the lateral condyle in this locked position, rendering motion almost completely impossible. For flexion to be initiated from a position of full extension, the knee must first be "unlocked." The role of locksmith in the closed kinetic chain is provided by the popliteus, which acts to

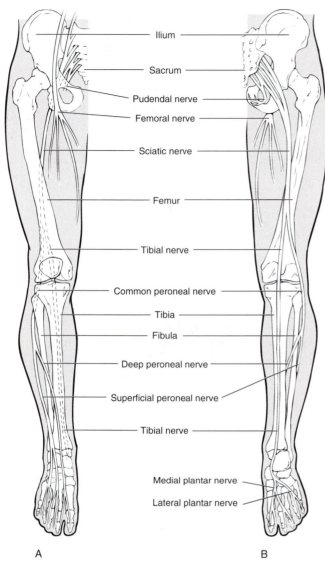

➤ FIGURE 15.4 Innervation of the knee. A, Anterior view. B, Posterior view.

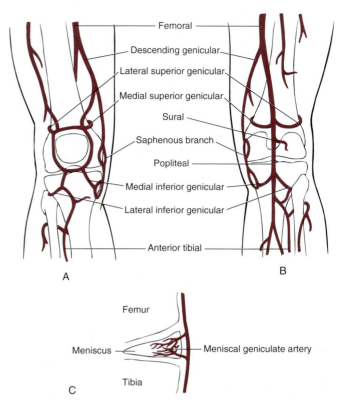

➤ FIGURE 15.5 Collateral circulation around the knee. A, Anterior view. B, Posterior view. C, Circulation to meniscus.

externally rotate the femur with respect to the tibia, thereby freeing the joint for motion.

Once the knee is unlocked from full extension, bony contact is diminished and motion in the transverse and frontal planes becomes freer. In an open kinetic chain, the popliteus causes internal rotation of the tibia on the femur. As the knee moves into flexion, the femur slides anteriorly on the tibia, and the menisci move posteriorly. During extension, the reverse occurs; the femur slides posteriorly on the tibia, and the menisci move anteriorly.

Rotation and Passive Abduction and Adduction

Rotational capability of the tibia with respect to the femur is maximal at approximately 90° of knee flexion. A few degrees of passive abduction and adduction are also permitted when the joint is positioned in the vicinity of 30° of flexion.

Knee Motion During Gait

During midstance of normal gait, the knee is flexed to about 20°, internally rotated approximately 5°, and slightly abducted. Knee motion during the swing phase includes about 70° of flexion, 15° of external rotation, and 5° of adduction. Gait is explained in more detail in Chapter 16.

Patellofemoral Joint Motion

During flexion and extension movements, the patella glides in the trochlear groove, primarily in a vertical direction with an excursion of as much as 8 cm. The patella also undergoes medial and lateral displacement as the tibia is rotated laterally and medially, respectively.

Tracking of the patella against the femur is dependent on the direction of the net force produced by the attached quadriceps. The vastus lateralis tends to pull the patella laterally in the direction of the muscle's action line, parallel to the femoral shaft. The IT band and lateral extensor retinaculum also exert a lateral force on the patella. Although there is considerable debate as to the role of the VMO, it seems to oppose the lateral pull of the vastus lateralis, thereby keeping the patella centered in the patellofemoral groove. If the magnitude of the force produced by the vastus lateralis exceeds that produced by the VMO, the patella is pulled laterally out of its groove during tracking. Mistracking of the patella during knee flexion/extension can be extremely painful and lead to several chronic patellofemoral conditions.

KINETICS OF THE KNEE

Because the knee is positioned between the body's two longest bony levers, the femur and the tibia, the potential for torque and force development at the knee is great. The key role played by the knee during weight-bearing also makes the knee subject to large forces during the gait cycle.

Forces at the Tibiofemoral Joints

Both compression and shear forces are created at the tibiofemoral joints during daily activities. Weight-bearing and tension development in muscles crossing the knee contribute to these forces, with compression dominating when the knee is fully extended. As knee flexion occurs and the angle at the joint increases to 90°, the shear component of joint force produced by weight-bearing increases. Shear at the knee, which causes a tendency for the femur to displace anteriorly on the tibial plateaus, must be resisted by the ligaments and other supportive structures crossing the knee. Because these structures can be stretched or even ruptured under such stress, activities like deep knee bends and full squats that require load-bearing during extreme knee flexion are not recommended.

Compressive force at the tibiofemoral joint can reach an estimated three times body weight during the stance phase of gait, increasing to around four times body weight during stair climbing. During sport participation, knee forces are undoubtedly greater, although quantitative estimates are lacking. It is also well known that tension in the knee extensors increases lateral stability of the knee, with tension in the knee flexors contributing to medial stability.

The menisci assist with force absorption at the knee, bearing as much as an estimated 45% of the total load (9). The medial two-thirds of each meniscus has an internal structure particularly well-suited to resisting compression. The menisci also serve to distribute force from the femur over a broader area, thus reducing the magnitude of joint stress. Tibiofemoral joint stress is an estimated three times higher during weight-bearing when the menisci have been removed. Because the menisci also serve to protect the articulating bone surfaces from wear, knees that have undergone complete or partial meniscectomies may still function adequately, but are more likely to develop degenerative conditions.

Forces at the Patellofemoral Joint

Compressive force at the patellofemoral joint has been found to be half the body weight during normal walking gait, increasing up to more than three times body weight during stair climbing. The squat exercise, known for being particularly stressful to the knee complex, produces a patellofemoral joint reaction force more than seven times body weight. Given the small contact area between the articulating bone surfaces, the transmitted stress at the patellofemoral joint during such maneuvers is high. The point of application of the resultant contact force moves superiorly as the knee goes through 20 to 90° of flexion (10).

PREVENTION OF KNEE INJURIES

Prevention of knee injuries must focus on a well-rounded physical conditioning program, because many of the muscles that move the knee also move the hip. Although much debate continues as to the effectiveness of prophylactic knee braces (see Chapter 3, Prophylactic Knee Braces), recent rule changes and improved shoe design have contributed significantly to a reduction of injuries at the knee.

Physical Conditioning

The development of a well-rounded physical conditioning program is the key to injury prevention. Exercises should include flexibility and muscular strength, endurance, and power, as well as speed, agility, balance, and cardiovascular fitness. Stretching exercises should focus on the quadriceps, hamstrings, gastrocnemius, IT band, and adductors. Because many of these muscles contribute to knee stability, strengthening programs should also focus on these muscle groups. Specific exercises to prevent injury to the musculature that moves the knee are provided in **Field Strategy 15.1**. Additional exercises for muscles that cross the hip region were demonstrated in Field Strategy 14.1. Many of these exercises can be supplemented with tubing to add resistance to the exercise.

Rule Changes

Rule changes in contact sports, particularly football, have significantly reduced injuries to the knee region. Modifications in acceptable techniques that prohibit blocking at or below the knee, and blocking from behind, have reduced traumatic injuries. Proper training methods on correct technique should continue throughout the season to ensure compliance with specific rules designed to prevent injury.

Shoe Design

In Chapter 3, changes in shoe design were discussed. In field sports, shoes may have a flat-sole, long cleat, short cleat, or a multicleated design (see Figure 3.18). The cleats should be properly positioned under the major weight-bearing joints of the foot, and should not be felt through the sole of the shoe. Research has shown that shoes with the longer irregular cleats placed at the peripheral margin of the sole with a number of smaller pointed cleats in the middle produce higher torsional resistance and are associated with a significantly higher ACL injury rate when compared to shoe models with flat cleats and screw-in cleats, or with pivot disc models (11). In football, a cleated shoe with a higher number of shorter, broader cleats can

FIELD STRATEGY 15.1   EXERCISES TO PREVENT INJURY AT THE KNEE

A. **Hamstrings stretch, seated position**. Place the leg to be stretched straight out with the opposite foot tucked toward the groin. Reach toward the toes until a stretch is felt.

B. **Quadriceps stretch, prone position**. Push the heel toward the buttocks, then raise the knee off the floor until tension is felt.

C. **Iliotibial band stretch, supine position**. With the trunk stabilized, adduct the leg to be stretched over the other leg and allow gravity to passively stretch the IT band.

D. **Iliotibial band stretch, standing position**. Cross the limb to be stretched behind the other, extending and adducting the hip as far as possible.

E. **Closed-chain exercises**:
   1. Step-ups, step-downs, and lateral step-ups
   2. Squats (Never below 85–90°)
   3. Leg press
   4. Lunges

F. **Open-chain exercises**:
   1. Knee extension (quadriceps)
   2. Knee flexion (hamstrings)

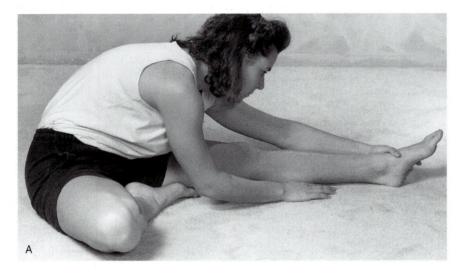

A

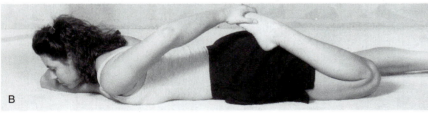

B

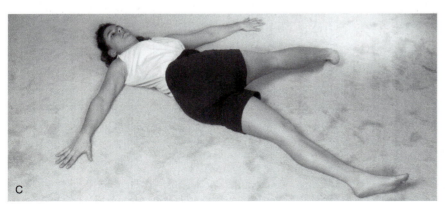

C

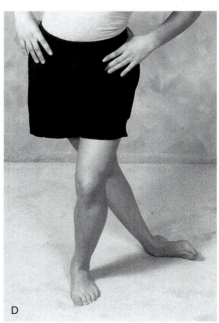

D

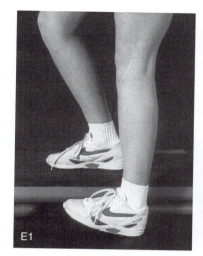
E1

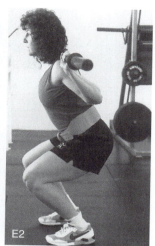
E2

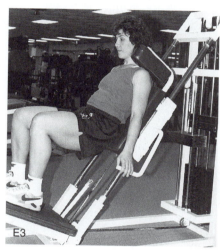
E3

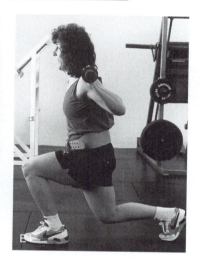

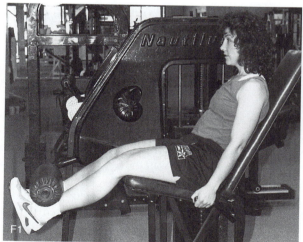
F1

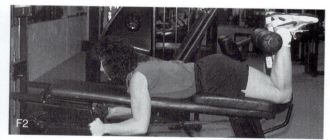
F2

prevent the foot from becoming fixed to the ground, yet still allow for good traction on running and cutting maneuvers.

CONTUSIONS

 A basketball player fell on the knee and felt an intense pain on the anterior of the joint. There is palpable pain on either side of the patellar tendon, but not directly on the tendon. When the knee is moved into full extension, pain significantly increases. What condition may be present, and how will you manage the injury?

Contusions resulting from compressive forces (i.e., a kick or falling on the knee) are common at the knee. General signs and symptoms include localized tenderness, pain, swelling, and ecchymosis. If swelling is extensive, other injuries may be obscured. For example, being kicked on the medial aspect of the tibia may appear as a contusion, when in fact the impact may have caused an avulsion fracture of the MCL or an epiphyseal injury in an adolescent. Extreme point tenderness and positive findings on any of the special tests should indicate a more serious injury, and referral to a physician is indicated.

Fat Pad Contusion

The infrapatellar fat pad may become entrapped between the femur and tibia, or inflamed during arthroscopy, leading to a tender, puffy, fat pad contusion.

➤ SIGNS AND SYMPTOMS

Signs and symptoms include locking, catching, giving way, palpable pain on either side of the patellar tendon, and extreme pain on forced extension.

➤ MANAGEMENT

After a full assessment to rule out fracture and major ligament damage, initial treatment includes ice, compression, elevation, rest, and nonsteroidal anti-inflammatory drugs (NSAIDs). Sport activity is usually not limited. The area, however, should be protected to prevent further insult.

Peroneal Nerve Contusion

The common peroneal nerve leaves the popliteal space and winds around the fibular neck to supply motor and sensory function to the anterior and lateral compartments of the lower leg (see Figure 15.4). A kick or blow to the posterolateral aspect of the knee can contuse this nerve, leading to temporary or permanent paralysis. The nerve may also be injured by prolonged compression from a knee brace or elastic wrap, prolonged squatting (e.g., baseball or softball catcher), or by traction due to a varus stress or hyperextension at the knee.

➤ SIGNS AND SYMPTOMS

In a mild injury, an immediate "shocking" feeling of pain may radiate down the lateral aspect of the leg and foot. If the actual nerve is not damaged, tingling and numbness may persist for several minutes. In severe cases where the nerve is crushed, initial pain is not immediately followed by tingling or numbness. Rather, as swelling increases within the nerve sheath, muscle weakness in dorsiflexion or eversion, and loss of sensation on the dorsum of the foot, particularly between the great and second toes, may progressively occur days or weeks later.

➤ MANAGEMENT

Treatment involves standard acute care for contusions. If the condition does not rapidly improve, however, carefully monitor any sensory changes or motor weakness as previously indicated, and refer the individual to a physician at the first sign of change.

 The basketball player probably contused the infrapatellar fat pad during the fall onto the knee. After assessing for a possible fracture, apply ice with compression. Rest and activity modification, along with NSAIDs when appropriate, should be sufficient to address the injury.

BURSITIS

 A cyclist is complaining of pain on the proximal, medial tibia just distal to the knee joint. It has been bothersome for nearly 2 weeks, especially after he completes his workout. What structure may be inflamed? Are there any factors which may contribute to this condition?

Bursitis may be caused by direct trauma, overuse, infections, metabolic abnormalities, rheumatic afflictions, and **neoplasms** (tumors). Compressive forces from a direct blow can be associated with a grossly distended, warm bursal sac filled with bloody effusion, called a hemobursa. Repeated insult can lead to the more common chronic bursitis. Here, the bursal wall thickens and when filled with fluid, appears distended.

Abrasions or penetrating injuries can lead to infected bursitis caused by bacteria entering the broken skin. This condition differs from acute bursitis because of the localized intense redness, increased pain, enlarged regional lymph nodes, spreading cellulitis, and subsequent fever and malaise.

 *If infection is suspected, immediate referral to a physician is warranted for proper cleansing, irrigation, and closure (often with a drain). The infection can enter the lymph system, causing **pyarthrosis**, or suppurative arthritis, at the knee.*

With the exception of puncture wounds, the suprapatellar bursa is rarely injured by direct trauma. It may, however, become enlarged and inflamed secondary to inflammation in the knee joint capsule.

Because of its location, the prepatellar bursa is commonly injured by compressive forces **(Figure 15.6)**. Swelling may occur immediately or over a 24-hour period, obscuring the visible outline of the patella. Direct pressure over the bursa, and passive flexion of the knee, lead to considerable pain. With chronic prepatellar bursitis, the condition may remain asymptomatic, except for mild discomfort when firm pressure is applied directly over the bursa.

Whereas the prepatellar bursa is injured more frequently by direct blows and shearing forces, as when an athlete dives for a loose ball on a basketball floor, inflammation of the deep infrapatellar bursa is usually caused by overuse and subsequent friction between the patellar tendon and structures behind it (fat pad and tibia). Because this bursa lies posterior to the patellar tendon, inflammation of the bursa is often confused with Osgood-Schlatter's

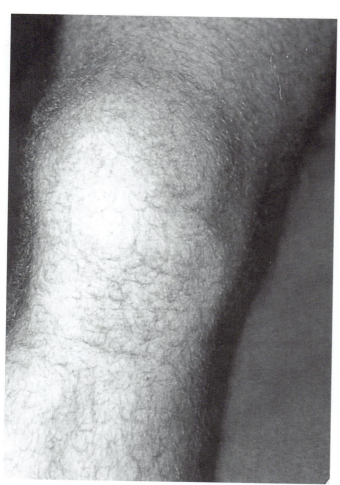

➤ **FIGURE 15.6 Prepatellar bursitis.** The prepatellar bursa is commonly injured by compression from a direct blow, or during a fall on a flexed knee. When injured, the bursa appears grossly distended and swollen.

disease in adolescents, and patellar tendinitis in older individuals. In extension, the fat pad is squeezed between the patellar tendon and tibia, and often extends beyond the sides of the tendon. Careful palpation over the distal patellar tendon and noting the specific area of tenderness determines which condition is present. In flexion, bursitis would be indicated by pain deep to the patellar tendon. In extension, pain palpated on either side of the patellar tendon would indicate a fat pad contusion.

Inflammation of the pes anserine bursa typically develops from friction, but may also occur in direct trauma. It is often seen in runners, cyclists, and swimmers who are subjected to excessive valgus stress at the knee, or in individuals who have tight hamstrings. Initial symptoms include point tenderness beneath the pes tendons (usually 2 cm below the joint line), localized swelling, pain aggravated by flexion of the knee, and crepitation. To avoid recurrence, the athlete should begin an extensive flexibility program for the hamstrings and gastrocnemius-soleus complex.

The term Baker's cyst identifies almost any synovial herniation of the posterior joint capsule, or bursitis on the posterior aspect of the knee. With no obstruction posteriorly, internal derangement injuries (i.e., meniscal problems, cruciate ligament tears, or arthritis) commonly lead to joint effusion that expands into the bursal sac. The semimembranosus bursa is most commonly involved, as it often communicates with the joint capsule. A soft, tumorous mass can be palpated in the medial popliteal space, and may or may not be painful. A Baker's cyst does not pose a serious problem, although it may be bothersome during full flexion or extension of the knee.

➤ SIGNS AND SYMPTOMS

Common symptoms of bursitis include swelling (prepatellar bursitis) and pain in the prepatellar region (prepatellar bursitis), in the distal patellar tendon region (deep infrapatellar bursitis), in the proximal medial tibia (pes anserine bursitis), or over the medial joint line (tibial collateral ligament bursitis).

➤ MANAGEMENT

Treatment consists of ice therapy, a compressive wrap, NSAIDs, avoiding activities that irritate the condition, or total rest until acute symptoms subside. A protective foam, or doughnut pad, may protect the area from further insult.

 If the skin is broken during the initial injury, there is a risk of infection. The individual should be referred immediately to a physician, who may culture any aspirated fluid to detect bacteria, and subsequently prescribe medication.

Corticosteroid injections may be administered by the physician when other means of treatment have been ineffective in decreasing inflammation. Because these injections can weaken surrounding tendons or ligaments, they should not be injected close to these structures.

The cyclist has pes anserine bursitis. Tight hamstrings and excessive valgus stress placed on the knee during the pedaling motion can predispose an individual to this injury. After initial acute care, this individual should begin an extensive flexibility program for the hamstrings and gastrocnemius-soleus complex.

LIGAMENTOUS INJURIES

A football player set the right foot, then forcefully pushed off the right leg to evade an oncoming tackler. Suddenly the player was tackled from behind from the right rear side. The individual was slow in getting up but was able to limp off the field, bearing the majority of his weight only on his left leg and the toes of the right foot. There is extreme pain on the medial aspect of the knee but only mild swelling. What structures might have been damaged? What is your course of action?

Knee joint stability depends primarily on a static, passive system of support from its ligaments and capsular structures, rather than from an active, dynamic system from the surrounding muscles. Bones and menisci provide some additional stability via their shape and inherent stability when two adjoining structures are in a close packed position. The American Academy of Orthopaedic Surgeons (AAOS) classifies ligamentous injuries at the knee according to the functional disruption of a specific ligament, or amount of laxity **(Box 15.2)**, and direction of laxity, which identifies four straight instabilities and four rotary instabilities **(Table 15.3)**. Knowing the knee position at impact and the direction the tibia displaces or rotates reveals the damaged structures.

Unidirectional Instabilities

A straight plane (unidirectional) instability implies instability in one of the cardinal planes. For example, injury to the ACL or PCL results in instability in the sagittal plane, allowing for equal anterior or posterior **translation** (shifting) of the medial and lateral tibial plateaus on the femur, whereas injury to the MCL and LCL leads to valgus or varus instability in the frontal plane. This type of injury involves damage that is isolated to a single structure.

STRAIGHT MEDIAL INSTABILITY

In straight medial instability, or **valgus instability**, lateral forces cause tension on the medial aspect of the knee, potentially damaging the MCL and posteromedial capsular ligaments, as well as the PCL **(Figure 15.7)**.

➤ SIGNS AND SYMPTOMS

A grade I sprain is characterized by mild pain on the medial joint line, little to no joint effusion, full range of

---

> ➤➤ **BOX 15.2**

Signs and Symptoms of Ligament Failure

MINIMAL LIGAMENT FAILURE (<5 MM DISTRACTION)

- Less than one-third of the fibers are torn
- Mild swelling and pain are localized over the injury site (with the MCL, pain is in the proximal 1 to 2 inches)
- Active and passive ROM are normal; muscular strength is normal or slightly decreased
- No joint laxity is apparent during stress test
- Definite end feel is present

PARTIAL LIGAMENT FAILURE (5–10 MM DISTRACTION)

- One-third to two-thirds of the ligament has been damaged, with microtears present
- Localized swelling and joint effusion may be due to deep capsular tears, meniscal damage, or cruciate ligament damage
- Pain is sharp and may be either transient or lasting
- Individual may complain of instability and an inability to walk with the heel on the ground
- ROM is decreased initially by pain and hamstring muscle spasm, later by soft tissue swelling or effusion
- Inability to fully extend the knee actively
- Visible translation of the tibia during stress tests

COMPLETE LIGAMENT FAILURE (>10 MM DISTRACTION)

- More than two-thirds of the ligament has been ruptured
- Swelling is diffuse, indicating severe capsular tear and damage to intracapsular structures
- Pain is initially sharp, and often disappears within a minute
- Individual is aware of the feeling of instability or the knee giving way
- Significant loss of ROM
- Visible distraction greater than 10 mm during stress testing that may appear as a subluxation

---

motion that may include some discomfort, and a stable joint when doing the valgus stress test. A positive valgus test in 30° of flexion with a positive end feel indicates at least a grade 2 injury to the middle third of the capsular ligament and MCL. The individual may be unable to fully extend the leg, and will often walk on the ball of the foot, unable to keep the heel flat on the ground. Often there is no significant intra-articular effusion in a grade 3 MCL injury, but if this is found, injuries to the cruciate ligaments, patella, or meniscus should be assessed. A grade 3 injury will have a positive valgus test with a soft or even absent end point, owing to a complete tear of the MCL, usually at the femoral attachment.

STRAIGHT LATERAL INSTABILITY

Straight lateral instability, or **varus instability**, results from medial forces that produce tension on the lateral compartment, damaging the LCL, lateral capsular liga-

TABLE 15.3 CLASSIFICATION OF KNEE INSTABILITY AND STRUCTURES INJURED

Instability	Tests Used to Assess Instability	Possible Structures Injured if Test Is Positive
Straight valgus (medial)	Abduction (valgus) stress with knee in full extension	1. Medial collateral ligament 2. Oblique popliteal ligament 3. Posteromedial capsule 4. Anterior cruciate ligament 5. Posterior cruciate ligament 6. Medial quadriceps expansion 7. Semimembranosus muscle
	Abduction (valgus) stress with knee slightly flexed (20 to 30°)	1. Medial collateral ligament 2. Oblique popliteal ligament 3. Posterior cruciate ligament
Straight varus (lateral)	Adduction (varus) stress with knee in full extension	1. Lateral collateral ligament 2. Posterolateral capsule 3. Arcuate-popliteus complex 4. Biceps femoris tendon 5. Anterior cruciate ligament 6. Posterior cruciate ligament 7. Lateral gastrocnemius muscle
	Adduction (varus) stress with knee slightly flexed (20 to 30°) and tibia laterally rotated	1. Lateral collateral ligament 2. Posterolateral capsule 3. Arcuate-popliteus complex 4. Iliotibial band 5. Biceps femoris tendon
Straight anterior	Anterior drawer test (90° knee flexion)	1. Anterior cruciate ligament (anteromedial bundle) 2. Posterolateral and posteromedial capsule 3. Deep medial collateral ligament 4. Iliotibial band 5. Oblique popliteal ligament 6. Arcuate-popliteus complex
	Lachman's test Modified Lachman's test	1. Anterior cruciate ligament (anteromedial bundle) 2. Oblique popliteal ligament 3. Arcuate-popliteus complex
Straight posterior	Posterior sag (gravity) test Posterior drawer sign Reverse Lachman's test	1. Posterior cruciate ligament (anterolateral bundle) 2. Arcuate-popliteus complex 3. Oblique popliteal ligament 4. Anterior cruciate ligament
Anteromedial rotary	Slocum drawer test (tibia internally rotated)	1. Medial collateral ligament 2. Oblique popliteal ligament 3. Posteromedial capsule 4. Anterior cruciate ligament
Anterolateral rotary	Slocum drawer test (tibia externally rotated) Lateral pivot shift test Jerk test Slocum ALRI Crossover test Flexion-rotation drawer test	1. Anterior cruciate ligament 2. Posterolateral capsule 3. Arcuate-popliteus complex 4. Lateral collateral ligament 5. Iliotibial band
Posteromedial rotary	Posteromedial drawer test Posteromedial pivot shift test	1. Posterior cruciate ligament 2. Oblique popliteal ligament 3. Medial collateral ligament 4. Semimembranosus muscle 5. Posteromedial capsule 6. Anterior cruciate ligament
Posterolateral rotary	Posterolateral drawer test External rotation recurvatum test	1. Posterior cruciate ligament 2. Arcuate-popliteus complex 3. Lateral collateral ligament 4. Biceps femoris tendon 5. Posterolateral capsule 6. Anterior cruciate ligament

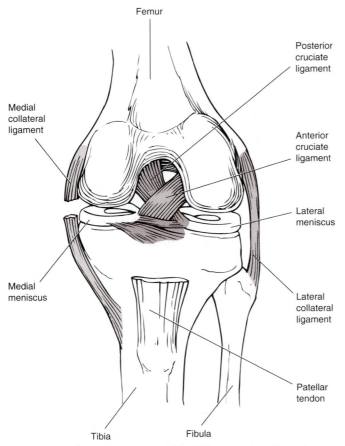

➤ **FIGURE 15.7 Valgus instability**. When a valgus force is applied to the knee, the tibial collateral ligament and medial capsular ligaments are damaged, leading to valgus laxity.

ments, PCL, and joint structures **(Figure 15.8)**. This isolated injury is rare because the biceps femoris, IT band, and popliteus provide a strong stabilizing effect. In wrestling, however, the opponent is often between the individual's legs and is able to deliver an excessive varus force that can lead to injury.

➤ SIGNS AND SYMPTOMS

Damage to the LCL follows general signs and symptoms associated with an MCL sprain. Occasionally, the individual may hear or feel a pop, accompanied by sharp lateral pain. Swelling will be minimal because the ligament is not attached to the joint capsule. Instability will be subtle because other structures are intact, but a positive varus test in 30° of flexion should confirm damage to the ligament. If tenderness is detected on the head of the fibula, an avulsion fracture or peroneal nerve injury may be present, although these injuries are usually associated with more severe knee injuries (12).

STRAIGHT ANTERIOR INSTABILITY

With straight anterior instability, both tibial plateaus sublux anteriorly an equal amount when an anterior drawer test is performed. This translation is resisted by the ACL.

Isolated anterior instability is rare. Instead, an anteromedial or anterolateral laxity usually occurs. Damage to the ACL commonly occurs during a cutting or turning maneuver, landing, or sudden deceleration **(Figure 15.9)**. The rate of ACL injuries is higher in women, particularly for those in jumping and pivoting sports. Several theories have been put forth to explain this phenomenon **(Box 15.3)**. Recent research has begun to look at muscle strength imbalance between the hamstrings and quadriceps. During a landing/deceleration maneuver, flexion moments are occurring at the hip and knee. Simultaneous eccentric contractions of the quadriceps to stabilize the knee, and the hamstrings to stabilize the hip, decelerate the horizontal velocity of the body. The hamstrings also act to neutralize the tendency of the quadriceps to cause anterior tibial translation. If the muscles are unable to meet the demand of stabilization, inert internal tissues, such as ligaments, cartilage, and bone, are at risk for injury. Therefore, a deficit in eccentric hamstrings strength relative to eccentric quadriceps strength could predispose an athlete to an ACL injury.

➤ SIGNS AND SYMPTOMS

Pain can range from minimal and transient to severe and lasting. It may be described as being deep in the knee, but is more often felt anterior on either side of the patellar

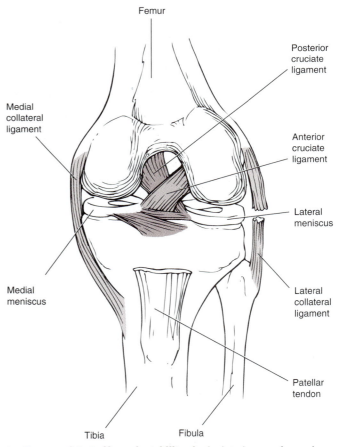

➤ **FIGURE 15.8 Varus instability**. An isolated varus force damages the fibular collateral ligament, leading to varus laxity.

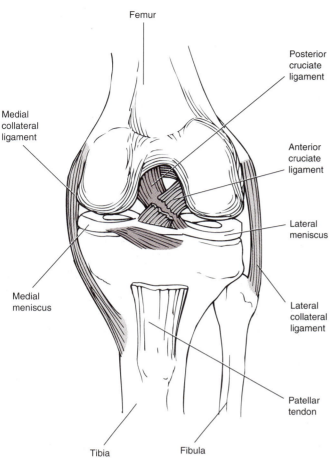

Femur

Posterior
cruciate
ligament

Medial
collateral
ligament

Anterior
cruciate
ligament

Lateral
meniscus

Medial
meniscus

Lateral
collateral
ligament

Patellar
tendon

Tibia   Fibula

➤ FIGURE 15.9 **Anterior instability**. When changing directions during deceleration, as occurs in basketball, the anterior cruciate ligament can be damaged.

tendon or laterally on the joint line. In about 80% of all ACL injuries, patients experience a popping, snapping, or tearing sensation, and a similar percentage note a rapid onset of swelling (hemarthrosis), usually within 3 hours. Weight-bearing leads to a feeling of the knee giving way or "just not feeling right." The high incidence of damage to other internal structures necessitates immediate referral to a physician.

STRAIGHT POSTERIOR INSTABILITY

In straight posterior instability, the medial and lateral tibial plateaus have equal translation posteriorly in a neutral position without rotation. The PCL, along with the arcuate complex and oblique popliteal ligament, provides nearly all resistance to prevent this motion. Hyperextension is the most common mechanism for injury, although the PCL can also be damaged during a fall on a flexed knee with the foot plantar flexed, resulting in a blow to the tibial tubercle that drives the tibia posteriorly **(Figure 15.10)**.

➤ SIGNS AND SYMPTOMS

In milder cases, intense pain and a sense of stretching are felt in the posterior aspect of the knee. In a total rupture,

a characteristic pop or snap is felt and heard. Effusion and hemarthrosis occur rapidly, and the individual is acutely aware of swelling. Knee extension is limited because of the effusion and stretching of the posterior capsule and gastrocnemius. A positive posterior sag (gravity) test or reverse Lachman's test confirms damage to the PCL. When the PCL is torn, the extensor mechanism, including the patella and patellar tendon, forcefully holds the tibia in a reduced position, which results in increased patellofemoral pressure. Increased patellofemoral loading is also caused by a vector change resulting from posterior tibial displacement, which may explain complaints of patellofemoral pain in individuals with PCL-deficient knees.

Multidirectional Instabilities

Whereas unidirectional instability involves damage that is isolated to a single structure, a multidirectional instability involves injury to multiple structures (e.g., the ACL and MCL). This injury is also called a multiplane or rotary instability.

ANTEROMEDIAL ROTARY INSTABILITY

Anteromedial rotary instability (AMRI) results from anterior external rotation of the medial tibia condyle on

---

➤➤ BOX 15.3

Possible Factors Influencing Increased Rate of ACL Injuries in Women

INTRINSIC FACTORS
- Ligament size
- Ligament laxity
- Intercondylar notch dimensions
- Limb alignment (wider pelvis, femoral anteversion, genu valgum, and external tibial torsion)
- Estrogen and estrogen receptors
- Cruciate-dependent knee

EXTRINSIC FACTORS
- Level of skill
- Level of experience
- Shoe-floor friction
- Ankle prophylactic braces
- Stylistic differences in sport play
    Plant and cut
    Straight-leg landing
    One-step stop landing with the knee hyperextended
    Pivoting with sudden deceleration
- Muscle strength imbalance (eccentric hamstrings strength relative to eccentric quadriceps strength)

Adapted from Moul (11), pages 118-121 and Moeller and Lamb (13), pages 41-48.

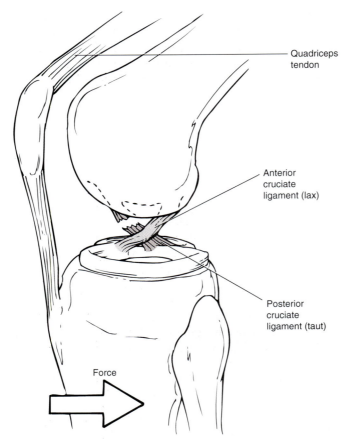

Quadriceps
tendon

Anterior
cruciate
ligament (lax)

Posterior
cruciate
ligament (taut)

Force

➤ FIGURE 15.10 **Posterior instability**. During hyperextension of the knee or when the knee is flexed and the tibia is driven posterior, the posterior cruciate ligament can be damaged.

the femur, leading to damage of the medial compartment ligaments and the oblique popliteal ligament **(Figure 15.11)**. This instability can be accentuated by a tear of the medial meniscus and ACL. Although referred to as the "unhappy triad," the MCL is the primary ligamentous restraint to this motion. With anteromedial rotary instability, valgus stress testing at 0 and 30° of flexion is positive. In addition, there is increased anterior translation of the medial tibial plateau when a Slocum drawer test or Lachman's test is performed with the tibia externally rotated.

ANTEROLATERAL ROTARY INSTABILITY

Anterolateral rotary instability (ALRI) is characteristic of an anterior internal subluxation of the lateral tibial condyle on the femur. The ACL is the primary structure damaged by this instability, but the IT band and lateral capsule ligaments can also be damaged. The injury is typically caused by a sudden deceleration and cutting maneuver, and is the most frequent rotatory instability at the knee. With anterolateral instability, the Slocum drawer test with the tibia internally rotated, jerk test, Slocum ALRI test, crossover test, and flexion-rotation drawer test show increased anterior translation of the lateral tibial plateau.

POSTEROMEDIAL ROTARY INSTABILITY

In posteromedial rotary instability (PMRI), the medial tibial plateau shifts posteriorly on the femur and opens medially. This is a severe injury and is indicative of damage

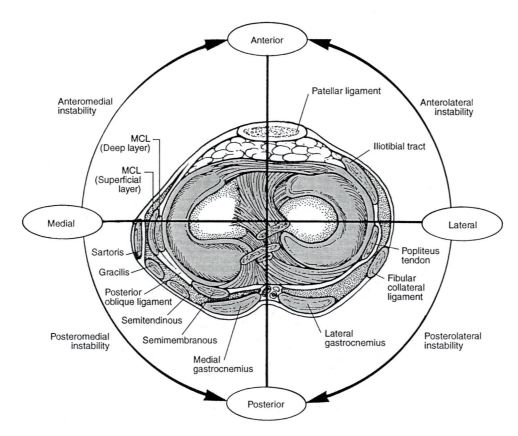

Anterior

Anteromedial
instability

Patellar ligament

Anterolateral
instability

MCL
(Deep layer)

MCL
(Superficial
layer)

Iliotibial tract

Medial

Lateral

Sartoris

Gracilis

Popliteus
tendon

Posterior
oblique ligament

Fibular
collateral
ligament

Semitendinous

Semimembranous

Lateral
gastrocnemius

Medial
gastrocnemius

Posteromedial
instability

Posterolateral
instability

Posterior

➤ FIGURE 15.11 **Instabilities at the knee**. MCL = medial collateral ligament. Adapted with permission from Magee DJ: Orthopedic Physical Assessment, 3rd ed. Philadelphia: WB Saunders, 1997:535.

to the superficial MCL, posteromedial capsule, oblique popliteal ligament, and both cruciate ligaments. Injury of the posteromedial capsule is suspected if joint space opening and a soft end point are apparent on valgus stress at 0°. The posteromedial drawer test and posteromedial pivot shift test will be positive.

POSTEROLATERAL ROTARY INSTABILITY

In posterolateral rotary instability (PLRI), there is a greater posterior translation of the lateral tibial plateau, as compared with the medial tibial plateau, when a posterior drawer force is applied. This injury is often caused by a sudden anteromedial force that brings the knee joint from near-full extension into hyperextension, resulting in rupture to the posterolateral structures. These structures include the PCL, arcuate-popliteal complex, posterolateral capsule, and LCL. Injury of the posterolateral capsule is suspected if joint space opening and a soft end point are apparent on varus stress at 0 and 30°. Additionally, the posterolateral drawer and external rotation recurvatum tests are positive.

Knee Dislocations

Knee dislocations and less severe multiple-ligament injuries make up about 20% of all grade III knee ligament injuries. Frequent two-ligament injuries include the ACL-MCL (most common), PCL-MCL, ACL-LCL, and ACL-PCL. Damage to only two ligaments does not result in enough translation of the joint to cause neurovascular injury. The exception is injury to the LCL and a cruciate ligament that results in enough lateral opening to damage the peroneal nerve, as noted earlier.

To dislocate the knee, at least three ligaments must be torn. Most often, this involves the ACL, PCL, and one collateral ligament. Although dislocations may occur in any direction, the most common is in an anterior or posterior direction. As with any dislocation, additional damage can occur to other joint structures, including the ligaments, capsular structures, menisci, articular surfaces, tendons, and neurovascular structures. Associated injuries include vascular damage in 20 to 40% of all knee dislocations and nerve damage in 20 to 30%. Posterior knee dislocations are associated with the highest incidence of damage to the popliteal artery, with posterolateral rotary dislocations having the highest incidence of nerve injury (5).

➤ SIGNS AND SYMPTOMS

An athlete may describe a severe injury to the knee and hearing a loud pop. Deformity of the knee may be present if the knee dislocated and remained unreduced. Unfortunately, knee dislocations often reduce spontaneously, making identification difficult. Swelling occurs within the first few hours, but may not be large due to an associated capsular injury and extravasation of the hemarthrosis. It is critical to identify the dislocated knee by the ligamentous structures that have been disrupted. If a vascular injury is present and left untreated, or not repaired within 8 hours after injury, there is an 86% amputation rate. If surgery is completed within 6 to 8 hours, the amputation rate drops to 11%. Associated nerve injury has a poor prognosis, regardless of the treatment (5).

Management of Ligament Injuries

Injuries involving minimal ligament failure are managed conservatively with ice application, compression, elevation, and protected rest until acute symptoms subside. A compression wrap, consisting of an inverted horseshoe around the patella secured by an elastic wrap, can be used with a knee immobilizer to reduce swelling. Cryotherapy and NSAIDs are used to reduce pain and inflammation. In suspected ACL injuries, radiographs should be obtained to rule out an associated intra-articular fracture. Avulsion fractures of the tibial eminence may occur, particularly in adults over 35 who have some associated osteopenia. Magnetic resonance imaging (MRI) is not generally used to diagnose an ACL injury, although it may be used to determine an associated meniscal tear, which is known to occur in 50 to 70% of patients with ACL tears (14).

In consultation with the team physician, a moderate injury with partial ligament failure is managed with ice, compression, elevation, and protected rest for 24 to 72 hours. Crutches are used until the individual walks without a limp. Progression to partial weight-bearing with heel-to-toe gait can begin as tolerated. Rehabilitation should be initiated as soon as acute symptoms subside. Range-of-motion exercises should include assisted knee flexion and knee extension. Isometric exercises of the quadriceps and straight leg raises in all directions should progress to resisted exercises throughout the full range of motion. Closed chain strengthening exercises and maintenance of range of motion can be supplemented by cardiovascular exercises as tolerated.

In injuries in which isolated complete ligament failure has occurred, or when more than one major ligament is involved, the team physician may determine that surgical repair is necessary. Surgical reconstruction is based on the degree of laxity, sport-specific demands, hours per week of activity, intensity of activity, frequency of instability, associated repairable meniscal tear, and side-to-side differences measured by maximum manual testing with a KT-1000 arthrometer. Reconstruction is usually delayed at least 3 weeks postinjury to allow for swelling to decrease and range of motion to increase. **Field Strategy 15.2** lists management and rehabilitation of a mild ACL injury.

 The football player reported a sharp pain on the anteromedial knee after being tackled from the rear. He was unable to put any weight on the right heel when he limped off the field. You should suspect a possible MCL and ACL injury. After

FIELD STRATEGY 15.2 MANAGEMENT OF AN ANTERIOR CRUCIATE INJURY

PHASE 1
A. PRICE. Ice, elevation, compression wrap, and rest with a knee immobilizer to reduce swelling
B. Use crutches if the individual cannot bear weight without pain
C. Range-of-motion exercises within pain-free limits:
- Heel slides
- Prone knee flexion assisted with the opposite leg
- Passive knee extension in a supine or seated position
D. Strengthening exercises:
- Bent leg raises in all directions
- Multiangle isometric exercises for the quadriceps, hamstrings, and hip adductors
E. Cardiovascular fitness. UBE and unilateral leg cycling

PHASE 2
A. Range of motion. Continue exercises to regain full range of motion
B. Unilateral balance activities. See Field Strategy 16.1, and progress as tolerated
C. Strengthening exercises:
- Do slow, controlled, eccentric closed-chain exercises, such as two-legged squats to 60°, step-ups, step-downs, and lateral step-ups
- Calf raises (seated position) can progress to standing position when pain free
- Straight leg raises in all directions with tubing added as tolerated

PHASE 3
A. Range of motion. Maintain full range of motion and flexibility in the lower extremity
B. Strengthening:
- Hip leg press and squats
- Toe raises with weights
- Lunges
- Isokinetic open- and closed-chain exercises
C. Cardiovascular fitness:
- Bilateral minimal tension cycling if 110–115° of knee flexion is present. Avoid full knee extension
- Pool running, swimming with a flutter kick, jogging in place on a trampoline, and power walking

PHASE 4
A. Balance and proprioception. Continue exercises from above
B. Functional activities:
- Running drills, e.g., circles, figure-eights, cross-over steps (kariocas), jumping with double limb/single limb progressing from standing in place, front to back, to diagonals
- Multidirectional high-speed balance drills are added after the individual can run 2 to 3 miles
- Jumping, bounding, and skipping (plyometrics)
- Slide board

standard on-site acute care, this individual should be fitted with crutches and referred to a physician for follow-up care.

MENISCAL INJURIES

A 37-year-old tennis player is complaining of mild swelling and tenderness on the medial joint line. Slight joint effusion is present, and pain can be elicited with rotation of the tibia on the femur, and during extreme knee flexion. What injury may be present? How will you manage this injury?

Menisci, which become stiffer and less resilient with age, are injured in similar manners as ligamentous structures. In addition to compression and tensile forces, shearing forces caused when the femur rotates on a fixed tibia trap the posterior horns of both menisci, leading to some tearing. Tears are classified according to age, location, or axis of orientation, and include longitudinal, bucket-handle, horizontal, and parrot-beak. Peak incidence of injuries has been found to occur in men between the ages of 21 and 40, and in girls and women between the ages of 11 and 20, and again between 61 and 70 (15). Medial meniscus damage is more common than lateral meniscus damage.

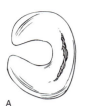 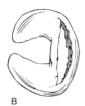 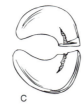 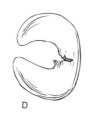

A   B   C   D

▶ **FIGURE 15.12 Meniscal tears**. A, Longitudinal. B, Bucket-handle. C, Horizontal. D, Parrot-beak.

Longitudinal tears result from a twisting motion when the foot is fixed and the knee flexed (**Figure 15.12A**). This action produces compression and torsion on the posterior peripheral attachment. The tear can be partial, affecting only the peripheral segment of the meniscus, or a complete tearing of the inner substance of the meniscus. A "**bucket-handle**" tear occurs when an entire longitudinal segment is displaced medially toward the center of the tibia (**Figure 15.12B**). This tear can lead to locking of the knee at about 10° flexion; however, this occurs in only about 40% of complete meniscal tears. Horizontal cleavage tears result from degeneration, and often affect the posterior medial portion of the meniscus (**Figure 15.12C**). With age, shearing forces from rotational motions tear the inner substance of the meniscus. If detached, momentary locking, associated pain, and instability may occur. A parrot-beak tear is seen in adolescents with a history of previous trauma, or some cystic pathology that makes the meniscus more fixed at its periphery (**Figure 15.12D**). Two tears commonly occur in the middle segment of the lateral meniscus, leading to the characteristic shape of a parrot's beak.

▶ SIGNS AND SYMPTOMS

Meniscal injuries are difficult to assess because they are not innervated by nociceptors, and only the outer 10 to 33% is supplied by blood (5). Localized pain and joint-line tenderness near the collateral ligament are probably the most common findings. Anterior joint-line pain rarely reflects meniscal pathology unless a bucket-handle or ruptured bucket-handle tear is present. Because the meniscal periphery is attached to the synovial lining, tensile forces may cause synovial inflammation and slight joint effusion to occur more than 12 hours after the initial injury. Pain will occur on rotation and extreme flexion of the knee, e.g., duck walk or deep knee squats. A chronic degenerative meniscal tear often results from multiple episodes of minimal trauma leading to almost no pain, disability, or swelling, though atrophy of the quadriceps may be present. Chronic tears in the absence of degeneration have point tenderness only over the site of the lesion. The individual may experience a popping, grinding, or clicking sensation that can lead to the knee buckling or giving way. Special tests used to identify meniscal injuries include McMurray's test, Apley's compression test, and the "bounce home" test.

▶ MANAGEMENT

Initial treatment depends on the extent of damage. Mild cases are managed with standard acute care—ice, compression, elevation, protected rest, NSAIDs, and crutches as needed. Isometric strengthening exercises can be initiated when swelling has subsided. **Field Strategy 15.3** summarizes the initial management and suggested rehabilitation exercises for a mild meniscal injury.

 If joint effusion is extensive, immediate referral to a physician is warranted to aspirate the fluid, if necessary. Immediate referral is also necessary if the knee is locked and cannot be spontaneously reduced, as surgical intervention is needed.

Bucket-handle tear segments can be surgically excised without removing the total meniscus, although regeneration of the centrally displaced portion will not occur. Arthroscopic meniscetomy is done as an outpatient procedure performed under local anesthesia, with return to function following partial meniscetomy within 2 to 6 weeks. Total meniscetomy increases rotary instability and can lead to arthritis.

 The tennis player had mild joint effusion and pain on the medial joint line that increased with rotation and extreme flexion of the knee. This suggests a possible chronic meniscal tear. This individual should be referred to a physician.

PATELLAR AND RELATED INJURIES

 A cross-country runner is complaining of an aching pain on the lateral side of the patella that increases during the workout, particularly when running downhill. Slight effusion is present in the patellofemoral joint, and pain is elicited over the lateral patellar border. Intense pain is felt when the patella is pushed downward into the patellofemoral groove. What factors may contribute to this condition? What long-term management should be considered after acute symptoms have subsided?

The patellofemoral joint is the region most commonly associated with anterior knee pain. Patellar tracking disorders and instability within the joint, along with obesity, direct trauma, and repetitive motions, all contribute to a variety of injuries. Patellofemoral pain may be classified into mechanical causes (such as patellar subluxation or dislocation), inflammatory causes (prepatellar bursitis, patellar tendinitis), and other causes (reflex sympathetic dystrophy, tumors).

The main dynamic stabilizer is the quadriceps mechanism. More accurately called the **extensor mechanism**, this is made up of the vastus lateralis, vastus intermedius,

---

FIELD STRATEGY 15.3   MANAGEMENT OF A PARTIAL MENISECTOMY

PHASE 1

A. PRICE. Ice, elevation, compression, and bracing to reduce swelling. Use crutches if needed

B. Range-of-motion exercises within pain-free limits:
- Heel slides
- Supine wall slides
- Prone knee flexion assisted with the opposite leg
- Passive knee extension in a supine or seated position

PHASE 2

A. Range of motion. Continue exercises as tolerated

B. Unilateral balance activities (see Field Strategy 16.1)

C. Strengthening exercises. Include:
- Multiangle isometric exercises for the quadriceps, hamstrings, and hip adductors
- Straight-leg raises in all directions. Add tubing or ankle weights in later stages
- Short-arc quadriceps extension exercises. Place a pillow or bolster under the knee to support the knee at 45° flexion. Extend the knee, and hold for 10 seconds. Add ankle weights to increase resistance
- Toe raises from a seated position can progress to standing position when pain-free
- Straight leg raises in all directions with tubing added as tolerated

D. Cardiovascular fitness
- UBE, and stationary cycling with bilateral minimal tension if 115–120° of knee flexion is present. Avoid full knee extension

PHASE 3

A. Range of motion. Maintain full range of motion and flexibility in the lower extremity

B. Strengthening:
- Hip leg press and squats
- Toe raises with weights
- Lunges
- Isokinetic open- and closed-chain exercises

C. Cardiovascular fitness:
- Pool running, swimming with a flutter kick, jogging on a trampoline, and power walking

PHASE 4, RETURN TO ACTIVITY

A. Maintain range of motion, flexibility, strength, and balance

B. Functional activities. Same as those listed in Field Strategy 15.2

---

vastus medialis, and rectus femoris, all of which are innervated by the femoral nerve. The vastus medialis (VM) has two heads, the superior longus head (VML), and the more inferior obliquus head (VMO). The VMO fibers approach the patella at a 55° angle. Although the VMO is incapable of producing knee extension, it provides a dynamic restraint to forces that would laterally displace the patella. Atrophy of this muscle is nearly always evident in patellofemoral dysfunction. The pes anserinus muscle group and biceps femoris also affect patellar stability, because they control tibial internal and external rotation, which can significantly influence patellar tracking.

The static stabilizers include the more anteriorly projected lateral aspect of the femoral sulcus, the extensor retinaculum, IT band, quadriceps tendon, and patellar tendon. Oblique condensations of the retinacula produce the patellofemoral ligament and medial and lateral patellotibial ligaments **(Figure 15.13)**. The structures that resist medial

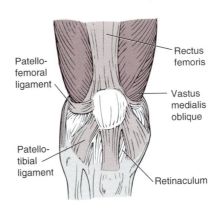

➤ **FIGURE 15.13 Extensor mechanism.** The extensor mechanism is composed of dynamic and static stabilizers. Working together, they combine rolling and gliding motions to place the femur and patella in specific positions to effect the deceleration mechanism of the patellofemoral articulation to provide stability and function at the knee.

displacement of the patella (lateral retinaculum and IT band) are thicker and stronger than the soft-tissue structures that resist laterally displacing forces (medial retinaculum and lateral aspect of femoral sulcus). The patellar tendon resists superiorly displacing forces on the patella, whereas the quadriceps tendon resists inferior displacement of the patella. Both medial and lateral retinacula assist in knee extension even though the patellar tendon may be ruptured.

Deficiencies in stabilization of the extensor mechanism can be caused by several abnormalities of the patellofemoral region **(Box 15.4)**, all of which can lead to anterior knee pain. Each condition can be counterbalanced in a healthy knee by the triangular shape of the patella, depth of the patellofemoral groove, and limiting action of the static ligamentous structures. Failure of medial structures to restrain the patella in a balanced position, or the presence of bony anomalies, can result in lateral tilting or lateral excursion of the patella, which in turn leads to patellofemoral **arthralgia**, or severe joint pain.

Patellofemoral Stress Syndrome

Patellofemoral stress syndrome, also called lateral patellar compression syndrome, is pain in the patellofemoral joint without documented instability. The condition often occurs when either the VMO is weak or the lateral retinaculum that holds the patella firmly to the femoral condyle is excessively tight. Pain results when a tense lateral retinaculum passes over the trochlear groove, or when increased patellofemoral stresses are transferred from the articular cartilage to pain fibers in the subchondral bone.

➤ SIGNS AND SYMPTOMS

The individual may report a dull, aching pain in the anterior knee made worse by squatting, sitting in a tight space with the knee flexed, and descending stairs or slopes.

➤➤ **Box 15.4**

Causes of Patellofemoral Pain

- Patellar instability due to:
  Abnormally shaped medial patellar facet
  Shallow patellofemoral (trochlear) groove
  Variable length and width of the patellar tendon
  Patella alta (high-riding patella)
- Weak VMO or VMO dysplasia
- Hypermobility of the patella due to:
  Muscle atrophy after an injury
  Tightness of the lateral retinaculum, IT band, and hamstrings
- Anatomical malalignment due to:
  Shallow patellofemoral groove
  Excessive femoral anteversion or external tibial rotation
  Genu valgum or genu recurvatum
  Increased Q-angle
  Excessive foot pronation
- Plica syndromes and repetitive minor trauma

Point tenderness can be located over the lateral facet of the patella, with intense pain and crepitus elicited when the patella is manually compressed into the patellofemoral groove. Synovial inflammation may also be present.

➤ MANAGEMENT

Treatment involves standard acute care and NSAIDs. The entire lower extremity should be assessed for gait characteristics, flexibility, and strength of the proximal and distal portions. Note decreased rotation or strength in the lateral rotators of the hip, and tightness in the hamstrings, quadriceps, and Achilles tendon. The McConnell taping technique uses passive taping of the patella to correct patellar position and tracking during knee motion. Other patellofemoral support devices, such as those demonstrated in Chapter 3, are also used to prevent lateral displacement of the patella.

Rehabilitation should focus on recruiting the VMO, normalizing patella mobility, and increasing flexibility and muscle control of the lower extremity. Resisted terminal knee extension exercises, straight leg raises in hip flexion and adduction, and quadriceps isometric, isotonic, and high-speed isokinetic exercises in a 60 to 90° arc may be performed. If the VMO is not monitored through the use of biofeedback devices, however, proper recruitment is difficult to determine. Closed-chain exercises are often preferred because of the decrease in patellofemoral compression forces. Examples of closed kinetic chain exercises include knee flexion in 30 to 70°, and lateral steps up from 1 to 8″ to allow eccentric and concentric movements. Eccentric quadriceps strengthening is emphasized because the quadriceps muscle is an important decelerator. Strengthening of the hip muscles to prevent adduction and internal rotation is critical to allow for the progression of closed-chain exercises. Restoring proprioception is also critical to reestablishing neuromuscular control. Weight training programs that load the patellofemoral joint, such as bent-knee exercises, should be avoided.

Chondromalacia Patellae

Chondromalacia patellae is a true degeneration in the articular cartilage of the patella, which results when compressive forces exceed the normal physical range, or when alterations in patellar excursion produce abnormal shear forces that damage the articular surface. Because articular cartilage does not contain nerve endings, chondromalacia should not be considered the true source of anterior knee pain. (Chrondromalacia is a surgical finding that represents areas of hyaline cartilage trauma or aberrant loading, but is not the cause of pain.) The medial and lateral patellar facets are most commonly involved. The condition is confirmed when pain results from Clarke's test and Waldron's test. Chondromalacia has four stages **(Figure 15.14)**:

➤ MANAGEMENT

Asymptomatic chondromalacia does not require treatment. If the condition becomes symptomatic, follow stan-

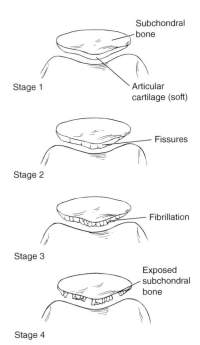

➤ FIGURE 15.14 **Four stages of chondromalacia patellae.** Stage 1 involves softening or blistering of the cartilage. Stage 2 reveals fissures in the cartilage. Stage 3 is reached when fibrillation of the cartilage occurs, causing a "crab-meat" appearance. Stage 4 reveals cartilage defects with subchondral bone exposed.

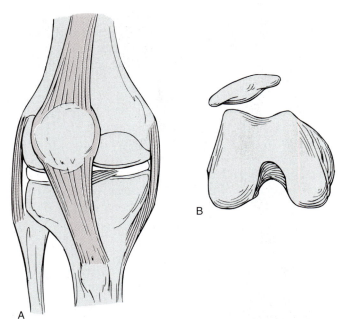

➤ FIGURE 15.15 **Dislocated patella**. A dislocated patella often displaces laterally and is accompanied by an audible pop and violent collapse of the knee following deceleration involving a cutting maneuver. A, Anterior view. B, Skyline view.

dard acute care protocol. Most individuals respond well to mild anti-inflammatory medication, quadriceps strengthening, and a hamstring flexibility program. All resisted exercises with knee extension from a fully flexed position, crouches, and deep knee-bends should be avoided, since these positions may aggravate the condition. A knee sleeve with a patellar cutout may be helpful. If this does not reduce the symptoms, surgical intervention may be necessary, such as arthroscopic patellar debridement, lateral retinacular release, extensor mechanism realignment, or elevation of the tibial tubercle to relieve patellar compression forces.

Patellar Instability and Dislocations

Patellar instability occurs when the patella has normal or abnormal alignment in the trochlear groove, but is displaced by internal or external forces. Displacement can range from microinstability to subluxation or gross dislocation. In a subluxation, there is transient partial displacement of the patella from the femoral trochlea. It may occur acutely, as in a patellar dislocation, or be intermittent with spontaneous reduction of the displacement. The athlete may or may not have a history of complete dislocation or patellofemoral pain, but will report a feeling of the patella slipping when cutting, twisting, or pivoting. Joint effusion may develop, but it improves rapidly when the individual resumes activity. Chronic subluxations produce less swelling, pain, and disability. The condition is verified by observing patellar position during active knee flexion and extension, and with a positive patellar apprehension test. An individual with patellofemoral stress syndrome will not

be apprehensive with this test, whereas one with patellar pain due to subluxation will resist any attempt to displace the patella laterally.

Acute patellar subluxations and dislocations appear the same, and generally occur during deceleration with a cutting maneuver **(Figure 15.15)**. Distinguishing one from the other depends on patient history. With a dislocation, the patient reports that the kneecap moved and had to be pushed back into place; with a subluxation, the patient reports that the kneecap slipped out, then went back into place spontaneously. Nearly all medial muscular and retinaculum attachments are torn from the medial aspect of the patella, leading to an audible pop and violent collapse of the knee. Localized tenderness may also occur along the medial extensor retinaculum or at the adductor tubercle, which is the origin of the medial patellofemoral ligament. There may also be localized tenderness along the peripheral edge of the lateral femoral condyle where impaction from the patella occurs with flexion of the knee. Typically, a traumatic displacement has acute effusion associated with a hemarthrosis. A dislocation without acute effusion should signal chronic laxity; the tissues are so lax that the patella moves in and out of the groove without traumatizing surrounding tissues. Palpate the area to assess any defects in the medial retinaculum and VMO before they are obscured by swelling. Occasionally, a fracture of the patella or lateral femoral condyle also occurs, resulting in a loose, bony fragment in the joint.

➤ MANAGEMENT

Immediate treatment includes ice, elevation, immobilization, and immediate referral to a physician.

After the physician reduces the dislocation, aspiration of the hemarthrosis may be indicated for comfort or to search for fat in the blood secondary to an osteochondral fracture. Immobilization of a first-time dislocation is only needed to control acute symptoms, followed by an extensive rehabilitation program and functional patellar bracing. While immobilized, isometric quadriceps exercises and straight leg raises can be performed. When immobilization is removed, a full rehabilitative program to strengthen the dynamic stabilizers of the patellofemoral joint, particularly the VMO, and a flexibility program for the hamstrings and IT band should be initiated. A knee sleeve with lateral pad to restrict lateral excursion and activity modification may be helpful. Most individuals with patellofemoral tracking disorders and instability can improve and return to activity without surgical intervention. However, an obvious disruption of the VMO insertion into the medial patellar edge, or a rupture of the medial patellofemoral ligament from the adductor tubercles, does best with early surgical repair.

Patella Plica Syndrome

The patella plica shelf is a fold in the synovial lining that projects into the joint cavity. This congenital abnormality is a remnant of the embyologic walls that divide the knee into medial, lateral, and suprapatellar pouches. It is typically crescent shaped and extends from the infrapatellar fat pad medially (medial plica), loops around the femoral condyle, crosses under the quadriceps tendon in the suprapatellar region (suprapatellar plica), then passes laterally over the lateral femoral condyle to the lateral retinaculum (**Figure 15.16**). Normally, a synovial plica remains asymptomatic until traumatized by a direct blow to the capsule, or becomes inflamed and thickened from overuse due to friction caused as the plica bow-strings across the medial

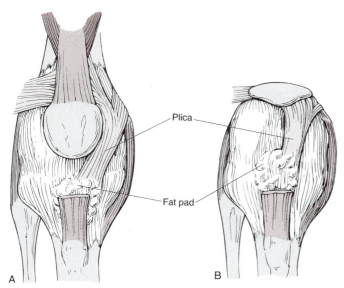
Plica

Fat pad

A   B

➤ **FIGURE 15.16 Patella plica**. The patella plica is a fold in the synovial lining of the knee joint that can become inflamed and thickened by trauma where it extends over the femoral condyle, or by microtrauma from overuse. A, Fully extended. B, 90° flexed.

femoral condyle. This bow-stringing results in two reservoirs for synovial fluid: a suprapatellar reservoir and the cavity of the knee joint itself.

➤ SIGNS AND SYMPTOMS

Anterior knee pain comes on gradually and is aggravated by quadriceps exercises. In about 25% of the cases, there is a positive "movie-goer's sign" (pain with prolonged sitting). As the individual stands and begins to walk, a sharp pain is felt for 8 to 10 steps, then disappears. The pain is caused by the plica being maximally stretched and impinged within the patellofemoral joint. As the articularis genus muscle contracts several times, it elevates the plica enough to prevent further impingement. Occasionally, adhesions present in the plica lead to a distinctive pop or snap as the individual extends the knee, or pseudolocking may occur over the medial patellofemoral joint, mimicking a torn meniscus. Assessment reveals slight joint effusion, palpable pain, and crepitus in the medial and lateral retinacular regions, particularly along the edge of the medial femoral condyle with the knee flexed at 45°. The test for medial synovial plica and the stutter test will be positive.

➤ MANAGEMENT

Treatment is symptomatic with ice therapy, NSAIDs, activity modification, phonophoresis, and an external patellar support device. The condition may improve with hamstring stretching, heelcord stretching, and VMO strengthening exercises, especially if the VMO is dysplastic (abnormally developed). If the condition warrants, the plica shelf can be removed arthroscopically.

Patellar Tendinitis (Jumper's Knee)

The patellar tendon frequently becomes inflamed and tender from repetitive or eccentric knee extension activities; these occur in running and jumping, hence the name "jumper's knee." Patellar subluxation, patellofemoral stress syndrome, and other conditions can also overload the patellar tendon, predisposing an athlete to this condition (see Box 15.4). These should be differentiated from tendinitis.

➤ SIGNS AND SYMPTOMS

Initially, pain after activity is concentrated on the inferior pole of the patella, but it also occurs at the insertion of the patellar tendon into the tibial tubercle (**Figure 15.17**). As the condition progresses, pain is present at the beginning of activity, subsides during warm-up, then reappears after activity. Increased pain is often reported while ascending and descending stairs or after prolonged sitting. Eventually, pain is present both during and after activity, and can become too severe for the individual to participate. Examination reveals point tenderness at the inferior pole of the patella, and less commonly over the body of the patellar tendon (**Box 15.5**). Pain can be elicited during passive knee flexion beyond 120° and during resisted knee extension. It is also common to find tightness in the hamstrings, quadriceps, and heelcord, with weakness in the ankle dorsiflexors. Chronic tendinitis may occasionally lead

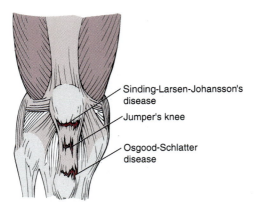

Sinding-Larsen-Johansson's disease

Jumper's knee

Osgood-Schlatter disease

➤ **FIGURE 15.17 Patellar tendon conditions**. Patellar tendon conditions may involve Sinding-Larsen-Johansson's disease, patellar tendinitis, or Osgood-Schlatter disease. The location of pain will typically define which problem is present.

to cystic changes at the distal pole of the patella, or ectopic calcification and nodule formation in the tendon.

➤ **MANAGEMENT**

Immediate treatment involves standard acute care and NSAIDs. **Field Strategy 15.4** summarizes the management of patellar tendinitis.

Osgood-Schlatter Disease

Osgood-Schlatter disease (OSD) is a traction-type injury to the tibial apophysis where the patellar tendon attaches onto the tibial tubercle. OSD typically develops in girls between the ages of 8 and 13, and in boys between ages 10 and 15 at the beginning of their growth spurt. It is estimated the condition occurs in 21% of adolescent athletes as compared to 4.5% of age-matched nonathletes (16).

> ➤➤ **BOX 15.5**
>
> ### Signs and Symptoms of Patellar Tendinitis
> - Initially, pain after activity is concentrated on the inferior pole of the patella or the distal attachment of the patellar tendon on the tibial tubercle
> - As the condition progresses, pain is present at the start of activity, subsides with warm-up, then reappears after activity
> - Pain is present while ascending and descending stairs
> - Pain occurs on passive knee flexion beyond 120°, and during resisted knee extension

The condition has been more common in boys, but the ratio may be equalizing with girls' increased participation in sports.

➤ **SIGNS AND SYMPTOMS**

Assessment of the condition is usually straightforward. Patients point to the tibial tubercle as the source of pain, and the tubercle appears enlarged and prominent. They report that pain generally occurs during activity and is relieved with rest. Point tenderness can be elicited directly over the tubercle, but range of motion is usually not affected. Pain is present at the extremes of knee extension and forced flexion. Severity is usually rated in three grades depending on the duration of pain **(Table 15.4)**.

➤ **MANAGEMENT**

Treatment is symptomatic and self-limiting, but it may take 12 to 24 months to run its course. In most cases, activity is unrestricted unless pain is disabling. Shock-absorbent insoles in sports shoes may decrease peak stress

FIELD STRATEGY 15.4   MANAGEMENT OF PATELLAR TENDINITIS

- Rest 2–3 weeks to allow symptoms to subside
- Other modalities that may be used in the early stages of healing include heat therapy, electrical stimulation, phonophoresis, iontophoresis, and ultrasound
- Transverse friction massage for 6 to 8 minutes may help facilitate healing
- Initiate early flexibility exercises for the gastrocnemius-soleus complex, quadriceps, and hamstrings
- Aquatic therapy in early stages can reduce gravitational forces
- Progressive resistance strengthening exercises may include:
  Straight-leg raises in all directions
  Short-arc knee extension exercises
  One-quarter knee squats
  Eccentric strengthening exercises for the quadriceps and dorsiflexors, such as drop squats (i.e., landing from a jump). Focus on the deceleration between the upward and downward phase. Increase deceleration as tolerated by the patient
- Cardiovascular fitness should be maintained with exercises that do not involve powerful knee extension (i.e., UBE, swimming, stationary bike with minimal tension)
- In the later stages, plyometrics may be incorporated (i.e., single-leg hop, double-leg hop, single-leg vertical jump, and bounding)
- A patellofemoral knee sleeve may reduce mobility of the patellar tendon during activity

TABLE 15.4	GRADES OF OSGOOD-SCHLATTER DISEASE
Grade	Characteristics
1	Pain after activity that resolves within 24 hours
2	Pain during and after activity that does not hinder performance and resolves within 24 hours
3	Continuous pain that limits sport performance and daily activities

Reprinted with permission from Wall EJ. Osgood-Schlatter disease: Practical treatment for a self-limiting condition. Phys Sportsmed 1998; 26(3):30.

on the tendon and tubercle. Icing the knee for 20 minutes after activity may also be beneficial, as are hamstrings and quadriceps stretching. Wrestling gel pads, basketball knee pads, or an Osgood-Schlatter pad may protect the tibial tubercle when kneeling and prevent repeated contusions to the sensitive area. The condition rectifies itself with closure of the apophysis, but a small percentage of individuals develop a painful ossicle, which can necessitate surgical excision. Others may develop painful kneeling as adults.

Sinding-Larsen-Johansson's Disease

A similar condition to OSD is **Sinding-Larsen-Johansson's (SLJ) disease**, in which pain, swelling, and tenderness result from excessive strain on the inferior patellar pole at the origin of the patellar tendon. The condition is usually seen in children 8 to 13 years old (17).

➤ SIGNS AND SYMPTOMS

The onset of pain over the inferior patellar pole is gradual and seen in children involved in running and jumping sports. The condition is often missed unless the clinician palpates the inferior patellar pole with the patient's knee extended and the patellar tendon relaxed. Repeating the exam with the knee flexed at 90° should reveal diminished tenderness as the patellar tendon becomes taut.

➤ MANAGEMENT

Treatment is symptomatic and similar to that for Osgood-Schlatter disease. Symptoms generally resolve quickly with standard acute care, NSAIDs, and activity modification.

Extensor Tendon Rupture

Extensor tendon ruptures can occur at the superior or inferior pole of the patella, tibial tubercle, or within the patellar tendon itself. Ruptures result from powerful eccentric muscle contractions, or in conjunction with severe ligamentous disruption at the knee. The rupture may be partial or total.

➤ SIGNS AND SYMPTOMS

A partial rupture will produce pain and muscle weakness in knee extension. If a total rupture occurs distal to the patella, assessment will reveal a high-riding patella, a palpable defect over the tendon, and an inability to do knee

extension or perform a straight-leg raise. If the quadriceps tendon is ruptured from the superior pole of the patella and the extensor retinaculum is still intact, knee extension is still possible, although it will be weak and painful. Individuals with a history of prior corticosteroid injections, anabolic steroid abuse, or use of systemic steroids are at a greater risk for tendon ruptures. Steroid use can cause softening or weakening of collagen fibers in the muscle tendon, predisposing the tendon to premature rupture.

➤ MANAGEMENT

 Immediate treatment involves standard acute care, use of a knee immobilizer, fitting the athlete for crutches, and immediate referral to a physician.

Treatment depends on the location and displacement of any bony fragment. In partial ruptures involving a shredded tendon, wiring through the patella may be necessary to relieve tension on the healing tendon. In total ruptures, surgical repair is necessary.

 The cross-country runner complained of lateral patellofemoral pain that increased when running down hills. Precipitating factors that increase stress on the patellofemoral region include patellar instability, a weak VMO, hypermobility of the patella, and anatomical malalignment conditions. After standard acute care, a total assessment of the lower extremity should be conducted to address deficiencies in muscle strength or biomechanical problems that contributed to the condition.

ILIOTIBIAL BAND FRICTION SYNDROME

 After an evening practice session on the third day of preseason, a lacrosse player is complaining of a sharp ache over the lateral epicondyle of the femur that has progressively gotten worse since the start of the week. While talking to the athlete, you learn that the daily double sessions have concentrated on technique drills and conditioning exercises. You also notice that both feet of the athlete are extremely pronated and he is bowlegged (genu varus). What actions might you suggest to this athlete to reduce the pain and correct the injury?

A condition common in runners, cyclists, weight lifters, and volleyball players is iliotibial (IT) band friction syndrome. The IT band continues the line of pull from the tensor fasciae latae and gluteus maximus muscle. The deep fibers are associated with the lateral intermuscular septum. The distal fibers become thicker at their attachment on Gerdy's tubercle adjacent to the tibial tubercle on the lateral proximal tibia. The band drops posteriorly behind the lateral femoral epicondyle with knee flexion, then snaps

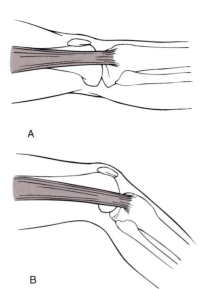

➤ FIGURE 15.18 **Iliotibial band**. The iliotibial band drops posteriorly behind the lateral femoral epicondyle during knee flexion, then snaps forward over the epicondyle during extension. Malalignment problems or constant irritation can inflame the iliotibial band, or lead to bursitis. A, Extension. B, Flexion.

forward over the epicondyle during extension **(Figure 15.18)**. Weight-bearing increases compression and friction forces over the greater trochanter and lateral femoral condyle. Individuals with a malalignment problem are predisposed to this condition **(Box 15.6)**.

➤ SIGNS AND SYMPTOMS

Initially, pain is present only after running a certain mileage, typically late in the run, but as the condition progresses, occurs earlier and earlier, and may occur while running uphill and downhill, and while climbing stairs **(Box 15.7)**. It is particularly intense on weight-bearing from foot strike through midstance. It is during this part of the gait cycle that the IT band is most compressed between the lateral femoral epicondyle and greater trochanter of the femur. Point tenderness is localized over the lateral femoral condyle about 2 to 3 cm above the lateral joint line, and occasionally radiates distally to the tibial attachment or proximally up the thigh. Positive Noble's and Ober's compression tests confirm the condition.

➤ MANAGEMENT

Immediate treatment involves standard acute care and NSAIDs. **Field Strategy 15.5** explains the management of IT band friction syndrome.

 The lacrosse player has IT band friction syndrome. The double sessions, coupled with the preexisting genu varus and pronated feet, have added strain to the IT band. After controlling inflammation, an extensive flexibility program for the IT band should be initiated.

FRACTURES AND ASSOCIATED INJURIES

 A 20-year-old golfer is complaining of an aching, diffuse pain in his right knee. He remembers tripping over a tree root several weeks ago and falling forward on his knees with the right leg internally rotated, and the foot plantar flexed and inverted. He iced the knee for a couple of days and it appeared to be better, but now it feels like the knee is giving way. It feels better when he walks with the right leg externally rotated, but it really hurts when he pushes off the leg to change direction. What may have happened to this individual?

Traumatic fractures about the knee area are rare in sports competition, except for high-velocity sports, such as motorcycling and auto racing. These fractures are usually associated with multiple trauma. Other more common fractures and associated bony conditions, however, can occur with regular sport participation. Displaced and undisplaced fractures of the femoral shaft were discussed in Chapter 14 and will not be discussed here.

Avulsion Fractures

Avulsion fractures are caused by direct trauma, excessive tensile forces from an explosive muscular contraction, re-

FIELD STRATEGY 15.5 **MANAGEMENT OF ILIOTIBIAL BAND FRICTION SYNDROME**

- Ice, compression, elevation, NSAIDs, and rest until acute symptoms subside
- Stretch hip abductors, flexors, and lateral thigh muscles
- Foot orthotics may correct some structural problems
- Non-weight-bearing strengthening exercises, such as leg lifts and isometric exercises for knee flexion, extension, hip abduction, and adduction can be initiated when pain-free, followed by concentric and eccentric strengthening of the hip and thigh muscles
- Hill running should be avoided until asymptomatic
- Running or training should be modified to the point of little or minimal pain during activity
- Cardiovascular fitness can be maintained with swimming
- Ice massage before and after running may be helpful
- Steroid injections may be used in resistant cases
- Full return to participation should be gauged on pain-free completion of all functional tests

petitive overuse, or a tensile force that pulls a ligament from its bony attachment. For example, getting kicked on the lateral aspect of the knee may avulse a portion of the lateral epicondyle, or the tibial tubercle may be avulsed when the extensor mechanism pulls a fragment away.

➤ **SIGNS AND SYMPTOMS**

The individual has localized pain and tenderness over the bony site. In some instances, a fragment may be palpated. If a musculotendinous unit is involved, muscle function will be limited. When the anterior cruciate is involved, the bony fragment may lodge in the joint, causing the knee to "lock."

➤ **MANAGEMENT**

Treatment involves standard acute care and application of a knee immobilizer. The athlete should be immediately referred to a physician for further care. If necessary, the athlete should be fitted for crutches and instructed to use a non-weight-bearing gait en route to the physician.

Epiphyseal and Apophyseal Fractures

Adolescents in contact sports are particularly susceptible to epiphyseal fractures in the knee region. A shearing force across the cartilaginous growth plate may lead to a disruption of growth and a shortened limb.

TIBIAL TUBERCLE FRACTURES

The tibial tubercle, a common site for apophyseal fractures in boys, may occur as a result of Osgood-Schlatter disease. The typical patient is a muscular, well-developed athlete who has almost reached skeletal maturity, and almost always is involved in a jumping sport, most commonly basketball (18). These fractures usually result from forced flexion of the knee against a straining quadriceps contraction, or a violent quadriceps contraction against a fixed foot.

➤ **SIGNS AND SYMPTOMS**

The individual will have pain, ecchymosis, swelling, and tenderness directly over the tubercle, and will have difficulty going up and down stairs. When the fracture extends from the tubercle to the tibial epiphysis (type II), or through the secondary epiphysis and into the joint (type III), quadriceps insufficiency makes knee extension painful and weak. With larger fractures involving extensive retinacular damage, the patella rides high, and knee extension will be impossible.

➤ **MANAGEMENT**

Treatment involves standard acute care and application of a knee immobilizer. The athlete should be immediately referred to a physician for further care. If necessary, the athlete should be fitted for crutches and instructed to use a non-weight-bearing gait en route to the physician. Displaced fractures will need open reduction and internal fixation.

DISTAL FEMORAL EPIPHYSEAL FRACTURES

Fractures to the distal femoral epiphysis are 10 times more common than proximal tibial fractures, and are more serious because of possible arterial damage to the growth plate. They may occur at any age, but are often seen in boys aged 10 to 14. These fractures occur when a varus or valgus stress is applied on a fixed, weight-bearing foot, as when someone falls on the outer aspect of the knee while the foot is planted.

➤ **SIGNS AND SYMPTOMS**

The individual complains of pain around the knee and is unable to bear weight on the injured leg.

➤ **MANAGEMENT**

Treatment involves standard acute care and application of a knee immobilizer or vacuum splint. The athlete should be immediately referred to a physician for further care.

Undisplaced type I fractures are usually treated with closed reduction and casting, with use of crutches and protective weight-bearing for 4 weeks, followed by rehabilitation to restore motion and strength. This fracture has a history of fairly good resolution, although it may take weeks to occur. More serious fractures will require internal fixation and may result in angular or leg-length discrepancy.

Stress Fractures

The femoral supracondylar region, medial tibial plateau, and tibia tubercle are common regions for stress fractures. These fractures occur when:

- Load on the bone is increased (jumping or another high-impact activity)
- The number of stresses on the bone increase (e.g., changes in training intensity, duration, frequency, or running surface, or unevenly worn shoes)
- The surface area of the bone that receives the load is decreased (during the normal process of bone repair, certain portions of the bone remain immature and less able to tolerate stress for a period of time)

➤ SIGNS AND SYMPTOMS

The individual will complain of localized pain before and after activity that is relieved with rest and non-weight-bearing. In a stress fracture of the medial tibial plateau, pain runs along the anteromedial aspect of the proximal tibia just below the joint line. Localized tenderness and edema will be present, but initial radiographs of the stress fracture may be negative. As the condition progresses, pain becomes more persistent. Follow-up radiographs 3 weeks postinjury may then show periosteal new bone development. Early bone scans are highly recommended.

➤ MANAGEMENT

Once identified as a stress fracture, treatment involves rest, crutches, or casting.

Chondral and Osteochondral Fractures

A chondral fracture is a fracture involving the articular cartilage at a joint. An osteochondral fracture involves the articular cartilage and underlying bone **(Figure 15.19)**. These fractures result from compression from a direct blow to the knee causing shearing or forceful rotation. A substantial amount of articular surface on the involved bone can be damaged.

➤ SIGNS AND SYMPTOMS

The individual will usually feel a painful "snap" and report considerable pain and swelling within the first few hours after injury. Displaced fractures can cause locking of the joint, and produce crepitation during range of motion.

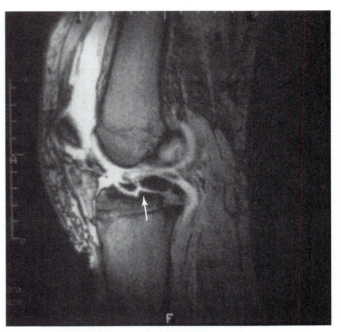

➤ **FIGURE 15.19   Osteochondral fracture**. This traumatic osteochondral fracture involves the articular cartilage and subchondral bone on the medial epicondyle of the tibia.

➤ MANAGEMENT

Following standard acute care and immobilization in a vacuum splint, the athlete should be immediately referred to a physician for further care.

Aspiration of the joint often yields bloody fluid containing fat. MRIs may be indicated because some fractures may not appear on standard radiographs. Small fragments can be removed during arthroscopic surgery. Internal fixation is necessary with larger fragments. Following surgery, range-of-motion exercises are performed to improve articular cartilage nutrition, limit joint adhesions, and prevent muscular atrophy.

Osteochondritis Dissecans

Osteochondritis dissecans (OCD) occurs when a fragment of bone adjacent to the articular surface of a joint is deprived of its blood supply, leading to avascular necrosis. The avascular bone fragment may be in its normal anatomical location with a smooth articular surface (stable), or the lesion may displace and form a loose body within the joint space, leaving a defect in the articular cartilage (unstable) **(Figure 15.20)**. The cartilage remains healthy even if the fragment is loose, since cartilage is nourished by synovial fluid rather than by a direct blood supply. However, repetitive trauma and the loss of mechanical support may cause the cartilage to undergo softening and degenerative changes. Although found in other joints, it more commonly affects the knee joint, particularly in males ages 10 to 20. Causes include direct and indirect trauma, skeletal abnormalities associated

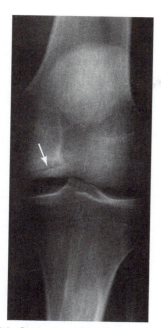

➤ **FIGURE 15.20** **Osteochondritis dissecans**. Osteochondritis dissecans occurs when a fragment of bone adjacent to the articular surface of a joint is deprived of its blood supply, leading to avascular necrosis. In this patient, a portion of the medial epicondyle of the femur is damaged.

with endocrine dysfunction, a prominent tibial spine that impacts the medial femoral condyle, and generalized ligamentous laxity. Common sites include the medial femoral condyle (80 to 85% of cases), the lateral femoral condyle (10 to 15% of cases), and the patella (5% of cases) (19).

➤ SIGNS AND SYMPTOMS

The most common symptom is an aching, diffuse pain, or swelling, with activity. Knee locking or giving way may develop as the disease progresses. Pain increases with strenuous activity and twisting motions, especially internal rotation of the tibia, which causes the medial tibial spine to strike the lateral aspect of the medial femoral condyle (the site of most OCD lesions). As a result, the athlete will walk with the affected leg externally rotated. Some individual with lesions of the lateral femoral condyle feel a painful "clunk" with knee flexion and extension. Individuals with OCD of the patella usually present with retropatellar pain and crepitus. Thigh circumference may be diminished due to muscle disuse atrophy.

➤ MANAGEMENT

Following standard acute care and immobilization with a knee immobilizer or vacuum splint, the athlete should be immediately referred to a physician for further care.

Treatment depends on the age of the individual **(Table 15.5)**, size and location of the lesion, and the radiographic appearance of the fragment and articular cartilage. Individuals in categories 1 and 2 (those <20 years of age) are treated nonsurgically if the fragment has not separated.

TABLE 15.5	CLASSIFICATION OF OSTEOCHONDRITIS DISSECANS	
Category	**Age Group**	**Prognosis**
1	Girls <11 and boys <13	Excellent, due to open physes
2	Women 12–20 and men 14–20	Fair to good, due to near skeletal maturity
3	All women, and men >20	Poor, with tendencies toward fragment instability, loose body formation, and degenerative joint disease

Adapted from Ralston BM, et al. (19), page 79.

A soft knee immobilizer is worn, and activity is restricted for 1 to 2 weeks, with minimal weight-bearing to control pain and initiate healing. Activities are then modified for 6 to 12 weeks; younger patients generally require a shorter period of activity modification than older patients. Rapid or strenuous movement of the lower extremities should be avoided, especially high-impact activities such as running, cutting, and jumping. Plain radiographs usually reveal evidence of healing between 3 and 6 months after treatment. Full activity may be permitted once the following criteria are met:

- The patient is pain-free
- Physical examination is normal, including full ROM, and no joint effusion or tenderness is present
- Radiographic evidence of healing is present, as noted by the disappearance of the radiolucent line that outlined the fragment

If the patient is older than 20 years of age, or the fragment is unstable (regardless of the patient's age) or is a chronic lesion that does not respond to conservative measures, internal fixation or removal of the fragment is indicated. Older individuals do not heal as well because degenerative joint changes may have already developed within the joint. For OCD lesions of the patella, conservative management is often unsuccessful, necessitating early surgical intervention to excise the fragment. For these individuals, brief postsurgical immobilization followed by activity limitations usually bring about gradual healing.

Patellar Fractures

Stress fractures of the patella are rare and typically involve the inferior pole of the patella. Traumatic fractures may be transverse, stellate or comminuted, or longitudinal. Displaced patellar fractures, which are generally associated with disruption of the quadriceps retinaculum, require open reduction and internal fixation. These fractures occur as a result of a fall onto the knee, a direct blow to the knee, or an eccentric contraction of the quadriceps that overloads the intrinsic tensile strength of the bone, as occurs in jumping activities. Patellar fracture is also a rare complication of ACL reconstruction using a bone-patella tendon-bone **autogenous** (from within the body) graft. These fractures occur an average of 7 weeks postsurgery and result from external trauma, a rapid flexion movement while preventing a fall backward, or a twisting maneuver (20). A **bipartite** (having two parts) patella, although not a fracture, is present in 1 to 4% of patients, and is more common in males. It is typically seen on the superolateral corner of the patella and will have rounded rather than sharp edges. The individual will lack point tenderness over the area and can maintain knee extension, which differentiates the condition from a true fracture.

➤ SIGNS AND SYMPTOMS

Generally, 2 mm of articular incongruity signifies a displaced fracture, which will produce diffuse extra-articular swelling on and about the knee. A portion of the patella is retracted proximally, and there will be a visible and palpable defect between the fragments, which are mobile. A straight-leg raise will be impossible to perform.

➤ MANAGEMENT

Initial treatment will involve ice, elevation, immobilization in a knee immobilizer, and immediate referral to a physician.

Radiographs are needed for verification. Nondisplaced patellar fractures are treated nonoperatively with either a long-leg cylinder cast or knee immobilizer for 4 to 6 weeks. Partial weight-bearing is then allowed, and a full rehabilitation program initiated. In a displaced fracture with major disruption to the extensor mechanism, surgery is indicated.

The golfer has osteochondritis dissecans. The position of the leg (internal rotation of the tibia) during the fall caused the medial tibial spine to strike the lateral aspect of the medial femoral condyle (the most common site for OCD lesions). As a result, it felt better to walk with the affected leg externally rotated. The sensation of the knee giving way, and the pain on twisting motions, are also key symptoms that signal the need for referral to a physician for assessment.

ASSESSING THE KNEE COMPLEX

A volleyball player is complaining of anterior knee pain over the lateral patella. It feels like the patella is slipping while cutting, twisting, pivoting, and squatting during play, but there is little pain or swelling. Knowing that the knee is a complex joint, why can't you limit the assessment to only the knee region?

The lower extremity works as a unit to provide motion. Several biomechanical problems at the foot directly affect strain on the knee. The knee plays a major role in supporting the body during dynamic and static activities, and referred pain from the hip and lumbar spine may also be involved. Assessment of the knee complex must therefore encompass an overview of the entire lower extremity. **Field Strategy 15.6** lists the basic components of a knee assessment. Refer back to Table 15.3 for a summary of the various knee instabilities, tests used, and the injured structures indicated by the various positive tests. Table 15.6 (later in the chapter) will summarize other specific special tests for the knee and patella region.

HISTORY

What information should be gathered from the volleyball player who is complaining of the patella slipping during practice? What questions can help identify the main components of the primary complaint?

Many conditions at the knee are related to family history, age, congenital deformities, mechanical dysfunction, and recent changes in training programs, surfaces, or foot attire. You should begin by gathering information on the mechanism of injury, associated symptoms, the progression of the symptoms, any disabilities that may have resulted from the injury, and related medical history. Injuries seldom occur in an absolute frontal or sagittal plane. Instead, most injuries involve a fixed, weight-bearing foot with the athlete trying to change directions or pivoting away from an opponent. These acute, non-contact-related injuries most likely involve a rotational stress on the knee, which may injure several structures.

Sprains of the collateral ligaments usually result in pain directly over the injury site. Injury to the ACL may be described as "deep in the knee" or "under the kneecap," whereas pain associated with a PCL tear is located in the posterior knee near the proximal attachment of the gastrocnemius. Unlike ACL injuries, PCL injuries usually do not cause incapacitating pain, but rather produce vague symptoms such as unsteadiness or insecurity of the knee. Menisci injuries often present pain directly over the joint line. The athlete may also describe an associated pop or snap at the time of injury. After ruling out a possible patellar dislocation or fracture, these sounds usually indicate a tear of one of the cruciate ligaments. Symptoms such as locking of the knee may indicate a meniscal tear. "Giving way" may indicate a patellar subluxation or internal derangement of the knee itself. Pain following prolonged periods of sitting, the "movie-goer's" or "theater" sign, is usually indicative of prolonged pressure being placed on one of the patellar facets. Individuals who have symptoms of patellar instability may have had a dislocation or recurrent subluxation. In addition to general questions covered in Chapter 4, specific questions related to the knee can be seen in **Field Strategy 15.7**.

The volleyball player reported a long history of anterior knee pain throughout her career. Four years ago, she dislocated her patella while skiing.

FIELD STRATEGY 15.6 KNEE EVALUATION

HISTORY

- Primary complaint including:
  - Current nature, location, and onset of the condition
- Mechanism of injury
  - Cause of stress; position of hip, knee, and ankle; direction of force
  - Changes in training, equipment, running technique, or shoes
- Characteristics of the symptoms
  - Evolution of the onset, nature, location, severity, and duration of pain and weakness
- Disability resulting from the injury
- Related medical history
  - Previous injuries in the area, congenital abnormalities, or family history

OBSERVATION AND INSPECTION

- Observation should analyze general posture and gait (see Field Strategy 15.8)
- Inspection at the injury site for deformity, swelling, discoloration, hypertrophy or muscle atrophy, visible congenital deformity, or surgical incision or scars

PALPATION

- Bony structures, to determine a possible fracture
- Soft tissue structures, to determine skin temperature, swelling, point tenderness, crepitus, deformity, muscle spasm, cutaneous sensation, and pulse

FUNCTIONAL TESTS

- Active range of motion
- Passive range of motion
- Resisted manual muscle testing

STRESS TESTS (REFER TO TABLES 15.3 AND 15.6.)

NEUROLOGIC TESTS

- Myotomes
- Reflexes
- Dermatomes

SPORT-SPECIFIC FUNCTIONAL TESTS

After an extensive rehabilitation program, she was able to return to sport participation and wore a patellofemoral brace. The patellofemoral joint began to hurt about 2 months ago when she started a new strength-training program that involved heavy lifting. Since then, the knee has occasionally been swollen and the outside of the patella tends to be very tender, but ice and NSAIDs have helped to make it feel better.

OBSERVATION AND INSPECTION

 In which position(s) do you want to observe this individual? Should you do a posture and gait analysis? Why? What specific congenital anomalies might contribute to pain at the knee?

Both legs should be clearly visible to check symmetry, any congenital deformity, swelling, discoloration, hypertrophy, muscle atrophy, or previous surgical incisions. The individual should wear running shorts to allow full view of the entire lower extremity. Ask the individual to bring the shoes normally worn when pain is present. Inspect the sole, heel box, and general condition of the shoe for unusual wear, which would indicate a biomechanical abnormality that may be affecting the knee.

Place the injured knee on a folded towel or pillow at 30° flexion to relieve any strain on the joint structures. Inspect the injury site for obvious deformities, discoloration, swelling, or scars that might indicate previous surgery, and note the general condition of the skin. Swelling proximal to the patella may indicate suprapatellar bursitis or quadriceps involvement. Swelling distal to the patella may indicate patellar tendinitis, fat pad contusion, or internal derangement. Posterior swelling may indicate a Baker's cyst, gastrocnemius strain, or venous thrombosis. Medial swelling over the pes anserine may indicate bursitis or tendinitis. Girth measurements can be taken at the joint line to determine presence of swelling. Measurements are then taken at 2-inch increments (1-inch for smaller athletes) above the superior pole of the patella to measure atrophy. Compare the affected limb with the unaffected

FIELD STRATEGY 15.7   DEVELOPING A HISTORY OF THE INJURY

CURRENT INJURY STATUS

1. Where is the pain (or weakness) located? How severe is the pain (weakness)? What type of pain is it (dull ache [degenerative problem], stabbing or sharp [mechanical problem], or pain in the morning [arthritic condition])?
2. Did the pain come on suddenly (acute) or gradually (overuse)? Was the pain greatest when the injury first occurred, or did it get worse the second or third day?
3. (If acute, ask:) What were you doing at the time of the injury? What position was the knee in when the injury occurred? From what direction, if any, did the traumatic force come from? Was the foot fixed during impact? (If chronic, ask:) What different activities have you been doing in the last week? (Look for changes in technique, frequency, duration, intensity, or changes in shoes, equipment, or running surface.)
4. Did you hear any sounds during the incident? Any snaps, pops, or cracks (ligament rupture, patellar dislocation, or osteochondral fracture)? Can you bear weight on the leg or balance on the leg? Did you notice any swelling, discoloration, muscle spasms, or numbness with the injury?
5. What actions or motions bring on the pain? Is it worse in the morning, during activity, after activity, or at night? Does it wake you up at night? When the pain sets in, how long does it last?
6. Are there certain activities you are unable to perform because of the pain? Which ones?
7. How old are you? (Remember that many problems are age-related.) Which leg is dominant?

PAST INJURY STATUS

1. Have you ever injured your knee before? When? How did that occur? What was done at the time of injury? Did you have any difficulty returning to your full functional status?
2. Have you had any medical problems recently? (Look for possible referred pain from the lumbar spine, hip, or ankle.) Are you on any medication? Do you have any musculoskeletal problems elsewhere in the body? What shoes do you wear?

---

limb. Quadriceps atrophy is usually a sign of a chronic injury.

Faulty posture or congenital abnormalities can also increase stress on any joint. In an ambulatory patient, complete your observations with a thorough postural exam. Observe the alignment of the femur on the tibia. Normally, the angle between the femoral and tibial shafts ranges from 180 to 195°. An angle <180° is called genu valgus ("knock knee"); an angle >195° is called genu varum ("bowlegs"). Hyperextension, or posterior bowing of the knee, is called **genu recurvatum**. Observe patella alignment for any abnormalities **(Box 15.8)**. The high-riding patella exposes the infrapatellar fat pad leading to a double hump when viewed from the lateral side ("camel sign"). Although some malalignments may be observed during a postural exam, radiographs are often required for definitive diagnosis.

With the individual sitting on the examination table, observe whether the tibial tubercles are directly below the patella, or are displaced laterally more than 10°, indicating an increased tubercle sulcus angle. Lateral displacement of the tubercle suggests bony patellofemoral malalignment and a predisposition to lateral patellar tracking. Ask the individual to actively extend and flex the knee, and observe the dynamic tracking of the patella. Palpate the patella

for crepitus during the movement, and compare to the contralateral knee. Although asymptomatic crepitus is common in certain individuals, symptomatic crepitus in the injured knee may indicate articular cartilage damage on the patella or trochlea.

After a static postural exam **(Field Strategy 15.8)**, observe the individual walking from anterior, posterior, and lateral views. Ask the individual to do a deep knee squat, and to ascend, and descend stairs. Note any abnor-

---

▶▶ **BOX 15.8**

Patellar Abnormalities

Patella alta	High-riding patella caused by a long patellar tendon
Patella baja	Low-riding patella caused by a short patellar tendon
Squinting patella	Medial-riding patella caused by hip anteversion (internal rotation of the femur) or internal tibial rotation
"Frog-eyed" patella	Lateral-riding patella caused by hip retroversion (external rotation of the femur) or external tibial rotation

FIELD STRATEGY 15.8 POSTURAL ASSESSMENT OF THE KNEE REGION

ANTERIOR VIEW

1. Both thighs should look the same. Ask the person to contract the quadriceps. Check for hypertrophy or atrophy. Check for genu valgus (knock-kneed), genu varus (bow-legged), or tibial torsion. Women tend to be more prone toward genu valgus.
2. Both patellae should be at the same height and face straight forward. The Q-angle should appear to be bilaterally equal. If there is swelling at the knee, is it intra-articular (diffuse with patella floating high) or extra-articular (localized with the outline of the patella obscured)? Are the fibular heads level?
3. The medial and lateral malleoli should be level as compared to the opposite foot. Both feet should be angled equally. Tibial torsion may result in the foot either pointing inward ("pigeon toes"), or slightly lateral. Check for supination or pronation of the feet.
4. Check the skin for normal contours, discolored lesions, bruising, ecchymosis, and scars indicating a previous injury or surgery. Note any signs of circulatory impairment or varicose veins.
5. Ask the individual to do a deep knee squat, and observe how posture is affected.

POSTERIOR VIEW

1. Are the gluteal and knee folds level? Do the hamstrings and calf muscles have equal bulk? Check the popliteal fossa for abnormal swelling that may indicate a Baker's cyst.
2. Does the Achilles tendon go straight down to the calcaneus? If it appears to angle laterally, excessive pronation of the foot may affect forces at the knee.

LATERAL VIEW

1. The knees should be slightly flexed (0 to 5°) with the plum line passing through the center of the knee. Women may be prone to genu recurvatum (hyperextended knees), leading to lordosis. If joint swelling is present, the involved knee may assume a position of 15 to 25° of flexion.
2. Check the level of the tibial tubercle for possible Osgood-Schlatter disease. If patella alta is present, the infrapatellar fat pad may become more prominent (camel's sign).

SEATED POSITION; ANTERIOR AND LATERAL VIEWS

1. The patellae should face forward and rest on the distal femur. With patella alta, the patella will rest on the anterior surface of the femur. Laterally displaced patellae give the appearance of "frog's eyes" or "grasshopper's eyes," and may lead to patellofemoral problems.
2. Ask the person to extend both knees, and note tibial movement and patella tracking.

malities in gait, favoring one limb, tibial torsion, increased Q-angle, or an inability to perform a fluid motion.

 The volleyball player appears to have genu valgus with femoral anteversion, external tibial torsion, and patella alta. Swelling is present on the lateral aspect of the patellofemoral joint.

PALPATION

 With pain and swelling centered on the lateral patella, where should you begin to palpate the various structures? During palpation, what factors are you looking for?

Bilateral palpation can determine temperature, swelling, point tenderness, crepitus, deformity, muscle spasm, and cutaneous sensation. Vascular pulses can be taken at the popliteal artery in the posterior knee, the posterior tibial artery behind the medial malleolus, and the dorsalis pedis artery in the dorsum of the foot. Before palpating for tenderness, which may lead to additional pain and apprehension, evaluate patella mobility. With the individual supine, perform the patellar tilt test. Grasp the patella, push down on the medial edge, and attempt to rotate the patella in the coronal plane to determine if the lateral patellar tilt can be corrected to "neutral" (when the patella's anterior surface comes parallel to the surface of the examination table). Then, while holding the patella in a corrected or neutral position, attempt to displace the patella first medially and then laterally. Medial glide of the patella stresses the lateral patellar retinaculum and the other soft tissue restraints. Lateral glide stresses the medial patellar retinaculum, the VMO, and the knee's medial joint capsule. The patella should move half its width (one to two quadrants of the size of the patella) in both directions with an end

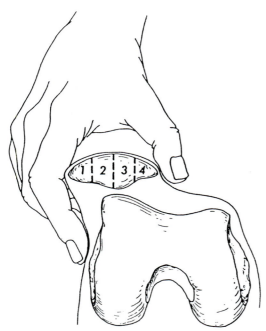

➤ FIGURE 15.21 **Patellar glide**. Passive lateral glide of the patella demonstrating subluxation to its second quadrant. Hypomobility is manifested by less than one quadrant of displacement; three or more quadrants (greater than one-half of patellar width) is considered hypermobile. Reprinted with permission from Jackson DW (ed.): The Anterior Cruciate Ligament: Current and Future Concepts. New York: Raven Press, 1993:358.

feel of tissue stretch (**Figure 15.21**). If lateral displacement produces apprehension or reproduces symptoms of a subluxation (apprehension test), the test is considered positive, indicating patellar instability. Movement of one quadrant or less is called a **hypomobile patella**; movement of three or more quadrants is a **hypermobile patella**, indicating laxity of the restraints. A hypermobile lateral glide may predispose the athlete to a laterally subluxating or dislocating patella. Comparing superior and inferior patellar glide can sometimes reveal side-to-side differences, especially in individuals who have undergone surgery. Compare with the other patella, and note any asymmetry.

Palpate proximal to distal, leaving the most painful area till last. With the individual non-weight-bearing, place a pillow under the knee to relax the limb. You may need to change knee position to palpate certain structures more effectively. For example, meniscal lesions are best palpated at 45°; the joint line is more prominent at 90°. Externally rotating the knee exposes the anteromedial border of the medial meniscus; internally rotating the knee exposes the lateral meniscus.

Extreme pain or point tenderness during palpation of bony structures may indicate a fracture. Compression, distraction, and percussion may also be used to detect fracture. For example, compression at the distal tibia and fibula causes distraction at the proximal tibiofibular joint. Percussion or tapping on the malleoli, or use of a tuning fork, may also produce positive signs at the fracture site.

If you suspect a fracture, put the joint in a knee immobilizer, or activate EMS if a traction splint is necessary. Assess circulatory and neural integrity distal to the fracture site, and take vital signs. The individual should be immediately referred to a physician for further care.

Anterior Palpation

1. Quadriceps muscles, adductor muscles, and sartorius
2. Patellar surface, edges, and retinaculum
3. Patellar tendon, fat pad, tibial tubercle, medial and lateral tibial plateaus, and bursa. With the knee extended, the infrapatellar fat pad can be palpated on the medial and lateral sides of the patellar tendon
4. Patella plica (medial to the patella, with the knee flexed at 45°)
5. Medial femoral condyle and epicondyle, and medial collateral ligament
6. Pes anserinus
7. Iliotibial band, lateral femoral condyle and epicondyle, lateral collateral ligament, and head of fibula. The lateral collateral ligament can be further palpated by having the individual place the foot of the affected limb on the knee of the unaffected leg while palpating the lateral joint line
8. With the knee flexed at 90°, palpate the tibiofemoral joint line, medial and lateral tibial plateaus, medial and lateral femoral condyles, and adductor muscles

Posterior Palpation with Knee Slightly Flexed

1. Popliteal fossa for Baker's cyst and popliteal artery
2. Popliteus muscle in posterolateral corner
3. Hamstring muscles and gastrocnemius

Palpation for Swelling

Two special tests are used to determine if the swelling is intra-articular or extra-articular. Intra-articular swelling feels heavy and mushy because blood is often mixed with the synovial fluid. Extra-articular swelling is light and fluid, and can easily be moved between the fingers from one side to the another.

BRUSH OR STROKE TEST (MILKING) FOR JOINT SWELLING

This test differentiates between synovial thickening and joint effusion. With effusion, the knee will assume a resting position of 15 to 25° of flexion, which allows the synovial cavity the maximum capacity for holding fluid. Beginning below the medial joint line, stroke 2 or 3 times toward the individual's hip, moving proximal to the suprapatellar pouch (**Figure 15.22A**). With the opposite hand,

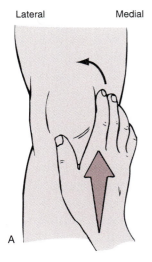

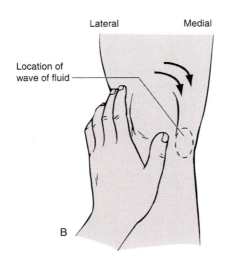

Lateral   Medial

Location of
wave of fluid

Lateral   Medial

A

B

➤ **FIGURE 15.22 Assessment of joint swelling.**
A, To assess joint swelling, stroke the medial side
of the knee several times, toward the hip. B, With
the opposite hand, stroke down the lateral side of
the patella, and note any wave of fluid as it moves
to the medial side of the joint.

stroke down the lateral side of the patella **(Figure 15.22B)**. With effusion, you should observe a wave of fluid pass to the medial side of the joint and bulge just below the medial, distal portion of the patella.

PATELLAR TAP ("BALLOTABLE PATELLA") TEST

With the leg relaxed, push the patella downward into the patellofemoral groove **(Figure 15.23)**. If swelling is intra-articular, the fluid under the patella will cause it to rebound, exhibiting the outlines of the floating patella. If the swelling is extra-articular, a click or definite stopping point will be felt when the patella strikes the patellofemoral groove. The outline of the patella will usually be obscured by extra-articular swelling, seen typically with a ruptured bursa.

 Mild pain is present over the medial retinaculum, but moderate pain was elicited over the lateral aspect of the patella and lateral trochlea. A hypermobile lateral glide was noted, but the athlete

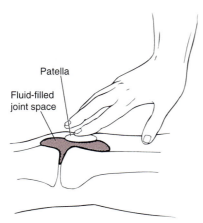

Patella

Fluid-filled
joint space

➤ **FIGURE 15.23 Patellar tap test.** To perform the patellar tap ("ballotable patella") test, the leg should be relaxed. Gently push the patella downward into the groove. If joint effusion is present, the patella will rebound and float back up.

was very apprehensive about the displacement, stating that it hurt and felt like it was going out.

PHYSICAL EXAMINATION TESTS

 Pain and swelling are localized on the lateral patellofemoral joint. What special tests can be performed to determine if the injury is muscular, capsular, or ligamentous?

Perform special tests with the injured athlete in a comfortable position, preferably supine. Pain and muscle spasm can restrict motion and cause an inaccurate result. Do not force the limb through any sudden motions. It may be necessary to place a rolled towel under the knee to relieve strain on the joint structures.

Functional Tests

The athletic trainer should determine the available range of motion in knee flexion/extension, and medial/lateral rotation of the tibia on the femur. Bilateral comparison with the noninjured knee is critical to determine normal or abnormal movement.

ACTIVE MOVEMENTS

Active movements can first be performed with the individual sitting with the leg flexed over the end of the table, then repeated in a prone or supine position. Stabilize the thigh and as always, perform the most painful movements last to prevent painful symptoms from overflowing into the next movement. The movements listed below can be assessed. The numbers in parentheses are normal ranges of motion for each movement.

- Knee flexion (0 to 135°)
- Knee extension (0 to 15°)
- Medial rotation of the tibia on the femur (20 to 30°) with the knee flexed at 90°

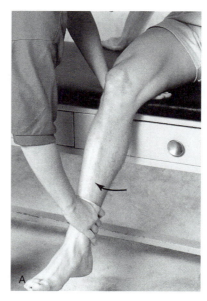

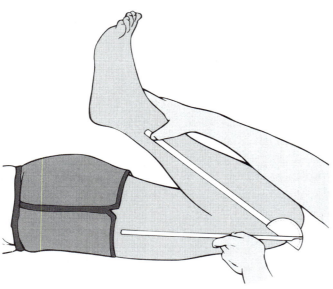

➤ FIGURE 15.24 **Goniometry measurement for knee flexion and extension**. Center the fulcrum over the lateral epicondyle of the femur. Align the proximal arm along the femur, using the greater trochanter for reference. Align the distal arm in line with the lateral malleolus.

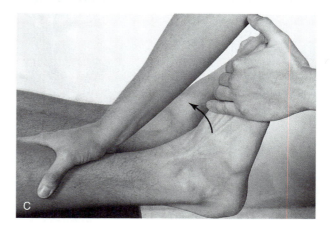

- Lateral rotation of the tibia on the femur (30 to 40°) with the knee flexed at 90°

Measuring range of motion at the knee with a goniometer is demonstrated in **Figure 15.24**.

PASSIVE RANGE OF MOTION

If the individual is able to perform full range of motion during active movements, apply gentle pressure at the extremes of motion to determine end feel. End feel for flexion is tissue approximation; for extension, and medial and lateral rotation, it is tissue stretch. Patellar motion should be performed passively, prior to palpation for point tenderness, with medial and lateral movement compared to the unaffected patella.

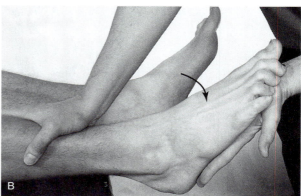

RESISTED MUSCLE TESTING

Stabilize the hip and perform all resisted muscle testing in a seated position except hamstring testing, which is done prone. To isolate the biceps femoris, place the tibia in external rotation and perform knee flexion against resistance. Internal tibial rotation and knee flexion test the medial hamstrings. As the quadriceps extend the knee, observe any abnormal tibial movement or excessive pain from patellar compression. **Figure 15.25** demonstrates motions that should be tested.

➤ FIGURE 15.25 **Resisted manual muscle testing**. A, Knee extension (L3). B, Ankle plantar flexion (S1). C, Ankle dorsiflexion (L4). D, Knee flexion (S1 and S2). Myotomes are listed in parentheses.

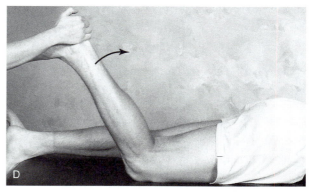

Stress Tests

From information gathered during the history, observation, inspection, and palpation, determine which tests will most effectively assess the condition. Perform only those tests you believe to be absolutely necessary. If you suspect anterior cruciate ligament damage, perform the tests for anterior cruciate instability first because swelling, joint effusion, and muscle spasm may occlude the extent of instability if performed later. Possible structures injured with the various positive tests for unidirectional and multidirectional instability were listed in Table 15.3 and will not be repeated here, except where necessary to explain the test. **Table 15.6** lists stress tests for other structures at the knee.

STRAIGHT ANTERIOR INSTABILITY
Anterior Drawer Test

With the patient supine, the hip is flexed at 45° and the knee is flexed at 90°. The foot is stabilized by placing it under your thigh to prevent any tibial rotation. In this position, the ACL is nearly parallel to the tibial plateau. Place both thumbs on either side of the patellar tendon to palpate the anteromedial and anterolateral joint line, and determine anterior translation as the tibia is drawn forward on the femur. The fingers are placed in the popliteal fossa to ensure that the hamstrings are relaxed. A step-off at the medial tibial plateau should first be palpated to ensure the proper starting position (see posterior drawer test). While palpating the joint line, apply an alternating anterior (anterior drawer) and posterior (posterior drawer) displacement force on the proximal tibia **(Figure 15.26A)**. Stability can be visualized from a lateral view or palpated with the thumb at the joint line. The knee is tested with the foot in neutral rotation, external rotation, and then in internal rotation. The amount of translation and end point are compared with the contralateral knee. The clinician should be aware

TABLE 15.6	OTHER STRESS TESTS FOR THE KNEE
Structure	**Stress Tests**
Meniscal tears	McMurray's test Apley's compression/distraction test "Bounce home" test
Proximal tibiofibular syndesmosis	Tibiofibular translation test
ITB friction syndrome	Noble's compression test Ober's test
Synovial plica	Test for medial synovial plica Stutter test
Patellar subluxation/dislocation	Apprehension test
Patellar articular cartilage	Patellar compression or grind test
Chondromalacia patella	Clark's sign Waldron test

that the anterior drawer test is not as effective as the Lachman's test for a variety of reasons **(Box 15.9)**.

Lachman's Test

A modification of the drawer test is Lachman's test, which tends to isolate the posterolateral bundle of the ACL. With the patient in a supine position, place the knee joint at 20 to 30°, and stabilize the femur with one hand. With the knee in slight flexion, the ACL is the primary restraining force that prevents anterior translation, because the secondary restraints are relaxed. Place the other hand over the proximal tibia, and displace the tibia anteriorly **(Figure 15.26B)**. If the athlete has heavy, muscular legs, or the clinician has small hands, a small support, such as a pillow or tightly rolled towel, can be placed under the femur. A

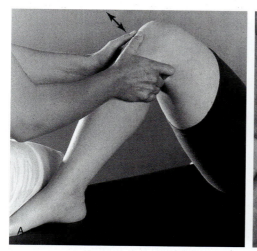
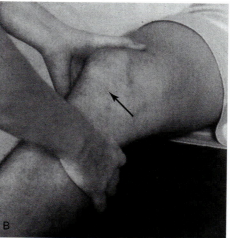

➤ **FIGURE 15.26 Anterior cruciate ligament tests**. A, Drawer test. With the knee flexed, apply an anterior and posterior displacement force on the proximal tibia. B, Lachman's test. With one hand stabilizing the femur, apply firm pressure on the posterior proximal tibia in an attempt to move the tibia anteriorly.

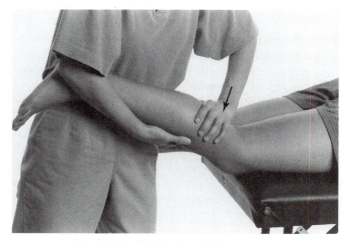

➤ **FIGURE 15.27 Modified Lachman's test**. A downward pressure is applied on the proximal posterior tibia. Note any anterior translation.

positive sign results in a "mushy" or soft end feel when the tibia is moved anterior in relation to the femur. With the tibia in slight internal rotation, anterior displacement indicates additional damage to the IT band, and anterior and middle lateral capsule. With the tibia in slight external rotation, anterior displacement indicates damage to the ACL, MCL, and medial meniscus.

Modified Lachman's Test

This test is used to differentiate abnormal tibiofemoral glide, caused by tears of the ACL, from glide caused by PCL deficiencies. It may also be used by clinicians with small hands, since the weight of the femur is supported by the examination table. With the athlete in a prone position and the knee flexed at 30°, the examiner supports the tibia with one hand while palpating either side of the joint line. The other hand then applies a downward pressure on the proximal portion of the posterior tibia **(Figure 15.27)**. The clinician notes any anterior tibial displacement. Positive anterior translation found with an anterior drawer, Lachman's test, or modified Lachman's test indicates a tear of the ACL. Positive anterior translation with the anterior drawer test or Lachman's test, and a negative modified Lachman's test, indicates a tear in the PCL.

STRAIGHT POSTERIOR INSTABILITY
Posterior Sag (Gravity) Test

The true posterior sag test is performed in a supine position with the hips flexed at 45° and the knees flexed at 90°. When viewed laterally, a loss of tibial tubercle prominence in a PCL-deficient knee is evident when the tibia falls back or sags on the femur due to gravitational forces.

The posterior displacement, however, is more noticeable when the hips and knees are both flexed at 90°. The clinician holds both relaxed legs distally to prevent manual reduction of the tibia. The clinician then moves to the side of the athlete and looks for the position of the tibia as it sags back on the femur, if the posterior cruciate ligament is torn **(Figure 15.28A)**. This maneuver is called Godfrey's sign. It is important to note the sag, because it may produce a false-positive Lachman's test if the sag goes unnoticed.

Posterior Drawer Test

The patient is positioned in the same position listed for the anterior drawer test. The clinician first observes the resting position of the tibial plateau in relation to the femoral condyles. With the knee flexed 90°, the medial tibial plateau normally lies approximately 1 cm anterior to the medial femoral condyle. This can be felt by running the thumb or index finger down the medial femoral condyle toward the tibia. In a PCL-deficient knee, however, this relationship will not be present. The clinician then applies a posteriorly directed force to the tibia (see Figure 15.26A). The knee is tested with the foot in neutral position, external rotation, and then in internal rotation. Truly isolated PCL tears often produce only minimal posterior translation when the secondary restraints of the knee, particularly the posterior capsule and the posteromedial and posterolateral structures, are intact.

False-negative results can occur with a displaced bucket-handle meniscal tear, hamstring or quadriceps spasm, or hemarthrosis.

Reverse Lachman's Test

Positioning is identical to the modified Lachman's test. With the athlete prone and the knee flexed to 20 to 30°, the clinician holds the distal femur to the table and grasps the proximal tibia **(Figure 15.28B)**. Using the hand

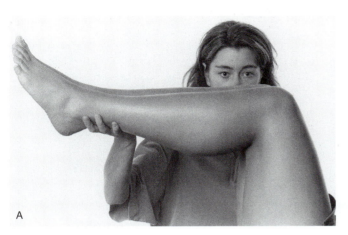

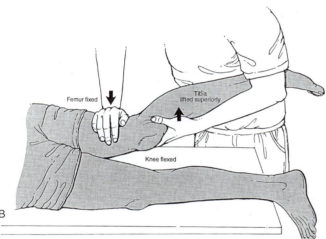

➤ **FIGURE 15.28 Posterior cruciate ligament tests**. A, Posterior sag (gravity) test. Flex both hips and knees. Look from the side and compare the anterior contours of both legs. If one leg sags back and the prominence of the tibial tubercle is lost, the posterior cruciate may be damaged (Godfrey's sign). B, Reverse Lachman's test. With the femur stabilized with one hand, the other hand lifts the tibia up (superiorly), noting any posterior translation and the quality of the end feel.

on the femur to stabilize the thigh and ensure that the hamstrings are relaxed, the clinician lifts the proximal tibia posteriorly (up), noting the amount of translation and quality of end point. A false-positive test may occur if the ACL is torn, allowing gravity to cause an anterior shift of the tibia. The test is not as sensitive for detecting a torn PCL, because the PCL functions more at 90° of knee flexion.

STRAIGHT VALGUS INSTABILITY
Abduction (Valgus Stress) Test

With the individual supine and leg extended, place the heel of one hand on the lateral joint line. The other hand stabilizes the distal lower leg. Apply a lateral force (valgus stress) at the joint line with the lower leg stabilized in slight lateral rotation **(Figure 15.29A)**. If positive (i.e., the tibia abducts), primary damage occurs to the structures of the medial joint capsule. To isolate the tibial collateral ligament, flex the knee at 30° and repeat the valgus stress.

STRAIGHT VARUS INSTABILITY
Adduction (Varus Stress) Test

The knee is placed in the same position as for the abduction test, but a medial force (varus stress) is applied at the knee joint **(Figure 15.29B)**. Laxity in full extension indicates major instability and damage to the fibular collateral ligament, popliteus, and posterolateral capsule. When testing at 20 to 30° of flexion, the true test for one-plane lateral instability, a positive test indicates damage to the fibular collateral ligament.

ANTEROMEDIAL ROTARY INSTABILITY (AMRI)
Slocum Drawer Test

This is performed in the same position as the anterior drawer test, but with the tibia externally rotated 15° **(Figure 15.30A)**. In this position, when an anterior drawer force is applied, the majority of anterior translation occurs on the medial side of the knee. If the amount of anterior translation is the same or increases, AMRI is present, indicating injury to the MCL, oblique popliteal ligament, posteromedial capsule, and the ACL (posteromedial corner).

ANTEROLATERAL ROTARY INSTABILITY (ALRI)
Slocum Drawer Test

This is also performed in the same position as the anterior drawer test, with the tibia internally rotated 25 to 30° **(Figure 15.30B)**. In this position, the majority of anterior translation occurs on the lateral side of the knee. If the anterior translation increases or does not decrease, ALRI is present.

Lateral Pivot Shift Test

This test duplicates the anterior subluxation/reduction phenomenon that occurs during functional activities in ACL-deficient knees. During the test, the tibia moves away from the femur on the lateral side (but rotates medially) and moves anteriorly in relation to the femur. While

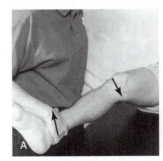
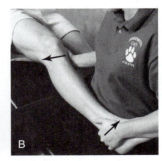

➤ **FIGURE 15.29 Valgus and varus stress tests**. A, Valgus stress test. With the knee flexed at 30°, apply a gentle valgus stress at the knee joint while moving the lower leg laterally. Repeat the test with the knee fully extended. B, Varus stress test. With the knee flexed at 30°, apply a varus stress at the knee joint while moving the lower leg medially. Repeat the test with the knee fully extended.

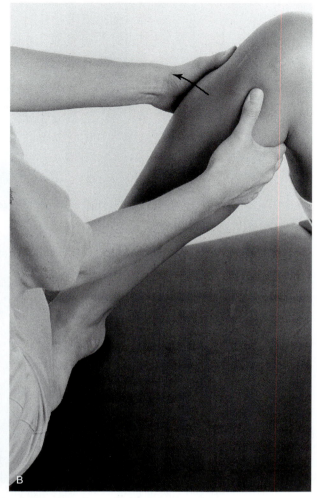

➤ FIGURE 15.30 Slocum drawer test. A, An anterior drawer force is applied for anteromedial rotary instability with the tibia externally rotated 15°. B, Anterolateral rotary instability is tested with the tibia internally rotated 25 to 30°.

supine, the hip is flexed at 30° with no abduction. One hand is placed behind the head of the fibula, and the other hand holds the foot while internally rotating the lower leg about 20°. A valgus force is applied to the knee while maintaining the internal rotation; the knee is moved from extension into flexion **(Figure 15.31)**. With a torn ACL, the femur displaces posteriorly when the knee is placed in 10 to 20° of flexion. As the knee continues to flex, the ITB changes its angle of pull from that of an extensor to that of a flexor. When the knee reaches 30 to 40° of flexion, the ITB causes the tibia to reduce or slide backward, resulting in a noticeable "clunk." This test is highly accurate for detecting acute and chronic ACL injuries.

➤ FIGURE 15.31 Lateral pivot shift test. With the hip flexed and abducted 30° and relaxed in slight medial rotation, place the heel of the hand behind the head of the fibula. The other hand grasps the distal tibia while maintaining 20° of internal tibial rotation. Apply a valgus force while the knee is slowly flexed. When the knee reaches 30 to 40° of flexion, the ITB causes the tibia to reduce or slide backward, giving a noticeable "clunk." Reprinted with permission from Magee DJ: Orthopedic Physical Assessment, 3rd ed. Philadelphia: WB Saunders, 1997.

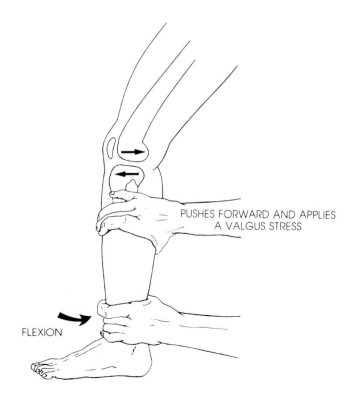

PUSHES FORWARD AND APPLIES A VALGUS STRESS

FLEXION

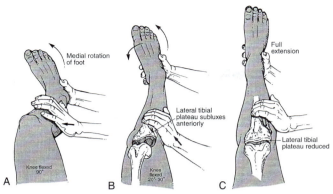

> FIGURE 15.32 **Jerk test**. A, With the knee flexed to 90°, one hand is placed behind the head of the fibula to produce internal tibial rotation. B, At 20 to 30°, the lateral tibial plateau subluxes anteriorly. C, At full extension, the lateral tibial plateau reduces.

Jerk Test

Similar to the lateral pivot shift maneuver, the jerk test is performed in the same position, except that the patient's hip is flexed at 45°. First, flex the knee to 90°. The leg is then extended, maintaining medial rotation and a valgus stress **(Figure 15.32)**. If positive, at approximately 20 to 30° of flexion, the tibia will jerk (shift) forward, causing a subluxation of the lateral tibial plateau. If the leg continues into further extension, it spontaneously reduces. Although not as sensitive as the lateral pivot shift test, a positive jerk test indicates injury to the ACL, posterolateral capsule, arcuate-popliteus complex, LCL, and IT band.

Slocum ALRI Test

Although this is not as sensitive as the pivot shift test, it aids in relaxing the hamstring muscles and is easier to perform on heavy or tense individuals. The individual is placed in a side-lying position (approximately 30° from supine) with the pelvis rotated posteriorly. The bottom leg is the uninvolved leg. With the involved foot stabilizing the tibia, a valgus force is applied to the knee while the knee is flexed at 25 to 45° **(Figure 15.33)**. During this range, a subluxation of the tibia is reduced with a noticeable "clunk."

Crossover Test

The individual is asked to bear weight on the involved limb and step across with the uninvolved leg **(Figure 15.34)**. Because the foot of the weight-bearing leg remains fixed, the lateral femoral condyle is allowed to displace posteriorly relative to the tibia in the presence of laxity in the lateral capsular restraints. An alternate method is to gently step on the involved foot and ask the patient to rotate the upper torso away from the injured leg approximately 90° from the fixed foot. Then, the individual is asked to contract the quadriceps muscles, producing the same symptoms and testing the same structures as in the lateral pivot shift test.

Flexion-Rotation Drawer Test

This test may be used in an acute injury and tends to be more sensitive than the other ALRI tests. With the

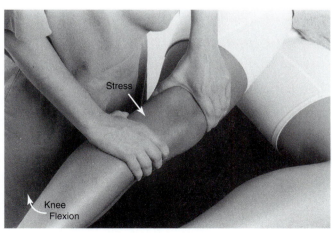

> FIGURE 15.33 **Slocum ALRI test**. With the uninvolved leg on the bottom, apply a valgus force to the top, injured knee while the knee is flexed at 25 to 45°. During this range, a subluxation of the tibia is reduced with a "clunk."

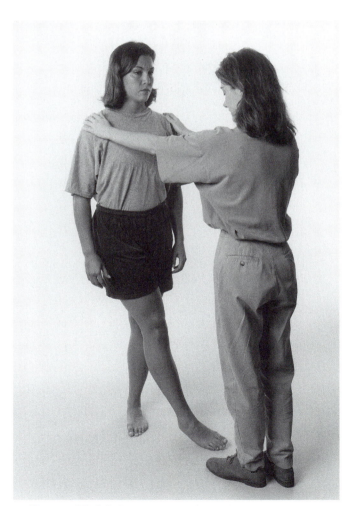

> FIGURE 15.34 **Crossover test**. Stepping across the injured leg will determine ALRI (illustrated here). Stepping behind the injured leg can determine AMRI.

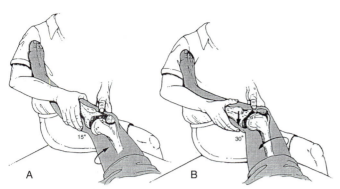

▶ **FIGURE 15.35 Flexion-rotation drawer test**. Flexion from (A) and (B) results in a posterior reduction of the subluxed tibia and medial rotation of the femur. Positive results correlate with ACL damage.

patient supine, the clinician holds the patient's ankle between the clinician's trunk and arm, with the hands around the tibia **(Figure 15.35)**. The knee is then flexed to 20 to 30° while maintaining the tibia in neutral rotation. The tibia is then pushed posteriorly, as in a posterior drawer test. This movement reduces the subluxation of the tibia, indicating a positive test for ALRI. If the tibia is alternately pushed posteriorly and released, and the femur is allowed to rotate freely, the reduction and subluxation are seen and felt as the femur rotates medially and laterally.

POSTEROMEDIAL ROTARY INSTABILITY (PMRI)
Posteromedial Drawer Test

With the patient supine, the knee flexed to 80 to 90°, and the hip flexed at 45°, the clinician medially rotates the patient's foot and sits on the foot to stabilize it. The tibia is then pushed posteriorly. If the tibia displaces or rotates posteriorly on the medial aspect an excessive amount relative to the normal knee, the test is positive.

Posteromedial Pivot Shift Test

With the patient supine, the clinician passively flexes the knee more than 45° while applying a varus stress, compression, and medial rotation of the tibia. In a positive test, these movements cause subluxation of the medial tibial plateau posteriorly. The clinician then moves the knee into extension. At about 20 to 40° of flexion, the tibia shifts into the reduced position.

POSTEROLATERAL ROTARY INSTABILITY (PLRI)
Posterolateral Drawer Test

The athlete is in the same position as the posteromedial drawer test, but with the foot laterally rotated. The tibia is then pushed posteriorly. If the tibia displaces or rotates posteriorly on the lateral aspect an excessive amount relative to the normal knee, this indicates PLRI, but only if the PCL is torn.

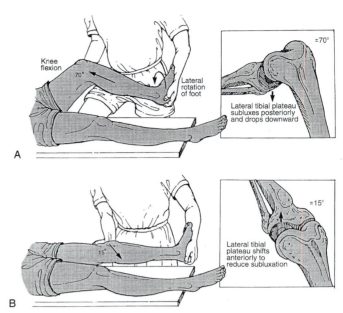

▶ **FIGURE 15.36 Reverse pivot shift test**. A, A flexed position with lateral rotation causes the lateral tibial tubercle to sublux. B, As the knee extends, the lateral tibial tubercle reduces.

Reverse Pivot Shift Test

The reverse pivot shift test discerns combination injuries from an isolated PCL injury. Lift the individual's leg, and stabilize it with one hand on the heel. The other hand supports the lateral calf, with the palm on the proximal fibula. In the first part of the test, the individual's knee is flexed to 70 to 80° and the foot is externally rotated, causing the tibia on the injured side to sublux posteriorly **(Figure 15.36A)**. Next, extend the leg while applying valgus stress to the knee **(Figure 15.36B)**. The test is positive if the subluxation reduces.

External Rotation Recurvatum Test

With the patient supine and the lower limbs relaxed, the clinician gently grasps the big toes of each foot and lifts both feet off the table **(Figure 15.37)**. The patient is told to keep the quadriceps relaxed. While elevating the legs, the clinician watches the tibial tubercles. With a positive test, the affected knee goes into relative hyperextension on the lateral aspect, with the tibia and tibial tubercle rotating laterally. The affected knee appears to have genu varum with damage to the posterior cruciate and lateral collateral ligaments, the arcuate ligament complex, the posterolateral joint capsule, and the biceps femoris.

TESTS FOR MENISCAL LESIONS
McMurray's Test

With the individual supine, flex the knee completely against the chest, externally rotate the tibia, and slowly extend the knee and hip **(Figure 15.38)**. You are attempting to trap the displaced posterior horn of the medial meniscus in the joint, producing an audible and palpable click or thud. Return to the starting position. With internal rotation and extension of the knee and hip, the posterior horn of the lateral meniscus is trapped. Each test is repeated several times.

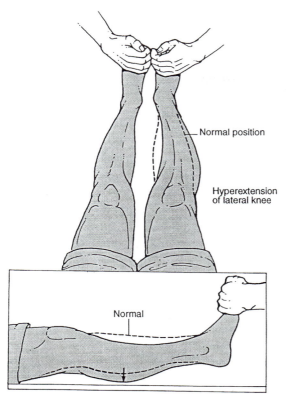

➤ **FIGURE 15.37 External rotation recurvatum test.** Grasp the big toes of each foot, and lift both feet off the table. Make sure the athlete keeps the quadriceps relaxed. With a positive test, the affected knee will become hyperextended on the lateral aspect, with the tibia and tibial tubercle rotating laterally.

Apley's Compression/Distraction Test

In a prone position with the knee flexed at 90°, stabilize the thigh and rotate the leg by applying downward compression in a medial and lateral direction **(Figure 15.39A)**. The test is positive if pain is produced. This compression test may or may not produce a positive sign, even though a meniscal tear is present. Pain should be relieved by repeating the test with the joint distracted **(Figure 15.39B)**. If rotation with distraction produces pain, the lesion is probably ligamentous.

"Bounce Home" Test

With the athlete supine with the knee fully flexed, the clinician cups the heel of the involved leg in one hand. The knee is then passively allowed to extend. If extension is not complete, or a rubbery end feel ("springy block") is present, there may be a torn meniscus present.

TESTS FOR TIBIOFIBULAR INSTABILITY
Proximal Tibiofibular Syndesmosis Test

With the athlete supine and the knees flexed at about 90°, stabilize the tibia with one hand while the other hand grasps the proximal fibular head. Attempt to displace the fibular head anteriorly, then posteriorly. A positive test is indicated by any perceived movement of the fibula on the tibia. An anterior shift indicates damage to the proximal posterior tibiofibular ligament; posterior displacement indicates damage to the proximal anterior tibiofibular ligament.

PLICA TESTS
Mediopatellar Plica Test

With the individual supine, the clinician flexes the affected knee to 30°. The clinician then moves the patella medially in an effort to cause pain, indicating a positive test. The pain is caused by pinching the edge of the plica between the medial femoral condyle and the patella.

Plica "Stutter" Test

This is done with the individual seated on the edge of the examination table with both knees flexed to 90°. With a finger placed over the patella, the patient is asked to extend the knee slowly. If the test is positive, the patella stutters or jumps somewhere between 45 and 60° of flexion (0° being full extension). The test is effective only if there is no joint swelling.

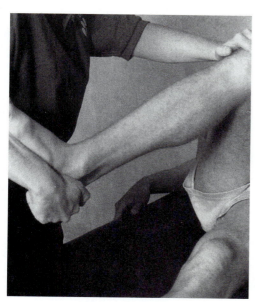

➤ **FIGURE 15.38 McMurray's test.** With the hip and knee flexed, stabilize the lower leg with one hand, and laterally rotate the tibia. Place the other hand over the anterior knee with the fingers on the joint line. Slowly extend the leg. If there is a loose body in the medial meniscus, this action will cause a snap or click. Internally rotating the leg and repeating the test with the thumb over the lateral joint line will test for lateral meniscus damage.

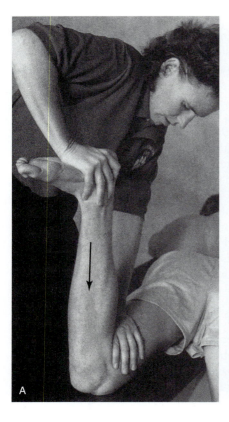

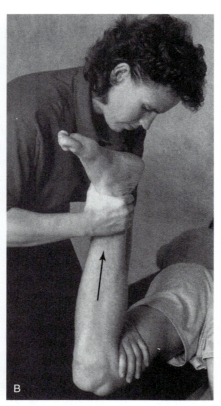

➤ FIGURE 15.39 **Apley's test**. A, Apley's compression test. If rotation and compression cause pain, meniscal damage may be present. B, Apley's distraction test. If rotation and distraction cause pain, ligamentous damage may be present.

Hughston's Plica Test

With the individual supine, the clinician flexes the knee and medially rotates the tibia with one arm and hand. The other hand presses the patella medially while palpating the medial femoral condyle with the fingers of the same hand. The individual's knee is passively flexed and extended while the clinician feels for "popping" of the plica band under the fingers, which indicates a positive test.

TESTS FOR PATELLOFEMORAL DYSFUNCTION
Patella Compression or Grind Test

To assess articular pain due to irritation of subchondral bone, compress the patella in the trochlea at various degrees of flexion. Normally, the patella enters the trochlea at 10 to 15° of knee flexion, so pressure applied in full extension does not directly produce articular compression between the patella and trochlea. Place a rolled towel under the knee, flexing it at about 20°. Compress the patella into the patellofemoral groove **(Figure 15.40A)**. In this position, the distal portion of the patella is articulating; pain with compression in this range suggests a lesion in the distal patellar or proximal trochlear area. Conversely, as knee flexion increases, the patella is drawn distally in the trochlea, causing the area of articulation to be more proximal on the patella; pain with compression in flexion suggests a more proximal patellar lesion. The test is positive if pain is felt or a grinding sound is heard, indicating pathology of the patellar articular cartilage.

Clarke's Sign

Using the web of your hand, place the hand just proximal to the superior pole of the patella **(Figure 15.40B)**. Ask the individual to contract the quadriceps while you gently push downward. If the individual can hold the con-

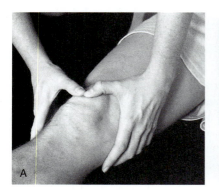

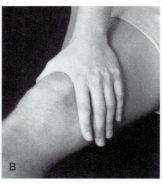

➤ FIGURE 15.40 **Patellofemoral dysfunction**. A, Patella compression or grind test. Pain on compression of the patella into the groove indicates pathology of the patella articular cartilage. B, Clarke's sign. Apply slight compression just proximal to the superior pole of the patella, and ask the individual to contract the quadriceps. The test is positive for chondromalacia patella if the individual has pain or is unable to hold the contraction.

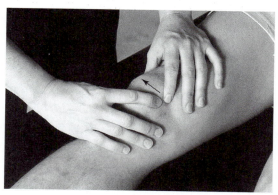

➤ FIGURE 15.41 Patellar apprehension test. Gently displace the patella laterally. The test is a positive sign for subluxating patella if the individual shows apprehension.

traction without pain, the test is negative. If the individual has pain and is unable to hold the contraction, the test is positive for chondromalacia patellae. This test can elicit pain in any individual if the pressure is significant. Therefore, it is imperative to repeat the procedure several times with increasing pressure in full knee extension, and at 30°, 60°, and 90° of knee flexion.

Waldron Test

Palpate the patella while the individual does several slow deep knee bends. Note any crepitus, pain, "catching," or improper tracking of the patella. If any of these signs or symptoms occur simultaneously, the test is positive for chondromalacia patellae.

Patellar Apprehension Test

With the knee in a relaxed position, push the patella laterally (Figure 15.41). If the individual voluntarily or involuntarily shows apprehension, it is a positive test for a subluxating patella.

TESTS FOR ILIOTIBIAL BAND FRICTION SYNDROME
Noble Compression Test

This test is used with Ober's test to determine if IT band friction syndrome is present near the knee (Figure 15.42A). The individual is supine on a table with the hip and knee flexed at 90°. The individual slowly lowers the leg and extends the knee. Apply pressure with the thumb directly over, or 1 to 2 cm proximal to, the lateral epicondyle of the femur. As the knee moves to 30° of knee flexion, the individual will report severe pain similar to that caused during activity.

Ober's Test

The individual lies on the side with the lower leg slightly flexed at the hip and knee for stability. Stabilize the pelvis with one hand to prevent the pelvis from shifting posteriorly during the test. Passively abduct and slightly extend the hip so the IT band passes over the greater trochanter (Figure 15.42B). Although the original Ober's test called for the knee to be flexed at 90°, the IT band has a greater stretch if the knee is extended. Slowly lower the upper leg. If the IT band is tight, the leg will remain in the abducted position.

Neurologic Assessment

Assess neurologic integrity with isometric muscle testing of the myotomes, reflex testing, and sensation in the segmental dermatomes and peripheral nerve cutaneous patterns.

MYOTOMES

Isometric muscle testing should be performed in the following motions to test specific segmental myotomes: hip flexion (L_1, L_2); knee extension (L_3); ankle dorsiflexion (L_4); toe extension (L_5); ankle plantar flexion, foot eversion, or hip extension (S_1); and knee flexion (S_2).

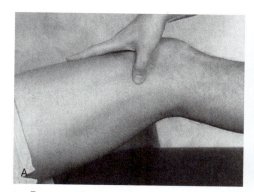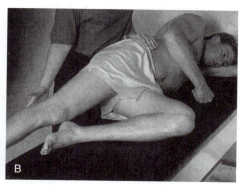

➤ FIGURE 15.42 Tests for iliotibial band friction syndrome. A, Noble compression test. Flex the hip and knee at 90° and apply thumb pressure over the lateral epicondyle of the femur as the leg is extended. Pain at or near 30° flexion indicates ITB syndrome. B, Ober's test. Passively abduct and slightly extend the hip. Slowly lower the extended leg. If the ITB is tight, the leg will remain in the abducted position.

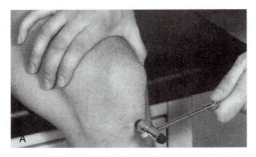

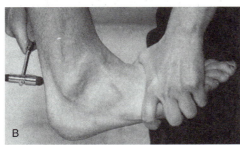

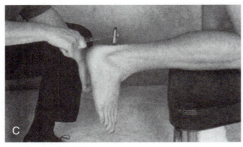

➤ **FIGURE 15.43 Reflex testing.** A, The patellar reflex. B, The Achilles reflex. C, Alternate position for the Achilles reflex.

REFLEXES

Reflexes in the lower leg region include the patella (L_3, L_4) and Achilles tendon reflex (S_1) **(Figure 15.43)**. To test the patellar reflex, flex the knee at 90° (seated), and strike the tendon with the flat end of the reflex hammer using a crisp, wrist-flexion action. A normal reflex exhibits a slight jerking motion in extension. To test the Achilles tendon reflex, slightly dorsiflex the ankle to place the tendon on stretch, and tap the tendon with the flat end of the reflex hammer. An alternate position is to have the individual lie prone on a table, or place the knee on a chair with the foot extended beyond the edge. A normal reflex should elicit a slight plantar-flexion jerk.

CUTANEOUS PATTERNS

In testing cutaneous sensation, run a sharp and dull object over the skin, e.g., blunt tip of taping scissors versus flat edge of taping scissors. With eyes closed or looking away, ask if the individual can distinguish sharp and dull. The segmental nerve dermatome patterns for the knee are demonstrated in **Figure 15.44**. The peripheral nerve cutaneous distribution patterns are demonstrated in **Figure 15.45**.

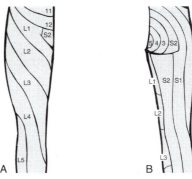

➤ **FIGURE 15.44 Segmental nerve dermatome patterns.** A, Anterior view. B, Posterior view.

Sport-Specific Functional Tests

Functional tests should be performed before clearing the individual for return to participation. These tests should be performed pain-free, without a limp or antalgic gait. Examples of functional tests include forward running, cross-over stepping, running figure-eights or V-cuts, side-step running, and karioca running. When appropriate, functional braces or protective supportive devices should be used to prevent reinjury.

 During special tests, you found increased pain and weakness during active and resisted knee extension, but neurologic assessment was normal. Increased pain and agitation were elicited during the Waldron and patellar apprehension tests. If you determined the individual may have chronic patellar subluxation, you are correct. This individual should be referred to a physician to determine if any long-term damage has occurred to the articular surface of the patella and trochlea.

REHABILITATION OF KNEE INJURIES

 What major components must be included in a knee rehabilitation program? How will you determine when an individual can return to sport participation?

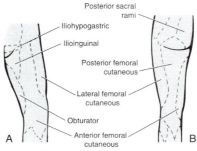

Posterior sacral rami
Iliohypogastric
Ilioinguinal
Posterior femoral cutaneous
Lateral femoral cutaneous
Obturator
Anterior femoral cutaneous

➤ **FIGURE 15.45 Peripheral nerve sensory distribution patterns.** A, Anterior view. B, Posterior view.

A rehabilitation program attempts to minimize inflammation and the effects of immobilization by initiating early mobilization and controlled movement to allow healing tissues to be stressed gradually and progressively until normal joint function is restored. The rehabilitation program should restore motion and proprioception, maintain cardiovascular fitness, and improve muscular strength, endurance, and power, predominantly through closed-chain exercises. Sample exercise programs for specific injuries were listed in Field Strategies 15.1–15.5.

Restoration of Motion

After most knee injuries, some loss of motion will occur. Passive range-of-motion exercises can begin on the first day after injury. There has been some concern about the use of continuous passive motion (CPM) machines (see Figure 6.18) following autogenous patellar tendon reconstruction of the ACL, because of potential damage to the graft. The literature does support the early use of the CPM in this population (21). The unit moves the knee through a protected range of motion to stimulate the intrinsic healing process (Box 15.10). When a CPM machine is not needed, range-of-motion exercises such as the supine wall slide, heel slide, assisted knee flexion and extension, half squats, or PNF stretching exercises can be performed (Figure 15.46). Extension is usually the most difficult motion to restore, and it is critical in achieving normal gait. Place the athlete prone with the thigh resting on the table. The lower leg is extended off the end of the table. A weight can be added on the distal tibia so a gradual stretch is achieved. Following the exercise bout, the knee can be iced in the supine position with the heel elevated to assist with extension.

In addition to active and passive range-of-motion exercises at the tibiofemoral joint, stretching exercises to improve passive glide of the patellofemoral joint, particularly medial glide, can stretch tight lateral structures to correct patellar positioning and tracking (Figure 15.47). Normal passive glide of the patellofemoral joint should be restored

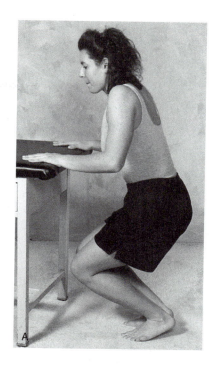

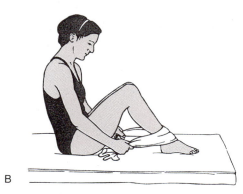

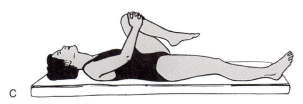

➤ FIGURE 15.46 Range-of-motion exercises. A, Half squat. B, Assisted heel slide. C, Assisted knee flexion.

before full flexion exercises, resisted exercises, or bicycling is initiated.

Restoration of Proprioception and Balance

Proprioception and balance must be regained to return safely to sport participation. In the early stages following injury, when weight-bearing is allowed, closed-chain exercises such as shifting one's weight while on crutches,

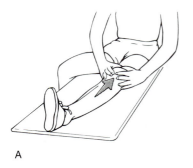

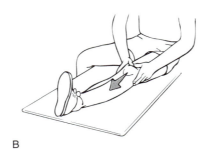

A   B

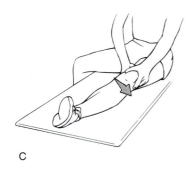

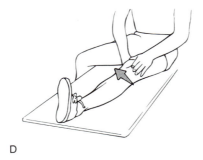

C   D

➤ FIGURE 15.47 Patellar self-mobilization.
A, Proximal. B, Distal. C, Medial. D, Lateral.

straight-leg raises, bilateral minisquats, or use of a BAPS board with support may be helpful. As balance improves, unassisted use of the BAPS board, closed-chain exercises, running in place on a minitramp, or use of a slide board may be incorporated along with other closed-chain exercises used to develop strength (see below).

Muscular Strength, Endurance, and Power

Early emphasis is placed on strengthening the quadriceps femoris musculature, particularly the vastus medialis and vastus medialis oblique (VMO). These muscles aid in the stabilization of the patella superiorly and medially. Isometric contractions, called quad sets, are performed at, or near, 0°, 45°, 60°, and 90° flexion. Isometric hip adduction exer-

cises are also used to recruit the VMO, and can be performed by squeezing a rolled towel between the knees in a seated position. Open-chain exercises may include straight-leg raises in all directions, supplemented by ankle weights or tubing to increase resistance. Knee extension and knee flexion exercises may be done with free weights or on several commercially available isotonic or isokinetic machines.

Closed-chain exercises performed during weight-bearing may include terminal knee extension (**Figure 15.48**), step-ups, step-downs, lateral step-ups, minisquats from 0 to 40°, leg presses on a machine from 0 to 60°, or use of a stepping machine or stationary bicycle. Several of these exercises were illustrated in Field Strategy 15.1. Closed-chain exercises can be made progressively more

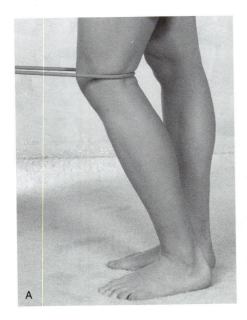

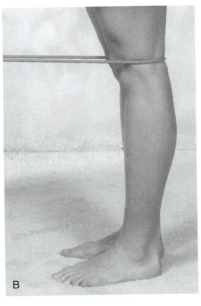

A   B

➤ FIGURE 15.48 Closed chain terminal extension. A, Starting position. B, Ending position.

difficult by increasing the resistance or speed of movement or by changing the individual's visual feedback (looking at the ceiling, looking at the floor, or closing the eyes). It is critical to ensure proper performance of closed-chain exercises. For example, when doing a minisquat or leg press, if the hip is not strong enough to control adduction and internal rotation, the knee will assume a valgus alignment with the foot pronated. This leads to an increased Q-angle, predisposing the athlete to patellofemoral pain.

Plyometric jumping in the later stages of rehabilitation can use small boxes and directional changes to improve power and proprioceptive function. Because of the increased eccentric contraction and the associated muscle microtrauma that results from the power maneuvers, these exercises should only be performed two or three times weekly (21).

Cardiovascular Fitness

Cardiovascular fitness exercises can begin immediately after injury with use of UBE or hydrotherapeutic exercise. Running in water and performing sport-specific exercises in deep water can allow the individual to maintain sport-specific functional skills in a non-weight-bearing position. When range of motion is adequate, a stationary bicycle may be used. The seat should be adjusted so the knee is flexed 15 to 30°. The individual should be instructed to pedal with the ball of the foot, using toe clips, and to pull through the bottom of the stroke. A low-to-moderate workload is recommended to reduce patellofemoral compressive forces. Other exercises, such as walking, light jogging, and functional activities can progress as tolerated.

 The rehabilitation program should restore motion and proprioception, maintain cardiovascular fitness, and improve muscular strength, endurance, and power. The individual can return to sport participation after completing all functional tests pain-free, and must be cleared by the supervising physician. These tests might include timed sprints, shuttle runs, agility runs, karioca runs, and hop or vertical jump tests.

Summary

1. The knee (tibiofemoral joint) functions primarily as a modified hinge joint with some lateral and rotational motions allowed.

2. The cruciate ligaments are intracapsular and extrasynovial. They prevent anterior and posterior translation of the tibia on the femur. The ACL is frequently subject to deceleration injuries, with internal tibial torque being the most dangerous loading mechanism, particularly when combined with an anterior tibial force. The shorter and stronger PCL is considered to be the primary stabilizer of the knee.

3. The collateral ligaments prevent valgus (medial) and varus (lateral) stress at the knee.

4. The menisci aid in lubrication and nutrition of the joint, reduce friction during movement, provide shock absorption by dissipating stress over the articular cartilage, improve weight distribution, and help the capsule and ligaments prevent hyperextension.

5. Tracking of the patella against the femur is dependent on the direction of the net force produced by the attached quadriceps. Factors such as patellar instability, a weak VMO, hypermobility of the patella, anatomical malalignment conditions, plica syndromes, or repetitive minor trauma can lead to chronic patellofemoral pain.

6. Because of its location, the prepatellar bursa is the bursa most commonly injured by compressive forces. The deep infrapatellar bursa, on the other hand, is often inflamed by overuse, and subsequent friction between the infrapatellar tendon and structures behind it (fat pad and tibia).

7. A straight plane instability implies instability in one of the cardinal planes. Injury of multiple structures in different planes is called a rotary instability.

8. Isolated anterior instability is rare. Instead, an anteromedial or anterolateral laxity usually occurs. The rate of ACL injuries is higher in women, due partially to a muscle strength imbalance, and both intrinsic and extrinsic factors.

9. Menisci become stiffer and less resilient with age. Tears are classified according to age, location, or axis of orientation, and include longitudinal, bucket-handle, horizontal, and parrot-beak. Because the menisci are not innervated by nociceptors, synovial inflammation and joint effusion may not develop for more than 12 hours after the initial injury.

10. Patellofemoral stress syndrome often occurs when either the VMO is weak or the lateral retinaculum that holds the patella firmly to the femoral condyle is excessively tight. This condition is much more common than chondromalacia patellae, which is a true degeneration in the articular cartilage of the patella.

11. Adolescents are particularly prone to Osgood-Schlatter disease, Sinding-Larsen-Johansson's disease, and fractures to the distal femoral epiphysis.

12. Pain in the knee region can be referred from the lumbar spine, hip, or ankle.

13. A rehabilitation program should minimize inflammation and the effects of immobilization by initiating early mobilization and controlled movement to allow healing tissues to be stressed gradually and progressively until normal joint function is restored.

14. Refer the individual to a physician if any of the following conditions are suspected:
    - Obvious deformity suggesting a dislocation or fracture
    - Significant loss of motion or locking of the knee

- Excessive joint swelling
- Gross joint instability
- Reported sounds, such as popping, snapping, or clicking, or giving way of the knee
- Possible epiphyseal injuries
- Abnormal or absent reflexes
- Abnormal sensations in either segmental dermatomes or peripheral cutaneous patterns
- Absent or weak pulse
- Weakness in a myotome
- Any unexplained or chronic pain that disrupts an individual's play or performance

References

1. VanMechelen W. Running injuries: A review of the epidemiological literature. Sports Med 1992;14(5):320-335.
2. Hickey GJ, Fricker PA, McDonald WA. Injuries of young elite female basketball players over a six-year period. Clin J Sport Med 1997; 7(4):252-256.
3. Aagaard H, Jörgenson U. Injuries in elite volleyball. Scand J Med Sci Sports 1996;6(4):228-232.
4. Markolf KL, et al. Combined knee loading states that generate high anterior cruciate ligament forces. J Orthop Res 1995;13(6):930-935.
5. Irrgang JJ, Safran MR, Fu FH. The knee: Ligamentous and meniscal injuries. In: Athletic Injuries and Rehabilitation. Edited by Zachazewski JE, Magee DJ, Quillen WS. Philadelphia: WB Saunders, 1996.
6. Starkey C, Ryan JL. Evaluation of Orthopedic and Athletic Injuries. Philadelphia: FA Davis Company, 1996.
7. Hahn T, Foldspang A. The Q angle and sport. Scand J Med Sci Sports 1997;7(1):43-48.
8. Schulthies SS, Francis RS, Fisher AG, Van de Graaff KM. Does the Q angle reflect the force on the patella in the frontal plane? Phys Ther 1995;75(1):24-30.
9. Shrive NG, Phil D, O'Connor JJ, Goodfellow JW. Load-bearing in the knee joint. Clin Orthop 1978;131:279-287.
10. Singerman R, Berilla J, Davy DT. Direct in vitro determination of the patellofemoral contact force for normal knees. J Biomech Eng 1995;117(1):3-14.
11. Moul JL. Differences in selected predictors of anterior cruciate ligament tears between male and female NCAA Division I collegiate basketball players. J Ath Train 1998;33(2):118-121.
12. Fadale PD, Hulstyn MJ. Common athletic knee injuries. Clin Sports Med 1997;16(3):479-499.
13. Moeller JL, Lamb MM. Anterior cruciate ligament injuries in female athletes: Why are women more susceptible? Phys Sportsmed 1997;25(4):31-48.
14. Bach BR Jr. Acute knee injuries: When to refer. Phys Sportsmed 1997;25(5):39-50.
15. Cooper DE, Arnoczky SP, Warren RF. Athroscopic meniscal repair. Clin Sports Med 1990;9(3):589-607.
16. Wall EJ. Osgood-Schlatter disease: Practical treatment for a self-limiting condition. Phys Sportsmed 1998;26(3):29-34.
17. Thein LA. The child and adolescent athlete. In: Athletic Injuries and Rehabilitation. Edited by Zachazewski JE, Magee DJ, Quillen WS. Philadelphia: WB Saunders, 1996.
18. Stanitski C, Sherman C. How I manage physeal fractures about the knee. Phys Sportsmed 1997;25(4):108-121.
19. Ralston BM, et al. Osteochondritis dissecans of the knee. Phys Sportsmed 1996;24(6):73-84.
20. Brownstein B, Bronner S. Patella fractures associated with accelerated ACL rehabilitation in patients with autogenous patella tendon reconstructions. JOSPT 1997;26(3):168-171.
21. Weber MD, Ware AN. Knee rehabilitation. In: Physical Rehabilitation of the Injured Athlete. Edited by Andrews JR, Harrelson GL, Wilk KE. Philadelphia: WB Saunders, 1998.

Lower Leg, Ankle, and Foot Conditions

OBJECTIVES

1. Identify the important bony and soft tissue structures of the lower leg, ankle, and foot.

2. Describe the various ligamentous structures that support the lower leg, ankle, and foot.

3. Explain the function of the plantar arches and their role in supporting and distributing body weight.

4. Describe the motions of the foot and ankle, and identify the muscles that produce them.

5. Explain what forces produce the loading patterns responsible for injury to the lower leg, ankle, and foot.

6. List basic principles in the prevention of injuries to the lower leg, ankle, and foot.

7. List common toe and foot conditions, and describe their management.

8. Differentiate between grade I, grade II, and grade III ankle sprains, and describe the management of medial and lateral ankle sprains.

9. Identify common sites for tendon injuries, and describe their management.

10. List the signs and symptoms of common overuse injuries of the lower leg, ankle, and foot, and describe their management.

11. Describe common vascular and neural disorders that may occur in the lower leg, ankle, and foot.

12. Identify common sites for stress and avulsion fractures, and describe their associated signs and symptoms.

13. Explain the management of the fractures in the lower leg, ankle, and foot.

14. Explain a thorough assessment of the lower leg, ankle, and foot.

15. Describe general rehabilitation exercises for the region.

ecause of the essential roles played by the lower leg, ankle, and foot in all sport activities, injuries to the region are common. Sport participation often places both acute and chronic overloads on the lower extremity, leading to sprains, strains, fractures, and overuse injuries. Volleyball and basketball players, in particular, sustain a high incidence of injury to this region (1–4). Among snowboarders, fractures of the lateral process of the talus are becoming an increasingly common injury (5).

This chapter begins with an anatomical review and biomechanical overview of the lower leg, ankle, and foot. Next, prevention of injuries will be followed by discussion on specific sports injuries and their management. Finally, a step-by-step injury assessment of the region will be presented, and examples of rehabilitative exercises will be provided.

ANATOMICAL REVIEW OF THE LOWER LEG, ANKLE, AND FOOT

The lower leg, ankle, and foot provide a foundation of support for the upright body, enabling propulsion through space, adaptation to uneven terrain, and absorption of shock. Discussion of the anatomical structures that contrib-

ute to these abilities begins with bone and ligamentous structures of the leg in the three major regions of the foot—the forefoot, midfoot, and hindfoot **(Figure 16.1)**. Next, the plantar arches are discussed, and finally, the muscles, nerves, and blood vessels of the region.

Forefoot

The forefoot is composed of 5 metatarsals and 14 phalanges, along with numerous joints. Together they work with the midfoot region to form interdependent longitudinal and transverse arches to support and distribute body weight throughout the foot.

METATARSOPHALANGEAL AND INTERPHALANGEAL JOINTS

The metatarsophalangeal (MTP) joint is a condyloid joint with a close-packed position in full extension. The proximal interphalangeal (PIP) and distal interphalangeal (DIP) joints are hinge joints with a close-packed position also in full extension (Figure 16.1). Numerous ligaments reinforce both sets of joints. Each MTP joint is surrounded by an articular and fibrous joint capsule, the plantar side

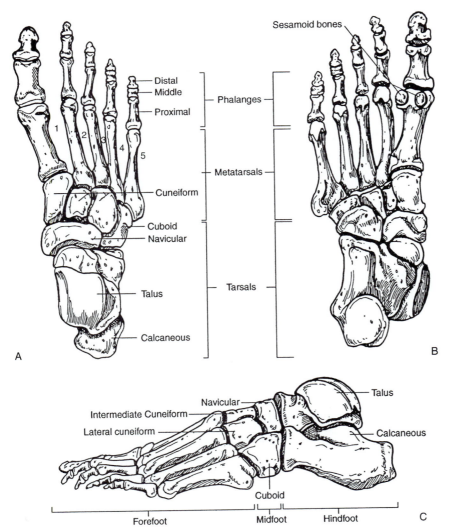

► FIGURE 16.1 **Bones of the foot**. A, Superior view. B, Medial view. C, Lateral view.

of which is reinforced by the plantar fascia and thickened portions of the capsule, the plantar ligament. The medial and lateral joint capsule are reinforced by collateral ligaments. The PIP and DIP joints are reinforced by the plantar and dorsal joint capsule and collateral ligaments. The toes function to smooth the weight shift to the opposite foot during walking and help maintain stability during weight-bearing by pressing against the ground when necessary. The first digit is referred to as the hallux, or "great toe," and is the main body stabilizer during walking or running.

The first MTP joint has two sesamoid bones, located on the plantar surface of the joint to share in weight-bearing. The sesamoid bones serve as anatomical pulleys for the flexor hallucis brevis muscle, and protect the flexor hallucis longus muscle tendon from weight-bearing trauma as it passes between the two bones.

TARSOMETATARSAL AND INTERMETATARSAL JOINTS

The deep transverse metatarsal ligament interconnects all five metatarsals. Both the tarsometatarsal (TM) and intermetatarsal (IM) joints are of the gliding type with the close-packed position in supination. These joints enable the foot to adapt to uneven surfaces during gait.

Midfoot

The midfoot region encompasses the navicular, cuboid, and three cuneiform bones, and their articulations. The navicular, like its counterpart in the wrist, the scaphoid, helps to bridge movements between the hindfoot and forefoot.

TRANSVERSE TARSAL JOINT

The transverse tarsal (or midtarsal) joint consists of two side-by-side articulations—the calcaneocuboid joint on the lateral side, and the talonavicular on the medial side. These two joints are collectively called the transverse tarsal joint because they are adjacent and they function as a unit.

The calcaneocuboid (CC) joint is a saddle-shaped joint with a close-packed position in supination. The joint is nonaxial and permits only limited gliding motion. It is supported by the bifurcate ligament, the plantar and dorsal calcaneocuboid ligaments, and long plantar ligament. The most important of these, the long plantar ligament, extends inferiorly between the calcaneus and the cuboid, then continues distally to the base of the second, third, and fourth metatarsals, contributing significantly to transverse tarsal joint stability.

Because the talus moves simultaneously on the calcaneus and navicular, the term talocalcaneonavicular joint (TCN) is often used to describe the combined action of the talonavicular and subtalar joint. The TCN is a modified ball-and-socket joint with a close-packed position in supination. Movements at the joint include gliding and

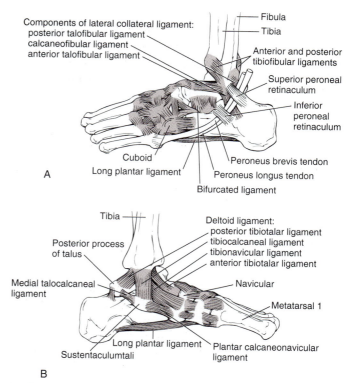

rotation. Three ligaments support the joint—the plantar calcaneonavicular (spring) ligament inferiorly, deltoid ligament medially, and the bifurcate ligament laterally **(Figure 16.2)**.

Because the subtalar joint is mechanically linked to the TCN and transverse tarsal joints, any motion at the subtalar joint produces like motions at the transverse tarsal joints. For example, when the TCN is fully supinated and locked, the midfoot region is also supinated and rigid. When the TCN is pronated and loose packed, the midfoot region is also mobile and loose.

➤ **FIGURE 16.2 Ligaments supporting the midfoot and hindfoot region.** A, Lateral view. B, Medial view.

OTHER MIDTARSAL JOINTS

The remaining joints of the midfoot region include the cuneonavicular, cuboideonavicular, cuneocuboid, and the intercuneiform. These joints provide gliding and rotation for the midfoot with a close-packed position in supination. They are bound together by several ligaments. When the midfoot (TCN) is locked in supination, these joints function in a compensatory manner to pronate the forefoot and increase stability. When the hindfoot is pronated, these joints supinate the forefoot to keep the foot flat on the surface.

Hindfoot

The hindfoot includes the calcaneus and talus. Rising off the anteromedial surface of the calcaneus is the **sustentaculum tali** that largely supports the talus. On the inferior surface of the sustentaculum tali is a groove through which the flexor hallucis longus tendon passes. The peroneal tubercle projects out of the lateral side of the calcaneus and splits the two peroneal tendons as they course inferior to the lateral malleolus. The peroneus brevis tendon runs superior to the tubercle, with the peroneus longus running inferior to the tubercle. The talus is saddle-shaped and serves as the critical link between the foot and ankle. It has several functional articulations, the two most important being the talocrural joint and the subtalar joint. Both serve a unique role in the integrated function of the lower leg, ankle, and foot.

TALOCRURAL JOINT

The talocrural (ankle) joint is a uniaxial, modified synovial hinge joint formed by the talus, the tibia, and the lateral malleolus of the fibula (Figure 16.3). The concave end of the weight-bearing tibia mates with the convex superior surface of the talus to form the roof and medial border of the ankle mortise. The fibula assists with weight-bearing, supporting approximately 17% of the load on the leg (6), serves as a site for muscle and ligamentous attachments, and forms the lateral border of the ankle mortise. The lateral malleolus extends farther distally than the medial malleolus, and hence eversion is more seriously limited than inversion. The dome of the talus is wider anteriorly than posteriorly. The joint's close-packed position is therefore maximum dorsiflexion.

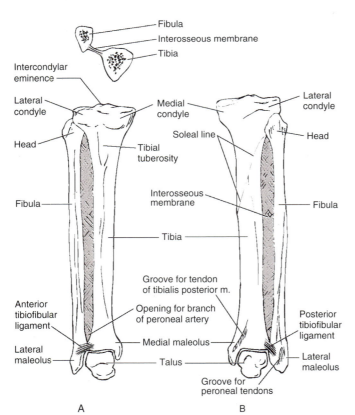

➤ **FIGURE 16.3 Bones of the lower leg**. Little motion occurs at the proximal tibiofibular joint, but the distal tibiofibular joint forms the mortise for the talocrural (ankle) joint. The interosseous membrane joins the full lengths of the tibia and fibula. A, Anterior view. B, Posterior view.

TABLE 16.1	**LIGAMENTS OF THE TALOCRURAL JOINT**	
	Proximal Attachment	Distal Attachment
Medial Collateral Ligaments		
Anterior tibiotalar (ATT)	Anteromedial aspect of medial malleolus	Superior portion of medial talus
Tibiocalcaneal (TC)	Apex of medial malleolus	Calcaneous directly below medial malleolus
Posterior tibiotalar (PTT)	Posterior aspect of medial malleolus	Posterior portion of the talus
Tibionavicular (TN)	Distal and slightly posterior to ATT	Medial aspect of the navicular
Lateral Collateral Ligaments		
Anterior talofibular (ATF)	Anterolateral surface of lateral malleolus	Talus near the sinus tarsi
Calcaneofibular (CF)	Posterior apex of lateral malleolus	Courses 133° inferiorly and posteriorly to attach on calcaneus
Posterior talofibular (TPF)	Posterolateral border of lateral malleolus	Posterior talus and calcaneus

Although the joint capsule is thin and especially weak anteriorly and posteriorly, a number of strong ligaments cross the ankle and enhance stability (Table 16.1). The four separate bands of the medial collateral ligament, more commonly called the deltoid ligament, cross the ankle medially. The anterior tibiotalar (ATT) and tibionavicular (TN) ligaments are taut when the subtalar joint is plantarflexed, whereas the tibiocalcaneal (TC) and posterior tibiotalar (PTT) ligaments are taut during dorsiflexion. Forces producing stress on the medial aspect of the ankle typically cause an avulsion fracture of the medial malleolus rather than tearing the deltoid ligament. The lateral side of the ankle is supported by three ligaments. The anterior talofibular (ATF) ligament is taut and resists inversion during plantar flexion, and limits anterior translation of the talus on the tibia. The calcaneofibular (CF) ligament is taut in the extreme range of dorsiflexion, and is the primary restraint of talar inversion within the midrange of motion. The posterior talofibular (PTF) ligament is the strongest of the lateral ligaments and limits posterior displacement of the talus on the tibia. The relative weakness of these lateral ligaments as compared to the deltoid ligament, coupled with the fact of less bony stability laterally than medially, contributes to a higher frequency of lateral ankle sprains.

SUBTALAR JOINT

As the name suggests, the subtalar joint lies beneath the talus, where facets of the talus articulate with the susten-

$\overline{X} = 7°$

$\overline{X} = 41°$

$\overline{X} = 23°$

➤ **FIGURE 16.4 Subtalar joint**. The axis of rotation at the subtalar joint lies oblique to the sagittal and frontal planes.

taculum tali on the superior calcaneus. Obliquely crossing the talus and calcaneus is the tarsal canal, a sulcus that allows for the attachment of an intra-articular ligament. Because no muscles attach to the talus, the stability of the subtalar joint is derived from several small ligaments. The talocalcaneal interosseous ligament lies in the tarsal canal and divides the subtalar joint into two articular cavities, serves as an axis for talar tilt, and contributes substantially to joint stability, particularly during supination. Four small talocalcaneal ligaments form interconnections between the talus and calcaneus, with added support from the calcaneofibular ligament and the tibiocalcaneal fascicle of the deltoid ligament. The close-packed position for the joint occurs under vertical loading with internal rotation.

Motion at the subtalar joint involves "male" ovoid bone surfaces sliding over reciprocally shaped "female" ovoid bone surfaces. The joint functions basically as a uniaxial hinge joint with the axis aligned in an oblique direction **(Figure 16.4)**. The orientation of the subtalar joint axis varies appreciably among individuals.

Tibiofibular Joints

The tibia and fibula articulate at both proximal and distal ends (Figure 16.3). The proximal, or superior, tibiofibular joint is a plantar synovial joint that is tightly reinforced with anterior and posterior ligaments. The inferior, or distal, tibiofibular joint is a syndesmosis, where dense fibrous tissue binds the bones together. There is no joint capsule, but the joint is supported by the anterior and posterior tibiofibular ligaments, as well as by an extension of the interosseous membrane, the crural interosseous (CI) ligament. This structural arrangement allows for some rotation and slight abduction (spreading), while still main-

taining joint integrity. The CI ligament is of such strength that strong lateral stresses will often fracture the fibula rather than tear the membrane, although excessive eversion or dorsiflexion can result in sufficient widening of the ankle mortise to injure the ligaments supporting the syndesmosis.

Plantar Arches

The bones and supporting ligamentous structures in the tarsal and metatarsal regions of the foot form interdependent longitudinal and transverse arches **(Figure 16.5)**. They function to support and distribute body weight from the talus through the foot, through changing weight-bearing conditions and over varying terrains. The longitudinal

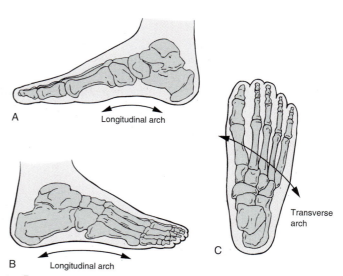

➤ **FIGURE 16.5 Arches of the foot**. A, Medial view. B, Lateral view. C, Dorsal view.

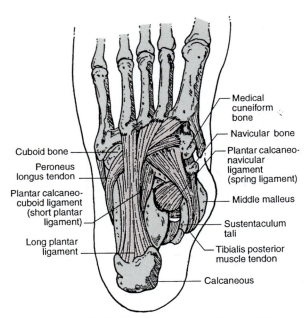

> **FIGURE 16.6 Medial longitudinal arch**. The medial longitudinal arch is supported by the calcaneonavicular (spring) ligament, short plantar ligament, long plantar ligament, plantar aponeurosis, and the tibialis posterior muscle tendon.

arch runs from the anterior, inferior calcaneus to the metatarsal heads. Because the arch is higher medially than laterally, the medial side is usually the point of reference, with the navicular bone serving as the point of reference between the anterior and posterior ascending spans.

The transverse arch runs across the anterior tarsals and metatarsals. The foundation of the arch is the medial

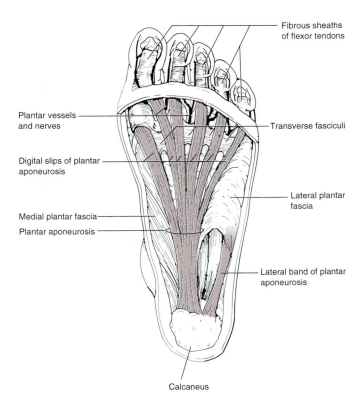

> **FIGURE 16.7 Plantar fascia**. The plantar fascia stores mechanical energy each time the foot deforms during the weight-bearing phase of the gait cycle.

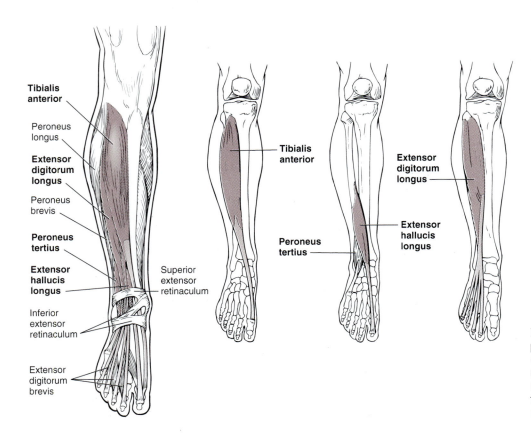

> **FIGURE 16.8 Anterior compartment muscles**. The anterior compartment of the leg (bolded muscles) contains the tibialis anterior, extensor digitorum longus, extensor hallucis longus, and peroneus tertius.

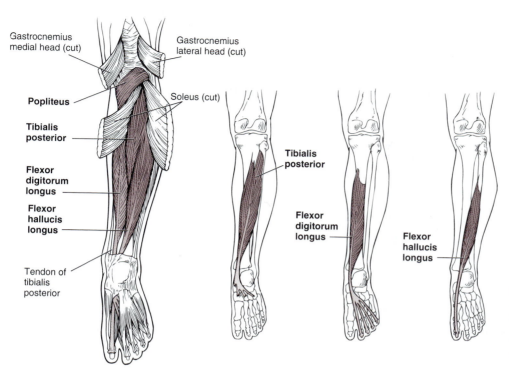

Gastrocnemius medial head (cut)

Gastrocnemius lateral head (cut)

Popliteus

Soleus (cut)

Tibialis posterior

Flexor digitorum longus

Flexor hallucis longus

Tendon of tibialis posterior

Tibialis posterior

Flexor digitorum longus

Flexor hallucis longus

➤ **FIGURE 16.9 Deep posterior compartment muscles.** The muscles in the deep posterior compartment (bolded muscles) pass behind the medial malleolus to enter the foot and include the tibialis posterior, flexor digitorum longus, and flexor hallucis longus.

cuneiform, with the apex of the arch formed by the second metatarsal. At the level of the metatarsal heads, the arch is reduced, with all metatarsals aligned parallel to the weight-bearing surface for even distribution of body weight. Structural support is derived from the intermetatarsal ligaments and the transverse head of the adductor hallucis muscle.

The primary supporting structures of the plantar arches are, in order of importance, the calcaneonavicular (spring) ligament, long plantar ligament, plantar fascia (plantar aponeurosis), and the short plantar (plantar calcaneocuboid) ligament **(Figure 16.6)**. When muscle tension is present, the muscles of the foot, particularly the tibialis posterior, also contribute support to the arches and joints as they cross them.

The **plantar fascia**, or plantar aponeurosis, is a specialized, thick, interconnected band of fascia that covers the plantar surface of the foot, providing support for the longitudinal arch **(Figure 16.7)**. It has three distinct slips. The central slip extends from the posterior medial calcaneal tubercle and inserts into the distal plantar aspects of the proximal phalanges of each toe, where it attaches with deep transverse metatarsal ligaments. As the central slip courses down the length of the foot, it gives off two other slips, one deviating medially and the other laterally. During the weight-bearing phase of the gait cycle, the plantar fascia functions like a spring to store mechanical energy that is then released to help the foot push off from the surface. Stretching the Achilles tendon may elongate the plantar fascia, because both structures attach to the calcaneus.

Muscles of the Lower Leg and Foot

Thick sheaths of fascia divide the muscles of the leg into four compartments—the anterior, deep and superficial

posterior, and lateral compartments. The anterior compartment contains the tibialis anterior, extensor digitorum longus, extensor hallucis longus, and peroneus tertius **(Figure 16.8)**. These muscles can easily be remembered by using the mnemonic Tom, Dick, and Harry, too. Muscles

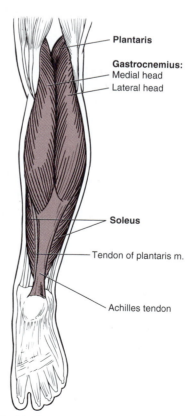

Plantaris

Gastrocnemius:
Medial head
Lateral head

Soleus

Tendon of plantaris m.

Achilles tendon

➤ **FIGURE 16.10 Superficial posterior compartment muscles.** The superficial compartment (bolded muscles) is composed of the gastrocnemius, soleus, and plantaris.

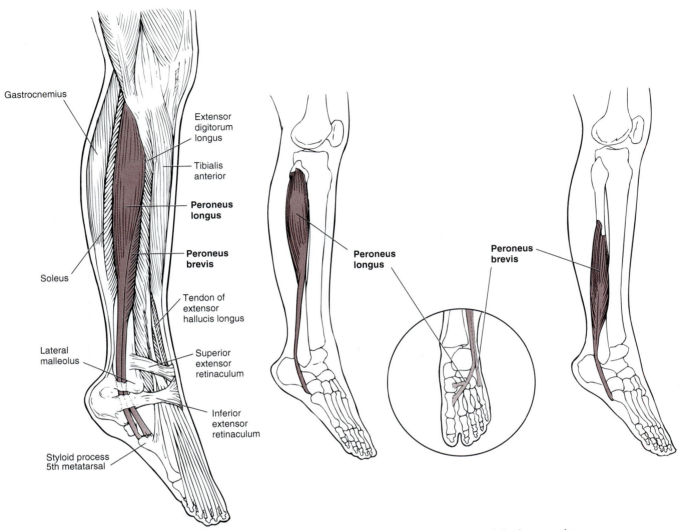

➤ FIGURE 16.11 **Lateral compartment muscles**. The lateral compartment of the leg contains the peroneus brevis and peroneus longus. Note that the peroneus tertius is an extension of the extensor digitorum longus, and is in the anterior compartment.

in the deep posterior compartment can also be remembered by the Tom, Dick, and Harry mnemonic; these include the tibialis posterior, flexor digitorum longus, tibialis posterior artery, tibial nerve, and flexor hallucis longus (**Figure 16.9**). The superficial posterior compartment contains the gastrocnemius, soleus and plantaris (**Figure 16.10**). The lateral compartment contains the peroneus longus and peroneus brevis (**Figure 16.11**).

The foot contains both intrinsic and extrinsic muscles (**Figure 16.12**). An intrinsic muscle has both attachments contained within the foot, while an extrinsic muscle has one attachment outside the foot. The attachments and primary actions of the major extrinsic muscles of the lower leg, ankle, and foot are summarized in **Table 16.2**.

Nerves of the Lower Leg, Ankle, and Foot

The sciatic nerve and its branches provide primary innervation for the lower leg, ankle, and foot (**Figure 16.13**). Traveling down the posterior aspect of the leg from the lumbosacral spine, the sciatic nerve branches into smaller nerves just proximal to the popliteal fossa. The major branches are the tibial nerve that innervates the posterior aspect of the leg, and the common peroneal nerve that spawns the deep and superficial peroneal nerves.

The tibial nerve (L_4–S_3) passes through the popliteal fossa and down the leg between the superficial and deep muscles in the posterior compartment of the leg. It continues medially behind the medial malleolus with the posterior tibial artery to become the medial and lateral plantar nerves. The saphenous nerve (L_2–L_4), which branches from the femoral nerve, supplies cutaneous innervation to the medial aspect of the ankle.

The common peroneal nerve passes laterally around the neck of the fibula to the anterolateral leg, where it splits into the deep and superficial peroneal nerves. The deep peroneal nerve (L_4–S_1) innervates the anterior compartment, containing the ankle dorsiflexors and toe extensors, then courses over the dorsum of the foot to innervate the skin between the first and second toes. The superficial

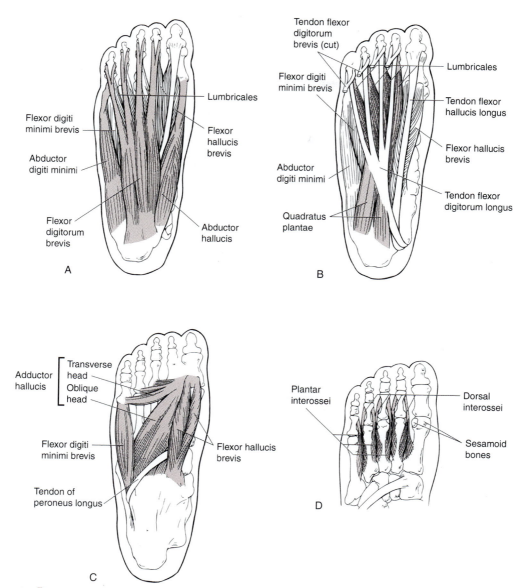

➤ FIGURE 16.12 **Intrinsic muscles of the foot**. A, Superficial layer. B, Second layer. C, Third layer. D, Fourth layer.

peroneal nerve (L_5–S_2) innervates the lateral compartment, containing the primary evertor muscles, and provides cutaneous innervation to the second through fourth toes. The sural nerve (L_4–S_2), a branch from both the common peroneal and tibial nerves, supplies cutaneous innervation to the lateral aspect of the ankle, heel, and foot. Given the extensiveness of the sciatic nerve supply to the lower extremity, it is no surprise that impingement of the sciatic nerve by a herniated disc in the lumbosacral region often results in pain, numbness, and/or impaired function in the foot and ankle region.

Blood Vessels of the Lower Leg, Ankle, and Foot

The blood supply to the lower leg, ankle, and foot enters the lower extremity as the femoral artery **(Figure 16.14)**. The femoral artery becomes the popliteal artery proximal and posterior to the knee, then branches into the anterior and posterior tibial arteries just distal to the knee. The anterior tibial artery becomes the dorsalis pedis artery to supply the dorsum of the foot. The posterior tibial artery gives off several branches that supply the posterior and lateral compartments, and the plantar region of the foot.

KINEMATICS OF THE LOWER LEG, ANKLE, AND FOOT

Kinematics is the study of spatial and temporal aspects of motion, which translates to movement, form, or technique. Evaluation of the kinematics of a particular movement can provide information about timing and sequencing of movement, which can then yield important clues for injury prevention. This section describes the kinematics of the lower leg, ankle, and foot, and identifies muscles responsible for specific movements.

TABLE 16.2   MAJOR MUSCLES OF THE FOOT AND LEG

Muscle	Proximal Attachment	Distal Attachment	Primary Action(s)	Nerve Innervation
Anterior Compartment				
Tibialis anterior	Upper two-thirds of lateral tibia and interosseous membrane	Medial surface of first cuneiform and first metatarsal	Dorsiflexion, inversion	Deep peroneal (L_4, L_5)
Extensor digitorum longus	Upper three-fourths of anterior fibula and interosseous membrane	2nd and 3rd phalanges of 4 lesser toes	Toe extension, dorsiflexion	Deep peroneal (L_5, S_1)
Extensor hallucis longus	Middle of anterior fibula and interosseous membrane	Dorsal surface of distal phalanx of great toe	Extension of great toe	Deep peroneal (L_5, S_1)
Peroneus tertius	Distal third of anterior fibula and interosseous membrane	Dorsal surface styloid process, 5th metatarsal	Eversion, dorsiflexion	Deep peroneal (L_5, S_1)
Lateral Compartment				
Peroneus longus	Proximal two-thirds of lateral fibula	Plantar surface of 1st cuneiform and 1st metatarsal	Eversion, plantar flexion	Superficial peroneal (L_5–S_2)
Peroneus brevis	Distal two-thirds of fibula	Lateral side of styloid process, 5th metatarsal	Eversion, plantar flexion	Superficial peroneal (L_5–S_2)
Posterior Deep Compartment				
Flexor digitorum longus	Posterior tibia	Distal phalanx of 4 lesser toes	Toe flexion, plantar flexion	Tibial (S_2, S_3)
Flexor hallucis longus	Distal two-thirds of posterior fibula	Distal phalanx of great toe	Flexion of the great toe, plantar flexion	Tibial (S_2, S_3)
Tibialis posterior	Upper two-thirds of tibia, fibula, and interosseous membrane	Cuboid, navicular, cuneiforms, and 2nd to 4th metatarsals	Inversion, plantar flexion	Tibal (L_4, L_5)
Popliteus	Lateral condyle of femur	Proximal portion of posterior tibia	Knee flexion, medial rotation of flexed leg	Tibial (L_4–S_1)
Posterior Superficial Compartment				
Gastrocnemius	Posterior medial and lateral condyles of femur	Calcaneal tuberosity via Achilles tendon	Plantar flexion, knee flexion	Tibial (S_1, S_2)
Soleus	Posterior proximal fibula and middle tibia	Calcaneal tuberosity via Achilles tendon	Plantar flexion	Tibial (S_1, S_2)
Plantaris	Posterior femur above lateral condyle	Calcaneal tuberosity via Achilles tendon	Plantar flexion, knee flexion	Tibial (S_1, S_2)

The Gait Cycle

The gait cycle requires a set of coordinated, sequential joint actions of the lower extremity. Despite variation in individual gait patterns, enough commonality exists in human gaits that one can describe the typical gait cycle (**Figure 16.15**). The gait cycle begins with a period of single-leg support in which body weight is supported by one leg while the other leg swings forward. The swing phase can be divided into the initial swing, midswing, and terminal swing. The period of double support begins with the contact of the swing leg with the ground or floor. As body weight transfers from the support leg to the swing leg, the swing leg undergoes a loading response and becomes the new support leg. A new period of single support then begins as the swing leg loses ground contact. The time through which body weight is balanced over the support leg is referred to as midstance. As the body's center of gravity shifts forward, the terminal stance phase of the support leg coincides with the terminal swing phase of the opposite leg.

Toe Flexion and Extension

Several muscles contribute to flexion of the second through fifth toes. These include the flexor digitorum longus, flexor digitorum brevis, quadratus plantae, lumbricals, and interossei. The flexor hallucis longus and brevis produce flexion of the hallux. Conversely, the extensor hallucis longus, extensor digitorum longus, and extensor digitorum brevis are responsible for extension and overextension of the toes.

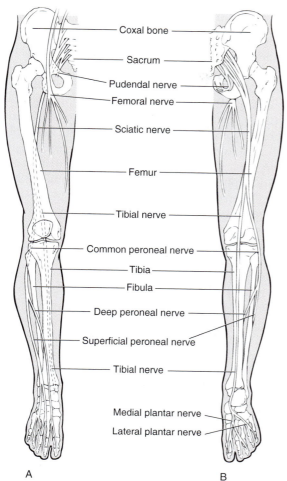

➤ FIGURE 16.13 **Nerve supply to lower leg, ankle, and foot.** Motor function to the lower leg is supplied by the sciatic nerve (L_4, L_5, S_1). Sensory innervation is supplied by the sciatic nerve and saphenous branch of the femoral nerve (L_2, L_3, L_4). A, Anterior view. B, Posterior view.

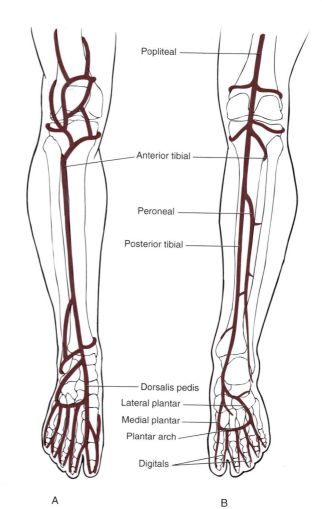

➤ FIGURE 16.14 **Blood supply to the leg, ankle, and foot region.** A, The dorsalis pedis artery is easily palpated in the midfoot region between the second and third tendons of the extensor digitorum longus. B, The posterior tibial artery can be palpated just posterior of the medial malleolus.

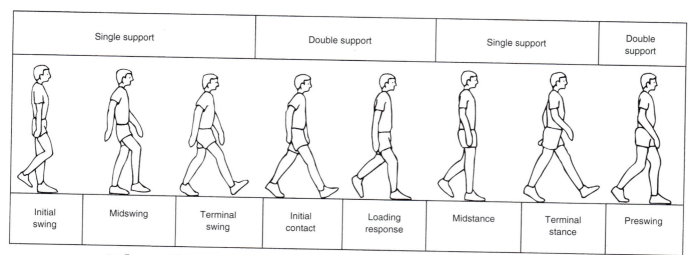

➤ FIGURE 16.15 **Gait.** The gait cycle consists of alternating periods of single-leg support and double-leg support.

Dorsiflexion and Plantar Flexion

Motion at the ankle occurs primarily in the sagittal plane, with ankle flexion and extension being termed dorsiflexion and plantar flexion, respectively **(Figure 16.16A)**. The medial and lateral malleoli serve as pulleys to channel the tendons of the leg muscles either posterior or anterior to the axis of rotation, thereby enabling their contributions to either plantar flexion or dorsiflexion. Muscles with tendons passing anterior to the malleoli, such as the tibialis anterior, extensor digitorum longus, and peroneus tertius, are dorsiflexors. Those with tendinous attachments running posterior to the malleoli contribute to plantar flexion. The major plantar flexors are the soleus, gastrocnemius, plantaris, and flexor hallucis longus, with assistance provided by the peroneal longus and brevis, and the tibialis posterior.

Inversion and Eversion

Rotations of the foot in the medial and lateral directions are termed inversion and eversion, respectively **(Figure 16.16B)**. These movements occur primarily at the subtalar joint, with secondary contributions from gliding movements at the intertarsal and tarsometatarsal joints. The tibialis posterior is the major inverter, with the tibialis anterior providing a minor contribution. Peroneus longus and peroneus brevis, with tendons passing behind the lateral malleolus, are primarily responsible for eversion, with assistance provided by the peroneus tertius.

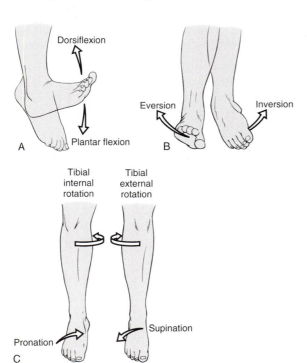

▶ **FIGURE 16.16 Motions of the leg and ankle**. A, Dorsiflexion and plantar flexion. B, Eversion and inversion. C, Supination of the subtalar joint results in external rotation of the tibia; pronation is linked with internal rotation of the tibia.

Pronation and Supination

The lower extremity moves through a cyclical sequence of movements during gait. Among these, the action at the subtalar joint during weight-bearing has the most significant implications for lower extremity injury potential. During heel contact with the support surface, the hindfoot is typically somewhat inverted. As the foot rolls forward and the forefoot initially contacts the ground, the foot is plantar flexed. This combination of calcaneal inversion, foot adduction, and plantar flexion, all at the subtalar joint, is known as **supination**. During weight-bearing at midstance, calcaneal eversion and foot abduction tend to occur, as the foot moves into dorsiflexion. These movements are known collectively as **pronation**. Supination of the subtalar joint also results in external rotation of the tibia, with pronation linked to internal tibial rotation **(Figure 16.16C)**.

Although a normal amount of pronation is useful in reducing the peak forces sustained during impact, excessive or prolonged pronation can lead to several overuse injuries including stress fractures of the second metatarsal and irritation of the sesamoid bones, plantar fasciitis, Achilles tendinitis, and medial tibial stress syndrome. Normal walking gait typically involves about 6 to 8° pronation, although individuals with **pes planus** (flat feet) may undergo as much as 10 to 12° (7).

KINETICS OF THE LOWER LEG, ANKLE, AND FOOT

Kinetics is the study of forces associated with motion. Because it is ultimately force that causes injury, understanding the kinetic aspects of lower leg, ankle, and foot function is an important foundation for understanding injury mechanisms.

Forces Commonly Sustained by the Lower Leg, Ankle, and Foot

During training, the bones of the lower extremity are subjected to a complex array of loading patterns, including tension, compression, bending, and torsion. During running, the foot sustains impact forces that can reach two to three times body weight; the magnitudes of the forces increase with gait speed. However, researchers have estimated strength of lower extremity bones to be two to four times that necessary to withstand the maximum stresses normally sustained during running (8).

Because repeated impact forces sustained during overtraining can produce stress fractures in the bones of the lower extremity, researchers have studied the factors associated with stress fracture incidence. In a study of infantry recruits, investigators found that thicker bones are generally more resistant to injury (9).

Women, who tend to have smaller bones than men, have also been found to incur more stress fractures than men, particularly in the tibia and metatarsals. Stress fractures are also common in runners, ballet dancers, and gymnasts, and are often secondary to decreased bone mineral density, or **osteopenia**. The **female athlete triad**, involving the simultaneous conditions of osteopenia, disordered eating, and amenorrhea (cessation of menses), is brought on by pressure placed on young women to achieve or maintain an unhealthy low body weight. The causal linkages among the components of the female athlete triad are not well understood, but appear to be related to low levels of circulating estrogen (10,11).

Foot Deformation During Gait

The structures of the foot are anatomically linked so the load is evenly distributed over the foot during weight-bearing. Approximately 50% of body weight is distributed through the subtalar joint to the calcaneus, with the remaining 50% channeled through the transverse tarsal joints to the forefoot (12). In normal individuals, the specific anatomical structure of the foot accounts for about 35% of the variance in plantar pressure during gait, with the remaining contribution from the dynamics of the gait cycle (13).

If the foot were a more rigid structure, each impact with the support surface would generate extremely large forces of short duration through the skeletal system. Because the foot is composed of numerous bones connected by flexible ligaments and restrained by flexible tendons, it deforms with each ground contact, thereby absorbing much of the shock and transmitting a much smaller force of longer duration up through the skeletal system.

The process of foot deformation during weight-bearing results in the storage of mechanical energy in the stretched tendons, ligaments, and plantar fasciae. As the tibia rotates forward over the talus during gait, additional energy is stored in the gastrocnemius and soleus as they develop eccentric tension. During the push-off phase, the stored energy in all of these elastic structures is released, contributing to the force of push-off, and actually reducing the metabolic energy cost of walking or running.

PREVENTION OF LOWER LEG, ANKLE, AND FOOT INJURIES

Preventing injuries should be a priority for all sport participants. Several steps can reduce the incidence or severity of injury. These include the use of appropriate protective equipment and footwear, and regular physical conditioning, including flexibility and strengthening exercises.

Protective Equipment

Chapter 3 discussed the use of protective braces and equipment for the lower leg, ankle, and foot. Shin pads can protect the anterior tibial area from direct impact by a ball, bat, stick, or a kick from a foot. Commercial ankle braces used to prevent or support a postinjury ankle sprain come in three categories: lace-up brace, semirigid orthrosis, or air bladder brace (see Figure 3.16). A lace-up brace can limit all ankle motions, whereas semirigid orthroses and air bladder braces limit only inversion and eversion. Ankle braces, in general, are more effective than taping the ankle to reduce injuries, are easier for the wearer to apply independently, do not produce some of the skin irritation associated with adhesive tape, provide better comfort and fit, are more cost-effective and comfortable to wear. Specific foot conditions can be padded and supported with a variety of products, including innersoles, semirigid orthotics, rigid orthotics, antishock heel lifts, heel cups, or commercially available pads and devices. Adhesive felt (Moleskin), felt, and foam can also be cut to construct similar pads to protect specific areas.

Physical Conditioning

Physical conditioning and strengthening of the body is one of the strongest defenses against injury. The foot and lower leg, however, are often neglected. A flexibility program should be completed prior to any sport participation. A tight Achilles tendon has been shown to predispose an individual to plantar fasciitis, Achilles tendinitis, and lateral ankle sprains. Strengthening exercises for the intrinsic and extrinsic muscles of the region should also be included. For example, to build strength in the foot, pick up marbles or dice with the toes and place them in a container close to the foot. Place a tennis ball between the soles of the feet and roll the ball back and forth from the heel to the forefoot. To increase strength in the lower leg muscles, secure a weight or a piece of elastic tubing around the forefoot, and move through the ranges of motion, doing three sets of 10 to 15 repetitions. Bilateral toe raises and heel raises may also be incorporated. **Field Strategy 16.1** demonstrates several exercises that can be used to prevent injuries to the lower leg, ankle, and foot.

Footwear

The demands of a particular sport require adaptations in shoe design and selection. In field sports, shoes may have a flat-sole, long cleat, short cleat, or a multicleated design (see Figure 3.18). Cleats should be positioned under the major weight-bearing joints of the foot, and should not be felt through the sole of the shoe. Shoe models with flat cleats, screw-in cleats, or pivot disc models have been shown to reduce the incidence of anterior cruciate ligament injuries when compared to shoes with the longer, irregular cleats. In individuals with arch problems, the shoe should include adequate forefoot, arch, and heel support. In all cases, individuals should select shoes based on the demands of the activity. In Chapter 3, shoe selection and guidelines for fitting shoes are discussed in detail. See Field Strategy 3.4 for review.

FIELD STRATEGY 16.1   EXERCISES TO PREVENT INJURY TO THE LOWER LEG

A. Foot Intrinsic Muscle Exercises

1. **Plantar fascia stretch.** Place a towel around the toes, and slowly overextend the toes. To stretch the Achilles tendon, dorsiflex the ankle.
2. **Towel crunches.** Place a towel between the plantar surfaces of the toes and feet. Push the toes and feet together, crunching the towel between the toes.
3. **Toe curls.** With the foot resting on a towel, slowly curl the toes under, bunching the towel beneath the foot. Variation: use two feet or a book or small weight on the towel for added resistance.
4. **Picking up objects.** Pick up small objects such as marbles or dice with the toes, and place in a nearby container, or use therapeutic putty to work the toe flexors.
5. **Shin curls.** Slide the plantar surface of the foot up the opposite shin, moving distal to proximal.
6. **Unilateral balance activities.** Stand on uneven surfaces with the eyes first open, then closed.
7. **BAPS board.** Seated position: roll the board slowly clockwise, then counterclockwise 20 times.

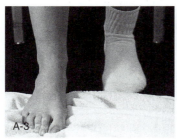

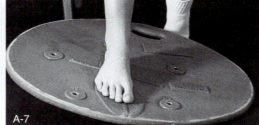

Continued

TOE AND FOOT CONDITIONS

A soccer player has an aching pain on the posterior calcaneus just above the attachment of the Achilles tendon. When he touches the tendon, it does not hurt, but when he reaches around the tendon and squeezes into the soft tissue area just anterior to the tendon, it really hurts. What may have caused this condition? How would the injury be managed?

Many individuals are at risk for toe and foot problems because of a leg length discrepancy, postural deviation, muscle dysfunction (such as muscle imbalance), or a malalignment syndrome (pes cavus, pes planus, pes equinus, hammer or claw toes) **(Figure 16.17)**. Pes cavus (high arch, rigid foot) and pes planus (flat foot, mobile foot), in particular, are associated with several common injuries **(Box 16.1)**. Skin conditions commonly found at the foot (e.g., calluses, corns, athlete's foot, plantars warts) are discussed in Chapter 27.

Toe Deformities

Most toe deformities are minor and can be treated conservatively. A few, however, require surgical intervention to correct serious structural malalignment.

HALLUS RIGIDUS

Degenerative arthritis in the first MTP joint, associated with pain and limited motion, is known as hallus

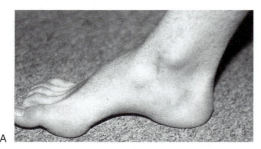

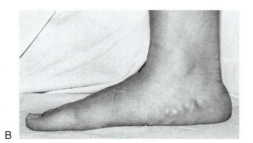

▶ **FIGURE 16.17 Common foot deformities.** A, Pes cavus. B, Pes planus.

FIELD STRATEGY 16.1   EXERCISES TO PREVENT INJURY TO THE LOWER LEG Continued   continued from page 496

B. Ankle/Lower Leg Muscle Exercises

1. **Ankle alphabet.** Using the ankle and foot only, trace the letters of the alphabet from A to Z, 3 times with capital letters, and 3 times with lowercase.
2. **Triceps surae stretch.** Keeping the back leg straight and heel on the floor, lean against a wall until tension is felt in the calf muscles (a). To isolate the soleus, bend both knees (b). Point the toes outward, straight ahead, and inward to stretch the various fibers of the Achilles tendon.
3. **Theraband or surgical tubing exercises.** Secure the Theraband or tubing around a table leg, and do resisted dorsiflexion, plantar flexion, inversion, and eversion.
4. **Unilateral balance exercises.** Balance on the opposite leg while doing Theraband exercises.
5. **BAPS board.** Standing position: Balance on the involved foot and repeat the process. Additional challenges, such as using no support, or dribbling with a basketball while balancing, can be added.

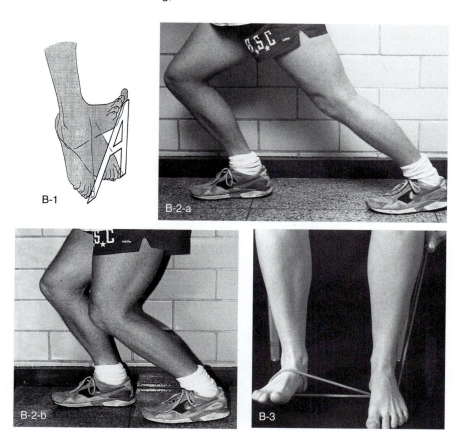

B-1

B-2-a

B-2-b

B-3

rigidus. Sports that involve running and jumping may predispose an individual to this condition.

➤ **SIGNS AND SYMPTOMS**

The individual will present with pain, loss of motion, and difficulty wearing shoes. A hallmark sign is restricted toe extension (dorsiflexion) due to a ridge of osteophytes that can be easily palpated along the dorsal aspect of the metatarsal head.

➤ **MANAGEMENT**

Conservative management includes wearing low-heeled shoes with adequate width and depth to accommodate the increased bulk of the joint. Individuals may also use a Morton's extension to their orthrosis, or a rigid insole or shoe to reduce stress across the joint. If conservative measures fail to resolve the symptoms within 6 months, surgery is indicated.

HALLUS VALGUS

Prolonged pressure against the medial aspect of the first MTP joint can lead to thickening of the medial capsule and bursa (bunion), resulting in a severe valgus deformity of the great toe **(Figure 16.18)**. Although the condition

➤➤ Box 16.1

Common Injuries Associated with Foot Deformities

Pes Cavus
Plantar fasciitis
Metatarsalgia
Stress fractures of the tarsals and meta-tarsals
Peroneal tendinitis
Sesamoid disorders
Iliotibial band friction syndrome

Pes Planus
Tibialis posterior tendinitis
Achilles tendinitis
Plantar fasciitis
Sesamoid disorders
Medial tibial stress syndrome
Patellofemoral pain

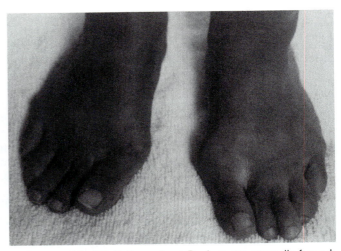

➤ **FIGURE 16.18 Hallus valgus.** Bunions are generally formed by constantly rubbing the medial aspect of the MTP joint of the great toe against the inside of the shoe. The toe then shifts laterally, forming the hallux valgus deformity.

may be caused by heredity, metatarsus pimus varus, pes planus, rheumatoid arthritis, and neurologic disorders, the most common cause is wearing poorly fitted shoes with a narrow toe box (14).

➤ SIGNS AND SYMPTOMS

Many individuals with the deformity are asymptomatic. Those with symptoms complain of pain over the MTP joint, and have difficulty wearing shoes because of the medial prominence and associated overlapping toe deformity.

➤ MANAGEMENT

Treatment varies depending on the degree of deformity and severity of symptoms. Wide, soft shoes with a broad toe box and sufficient insole padding are critical for comfort. Orthoses that support the longitudinal arch and redistribute the pressure areas may also provide some relief. If conservative measures fail, surgery is indicated.

CLAW, HAMMER, AND MALLET TOE

Other lesser toe deformities may be congenital (**Figure 16.19**), but more often develop because of improperly fitted shoes, neuromuscular disease, arthritis, or trauma. A **hammer toe** is extended at the MTP joint, flexed at the PIP joint, and hyperextended at the DIP joint. **Claw toe** involves hyperextension of the MTP joint and flexion of the DIP and PIP joints. A **mallet toe** is in neutral position at the MTP and PIP joints, but flexed at the DIP joint.

➤ SIGNS AND SYMPTOMS

All three conditions can lead to painful callus formation on the dorsum of the IP joints. This pressure against

the shoe and under the metatarsal head, particularly the second toe, is caused by the retrograde pressure on the long toe.

➤ MANAGEMENT

These conditions are difficult to treat conservatively. A metatarsal pad may help control symptoms, but surgery may be necessary. Soft-tissue surgery may involve tendon lengthening, capsulotomy, and/or ligament release. For more significant deformities, resection of the head of the proximal phalanx is often necessary to treat the condition.

Turf Toe

Turf toe, or a sprain of the plantar capsular ligament of the first MTP joint, results from forced hyperextension or hyperflexion of the great toe (i.e., jamming the toe into the end of the shoe). Hyperextension causes the sesamoids to be drawn forward to bear weight under the first metatarsal head. Repetitive overload leads to injury, particularly when associated with a valgus stress.

➤ SIGNS AND SYMPTOMS

The individual will have pain, tenderness, and swelling on the plantar aspect of the MTP joint of the great toe. Extension of the great toe will be extremely painful. Because the sesamoid bones are located in the tendons of the flexor hallucis brevis, this condition is sometimes associated with tearing of the flexor tendons, fracture of the sesamoid

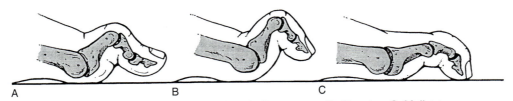

➤ **FIGURE 16.19 Toe deformities.** A, Hammer toe. B, Claw toe. C, Mallet toe.

bones, bone bruises, and osteochondral fractures in the metatarsal head.

➤ MANAGEMENT

Initial treatment for mild sprains involves ice therapy, NSAIDs, rest, and protection from excessive motion. Taping to limit motion at the MTP joint, a metatarsal pad to lower stress on the first metatarsal, or use of a rigid shoe or a rigid metal or plastic forefoot plate may be helpful. In moderate to severe cases, the athlete may need to be restricted from play until symptoms disappear (usually in 3 to 6 weeks).

Reverse Turf Toe (Soccer Toe)

Because of forced hyperflexion of the MTP joint while kicking an instep ball strike, soccer players often irritate the dorsal capsular structures of the first MTP joint. The condition can be acute or chronic, and demonstrates similar signs and symptoms as the traditional turf toe, except pain is noted dorsally over the joint and passive flexion of the toe is painful. Treatment is also similar with the exception of taping, which should limit flexion, rather than extension, of the MTP joint.

Ingrown Toenail

Though ingrown toenails are common, they are preventable with proper hygiene and nail care. The toenail length should be long enough to extend beyond the underlying skin, but short enough so as not to push into the toe box of the shoe. The toenails should be trimmed straight across to prevent the edges from growing under the skin on the side of the nail. In addition, properly fitted shoes and socks should be worn. Improper cutting of the nail, improper shoe size, and constant sliding of the foot inside the shoe can traumatizes the nail, causing its edge to grow into the lateral nail fold and surrounding skin. The nail margin reddens and becomes very painful. If a fungal or bacterial infection is present, the condition is called **paronychia**. Two methods to treat this condition are discussed in **Field Strategy 16.2**.

 FIELD STRATEGY 16.2 MANAGEMENT OF AN INGROWN TOENAIL

METHOD 1

- Soak the involved toe in hot water (108 to 116°) until the nail bed is soft (usually 10 to 15 minutes)
- Lift the edge of the nail, and place a small piece of cotton or tissue under the nail to elevate the nail out of the skinfold (Figure A)
- Apply antiseptic to the area and cover with a sterile dressing
- Repeat the procedure daily, keeping the area clean and dry

 If a purulent infection is present, refer to a physician for antibiotics and drainage of the infection.

METHOD 2

- Soak the toe as above, and cut a V in the center of the nail (Figure B)
- As the nail grows, its edges will pull toward the center, drawing the nail edges from under the skin
- Apply an antiseptic, cover with a sterile dressing, and keep the area clean and dry

 If a purulent infection is present, refer to a physician for antibiotics and drainage of the infection.

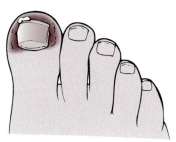

A

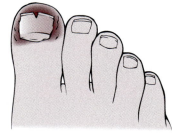

B

Metatarsalgia

General discomfort around the metatarsal heads is called **metatarsalgia**, or Morton's metatarsalgia. Constant overloading of the transverse ligaments leads to flattening of the transverse arch, resulting in callus formation over the middle three metatarsal heads, particularly the second. Although often related to sport participation **(Box 16.2)**, other factors such as age, arthritic disease, gout, diabetes, circulatory disease, and some neurologic conditions can also predispose an individual to metatarsal pain. Treatment involves reducing the load on the metatarsal heads through activity modification, footwear examination, metatarsal pads or bars, and strengthening the intrinsic muscles of the foot.

Bunions

Bunions are found on the medial aspect of the MTP joint of the great toe, but can occur on the lateral aspect of the fifth toe (called a bunionette or tailor's bunion). Pronation of the foot, prolonged pronation during gait, contractures of the Achilles tendon, arthritis, and generalized ligamentous laxity between the first and second metatarsal heads can produce a thickening on the medial side of the first metatarsal head as it is constantly rubbed against the inside of the shoe.

➤ SIGNS AND SYMPTOMS

As the condition worsens, the great toe may shift laterally and overlap the second toe, leading to a rigid, nonfunctional hallux valgus deformity (see Figure 16.18). This condition is exacerbated by high heels and pointed toe boxes in shoes, factors that account for the higher incidence of the condition in women.

➤ MANAGEMENT

Once the deformity occurs, little can be done. Strapping the great toe as closely to proper anatomical position as possible, and wearing wider shoes, can provide some relief, but surgical correction is indicated in severe cases.

Retrocalcaneal Bursitis

External pressure from a constrictive heel cup, coupled with excessive pronation or a varus hindfoot, can lead to swelling, erythema, and irritation of the retrocalcaneal bursa located between the Achilles tendon and calcaneus **(Figure 16.20)**. The posterior calcaneal bursa may also be irritated.

➤ SIGNS AND SYMPTOMS

Pain is elicited when you reach around the Achilles tendon to palpate the soft tissue just anterior to the tendon, and the skin may be thickened, especially on the lateral side. Active plantar flexion during push-off compresses the bursa between the tendon and bone.

➤ MANAGEMENT

Initial treatment involves ice therapy, NSAIDs, stretching exercises for the Achilles tendon, shoe modification, or a heel lift to relieve external pressure on the bursa. Occasionally, an inflamed bursa can lead to a dramatic, large mass referred to as a "pump bump," common in female figure skaters and runners (runner's bump). This bump may be related to an underlying bony spur caused by frequent microtrauma or microavulsions surrounding the distal attachment of the Achilles tendon.

 The soccer player may have retrocalcaneal bursitis. Ice therapy, NSAIDs, a heel lift, shoe modifications, and increasing the flexibility of the Achilles tendon may alleviate some of the symptoms.

CONTUSIONS

 A distance runner is complaining of heel pain during heel strike when he runs on black-top roads

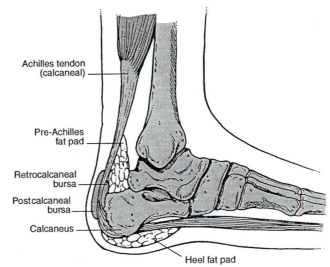

Achilles tendon (calcaneal)

Pre-Achilles fat pad

Retrocalcaneal bursa

Postcalcaneal bursa

Calcaneus

Heel fat pad

➤ **FIGURE 16.20 Retrocalcaneal bursa.** The retrocalcaneal bursa is commonly inflamed when it is pinched between the Achilles tendon and calcaneus during plantar flexion.

or walks barefoot. You notice that his shoes appear to be very old and worn. What injury might be present? If the condition goes untreated, what possible complication may result?

Contusions of the foot and leg result from direct trauma, such as dropping a weight on the foot, or being stepped on, kicked, or hit by a speeding ball or implement. Many of these injuries are minor and easily treated with immediate ice therapy, compression, elevation, and rest. However, a few injuries can result in complications, such as excessive hemorrhage, periosteal irritation, nerve damage, or damage to tendon sheaths, leading to tenosynovitis.

Foot Contusions

Compression on the midfoot can be quite painful, and can damage the extensor tendons or lead to a fracture of the metatarsals or phalanges. With weight-bearing, contusions of the plantar aspect of the forefoot may result from a loose cleat or spike irritating the ball of the foot. Repairing or replacing the object, along with ice therapy to reduce immediate hemorrhage and discomfort, is usually sufficient to remedy the situation.

A contusion to the hindfoot, called a **heel bruise**, can be more serious. Elastic adipose tissue lies between the thick skin and the plantar aspect of the calcaneus to cushion and protect the inferior portion of the calcaneus from trauma. It is constantly subjected to extreme stress in running, jumping, and changing directions. Excessive body weight, age, poorly cushioned or worn-out running shoes, increases in training, and hard, uneven training surfaces can predispose an individual to this condition. Walking barefoot is particularly painful. Ice treatments to minimize pain and inflammation, followed by regular use of a heel cup or doughnut pad, can minimize the condition. Despite excellent care, the condition may persist for months.

Lower Leg Contusions

Contusions to the gastrocnemius result in immediate pain, weakness, and partial loss of motion. Hemorrhage and muscle spasm quickly lead to a tender, firm mass that is easily palpable. When applying ice, keep the muscle on static stretch to decrease muscle spasm. If the condition does not improve in 2 to 3 days, ultrasound may be used under the direction of a physician to assist in breaking up the hematoma.

A contusion to the tibia, commonly called a **shin bruise**, may occur in soccer, field hockey, baseball, softball, or football, where the lower leg is often subjected to high-impact forces. The shin is particularly void of natural subcutaneous fat, and is thus vulnerable to direct blows that irritate the periosteal tissue around the tibia. Participants should always wear appropriate shin guards to protect this highly vulnerable area. Although painful, the condition can be managed effectively with ice, compression, elevation, and rest. A doughnut pad over the area and additional shin

protection can allow the individual to participate within pain tolerance levels.

Acute Compartment Syndrome

An acute compartment syndrome occurs when there is a rapid increase in tissue pressure within a nonyielding anatomical space that leads to increased local venous pressure and obstructs the neurovascular network. In the lower leg, it tends to be caused by a direct blow to the anterolateral aspect of the tibia, or by a tibial fracture. The anterior compartment is particularly at risk, as it is bounded by the tibia medially, the interosseous membrane posteriorly, the fibula laterally, and a tough fascial sheath anteriorly. Although an acute compartment syndrome occurs less frequently than the more common chronic compartment syndrome, the acute syndrome is considered a medical and surgical emergency because of the compromised neurovascular functions.

➤ SIGNS AND SYMPTOMS

Signs and symptoms include a recent history of trauma, excessive exercise, a vascular injury, or prolonged, externally applied pressure. The increasing severe pain and swelling appear to be out of proportion to the clinical situation. A firm mass, tight skin (because it has been stretched to its limits), loss of sensation on the dorsal aspect between the great toe and second toe, and diminished pulse at the dorsalis pedis are all late and dangerous signs. A normal pulse, however, does not rule out the syndrome. Acute compartment syndrome can produce functional abnormalities within 30 minutes of onset of hemorrhage. Immediate action is necessary, because irreversible damage can occur within 12 to 24 hours.

➤ MANAGEMENT

Immediate care involves ice and total rest. Compression is not recommended because the compartment is already unduly compressed and additional external compression will only hasten the deterioration. Furthermore, the limb must not be elevated, as this decreases arterial pressure and further compromises capillary filling. Referral to a physician for immediate care is absolutely necessary.

If numbness in the foot is present, an intercompartmental pressure is taken using either a slit-catheter or the solid-state intracompartment catheter. If the pressure ranges between 30 and 40 mm Hg (normal range is 0 to 10 mm HG), the patient is watched carefully and repeated measurements are taken until symptoms subside. If the pressure ranges from 40 to 60 mm Hg, a surgical release of the fascia (fasciotomy) is required to prevent permanent tissue damage.

The runner may have a heel bruise. You might recommend new shoes with better padding in the heel, or wearing a heelcup to absorb the impact forces during running. If the condition continues

to progress unabated, a stress fracture or bone spur may result.

FOOT AND ANKLE SPRAINS

 A lacrosse player stepped in a hole, inverting the ankle. Although she stayed off the ankle and iced it during the night, the ankle appeared swollen and discolored the next morning, and continued to hurt on weight-bearing. How will you manage this condition?

Sprains to the foot and ankle region are common in sports, particularly for those individuals who play on badly maintained fields. In many sports, cleated shoes become fixed to the ground while the limb continues to rotate around it. In addition, the very nature of changing directions places an inordinate amount of strain on the ankle region. Other methods of injury include stepping in a hole, stepping off a curb, stepping on an opponent's foot, or rolling the foot off the surface.

Toe and Foot Sprains and Dislocations

Sprains and dislocations to the MP and IP joints of the toes may occur by tripping or stubbing the toe. Varus and valgus forces more commonly affect the first and fifth toes, rather than the middle three. Pain, dysfunction, immediate swelling, and, if dislocated, gross deformity are clearly evident.

 Radiographs should be taken to rule out possible fracture, but closed reduction and strapping to the next toe for 10 to 14 days are usually sufficient to remedy the problem.

Midfoot sprains often result from severe dorsiflexion, plantar flexion, or pronation. Although the condition is seen in basketball and soccer players, it is more frequent in activities where the foot is unsupported, such as in gymnastics or dance where slippers are typically worn, or in track athletes who wear running flats. Pain and swelling is deep on the medial aspect of the foot, and weight-bearing may be too painful. Depending on the location and severity

of pain, adequate strapping, arch supports, and limited weight-bearing are warranted during the acute stage. If the condition does not improve, refer the individual to a physician to rule out a possible avulsion fracture at the tarsal joints. Reconditioning exercises should include range of motion and strengthening for the intrinsic muscles of the foot.

Mechanisms of Injury for Ankle Sprains

Ankle sprains are the most common injury in recreational and competitive athletes. They are classified as grade I (first-degree), grade II (second-degree), and grade III (third-degree), based on the progression of anatomical structures damaged and the subsequent disability **(Table 16.3)**. In basketball, ankle sprains comprise more than 45% of all injuries, and in soccer up to 31% of all injuries are ankle sprains (15).

Ankle sprains are generally caused by severe medial (supination or inversion) and lateral (pronation or eversion) rotation motions, and may or may not also be coupled with plantar flexion or dorsiflexion. Excessive supination of the foot (adduction, inversion, and plantar flexion) results when the plantar aspect of the foot is turned inward toward the midline of the body, commonly referred to as an inversion sprain. Excessive pronation (abduction, eversion, and dorsiflexion) results when the plantar aspect of the foot is turned laterally, referred to as an eversion sprain.

Lateral Ankle Sprains

Acute inversion sprains often occur while changing directions rapidly. Interestingly, injury typically involves the unloaded foot and ankle (or, more accurately, just at the moment of loading) with a plantar flexion and inversion force. In plantar flexion, the anterior talofibular ligament (ATFL) is taut and the calcaneofibular ligament (CFL) is relatively loose, whereas in dorsiflexion the opposite is true. The medial and lateral malleoli project downward over the talus to form a mortise-tenon joint. The lateral malleolus projects farther downward than the medial, thus limiting lateral talar shifts. As stress is initially applied to the ankle

TABLE 16.3	MECHANISMS OF COMMON ANKLE SPRAINS AND RESULTING LIGAMENT DAMAGE		
Mechanism	**1st (Mild)**	**2nd (Moderate)**	**3rd (Severe)**
Inversion and plantar flexion	Anterior talofibular stretched	Partial tear of anterior talofibular with calcaneofibular stretched	Rupture of anterior talofibular and calcaneofibular with posterior talofibular and tibiofibular torn
Inversion	Calcaneofibular stretched	Calcaneofibular torn, anterior talofibular stretched	Rupture of calcaneofibular, and anterior talofibular with posterior talofibular stretched
Dorsiflexion	Tibiofibular stretched	Partial tear of tibiofibular	Rupture of tibiofibular
Eversion	Deltoid stretched or an avulsion fracture of medial malleolus	Partial tear of deltoid and tibiofibular	Rupture of deltoid, and interosseous membrane with possible fibular fracture above syndesmosis

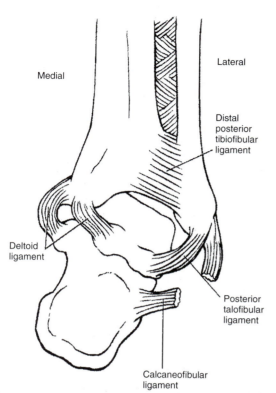

➤ **FIGURE 16.21 Inversion ankle sprain.** During inversion, the medial malleolus acts as a fulcrum to further invert the talus, leading to stretching or tearing of the calcaneofibular ligament.

during plantar flexion and inversion, the ATFL first stretches. If the strain continues, the ankle loses ligamentous stability in its neutral position. The medial malleolus acts as a fulcrum to further the inversion, and stretches or ruptures the CFL **(Figure 16.21)**. The overlying inner wall of the peroneal tendon sheath lies adjacent to the calcaneofibular ligament, and can absorb some strain to prevent injury to this ligament. If the peroneal muscles are weak, however, they are unable to stabilize the joint, leading to tearing of the calcaneofibular ligament. With severe injuries, the posterior talofibular ligament (PTFL) is also involved. As the ankle joint becomes unstable, the talus can pinch the deltoid ligament against the medial malleolus, which leads to injury on both sides of the ankle joint.

➤ SIGNS AND SYMPTOMS

The individual will usually report a cracking or tearing sound at the time of injury. With a grade I injury, the individual can bear weight immediately after injury. Pain and swelling are mild. With a grade II injury, swelling and tenderness will be localized over the ATFL and may extend over the CFL, and the individual can bear some weight. If no fracture is involved, bony tenderness will only be found at the ligamentous attachments. A complete tear of one or more of the ligaments is considered a grade III sprain. Swelling and ecchymosis will be rapid and diffuse, and the individual will demonstrate functional and clinical instability. Immediate assessment should distinguish the severity of injury, because swelling may soon obscure the level of instability. **Table 16.4** summarizes signs and symptoms of the various grades of ankle sprains.

Degree	Signs and Symptoms
TABLE 16.4	**SIGNS AND SYMPTOMS OF A LATERAL ANKLE SPRAIN**
1st	Pain and swelling on anterolateral aspect of lateral malleolus Point tenderness over ATFL No laxity with stress tests
2nd	Tearing or popping sensation felt on lateral aspect; pain and swelling on anterolateral and inferior aspect of lateral malleolus Painful palpation over ATFL and CFL May also be tender over PTFL, deltoid ligament, and anterior capsule area Positive anterior drawer and talar tilt test
3rd	Tearing or popping sensation felt on lateral aspect with diffuse swelling over entire lateral aspect with or without anterior swelling Can be very painful or absent of pain Positive anterior drawer and talar tilt test

➤ MANAGEMENT

After assessment for possible fracture and ligamentous damage, initial treatment should consist of ice therapy, compression (with or without a horseshoe pad), elevation, and restricted activity. If the individual is unable to bear weight, crutches should be used.

 Moderate to severe sprains should be referred immediately to a physician.

Radiographs can determine damage to the syndesmosis or detect an osteochondral fracture to the dome of the talus. **Field Strategy 16.3** summarizes the management of lateral ankle sprains.

Because lateral ankle sprains are so common, there may be a tendency to view all injuries around the ankle as "ankle sprains." Several aspects of the athlete's symptoms, including the inability to recall or describe a specific mechanism of injury, should lead to clinician to question the possibility of other injuries such as a syndesmosis sprain, peroneal tendon injury, loose body, or osteochondral fracture **(Box 16.3)**.

➤➤ **BOX 16.3**

Signs and Symptoms That Indicate a More Serious Underlying Condition Other Than a Lateral Ankle Sprain

- Inability to recall or describe the exact mechanism of injury
- Inability to bear any weight on the foot and ankle
- Any deformity to the foot and ankle
- Severe midfoot swelling or any blistering of skin (suggesting significant skin stretching caused by associated joint subluxation, dislocation, or fracture)
- In a chronic setting, the primary complaint of pain rather than instability
- Persistent pain exceeding 3 to 4 weeks postinjury

FIELD STRATEGY 16.3   MANAGEMENT ALGORITHM FOR LATERAL ANKLE SPRAIN

Apply crushed ice packs directly to the skin as quickly as
possible following the injury, for 30 minutes
↓
Do not place a towel or elastic wrap (dry or wet) between the crushed ice pack
and skin (reduces effectiveness of treatment)
↓
Elevate foot and ankle 6–10 inches above level of the heart
↓
After initial ice treatment:
-remove ice pack
-replace compression wrap
-continue elevation
↓
Apply a horseshoe pad and open basket weave
with tape and/or elastic wrap to protect the area
↓
Instruct athlete to reapply crushed ice pack regularly until going to bed:
-every 2 hours
-every hour if active between applications
(crutch walking, showering)
↓
If limping:
-fit with crutches
-reassess in the morning
-start rehabilitation

*If fracture is suspected, refer to physician (a short walking
cast may need to be applied).*

Medial Ankle Sprains

Eversion ankle sprains involve injury to the medial, deltoid-shaped talocrural ligaments (deltoid ligament). Although an isolated injury to the deltoid ligament (DL) may result from forced dorsiflexion and eversion, such as landing from a long jump with the foot abducted, or landing on another player's foot, these account for less than 10% of all injuries (15). Most injuries to the DL are associated with a fibula fracture, syndesmotic injury, or severe lateral ankle sprain. Individuals with pronated or hypermobile feet tend to be at a greater risk for eversion injuries.

The talar dome is wider anteriorly than posteriorly. During dorsiflexion, the talus fits more firmly in the mortise supported by the distal anterior tibiofibular ligament. With excessive dorsiflexion and eversion, the talus is thrust laterally against the longer fibula, resulting in either a mild sprain to the DL or, if the force is great enough, a lateral malleolar fracture. If the force continues after the fracture occurs, the deltoid ligament may be ruptured, or may remain intact, avulsing a small bony fragment from the medial malleolus and leading to a bimalleolar fracture. In either case, the distal anterior tibiofibular ligament and interosseous membrane may be torn, producing total instability of the ankle joint and eventual degeneration **(Figure 16.22).**

➤ SIGNS AND SYMPTOMS

Signs and symptoms of an isolated medial sprain depend on the severity of injury. In mild to moderate injuries, the individual will often be unable to recall the mechanism of injury. There may be some initial pain at the ankle when it was everted and dorsiflexed, but as the ankle returns to its normal anatomical position, pain often subsides and the athlete continues to play. In attempts to run or put pressure on the area, pain will intensify but the individual may not make the connection between the pain and the earlier injury. Swelling may not be as evident as a lateral sprain because hemorrhage occurs deep in the leg and is not readily visible. Swelling may occur just posterior to the lateral malleolus, between it and the Achilles tendon. Point tenderness can be elicited over the DL and distal anterior tibiofibular ligaments, and the anterior and posterior joint lines. In severe injuries, passive motion may be pain-free in all motions except dorsiflexion. With fractures of the malleoli, pain will be evident over the fracture site and will increase with any movement of the mortise. Percussion and heel strike will produce increased pain.

➤ MANAGEMENT

Initial management is the same as for a lateral ankle sprain. Use appropriate immobilization with a rigid posterior or

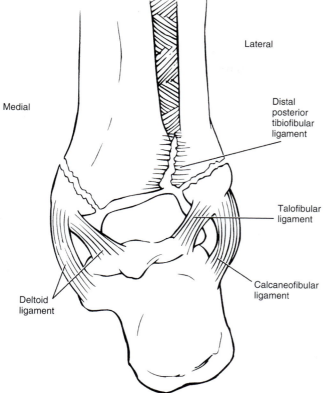

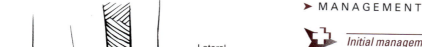

➤ FIGURE 16.22 **Eversion ankle sprain.** During a severe eversion ankle sprain, the lateral malleolus can fracture, the deltoid ligament can avulse the medial malleolus, and the distal tibiofibular joint can be disrupted.

vacuum splint. Referral to a physician is warranted because surgical repair is generally indicated when a fracture or ligamentous disruption of the syndesmosis is involved.

Syndesmosis Sprain

Injury to the distal tibiofibular syndesmosis often goes undetected, resulting in a longer recovery time and greater disability than the more frequent lateral ankle sprain. The mechanism of injury differs from that of an inversion sprain. Often, the foot is dorsiflexed and externally rotated.

➤ SIGNS AND SYMPTOMS

The area of maximum point tenderness is usually higher, between the tibia and fibula. The most commonly injured ligament, and a source of anterolateral ankle impingement, is the anterior inferior tibiofibular ligament (AITFL); the least injured ligament is the posterior inferior tibiofibular ligament (PITFL) (16). Assessment rests on four specific tests, including (1) stabilizing the lower leg with one hand while applying an external rotation force to the ankle (external rotation test), (2) compressing the proximal tibia and fibula while asking about pain at the ankle (squeeze test), (3) syndesmosis ligament palpation, and (4) passive dorsiflexion test.

➤ MANAGEMENT

Initial management is the same as for a lateral ankle sprain. Referral to a physician is warranted for radiographic confirmation to assess for fractures, bony avulsions (10 to 50% occur off the tibia), and more importantly the mortise alignment of the tibia, talus, and fibula.

Without fracture or ligament tears, treatment usually involves stabilization with a fracture brace for 3 to 4 weeks, then a stirrup brace for an additional 6 weeks, cold therapy until swelling is reduced, weight-bearing initially with crutches, and weaning off of the crutches as tolerated. Sports participation may be delayed for up to 3 months after the initial treatment begins. If the injury involves no fracture but there is widening of the joint mortise on stress radiographs, surgery is recommended.

Subtalar Sprain

The ligaments associated with the lateral subtalar joint are the CFL (spanning both the ankle and subtalar joints), the inferior extensor retinaculum, the lateral talocalcaneal ligament (TCL), the cervical ligament (just anterior to the TCL), and the interosseous ligament.

➤ SIGNS AND SYMPTOMS

The athlete will often complain of the sensation of the ankle "turning inward" or "turning over" during sports participation. Individuals with this problem consistently watch the ground when they walk and are uncomfortable when running on uneven surfaces. Assessment of chronic subtalar instability varies only slightly from ankle instability; the conditions may coexist. The anterior drawer test should be negative in isolated subtalar instability but positive with ankle instability; however, a subtle finding with subtalar instability is increased rotation of the calcaneus under the talus on the anterior drawer test. The definitive diagnosis can only be made with stress radiographs.

➤ MANAGEMENT

Conservative treatment is similar to a lateral ankle sprain: standard acute care, strengthening of the peroneals, stretching the heel cord, proprioceptive training, and use of a brace if needed. Chronic instability may necessitate surgical repair.

Subtalar Dislocation

Another serious sprain that involves the subtalar joint results from a fall from a height (as in basketball or volleyball). The foot lands in inversion, disrupting the interosseous talocalcaneal and talonavicular ligaments. If the foot lands in dorsiflexion and inversion, the CFL will also be ruptured. When the dislocation occurs, the injury is better known as "basketball foot."

➤ SIGNS AND SYMPTOMS

Extreme pain and total loss of function is present. Gross deformity at the subtalar joint may not be clearly visible. The foot may appear pale and feel cold to the touch if neurovascular damage is present. The individual may also show signs of shock.

➤ MANAGEMENT

Because of the potential for peroneal tendon entrapment and neurovascular damage, leading to reduced blood supply to the foot, this dislocation is considered a medical emergency. Activate EMS and assess neurovascular function. The lower leg should be immobilized with a vacuum splint in the position found, and transported immediately to the nearest medical facility.

Upon seeing the swollen ankle the next day, reassess it for possible fracture, control the inflammatory stage with continued ice therapy, apply a horseshoe pad or open basketweave strapping and an elastic wrap for compression, and fit the individual with crutches. If pain persists, refer the individual to a physician.

STRAINS OF THE FOOT AND LOWER LEG

A middle-aged tennis player reports pain and swelling behind the medial malleolus, and pain in the arch when arising in the morning. You notice that the individual has pes planus. During resisted muscle testing, plantar flexion and inversion are weak. What muscle is involved in this injury, and how will you manage the condition?

Injury to the musculotendinous unit may involve simple inflammation of the tendon (tendinitis), inflammation between the tendon and its surrounding sheath (tenosynovitis), muscle cramps, muscle strains, or acute rupture of the muscle or tendon. Because many of these condition can occur as both an acute injury and a chronic condition, each will be covered in this section.

Strains and Tendinitis

Muscle strains seldom occur in the lower extremity, except in the gastrocnemius-soleus complex. Instead, injury occurs to the musculotendinous junction or to the tendon itself. Most of the tendons in the lower leg have a synovial sheath surrounding the tendon, except the Achilles tendon, which has a peritendon sheath that is not synovial. Several factors can predispose an athlete to tendinitis **(Box 16.4)**. Common sites for tendon injuries include the:

- Achilles tendon just proximal to its insertion into the calcaneus
- Tibialis posterior just behind the medial malleolus
- Tibialis anterior on the dorsum of the foot just under the extensor retinaculum
- Peroneal tendons just behind the lateral malleolus and at the distal attachment on the base of the fifth metatarsal

> ➤➤ **Box 16.4**
>
> ## Predisposing Factors for Tendinitis in the Lower Leg
>
> - Training errors that include:
>   Lack of flexibility in the gastrocnemius-soleus muscles
>   Poor training surface or sudden change from soft to hard surface or vice versa
>   Sudden changes in training intensity or program (adding hills, sprints, or distance)
>   Inadequate work-rest ratio that may lead to early muscle fatigue
>   Returning to participation too quickly following injury
> - Direct trauma
> - Infection from a penetrating wound into the tendon
> - Abnormal foot mechanics producing friction between shoe, tendon, and bony structure
> - Poor footwear that is not properly fitted to foot

➤ SIGNS AND SYMPTOMS

Common signs and symptoms include a history of morning stiffness following a period of inactivity, localized tenderness over the tendon, possible swelling or thickness in the tendon and peritendon tissues, pain with passive stretching, and pain with active and resisted motion.

➤ MANAGEMENT

Treatment for muscle strains, tendinitis, or peritendinitis is conservative for the majority of cases. If mechanical problems are present, they should be addressed first so recovery can occur. Early exercises should be within the levels of pain tolerance, and should not be too strenuous. Ice massage, active range-of-motion (AROM) exercises with elastic tubing for resistance, stretching of the Achilles tendon, and eccentric calf exercises are recommended during the early phase of rehabilitation.

FOOT STRAINS

Foot strains caused by a direct blow or chronic overuse frequently affect the intrinsic and extrinsic muscles of the foot. Tenosynovitis is caused by friction and subsequent irritation between the tendon and its surrounding sheath. The tibialis anterior and the toe extensor tendons may be injured as a result of having the feet repeatedly stepped on, or by having the shoe laces tied too tightly.

➤ SIGNS AND SYMPTOMS

Pain, localized edema, inflammation, and adhesions may be present. During assessment, the involved tendon(s) will have pain on passive stretching, and active and resisted motion. Palpation over the tendon during active motion may reveal a sound similar to that heard when crunching a snowball together; hence the sound is called "**snowball**" crepitation.

➤ MANAGEMENT

Treatment involves ice therapy, NSAIDs, and strapping to limit active motion of the tendon. Range-of-motion and strengthening exercises should be started after acute pain has subsided.

PERONEAL TENDON STRAINS

Peroneal tendon strains may be acute or chronic. Common mechanisms include forceful passive dorsiflexion, as occurs when a skier catches the tip of the ski and falls forward; exploding off a slightly pronated foot, as when a football player is in a three-point stance and makes a forward surge; or by being kicked from behind in the vicinity of the lateral malleolus. The retinaculum that holds the tendons in place on the posterior aspect of the lateral malleolus gives way; the tendons slip forward over the lateral malleolus, but usually return spontaneously. This condition can be overlooked or confused with an ankle sprain because it, too, gives a feeling of instability and pain over the lateral malleolus.

➤ SIGNS AND SYMPTOMS

A cracking sensation followed by intense pain and an inability to walk will be reported. Swelling and tenderness are localized over the posterior, superior aspect of the lateral malleolus, rather than the anterior, inferior aspect, as in an inversion ankle sprain. A hallmark symptom is extreme discomfort or apprehension during attempted eversion of the foot against resistance. If done immediately after injury, the dislocated tendons may be palpated during resisted dorsiflexion and eversion; however, this may soon be obscured with swelling. In a chronic injury, the athlete complains primarily of instability, a "giving way," or slippage around the ankle, with little discomfort.

➤ MANAGEMENT

Treatment involves standard acute care. Acute injuries may respond to cast immobilization. External padding and strappings may also help stabilize the tendons, but due to the high rate of recurrence in the athletically active population, surgery is often still required.

TIBIALIS POSTERIOR STRAIN AND RUPTURE

Acute strains to the tibialis posterior tendon often occur as it courses behind the medial malleolus. In middle-aged athletes, the tibialis posterior is the foot tendon most at risk for tenosynovitis and possible rupture (14). Unfortunately, the problem is frequently missed because progressive pronation is insidious and relatively painless.

➤ SIGNS AND SYMPTOMS

With tenosynovitis, the individual will complain of pain, tenderness, and swelling behind the medial malleolus, often accompanied by an aching discomfort in the medial longitudinal arch. Weakness will be evident in plantar flexion and inversion. If the tendon ruptures, a painful pop can be felt, resulting in a flatfoot deformity (acquired pes planus).

➤ MANAGEMENT

Early treatment will depend on the severity of injury, and may include standard acute care, NSAIDs, restricted activity, and a medial shoe wedge. With moderate to severe cases, the athlete should be referred to a physician. The physician may recommend cortisone injections into the tendon sheath. In chronic cases involving a partial tear of the tendon, painful, palpable nodular scar tissue may build up in the tendon sheath, requiring surgical debridement.

GASTROCNEMIUS MUSCLE STRAIN

Strains to the medial head of the gastrocnemius are often seen in tennis players over 40, hence the nickname "tennis leg." Common mechanisms are:

- Forced dorsiflexion while the knee is extended
- Forced knee extension, while the foot is dorsiflexed
- Muscular fatigue with fluid-electrolyte depletion and muscle cramping

If related to muscle cramping, the strain is commonly attributed to dehydration (particularly in the heat), electrolyte imbalance, or prolonged muscle fatigue that stimulates cramping followed by an actual tear in the muscle fibers. For some, acute spasms may awaken them in the night following a day of strenuous exercise. Acute cramps are best treated with ice, pressure, and slow stretch of the muscle as it begins to relax. Prevention of this condition involves adequate water intake during strenuous activity and a regular stretching program for the gastrocnemius-soleus complex. When participation may extend over 2 hours in hot weather, increased water intake with a weak electrolyte solution should be ensured during and after strenuous activity.

➤ SIGNS AND SYMPTOMS

In an acute strain, the individual experiences a sudden, painful tearing sensation in the calf muscles, primarily at the musculotendinous junction between the muscles and Achilles tendon, or in the medial head of the gastrocnemius muscle **(Figure 16.23)**. Immediate pain, swelling, loss of function, and stiffness are common. Later, ecchymosis will progress down the leg into the foot and ankle.

➤ MANAGEMENT

Acute care consists of ice therapy and compression to control inflammation, restricted activity, gentle stretching of the gastrocnemius, heel lifts, and a progressive strengthening program. In more severe cases, immobilization and non-weight-bearing may be necessary to allow the muscle to heal fully.

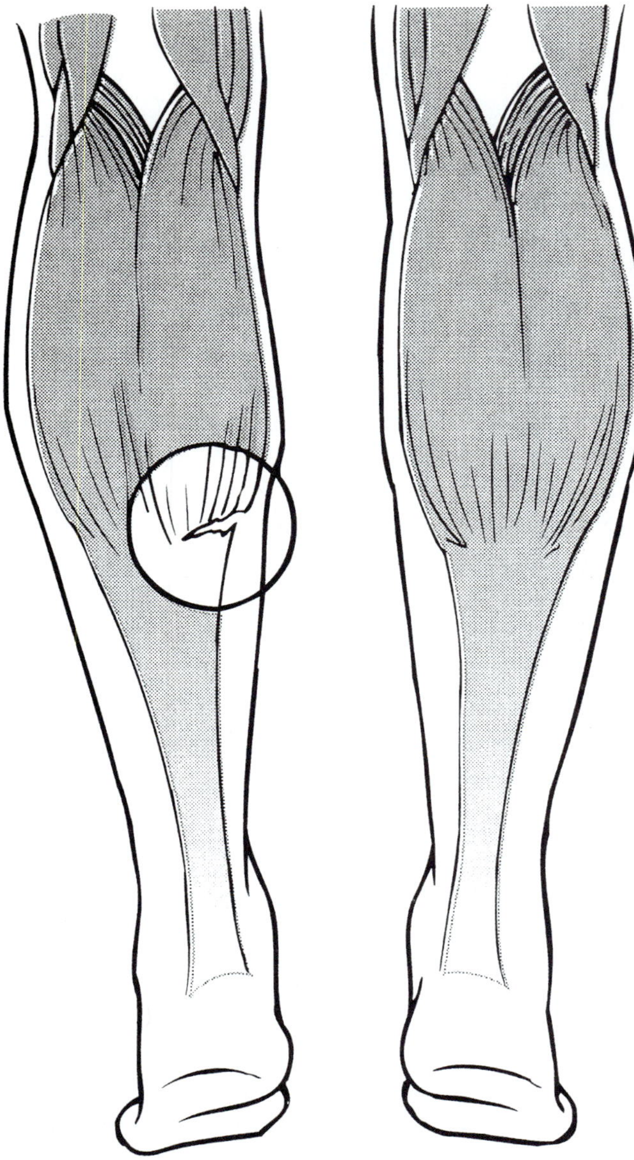

► FIGURE 16.23 Gastrocnemius muscle strain. The medial head of the gastrocnemius muscle is commonly strained in individuals over 40 years of age. A defect can often be palpated at the musculotendinous junction.

ACHILLES TENDINITIS

Achilles tendinitis is the most common tendinitis. Risk factors include tight heel cords, foot malalignment deformities, a recent change in shoes or running surface, a sudden increase in workload (e.g., distance, intensity) or change in exercise environment (e.g., excessive hill climbing or impact-loading activities—jumping, changing running surfaces, or changing footwear). The tendon is relatively avascular about 0.8 inches (2 cm) above its distal insertion into the calcaneus, which is the site of most torque on the tendon. This area is highly vulnerable to partial tears, with secondary nodule formation and degenerative cysts seen in tendinosis (a degenerative change secondary to chronic, repetitive activity, in which no evidence of inflammatory cells is present).

► SIGNS AND SYMPTOMS

Acute signs and symptoms include an aching or burning pain in the posterior heel, which increases with passive dorsiflexion and resisted plantar flexion, such as going up onto the toes. Point tenderness and crepitus can be elicited at the bony insertion, or 1 to 3 cm above the insertion. There can also be associated retrocalcaneal bursitis. Palpation may reveal local nodules either within the tendon, which moves during dorsiflexion and plantar flexion, or the periotendon, which does not move during these motions.

Chronic signs and symptoms can include pain that is worse after exercise, and may become constant. The tendon often becomes thickened, and pain is localized on the posterolateral heel. The gastrocnemius-soleus complex is tight, which may be due to tendon adhesions, muscle spasm, or inflexibility. Radiographs usually show a prominent posterior, superior calcaneus (Haglund deformity), and calcific spurring often occurs at the bone-tendon interface. Pathologically, the tendon demonstrates chronic degeneration rather than inflammation.

► MANAGEMENT

Acute treatment involves ice therapy, NSAIDs, activity modification, and correcting the training error. In moderate to severe cases, complete restriction of activity may be necessary for 3 weeks. Active stretching of the Achilles tendon before and after activity, along with a full strengthening program for the gastrocnemius-soleus complex including eccentric loading, is initiated immediately after acute pain has subsided. Heel lifts and a short period of cross-training may be helpful. In chronic cases where conservative treatment does not resolve symptoms, surgery may be necessary.

ACHILLES TENDON RUPTURE

Acute rupture of the Achilles tendon is probably the most severe acute muscular problem in the lower leg. It is more commonly seen in individuals 30 to 50 years old (17). The usual mechanism is a push-off of the forefoot while the knee is extending, a common move in many propulsive activities. Tendinous ruptures usually occur 1 to 2 inches proximal to the distal attachment of the tendon on the calcaneus (Figure 16.24).

► SIGNS AND SYMPTOMS

The individual hears and feels a characteristic "pop" in the posterior ankle and reports a feeling of being shot or kicked in the heel. Clinical signs and symptoms include a visible defect in the tendon, inability to stand on tiptoes or even balance on the affected leg, swelling and bruising around the malleoli, excessive passive dorsiflexion, and a positive Thompson's test (see Figure 16.34). Because the peroneal longus, peroneal brevis, and muscles in the deep posterior compartment are still intact, the individual may limp or walk with the foot and leg externally rotated, since this does not require push-off with the superficial calf muscles.

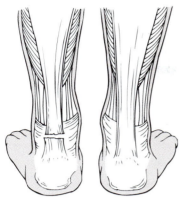

➤ FIGURE 16.24 **Achilles tendon rupture**. The Achilles tendon is often ruptured 1 to 2 inches proximal to its distal attachment. The individual will hear and feel a characteristic "pop" sensation similar to being kicked in the tendon.

➤ MANAGEMENT

A compression wrap should be applied from the toes to the knee. The leg and foot can be immobilized in a posterior splint, and the individual should be referred immediately to an orthopedist.

Nonoperative treatment offers excellent functional results for partial tears in older, noncompetitive individuals. In delayed diagnosis or in highly competitive individuals, surgical repair provides better push-off strength and prevents overelongation of the tendon, thus lowering the risk for reinjury. The course of action depends on the supervising physician, but either way, full range of motion and strength may not be achieved until 6 months after the injury.

The middle-aged tennis player has tenosynovitis of the tibialis posterior. Pes planus, along with weakness in plantar flexion and inversion, should have helped identify the muscle involved. After following standard acute care, you might suggest getting shoes with better arch support or strapping the arch with a figure-eight technique. If the condition does not improve, refer the individual to a physician.

OVERUSE CONDITIONS

A slightly overweight novice runner reports excruciating pain in the anteromedial hindfoot while running and upon arising in the morning, but it disappears within 5 to 10 minutes. What condition may be present? How will you manage this injury?

Repetitive microscopic injury to tendinous structures can lead to chronic inflammation that overwhelms the tissue's ability to repair itself. Other factors, such as faulty biomechanics, poor cushioning or stiff-soled shoes, or excessive downhill running, can also inflame the tendons. Several overuse conditions are common in specific sports, such as plantar fasciitis in running; medial tibial stress syndrome

(shin splints) in football, dance, or running; and exertional compartment syndrome in soccer or distance running. Many individuals complain of vague leg pain, but will have no history of a specific injury that caused the pain, differentiating this from an acute muscle strain. A common complaint is pain caused by activity.

Plantar Fasciitis

Plantar fasciitis is the most common hind foot problem in runners (18). Excessive tightness of the Achilles tendon, excessive or prolonged pronation, pes cavus, or obesity can overload the plantar fascia's origin on the anteromedial aspect of the calcaneus during weight-bearing activities. In a chronic condition, entrapment of the first branch of the lateral plantar nerve can contribute to the pain syndrome.

➤ SIGNS AND SYMPTOMS

The individual will report pain on the plantar, medial heel that is worse after rest and with the first few steps in the morning, but diminishes within 5 to 10 minutes (**Box 16.5**). Pain and stiffness are related to muscle spasm and splinting of the fascia secondary to inflammation. Normal muscle length is thus not easily attained, and it leads to additional pain and irritation. Point tenderness is elicited over the medial tubercle of the calcaneus, and increases with passive toe extension. If the lateral plantar nerve is involved, tenderness will also be noted at the proximal, superior abductor hallucis muscle.

➤ MANAGEMENT

Treatment involves standard acute care. After the inflammatory stage has ended, therapeutic modalities used to alleviate symptoms may include ice, deep friction massage, ultrasound, and electrical muscle stimulation. Achilles tendon stretching exercises, stretching of the toe flexor tendons, strengthening of the intrinsic muscles, NSAIDs, and a soft heel lift may be helpful. A Moleskin plantar fascia strap or figure-eight arch strapping is an effective means of support; circular strips of tape around the foot are contraindicated because they may overstretch the fascia and prolong recovery. **Field Strategy 16.4** highlights the management of plantar fasciitis.

➤➤ **Box 16.5**

Signs and Symptoms of Plantar Fasciitis

- Pain with first steps in the morning, particularly in the proximal, plantar, medial heel
- Point tenderness over or just distal to the medial calcaneal tubercle
- Pain may radiate up the medial side of the heel, and occasionally across the lateral side of the foot
- Passive extension of the great toe and dorsiflexion of the ankle will increase pain and discomfort
- Pain increases with weight-bearing
- Pain is relieved with activity, but recurs after rest

FIELD STRATEGY 16.4   MANAGEMENT OF PLANTAR FASCIITIS

- Immediate ice therapy and NSAIDs
- Use a shock-absorbing soft heel pad or soft plantar arch pad
- Figure-eight arch strapping or night splints may relieve acute symptoms
- Aggressive Achilles tendon stretching for 2 to 4 minutes, three to four times a day, with toes straight ahead, toes in, and toes out
- Gentle isometric contractions for intrinsic muscles of the foot, initially
- Progress to AROM exercise within pain-free ranges—toe curls, marble pick-up, towel crunches, and towel curls
- Strengthen intrinsic and extrinsic muscles of leg
- Maintain body fitness and strength, and aerobic fitness, with non-weight-bearing activities
- Physician may administer cortisone injections into the plantar fascia aponeurosis

Medial Tibial Stress Syndrome (MTSS)

Medial tibial stress syndrome is a periostitis (inflammation of the periosteum) along the posteromedial tibial border, usually in the distal third, not associated with a stress fracture or compartment syndrome. Although originally thought to be related to stress along the posterior tibialis muscle and tendon causing myositis, fasciitis, and periostitis, it is now believed to be related to periostitis of the soleus insertion along the posterior medial tibial border. The soleus makes up the medial third of the heel cord as it inserts into the calcaneus. With excessive pronation or prolonged pronation of the foot, it causes an eccentric contraction of the soleus, resulting in the periostitis that produces the pain. Other contributing factors include recent changes in running distance, speed, form, stretching, footwear, or running surface.

▶ SIGNS AND SYMPTOMS

Typically seen in runners or jumpers, the pain may occur at any point in the workout and is characterized as a dull ache. As activity progresses, pain diminishes only to recur hours after activity has ceased. In later stages, pain will be present before, during, and after activity, and may restrict performance. Point tenderness will be elicited in a 3 to 6 cm area along the distal posteromedial tibial border. Pain is aggravated by resisted plantar flexion or standing on tip-toe. There is often an associated varus alignment of the lower extremity, including a greater Achilles tendon angle (Box 16.6).

▶ MANAGEMENT

Five to seven days of rest is essential to relieve acute symptoms. Other modalities (cryotherapy, NSAIDs, cortisone injections, heel pads, casting, crutches, and activity modification) have not been shown to be as effective as rest alone. Pain-free stretching of both the anterior and posterior musculature will help improve joint mobility, increase muscle and tendon strength and coordination, and aid the musculoskeletal system in adapting to the physical demands of a specific sport. If the condition does not improve, possible stress fractures to the tibia should be ruled out through appropriate radiograph or scanning proce-

dures. Analysis of the individual's running motion, foot alignment, running surface, and footwear may prevent recurrence. **Field Strategy 16.5** summarizes the management of MTSS.

Exertional Compartment Syndrome

Exertional compartment syndrome (ECS) is characterized by exercise-induced pain and swelling that is relieved by rest. The compartments most frequently affected are the anterior (50 to 60%) and deep posterior (20 to 30%). The remaining 10 to 20% are divided evenly among the lateral, superficial posterior, and the "fifth" compartment around the tibialis posterior muscle (19). Whereas acute ECS generally occurs in relatively sedentary people who undertake strenuous exercise, chronic ECS is usually seen in well-conditioned athletes younger than 40 (20).

▶ SIGNS AND SYMPTOMS

The typical history of chronic ECS is exercise-induced aching leg pain and a sense of fullness, both over the involved compartment. These symptoms are almost always

---

▶▶ BOX 16.6

Signs and Symptoms of Medial Tibial Stress Syndrome

- Dull pain begins at any point in the workout; occasionally may be sharp and penetrating
- Pain occurs along posteromedial border of tibia in a 3 to 6 cm area, usually in distal third
- Pain is relieved with rest, but may recur hours after activity stops
- In experienced runners, condition is usually secondary to mechanical abnormalities:
  - Increased Achilles tendon angle (during stance phase and while running)
  - Greater Achilles tendon angle between heel strike and maximal pronation
  - Greater passive subtalar motion in inversion and eversion
- Pain is aggravated by active plantar flexion

FIELD STRATEGY 16.5   MANAGEMENT OF MEDIAL TIBIAL STRESS SYNDROME

- 5 to 7 days of rest is essential
- Ice, compression, elevation, and NSAIDs may help relieve acute symptoms
- Determine if there is a possible stress fracture present
- Evaluate and correct any foot malalignment or problems in technique
- Change running surface and possibly shoes
- Increase flexibility in muscles in anterior and posterior compartment
- Increase strength in all muscles of lower leg and foot

relieved with rest, usually within 20 minutes of exercise, only to recur if exercise is resumed. Bilaterality is common. Activity-related pain begins at a predictable time after starting exercise or after reaching a certain level of intensity. Many individuals with anterior compartment involvement describe mild foot drop or paresthesia (or both) on the dorsum of the foot, and demonstrate fascial defects or hernias, usually in the distal third of the leg over the intramuscular septum.

Evaluation should be performed after the individual has exercised strenuously enough to reproduce the symptoms. The exercise will produce swelling and tenderness in the involved compartments, and increased leg girth. Tenderness, if present, may be located in the midthird of the tibia, although many individuals will have no focal pain. Vibration with a tuning fork will produce no pain, as one would typically see in a stress fracture. Likewise, pain will not be present in the distal leg, which corresponds with MTSS. To confirm the diagnosis, intracompartmental pressure must be measured (see Anterior Compartment Syndrome).

➤ MANAGEMENT

Treatment involves assessing extrinsic factors (e.g., training patterns, technique, shoe design, and training surface) and intrinsic factors (e.g., foot alignment—especially hindfoot pronation, muscle imbalance, and flexibility). In minor conditions, ice massage, NSAIDs, and occasionally diuretics may assist, along with stretching and strengthening the involved compartment muscles, orthotics, and activity modification. If symptoms persist for 3 months, fasciotomy is recommended; unlike a fasciotomy for acute ECS, this may be limited to complete release of the involved compartments.

The runner may have plantar fasciitis. As part of the assessment, check foot alignment, gait, and shoes for problems that may have contributed to the condition. Stretching of the toe flexors and Achilles tendon should be a major part of the treatment plan.

VASCULAR AND NEURAL DISORDERS

An ice hockey player is complaining of bilateral numbness in the posterolateral aspect of the leg along the Achilles tendon for the past 2 to 3 weeks. There was no history of trauma to the ankle, but he admits that, in order to provide better support for the ankles, he routinely spiraled his laces tightly around the proximal portion of each ice hockey boot, then applied several circular bands of white tape to hold them in place. Could this technique impair the vascular or neural function of the lower leg? How will you manage this situation?

Vascular and neural disorders of the lower leg are rare in sports, but can occur. Vascular disorders typically involve occlusion of venous blood in the calf region, whereas neural involvement typically affects the distal ankle and foot region. In either case, any change in circulation, sensation, or function should trigger referral to a physician for follow-up assessment and care.

Venous Disorders

By way of contraction of smooth and skeletal muscles, blood within the superficial venous system, as well as the deep venous system, is pushed or "milked" back to the heart and lungs for elimination or metabolism. In some instances, particularly during inactivity following fracture or surgery, prolonged bed rest, and increasing age, this system becomes inefficient, leading to a reduced blood flow. The accumulated blood products may form a clot that can grow in size, depending on the vessel in which it is contained, causing partial or complete blockage, called a deep-vein thrombosis (DVT). The deep calf veins are most frequently involved, but the popliteal, superficial femoral, and ileofemoral vein segments are also commonly involved. In sports, skate lace tightness can lead to the development of venous thrombosis in the calf region. An **embolism** occurs when a loosened thrombus circulates from a larger vessel to a smaller one, subsequently obstructing circulation. When the obstruction occurs in the veins of the lungs, it is called a pulmonary embolism.

➤ SIGNS AND SYMPTOMS

DVT is typically asymptomatic and may not become apparent until a pulmonary embolism occurs. The most reliable signs are paresthesia in the area, chronic swelling and edema in the involved extremity, engorged veins, ecchymosis formation with a blue hue, and a positive Homan's sign (see Figure 16.35).

➤ MANAGEMENT

Immediate referral to a physician is warranted.

Treatment will involve anticoagulant therapy, leg elevation, and ambulation in individuals who are clinically stable and for whom it is medically indicated. Functional neuromuscular stimulation of the gastrocnemius and tibialis anterior may help activate the physiologic muscle pump while moving venous blood back to the central circulation to prevent deep venous thrombosis.

Neurologic Conditions

Impingement of nerves in the lower leg and foot is rare, but does happen. Three such conditions involve the compression of the interdigital nerves as they bifurcate at the metatarsal heads (plantar interdigital neuroma), the posterior tibial nerve beneath the flexor retinaculum and behind the medial malleolus (tarsal tunnel syndrome), and the sural nerve as it courses behind the lateral malleolus and into the lateral aspect of the foot.

PLANTAR INTERDIGITAL NEUROMA

A plantar interdigital neuroma (Morton's neuroma) is a common source of forefoot pain, especially in middle-aged women, and is sometimes bilateral. Trauma or repetitive stress caused by tight-fitting shoes or a pronated foot can lead to abnormal pressure on the plantar digital nerves as they are compressed between the metatarsal heads and transverse intermetatarsal ligament. It typically occurs at the web space between the third and fourth metatarsals (second and third intermetatarsal spaces) and, to a lesser extent, between the second and third metatarsals **(Figure 16.25)**.

➤ SIGNS AND SYMPTOMS

The individual may initially describe a sensation of having a stone in the shoe that worsens when standing. Tingling or burning, radiating to the toes, along with intermittent symptoms of a sharp shock-like sensation into the involved toes, is commonly reported. Pain subsides when activity is stopped or when the shoe is removed. In fact, the desire to remove the shoe and massage the foot is a classic indicator of a neuroma. The clinician may be able to palpate a painful mass, and elicit pain by palpating between the metatarsal heads, or sense a palpable click with lateral compression of the metatarsal heads.

➤ MANAGEMENT

Conservative management involves placing a metatarsal pad just proximal to the metatarsal heads and wearing a broad, soft-soled shoe with a low heel. However, local corticosteroid injections or surgical incision may be necessary to remedy the situation.

TARSAL TUNNEL SYNDROME

Tarsal tunnel syndrome occurs when the posterior tibial nerve or one of its branches becomes constricted

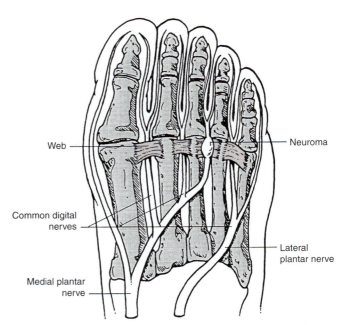

➤ FIGURE 16.25 **Plantar's neuroma**. Plantar's neuroma (Morton's neuroma) is caused by pinching of the interdigital nerve between the metatarsal heads. While weight-bearing in shoes, the individual will have an agonizing pain on the lateral side of the foot, which will be relieved when barefoot.

beneath the fibrous roof of the flexor retinaculum of the foot **(Figure 16.26)**. Entrapment most often occurs at the anterior, inferior aspect of the canal where the nerve winds around the medial malleolus. The lateral plantar nerve branch tends to be more frequently affected than the medial branch. The condition is often linked to excessive pronation or an excessive valgus deformity that leads to stress or traction on the nerve with impingement.

➤ SIGNS AND SYMPTOMS

Clinically, the individual will complain of pain at the medial malleolus radiating into the sole and heel (particularly with entrapment of the lateral plantar nerve), pares-

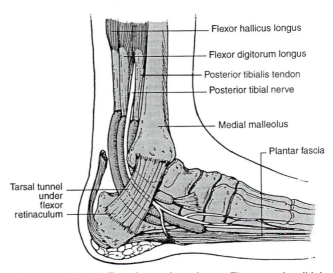

➤ FIGURE 16.26 **Tarsal tunnel syndrome**. The posterior tibial nerve can become constricted beneath the tarsal tunnel roof formed by the flexor retinaculum.

thesia (abnormal sensation), dysesthesia (impaired sensation), and hyperesthesia (heightened sensation) in the distribution of the posterior tibial nerve. One of the most reliable signs is a positive Tinel's sign (tingling elicited by tapping along the course of the nerve).

➤ MANAGEMENT

Conservative management involves rest, NSAIDs, orthoses (especially in athletes with hyperpronation), and gradual return to activity. A one-time injection of cortisone and lidocaine without epinephrine may be given into the tarsal tunnel, but if symptoms persist and other causes of heel pain are eliminated, surgical release may be necessary (14).

SURAL NERVE ENTRAPMENT

The sural nerve, formed from branches of the tibial and peroneal nerves, provides cutaneous innervation to the lateral lower leg and foot. It passes distally along the lateral margin of the Achilles tendon to emerge from the fascia of the leg proximal to the lateral malleolus. After providing lateral calcaneal branches to the ankle and heel, the nerve passes behind the lateral malleolus and continues along the lateral border of the foot to extend to the fifth toe as the lateral dorsal cutaneous nerve. In addition to being vulnerable to compression from tight-fitting skates, boots, and shoes, the nerve can be irritated by fibrous adhesions that result from repetitive inversion ankle injuries, or ganglia that may form in the peroneal tendon sheath. Peripheral sural nerve neuropathy related to diabetes may also be a cause of paresthesia in this area.

➤ SIGNS AND SYMPTOMS

Symptoms of sural nerve involvement include numbness in the affected area with decreased temperature sensation along the dorsolateral aspect of the foot, a burning sensation, local tenderness over the sural nerve itself, and reproduction of the symptoms by compression over the nerve (positive Tinel's sign).

➤ MANAGEMENT

Conservative treatment may be as simple as changing the lacing of the skates, boots, or shoes. Surgical intervention, however, may be necessary to correct the problem.

The ice hockey player may have compressed the sural nerve with the tight laces and tape. This individual should be referred to a physician to determine the extent of injury to the nerve, and encouraged to change the way he laces his boots.

FRACTURES

A softball player sprained the right ankle a week ago. After standard acute care and partial weight-bearing, the swelling and pain have significantly decreased around the lateral malleolus,

but pain is still present on the styloid process of the fifth metatarsal. What additional injury may be present?

Fractures in the foot and lower leg region seldom result from a single traumatic episode. Often, repetitive microtraumas lead to apophyseal or stress fractures. Tensile forces associated with severe ankle sprains can lead to avulsion fractures of the fifth metatarsal, or severe twisting can lead to displaced and undisplaced fractures in the foot, ankle, or lower leg. A combination of forces can lead to a traumatic fracture–dislocation. General assessment techniques used to determine a possible fracture can be seen later in the chapter in Field Strategy 16.6.

Freiberg's Disease

Freiberg's disease is a painful avascular necrosis of the second, or rarely, third metatarsal head, often seen in active adolescents aged 14 to 18 before closure of the epiphysis. Although not specifically a sport injury, it can lead to diffuse pain in the forefoot region. Early detection is best treated by a metatarsal pad or bar to unload the involved metatarsal head, and activity modification to eliminate excessive running and jumping. If pain persists and deformity develops with degenerative osteophytes, surgical resection of the distal metatarsal head may be necessary.

Sever's Disease

Sever's disease, or calcaneal apophysitis, is frequently seen in 8 to 13-year-old athletes and is associated with growth spurts, tight heel cords, poor hamstring flexibility, and other biomechanical abnormalities contributing to poor shock absorption (forefoot varus, hallux valgus, pes cavus, pes planus, and more commonly, forefoot pronation). Because the apophyseal plate is vertically oriented, it is particularly susceptible to shearing stresses from the gastrocnemius. Hard surfaces, poor-quality or worn-out athletic shoes, being kicked in the region, or landing off-balance may also precipitate the condition.

➤ SIGNS AND SYMPTOMS

The individual will complain of unilateral or bilateral, intermittent or continuous, posterior heel pain that occurs with activity shortly after beginning a new sport or season. Although gait may be normal, the child may walk with a limp or exhibit a forceful heel strike. Point tenderness can be elicited at or just anterior to the insertion of the Achilles tendon along the posterior border of the calcaneus. Mediolateral compression (the "squeeze test") of the calcaneus over the lower one-third of the posterior calcaneus elicits pain, as does standing on the tiptoes (positive Sever's sign). Heel cord flexibility is tested by passive dorsiflexion of the foot with the knee extended. It is often reduced to less than 10°, and testing may elicit increased pain (21). Other conditions that may also lead to heel pain should be ruled out prior to determining the treatment plan (**Box 16.7**).

Differential Diagnosis of Heel Pain in Young Athletes

- Plantar fasciitis
- Heel fat pad syndrome
- Achilles tendinitis/strain
- Retrocalcaneal bursitis
- Calcaneal stress fracture
- Calcaneal exostosis
- Contusion
- Infection
- Tarsal coalition
- Tarsal tunnel syndrome

▶ MANAGEMENT

Following standard acute care, the athlete should be referred to a physician for further care.

The condition usually resolves itself with closure of the apophysis. Until then, rest, ice, NSAIDs, heel lifts, heel cups, strapping the foot in slight plantar flexion to relieve some strain on the Achilles tendon, and activity modification will usually relieve symptoms. Heel cord flexibility and strengthening exercises of the dorsiflexors are recommended.

Stress Fractures

Stress fractures are often seen in running and jumping, particularly after a significant increase in training mileage, or a change in surface, intensity, or shoe type. Women with amenorrhea (absence of menses) and oligomenorrhea (infrequent menses or menses with scant blood flow) have a higher incidence of stress fractures of the foot and leg during sport activity; however, women who use oral contraceptives tend to have significantly fewer stress fractures than do nonusers (22). The neck of the second metatarsal is the most common location for a stress fracture, although it is also seen on the fourth and fifth metatarsals.

The two sesamoid bones of the great toe are often fractured as a result of constant weight-bearing on a hyperextended great toe, or because of prolonged pronation during running. Individuals with pes cavus or tight plantar fascia are predisposed to this injury because of the large tensile forces placed on the bones. Pain and swelling will be present on the ball of the foot, and the individual will be unable to roll through the foot to stand on the toes. Radiographs may be inconclusive, because it is common for sesamoid bones to be bipartite (having two parts).

Stress fractures of the navicular are seen in jumpers, ballet dancers, and equestrians due to the nature of foot positions, and the motions and inevitable stresses produced in the midfoot. Often seen in young men, this fracture is difficult to assess. A high degree of suspicion is required when an individual complains of generalized foot pain on the dorsomedial aspect of the midfoot brought on by activ-

ity and relieved with rest. In advanced stages, overlying swelling and pain on walking become evident.

Stress fractures of the calcaneus produce significant pain on heel strike. There is often a history of a substantial increase in the individual's activity level, particularly in distance runners. Palpation will reveal maximum pain on the medial and lateral aspects of the plantar-calcaneal tuberosity. Squeezing the calcaneus will also produce pain.

Stress fractures of the tibia and fibula result from repetitive stress to the leg that lead to muscle fatigue. The resulting loss in shock absorption increases stress on the bone and periosteum. In the tibia, most stress fractures occur at the junction of the middle and distal thirds, the posterior medial tibial plateau, or just distal to the tibial tuberosity. Fibular stress fractures usually occur in the distal metadiaphyseal region.

▶ SIGNS AND SYMPTOMS

Pain from a stress fracture begins insidiously, increasing with activity and decreasing with rest; pain is usually limited to the fracture site. Pain can be elicited with percussion, a tuning fork, or ultrasound. Encircling the forefoot (metatarsal and tarsal fractures) or calcaneus (calcaneal fracture) with the hand and squeezing the fingers together produce added discomfort.

▶ MANAGEMENT

Following standard acute care, the athlete should be referred to a physician for further care.

Frequently, radiographs are negative early, but periosteal reaction or cortical thickening can be seen 2 to 4 weeks later. Bone scans usually reveal the presence of a fracture long before it becomes evident on radiography **(Figure 16.27)**.

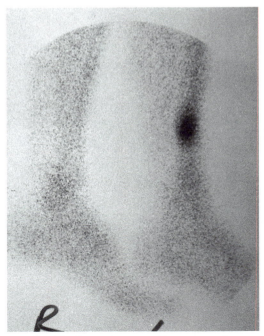

▶ **FIGURE 16.27 Stress fractures**. Bone scans detect stress fractures long before the fractures become apparent on x-rays.

Treatment consists of rest until symptoms disappear (generally 4 to 8 weeks or longer), ice therapy, NSAIDs, stretching and strengthening exercises, and correcting any mechanical abnormalities that may have contributed to the condition. Protected weight-bearing, a stiff shoe, a rigid orthrosis, or a walking cast may be indicated in fractures of the metatarsals, calcaneus, or tibia. Wearing stiff-soled shoes or a heel cup may be helpful with stress fractures of the sesamoid bones and calcaneus, respectively. The individual should be completely asymptomatic before returning to participation.

Avulsion Fractures

Avulsion fractures may occur at the site of any ligamentous or tendinous attachment. Severe eversion ankle sprains may cause the deltoid ligament to avulse a portion of the distal medial malleolus rather than tearing the ligament. Inversion ankle sprains can provide sufficient overload to cause the plantar aponeurosis or peroneus brevis tendon to be pulled from the bone, avulsing the base of the fifth metatarsal, the so-called dancer's fracture. If the styloid process is avulsed, it is called a Type 2 fracture and has an excellent prognosis, with healing occurring within 4 to 6 weeks.

A much more complicated avulsion fracture seen in sprinters and jumpers involves a Type I transverse fracture into the proximal shaft of the fifth metatarsal at the junction of the diaphysis and metaphysis, called a **Jones fracture (Figure 16.28)**. It is often overlooked in conjunction with a severe ankle sprain that involves plantar flexion and a strong adduction force to the forefoot. Because of low vascularization and high stresses at this site, Jones fractures are associated with a poor outcome; nonunions and delayed unions are common.

▶ MANAGEMENT

Following standard acute care, the athlete should be referred to a physician for further care.

Treatment usually involves non-weight-bearing immobilization for a minimum of 4 weeks, followed by use of a walking cast or orthrosis for an additional 4 weeks. Athletic activity should be avoided until clinical and radiographic evidence of union appears, typically by 8 to 12 weeks. Failure to heal by 12 weeks is not uncommon; at this point, surgery with bone grafting and internal fixation may be necessary (23).

Osteochondral Fracture of the Talus

Severe ankle sprains can impinge the dome of the talus against the malleoli, leading to a fracture of the cartilaginous cover. Anterolateral fractures result from forceful inversion and dorsiflexion; posteromedial fractures result from forceful inversion and plantar flexion **(Figure 16.29)**.

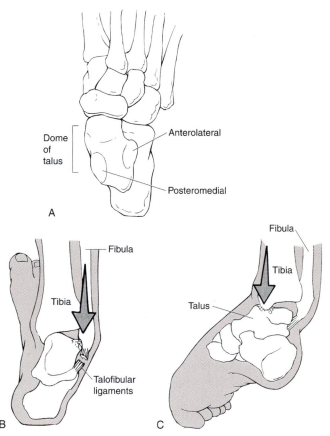

▶ FIGURE 16.29 **Osteochondral fractures**. A, A severe ankle injury that can fracture a portion of the cartilaginous cover on the dome of the talus is called an osteochondral fracture. B, Forceful inversion of a dorsiflexed ankle can produce damage to the anterolateral talar dome. C, Forceful inversion of a plantar flexed ankle can produce damage to the posteromedial aspect of the dome.

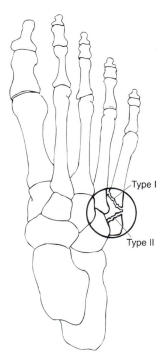

▶ FIGURE 16.28 **Avulsion fractures**. A Type I transverse fracture into the proximal shaft of the 5th metatarsal is often overlooked in an inversion ankle sprain, resulting in a nonunion fracture. A Type II fracture involves the styloid process of the 5th metatarsal.

The fragment may remain nondisplaced or may float freely in the joint. Osteochondritis dissecans of the talus can develop if the fragment, particularly one of the corners, floats freely in the ankle joint, thus losing its blood supply.

➤ SIGNS AND SYMPTOMS

Symptoms may be nonspecific, and include a deep, aching pain aggravated by activity; ankle swelling; stiffness; occasional crepitus; clicking; and locking (if displaced). Passive plantar flexion and palpation of the anterolateral and posteromedial corner of the talus will elicit point tenderness, or a palpable lesion or crepitus may be felt on the corners.

➤ MANAGEMENT

If pain and joint effusion persist after an inversion ankle sprain or ankle fracture, or if symptoms return after an asymptomatic period, suspect a more serious underlying condition, and immediately refer the athlete to a physician.

Limited weight-bearing, and/or immobilization, and NSAIDs are used to treat undisplaced fractures. In displaced fractures, arthroscopic excision or repair is usually necessary.

Displaced Fractures and Fracture Dislocations

Severe fractures result from direct compression in acute trauma (e.g., falling from a height or being stepped on), or from combined compression and shearing forces, as occurs during a severe twisting action. Because of the proximity of major blood vessels and nerves, many displaced and undisplaced fractures necessitate immediate immobilization and referral to the nearest trauma center.

FOREFOOT FRACTURES

Phalangeal fractures are caused by an axial load (jamming the toe into an immovable object) or direct trauma (crushing injury). With the exception of a fracture to the great toe, most are minor injuries. Swelling, ecchymosis, and pain are present; the individual is able to walk, but may have problems with footwear. Most tenderness resolves in 3 to 4 weeks. If the bony fragment is nondisplaced, buddy padding, splinting, and wearing a wooden shoe or a shoe with a wide toe box may help.

Metatarsal fractures are classified according to their anatomical location (neck, shaft, or base). A single fracture tends to be minimally displaced because of the restraining forces of the intermetatarsal ligaments. Swelling and pain are localized over the fracture site; pain increases with weight-bearing.

TARSAL FRACTURES

A **LisFranc injury** involves disruption of the tarsometatarsal joint, with or without an associated fracture. The typical mechanism is a severe twisting injury, as when a football player falls onto the heel of another player's plantar-flexed foot, causing an axial load along the metatarsals. The first metatarsal is typically dislocated from the first cuneiform, while the other four metatarsals are displaced laterally, usually in combination with a fracture at the base of the second metatarsal (24). Since blood supply to the forefoot can be compromised by the dislocation and subsequent swelling, a compartment syndrome can develop and create a serious injury. If assessed shortly after the injury, it may appear unremarkable until massive swelling sets in. A history of severe midfoot pain, paresthesia, or swelling along the midfoot region with variable flattening of the arch or abduction of the forefoot should signal a serious condition.

The talus is often fractured in a hyperdorsiflexion injury. A fracture of the lateral process of the talus and neck of the talus, which is rare, is caused by acute hyperdorsiflexion with inversion, which leads to severe hindfoot pain and moderate to severe edema, tenderness, and ecchymosis. Because of the potential devastating complication of avascular necrosis of the talus, talar neck fractures need immediate immobilization and referral to a physician. Posterior fractures of the talus are seen in individuals aged 15 to 30, particularly in those sports requiring forced plantar flexion of the foot, such as ballet or soccer, and may be either acute or stress-related. Posterior pain is present when jumping, running, or kicking with the instep of the foot, and is increased on forced plantar flexion and resisted great toe flexion, stemming from the close proximity of the flexor hallucis longus tendon to the fractured process.

Traumatic fractures of the calcaneus are rare, but when they occur, are commonly caused by high-energy axial loads. Occasionally, fractures will occur at the anterior process either by forceful plantar flexion and adduction, or by compression. Nearly 75% of all calcaneus fractures extend into the subtalar joint. Symptoms include severe heel pain, an inability to walk, and palpable, intense pain directly over the process, located just distal to the sinus tarsi. Initial treatment of intra-articular fractures includes immobilization in a bulky dressing and splint, with ice and elevation to control edema.

TIBIA–FIBULA FRACTURES

With inversion sprains, the medial malleolus is typically fractured at the level of the talar dome, or the injury may occur as a spiral fracture at the distal tibial metaphysis. Eversion and dorsiflexion injuries lead to spiral or comminuted fractures of the lateral malleolus. With lateral malleolar fractures, the risks are high for a bimalleolar fracture when the deltoid ligament avulses the medial malleolus (see Figure 16.22). Often a crack will be heard, and the individual is unable to bear weight on the injured extremity due to intense pain. Deformity may or may not be present.

A **Maisonneuve fracture** is an external rotation injury of the ankle with an associated fracture of the proximal third of the fibula; this injury is often missed, resulting in long-term disability. The typical mechanism is external rotation of the foot. The athlete will present with tenderness over the deltoid ligament and the fracture site on the proximal fibula. Any proximal fibular tenderness after a twisting injury calls for radiographs of the ankle, and the tibia and fibula. Often, a high fibula fracture requires open reduction and internal fixation between the distal fibula and tibia to maintain the bones' normal relationship while ligament healing occurs. The screws are generally removed 8 to 12 weeks after surgery.

Nearly 60% of all tibial fractures involve the middle and lower third of the tibia. The majority are closed (25). Whether open or closed, this fracture is associated with complications such as delayed union, nonunion, or malunion. The most common cause of an isolated tibial fracture is torsional force resulting in either a spiral or oblique fracture of the lower third of the tibia. Gross deformity, gross bone motion at the suspected fracture site, crepitus, immediate swelling, extreme pain, or pain with motion should signal immediate action.

ANKLE FRACTURE–DISLOCATIONS

Fracture–dislocations are usually caused by landing from a height with the foot in excessive eversion or inversion, or by being kicked from behind while the foot is firmly planted on the ground. The foot will typically be displaced laterally at a gross angle to the lower leg, and extreme pain will be present. This position can compromise the posterior tibial artery and nerve.

➤ MANAGEMENT OF DISPLACED FRACTURES AND FRACTURE–DISLOCATIONS

Management of lower leg, ankle, and foot fractures involves removing the shoe and sock to expose the injured area. If a fracture is suspected, the athletic trainer can perform percussion, compression, and distraction prior to any movement of the limb. Depending on the site, techniques listed in Field Strategy 16.6 may be helpful. The athletic trainer

should also assess the neurovascular integrity of the limb before and after immobilization by taking a distal pulse at the posterior tibial artery, dorsalis pedis artery, or blanching the toenails to determine capillary refill. The athletic trainer should note the skin color of the foot and toes and feel the toes for warmth. The pulp of the fingers can be stroked across the top of the distal metatarsal heads, and the individual can be asked if he or she can feel the finger. Repeat this action with the fingernail. Because shock is possible in serious traumatic fractures, activate EMS to immobilize and transport the individual to the nearest medical facility. Suspected disruption of the tarsometatarsal joint (LisFranc fracture) and fractures with suspected neurovascular compromise should be immobilized in a noncircumferential bulky splint to prevent complications from further compression.

If the great toe is fractured, a walking cast with a toe plate, or a wooden shoe and crutches, is helpful; if displaced, surgery may be necessary to prevent osteoarthritis. Metatarsal fractures are treated with a short slipper cast or wooden shoe for 6 weeks, with weight-bearing as tolerated. A nondisplaced Lisfranc injury can be treated in a short-leg nonwalking cast for 6 weeks, followed by 6 weeks in a short-leg walking cast. Most injuries, however, require open reduction and internal fixation. Nondisplaced extra-articular calcaneal fractures can be treated with a short-leg cast or walking boot for about 6 weeks. Most displaced fractures must be surgically repaired, but patients typically experience residual stiffness of their subtalar joint that can adversely affect future athletic performance.

Nondisplaced malleoli fractures are treated conservatively with cast immobilization for 4 to 6 weeks, followed by a functional brace until completely healed. Displaced fractures involving joint stability require surgical intervention with open reduction and internal fixation. Healing after surgery usually takes 2 to 3 months or longer, followed by extensive rehabilitation. Internal fixation with plates

---

FIELD STRATEGY 16.6   DETERMINE A POSSIBLE FRACTURE IN THE LOWER LEG AND FOOT

- **Percussion.** Tapping on the head of the fibula or tibial shaft, can be used to detect a fracture of the malleolus. Tapping on the ends of the toes along the long axis of the bone may detect a phalangeal fracture.
- **Bump test.** Strike the bottom of the heel with the palm to drive the talus into the mortise. Increased pain may indicate an osteochondral fracture, malleolar fracture, or increased mortise spread.
- **Squeeze test.** Compress the tibia and fibula together just distal to the knee. This causes the distal malleoli to distract. Increased pain distally may indicate a fracture.
- **Circumferential squeeze test.** Encircle the midfoot with the hand, and slowly squeeze the metatarsal heads. Increased pain may indicate a tarsal or metatarsal fracture.
- **Vibration.** Place a vibrating tuning fork near the suspected fracture site. Increased localized pain is a positive sign.
- **Compression/Distraction.** Compress the ends of the toes and metatarsals along the long axis of the bone. Follow this with distraction along the long axis. If a fracture is present, compression should increase pain, but distraction should decrease pain. If distraction increases pain, the injury may be a joint sprain.

and screws is often necessary to stabilize tibial fractures; however, there is a high rate of infection (44%) as a complication of internal fixation (25).

 The softball player has a possible avulsion fracture of the styloid process of the fifth metatarsal, caused by an associated injury to the peroneus brevis. This individual should be referred to a physician for further assessment and treatment.

ASSESSMENT OF THE LOWER LEG, ANKLE, AND FOOT

 A football lineman reports an aching pain on the posterior heel just proximal to the calcaneus. Pain increases when he touches the Achilles tendon and when he stands on tiptoes. Can you limit the assessment to only the foot, or should you assess the entire lower leg? How will you proceed?

Although pain, discomfort, or weakness may occur at a specific site, the lower extremities work as a unit to provide a foundation of support for the upright body, propulsion through space, absorption of shock, and adaptation to varying terrains. Assessment must therefore include the entire lower extremity, to evaluate how the body segments work together to provide motion. Always enter the assessment with an open mind because pain may be referred to the lower leg, ankle, and foot from conditions in the lumbar spine, sacrum, hip, or knee. Keep this in mind as you progress through the assessment. **Field Strategy 16.7** summarizes a complete evaluation for the lower leg, ankle, and foot.

FIELD STRATEGY 16.7   LOWER LEG, ANKLE, AND FOOT EVALUATION

HISTORY

- Primary complaint including:
  - Current nature, location, and onset of the condition
- Mechanism of injury
  - Cause of stress; position of hip, knee, and ankle; direction of force
  - Changes in kicking style, equipment, running techniques, or conditioning modes
- Characteristics of the symptoms
  - Evolution of the onset, nature, location, severity, and duration of pain and weakness
- Disability resulting from the injury
- Related medical history
  - Previous injuries in the area, congenital abnormalities, or family history

OBSERVATION AND INSPECTION

- Observation should analyze general posture and gait (see Field Strategy 16.9)
- Inspection at the injury site for deformity, swelling, discoloration, hypertrophy or muscle atropy, visible congenital deformity, or surgical incision or scars

PALPATION

- Bony structures, to determine a possible fracture
- Soft tissue structures, to determine skin temperature, swelling, point tenderness, crepitus, deformity, muscle spasm, cutaneous sensation, and pulse

FUNCTIONAL TESTS

- Active range of motion
- Passive range of motion

RESISTED MANUAL MUSCLE TESTING

STRESS TESTS

- Anterior drawer test
- Talar tilt
- External rotation (Kleiger's) test
- Thompson's test for Achilles tendon rupture
- Homan's test

NEUROLOGIC TESTS

- Myotomes
- Reflexes
- Dermatomes

SPORT-SPECIFIC FUNCTIONAL TESTS

HISTORY

What information do you need from the football player complaining of pain at the Achilles tendon? How will you phrase the questions to identify the main components of the primary complaint?

Many conditions in the lower leg, ankle, and foot are related to family history, congenital deformities, poor technique, and recent changes in the training program, surface, or foot attire. Begin by asking questions related to the mechanism of injury, associated symptoms, the progression of the symptoms, any disabilities that may have resulted from the injury, and related medical history. For example, an acute onset should lead one to suspect bony trauma or an acute ankle sprain until ruled out. A gradual onset of pain may signal inflammation from overuse of a muscle or the plantar fascia, or the development of a stress fracture. Pay particular attention to recent changes in the distance, duration, or intensity of training. Each component can lead to overuse injuries. Medial heel pain may indicate plantar fasciitis or a heel spur, if in the middle of the plantar heel area. Pain in the medial arch can be a sign of a fallen medial longitudinal arch, or tarsal tunnel syndrome. Pain around either malleolus may indicate an ankle sprain. Pain poste-

rior to the lateral malleolus can signify a peroneal tendinitis, subluxation, or dislocation, or sural nerve entrapment. Pain posterior to the medial malleolus may reflect tendinitis or rupture of the tibialis posterior. In addition to general questions discussed in Chapter 4, specific questions related to the lower leg, ankle, and foot are listed in **Field Strategy 16.8**.

The football player has had posterior heel pain off and on for the past 2 years. This week has been particularly painful because he has been trying to break in new cleats with the running and sprinting drills. He has been icing both heels after each practice and taking over-the-counter NSAIDs to help alleviate the symptoms, but the pain persists.

OBSERVATION AND INSPECTION

Think about the position(s) in which you want to observe this individual. Would a posture and gait analysis help? Why? What specific malalignment conditions might contribute to pain in the foot, ankle, or leg?

FIELD STRATEGY 16.8 DEVELOPING A HISTORY OF A LOWER LEG, ANKLE, OR FOOT INJURY

CURRENT INJURY STATUS

1. Where is the pain (or weakness) located? How severe is the pain (weakness)? Does the pain radiate? (Hip pain may be referred pain, so ask additional questions if you suspect a visceral, low back, lumbar, or knee problem.)
2. Did the pain come on suddenly (acute) or gradually (overuse)? Was the pain greatest when the injury first occurred, or did it get worse the second or third day?
3. (If acute, ask:) What were you doing at the time of the injury? What position was the leg in when the injury occurred? (If chronic, ask:) What different activities have you been doing in the last week? (Look for changes in technique, frequency, duration, intensity, or changes in shoes, equipment, or running surface.)
4. Did you hear any sounds during the incident? Has the joint ever locked on you (possible talar dome lesion)? Can you bear weight on the leg or balance on the leg? Did you notice any swelling, discoloration, muscle spasms, or numbness with the injury?
5. What actions or motions bring on the pain? It is worse in the morning, during activity, after activity, or at night? Does it wake you up at night? When the pain sets in, how long does it last?
6. Are there certain activities you are unable to perform because of the pain? Which ones?
7. Do you stand, sit, or walk on uneven surfaces for long periods? What shoes do you wear when the pain sets in? (Check heel height, wear pattern, and internal arch and heel padding.)
8. How old are you? (Remember that many problems are age-related.) Which leg is dominant?

PAST INJURY STATUS

1. Have you ever injured your leg, ankle, or foot before? How did that occur? What was done for the injury? Did you have any difficulty returning to your full functional status?
2. Have you had any medical problems recently? (Look for problems that may refer pain to the area.) Are you on any medication? Do you have any musculoskeletal problems elsewhere in the body? (This may cause changes in gait or technique that transfer abnormal forces to structures in the lower limb.)

Both lower legs should be clearly visible to denote symmetry, any congenital deformity, swelling, discoloration, hypertrophy, muscular atrophy, or previous surgical incisions. The individual should wear running shorts to allow full view of the lower extremity. Ask the athlete to bring along the shoes normally worn when pain is present. Inspect the sole, heel box, toe box, and general condition of the shoes for unusual wear, indicating a biomechanical abnormality.

In an ambulatory patient, begin observations by completing a postural exam. Note any bilateral gross deformity, swelling, or redness in the toes, foot, or ankle. At the foot, note the presence or absence of an arch on weight-bearing and non-weight-bearing. A supple, or flexible, flat foot appears flattened when weight-bearing but produces an obvious arch when non-weight-bearing. In contrast, a rigid flat foot appears flattened on weight-bearing and non-weight-bearing. Is the foot in a pronated, neutral, or supinated position (see Box 16.1)? Specific areas to focus on in the lower extremity are summarized in **Field Strategy 16.9**.

Next, place the individual prone on a table with the knee extended and the feet over the end of the table. Observe the relationship of the rearfoot to forefoot alignment. After completing a static exam, observe the individual walking barefoot from anterior, posterior, and lateral views. Note any abnormalities in gait, favoring of one limb, heel-toe floor contact, and heel alignment. Have the individual put on shoes and any orthoses, and repeat the gait analysis to get a better perspective of the wear pattern. Inspect the injury site for obvious deformities, discoloration, edema, or scars that might indicate previous surgery, and note the general condition of the skin. Remember to compare the affected limb with the unaffected limb.

 The individual has bilateral redness and swelling over the Achilles tendon, and there is a slight hindfoot valgus deformity. With the exception of prolonged pronation on the right foot, gait appears normal. The new cleats he has been wearing have an extended tab on the posterior heel cup that appears to be very rigid.

PALPATION

 With pain centered on the Achilles tendon, think for a minute where you should begin to palpate the various structures. During palpation, what factors are you looking for?

 FIELD STRATEGY 16.9   POSTURAL ASSESSMENT OF THE LOWER LEG, ANKLE, AND FOOT

ANTERIOR VIEW

- The iliac crests should be level, with equal space between the arms and waist. Both thighs should look the same. Check for hypertrophy or atrophy. The patellae should be at the same height and facing straight forward
- The legs should be straight. The knees may be in genu valgus (knock-kneed) or genu varus (bow-legged)
- The medial and lateral malleoli should be level as compared to the opposite foot. Is there swelling in the ankle joint?
- Both feet should be angled equally. Tibial torsion may result in the foot either pointing inward ("pigeon toes"), or pointing slightly lateral. Check for supination or pronation of the feet. Both feet should have visible equal arches. Note any pes cavus (high arch), or pes planus (flatfoot). Are the feet splayed (widening of the forefoot)? Are the toes straight and parallel? Do the nails appear normal?
- Check the skin for normal contours, discolored lesions, exostosis or other bumps, corns, calluses, or scars indicating a previous injury or surgery. Note any signs of circulatory impairment or varicose veins

POSTERIOR VIEW

- The gluteal folds and knee folds should be level. The hamstrings and calf muscles should have equal bulk
- The Achilles tendons should go straight down to the calcaneus. If they appear to angle out, excessive pronation may be present. The heels should appear to be straight, with equal shape and position
- The lateral malleoli should extend slightly more distal than the medial malleoli, and the medial malleoli will be slightly more anterior than the lateral malleoli

LATERAL VIEW

- The knees should be slightly flexed (0 to 5°)
- The lateral malleolus should be slightly posterior to the center of the knee

NON-WEIGHT-BEARING VIEW

- Check for abnormal calluses, plantar warts, arches, and scars on the plantar side of the foot

With the athlete seated on an examination table, extend the foot and ankle beyond the table's edge. Perform bilateral palpation to determine temperature, swelling, point tenderness, crepitus, deformity, muscle spasm, and cutaneous sensation. Pulses can be taken at the posterior tibial artery behind the medial malleolus, and at the dorsalis pedis artery on the dorsum of the foot. Proceed proximal to distal, but palpate the most painful areas last. Allow the individual to sit on a table so you can perform bilateral palpation.

Anterior and Medial Palpation

1. Shaft of the tibia
2. Medial malleolus
3. Posterior tibial artery
4. Tibialis posterior, flexor digitorum longus, and flexor hallucis longus muscles and tendons
5. Deltoid ligament
6. Sustentaculum tali (one finger's width inferior to the medial malleolus)
7. Talar dome and neck (plantar flexion will expose this area)
8. Joint capsule
9. Tibialis anterior, extensor hallucis longus, extensor digitorum longus muscles and tendons, and dorsalis pedis artery
10. Navicular bone and tubercle of the navicular
11. Medial, middle, and lateral cuneiforms
12. Calcaneonavicular ligament (spring ligament)
13. Medial calcaneus
14. Plantar fascia
15. Head of first metatarsal, sesamoid bones, great toe
16. Second metatarsal and second toe

Anterior and Lateral Palpation

1. Head of the fibula, peroneal longus and brevis
2. Distal tibiofibular joint and ligament
3. Lateral malleolus
4. Anterior and posterior talofibular ligaments, calcaneofibular ligament, peroneal tubercle, and peroneal tendons
5. Sinus tarsi (indentation over the talus next to the muscle belly of the extensor digitorum brevis)
6. Joint capsule and dome of the talus (plantarflex the foot)
7. Cuboid bone
8. Styloid process of the fifth metatarsal, shafts of the third, fourth, and fifth metatarsals
9. Third through fifth toes

Posterior Palpation

1. Triceps surae and Achilles tendon
2. Calcaneus, calcaneal bursa, and retrocalcaneal bursa
3. Posterior aspect of heel pad and calcaneus

If a fracture is suspected, perform percussion, compression, and distraction prior to any movement of the limb. Examples of these techniques were provided earlier in the chapter in Field Strategy 16.6. These tests should be completed before a postural or gait analysis.

 You found increased pain and crepitus on palpation of the Achilles tendon and pain just anterior to the tendon in the soft tissue. Localized swelling and a slight increase in skin temperature are also present in that region. Fracture tests were negative.

PHYSICAL EXAMINATION TESTS

 Pain and swelling are localized on and slightly anterior to the Achilles tendon. What special tests can be performed to determine if the injury is to the tendon, bursa, or other soft-tissue structures that course through the area?

Special tests should be performed in a comfortable position with the individual lying on a table with feet hanging over the end or with the individual sitting. Bilateral comparison is used to assess normal level of function.

Functional Tests

The athletic trainer should determine the available range of motion in ankle dorsiflexion/plantar flexion, supination/pronation, toe flexion/extension, and toe abduction/adduction. As always, bilateral comparison is critical to determine normal or abnormal movement.

ACTIVE MOVEMENTS

Active movements are best performed with the individual sitting on a table with the leg flexed over the end of the table. Stabilize the thigh and knee. Perform those actions causing pain last to prevent any painful symptoms from overflowing into the next movement. The following movements listed below should be performed weight-bearing and non-weight-bearing. The number in parentheses are normal ranges of motion for each movement.

- Dorsiflexion of the ankle (20°)
- Plantar flexion of the ankle (30 to 50°)
- Pronation (15 to 30°)
- Supination (45 to 60°)
- Toe extension
- Toe flexion
- Toe abduction and adduction

PASSIVE RANGE OF MOTION

If the individual is able to perform full range of motion during active movements, apply gentle pressure at the extremes of motion to determine end feel. The end feel for

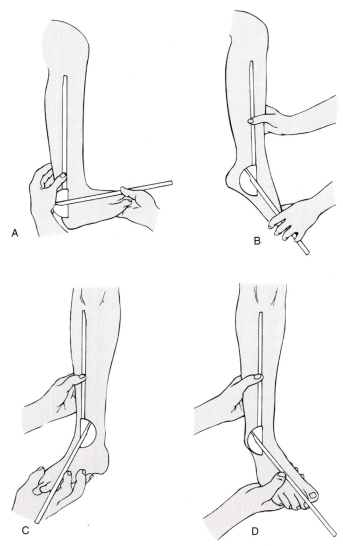

tions should be delayed until last. **Figure 16.31** demonstrates motions that should be tested.

Stress Tests

From information gathered during the history, observation, inspection, and palpation, determine which tests most effectively assess the condition. Only those tests deemed relevant should be used.

ANTERIOR DRAWER TEST

This test can assess collateral ligament integrity of the ankle. With the individual supine and the foot extended beyond the table, the athletic trainer should stabilize the tibia and fibula in one hand and cup the individual's heel in the other hand. To test both the anterior talofibular and deltoid ligaments, apply a straight anterior movement with slight dorsiflexion **(Figure 16.32A)**. If the entire dome of the talus shifts equally forward, it indicates both medial and lateral ligament damage. To isolate the anterior talofibular ligament and anterolateral capsule, apply a straight anterior movement with slight plantar flexion and inversion. A positive test will result in the lateral side of the talus shifting forward, indicating anterolateral rotary instability.

TALAR TILT

The calcaneofibular and deltoid ligaments are tested in the same position described for the anterior drawer test. Maintain the calcaneus in normal anatomical position (90° flexion). The talus is then slowly rocked between inversion and eversion **(Figure 16.32B)**. Inversion tests the calcaneofibular ligament, and eversion the deltoid ligament.

EXTERNAL ROTATION (KLEIGER'S) TEST

A variation of the talar tilt test for deltoid ligament instability is the external rotation, or Kleiger's, test. Stabilize the lower leg proximal to the distal tibiofibular syndesmosis, being careful not to compress the joint. With the foot in a neutral position, grasp the medial side of the foot and rotate the foot laterally (external rotation) **(Figure 16.33)**. If pain is felt over the medial joint line, it indicates damage to the deltoid ligament, whereas pain in the area of the lateral malleolus indicates injury to the syndesmosis.

THOMPSON'S TEST FOR ACHILLES TENDON RUPTURE

With the individual prone on a table, squeeze the calf muscles. A normal response is slight plantar flexion. A positive test, indicating a rupture of the gastrocnemius-soleus complex or Achilles tendon, is indicated by the absence of plantar flexion **(Figure 16.34)**. Always compare the amount of motion to the uninjured side, as some plantar

▶ **FIGURE 16.30 Goniometry measurement**. Ankle dorsiflexion (A) and plantar flexion (B). Center the fulcrum over the lateral malleolus. Align the proximal arm along the fibula using the head of the fibula for reference. Align the distal arm parallel to the midline of the 5th metatarsal. Pronation (C) and supination (D). Center the fulcrum over the anterior ankle midway between the malleoli. Align the proximal arm with the midline of the crest of the tibia. Align the distal arm with the midline of the 2nd metatarsal.

dorsiflexion, plantar flexion, pronation, supination, and toe flexion and extension is tissue stretch. If the individual is unable to perform full active movements, passive movement should then be performed to determine available range of motion and end feel. **Figure 16.30** demonstrates proper positioning for goniometry measurement at the ankle.

RESISTED MUSCLE TESTING

Stabilize the thigh, and perform all resisted muscle testing throughout the full range of motion. Begin with the muscle on stretch, and apply resistance throughout the full range of motion. Note any muscle weakness when compared to the uninvolved limb. As always, painful mo-

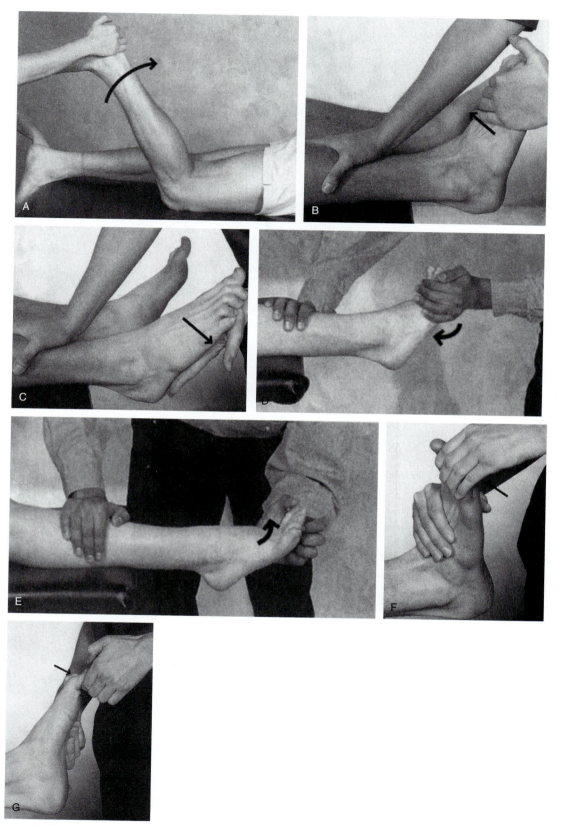

➤ **FIGURE 16.31 Resisted manual muscle testing.** A, Knee flexion (S_1 and S_2). B, Dorsiflexion (L_4). C, Plantar flexion (S_1). D, Pronation. E, Supination. F, Toe extension (L_5). G, Toe flexion. (Myotomes are listed in parentheses.)

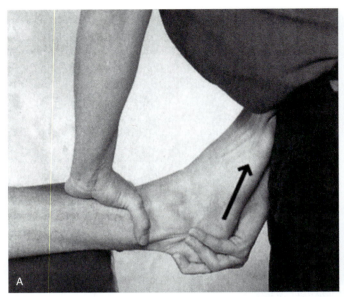

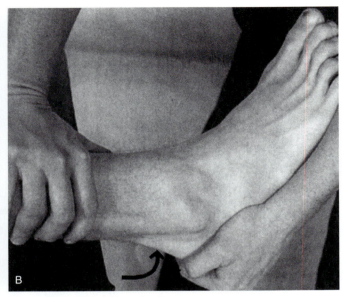

➤ FIGURE 16.32 **Stress tests for the ankle collateral ligaments**. A, Anterior drawer test. B, Talar tilt test.

flexion may occur if the plantaris muscle is intact. However, the magnitude of contraction will be significantly reduced when compared to the uninvolved leg.

HOMAN'S SIGN

To test for deep venous thrombosis, place the individual supine on a table. Passively dorsiflex the foot of the involved leg with the knee extended **(Figure 16.35)**. Pain

in the calf indicates a positive Homan's sign. Tenderness may also be elicited with palpation of the calf. In addition, pallor or swelling in the leg may be accompanied by an absence of the dorsalis pedis pulse.

Neurologic Assessment

Assess neurologic integrity with isometric muscle testing of the myotomes, reflex testing, and sensation in the segmental dermatomes and peripheral nerve cutaneous patterns.

MYOTOMES

Isometric muscle testing should be performed in the following motions to test specific segmental myotomes: knee extension (L_3), ankle dorsiflexion (L_4), toe extension (L_5); and ankle plantar flexion, foot eversion, or hip extension (S_1).

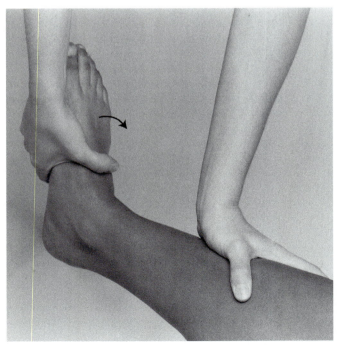

➤ FIGURE 16.33 **External rotation test**. Passively dorsiflex the ankle, and rotate the foot laterally. Pain in the area of the lateral malleolus indicates injury to the syndesmosis.

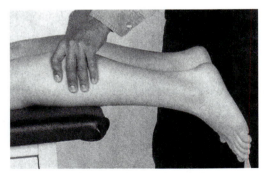

➤ FIGURE 16.34 **Thompson's test**. Do passive compression of the calf muscles. This should produce slight plantar flexion at the ankle. If no plantar flexion occurs, suspect a possible rupture of the gastrocnemius-soleus complex or the Achilles tendon.

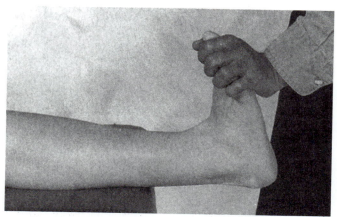

➤ FIGURE 16.35 **Homan's sign**. Passively dorsiflex the foot with the knee extended. Pain in the calf indicates a possible deep venous thrombosis.

REFLEXES

Reflexes in the lower leg region include the patella (L_3, L_4) and Achilles tendon reflex (S_1). These were discussed in Chapter 15 and demonstrated in Figure 15.27.

CUTANEOUS PATTERNS

In testing cutaneous sensation, run sharp and dull objects over the skin, i.e., the blunt tip and flat edge of taping scissors. With the eyes closed or looking away, ask if the individual can distinguish sharp and dull. The segmental nerve dermatome patterns for the foot and lower leg are demonstrated in **Figure 16.36**. The peripheral nerve cutaneous distribution patterns are demonstrated in **Figure 16.37**.

Sport-Specific Functional Tests

Functional tests should be performed pain-free before clearing any individual for return to competition. These may include any or all of the following:

- Squatting with both heels maintained on the floor
- Going up on the toes at least 20 times without pain
- Walking on the toes for 20 to 30 feet
- Balancing on one foot at a time
- Running straight ahead, stopping, and running backwards
- Running figure-eights with large circles, slowly decreasing in size
- Running at an angle sideways and making V-cuts
- Jumping rope for at least 1 minute
- Jumping straight up and going to a 90° squat

These activities are examples that can be used to test the integrity of injured anatomical structures. All should be performed pain-free and without a limp or antalgic gait.

 Pain increased with passive dorsiflexion, and active and resisted plantar flexion with the knee

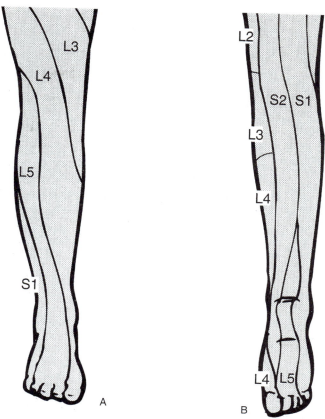

➤ FIGURE 16.36 **Dermatomes for the lower leg, ankle, and foot.** A, Anterior. B, Posterior.

extended. Palpation of the Achilles tendon elicited crepitus during resisted plantar flexion. All other tests were negative. This individual probably has Achilles tendinitis and retrocalcaneal bursitis that may have been aggravated by the rigid tab on the new cleats compressing into the tendon during repetitive plantar flexion.

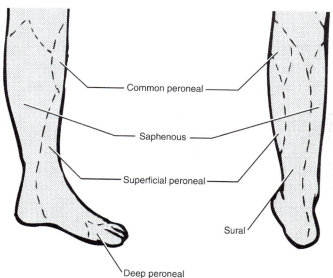

➤ FIGURE 16.37 **Peripheral nerve distribution in the lower leg, ankle, and foot.**

REHABILITATION

A heel lift was placed in the football player's new cleats, and the tab was cut from the shoe. After 2 days of rest and ice therapy, pain in the Achilles tendon has significantly improved. What exercises should now be included in the rehabilitation program?

Rehabilitation exercises for the lower leg, ankle, and foot can be initiated during the acute inflammatory phase so long as the condition is not further irritated. For example, while icing an ankle, the gastrocnemius and soleus can be passively stretched, or strengthening exercises for the foot intrinsic muscles can be started. Pain and swelling dictate the amount of exercise tolerated, and may necessitate restricted weight-bearing. The rehabilitation program should restore motion and proprioception, maintain cardiovascular fitness, and improve muscular strength, endurance, and power, predominantly through closed-chain exercises.

Restoration of Motion

Field Strategy 16.1 introduced several range-of-motion exercises that can be performed non-weight-bearing. For example, towel pulls stretching the Achilles tendon, writing the alphabet in large circles, picking up objects in the toes and combining the action with shin curls, and use of a BAPS board can all be done in a seated position. As pain subsides and weight-bearing is initiated, Achilles tendon stretches, toe raises, balance exercises, and use of the BAPS board can be completed in a standing position.

FIELD STRATEGY 16.10   REHABILITATION EXERCISES FOR THE LOWER LEG

A. **Phase one.** Control inflammation. Minimize inversion and eversion exercises to allow for healing. Dorsiflexion and plantar flexion should be performed within the limits of pain. Exercises should be combined with ice therapy or electrical stimulation, with elevation. Use those exercises listed in Field Strategy 16.1 as tolerated.
   1. Plantar fascia stretch
   2. Towel crunches
   3. Toe curls
   4. Picking up objects
   5. BAPS board in seated position
   6. Triceps surae stretch, non-weight-bearing
   7. Pool therapy or upper body ergometer (UBE) exercises for cardiovascular fitness
B. **Phase two.** As pain and tenderness subside, initiate inversion and eversion range of motion. Initiate strengthening exercises as tolerated. Include:
   1. Shin curls
   2. Ankle alphabet
   3. Triceps surae stretch, standing position
   4. Toe raises
   5. Theraband or tubing exercises in dorsiflexion, plantar flexion, inversion, and eversion
   6. Unilateral balance—BAPS board activities with support
   7. Pool therapy, UBE, and stationary bike (if tolerated) for cardiovascular fitness
C. **Phase three**
   1. Toe raises with weights
   2. Multi-axial ankle machine
   3. Squats and lunges
   4. Balance exercises with challenges, such as dribbling while balancing on one leg, doing Theraband exercises while balancing on one leg, or balancing on an uneven surface
   5. Straight-ahead jogging, if able to walk without a limp
D. **Phase four.** (Use external support for the ankle as needed.)
   1. Isokinetic exercises to work functional speeds
   2. Multi-angle plyometrics, including single- and double-limb jumping, front to front, side to side, and diagonals
   3. Side-to-side running
   4. Running backwards
   5. Jumping for height and distance (long jump)
   6. Slide board
   7. Gradual return to sport activity with protection

Restoration of Proprioception and Balance

Proprioception and balance must be regained to allow safe return to sport participation. Early exercises may include shifting one's weight while on crutches, doing bilateral minisquats, or using a BAPS board in a seated position. As balance improves, BAPS board exercises can progress to partial weight-bearing while supported by a table, and then to full-weight-bearing exercises. Running in place on a minitramp and use of a slide board are also closed-chain exercises that improve proprioception and balance.

Muscular Strength, Endurance, and Power

Early emphasis is placed on strengthening the foot's intrinsic muscles. Towel crunches were demonstrated in Field Strategy 16.1. As the condition allows, toe raises and Theraband or surgical tubing exercises are added. Use of a multi-axial ankle machine, toe raises with weights, squats and lunges, and isokinetic exercises will continue to strengthen the lower leg musculature. In later stages, jogging, running side to side, and multiangle plyometrics can assist the individual in returning gradually to sport participation.

Cardiovascular Fitness

Maintenance of cardiovascular fitness can begin immediately after injury with use of an upper body ergometer (UBE) or hydrotherapeutic exercise. Running in deep water and performing sport-specific exercises can provide mild resistance in a non-weight-bearing medium. When range of motion is adequate, a stationary bicycle may be used. Light jogging, running backwards, and running side-to-side should increase in intensity and duration to facilitate return to activity. **Field Strategy 16.10** lists several rehabilitation exercises that may be incorporated in a complete program for the lower leg.

In addition to exercises, the individual should be assessed for biomechanical anomalies, and appropriate orthotics should be fabricated to correct any malalignment. With ankle injuries, it may be necessary to provide external support to the ankle region. After the rehabilitation program is completed and the individual is cleared for full participation, a proper maintenance program of stretching and strengthening exercises should be provided.

 Flexibility and strengthening exercises for the gastrocnemius-soleus complex should be a priority in the rehabilitation program. In addition, the hindfoot valgus deformity should be further assessed to determine if orthoses are necessary.

Summary

1. The true ankle (talocrural) joint is the mortise-tenon joint between the tibia, fibula, and talus. Plantar flexion and dorsiflexion occur at this joint. Motion at the subtalar joint occurs in an oblique direction. The combination of calcaneal inversion, foot adduction, and plantar flexion is known as supination; calcaneal eversion, foot abduction, and dorsiflexion is known as pronation.

2. The primary supporting structures of the plantar arches are the spring (calcaneonavicular) ligament, long plantar ligament, plantar fascia (plantar aponeurosis), and the short plantar (plantar calcaneocuboid) ligament. In addition, the tibialis posterior provides some support.

3. Congenital abnormalities, leg length discrepancy, muscle dysfunction (such as muscle imbalance), or a malalignment syndrome (pes cavus, pes planus, pes equinus, hammer or claw toes) can predispose an individual to several chronic injuries.

4. Generalized forefoot pain may be due to intrinsic factors (excessive body weight, limited flexibility of the Achilles tendon, pronation, valgus heel, hammer toes, fallen metatarsal arch, pes planus, or pes cavus) or extrinsic factors (narrow toe box, improperly placed shoe cleats, repetitive jumping or running, or landing poorly from a height).

5. An acute anterior compartment syndrome is a medical emergency. Signs and symptoms include a recent history of trauma, a palpable firm mass in the anterior compartment, tight skin, and a diminished dorsalis pedis pulse.

6. Ankle sprains are classified as grade I, II, or III based on the progression of anatomical structures damaged and the subsequent disability. In lateral ankle sprains involving plantar flexion and inversion, the anterior talofibular ligament is first torn, followed by the calcaneal fibular ligament. In eversion ankle sprains, the deltoid ligament is injured; there may also be an associated avulsion fracture of one or both malleoli.

7. Common sites for tendon injuries include the Achilles tendon just proximal to its insertion into the calcaneus, the tibialis posterior just behind the medial malleolus, the tibialis anterior just under the extensor retinaculum, and the peroneal tendons behind the lateral malleolus or at the distal attachment on the styloid process of the fifth metatarsal.

8. Injury to the tibialis posterior will result in weakness in plantar flexion and inversion, and may lead to acquired pes planus.

9. Risk factors for Achilles tendinitis include a tight heel cord, foot malalignment deformities, a recent change in shoes or running surface, a sudden increase in workload (distance or intensity), or changes in the exercise environment (changing footwear, or excessive hill climbing or impact-loading activities, such as jumping).

10. Medial tibial stress syndrome is a periostitis along the posteromedial tibial border, usually in the distal third, not associated with a stress fracture or compartment syndrome. Signs and symptoms include point tenderness in a 3 to 6 cm area along the distal posteromedial tibial border, and pain and weakness with resisted plantar flexion or standing on tiptoe.

11. Exertional compartment syndrome is characterized by exercise-induced pain and swelling that are relieved by rest. The anterior compartment is most frequently affected, and if so, mild foot drop or paresthesia (or both) may be present. Fascial defects or hernias may also be present in the distal third of the leg over the anterior intramuscular septum.

12. Nerve impingement may involve the interdigital nerves as they bifurcate at the metatarsal heads (plantar interdigital neuroma), the posterior tibial nerve beneath the flexor retinaculum and behind the medial malleolus, or the sural nerve as it courses behind the lateral malleolus into the lateral foot.

13. Fractures of the lower leg, ankle, and foot may involve:
    - Freiberg's disease (avascular necrosis of the second metatarsal head)
    - Sever's disease (calcaneal apophysis)
    - Stress fractures (neck of the second metatarsal is most common)
    - Avulsion fractures (styloid process of the fifth metatarsal, medial and lateral malleoli)
    - Osteochondral fractures (talar dome)
    - Displaced fractures or fracture–dislocations

14. Pain may be referred to the lower leg, ankle, and foot from the lumbar spine, hip, or knee.

15. Conditions that warrant special attention include:
    - Obvious deformity suggesting a dislocation, fracture, or ruptured Achilles tendon
    - Significant loss of motion or weakness in a myotome
    - Excessive joint swelling
    - Possible epiphyseal or apophyseal injuries
    - Abnormal reflexes or sensation, or absent or weak pulse
    - Gross joint instability
    - Any unexplained pain

16. Functional tests should be performed pain-free without limp or antalgic gait before clearing any individual for reentry into competition. In addition, the individual should have bilaterally equal range of motion, strength, proprioception, and a high cardiovascular fitness level before being allowed to return to activity. When necessary, protective equipment or braces should be used to prevent reinjury.

References

1. Aagaard H, Jörgenson U. Injuries in elite volleyball. Scand J Med Sci Sports 1996;6(4):228-232.
2. Bahr R, Bahr IS. Incidence of acute volleyball injuries: A prospective cohort study of injury mechanisms and risk factors. Scand J Med Sci Sports 1997;7(3):166-171.
3. Briner WW, Kacmar L. Common injuries in volleyball. Mechanisms of injury, prevention and rehabilitation. Sports Med 1997;24(1):65-71.
4. Hickey GJ, Fricker PA, McDonald WA. Injuries of young elite female basketball players over a six-year period. Clin J Sports Med 1997;7(4):252-256.
5. McRory P, Bladin C. Fractures of the lateral process of the talus: A clinical review. "Snowboarder's ankle." Clin J Sports Med 1996;6(2):124-128.
6. Wang Q, et al. Fibula and its ligaments in load transmission and ankle joint stability. Clin Orthop 1997;(330):261-270.
7. Renstrom P, Johnson RJ. Overuse injuries in sports: A review. Sports Med 1985;2(5):316-333.
8. Klein P, Mattys S, Rooze M. Moment arm length variations of selected muscles acting on talocrural and subtalar joints during movement: An in vitro study. J Biomech 1996;29(1):21-30.
9. Milgrom C, et al. The area moment of inertia of the tibia: A risk factor for stress fractures. J Biomech 1989;22(11/12):1243-1248.
10. Bennell KL, et al. Skeletal effects of menstrual disturbances in athletes. Scand J Med Sci Sports 1997;7(5):261-273.
11. Benson JE, et al. Nutritional aspects of amenorrhea in the female athlete triad. Int J Sport Nutr 1996;6(2):134-135.
12. Norkin CC, Levangie PK. Joint structure and function: A comprehensive analysis. Philadelphia: FA Davis, 1992.
13. Cavanagh PR, et al. The relationship of static foot structure to dynamic foot function. J Biomech 1997;30(3):243-250.
14. Coady CM, Gow N, Stanish W. Foot problems in middle-aged patients: Keeping active people up to speed. Phys Sportsmed 1998;26(5):31-42.
15. Clanton TO, Porter DA. Primary care of foot and ankle injuries in the athlete. Clin Sports Med 1997;16(3):435-466.
16. Alonso A, Khoury L, Adams R. Clinical tests for ankle syndesmosis injury: Reliability and prediction of return to function. JOSPT 1998;27(4):276-284.
17. Brown DE. Ankle and leg injuries. In: The Team Physician's Handbook. Edited by Mellion MB, Walsh WM, and Shelton GL. Philadelphia: Hanley & Belfus, 1997.
18. Middleton JA, Kolodin EL. Plantar fasciitis Heel pain in athletes. J Ath Train 1992;27(1):70-75.
19. Davey JR, Rorabeck CH, Fowler PJ. The tibialis posterior muscle compartment: An unrecognized cause of exertional compartmental syndrome. Am J Sports Med 1984;12(5):391-397.
20. Edwards P, Myerson MS. Exertional compartment syndrome of the leg: Steps for expedient return to activity. Phys Sportsmed 1996;24(4):31-46.
21. Madden CC, Mellion MB. Sever's disease and other causes of heel pain in adolescents. Am Fam Phys 1996;54(6):1995-2000.
22. Blue JM, Matthews LS. Leg injuries. Clin Sports Med 1997;16(3):467-478.
23. Yu WD, Shapiro MS. Fractures of the fifth metatarsal: Careful identification for optimal treatment. Phys Sportsmed 1998;26(2):47-64.
24. Thompson E, Cordas M Jr. Fracture-dislocations you can't afford to miss. Phys Sportsmed 1996;24(6):37-42.
25. Garl TC, et al. Tibial fracture in a basketball player: Treatment dilemmas and complications. Phys Sportsmed 1997;25(6):41-53.

Special Considerations

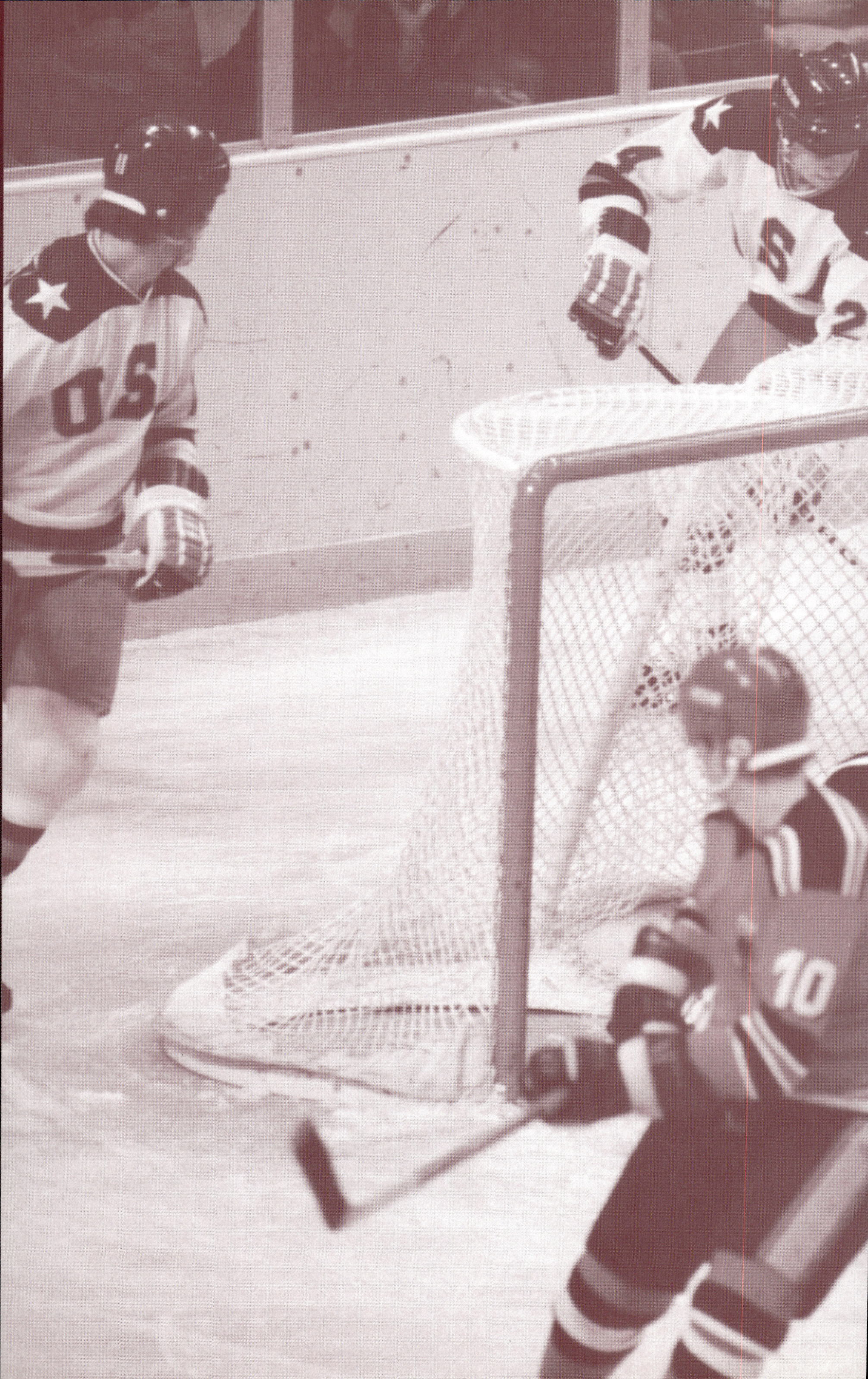

SECTION VI

CHAPTER **17**

Environmental Conditions

OBJECTIVES

1. Describe how heat-regulating mechanisms are activated, and explain the methods used to generate heat via internal and external sources.

2. Demonstrate measurement of the heat stress index using a sling psychrometer.

3. Explain methods used to prevent heat illness.

4. Identify the signs and symptoms of heat-related conditions, and describe their management.

5. Describe how the body generates internal heat during cold ambient temperatures.

6. Differentiate between frostbite and systemic cooling, and describe the management of each.

7. Describe what impact high altitude and poor air quality have on exercise and sport performance.

8. Explain what steps should be taken if you are caught outdoors during lightning or a thunderstorm.

E nvironmental conditions affect even the best-conditioned athlete. Athletic contests are often held on hot, humid days, or in cold, windy conditions where hyperthermia and hypothermia, respectively, may affect performance. In addition, exercising during thunderstorms that produce lightning can be extremely dangerous. These environmental conditions, in addition to altitude and air quality, will be discussed in this chapter.

HEAT-RELATED CONDITIONS

 It is early August and the soccer team is reporting back for the fall season. What measures can you take to decrease the risk of heat illness during this preseason practice period?

The process by which the body maintains body temperature is called **thermoregulation**, which is primarily controlled by the **hypothalamus**, a region of the diencephalon

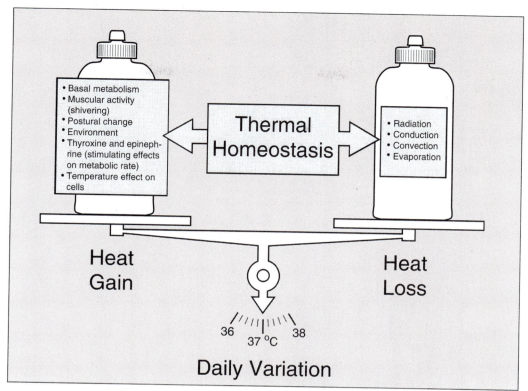

➤ FIGURE 17.1 Thermal homeostasis. Homeostasis is achieved when internal heat production and heat loss are properly balanced to maintain a relatively constant body core temperature.

forming the floor of the third ventricle of the brain. **Hyperthermia**, or elevated body temperature, occurs when internal heat production exceeds external heat loss **(Figure 17.1)**. The hypothalamus gland maintains **homeostasis**, or a state of equilibrium within the body, by initiating cooling or heat-retention mechanisms to achieve a relatively constant body core temperature between 36.1° and 37.8°C (97° to 100°F). The body core, encompassing the skull, thoracic, and abdominal area, contains the vital organs of the body. Heat-regulating mechanisms such as perspiring or shivering are activated by two means: (1) stimulation of peripheral thermal receptors in the skin, and (2) changes in blood temperature as it flows through the hypothalamus.

Internal Heat Regulation

During exercise, the body gains heat either from external sources (environmental temperatures) or internal processes **(Figure 17.2)**. Much of the internal heat is generated during muscular activity through energy metabolism. From shivering alone, the total metabolic rate can increase three-fold to fivefold. During sustained vigorous exercise, the metabolic rate can increase 20 to 25 times above the resting level. This theoretically can increase core temperature by about 1°C (1.8°F) every 5 to 7 minutes (1). During exercise, the circulatory system must deliver oxygen to the working muscles and deliver heated blood from deep tissues (core) to the periphery (shell) for dissipation. The increased

blood flow to the muscles and skin is made possible by increasing cardiac output and redistributing regional blood flow (i.e., blood flow to the visceral organs is reduced). As exercise begins, heart rate and cardiac output increase while superficial venous and arterial blood vessels dilate to divert warm blood to the skin surface. Heat is dissipated when the warm blood flushes into skin capillaries. This is evident when the face becomes flushed and reddened on a hot day or after exercise. When the individual is in a resting state and the air temperature is below 30.6°C (87°F), about two-thirds of the body's normal heat loss occurs as a result of conduction, convection, and radiation. As air temperature approaches skin temperature and exceeds 30.6°C, evaporation becomes the predominant means of heat dissipation.

RADIATION

Radiation is the loss of heat from a warmer object to a cooler object in the form of infrared waves (thermal energy) without physical contact. Usually, body temperature is warmer than the environment and radiant heat is dissipated through the air to surrounding solid, cooler objects. When the temperatures of surrounding objects in the environment exceed skin temperature, such as the sun or hot artificial turf, radiant heat is absorbed. Participating in a shaded area is an example of how the effects of radiant heat can be controlled during activity.

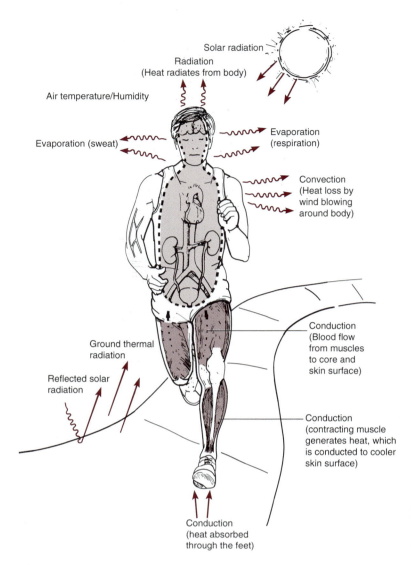

➤ FIGURE 17.2 Heat gain and heat loss. Heat produced within working muscles is transferred to the body's core and skin. During exercise, body heat is dissipated into the surrounding environment by radiation, conduction, convection, and evaporation. Straight lines represent heat gain, and wavy lines indicate heat loss.

CONDUCTION

Conduction is the direct transfer of heat through a liquid, solid, or gas from a warm object to a cooler object. For example, a football player can absorb heat through the feet simply by standing on hot artificial turf. The rate of conductive heat loss depends on the temperature gradient (difference) between the skin and surrounding surfaces, and the thermal qualities of those surfaces. For example, heat loss in water can be considerable.

CONVECTION

Convection depends on conduction from the skin to the water or air next to it. The effectiveness of heat loss by convection is dependent on how fast the air (or water) next to the body is exchanged once it becomes warmer. If air movement is slow, air molecules next to the skin are warmed and act as insulation. In contrast, if warmer air molecules are continually replaced by cooler air molecules, as occurs on a breezy day or in a room with a fan, heat loss increases as the air currents carry heat away. Convec-

tion cools the body as air currents pass by while running or cycling. For example, air currents at 4 miles an hour are about twice as effective for cooling as air moving at 1 mile per hour. This is the basis of the wind-chill index (see Figure 17.5), which shows the equivalent still-air temperature for a particular ambient temperature at different wind velocities. In water, the body loses heat more rapidly by convection while swimming than while lying motionless.

EVAPORATION

Evaporation is the most effective heat loss mechanism used to cool the body. At rest, sweat glands assist thermoregulation by secreting unnoticeable amounts of sweat (about 500 mL/day). Sweat is a weak saline solution, largely water (99%), that evaporates when molecules in the water absorb heat from the environment and become energetic enough to escape as a gas. As core temperature rises during exercise or illness, peripheral blood vessels dilate and sweat glands are stimulated to produce noticeable sweat, which can amount to a loss of 1.5 to 2.5 liters of body water in

1 hour (2). On a hot, dry day, sweating is responsible for more than 80% of heat loss. Sweating itself does not cool the body; evaporation of the sweat does the cooling. The total sweat vaporized from the skin depends on three factors:

- The skin surface exposed to the environment
- The temperature and relative humidity of the ambient air
- The convective air currents around the body

Relative humidity is the most important factor in determining the effectiveness of evaporative heat loss. Relative humidity, the ratio of water in the ambient air to the total quantity of moisture that can be carried in air at a particular ambient temperature, is expressed in a percentage. For example, 65% relative humidity means that ambient air contains 65% of the air's moisture-carrying capability at the specific temperature. When humidity is high, the ambient vapor pressure approaches that of the moist skin, and evaporation is greatly reduced. Therefore, this avenue for heat loss is closed, even though large quantities of sweat bead on the skin and eventually roll off. This form of sweating represents a useless water loss that can lead to a dangerous state of dehydration and overheating.

In addition to heat loss through sweating, there is a basal level of body heat loss due to the continuous evaporation of water from the lungs, from the mucosa of the mouth, and through the skin. This averages about 350 mL of water as it seeps through the skin every day, and another 300 mL of water vaporized from mucous membranes in the respiratory passages and mouth. The latter is illustrated when you "see your breath" in very cold weather. In total, it is not uncommon for sport participants to lose 1.5 to 2.5 L/hr of water during exercise. This translates into a loss of 3 to 6 pounds of body weight per hour. During a 2- to 3-hour practice, an athlete could lose from 6 to 12 pounds of body weight. Although an individual may continually drink water throughout an exercise bout, less than 50% of the fluid lost will be replenished. This "voluntary dehydration" was recognized long ago and has been well characterized by researchers since then (2). This is why an athlete should drink as much fluid as possible prior to exercise, and before thirst is perceived during exercise. Just as important, it is also critical to drink beyond the perception of satisfying one's thirst to **hyperhydrate** (overhydrate) the body to prevent voluntary dehydration.

Measuring the Heat-Stress Index

The heat-stress index is a measure of ambient air temperature, humidity, and solar radiant energy. The most commonly used heat-stress index, the Wet-Bulb–Globe Temperature Index (WBGT), is calculated as follows:

$$WBGT = (0.1 \times DBT) + (0.7 \times WBT) + (0.2 \times GT)$$

Ambient temperature is measured by a dry-bulb thermometer (DBT), but does not take into account vapor pressure, which has a direct impact on the ability to evaporate sweat.

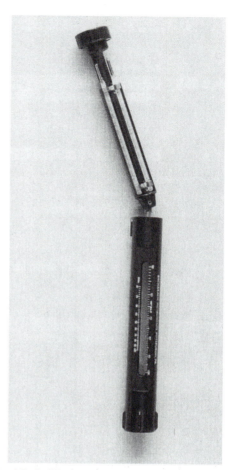

➤ **FIGURE 17.3 Sling psychrometer**. A sling psychrometer measures heat by exposing a dry-bulb and wet-bulb thermometer to rapid airflow, which can help determine safe participation levels on hot, humid days.

Wet-bulb temperature (WBT) is the temperature recorded by a thermometer with the mercury bulb surrounded by a wet wick, commonly called a sling psychrometer **(Figure 17.3)**. A sling psychrometer measures heat stress by exposing dry-bulb and wet-bulb thermometers to rapid airflow. Great differences in the recorded temperatures indicate a high rate of evaporation and low humidity. Smaller differences indicate a low rate of evaporation and high humidity. Globe temperature (GT) is the temperature recorded by a thermometer with a mercury bulb encased in a sphere painted black. The black globe absorbs radiant energy from the environment to measure this important factor that dry- and wet-bulb thermometers cannot. The top portion of **Table 17.1** lists recommendations for activities when temperature, humidity, and radiation are measured using the WBGT index. Guidelines for safe participation using only a sling psychrometer for measurement are listed in the lower portion of the table.

Factors That Modify Heat Tolerance

Several factors can affect one's tolerance to heat. Acclimatization and proper hydration are among the most critical in preventing heat illness.

TABLE 17.1   PARTICIPATION GUIDELINES IN HOT WEATHER

WBGT Range

°F	°C	Recommendations
80–84	26.5–28.8	Curtail active exercise for unacclimatized persons (yellow flag)
85–87	29.5–30.5	Curtail active exercise for all persons, except well-acclimatized persons (red flag)
88+	31.2+	Curtail all active exercise (black flag)

WBT (Sling Psychrometer) Range

°F	°C	Recommendations
60	15.5	No prevention necessary
61–65	16.2–18.4	Alert persons to symptoms of heat stress and the importance of adequate hydration
66–70	18.8–21.1	Insist that adequate water be ingested
71–75	21.6–23.8	Rest periods and water breaks every 20 to 30 minutes; place limits on intense exercise
76–79	24.5–26.1	Modify practice considerably, and curtail activity for unacclimatized individuals
80+	26.5+	Cancel practice

ACCLIMATIZATION

Exercising moderately during repeated heat exposures can result in physiological adaptation to a hot environment, which can improve performance and heat tolerance **(Box 17.1)**. In general, the major acclimatization occurs during the first week of heat exposure and is complete after 10 days. Only 2 to 4 hours of daily heat exposure is required. The first several sessions should be light and last about 15 to 20 minutes. Thereafter, exercise sessions can progressively increase in duration and intensity. Proper hydration is essential for the acclimatization process to be effective. Heat acclimatization is lost rapidly. As a general rule, 1 day of heat acclimatization is lost over 2 to 3 days without heat exposure, with the major benefits lost within 2 to 3 weeks after returning to a more temperate environment.

➤➤ BOX 17.1

Physiologic Changes Seen After 10 Days of Heat Exposure

- Decrease in heart rate and body temperature
- Increase in peripheral blood flow and plasma volume
- Sweating capacity is nearly doubled
- Sweat becomes more diluted (less salt is lost)
- Sweat is more evenly distributed over the skin surface
- The increased perspiration rate is sustained over a longer period of time

---

FLUID REHYDRATION

The primary objective of fluid replacement is to maintain plasma volume so that circulation and sweating occur at optimal levels. Dehydration progressively decreases plasma volume, peripheral blood flow, sweating, and stroke volume (quantity of blood ejected with each heartbeat), and leads to a compensatory increase in heart rate. The general deterioration in circulatory and thermoregulatory efficiency increases the risk of heat illness, impairs physiologic functions, and decreases physical performance. Thirst is not an adequate indicator of water needs during exercise, because an individual is already 1% dehydrated when thirst is perceived (3). Rather, thirst develops in response to increases in osmolality, blood sodium concentrations, and decreases in plasma volume due to dehydration. It is essential that an adequate water replacement schedule be strictly followed to prevent dehydration **(Table 17.2)**. Cold liquids, especially water, empty from the stomach and small intestines significantly faster than warm fluids. Gastric emptying rate can be retarded when ingested fluids contain even the smallest traces of salt or simple sugars, whether glucose, fructose, or sucrose. Several steps can be taken to ensure adequate hydration before, during, and after exercise **(Box 17.2)**.

To prevent dehydration, fluids must be ingested and absorbed by the body. Running through sprinklers or pouring water over the head may feel cool and satisfying, but it does not prevent dehydration. A standard rule is to drink until thirst is quenched and then drink a few more ounces. An easy method to determine if an athlete is drinking enough fluids is to have them monitor the color and volume

TABLE 17.2   RECOMMENDED FLUID INTAKE FOR A STRENUOUS 90-MINUTE EXERCISE BOUT

Weight Loss/lbs	Minutes Between Water Breaks	Fluid/break (oz)
8	No practice recommended	—
7½	No practice recommended	—
7	10	8 to 10
6½	10	8 to 9
6	10	8 to 9
5½	15	10 to 12
5	15	10 to 11
4½	15	9 to 10
4	15	8 to 9
3½	20	10 to 11
3	20	9 to 10
2½	20	7 to 8
2	30	8
1½	30	6
1	30	6
½	30	6

Strategies to Reduce the Risk of Dehydration

HEALTHY POPULATION

- Drink 8–12 cups (8 oz/cup) of fluid at least 24 hours prior to an event.
- Drink at least 16 oz of fluid 2 hours prior to exercise and again about 20 minutes before exercise.
- Have unlimited fluid available during exercise.
- When exercising an hour or more, drink at least 5–10 oz of fluid every 15–20 minutes. Drink beyond thirst.
- Drink cool fluids containing less than 8% carbohydrate.
- Use individual water bottles to accurately measure fluid consumption.
- Freeze fluid in plastic bottles prior to exercise, as they will thaw and stay cool during exercise sessions.
- Record pre- and postexercise weight with athletes in minimal, dry clothing.
- Replenish lost fluid with at least 24 oz of fluid for every pound of body weight lost.
- Avoid caffeine, alcohol, and carbonated beverages.

CHILDREN (IN ADDITION TO ABOVE)

- Allow for 10–14 days of acclimatization.
- Reduce intensity of prolonged exercise.

Adapted from American College of Sports Medicine (6), pages i–iv.

of their urine. An average adult's urine amounts to 1.2 quarts in a 24-hour period. Urination of a full bladder usually occurs four times each day. Within 60 minutes of exercise, passing a light-colored urine of normal to above-normal volume is a good indicator of adequate hydration. If the urine is dark yellow in color, is of a small volume, and has a strong odor, the athlete needs to continue drinking. However, ingesting vitamin supplements often result in a dark-yellow urine, so urine color, volume, and odor must all be considered when determining hydration status (2,3).

ELECTROLYTE REPLACEMENT

The minerals sodium, chloride, magnesium, and potassium are called electrolytes because they are dissolved in the body as electrically charged particles called ions. Electrolytes regulate fluid balance, nerve conduction, and muscle contractions. Ionic concentrations in sweat are greatly influenced by the rate of perspiration and acclimatization. Four liters of perspiration equals approximately a 5.8% loss of body weight; sweat contains high levels of sodium and chloride, but little potassium, calcium, or magnesium. These losses lower the body's sodium and chloride content by 5 to 7%, and potassium by less than 1.2% (4). Because the body loses more water than electrolytes, the ionic concentration of these minerals in the body fluids

rise. This illustrates that during periods of heavy perspiration, the need to replace body water is greater than replacing electrolytes. Any lost electrolytes are readily replenished by adding a slight amount of salt to food when the need exists, or by eating potassium-rich foods such as citrus fruits and bananas. A glass of orange juice or tomato juice replaces almost all the potassium, calcium, and magnesium excreted in about 3 L of sweat.

Electrolyte solutions are unnecessary for individuals with normal diets. However, for athletes demanding peak performance in competitions greater than 1 hour or during intense intermittent exercise, carbohydrate drinks may benefit performance (5). Commercial drinks may be used; however, they should be cooler than ambient temperature (between 15° to 22°C [59° to 72°F]), flavored to enhance palatability, range between 4 to 8% of multiple transportable carbohydrate, and contain a small amount of sodium (5,6). It is important to note that drinks favored during rest may not be favored during exercise. For example, during activity, athletes may favor water; after activity, they may prefer a flavored fluid. While maintaining hydration, the participant should avoid **diuretics** (substances that promote the excretion of urine) such as excessive amounts of protein, caffeinated drinks (soda, tea, coffee), chocolate, and alcoholic beverages.

CLOTHING

Light-colored, lightweight, porous clothing is preferred to dark, heavyweight, nonporous material. Cottons and linens readily absorb moisture. Evaporative heat loss occurs only when clothing is thoroughly wet and perspiration can evaporate. Changing into a dry shirt simply prolongs the time between sweating and cooling. Heavy sweat suits or rubberized plastic suits produce high relative humidity close to the skin and retard evaporation, severely increasing the risk of heat illness. Even when wearing only football helmets and loose-fitting, porous jerseys and shorts, 50% of the body surface of football players can be sealed, limiting evaporative cooling. Increased metabolic rate needed to carry the weight of their equipment, and increased temperature on artificial surfaces, also increase the risk of heat illness. To counter this, football players should initially practice in tee-shirts, shorts, and low cut socks. On hot, humid days, uniforms should not be worn, and if possible shoulder pads and helmets should be removed often to allow for radiation and evaporative cooling. Since much of the body's heat escapes through the head, helmets used in noncontact sports (cycling) should allow for adequate airflow and evaporation.

AGE

Children have a lower sweating capacity and a higher core temperature during exposure to heat when compared to adolescents and adults. This occurs even though children have a higher number of heat-activated sweat glands per unit of skin. Sweat composition also differs. Children excrete higher concentrations of sodium and chlorine, and lower concentrations of lactate and potassium. Therefore, children do not benefit from electrolyte beverages and should use only cool water for fluid replacement (7). In addition, children require a longer time to acclimatize to heat when compared to adolescents and young adults.

Aging can lead to a limited peripheral vascular response that can impair local vasodilation. There is also an apparent delayed onset in sweating with advancing age, as well as a blunted sweating response. This may be due to either a limitation in sweat gland output or to a dehydrated-limited sweat output if fluid replacement is insufficient. In addition, older athletes do not recover from dehydration as effectively as younger athletes, which may be related to a blunted thirst drive. This may make older athletes more prone to dehydration that could adversely affect the thermoregulatory capacity (1).

SEX

The general consensus is that women can tolerate the physiologic and thermal stress of exercise at least as well as men of comparable fitness and level of acclimatization; both sexes can acclimatize to a similar degree. Sweating, however, does differ. Although women possess more heat-activated sweat glands per unit of skin area than men, women sweat less than men. Women begin to sweat at higher skin and core temperatures, produce less sweat than men for a comparable heat-exercise load, and yet show a heat tolerance equivalent to men (1). Women probably rely more on circulatory mechanisms for heat dissipation, whereas men rely upon evaporative cooling. The production of less sweat to maintain thermal balance can provide women with significant protection from dehydration during work at a high ambient temperature.

USE OF DIURETICS AND OTHER SUPPLEMENTS

If individuals are taking diuretics or laxatives, they should be carefully observed for dehydration; these agents increase fluid loss, reduce plasma volume, and may adversely affect thermoregulation and cardiovascular function. Substances used to induce vomiting and diarrhea also lead to dehydration, and may cause excessive electrolyte loss with accompanying muscle weakness. Some nutritional supplements, such as creatine phosphate, require additional fluids to decrease the risk of heat cramps and other associated heat illnesses. Before athletes take supplements or medications, it is advisable that they be fully informed of the proper use and possible side effects of the substances.

PRACTICE SCHEDULES

On hot, humid days, reschedule workouts, practices, and competitions to early morning or evening hours to avoid the worst heat of the day (11:00 AM to 3:00 PM).

Allow for frequent water breaks (i.e., 10 minutes every half hour), shorten practices, and lessen the exercise intensity. Whenever possible, get the players out of the direct sunlight (shade trees and tents), and remove restrictive equipment (pads and helmets) frequently.

WEIGHT CHARTS

Measuring pre- and postexercise weight can decrease the risk of heat illness. A fluid loss equivalent to as little as 1% of body mass is associated with a significant increase in rectal temperature. For each liter of sweat-loss dehydration, the heart rate can increase by about 8 beats per minute with a corresponding decrease in cardiac output. When water loss reaches 4 to 5% (a value commonly seen among high school wrestlers), a definite impairment is noted in physical work capacity, physiologic function, and thermoregulation (1). A rule of thumb is that for every pound of water lost, 24 oz (3 cups) of fluid should be ingested, meaning that 150% of the fluid loss during exercise is replenished (4).

In addition to fluids, carbohydrates should also be ingested within 30 minutes postexercise, especially those with a high water content (melons, tomatoes). Even under the best circumstances, 24 hours will be needed to fully restore the fluids and muscle glycogen that is used during just 2 hours of strenuous exercise. Prior to the next exercise period, the athlete should ingest 3.5 to 4.5 grams of carbohydrates per pound of body weight each day. Alcohol should be avoided. Lost fluid should be replaced and weight normalized before the next episode of exercise (3). Recommended fluid intake to compensate for fluid loss is listed in Table 17.2.

Identifying Individuals at Risk

Healthy individuals at risk for heat illness include those poorly acclimated or conditioned, those inexperienced with heat illness, individuals with large muscle mass, children, wheelchair athletes, Special Olympians, and the elderly. Others at risk are listed in **Box 17.3**.

Heat Illnesses

If the signs and symptoms of heat stress (thirst, fatigue, lethargy, and visual disturbances) are not addressed, cardiovascular compensation begins to fail and a series of progressive complications, termed heat illness, can result. The various forms of heat illness, in order of severity, include heat cramps, heat exhaustion, and heat stroke. Although symptoms often overlap between the conditions, failure to take immediate action can result in severe dehydration and possible death.

HEAT CRAMPS

Heat cramps are painful, involuntary muscle spasms caused by excessive water and electrolyte loss during and

➤➤ Box 17.3

Individuals at Risk for Heat Illness

- Healthy individuals
  - Age extremes: children, elderly
  - Excessive muscle mass, large, or obese
  - Poorly acclimatized or poorly conditioned
  - Previous history of heat illness
  - Salt or water depletion
  - Sleep deprived
- Those with acute illnesses
  - Illnesses that involve fever
  - Gastrointestinal illnesses
- Those with chronic illnesses
  - Alcoholism and substance abuse (amphetamines, cocaine, hallucinogens, laxatives, diuretics, or narcotics)
  - Cardiac disease
  - Certain nutritional supplements (creatine phosphate)
  - Cystic fibrosis
  - Eating disorders
  - Medications (anticholinergics, antidepressants, antihistamines, diuretics, neuroleptics, and beta blockers)
  - Skin problems with impaired sweating (miliaria rubra or miliaria profunda)
  - Uncontrolled diabetes mellitus or hypertension
  - Using oil-based or gel-based sunscreens that block evaporative cooling
- Wheelchair athletes who:
  - Have a spinal cord injury (alters thermoregulation)
  - Limit water intake to avoid going to the bathroom

Adapted from Mellion (8), page 158.

after intense exercise in the heat. Paradoxically, the condition most frequently occurs in well-conditioned, acclimatized athletes who have overexerted themselves in hot weather and rehydrated only with water. Predisposing factors include lack of acclimatization, use of diuretics or laxatives, and sodium depletion in the normal diet. The condition can be prevented by ingesting copious amounts of water and increasing the daily intake of salt through a normal diet several days before the period of heat stress.

➤ SIGNS AND SYMPTOMS

Cramps commonly occur in the calf and abdominal muscles, but may involve muscles of the upper extremity. With heat cramps, body temperature is not usually elevated, and the skin remains moist and cool. Pulse and respiration may be normal or slightly elevated, and dizziness may be present.

➤ MANAGEMENT

Passive stretching of the involved muscle(s) and ice massage over the affected area is helpful. The athlete should also ingest enough cool fluids containing an electrolyte solution to drink beyond the point of satisfying his or her

thirst. The individual should be watched carefully, as this condition may precipitate heat exhaustion or heat stroke.

HEAT EXHAUSTION

Heat exhaustion usually occurs in unacclimatized individuals during the first few intense exercise sessions on a hot day. Those who wear protective equipment or heavy uniforms are also at greater risk, as evaporation through the material may be retarded. It is a "functional" illness and is not associated with organ damage. Exercise-induced heat exhaustion is caused by ineffective circulatory adjustments compounded by a depletion of extracellular fluid, especially plasma volume, owing to excessive sweating. Blood pools in the dilated peripheral vessels, which dramatically reduces the central blood volume necessary to maintain cardiac output.

➤ SIGNS AND SYMPTOMS

Thirst, headache, dizziness, mild anxiety, fatigue, a weak and rapid pulse (**tachycardia**), and low blood pressure in the upright position are common signs and symptoms. The individual may also appear ashen and gray, and have an uncoordinated gait and a small urine output (**Figure 17.4A**). Sweating may be reduced if the person is dehydrated, but body temperature generally does not exceed 39.5°C (103°F).

➤ MANAGEMENT

The athletic trainer should immediately move the person to a cool place, remove all equipment and unnecessary clothing, and rapidly cool the body. Cooling can be enhanced by sponging or toweling the individual with cool water or placing them in front of a fan/cool-mist machine. It is essential to administer copious amounts of cool fluids with a diluted electrolyte solution as quickly as possible. Elevating the legs to reduce postural hypotension can also be effective. Intravenous fluids may need to be administered if the dehydrated state is moderate to severe.

Physical activity should not be resumed until the individual has returned to the predehydrated state and has been cleared by a physician.

HEAT STROKE

Heat stroke is the least common but most serious heat illness. In football, heat stroke is second only to head injuries as the most frequent cause of death. The condition is also seen in dehydrated distance runners and wrestlers. Heat stroke is almost always preceded by prolonged strenuous physical exercise in individuals who are poorly acclimatized, or in situations where evaporation of perspiration is blocked. During exercise, metabolic heat continues to rise. Decreased blood plasma volume causes the heart to beat faster and work harder to pump blood through the circulatory system. The thermoregulatory system is overloaded, and the body's cooling mechanisms fail to dissipate the rising core temperature. The hypothalamus shuts down all

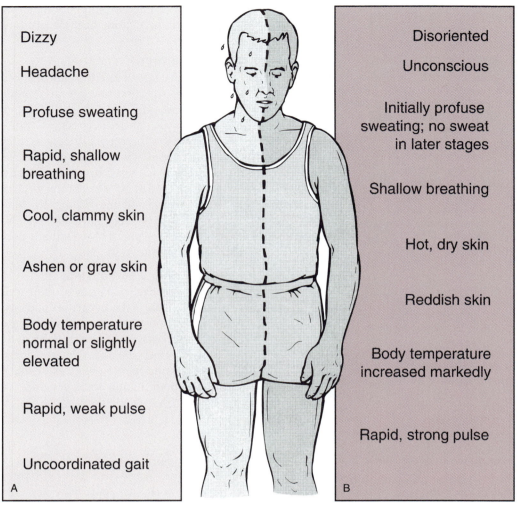

Dizzy

Headache

Profuse sweating

Rapid, shallow breathing

Cool, clammy skin

Ashen or gray skin

Body temperature normal or slightly elevated

Rapid, weak pulse

Uncoordinated gait

A

Disoriented

Unconscious

Initially profuse sweating; no sweat in later stages

Shallow breathing

Hot, dry skin

Reddish skin

Body temperature increased markedly

Rapid, strong pulse

B

▶ **FIGURE 17.4** **Signs and symptoms of heat exhaustion and heat stroke.** A, Heat exhaustion. B, Heat stroke.

heat-control mechanisms, including the sweat glands, to conserve water loss. This creates a vicious circle: as temperature increases, the metabolic rate increases, which in turn increases heat production. The skin becomes hot and dry. As the temperature continues to rise, permanent brain damage may occur. Core temperature can rise to 40.6°C (105°F), and has been known to reach 41.7° to 42.2°C (107° to 108°F). If untreated, death is imminent. Mortality is directly related to magnitude and duration of hyperthermia.

▶ SIGNS AND SYMPTOMS

The level of mental status impairment differentiates heat stroke from heat exhaustion. Initial symptoms include a feeling of burning up with a moderate level of confusion, disorientation, agitation, profuse sweating, and an unsteady gait. As the condition deteriorates, sweating ceases. The skin is hot and dry, and appears reddened or flushed **(Figure 17.4B)**. The individual will breathe deeply and have dilated pupils, giving the appearance of a glassy stare. As core temperature rises, the pulse becomes rapid and strong, as high as 150 to 170 beats per minute. The individual may become hysterical or delirious. Tissue damage by excessive body heat leads to vasomotor collapse, shallow breathing,

decreased blood pressure, and a rapid and weak pulse. Muscle twitching or seizures may occur just before the individual lapses into a coma.

▶ MANAGEMENT

The athletic trainer should immediately activate EMS. Move the athlete to a cool place, remove all equipment and unnecessary clothing, and rapidly cool the body. The most effective cooling method is ice water immersion (9). If ice water immersion is not available, other cooling methods should be used. These may include cool water immersion; wrapping in cool, wet towels; using fans; and applying crushed ice packs to the neck, axilla, and groin. Fans and cool-mist machines, though, have limited use in humid conditions. Core temperature should be measured every 10 minutes and should not fall below 38°C (101°F) to avoid hypothermia (10). Heat stroke victims usually require airway management, intravenous fluids, and in severe cases, circulatory support. Continue body cooling during transport to the nearest medical center.

Physical activity should not be resumed until the individual has returned to the predehydrated state and has been cleared by a physician.

TABLE 17.3   **MANAGEMENT OF HEAT-RELATED CONDITIONS**

Condition	Signs/Symptoms	Treatment
Heat cramps	Involuntary muscle spasms or cramps; normal pulse and respirations; profuse sweating and dizziness	Rest in cool place; massage cramp with ice and passive stretching; drink cool water with diluted electrolyte solution
Heat syncope	Weakness; fatigue; hypotension; blurred vision; fainting; elevated skin and core temperature	Place supine in cool place; elevate legs; give oral saline if conscious; record blood pressure and body temperature
Miliaria rubra and miliaria profunda	Pruritic, inflamed skin eruptions	Cool and dry affected skin; control infection; avoid reexposure until lesions have healed
Heat exhaustion	Thirst; headache; weakness; confusion; profuse sweating; skin is wet, cool, and clammy and may appear ashen; breathing is rapid and shallow; pulse is weak	Rest in cool place; remove equipment and clothing; execute rapid cooling of body; sponge or towel with cool water, or use fan; IV fluids; discontinue activity until thoroughly recovered and cleared by a physician
Heat stroke	Sweating ceases; irritability progresses to confusion and hysteria; unsteady gait; pulse is rapid and strong; skin is hot, dry, red or flushed; BP falls; convulsions; seizures; coma	ACTIVATE EMS; rest in cool place; rapidly cool body with ice water immersion or place crushed ice packs on the neck, axilla, and groin; transport immediately to the nearest medical center

Other Heat Conditions

Three other common conditions may occur as a result of exercising in the heat. These include heat syncope, miliaria rubra, and miliaria profunda. Although not usually life-threatening, they can be quite bothersome to a competitive athlete. **Table 17.3** lists the signs, symptoms, and immediate care for all heat-related conditions.

HEAT SYNCOPE

Heat syncope (fainting) or lightheadedness is usually seen at the end of a race in nonacclimated individuals who may or may not be under heat stress. It can also occur with prolonged standing or standing suddenly from a sitting or lying position. The athlete is maximally vasodilated; when activity stops, much of the blood volume pools in the lower extremities. As a result, the heart has too little venous return to pump an adequate supply of blood to the brain. Predisposing factors include dehydration, lack of acclimatization, ending the exercise bout without a cool-down, or moving quickly from the cold (such as a cold bath) into a hot sauna or whirlpool.

➤ SIGNS AND SYMPTOMS

Signs and symptoms include low blood pressure (hypotension), blurred vision, pallor, weakness or fatigue, and an elevated skin and core temperature.

➤ MANAGEMENT

Treatment involves placing the individual in a supine position and replacing any water deficit.

MILIARIA RUBRA AND MILIARIA PROFUNDA

Miliaria rubra (heat rash or prickly heat) is an inflamed, itchy (**pruritic**) skin eruption that arises when active sweat glands become blocked by organic debris. It is often seen in humid climates or in skin that is totally covered by clothing, which produces a highly humid environment. Treatment involves cooling and drying the skin, and treating the itching symptoms. Taking cool baths and applying topical antipruritics such as pramoxine and calamine lotion can provide relief. The rash usually subsides if a person avoids sweating for 1 or 2 days (11).

If miliaria rubra becomes generalized and prolonged, it is called miliaria profunda, and can lead to heat exhaustion since the sweat glands are occluded and can no longer produce sweat for evaporation. The lesions are truncal, noninflamed, and **papular** (small, confined, solid elevations on the skin). Individuals with profunda are less heat tolerant than the general population, and therefore, are at a higher risk for heat illnesses (12). The condition is managed in a similar manner as miliaria rubra.

💡 *Measures to prevent heat illness during preseason may include gradual acclimatization; scheduling practices in the early morning or evening hours; gradually increasing the intensity and length of the practice sessions; taking frequent, regular water breaks; wearing light-colored, lightweight, porous clothing; increasing salt intake at the dinner table; and increasing the general amount of fluids ingested during the day.*

COLD-RELATED CONDITIONS

 The weather for a scheduled field hockey game is forecast to be in the low 40s with winds gusting up to 25 miles per hour. What measures can be taken to prevent cold-related conditions?

Hypothermia, or reduced body temperature, occurs when the body is unable to maintain a constant core temperature. In cold weather, three primary heat-promoting mechanisms attempt to maintain or increase core temperature. The initial response is cutaneous vasoconstriction to prevent blood from shunting to the skin. Because the skin is insulated with a layer of subcutaneous fat, heat loss is reduced. The second response is to increase metabolic heat production by shivering, which is involuntary contraction of skeletal muscle, or to increase physical activity. During vigorous exercise, skeletal muscles can produce 30 to 40 times the amount of heat produced at rest. During gradual, seasonal changes, more of the hormone thyroxine is released by the thyroid gland, which serves as the third avenue to increase metabolic rate.

Due to their larger ratio of surface area to body mass, and a smaller amount of subcutaneous fat, children are more prone to heat loss during cold exposure than adults. Cold exposure also increases the risk for exercise-induced bronchospasm, which is seen increasingly in children. Women are less able to produce heat through exercise or shivering because of their lower ratio of lean body mass, although the additional subcutaneous fat does provide more tissue insulation. In cold, men tend to maintain lower heart rate, higher stroke volume, and higher mean arterial blood pressure than women, but there are no distinct differences in cold tolerance when genders are matched for aerobic fitness at the same relative workload.

Preventing Cold-Related Injuries

During cold weather, body heat is lost through respiration, radiation, conduction, convection, and evaporation. Although the body will attempt to generate heat through heat-producing mechanisms, this may be inadequate to maintain a constant core temperature. **Box 17.4** lists factors that contribute to cold injuries.

Several steps that can be taken to prevent heat loss are summarized in **Box 17.5**. The "layered principle" of clothing allows for several (three or more) thin layers of insulation rather than one or two thick ones. Fabrics should

---

➤➤ **BOX 17.4**

Predisposing Factors for Cold Injuries

- Inadequate insulation from cold and/or wind
- Restrictive clothing or arterial disease that prevents peripheral circulation, especially in the feet
- Diet lacking adequate carbohydrates or fat
- Presence of chronic metabolic disorders
- Spinal cord–injured person (cannot vasoconstrict peripheral arterioles in the skin, and has a blunted shivering response to cold)
- Preexisting fatigue or general weakness
- Use of alcohol, tobacco products (especially smoking tobacco), and other medications such as barbiturates, phenothiazines, reserpine, and narcotics
- Age (very young or old)
- Decreased circulation

➤➤ **BOX 17.5**

Reducing the Risk of Cold Injuries

- Check weather conditions, and consider possible deterioration.
- Identify individuals who may be susceptible to cold, and observe closely.
- Dress in several light layers.
- Wear windproof, dry, well-insulated clothing that allows for water evaporation; wool, polypropylene, or polyesters such as Capilene or Thermastat are recommended.
- Carry windproof pants and jacket if conditions warrant; keep your back to the wind.
- Wear well-insulated, windproof mittens, gloves, hats, and scarves.
- Wear well-insulated footwear that keeps feet dry.
- Avoid dehydration. Do not drink alcoholic beverages or snow because these worsen hypothermia.
- Carry nutritious snacks that predominantly contain carbohydrates.
- Eat small amounts of food frequently.
- Do not stand in one position for extended periods of time. Wiggle your toes and keep moving to bring warm blood to various areas of the body.
- Stay dry by wearing appropriate rain gear or protective clothing. If you get wet, change as soon as possible into dry clothing.
- Breath through your nose, rather than your mouth, to minimize heat and fluid loss.
- Watch the face, ears, and fingers for signs of frostbite.

---

be light, yet porous enough to allow free exchange of perspiration, and should not restrict movement. Fabrics may include wool, wool/synthetic blends, polypropylene, or treated polyesters such as Capilene and hollow polyesters such as Thermastat (13). Cotton has poor insulating ability that is markedly decreased when saturated with perspiration. Pile garments contain down, Dacron, Hollofil, Thinsulate, or Quallofil, and are more useful when worn during warm-up, time-outs, or during cool-down periods following exercise. Jackets with a hood and drawstring, and pants made of wind-resistant material, such as Gore-Tex, nylon, or 60/40 cloth, can protect against the wind.

A ski cap, face mask, and neck warmer can protect the face and ears from frostbite. Ski goggles can protect the eyes. They must be well ventilated to prevent fogging, and can also be treated with antifog preparations. Polypropylene gloves or, in extreme temperatures, woolen mittens can be worn with windproof outer mittens of Gore-Tex or nylon. Athletic shoes should be large enough to accommodate an outer pair of heavy wool socks. It is important to avoid getting wet, because heat loss can be increased by evaporation. The insulating ability of clothing can be decreased as much as 90% when saturated either with external moisture or condensation from perspiration. If weather conditions are bad enough, it is better to cancel the practice or event for the day.

Cold Conditions

People tend to adapt less readily to cold than to heat. Even inhabitants of cold regions show only limited evidence of adaptation, such as a higher metabolic rate. Like heat illness, cold injuries range from minor problems, such as Raynaud's syndrome, cold-induced bronchospasm, or frostbite to the more severe general systemic cooling, or hypothermia, which can be life-threatening. Cold emergencies occur in two ways. In one, the core temperature remains relatively constant but the shell temperature decreases. This results in localized injuries from frostbite. The second cold emergency occurs when both core temperature and shell temperature decrease, leading to general body cooling. All body processes slow down and systemic hypothermia results. If left unabated, death is imminent.

RAYNAUD'S SYNDROME

Raynaud's syndrome is seen in young athletes, especially women, and is characterized by bilateral episodes of spasms of the digital blood vessels in response to emotion or cold exposure. It can be caused by an underlying disease or anatomical abnormality, and can be a long-term complication of frostbite. However, its source is usually unknown. Initially during the ischemic phase, the affected digits (usually the fingers) become cold, pale, and numb. This is followed by **hyperemia** (increased blood within a body part) with redness, throbbing pain, and swelling. The condition is treated by warming the affected extremity. A physician should evaluate the individual to rule out an underlying condition. Smoking should be avoided, since this compromises circulation.

COLD-INDUCED BRONCHOSPASM

A condition seen frequently among today's youth is cold-induced bronchospasm. The condition is brought on by exposure to cold, dry air during cold-weather sports, such as cross-country skiing. Linked to exercise-induced bronchospasm (EIB), the athlete experiences difficulty breathing, manifested by shortness of breath, coughing, chest tightness, and wheezing. Attacks can be prevented by the use of bronchodilators or cromolyn sodium. Salmeterol, a more recent, long-acting bronchodilator, administered 30 to 60 minutes before exercise, appears to protect many athletes for up to 12 hours (13). Refer to Chapter 18 for more information on exercise-induced bronchospasm.

FROSTBITE INJURIES

Frostbite is caused by freezing soft tissue. Individuals who have cold urticaria (cold allergy) or Raynaud's syndrome are at higher risk for frostbite. Frostbite is classified on a continuum of three degrees **(Table 17.4)**. First degree, or superficial, frostbite involves the skin and underlying tissues, but the deeper tissues can be felt to be soft and pliable. If damage extends into the subcutaneous tissues,

TABLE 17.4	SIGNS AND SYMPTOMS OF FROSTBITE
First Degree	Skin is soft to touch and appears initially red, then white, and is usually painless. The condition is typically noticed by others first.
Second Degree	Skin is firm to touch but tissue beneath is soft and appears initially red and swollen. Diffuse numbness may be preceded by an itchy or prickly sensation. White or waxy skin color may appear later.
Third Degree	Skin is hard to touch and totally numb, and appears blotchy white to yellow-gray or blue-gray.

it is classified as second-degree frostbite. Third-degree, or deep, frostbite involves the tissues deep to the subcutaneous layers, and may result in complete destruction of the injured tissue. Damage depends on the depth of cold penetration resulting from the duration of exposure, temperature, and wind velocity. Areas commonly affected are the fingertips, toes (especially when wearing constricting footwear), earlobes, and tip of the nose.

► SIGNS AND SYMPTOMS

In superficial frostbite, the area may feel firm to touch, but the tissue beneath is soft and resilient. The skin initially appears red and swollen, and the individual complains of diffuse numbness that may or may not be preceded by an itchy or prickly sensation. If the frostbite extends into the subcutaneous or deep layers, the skin feels hard because it is actually frozen tissue. The area then turns white with a yellow or blue tint that looks waxy.

► MANAGEMENT

A person with superficial frostbite should be removed from the cold and taken indoors immediately and treated with careful, rapid warming of the area. Remove clothing, jewelry, or rings, and immerse the injured area in water heated to 39° to 42°C (102° to 108°F) for 30 to 45 minutes (13). A whirlpool is ideal, but if this is unavailable, use a basin large enough so the skin does not touch the sides of the container. Hot water should be avoided as this may cause burns. When the part is completely rewarmed, the affected area should be dried, and a sterile dressing applied to the injured area. If fingers or toes are involved, sterile dressings should be placed between the digits before covering. The entire area can be covered with towels or a blanket to keep it warm, and the individual should be transported to the nearest medical center with the affected limb slightly elevated.

Deep frostbite is best rewarmed under controlled conditions in a hospital. EMS should be activated to transport the individual. During transport, the individual should be kept warm, but active rewarming of the frozen part should not occur.

If the frostbite is severe, blisters may form over the area, and gangrene may develop within 2 to 3 weeks. Throbbing, aching pain, and burning sensations may last for weeks. The skin may remain permanently red, tender, and sensitive to reexposure to cold.

SYSTEMIC BODY COOLING (HYPOTHERMIA)

Hypothermia is more of a danger to athletes exposed to cold for long periods of time, such as long distance runners and Nordic ski racers, especially those who are slowing down late in a race because of fatigue or injury. Any injured or ill athlete who has been exposed to cold weather or cold water, however, is suspected of having hypothermia until proven otherwise.

Exposed surfaces on the hands, face, head, and neck lose most of the body heat through radiation. At 4.4°C (40°F), more than half of the body's generated heat can be lost from an uncovered head. At −15°C (5°F), up to 75% of the body's heat is lost through the head. Air movement coupled with cold produces a wind chill factor that causes heat loss from the body much faster than in still air. The faster the wind, the higher the wind chill factor **(Figure 17.5)**.

When core temperature falls below 34.4°C (94°F), essential biochemical processes begin to slow. Heart and respiration rates slow, cardiac output and blood pressure fall, and as the skin and muscles cool, shivering increases violently. Numbness sets in, and even the simplest task becomes difficult to perform. If core temperature continues to drop below 32°C (90°F), shivering ceases and muscles become cold and stiff. Cold diuresis (polyuria) occurs as blood is shunted away from the shell to the core in an effort to maintain vascular volume. This leads to excessive

Core Temperature		Signs and Symptoms
(°C)	(°F)	
35.5–37.2	96–99	Intense involuntary shivering.
32.8–35	91–95	Persistent violent shivering, difficulty with speech if conscious.
30–32.2	86–90	Shivering decreases and is replaced by muscular rigidity with jerky erratic movements. Thinking is clouded, and amnesia may be present.*
27.2–29.4	81–85	Loss of awareness of surroundings, irrational thinking, drifting into a stuporous state. Rigidity continues, and heart and respiration rates slow. Cardiac arrhythmias may be present.
25.6–26.7	78–80	Unconsciousness. Reflexes cease to function, and heartbeat is erratic.
<25.6	<78	Cardiac and respiratory centers fail. Edema and hemorrhage occur in lungs, leading to death.

TABLE 17.5   SIGNS AND SYMPTOMS OF HYPOTHERMIA

*Note: Rough handling can trigger cardiac arrest at or below 32°C (90°F).

excretion of urine by the kidneys. If intervention is not initiated, death is imminent. **Table 17.5** highlights the stages of systemic hypothermia.

▶ SIGNS AND SYMPTOMS

Hypothermia is divided into those with mild hypothermia (rectal temperature >32°C [90°F]) and those with moderate to severe hypothermia (rectal temperature <32°C [90°F]). In mild hypothermia, the individual is still shivering. The individual may appear clumsy, apathetic, or confused and has slurred speech, stumbles, and drops things. An individual who does not feel any sensation or pain, and is not shivering is likely to be colder than 32°C

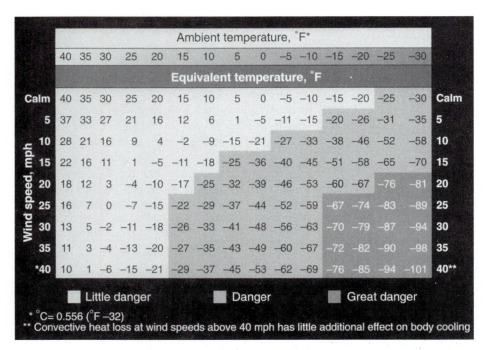

▶ FIGURE 17.5 Wind-chill index. From McArdle WD, Katch FI, and Katch VI. Exercise Physiology: Energy, Nutrition, and Human Performance. 4th ed. Baltimore: Williams & Wilkins, 1996:521.

(90°F). Movements will become jerky, and the individual will become unaware of his or her surroundings.

➤ MANAGEMENT

With mild hypothermia, the athletic trainer should activate EMS and carefully get the individual into a warm shelter. Rewarming of the individual can be accomplished by allowing him or her to shiver themselves warm inside a sleeping bag, or by using external rewarming devices such as hot water bottles or heating pads. Hot tubs can be used if available. The water should be around 43°C (110°F) (13). Hot (preferably noncaffeinated) drinks may be useful after the individual is partly rewarmed and able to swallow. The individual should continue to be rewarmed en route to the nearest medical facility. With moderate to severe hypothermia, on-the-site-rewarming should not be attempted. Once rewarming begins, serious electrolyte, metabolic, and cardiovascular changes occur that cannot be treated in the field. Prevent any further cooling, maintain the ABCs, and transport the individual to the nearest medical facility, because advanced life support is often necessary.

The effects of cold can be minimized by dressing in several layers of insulating clothing under the uniforms. Jackets with a hood and drawstring, and pants made of wind-resistant material can protect against the wind. Wool socks and gloves may also keep the player warm.

OTHER ENVIRONMENTAL CONDITIONS

Although it is not raining, you hear the rumble of thunder in the distance during a softball game. Should you alert the umpires to call the game, or would it be better to wait and see if any lightning is associated with the storm?

The ever-changing environment presents a unique challenge to athletic competition. Athletes must cope with heat, humidity, cold, rain, lightning, altitude, and air pollution, yet still expect to perform at their best. A basic understanding of these situations can help facilitate their performance.

Altitude Disorders

The percentage of oxygen in the atmosphere at an altitude of 10,000 ft is exactly the same as that at sea level. The density of air, however, decreases progressively as you ascend above sea level. The decreased partial pressure of ambient oxygen, or density of oxygen molecules, makes it more difficult to deliver oxygen to working muscles of the body, leading to a reduction in work capacity directly proportional to altitude. This will have little if any effect on short bursts of energy, but can have significant impact on sustained aerobic activities. Often individuals are unaware of the impact altitude exposure can have on their performance, and will compensate for this decrease in maxi-

mum oxygen uptake by hyperventilating or experiencing tachycardia (rapid heartbeats). As a result, stroke volume is reduced, and fewer red blood cells will be available to transport needed oxygen.

ACUTE MOUNTAIN SICKNESS

Altitude sickness, also called acute mountain sickness (AMS), is a disorder related to **hypoxia** (subnormal levels of oxygen in the blood and tissues) at high altitudes. Predisposing factors include cold temperatures, strenuous exercise, use of cigarettes or alcohol, individuals with respiratory infections or a blunted ventilatory response, women in the water-retaining phase of their menstrual cycle, and a family history of AMS. AMS, the mildest form of altitude sickness, arises after rapid ascent (<24 hours) to altitudes above 8200 feet (2500 meters). There is a time lag of 6 to 36 hours between arrival at the altitude and the onset of symptoms (12).

➤ SIGNS AND SYMPTOMS

The signs and symptoms are directly proportional to the rapidity of the ascent, and the duration and degree of physical exertion, and are inversely proportional to acclimatization and physical conditioning. Initial symptoms include headache, dizziness, fatigue, nausea, vomiting, anorexia, insomnia, dyspnea (labored breathing), decreased urine output, and tachycardia during physical exertion. Appetite suppression can be severe during the onset of a high-altitude stay, and can result in an average reduction in energy intake of about 40%, with an accompanying loss of body mass.

➤ MANAGEMENT

Acclimatization and physical conditioning can enhance altitude tolerance, reduce the severity of AMS, and decrease the physical performance decrements during the early stages of altitude sickness. In addition, diets high in carbohydrates (>70% of total Kcal) and low in salt can lessen the impact of AMS. If AMS occurs, treatment involves a reduction in altitude, physical rest, eating frequent small meals, avoiding alcohol, and taking acetaminophen for the headache. Recovery is normally seen within a few days with no residual affects.

HIGH-ALTITUDE PULMONARY EDEMA

For unknown reasons, some individuals experience a severe aspect of AMS at altitudes over 9000 ft called high-altitude pulmonary edema or HAPE. Individuals at greatest risk include those who ascent rapidly, perform strenuous exercise upon arrival, are obese, are male, and have a previous history of pulmonary edema (accumulation of fluid in the lungs) (12). HAPE may develop during the first exposure, but often develops after descent and re-ascent, or occurs the second night after ascent. The lungs accumulate fluid within the alveolar walls that may progress to pulmonary edema.

➤ SIGNS AND SYMPTOMS

Signs and symptoms include rapid breathing (**tachypnea**) and shortness of breath at rest, dry cough with substernal chest pains, headache, decreased concentration, fatigue, tachycardia, and abnormal breath sounds (**rales**) in the middle right lobe. Later, **cyanosis** (a bluish tinge of the skin due to deficient oxygenation of the blood), extreme weakness, a productive cough that produces blood frothy sputum, irrational behavior, and coma may occur.

➤ MANAGEMENT

It is imperative that these individuals return to a lower altitude quickly, and be given oxygen as soon as possible. The condition resolves rapidly.

HIGH-ALTITUDE CEREBRAL EDEMA

High-altitude cerebral edema (HACE) rarely occurs below 10,000 feet, and usually happens in people who ascend rapidly to significant altitudes. Several days after the onset of mild AMS, increased brain cell volume leads to a severe headache, nausea and vomiting, ataxia (incoordination), impaired judgment, inability to make decisions, irrational behavior, and in some cases, coma. The condition can result quickly in death, so an immediate descent is mandatory. High-flow supplemental oxygen or a portable hyperbaric bag should be used while descending, or if descent is delayed.

PREVENTING ALTITUDE ILLNESS

Acclimatization is the single most important factor in preventing the onset of altitude sickness. In general, the length of the acclimatization period needed depends on the altitude. Individuals who are native to areas of high altitude have a larger chest capacity, more alveoli, more capillaries that transport blood to tissues, and a higher red blood cell level. As a result, these individuals clearly have an advantage in endurance activities at higher altitudes. Training for aerobic activities (events lasting longer than 3 or 4 minutes) at altitudes above 6800 feet (2000 meters) requires acclimatization for 10 to 20 days for maximal performance. Highly anaerobic activities at intermediate altitudes do not require arrival in advance of the event (12). The benefits of acclimatization are probably lost within 2 to 3 weeks after returning to sea level.

Air Pollution and Exercise

Chemicals that make up air pollution are typically classified as either primary pollutants (those emitted directly into the environment) or secondary pollutants (those that develop from the interactions of the primary pollutants). Most primary pollutants essentially come from the combustion of petroleum-based fuels, and include carbon monoxide, sulfur oxides, nitrogen oxides, hydrocarbons, and particulates. Secondary pollutants include ozone, peroxyacetyl nitrate, sulfuric acid, aldehydes, and sulfates. Smog usually contains both primary and secondary pollutants. Certain individuals are more susceptible to the adverse effects of air pollution. Even subthreshold concentrations of air pollutants for healthy adults can compromise respiratory and cardiovascular function in children and the elderly. Others affected by air pollution include persons with respiratory disorders (asthma or chronic obstructive pulmonary disease), and persons with heart disease. Because of the complexity of air pollution, only a few chemicals will be discussed here.

CARBON MONOXIDE

The most frequent air pollutant is carbon monoxide, a colorless, odorless gas that reduces the ability of hemoglobin to transport oxygen, and restricts the release of oxygen at the cellular level. In smokers, carbon monoxide reduces both aerobic power and the ability to sustain strenuous, submaximal exercise. It not only interferes with maximal performance during exercise but can also impair attentiveness, decision making, and psychomotor, behavioral, or attention-related tasks, and may result in higher core temperatures during prolonged exercise. The major group at risk from carbon monoxide exposure includes individuals with cardiovascular disorders (e.g., angina pectoris, ischemic cardiovascular disease, intermittent claudication [ischemia of the muscles due to narrowing of the arteries]), pulmonary diseases (e.g., chronic bronchitis, emphysema), or anemia.

SULFUR OXIDES

Sulfur oxides are produced from burning coal or petroleum products. They include sulfur dioxide, sulfuric acid, and sulfate, with 98% of the sulfur released into the atmosphere being in the form of sulfur dioxide. By itself, sulfur dioxide has little effect on lung function in normal individuals, but it can be a potent bronchoconstrictor in asthmatics. Exposure to just a trace of this gas during brief periods of strenuous exercise (10 minutes) can produce a marked decrease in airway conductance in asthmatics. Asthmatics can prevent problems in breathing with a prior administration of disodium cromoglycate, or by breathing through the nose.

NITROGEN OXIDES

Nitrogen oxide is a combination of nitrogen and oxygen that develops from high-temperature combustion; it is seen in several forms—nitrous oxide, nitric oxide, nitrogen dioxide (NO_2), dinitrogen dioxide, dinitrogen pentoxide, and nitrate ions. Oxide levels in the air are particularly high during peak traffic periods, at airports, and in the smoke associated with cigarette smoking and fire fighting. High NO_2 levels (200 to 4000 parts per million [ppm]) can cause severe pulmonary edema and death. At lower concentrations (2 to 5 ppm), NO_2 increases airway resistance and reduces pulmonary diffusion capacity. Although normal ambient air concentration is generally less than 1 ppm, the elderly show a reduced tolerance to NO_2, and people with chronic obstructive pulmonary disease and other respiratory diseases have shown a reduced pulmonary function when exposed for 4 hours to 0.3 ppm to NO_2 (12).

OZONE

Ozone (triatomic oxygen) is a complex union of oxygen, nitrogen oxides, hydrocarbons, and sunlight, and is therefore designated a photochemical oxidant. Ozone is classified as either ground level or atmospheric. Atmospheric ozone is produced naturally and protects the earth from the sun's ultraviolet waves. The ozone that interferes with functional capacity is ground level, which stays close to the earth's surface and originates in automobile and factory emissions. Ground-level ozone is an irritant that can exacerbate existing respiratory conditions such as emphysema and asthma. The effects of ground-level ozone are normally short term, but they can diminish work production and may produce shortness of breath and early fatigue. When maximal exertion is required, ozone may lead to coughing, chest tightness, shortness of breath, pain during deep breaths, nausea, eye irritation, fatigue, and lowered resistance to lung infections.

Ozone levels are indexed as low, moderate, and high (Table 17.6). The ozone index for the day can be found on the weather page of most newspapers. Individuals who reside in regions of high ozone levels may become desensitized to the irritating effects of ozone after repeated exposures and thus develop no symptoms or changes in functional abilities.

PRIMARY PARTICULATES

Primary particulates include dust, soot, and smoke, all of which can impair pulmonary function when inhaled into the lungs. The fine dust from charcoal and cigarette smoke increases airway resistance and reduces forced expiratory volume. The fine dust can infiltrate the lungs, depending on the particle size, amount of air inspired and expired in a single breath (tidal volume), frequency of breathing, and whether the particle was inhaled nasally or orally. During strenuous exercise, the breathing rate significantly increases and breathing tends to be oral; therefore, it is likely that exercise increases the impact of these pollutants on breathing effectiveness.

Exercising in Thunderstorms

An environmental threat that is seldom discussed is participating under inclement weather conditions where rain, lightning, and thunderstorms are present. Most organized outdoor sport practices and competitions are held between 3:00 and 9:00 PM, peak periods for the development of thunderstorms and lightning.

INJURIES DUE TO LIGHTNING

Lightning poses a triple threat of injury: burns from the high temperature of the lightning strike, injury caused by the elicited mechanical forces activated by the intense levels of electricity (electromechanical forces), and from the resulting concussive forces that can propel objects through the air, causing blunt trauma (e.g., fracture, concussion). The most common burn from lightning is a Lichtenburg Figure, which resembles a feathering pattern on the skin. A Lichtenburg Figure is not actually a burn, but a pattern on the skin from the electron avalanche that strikes the body hit by lightning, causing a inflammatory dermal response (14). The pattern is transient and fades after 24 hours. Direct strikes are the most deadly, particularly when the person is in contact with metal (golf club, shoe cleats, belt buckle, bra clips, watch band, metal bleachers), with the burn normally appearing where the person's body is in contact with the metal object.

Electromechanical forces are developed through a lightning strike's amperage and duration, in addition to the body's resistance and relationship to the strike. The most common condition associated with a lightning strike is cardiac asystole (cardiac standstill) and respiratory arrest. Fortunately, the heart is likely to spontaneously restart if the victim is not experiencing respiratory arrest. Surprising, the most critical factor in determining morbidity and mortality associated with a lightning strike is the duration of apnea (cessation of breathing) rather than cardiac asystole. It is not uncommon for a person to become unconscious, or confused, or develop amnesia following a lightning strike. Other medical conditions that have been reported are: blunt trauma, including fractures and internal organ damage; brain lesions due to hypoxia caused by cardiac asystole; ruptured tympanic membranes; ocular problems, including hyphemas and fixed and dilated pupils; seizures; subdural and epidural hematomas; anterior compartment syndromes; and transitory lower extremity paralysis (14).

TREATMENT FOR LIGHTNING INJURIES

Lightning strikes claim the lives of about 100 people each year (15). If the person is conscious and has normal cardiorespiratory function, a secondary assessment should

TABLE 17.6	OZONE LEVELS
Level	Activity Precautions
Low	No precautions are necessary.
Moderate	Individuals with respiratory conditions should minimize outdoor exposure and decrease prolonged exercise or work.
High	Individuals with respiratory conditions should stay indoors. Individual without respiratory conditions should minimize outdoor exposure.

be conducted to determine if they have sustained burns, fractures, or other trauma.

 If not breathing and in cardiac arrest, activate EMS and begin immediate rescue breathing and CPR. Unless ruled out, always suspect a cervical spine injury, and treat accordingly. Any person struck by lightning should be immediately transported to the nearest medical facility.

LIGHTNING SAFETY POLICY

As discussed earlier, most organized outdoor sport practices and competitions are conducted between the hours of 3:00 and 9:00 PM, when risk of thunderstorms is greatest; 70% of all lightning injuries and fatalities occur in the afternoon (16). Thunderstorms can become threat-ening within 30 minutes of the first sign of thunder. All coaches, athletic trainers, athletic directors, athletic supervisors, managers, and athletes should understand how thunderstorms develop and why lightning strikes. The organization or institution should develop a policy within guidelines that can be implemented when conditions are favorable for thunderstorm and lightning activity. This lightning safety policy can decrease the risk of injury and death, and protect the organization or institution from litigation if the policy is referred to, and heeded **(Box 17.6)**.

 Thunder indicates lightning inside the storm, even though you cannot see it. Alert the umpires to the thunder and potential for lightning. A decision can then be made as to whether to call the game and seek shelter.

▶▶ Box 17.6

Lightning Safety Policy for all Outdoor Activities Including Swimming

- Check weather reports and be aware of potential thunderstorms in the area. Note: it does not need to be raining for lightning to strike.
- Have a nearby shelter available.
- Know how close the storm is to your location. Using the "flash-to-bang" method, count the seconds between seeing a lightning flash and hearing the thunder. Divide this number by 5. This is the approximate distance in miles the storm is away from you (sounds travels approximately 5 seconds a mile).
- If the lightning (flash) to thunder (bang) is within 30 seconds, all outdoor activities should end, and all participants should seek shelter (preferably in a sturdy building). If this type of shelter is not available, retreat to a car with a hard metal roof. Keep the windows rolled up.
- If no shelter or cars are available, crouch in a thick grove of small trees surrounding taller trees or in a ditch. Do not lie flat, crouch with only the feet in contact with the ground, wrapping your arms around your knees and lowering your head to minimize body surface area. Stay away from tall or individual trees, lone objects (poles), metal objects, standing pools of water, and open fields.
- Do not remain in a boat or continue to swim in open water.
- If you feel your hair stand on end or your skin tingle, immediately assume the crouched position.
- Do not use the telephone unless it is an emergency.
- Allow 30 minutes to pass after the last sound of thunder or flash of lightning before resuming outdoor activities.
- Persons struck by lightning do not carry a residual electrical charge. Therefore, artificial breathing and CPR are safe to perform on a victim of a lightning strike.

Adapted from Bennett (17), pages 251-252.

Summary

1. The body generates heat via cutaneous vasoconstriction and increasing the metabolic heat production by shivering or physical activity, and through the hormone thyroxine during gradual, seasonal changes. The body loses heat through respiration, radiation, conduction, convection, and evaporation.

2. During exercise, the body gains heat either from external sources (environmental temperatures) or internal processes.

3. At rest, about two-thirds of the body's normal heat loss occurs as a result of conduction, convection, and radiation. As air temperature approaches skin temperature and exceeds 30.6°C (87°F), evaporation becomes the primary means of heat dissipation.

4. Sweating places a high demand on the body's fluid reserves and can create a relative state of dehydration. If sweating is excessive and fluids are not continually replaced, plasma volume falls and core temperature may rise to lethal levels.

5. Acclimatization and proper hydration are among the most critical factors in preventing heat illness. Minerals lost through sweating generally can be replaced through the diet. With prolonged exercise, a small amount of electrolytes added to a rehydration beverage will replace fluids more effectively than drinking plain water.

6. To prevent dehydration, fluids must be ingested and absorbed by the body. Cold liquids, especially water, empty from the stomach and small intestines faster than warm fluids.

7. Heat cramps are caused by excessive water and electrolyte loss during and after intense exercise in the heat. Treatment involves passive stretching of the involved muscle(s) and ice massage over the affected area. The individual should also ingest enough fluids containing an electrolyte solution to drink beyond the point of satisfying his or her thirst.

8. Heat exhaustion is a functional illness and is not associated with organ damage. Treatment involves moving the individual to a cool place and rapidly cooling the body. The individual should also ingest enough fluids containing an electrolyte solution to drink beyond the point of satisfying his or her thirst. Intravenous fluids may need to be administered if the dehydrated state is moderate to severe.

9. Heat stroke signifies significant elevated core temperature and dehydration. Immediately activate EMS as the athlete may require airway management, intravenous fluids, and in severe cases, circulatory support. While waiting for EMS to arrive, the athlete should be moved to a cool place, and efforts should be made to rapidly cool the body. Ice water immersion is the most effective method to cool the body; however, the core temperature should not fall below 38°C (101°F) to avoid hypothermia. If conscious, the individual should drink copious amounts of fluid.

10. The principle of layering clothing allows for several thin layers of insulation. In addition, a ski cap, face mask, and neck warmer can protect the face and ears from frostbite.

11. Frostbite occurs when the core temperature remains relatively constant but the shell temperature decreases. Superficial frostbite is treated by moving the athlete indoors and rapidly rewarming the involved body part in water heated to 39° to 42°C (102° to 108°F) for 30 to 45 minutes. Deep frostbite is best rewarmed under controlled conditions in a hospital. EMS should be activated to transport the individual.

12. Hypothermia occurs when both core and shell temperatures decrease, leading to general body cooling. Treatment involves activating EMS to transport the individual immediately to the nearest medical facility. With mild hypothermia, the individual can be rewarmed; however, with moderate to severe hypothermia, on-site rewarming should not be attempted.

13. Altitude sickness may involve acute mountain sickness, high-altitude pulmonary edema, or high-altitude cerebral edema. The latter two can lead quickly to death, so oxygen therapy and immediate descent are mandatory.

14. Carbon monoxide, the most frequent air pollutant, interferes with the ability of hemoglobin to transport oxygen to the cellular level. Other air pollutants that can affect sport performance include sulfur oxides, nitrogen oxides, ozone, and primary particulates.

15. Lightning poses a double threat of injury: burns from the high temperature of the lightning strike, and concussive injuries caused by the elicited electromechanical forces.

16. Most thunderstorms occur between 3:00 and 9:00 PM. Schools and sport organizations should have a detailed lightning safety policy to prevent injury or death from storms.

References

1. McArdle WD, Katch FI, Katch VI. Exercise Physiology: Energy, Nutrition, and Human Performance. 4th ed. Baltimore: Williams & Wilkins, 1996.
2. Murray R. Dehydration, hyperthermia, and athletes: Science and practice. J Ath Train 1996;31(3):248-252.
3. Granjean AC, Reimers KJ. Sports nutrition. In: The Team Physician's Handbook. Edited by Mellion MB, Walsh WM, Shelton GL. Philadelphia: Hanley & Belfus, 1997.
4. Gatorade Sports Science Institute. Dehydration & Heat Injuries: Identification, Treatment, and Prevention. Chicago: Gatorade, 1997.
5. Shi X, Gisolfi CV. Fluid and carbohydrate replacement during intermittent exercise. Sports Med 1998;25(3):157-172.
6. American College of Sports Medicine. Position Stand on Exercise and Fluid Replacement. Med Sci Sports Exerc 1996;28(1):i-vii.
7. Myer F, Bar-Or D, MacDougall D, Heigenhauser G. Drink composition and electrolyte balance of children exercising in the heat. Med Sci Sport Exerc 1995;27(6):882-887.
8. Mellion MB, Shelton GL. Safe exercise in the heat and heat injuries. In: The Team Physician's Handbook. Edited by Mellion MB, Walsh WM, Shelton GL. Philadelphia: Hanley & Belfus, 1997.
9. Armstrong LE, et al. Whole-body cooling of hyperthermic runners: comparison of two filed therapies. Am J Emerg Med 1996;14(4):355-358.
10. Sandor RP. Heat illness: On-site diagnosis and cooling. Phys Sportsmed 1997;25(6):35-40.
11. Leshaw SM. Itching in active patients: Causes and cures. Phys Sportsmed 1998;26(1):47-53.
12. Montain SJ, Freund BJ. Environmental considerations for exercise. In: Athletic Injuries and Rehabilitation. Edited by Zachazewski JE, Magee DJ, Quillen WS. Philadelphia: WB Saunders, 1996.
13. Bowman WD. Safe exercise in the cold and cold injuries. In: The Team Physician's Handbook. Edited by Mellion MB, Walsh WM, Shelton GL. Philadelphia: Hanley & Belfus, 1997.
14. Walsh KM, et al. A survey of lightning policy in selected Division I colleges. J Ath Train 1997;32(3):206-210.
15. Cherington M, Yarnell P, Wappes JR. Lightning strikes: How to lower your risk. Phys Sportsmed 1997;25(5):129-130.
16. Uman MA. All About Lightning. New York: Dover Publications, 1996.
17. Bennett BL. A model lightning safety policy for athletics. J Ath Train 1997;32(3):251-253.

CHAPTER 18

Respiratory Tract Conditions

OBJECTIVES

1. Explain physiological factors associated with common respiratory tract conditions.

2. List the signs and symptoms of common upper respiratory tract conditions, including the common cold, sinusitis, pharyngitis, influenza, and allergic rhinitis.

3. Describe strategies that can be used to prevent the common cold.

4. List the signs and symptoms of lower respiratory tract conditions, including bronchitis, bronchial asthma, and exercise-induced bronchospasm.

5. Describe the management and treatment of common respiratory tract conditions.

6. Explain how to use a metered-dose inhaler, and a peak flow meter in the management of asthma.

Conditions of the respiratory tract are common in sport participants. Many factors such as fatigue, chronic inflammation from a localized infection, environmental factors (allergens, dust, smog), and psychological stress brought on by stressful life events can suppress resistance to these conditions. In this chapter, common upper respiratory tract infections and general respiratory conditions will be discussed.

UPPER RESPIRATORY TRACT INFECTIONS

 Athletes often contract colds and influenza during their competitive season. What strategies would you use to decrease the risk of getting a cold, or to decrease the severity of a cold?

Viral conditions are often referred to as upper respiratory infections (URIs). These conditions, although minor, can clearly impact one's performance. In this section, the common cold, sinusitis, pharyngitis, influenza, and allergic rhinitis (hay fever) will be discussed.

Common Cold

The average adult has from one to six colds each year, with human rhinoviruses (HRVs) accounting for 40 to 50% of these infections; the majority of them occur in the fall and spring months (1). The condition may be triggered by aspirin sensitivity, use of oral contraceptives, topical decongestant abuse, cocaine abuse, presence of nasal polyps or deviated septum, or allergic conditions. A cold can be quite contagious and can be transmitted by either person-to-person contact or airborne droplets. However, several strategies can be implemented to reduce the risk of getting a cold **(Box 18.1)**.

Upper respiratory symptoms usually begin 1 to 2 days after exposure and generally last 1 to 2 weeks, even though viral shedding and contagion can continue for 2 or 3 more weeks (2). Although many athletes feel that sport performance is hindered by a cold, a recent study of male and female athletes who underwent a resting pulmonary function test and submaximal exercise test while healthy and again at the peak of their illness, found no significant impairment of pulmonary function, maximum oxygen consumption, maximum heart rate, or rating of perceived exertion (3).

➤ SIGNS AND SYMPTOMS

Symptoms include a rapid onset of clear nasal discharge **(rhinorrhea)**, nasal itching, sneezing, nonproductive cough, and associated itching and puffiness of the eyes. Malaise (feeling lousy or tired), a mild sore throat, chills, and, in some cases, a low-grade fever may also be present. Although most cold symptoms are benign and confined to the upper respiratory tract, colds can lead to middle ear infections and bacterial sinusitis when airflow is obstructed by swollen nasal membranes.

➤ MANAGEMENT

Although there is no cure for the viral common cold, over-the-counter medications can alleviate or lessen symptoms. It is a well known that vitamin C supplements can decrease the duration of cold episodes and the severity of symptoms. Likewise, zinc gluconate in the form of throat lozenges has also been shown to decrease the duration of cold episodes and the severity of symptoms if started within 24 to 48 hours of onset (4). If environmental factors, allergens, bacterial infections, or stressful life events are the cause, treatment involves rest, reducing contributing factors, and using topical therapy delivered through pump sprays rather than systemic therapy. When compared to over-the-counter squeeze containers, pump sprays offer better dosage control and provide less irritation to the interior nose, particularly the septum. Topical medications may include antiasthmatic agents (cromolyn sodium, Nasalcrom), corticosteroids (beclomethasone, flunisolide), and anticholinergics (nasal ipratropium, atropine in saline). Observe caution when any of the preceding medications are used by competitive athletes, as any agent may be on the list of banned substances, particularly at high competitive levels.

Sinusitis

Sinusitis is an inflammation of the paranasal sinus caused by a bacterial or viral infection, an allergy, or environmental factors **(Figure 18.1)**. Sinusitis can be acute, lasting for less than 30 days; subacute, lasting 3 weeks to 2 months; or chronic, lasting longer than 2 months. The condition is often triggered by an obstruction of the passageway between the sinuses (ostium) due to local mucosal swelling and local insult, or mechanical obstruction. Local mucosal swelling may be secondary to an upper respiratory tract infection, allergy, or direct trauma. Mechanical obstruction may be caused by a deviated septum, concha bullosa (vesicle of serum or blood located on the concha inside the nose), or nasal masses from polyps or tumors.

➤ SIGNS AND SYMPTOMS

Nasal congestion, facial pain or pressure over the involved sinus, pain in the upper teeth, or pain and pressure behind the eyes (retro-orbital) will be present. Other symptoms may include purulent nasal discharge (anterior and posterior), palpable pain over the involved sinus, nighttime and daytime coughing, and in severe cases, perinasal and eyelid swelling, fever, and chills. Drainage with bacterial infections will most likely be dark colored, whereas other causes will usually be clear. Chronic sinusitis is character-

---

➤➤ BOX 18.1

Strategies to Reduce the Risk of Getting a Cold

- Avoid contact with individuals who have upper respiratory tract infections (URIs), particularly children, as they tend to have more frequent URIs.
- In the presence of individuals who have URIs, avoid touching objects or sharing objects that they have touched.
- Wash your hands frequently during cold season, and avoid touching your eyes and nose with your fingers. This will prevent many viruses from reaching the mucus membranes.
- Drink plenty of clear fluids (nonalcoholic).
- Although vitamin C supplements will not decrease the incidence of colds, they have been found to decrease the duration and severity of symptoms.
- Reduce environmental factors (dust, smog, allergens) that may predispose you to rhinitis.
- Reduce stress.
- If using a topical decongestant, follow the instructions carefully and do not prolong its use, as rebound rhinitis may occur. Use decongestants during the day and antihistamines at night because of their sedative effect.
- If cold symptoms are mild, exercise is safe. If symptoms include headache, fever, muscular aches, hacking productive cough, or loss of appetite, however, exercise should cease. Rest is best.

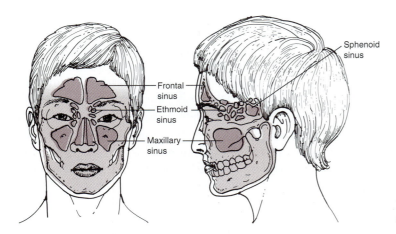

Sphenoid sinus

Frontal sinus

Ethmoid sinus

Maxillary sinus

➤ **FIGURE 18.1 Facial sinuses.** The frontal and ethmoid sinuses are more commonly involved in sinusitis.

ized by chronic nasal congestion, rhinorrhea or postnasal discharge accompanied by perinasal pressure, and headache not associated with migraine or muscle tension. The individual will often pinch the bridge of the nose to demonstrate the area of discomfort, or will report discomfort aggravated by eyeglasses.

➤ MANAGEMENT

Treatment involves controlling the infection, reducing mucosal edema, and allowing for nasal discharge. Oral antibiotics such as amoxicillin, penicillin, or erythromycin may be prescribed. Topical agents such as phenylephrine hydrochloride (Neo-Synephrine) or oxymetazoline hydrochloride (Afrin) can be used during the first 3 to 4 days of treatment to facilitate drainage. Longer use of decongestants can lead to a rebound effect, whereby excessive mucus production and edema are increased. In severe cases, surgical intervention may be necessary to drain the sinuses.

Pharyngitis (Sore Throat)

Pharyngitis may be caused by a viral, bacterial, or fungal infection of the pharynx, leading to a sore throat. The condition may result from a common cold, influenza, streptococcus infection, diphtheria, herpes simplex 1 and 2, Epstein-Barr virus, gonococcal bacteria, chlamydia, or candidiasis. If caused by the bacteria *Streptococcus pyogenes* (strep throat) and inadequately treated, peritonsillar abscess, scarlet fever, rheumatic fever, or rheumatic heart disease may result.

➤ SIGNS AND SYMPTOMS

The throat typically appears dark red, the tonsils appear red and swollen, and a pussy discharge may be present. Throat pain is aggravated by swallowing and may radiate along the distribution of the glossopharyngeal nerve (cranial nerve IX) to the ears. Other symptoms include rhinorrhea, swollen lymph glands, hoarseness, headache, cough, a low-grade fever, and malaise.

➤ MANAGEMENT

Treatment for streptococcal pharyngitis includes antibiotics such as penicillin or erythromycin (5). In cases not involving streptococcal pharyngitis, treatment involves bed rest, plenty of fluids, warm saline gargles, throat lozenges, and mild analgesics (aspirin, ibuprofen).

Influenza

Influenza, or "flu," is a specific viral bronchitis caused by *Hemophilus* influenza type A, B, or C. It often occurs in epidemic proportions, particularly in school-aged children. Immunization for the influenza type A and B viruses is available for individuals at high risk, including pregnant women; individuals with chronic illness, such as diabetes mellitus and disorders of the pulmonary or cardiovascular system; children; and those with immunocompromised systems. Individuals with a fever should not be immunized until the fever has passed.

➤ SIGNS AND SYMPTOMS

A fever of 39° to 39.5°C (102° to 103°F), chills, malaise, headache, general muscle aches, a hacking cough, and inflamed mucous membranes may be present. Rapid onset of symptoms can occur within 24 to 48 hours after exposure to the virus. Sore throat, watery eyes, sensitivity to light (photophobia), and a nonproductive cough may linger for up to 5 days. The cough may progress into bronchitis.

➤ MANAGEMENT

Initial treatment consists of rest, plenty of fluids, saltwater gargles, cough medication, and analgesics to control fever, aches, and pains.

 If the fever does not return to near normal within 24 hours, the individual should be seen immediately by a physician to rule out other infectious conditions.

Allergic Rhinitis (Hay Fever)

Allergic rhinitis (inflammation of the nasal mucous membranes) affects nearly 20% of all children and adults in the United States (6). The risk of rhinitis increases throughout childhood and adolescents, and peaks during the late 20s and early 30s. It is often divided into seasonal allergic rhinitis, or "hay fever," and perennial allergic rhinitis. Hay fever usually involves a specific period of symptoms in successive years caused by airborne pollens or fungus spores associated with that season. In contrast, perennial allergic rhinitis occurs year-round if the individual is continually exposed to allergens such as food (shellfish, bread mold), dust, and animal emanations (cat hair, feathers).

➤ SIGNS AND SYMPTOMS

Postnasal drainage leads to a chronic sore throat and bronchial infection. In addition, the phalangeal openings of the eustachian tubes can become blocked by swollen mucosa, enlarged lymphoid tissue, or exudate. Without normal airflow, increasing negative pressure in the middle ear results in fluid accumulation, leading to a partial hearing loss and recurrent middle ear infections.

Taking a complete history is the key to differentiating allergic rhinitis from other respiratory conditions. Questions should focus on the relationship of symptoms to seasons or exposures that trigger symptoms. For example, if symptoms increase outdoors, pollen may be the triggering agent; indoors it may be mold. In addition, certain geographical areas may have more environmental allergens than others. Athletes should try to limit exposure to allergens when participating in different environments. Allergy tests (skin or intradermal testing) may not be necessary if a history uncovers allergens to specific environmental factors.

➤ MANAGEMENT

Management involves limiting exposure to the allergen or irritant, suppressive medication to alleviate symptom severity, and specific hypersensitization to reduce responsiveness to unavoidable allergens. For example, if dust is an allergen, having bare floors, pillows, and mattresses encased in plastic covers, minimizing cloth curtains, and avoiding cluttered tabletops can reduce the amount of dust in a home. Antihistamine drugs (Benadryl, Tavist-1, Chlor-Trimeton) are effective agents in reducing symptoms of allergic rhinitis. In competitive athletes, however, drowsiness, lethargy, mucous membrane dryness, and occasional nausea and light-headedness may be unwanted side effects. Medications including ephedrine (Fedrine, Ephedd II, Efedron nasal jelly), isoephedrine, and phenylpropanolamine acting as mucosal decongestants can offset sedative effects of antihistamine agents. Cromolyn sodium can reduce the symptoms of allergic rhinitis and conjunctivitis. Observe caution when any of the preceding medications are used by competitive athletes, as any agent may be on the list of banned substances, particularly at high competitive levels.

 To prevent or reduce the severity of a cold, avoid contact with individuals who have upper respiratory infections, wash your hands frequently during cold season, drink plenty of clear fluids, take vitamin C supplements, and reduce stress.

GENERAL RESPIRATORY CONDITIONS

 A 15-year-old asthmatic would like to improve his cardiovascular endurance without triggering exercise-induced bronchospasm. What activities might be recommended and what guidelines should be followed in developing the exercise program?

General respiratory conditions may result from infection or irritation from inhaled particles and substances. Bronchitis, bronchial asthma, and exercise-induced bronchospasm (EIB), formerly called exercise-induced asthma (EIA), will be discussed here.

Bronchitis

Bronchitis is inflammation of the mucosal lining of the tracheobronchial tree resulting from infection or inhaled particles and substances, and may be acute or chronic. Acute bronchitis, commonly seen in sport participants, involves bronchial swelling, mucus secretion, and increased resistance to expiration. Coughing, wheezing, and large amounts of purulent mucus will be present. Once the stimulus is removed, the swelling decreases and airways return to normal.

Chronic bronchitis is characterized by individuals who have a productive daily cough for at least 3 consecutive months in 2 successive years. Irritation may result from cigarette smoke, air pollution, or infections. This condition can progress to increased airway obstruction, heart failure, and cellular changes in respiratory epithelial cells that may become malignant. Signs and symptoms included marked cyanosis, edema, large production of sputum, and abnormally high levels of carbon dioxide and low levels of oxygen in the blood. This condition is often seen simultaneously with emphysema.

Bronchial Asthma

Asthma is caused by a constriction of bronchial smooth muscles (bronchospasm), increased bronchial secretions, and mucosal swelling, all leading to an inadequate airflow during respiration (especially expiration) **(Figure 18.2)**. The condition is classified as intermittent, seasonal, or chronic. Intermittent asthma is usually of relatively short duration, occurring less than 5 days per month with extended symptom-free periods. Symptoms of seasonal asthma occur for prolonged periods only in response to exposure to seasonal inhalant allergens. Chronic asthma occurs daily or near daily with an absence of extended, symptom-free periods.

➤ SIGNS AND SYMPTOMS

Wheezing is a common sign that results from air squeezing past the narrowed airways. Because the airways cannot fill or empty adequately, the diaphragm tends to

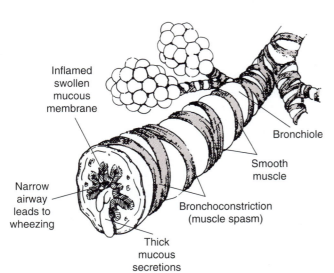

Inflamed
swollen
mucous
membrane

Bronchiole

Smooth
muscle

Narrow
airway
leads to
wheezing

Bronchoconstriction
(muscle spasm)

Thick
mucous
secretions

➤ FIGURE 18.2 **Bronchospasm**. An asthma attack is caused by bronchospasm that constricts the bronchiolar tubes. This spasm, combined with increased bronchial secretions and mucosal swelling, results in a characteristic loud wheezing sound heard during expiration.

flatten and the accessory muscles must work harder to enlarge the chest during inspiration. This increased workload leads to a rapid onset of fatigue when the individual can no longer hyperventilate enough to meet the increased oxygen need. Acute attacks may occur spontaneously, but are often provoked by a viral infection.

A large amount of thick, yellow or green sputum is produced by the bronchial mucosa. As dyspnea (difficult breathing) continues, anxiety, loud wheezing, sweating, rapid heart rate, and labored breathing are apparent. In severe cases, respiratory failure may be indicated by cyanosis, decreased wheezing, and decreased levels of consciousness.

➤ MANAGEMENT

Individuals diagnosed with asthma typically carry medication delivered by a compressor-driven nebulizer or inhaler, to alleviate the attack. The value of bronchodilators in children and young adults continues to be debated. Medications involve selective bronchodilators, aerosol corticosteroids, and cromolyn sodium, an antihistaminic drug that prevents the release of chemical mediators that cause bronchospasms and mucous membrane inflammatory changes. Once the attack has subsided, the lungs usually return to normal.

Exercise-induced Bronchospasm

Exercise-induced bronchospasm (EIB), formerly known as exercise-induced asthma (EIA), affects up to 90% of asthmatics and up to 35% of those without known asthma. Factors contributing to the severity of EIB include ambient air conditions (cold air, low humidity, pollutants);

duration, type, and intensity of exercise; exposure to allergens in sensitized individuals; overall control of asthma; poor physical conditioning; respiratory infections; time since the last episode of EIB; and any underlying bronchial hyperreactivity (7). Individuals suffering from allergies, sinus disease, or hyperventilation may be at increased risk for EIB, and those with bronchitis, emphysema, and other diseases affecting the bronchial tubes can exacerbate symptoms.

Despite its prevalence, the precise mechanisms responsible for EIB are still unknown. Theories include hyperventilation resulting in airway heat and water loss, carbon dioxide loss with hyperventilation, and release of chemical mediators causing bronchospasm. These theories, however, have not been substantiated. It is thought that breathing dry, cold air through the mouth stimulates bronchospasm. Thus, breathing through the nose or covering the nose and mouth when exercising in cold weather can warm and humidify the air, and lessen the onset of symptoms. Swimming in an indoor pool where the air is typically warm and humid may also prevent the onset of symptoms. Regardless of the mechanism, the amount of ventilation and the temperature of the inspired air during and after exercise are important factors in determining the severity of EIB. The greater the ventilations in cold, dry, air, the greater the risk of EIB. The more strenuous the exercise, the greater the ventilations.

Several questions can be used to help screen for EIB (**Box 18.2**). Recently, EIB has been diagnosed according to forced expiratory volume at 1 second (FEV_1) using a peak flowmeter device. Normally, individuals can have up to a 10% decrease in FEV_1, postexercise. When FEV_1 drops between 10 and 20%, however, the individual is considered to have mild EIB; 20 to 40% indicates moderate to severe, and more than 40% indicates severe EIB (8). **Field Strategy 18.1** describes the use of a peak flowmeter.

➤➤ Box 18.2

History Questions to Screen for EIB
- Have you ever been told that you have asthma or exercise-induced bronchospasm?
- Do you ever have chest pain or chest tightness during or following exercise?
- Do you ever wheeze during or after moderate exercise?
- Do you ever have shortness of breath during or after exercise?
- Do you ever have itching of the nose or throat, or sneezing episodes during or after exercise?
- Have you ever experienced stomach cramps after exercise?
- Have you ever missed work or school because of chest pain, chest tightness, coughing, wheezing, or prolonged shortness of breath?

FIELD STRATEGY 18.1   USE OF A PEAK FLOWMETER

1. Place the mouth on the mouthpiece of the peak flowmeter.
2. Make sure the red indicator is at the bottom of the scale before using unit.
3. Hold the meter vertically, making sure the fingers do not block the opening.
4. Inhale as deeply as possible, and tightly seal the lips around the mouthpiece.
5. Blow as hard and as fast as possible into the meter; this will cause the red indicator to move up the scale. The final position of the red indicator is the peak flow measurement.
6. Repeat steps 2 through 5 two more times, and take the highest value of the three measurements. This value is the peak flow measurement.

➤ SIGNS AND SYMPTOMS

Chest pain, chest tightness, or a burning sensation with or without wheezing; a regular dry cough; shortness of breath shortly after or during exercise; and stomach cramps after exercise are common signs and symptoms. EIB symptoms typically appear after 8 to 10 minutes of vigorous exercise and may worsen after activity is terminated. Episodes usually remit completely within 30 to 60 minutes and do not increase airway reactivity or induce long-term deterioration in lung function. An interesting facet of EIB is the occurrence in about half of individuals of a "refractory" period. Generally, if exercise is repeated within 1 hour of the first bout, bronchial narrowing recurs but is less severe than the previous episode. The refractory period can last from 40 minutes to 3 hours. Within this period, it may be possible to exercise longer and more strenuously without difficulty (9,10).

➤ MANAGEMENT

Management includes medications used in regular asthma treatment such as bronchodilators, cromolyn sodium, oral theophylline, and leukotriene modifiers zafirlukast and zileitron (7,10). However, athletes should check with the appropriate governing sport body to ensure the medication is legal for competition. **Field Strategy 18.2** provides guidelines for the use of a metered-dose inhaler.

Children and young adults who have asthma, and are physically fit and free of significant airway obstruction, respond to exercise similar to nonasthmatic individuals.

Activities such as tennis, running, and football are well tolerated if exercise includes a 5- to 10-minute stretching program followed by a 10- to 15-minute warm-up at 60% of maximum heart rate performed a half hour before more strenuous exercise. After warming up, athletes should pretreat themselves with two puffs of a short-acting inhaler to protect against an attack for 2 to 6 hours. Using an inhaler alone often does not allow for a full dose of medication to be delivered to the lungs. Adjuncts such as aeroflow chambers or Inspirease can be used with metered-dose inhalers to enhance the delivery and more evenly distribute the medication to the bronchial tubes and lungs. After exercise, a cool-down period of several minutes of stretching or less strenuous activity will allow a gradual rewarming of the airways and make postexercise symptoms less likely (10). **Field Strategy 18.3** presents a management algorithm for individuals with exercise-induced bronchospasm.

The asthmatic individual should be seen by a physician before starting an exercise program. In general, the program can include a 5- to 10-minute warm-up of moderate stretching, and 10 to 15 minutes of low-intensity exercise, keeping the pulse below 60% maximum heart rate. Use of a bronchodilator 15 minutes prior to exercise can also be used to delay symptoms for 2 to 6 hours. After exercise, a 10- to 30-minute cool-down period of stretching and less strenuous activity will allow for gradual rewarming of the airways.

FIELD STRATEGY 18.2   USE OF A METERED-DOSE INHALER

1. Remove cap and hold inhaler upright.
2. Shake inhaler.
3. Tilt head slightly backward, and exhale fully but do not force expired air.
4. Hold inhaler 1–2 inches (1–2 finger widths) from the open mouth.
5. Start to breath in slowly, and press down once on the inhaler.
6. Continue to breath in slowly for 3–5 seconds (the slower the breath, the better the absorption into the lungs).
7. Hold the breath for 10 seconds.
8. Repeat steps 4 through 7.

*Note adjuncts such as aeroflow chambers or Inspirease can also enhance delivery.

FIELD STRATEGY 18.3   MANAGEMENT ALGORITHM FOR EXERCISE-INDUCED BRONCHOSPASM

General Recommendations

- Consult a physician before beginning an exercise program
- Take medication for asthma as prescribed to achieve good overall control of asthmatic symptoms, including those caused by exercise and airborne allergens
- Use a peak flowmeter as directed by a physician
- Avoid exposure to air pollutants and allergens whenever possible
- Avoid exercise in the early morning hours, when the concentration of ragweed is highest

Exercise Routine

Use a bronchodilator prior to exercise

↓

Perform a 5- to 10-minute warm-up of moderate stretching, and work out slowly for another 10–15 minutes, keeping the pulse rate below 60% maximum heart rate (140 beats per minute)

↓

Increase the time and intensity of the workout as tolerated, especially if the activity is new

↓

Breathing:

- Breath slowly through the nose to warm and humidify the air. Exercise in a warm, humid environment such as a heated swimming pool
- In cold, dry environments, breathe through a mask or scarf. Alternatively, consider different locations and types of exercise during winter months, such as swimming, running, or cycling indoors

↓

Perform a gradual 10- to 30-minute cool-down after a vigorous workout. This:
- avoids rapid thermal changes in the airways
- can be achieved by slowing to a less intense pace while jogging, cycling, swimming, and stretching

Summary

1. Viral conditions are often referred to as upper respiratory infections or URIs.
2. The common cold is an acute viral infection that may be triggered by aspirin sensitivity, use of oral contraceptives, topical decongestant abuse, cocaine abuse, presence of nasal polyps or a deviated septum, and allergic conditions.
3. Sinusitis is an inflammation of the paranasal sinus caused by a bacterial or viral infection, an allergy, or environmental factors.
4. If pharyngitis is caused by the bacteria *Streptococcus pyogenes*, and if inadequately treated, peritonsillar abscess, scarlet fever, rheumatic fever, or rheumatic heart disease may result.
5. Hay fever may be seasonal (caused by airborne pollens and fungus spores associated with that season) or perennial (occurs year-round if continually exposed to allergens).
6. Bronchitis may be acute or chronic, and is characterized by bronchial swelling, mucus secretion and increased resistance to expiration.

7. Asthma is caused by a constriction of bronchial smooth muscles (bronchospasm), increased bronchial secretions, and mucosal swelling, all leading to inadequate airflow during respiration (especially expiration). Wheezing, a common sign of asthma, results from air squeezing past the narrowed airways. The condition is classified as intermittent, seasonal, or chronic, and is managed with bronchodilators, aerosol corticosteroids, and cromolyn sodium.
8. Exercise-induced bronchospasm (EIB) affects up to 90% of asthmatics and up to 35% of those without known asthma. Key signs are a dry, regular cough within 8 to 10 minutes of the start of moderate exercise, and stomach cramps after exercise.

References

1. Weidner TG, Gehlsen G, Schurr T, Dwyer GB. Effects of viral upper respiratory illness on running gait. J Ath Train 1997;32(4): 309-314.
2. Swain RA, Kaplan B. Upper respiratory infections: Treatment selection for active patients. Phys Sportsmed 1998;26(2):85-96.

3. Weidner TG, et al. Effect of a rhinovirus caused upper respiratory illness on pulmonary function test and exercise response. Med Sci Sports Exerc 1997;29(5):604-609.

4. Mossad SB, et al. Zinc gluconate lozenges for treating the common cold. Ann Intern Med 1996;125(2):81-88.

5. Mellion MB. Infections in athletes. In: The Team Physician's Handbook. Edited by Mellion MB, Walsh WM, Shelton GL. Philadelphia: Hanley & Belfus, 1997.

6. Ferguson BJ. Allergic rhinitis: Recognizing signs, symptoms, and triggering allergens. Postgrad Med 1997;101(5):110-116.

7. Rupp NT. Diagnosis and management of exercise-induced asthma. Phys Sportsmed 1996;24(1):77-87.

8. Randoph C. Exercise-induced asthma: Update on pathophysiology, clinical diagnosis, and treatment. Curr Prob Pediatr 1997;27(2): 53-77.

9. Tan RA, Sheldon SL. Exercise-induced asthma. Sport Med 1998; 25(2):1-6.

10. Disabella V, Sherman C. Exercise for asthma patients: Little risk, big rewards. Phys Sportsmed 1998;26(6):75-84.

CHAPTER 19

Gastrointestinal Conditions

OBJECTIVES

1. Explain the physiological factors associated with common gastrointestinal conditions.

2. List the common signs and symptoms associated with upper gastrointestinal conditions such as dysphagia, gastroesophageal reflux, dyspepsia (indigestion), peptic ulcers, gastritis, and gastroenteritis.

3. List the common signs and symptoms associated with lower gastrointestinal conditions such as diarrhea, constipation, and hemorrhoids.

4. Describe the general management of upper and lower gastrointestinal conditions.

5. List other factors that may not be related to an injury or condition specific to the upper or lower gastrointestinal tract, but may adversely affect the entire gastrointestinal tract.

The gastrointestinal (GI) tract extends from the mouth to the anus, and functions to absorb nutritional substances from ingested food and expel waste. It is important to note that, in an active population, exercise alone can induce both upper and lower gastrointestinal symptoms and problems. During exercise, up to 20% of the central blood volume is shunted away from the visceral organs to the working muscles. This can result in the reduction of normal intestinal blood flow by as much as 80% to maintain an adequate central blood volume (1). Exercised-induced shunting, as it is often called, can lead to decreased esophageal motility, erosive hemorrhagic gastritis, delayed gastric emptying, diarrhea, or intestinal bleeding. Dehydration, a high ambient temperature, and lack of acclimatization to exercise in the heat can all exacerbate this hypoperfusion of the GI tract. Nervous tension can also lead to indigestion, diarrhea, or constipation, and adversely affect sport participation. Many seemingly minor disorders, however, can be the first sign of more serious underlying conditions. If symptoms persist with any disorder, referral to a physician is warranted.

In this chapter, disorders affecting the upper gastrointestinal region will be discussed first, followed by disorders affecting the lower gastrointestinal region. Finally, other factors not specific to the upper or lower GI tract, but affecting the entire GI tract, will be presented.

UPPER GASTROINTESTINAL DISORDERS

 A young swimmer reports to practice with a mild fever, upset stomach, and abdominal cramps. He reported that during the previous night, he had diarrhea and felt nauseated, but did not vomit. What condition might be present, and how will you manage this situation?

Upper gastrointestinal (GI) disorders (i.e., stomach and above) are caused by local irritation due to a variety of factors, including stress and the ingestion of caffeine, alcohol, and tomato and citric acid products. This irritation can lead to nausea, **emesis** (vomiting), bloating, abdominal cramps, and heartburn. General management includes agents with **antacids** (acid neutralizers) and diet modification.

Dysphagia

Dysphagia, an inability or difficulty to swallow properly, is associated with labored swallowing actions. Predisposing factors include a narrowing of the esophagus, and paralysis or muscle spasms of the esophageal or pharyngeal muscles.

 Any athlete who exhibits dysphagia should discontinue activity, and be immediately referred to a physician for further evaluation.

Gastroesophageal Reflux

When gastric juice (which is extremely acidic) regurgitates into the esophagus, it is called gastroesophageal reflux. The condition is most likely to occur when an individual has eaten or drunk to excess, but is also caused by conditions that force abdominal contents superiorly, such as obesity, pregnancy, and running, which causes stomach contents to splash upward with each step (runner's reflux). With increasing exercise intensity, the frequency, amplitude, and duration of esophageal contractions decrease.

➤ SIGNS AND SYMPTOMS

Gastroesophageal reflux is associated with mild heartburn, a burning, radiating substernal pain. Gastroesophageal (GOR) disease, caused by a chronic exposure to gastric juices, occurs when reflux leads to physical complications such as severe heartburn and upper chest pain. Symptoms are so similar to those of a heart attack that many first-time sufferers are rushed to the nearest medical facility.

➤ MANAGEMENT

Initial management involves use of antacids 4 hours prior to exercise, and changes in diet, timing of meals prior to exercise, and activity modification.

Dyspepsia (Indigestion)

Dyspepsia, or indigestion, is associated with upper gastrointestinal pain with no identified etiology.

➤ SIGNS AND SYMPTOMS

Irregularly occurring symptoms can range from a sense of fullness after eating, to feeling as though something is lodged in the esophagus, to heartburn, nausea, vomiting, and loss of appetite. Pain and discomfort at the xiphoid region during digestion are the most common symptoms. Similar to peptic ulcers, dyspepsia can be caused by an excessive acid accumulation in the stomach, and overconsumption of alcohol.

➤ MANAGEMENT

Antacids 4 hours prior to exercise and activity modification may help with the discomfort.

 If symptoms persist, immediate referral to a physician is warranted to rule out more serious abdominal conditions or diseases.

Peptic Ulcers

Peptic ulcers generally occur at the lower end of the esophagus, in the stomach, or in the duodenum. Excessive production of gastric acid is usually a precursor, along with the consumption of excessive alcohol, spicy or salty foods, pepper or caffeinated drinks, and the use of tobacco products, particularly cigarettes and cigars. The resulting open lesion on the mucosal tissue is further exposed to the effects of gastric acid.

➤ SIGNS AND SYMPTOMS

The most common symptom is a gnawing epigastric pain that typically occurs within 1 to 3 hours of eating and is often relieved by eating again. Dyspepsia, nausea, vomiting, heartburn, and diarrhea may also be present. The danger with a peptic ulcer is perforation of the stomach wall followed by peritonitis and, perhaps, massive hemorrhage.

➤ MANAGEMENT

When taken on an empty stomach or 1 hour after a meal, antacids reduce acidity within 30 minutes and continue to reduce it for up to 3 hours.

 If over-the-counter antacids fail to reduce the pain and discomfort, the individual should be immediately referred to a physician. Hemorrhaging and perforations, which may be present, can result in an emergency situation. These individuals should be under a physician's supervision.

Gastritis

Gastritis occurs when the stomach lining becomes inflamed. It may be induced by anxiety, exercise-related hypoperfusion, nonsteroidal anti-inflammatory drugs (NSAIDs), or excessive consumption of alcohol.

➤ SIGNS AND SYMPTOMS

Vague stomach tenderness is often accompanied by nausea, vomiting, fever, and stomach pain.

➤ MANAGEMENT

Gastritis should be managed with an increase in clear fluids and physician referral. Drug therapy (antacids) may be contraindicated if gastric bleeding is present. If gastric bleeding does occur, exercise is contraindicated.

Gastroenteritis

The incidence of gastroenteritis, an acute inflammation of the mucous membrane of the stomach or small intestine, is second only to upper respiratory tract infections in adolescents and young adults (1). The condition may be caused by viral or bacterial infection, allergic reaction, medication, contaminated food (food poisoning), or emotional stress.

➤ SIGNS AND SYMPTOMS

In mild cases, increased secretion of hydrochloric acid in the stomach may lead to indigestion, nausea, flatulence (gas), and a sour stomach. In moderate to severe cases, abdominal cramping, diarrhea, fever, and vomiting can lead to fluid and electrolyte imbalance.

➤ MANAGEMENT

The condition is often self-limiting and usually clears in 2 to 3 days. Treatment includes eliminating irritating foods from the diet, avoiding factors that bring on anxiety and stress, and avoiding dehydration by drinking clear fluids or electrolyte-containing fluids (e.g., sport drinks). Antimotility drugs (e.g., Imodium, Lomotil, Diasorb) reduce movement in the small intestines, and may be effective for abdominal cramps and diarrhea, but may also prolong some infections. Return to competition will be limited only by the hydration status, infective nature of the problem, complexity of the symptoms (i.e., frequent diarrhea), and reconditioning.

The young swimmer had a mild fever, upset stomach, abdominal cramps, diarrhea, and nausea. He may have gastroenteritis. The athlete should be isolated from the team, and encouraged to rest and increase the intake of clear fluids or electrolyte-containing fluids. If the condition does not improve in 2 days, he should be seen by a physician.

LOWER GASTROINTESTINAL DISORDERS

A distance runner has reported the consistent need to stop and have a bowel movement while training. Is this normal for runners? What can be done about the situation?

Lower GI disorders occur distal to the stomach. Common symptoms associated with lower GI problems include diarrhea, constipation, rectal bleeding, and hemorrhoids. Many lower GI disorders are managed by increasing dietary fiber and avoiding irritating foods.

Diarrhea

Anxiety and precompetition jitters commonly result in "nervous diarrhea." **Diarrhea**, a common and troublesome disorder, is characterized by abnormally loose, watery stools. This is caused by food residue running through the large intestine before that organ has had sufficient time to absorb the remaining water. Prolonged diarrhea can lead to dehydration and depletion of electrolytes, particularly sodium, bicarbonate, and potassium. Common among runners, runner's diarrhea or runner's trots is caused by increased intestinal motility that can lead to several patterns of bowel dysfunction **(Box 19.1)**. If this is a known problem, the athlete should do light exercise before competition to help empty the bowels, and drink extra water to maintain hydration.

➤ MANAGEMENT

Diarrhea may respond to certain antidiarrheal medications, which reduce intestinal movement, increase fluid absorption, modify intestinal bacteria, or reduce inflammation associated with diarrhea. Pepto-Bismol, loperamid (Imodium), or diphenoxylate with atropine (Lomotil) may help; however, these products should not be used on a regular basis. An attempt should be made to defecate at a regular daily time, taking advantage of the morning **gastrocolic reflex** (propulsive reflex in the colon that stimulates defecation). Peristalsis and defecation can be stimulated by drinking coffee or tea, having a light meal before competition, and then jogging to stimulate the gastrocolic reflex. Exercise, specifically more than what the body is accus-

---

➤➤ **Box 19.1**

Patterns of Bowel Dysfunction Found in Runners

1. Nervous diarrhea prior to competition
   - More common in women
   - Occurs in runners with:
     - Irregular bowel function when not running
     - History of lactose intolerance
2. The need to stop and have a bowel movement while training
   - More common in men during the first few miles of a run
   - Occurs in runners:
     - With irregular bowel function
     - Who eat prior to running
     - Who do a morning run before breakfast
3. Cramps and diarrhea without blood in the stool, after hard running
   - Common in runners; associated with severe lower abdominal cramps, nausea, and vomiting
4. Cramps and diarrhea with blood in the stool, after hard running
   - Associated with diarrhea, severe lower abdominal cramps, and rectal bleeding

tomed to, increases intestinal activity. Therefore, athletes may want to:

- Immediately decrease the level of training and competition by 20 to 40% in both mileage and intensity until the episode passes, then build back up slowly.
- Eliminate foods that trigger bowel irritation, including dairy products if lactose intolerance is involved, excessive juices, fresh fruits, raisin and other dried fruits, beans, and lentils.
- Limit the amount of sugar-free gum and hard candies that contain sorbitol, which can cause diarrhea.
- Improve hydration before and during exercise to increase plasma volume and decrease intestinal mucosal ischemia.

Athletes on a low-fiber diet may benefit from adding fiber to absorb excess fluids. In contrast, athletes on a high-fiber diet may benefit by reducing fiber to decrease stimulation of intestinal motility. To identify food triggers, the athlete should keep a food/diarrhea chart. Take away any suspected food for a few days, then eat a big portion and observe changes in bowel movements. Food usually moves through the intestines in 2 to 4 days. A simple way to identify your body's "transit time" is to eat corn, sesame seeds, or beets, foods that can be seen in the feces. An increase in clear liquids 24 to 48 hours should be followed by a readjustment to a regular diet (1,2).

Constipation

Infrequent or incomplete bowel movements (constipation) is not a disease but rather a description of symptoms that may indicate a more serious underlying condition. Potential causes include lack of fiber in the diet, improper bowel habits, lack of exercise, emotional distress, diabetes mellitus, pregnancy, laxative abuse, and drug effects (diuretics, bile acid binders, calcium supplements, aluminum antacids, antidepressants, antihistamines, antihypertensives, antispasmodics, and narcotic pain relievers) (3,4).

➤ MANAGEMENT

Management depends on the origin. Athletes who have a low-fiber diet should gradually increase the intake of high-fiber foods. Fiber absorbs water and makes feces softer and easier to eliminate. Bran cereals are the richest fiber foods, superior to salads and many vegetables and fruits. Increasing daily exercise, particularly aerobic exercise, and ensuring adequate fluid intake can alleviate symptoms. Laxatives or suppositories are useful, but should be used sparingly and only for short-term treatment. Laxatives stimulate and promote bowel emptying. They work by holding water and swelling in the intestines, while stool softeners work by mixing fat and water into fecal matter. Some common over-the-counter stool softeners include Dulcolax, Senokot, Metamucil, and Citrucel.

In addition to medications, drinking warm clear fluids (e.g., juice, soda, broth), particularly in the morning, can stimulate bowel activity. The body naturally wants to defecate about a half hour after consuming a warm beverage in the morning. Time should be allotted to relax and honor this urge. Drink plenty of fluids throughout the day, but no more than a half cup of prune juice. You can determine if you are drinking enough fluids if you urinate every 2 to 4 hours, and the urine is light colored like lemonade, not dark like apple cider. In chronic constipation, surgical intervention may be necessary.

Hemorrhoids

Hemorrhoids are dilations of the venous plexus surrounding the rectal and anal area. They are most common during pregnancy, and in those over age 30. The dilated sacs become exposed if they protrude internally into the rectal and anal canals (polyps), or externally around the anal opening. Several factors increase the incidence of hemorrhoids, including constipation, diarrhea, straining during physical exertion, pelvic congestion, enlargement of the prostate, uterine fibroids, rectal tumors, varicose veins, and pregnancy.

➤ SIGNS AND SYMPTOMS

Pain, itching, and passing small amounts of bright red blood upon defecation, separate from the feces, are the most common signs and symptoms.

➤ MANAGEMENT

The condition will normally heal within 2 to 3 weeks. Medicated rectal anesthetic preparations can be used to relieve pain, itching, and irritation. Forms include suppository, cream, ointment, and aerosol foam. Preparation-H, Proctofoam, Tucks Pads, and Tronolane are all over-the-counter rectal preparations. Pain or swelling can also be relieved by following suggestions listed in **Box 19.2**.

➤➤ **Box 19.2**

Reducing the Inflammation of Hemorrhoids

- Take warm sitz baths for 15 minutes several times a day, especially after bowel movements.
- Use stool softeners to prevent constipation, and products to ease friction (i.e., petroleum jelly applied around the anus).
- Increase fiber in the diet by adding unprocessed bran to breakfast cereals, and eating other high-roughage food.
- Drink plenty of water and other clear fluids.
- Do not ignore the urge for bowel movements, as delay builds up pressure in the rectum and increases the chance of constipation and development of hemorrhoids.
- Exercise to promote good abdominal muscle tone.
- Avoid pushing too hard or too long during bowel movements.

If these suggestions are not successful, immediate physician referral is indicated. Prescribed nitroglycerin ointment applied over the inflamed area has been found to relieve hemorrhoid pain in about 5 minutes (5). In severe cases, however, surgery may be necessary.

Athletes who participate in contact or collision sports (e.g., boxing, football, and ice hockey) may normally experience small amounts of blood on defecation. In many endurance runners, blood in fecal material is caused by gastrointestinal bleeding and is quite common and normal. This bleeding can lead to iron-deficiency anemia, discussed in Chapter 25 with concerns of the female athlete. If moderate amounts of blood are mixed with feces, however, a full evaluation by a physician should be conducted.

The runner's condition is not unusual. Find out if there is a history of irregular bowel function, eating prior to running, or running before breakfast. A high-fiber diet, an increase in daily exercise and fluid intake, and over-the-counter antimotility medication may be recommended. If the condition continues, the individual should see a physician to rule out other conditions.

OTHER GASTROINTESTINAL PROBLEMS

Three hours after eating a pregame meal, several members of a softball team develop stomach cramping, nausea, and diarrhea. With these signs and symptoms, how will you manage the condition? What detrimental effects, if any, will this situation have on the players' performance?

Certain factors, though they may not be related to an injury or condition specific to the upper or lower gastrointestinal tract, may affect the entire GI tract. Anxiety and stress, vomiting, and food poisoning are three such conditions.

Anxiety and Stress Reaction

Performance anxiety and pregame stress are common in competing athletes. Upper GI tract function can be affected through decreased acid secretion in the stomach, slowed intestinal motility, or decreased blood flow. Continued anxiety can lead to hypersecretion of stomach acids, increased motility, or decreased transit time.

➤ SIGNS AND SYMPTOMS
Common symptoms include a dry mouth, dyspepsia, gastroesophageal reflux, heartburn, abdominal cramping, or diarrhea.

➤ MANAGEMENT
Treatment involves reassurance and education about the body's processes; relaxation techniques such as deep breathing, passive and active relaxation, soothing music,

smiling, and therapeutic massage; and behavior modification using cognitive restructuring, concentration skills, confidence training, coping rehearsal, imagery, and positive self-talk. Many of these intervention strategies were discussed in Chapter 7.

Vomiting

Vomiting involves the oral ejection of stomach contents from reverse peristaltic contractions of voluntary and involuntary muscles. It is often preceded by a watering mouth and nausea. It often results from the intake of irritating foods and other intestinal irritants, stress, excessive alcohol or other drug consumption, or food poisoning.

➤ MANAGEMENT
Vomiting is best managed by first comforting the athlete and maintaining a clear airway. The mouth should be rinsed and monitored for repeated vomiting, followed by the administration of antinausea medication and clear fluids to prevent dehydration.

If food poisoning is expected or if blood is found in the vomit, an immediate physician referral is necessary. Vomiting can also be an early sign of pregnancy, particularly if it occurs in the morning hours.

Food Poisoning

The most common cause of food poisoning is contaminated food. However, food poisoning can also stem from insecticides or infectious organisms (bacteria from the salmonella group, certain staphylococci, streptococci, or dysentery bacilli) from food that is undercooked or decomposed.

➤ SIGNS AND SYMPTOMS
Food poisoning includes varying levels of abdominal gas and pain, nausea, vomiting, low-grade fever, and diarrhea. These signs and symptoms can begin 1 to 6 hours after ingestion of contaminated foods, and may last for 1 to 3 days. Dehydration from the vomiting and diarrhea can lead to weakness, fatigue, and an increased risk of heat illness.

➤ MANAGEMENT
Mild symptoms are treated conservatively with rapid replacement of fluids and electrolytes, and administration of an antidiarrheal agent. If tolerated, light fluids, broth, or bouillon with a small amount of salt, poached eggs, or bland cereals may be given.

Severe cases require activation of EMS. Fluids must be replaced intravenously, and pumping of the stomach contents may be necessary. If possible, samples of the vomitus should accompany the individual who is transported to the nearest medical facility. This can aid in identifying the food responsible for the poisoning.

Within 3 hours of eating the pregame meal, the softball players had abdominal cramps, nausea, and diarrhea. Because of the number of players exhibiting the same signs and symptoms, you should suspect food poisoning. The management plan includes administration of an antidiarrheal agent, drinking clear fluids, and rest. Frequent diarrhea can decrease athletic performance because of dehydration that leads to weakness, fatigue, and an increased risk of heat illness.

Summary

1. Exercise-induced shunting can lead to decreased esophageal motility, erosive hemorrhagic gastritis, delayed gastric emptying, diarrhea, or intestinal bleeding. Dehydration, high ambient temperatures, and lack of acclimatization can all exacerbate hypoperfusion of the GI tract.

2. Many upper GI tract disorders are caused by irritation due to stress or the ingestion of caffeine, alcohol, or tomato and citric acid products, leading to nausea, vomiting, bloating, abdominal cramps, and heartburn.

3. Gastroesophageal reflux is associated with the regurgitation of gastric juices into the esophagus. Dyspepsia, or indigestion, is associated with upper gastrointestinal pain with no identified etiology. Both are treated with antacids taken 4 hours prior to exercise.

4. Peptic ulcers generally occur at the lower end of the esophagus, in the stomach, or in the duodenum. Antacids may reduce or neutralize stomach acids and prevent them from moving into the esophagus, reducing heartburn and discomfort.

5. Gastroenteritis is second in incidence only to upper respiratory tract infections in adolescents and adults, and is caused by viral or bacterial infection, allergic reaction, medication, contaminated food, or emotional stress. The condition is self-limiting and usually clears in 2 to 3 days. Treatment includes eliminating irritating foods from the diet, avoiding factors that bring on anxiety and stress, and avoiding dehydration.

6. Diarrhea, common among runners, is caused by increased intestinal motility. Antidiarrheal medications reduce intestinal movement, increase fluid absorption, modify intestinal bacteria, or reduce inflammation associated with diarrhea. If this is a known problem, the athlete should try to defecate before exercise, and should not eat prior to running.

7. Hemorrhoids are dilations of the venous plexus surrounding the rectal and anal area. Pain, itching, and passing small amounts of bright red blood upon defecation, separate from the feces, are the most common signs and symptoms. Medicated rectal anesthetic preparations can be used to relieve pain, itching, and irritation. The condition will normally heal within 2 to 3 weeks.

8. Anxiety and stress can lead to decreased acid secretion in the stomach, slower intestinal motility, or decreased blood flow. Continued anxiety can lead to hypersecretion of stomach acids, increased motility, or decreased transit time. Treatment involves reassurance and education about the body's processes, relaxation techniques, and behavior modification.

9. Vomiting may be caused by irritating foods and other intestinal irritants, stress, excessive alcohol or drug consumption, or food poisoning. Although it often can be treated conservatively with antinausea medication and clear fluids to prevent dehydration, it may be an early sign of pregnancy, particularly if it occurs in the morning hours. Persistent vomiting signals a more serious condition, in which case immediate referral to a physician is warranted.

References

1. Torres JL, Mellion MB. Gastrointestinal problems. In: The Team Physician's Handbook. Edited by Mellion MB, Walsh WM, Shelton GL. Philadelphia: Hanley & Belfus, 1997.

2. Clark N. Process of elimination. Am Fitness 1998;16(3):58-59.

3. Martin M, Yates WN. Therapeutic Medications in Sports Medicine. Baltimore: Williams & Wilkins, 1998.

4. Consumers Union. Pillbox: Laxatives and alternatives. Consumer Reports Health 1998;10(4):8-9.

5. Men's Health. Fast relief from a pain in the butt. Men's Health 1997;12(9):144.

20

The Diabetic Athlete

OBJECTIVES

1. Explain how insulin regulates blood glucose levels.

2. Explain the physiological basis of diabetes.

3. List and describe the four types of diabetes mellitus.

4. Describe what circulatory and neural complications can result from diabetes mellitus.

5. Contrast the signs and symptoms of insulin shock and diabetic coma.

6. Describe how to manage insulin shock and diabetic coma.

7. List nutritional recommendations for a type 1 and type 2 diabetic athlete.

8. List physical activities that are indicated and contraindicated for a physically active individual with diabetes.

Diabetes mellitus (DM) is a chronic metabolic disorder characterized by near or absolute lack of the hormone insulin, insulin resistance, or both. The disease affects approximately 15 million Americans, and ranks seventh among the leading causes of death in the United States. In addition, the disease can contribute to a variety of other major diseases, including heart disease and stroke. In fact, individuals with diabetes are twice as likely to develop these cardiovascular conditions as someone without diabetes (1). Several factors increase the risk and severity of diabetes, including heredity, increasing age, minority ethnicity, obesity, being female, stress, infection, a sedentary lifestyle, and a diet high in carbohydrates and fat.

THE PHYSIOLOGICAL BASIS OF DIABETES

Carbohydrates in human nutrition supply the body's cells with glucose to deliver energy to the body's systems. Upon eating, a person's blood glucose rises, stimulating the pancreas to release insulin. Under normal conditions, blood glucose ranges between 80 and 120 mg/dL. Insulin's main effect is to lower blood sugar levels, but it also stimulates amino acid uptake, fat metabolism, and influences protein synthesis in muscle tissue. Insulin lowers blood sugar by enhancing membrane transport of glucose (and other simple sugars) from the blood, into body cells, especially the skeletal and cardiac muscles (**Figure 20.1**). It does not accelerate glucose entry into

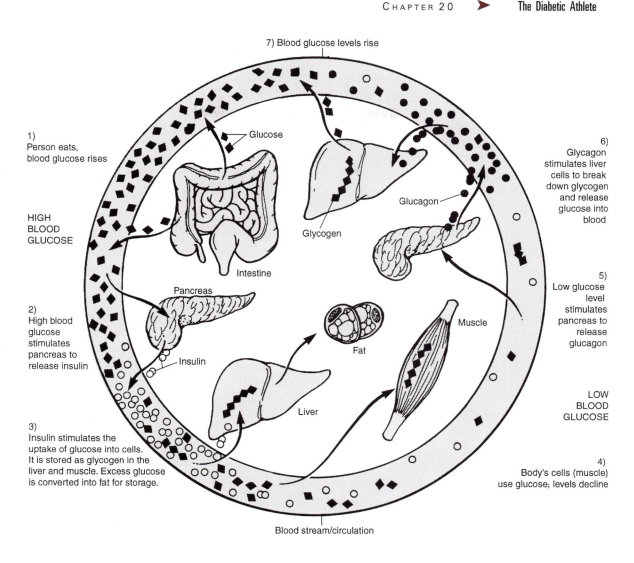

7) Blood glucose levels rise

1) Person eats, blood glucose rises

HIGH BLOOD GLUCOSE

2) High blood glucose stimulates pancreas to release insulin

3) Insulin stimulates the uptake of glucose into cells. It is stored as glycogen in the liver and muscle. Excess glucose is converted into fat for storage.

Glucose

Glycogen

Glucagon

Intestine

Pancreas

Insulin

Liver

Fat

Muscle

6) Glycagon stimulates liver cells to break down glycogen and release glucose into blood

5) Low glucose level stimulates pancreas to release glucagon

LOW BLOOD GLUCOSE

4) Body's cells (muscle) use glucose; levels decline

Blood stream/circulation

Glycogen

➤ **FIGURE 20.1 Maintaining a balance of blood glucose.** Insulin must be available to stimulate uptake of blood glucose into the body's cells. As the cells use glucose, blood levels decline and the liver responds by releasing glucagon into the bloodstream. Glucagon stimulates liver cells to break down stored glycogen and releases glucose into the blood, thereby raising the level of blood glucose to normal levels. (Adapted from Whitney EN, Rolfes SR. Understanding Nutrition. Belmont, CA: Wadsworth Publishing, 1999:105.)

liver, kidney, and brain tissue, all of which have easy access to blood glucose regardless of insulin levels. After glucose enters the target cells, insulin:

- Promotes the oxidation of glucose for ATP production
- Joins glucose together to form glycogen
- Converts glucose to fat for storage (particularly in adipose tissue)

As a general rule, energy needs are met first, then liver and muscle cells can assemble the excess single glucose cells into long, branching chains of glycogen for storage. The liver cells can also convert excess glucose to fat for export to other cells. High blood glucose levels return to normal as excess glucose is stored as glycogen (which can be converted back to glucose) and fat (which cannot be).

When blood glucose falls (as occurs between meals), other special cells of the pancreas respond by secreting glucagon into the blood. **Glucagon** raises blood glucose by stimulating the liver to dismantle its glycogen stores and release glucose into the blood for use by the body's cells. Epinephrine, another hormone, can also stimulate the liver cells to return glucose to the blood from liver glycogen. This "fight-or-flight" response is often triggered when a person experiences stress.

When insulin activity is absent or deficient as in diabetes, blood sugar remains high after a meal because glucose is unable to move into most tissue cells, causing blood glucose levels to increase to abnormally high levels. Increased osmotic blood pressure drives fluid from the cells into the vascular system, leading to cell dehydration. The excess glucose is passed into the kidneys, resulting in **poly-**

uria, a huge urine output of water and electrolytes that leads to decreased blood volume and further dehydration. Serious electrolyte losses also occur as the body rids itself of excess ketones. Since ketones are negatively charged ions, they carry positive ions out with them; as a result, sodium and potassium ions are lost. An electrolyte imbalance leads to abdominal pains, possible vomiting, and the stress reaction spirals. Dehydration stimulates the hypothalamic thirst centers, causing **polydypsia,** or excessive thirst. In response, the body shifts from carbohydrate metabolism to fat metabolism for energy. The final cardinal sign, **polyphagia,** refers to excessive hunger and food consumption, a sign that the person is "starving." Thus, although plenty of glucose is available, it cannot be used. In severe cases, blood levels of fatty acids and their metabolites rise dramatically, producing an excess of ketoacids, resulting in acidosis. Acetone, formed as a by-product of fat metabolism, is volatile and blown off during expiration, giving the breath a sweet or fruity odor. If the condition is not rectified with insulin injection, further dehydration and **ketoacidosis** result as the ketones begin to spill into the urine **(ketonuria).** If untreated, ketoacidosis disrupts virtually all physiological processes, including heart activity and oxygen transport. Severe depression of the nervous system leads to confusion, drowsiness, coma, and finally, death.

TYPES OF DIABETES

The National Diabetes Data Group and the World Health Organization recognize four types of diabetes mellitus: type 1, type 2, gestational diabetes mellitus (GDM), and diabetes secondary to other conditions. Each group is characterized by high blood glucose levels, or **hyperglycemia.** For individuals with symptoms of DM, such as excessive thirst and urination or unexplained weight loss, only an elevated fasting plasma glucose (FPG) >140 mg/dL, or a random venous plasma glucose >200 mg/dL is required to confirm the diagnosis. Because athletic trainers will most likely encounter physically active individuals with type 1 or type 2 DM, these conditions will receive more focus, and are compared in **Table 20.1.**

Type 1 Diabetes Mellitus

In type 1, the pancreas cannot synthesize insulin. As such, the individual must obtain insulin to assist the cells in taking up the needed fuels from the blood. The insulin must be injected; it cannot be taken orally because insulin is a protein and the gastrointestinal enzymes would digest it. Type 1 DM (formerly called insulin-dependent diabetes [IDDM] or juvenile diabetes) is considered to be an autoimmune disorder, and is one of the most frequent chronic childhood diseases. The onset is usually acute, developing over a period of a few days to weeks. More than 95% of individuals who develop type 1 DM are under 25 years of

age, with equal incidence in both sexes and an increased prevalence in the white population (2). A family history of type 1 DM or other endocrine disease is found in a small number of cases. The disease typically has an onset prior to age 30 in people who are typically not obese, however, it can begin at any age. Obese individuals generally have a more severe time balancing glucose levels, the effects of exercise on the metabolic state are more pronounced, and the management of exercise-related problems is more difficult.

Type 2 Diabetes Mellitus

Formerly called non-insulin-dependent diabetes (NIDDM) or adult-onset, type 2 DM is the most common form of diabetes (90 to 95% of all cases) (1,3). It is highly associated with a family history of diabetes, older age, obesity, and lack of exercise. It is also more common in women with a history of gestational diabetes, and in blacks, Native Americans, and Hispanics (2). Although the exact cause of type 2 DM is unknown, high blood glucose and insulin resistance are major contributing factors. The insulin resistance is related to an insulin secretory defect of the beta cells, which prohibit or limit the transfer of insulin across the

TABLE 20.1   COMPARISON OF TYPE 1 AND TYPE 2 DIABETES

	Type 1	Type 2
Former names	Juvenile-onset diabetes Insulin-dependent diabetes mellitus	Adult-onset diabetes Non-insulin-dependent diabetes mellitus
Age of onset	Usually before 30	Usually after 30
Type of onset	Abrupt (days to weeks)	Usually gradual (weeks to months)
Nutritional status	Almost always lean	Usually obese
Insulin production	Negligible to absent	Present, but may be in excess and ineffective due to obesity
Insulin	Needed for all patients	Necessary in only 20 to 30% of patients
Diet	Mandatory along with insulin for control of blood glucose	Diet alone is frequently sufficient to control blood glucose
High incidence	White population	Women with history of gestational diabetes Blacks Native Americans Hispanics
Family history	Minor	Common link

cellular membrane. As such, the individual may actually have higher-than-average insulin levels, but the cells respond less sensitively to it; that is, they become insulin resistant. Like type 1 DM, blood glucose rises too high (hyperglycemia). The high blood glucose stimulates the pancreas to make insulin, exhausting these cells and reducing their ability to make insulin. Therefore, type 2 DM appears to be a self-aggravating condition (1).

Onset is typically after age 40, but is also seen in obese children. Obesity, a major factor in adults, affects nearly 90% of adults with type 2 DM. Compared to normal-weight individuals, obese people require much more insulin to maintain normal blood glucose. More insulin is produced, but as body fat increases, insulin receptors are reduced in number and ability to function. Consequently, insulin resistance increases, and adipose and muscle tissues become less and less able to take up glucose. At some point, the body cannot supply enough insulin to keep up, and type 2 DM develops.

Gestational Diabetes Mellitus (GDM)

Gestational DM is an operational classification (rather than a pathophysiological condition) that identifies women who develop DM during **gestation** (pregnancy). The condition is associated with older age, obesity, and a family history of diabetes. Women who are diagnosed with DM before pregnancy are not included in this group. Women who develop type 1 DM during pregnancy and women with undiagnosed asymptomatic type 2 DM that is discovered during pregnancy are classified with GDM. Most women classified with GDM have normal glucose homeostasis during the first half of the pregnancy, but the mother's blood glucose rises due to hormones secreted during the later half of the pregnancy. As a result, the mother cannot produce enough insulin to handle the higher blood glucose, leading to hyperglycemia. The hyperglycemia usually resolves after delivery, but places the woman at risk for developing type 2 DM later in life.

Diabetes Secondary to Other Conditions

Types of DM from various known causes are grouped together to form the classification called "other specific types." The group includes those with genetic defects of beta-cell function (formerly called MODY or maturity-onset diabetes in youth) or with defects of insulin action and persons with pancreatic disease, hormonal disease, and drug or chemical exposure (3).

COMPLICATIONS OF DIABETES MELLITUS

 A diabetic basketball player has suddenly gotten very dizzy and is complaining of a headache, but is very hungry. You notice that the individual is sweating profusely, the skin appears pale and clammy, movement is somewhat clumsy, and the person appears to be swallowing an excessive number of times. You suspect low blood sugar or hypoglycemia. How will you manage this condition?

In types 1 and 2 DM, glucose fails to enter into the cells and accumulates in the blood, which can lead to both acute and chronic complications. **Figure 20.2** illustrates some of the metabolic consequences of untreated diabetes. Over the long term, these metabolic changes can lead to serious chronic complications. Chronically elevated blood glucose levels can damage the blood vessels and nerves, leading to circulatory and neural damage. Failure to adequately balance nutrition, exercise, insulin injections, and blood glucose levels can also cause a physically active individual to experience insulin shock or diabetic coma.

Circulatory Complications

Coronary heart disease (CHD), the most common form of cardiovascular disease, usually involves atherosclerosis and hypertension. Atherosclerosis is the accumulation of lipids and other materials in the arteries. The condition begins with the accumulation of soft fatty deposits along the inner arterial wall, especially at branch points. These deposits eventually enlarge and become hardened with minerals, forming plaque, which hardens and narrows the arteries. Blood platelets cause clots to form whenever an injury occurs. Under normal conditions, these clots form and dissolve in blood all the time, but with atherosclerosis, clots form faster than they are dissolved. In diabetics, atherolosclerosis tends to develop early, progress rapidly, and be more severe. More than 80% of people with diabetes die as a result of cardiovascular diseases, especially heart attacks (1). Complications in the capillaries may also lead to impaired kidney function and retinal degeneration with accompanying loss of vision. About 85% of people with diabetes have impaired kidney function, loss of vision, or both (1). Consequently, diabetes is the leading cause of kidney failure and blindness.

Nerve Complications

Diabetes also causes nerves to deteriorate. The initial symptom is often a painful prickling sensation in the arms and legs. Later, loss of sensation may occur in the hands and feet. Injuries to these area may go unnoticed, and infections can progress rapidly. With both circulatory impairment and loss of sensation, undetected injuries and infection may lead to aseptic necrosis of tissue **(gangrene)**, necessitating amputation of the limbs (most often the feet or legs). For this reason, it is critical that diabetics take very good care of their feet and visit a podiatrist regularly. To minimize trauma, use silica gel shoe inserts and wear cotton-polyester socks to prevent blisters, and keep the feet dry. All open wounds should be treated promptly,

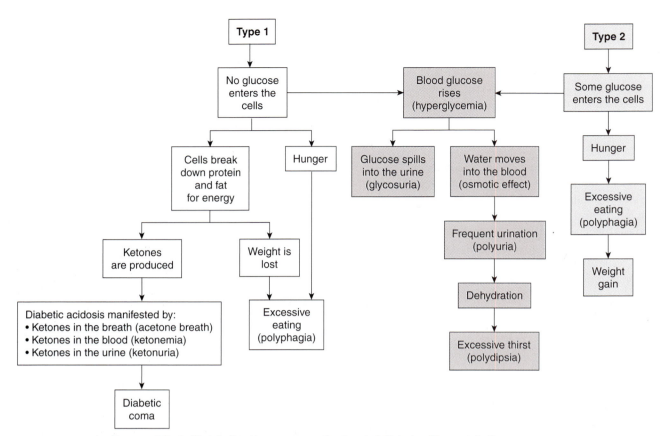

➤ **FIGURE 20.2 Metabolic consequences of untreated diabetes.** The metabolic consequences of type 1 diabetes are more rapid and severe than those of type 2. In type 1 diabetes, no insulin is available to allow glucose to enter the cells, resulting in a cascade of metabolic changes. In type 2 diabetes, some glucose enters the cells. Because the cells are not "starved" for glucose, the body does not shift into the metabolism of fasting (losing weight and producing ketones). (Adapted from Whitney EN, Rolfes SR. Understanding Nutrition. Belmont, CA: Wadsworth Publishing, 1999:579.)

cleaned daily, and carefully checked for infection. Nerve damage can also retard gastric emptying. When the stomach empties slowly after a meal, the person may experience a premature feeling of fullness. This can lead to bloating, nausea, vomiting, weight loss, and poor blood glucose control due to irregular nutrient absorption.

Hypoglycemia

Hypoglycemia, common in type 1 insulin-treated diabetics, can range from very mild lower levels of glucose (60–70 mg/dL) with minimal or no symptoms, to severe hypoglycemia with very low levels of glucose (<40 mg/dL) and neurologic impairment. Although hypoglycemia can occur with any individual, it is critical in a type 1 diabetic because the ability to recover from it is limited. Recovery is mediated by the release of epinephrine, norepinephrine, and glucagon (4). In a diabetic, hypoglycemia associated with insulin therapy may be related to errors in dosage, delayed or skipped meals, exercise, intensity of blood glucose control, variation in absorption of insulin from subcutaneous injection sites, variability of insulin binding, impairment

of counterregulation, and possibly the use of human insulin (3). When left untreated, this condition can lead to insulin shock.

Insulin Shock

Exercise lowers blood sugar, hence any exercise must be counterbalanced with increased food intake or decreased amounts of insulin. If blood glucose falls below normal levels, hypoglycemia results. Although any individual can experience hypoglycemia, it is particularly critical for the diabetic athlete to address the situation immediately.

➤ SIGNS AND SYMPTOMS

Contrary to the slow onset of a diabetic coma, hypoglycemia has a rapid onset. Signs and symptoms include dizziness; headache; intense hunger; aggressive behavior; pale, cold, and clammy skin; and profuse perspiration, salivation, drooling, and tingling in the face, tongue, and lips. Other observable signs may include a staggering gait, clumsy movements, confusion, and a general decrease in performance.

➤ MANAGEMENT

Since glucose levels in the blood are low compared to high levels of insulin, treatment focuses on getting 10 to 15 g of a fast-acting carbohydrate into the system quickly. This can be found in 4 ounces of regular cola or 6 ounces of ginger ale, 4 ounces of apple or orange juice, four packets of table sugar, two tablespoons of raisins, or five to seven Lifesavers (4,6). These should only be given to a conscious person who can swallow well. Chocolates, which contain a high level of fat, should not be used for treating a hypoglycemic reaction because the fat interferes with the absorption of sugar. If the person is unconscious or unable to swallow, roll the individual on his or her side, and pay close attention to the airway so saliva will drain out of the mouth, not into the throat or airway. Place sugar or honey under the tongue, as it will be absorbed through the mucous membrane. Recovery is usually rapid.

After initial recovery, the athlete should wait 15 minutes and check the blood sugar level. If the level is still below 70 mg/dL, or if there is no meter, and the athlete still has symptoms, another 10 to 15 g of carbohydrates are given. Repeat blood testing and treatment until the blood glucose level is normalized (4). Even when blood glucose has returned to normal, physical performance and judgment may still be impaired, or the individual may relapse if the quick sugar influx is quickly depleted. After the symptoms resolve, the individual should be instructed to have a good meal as quickly as possible to increase carbohydrates in the body.

Many diabetic athletes who experience repeated bouts of hypoglycemia have glucagon injection kits that contain a syringe prefilled with a diluting solution and a vial of glucagon powder. Once the solution and powder are mixed, they are injected into the upper arm, thigh, or buttock. Although the diabetic may instruct friends and family members on how to mix, draw up, and inject the glucagon, athletic trainers may not be included in the process. However, it is critical that athletic trainers know whether, and under what circumstances, a glucagon injection should be administered and when to activate EMS. The athletic trainer should be properly trained by the athlete's physician or designee, and permission to administer the solution should be documented.

Diabetic Coma

Without insulin, the body is unable to metabolize glucose, leading to hyperglycemia. As the body shifts from carbohydrate metabolism to fat metabolism, an excess of ketoacids in the blood can lower the blood pH to 7.0 (normal pH is 7.35 to 7.45), leading to a condition called diabetic ketoacidosis (DKA). This is manifested by ketones in the breath (acetone breath), ketones in the blood (ketonemia), and ketones in the urine (ketonuria).

➤ SIGNS AND SYMPTOMS

Symptoms appear gradually and often occur over several days. The individual becomes increasingly restless and confused, and will complain of a dry mouth and intense thirst. Abdominal cramping and vomiting are common. As the individual slips into coma, signs include dry, red, warm skin; eyes that appear deep and sunken; deep, exaggerated respirations; a rapid, weak pulse; and a sweet, fruity acetone breath, similar to nail polish remover.

➤ MANAGEMENT

 As the name implies, diabetic coma is a serious condition and is considered a medical emergency. It is usually not possible to tell with certainty whether an individual is in a diabetic coma or insulin shock (see previous section). Therefore, give the individual glucose or orange juice, if conscious. If recovery is not rapid, then a medical emergency exists, and EMS should be activated. The additional glucose will not worsen the condition, provided the individual is transported immediately. If the person is unconscious or semiconscious, nothing should be given orally. Instead, maintain an open airway, treat the person for shock, and activate EMS, who will deliver an IV solution of insulin to aid the athlete. **Field Strategy 20.1** *summarizes the management of insulin shock and diabetic coma.*

 An individual with low blood sugar needs to get sugar into the system quickly. Give table sugar, honey, sugared candy, orange juice, or a regular soda. Recovery should be rapid. Instruct the individual to have a good meal as soon as possible, and watch the individual closely for any relapse.

NUTRITION AND EXERCISE RECOMMENDATIONS

 A junior high athlete has been diagnosed with diabetes mellitus. What recommendations would you suggest pertaining to nutrition and exercise for this individual?

Controlled diabetes rests on a balance of glucose levels, insulin production, nutrition, and exercise. Prior to any exercise program, a physician should be consulted about diet, and normal blood glucose (BG) levels should be documented, as strenuous exercise is contraindicated for some diabetics. With the advent of blood glucose self-monitoring, exercise is encouraged if certain precautions are followed. Blood glucose levels should be taken 30 minutes before and 1 hour after exercise to see how exercise affects BG. This allows for better regulation of food intake and insulin dosage.

Nutritional Recommendations for Type 1 Diabetes

Normally, the body secretes a constant, baseline amount of insulin at all times and secretes more as blood glucose rises following meals. Individuals with type 1 diabetes must learn to adjust their insulin doses and schedule of adminis-

FIELD STRATEGY 20.1   MANAGEMENT ALGORITHM FOR DIABETIC EMERGENCIES

Look for a medic alert tag
↓
Is the person conscious?
Yes   No
↙   ↘

Administer 10–15 g of fast-acting
carbohydrate:
- 4 oz of regular cola
- 6 oz of ginger ale
- 4 oz of apple or orange juice
- 4 packets of table sugar
- 2 tablespoons of raisins
- 5–7 Lifesavers or other sugared candy
↓
Does the individual show signs of
improvement after the initial
carbohydrates?
Yes   No
↘

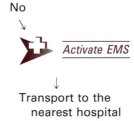 *Activate EMS*

Roll the individual on his or her side
so saliva will drain out of the mouth
↓
Maintain an open airway
↓
Place sugar or fast-acting
carbohydrates under the tongue
↓
Do not give liquids
↓
Transport to the hearest hospital

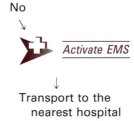 *Activate EMS*
↓
Transport to the
nearest hospital
↓
Wait 15 minutes and check the blood
sugar level
↓
If the blood glucose level is still below
70 mg/dL, or if symptoms persist:
- give another 10–15 g carbohydrates
- repeat blood testing and treatment
  until blood glucose is normalized
↓
After the symptoms resolve:
The individual should eat a good meal
as soon as possible

---

tration to accommodate meals, physical activity, and health status. Recommendations for maintaining optimal nutritional status focus on controlling blood glucose levels, achieving a desirable blood lipid profile, controlling blood pressure, and preventing and managing complications from diabetes. The diet should provide a consistent daily intake of carbohydrates at each meal and snack to minimize fluctuations in blood glucose. A pregame meal should be ingested 1 to 3 hours prior to exercise, and the athlete should have about 10 to 15 grams of additional carbohydrate 30 minutes prior to moderate activity or about 20 to 30 grams of carbohydrate prior to vigorous activity (1). During intense exercise, 15 to 30 grams of carbohydrates should be

ingested every 30 minutes. A snack of carbohydrates should also follow the exercise period. Carbohydrates are readily available from fruits, fruit juices, yogurt, crackers, and other starches.

When exercise lasts for several hours, insulin requirements decrease, hence total insulin dosage should be decreased 20 to 50%. Injection administration is timed so that peak activity does not take place when high insulin levels are present (2 to 4 hours after injection). If this is not possible, due to rain delays in competition or other associated factors, the individual should eat a high carbohydrate snack like juice and crackers, or milk and cookies, about 30 minutes prior to the resumption of activity (5). In addition, food should always be available for supplemental feeding (e.g., in the locker room, on the bus, at half time, in the athletic training kit).

Nutritional Recommendations for Type 2 Diabetes

As with type 1 diabetes, an individual with type 2 diabetes must maintain near-normal blood glucose by delivering the same amount of carbohydrate each day, spaced evenly throughout the day. Eating too much carbohydrate at one time can raise blood glucose too high, stressing the already-compromised insulin-producing cells. Eating too little carbohydrate can lead to hypoglycemia. In addition, those who have elevated blood lipids may need to watch not only their carbohydrates, but also their fat intake. When an individual lowers fat intake, the percentage of calories from carbohydrates increases. A high-carbohydrate diet raises triglycerides and lowers HDL. For those individuals accustomed to a high-fat diet, complying with a low-fat diet may be difficult. When combined with regular exercise, even moderate weight loss (10 to 20 pounds) can improve blood glucose control and blood lipid profiles, help reverse insulin resistance, and reduce blood pressure (1).

Exercise Recommendations

Exercise is a critical component in managing diabetes. Aerobic exercise can decrease the requirements of insulin and increase the body's sensitivity to it. Exercise can also help attain and maintain ideal body weight and decrease the risk for hypertensive diseases, including cardiovascular and peripheral vascular disease, and slow the progression of diabetic **nephropathy** (kidney damage). It is recommended that all exercising diabetics should follow the guidelines listed in **Box 20.1.**

Despite the benefits of exercise, type 2 diabetics who have lost protective neural sensation should not participate in treadmill walking, prolonged walking, jogging, or step exercises. Recommended exercises include low-resistance walking, swimming, bicycling, rowing, chair exercises, arm exercises, and other non-weight-bearing exercises. Sports that require resistance strength training are permissible as long as there are no indications of retinopathy or nephropathy. Scuba diving, rock climbing, and parachuting are strongly discouraged.

The junior high school athlete should exercise and compete, but with caution and under the direct supervision of a physician. You might also recommend eating carbohydrates 1 to 3 hours prior to exercise, ingesting 15 to 30 grams of carbohydrates every 30 minutes during intense exercise, and adjusting his insulin dosage and requirements consistent with the level of exercise.

➤➤ **BOX 20.1**

Guidelines for Safe Exercise
- Have a routine medical examination, and be cleared for activity
- Develop a balanced program of diet and exercise under a physician's supervision
- Wear identification (bracelet, necklace) indicating that the athlete is a diabetic
- Eat at regular times throughout the day
- Avoid exercising at the peak of insulin action and in the evening when hypoglycemia is more apt to occur
- Adjust carbohydrate intake and insulin dosage prior to exercise
- Check blood glucose levels before, during (if possible), and after exercise
- Prevent dehydration by consuming adequate fluids before, during, and after exercise
- Have access to fast-acting carbohydrates during exercise to prevent hypoglycemia
- Avoid alcoholic beverages, or drink them in moderation
- Avoid smoking

Summary

1. Insulin is needed after carbohydrate ingestion to transfer glucose from the blood into the skeletal and cardiac muscles. It also promotes glucose storage in the muscles and liver in the form of glycogen. If little or no insulin is secreted by the pancreas, blood glucose bypasses the body cells and rises to abnormally high levels in the blood. The excess glucose is excreted in the urine, drawing large amounts of water and electrolytes with it, leading to weakness, fatigue, malaise, and increased thirst.

2. When glucose cannot enter the cells, the cells shift from carbohydrate metabolism to fat metabolism for energy, resulting in dehydration and ketoacidosis, which can depress cerebral function. Acetone, formed as a by-product of fat metabolism, is volatile and blown off during expiration, giving the breath a sweet or fruity odor.

3. There are four types of diabetes mellitus:
   - Type 1 (insulin-dependent) DM has an onset prior to age 30 in people who are not obese.
   - Type 2 (non-insulin-dependent) DM has an onset after age 40 and is the most common form of diabetes. It is highly associated with a family history of diabetes, older age, obesity, and lack of exercise.
   - Gestational DM occurs when the mother cannot produce enough insulin to handle the higher blood glucose due to hormones secreted during the later half of pregnancy. The condition usually resolves after delivery, but places the woman at risk for developing type 2 DM later in life.

- Diabetes secondary to other conditions includes individuals with genetic defects of beta-cell function or with defects of insulin action and persons with pancreatic disease, hormonal disease, and drug or chemical exposure.

4. Chronic diabetes can lead to atherosclerosis and coronary heart disease, kidney failure, blindness, and impaired neural function, whereby the individual may become unaware of injuries or infections of the hands and feet.

5. Severe hypoglycemia can lead to insulin shock, which has a rapid onset with dizziness; headache; intense hunger; aggressive behavior; pale, cold, and clammy skin; profuse perspiration, salivation, and drooling; and tingling in the face, tongue, and lips.

6. An individual will progress into a diabetic coma (hyperglycemia) over a long period of time. Common symptoms include a dry mouth, intense thirst, abdominal pain, confusion, and fever. Severe signs include deep respirations; rapid, weak pulse; dry, red, warm skin; and a sweet, fruity acetone breath.

7. Because it may be difficult to determine which condition is present, give a fast-acting carbohydrate to the individual. If the individual is in insulin shock, recovery is usually rapid. If recovery does not occur, activate EMS, and transport the individual immediately to the nearest medical facility.

8. A diabetic athlete should have a consistent daily intake of carbohydrates at each meal and snack to minimize blood glucose fluctuations. A pregame meal should be eaten 1 to 3 hours prior to exercise, and 10 to 15 grams of carbohydrates should be ingested 30 minutes prior to moderate activity; 20 to 30 grams prior to vigorous activity. In addition, 15 to 30 grams of carbohydrates should be ingested every 30 minutes during exercise.

9. Aerobic, low-resistance exercise is recommended for the diabetic athlete. The program should be established under the guidance of a supervising physician.

References

1. Whitney EN, Rolfes SR. Understanding Nutrition. Belmont, CA: Wadsworth Publishing, 1999.
2. Mayfield M. Diagnosis and classification of diabetes mellitus: New criteria. Am Fam Phys 1998;58(6):1355-1363.
3. National Institutes of Health. Diabetes in America. Washington, DC: National Institute of Diabetes and Digestive and Kidney Diseases, 1995.
4. Jimenez CC. Diabetes and exercise: The role of the athletic trainer. J Ath Train 1997;32(4):339-343.
5. Small E, Bar-Or O. The young athlete with chronic disease. Clin Sports Med 1995;14(3):709-726.
6. Seitzman A, Anderson C. Lower your risk for lows. Diabetes Forecast 1998;51(6):60-65.

CHAPTER 21

Common Infectious Diseases

OBJECTIVES

1. List the most common childhood diseases that can be prevented through early vaccinations.

2. Describe the characteristic lesions and associated symptoms of the more common childhood diseases.

3. Describe the mode of transmission, incubation period, common signs and symptoms, and treatment of infectious mononucleosis.

4. List the signs and symptoms of viral meningitis.

5. Differentiate the signs and symptoms of the more common sexually transmitted diseases (STDs).

6. State which STDs can be successfully treated and how.

7. List the five different classifications of hepatitis, and differentiate their modes of transmission.

8. Describe the early signs and symptoms of hepatitis, and identify how these symptoms progress in severity.

9. Identify the common signs and symptoms of AIDS.

10. Review the safety precautions that can be taken in an athletic training room to minimize the transmission of highly infectious diseases.

Although it is not the intention of this chapter to discuss all infectious diseases to which sport participants may be exposed, there are several common diseases that may confront the athletic trainer. For some of these childhood diseases, vaccines exist that can prevent infection in fully vaccinated children. However, in older populations, individuals may not have received necessary booster shots to prevent the onset of various illnesses. Chicken pox, mumps, measles (rubeola), rubella (German measles), and influenza are among the more common infections transmitted.

Sexually transmitted diseases (STDs) continue to be a major concern for health care providers working with teenagers and college students, most of whom are sexually active. Chlamydia, candidiasis, and trichomoniasis are common STDs that can affect sport performance. If diagnosed and treated early, they are more annoying than troublesome. There are, however, several serious STDs, such as hepatitis and acquired immunodeficiency syndrome (AIDS), that deserve special attention.

This chapter will address the signs and symptoms, identification, and treatment of common childhood diseases, STDs, and other common infectious conditions such as mononucleosis. Although definitive diagnosis and treatment will be done by a physician, it is critical that the athletic trainer initially recognize a potential condition and make immediate referral to the primary care physician or team physician.

COMMON CHILDHOOD DISEASES

 A male swimmer is complaining of a swollen throat, difficulty in swallowing, and a mild fever. There are also notable irregular, brownish-pink spots around the hairline and extending down the neck onto the shoulders and arms. In taking a history of the problem, what questions might you ask this athlete to determine a possible cause of the condition?

Today most bacterial and viral infectious childhood diseases are prevented through a series of early vaccinations given between birth and 18 months. Booster shots are given upon entry into school (ages 4 to 6) and again in adolescence (ages 11 to 12 and/or 14 to 16). To maintain immunity to diphtheria and tetanus, booster vaccinations should be given every 10 years. Hepatitis, because of its bloodborne transmission and its significance to athletic trainers, will be discussed in more detail later in the chapter.

Bacterial Childhood Diseases

In the United States, infants are immunized against diphtheria, tetanus, and pertussis (DTP) and *Haemophilus influenzae* type b (Hib). Despite this, a few cases of diphtheria and tetanus are reported each year in nonimmunized or partially immunized adults. Hib is one of the leading causes of invasive bacterial disease in children under 5 years of age, and is the leading cause of meningitis in this age group (1).

DIPHTHERIA

Diphtheria, caused by the organism *Corynebacterium diphtheriae*, invades the upper respiratory region. The organism irritates the tissue producing a pseudomembrane (false membrane).

➤ SIGNS AND SYMPTOMS

The characteristic symptom is a thick, patchy, gray membrane that forms over the mucous membranes of the pharynx, larynx, tonsils, soft palate, and nose. Other symptoms include fever, sore throat, a rasping cough, hoarseness, and enlarged tender cervical lymph nodes. If untreated, the pseudomembrane, along with swelling, may occlude the air passages, leading to death by suffocation, or the infection may spread throughout the body, leading

to death from its adverse effects on the heart, nerves, and kidneys. Transmission is by direct contact, droplet spread, and indirect contact with articles soiled with discharges from infected persons.

➤ MANAGEMENT

 Immediate referral to a physician is warranted. Treatment involves the administration of a diphtheria antitoxin and antibiotics to destroy the organism.

TETANUS

The tetanus bacillus, *Clostridium tetani*, grows in the absence of oxygen (anaerobically) in soil, dust, feces, and saliva. Tetanus spores invade the body, usually through a puncture wound, or through lacerations, burns, trivial or unnoticed wounds, or by injected contaminated street drugs.

➤ SIGNS AND SYMPTOMS

Abdominal rigidity is usually followed by painful muscle contractions, primarily of the masseter and neck muscles, although the trunk muscles may also be involved. Contractions of the neck and facial muscles lead to locked jaw, and a grinning expression. Other symptoms include tachycardia, profuse sweating, and low-grade fever.

➤ MANAGEMENT

 Because of the serious nature of tetanus, all wounds should be thoroughly cleansed following standard protocol (see Chapter 5). In puncture wounds, bite wounds, and more significant lacerations or burns, a booster shot is recommended as soon as possible (within 72 hours) if the time from the previous booster is greater than 5 years. If the tetanus antitoxin is administered before the toxin becomes attached to nerve tissue, the toxin will be neutralized.

PERTUSSIS (WHOOPING COUGH)

Pertussis is caused by the bacillus *Bordetella pertussis*. It is an extremely contagious respiratory infection common to children, yet remains the most common of all diseases preventable by routine childhood immunization (2).

➤ SIGNS AND SYMPTOMS

There are three stages of whooping cough: catarrhal (insidious), paroxysmal (sudden and periodic), and convalescent. The catarrhal state begins with an insidious onset of an irritating cough, particularly at night, which may be accompanied by anorexia, sneezing, listlessness, conjunctivitis, and a low-grade fever. The cough becomes progressively more irritating, violent, and eventually paroxysmal within 1 to 2 weeks. The repeated episodes of violent coughing are interspersed with inhalations that feature a crowing or high-pitched whoop. In older children and in adults, the whoop may be absent, but persistent coughing spells are present. These attacks frequently end with the expulsion of clear mucus followed by vomiting caused by choking on mucus. The coughing can be violent enough to cause a nosebleed, detached retina, and hernia. The child is also highly susceptible to secondary infections during this stage, such as otitis media (middle ear infection), pneumonia, or encephalopathy (brain damage). This stage lasts between 2 and 4 weeks. The final stage, the convalescent stage, may last 1 to 2 months, with even a mild upper respiratory infection triggering symptoms.

➤ MANAGEMENT

Immediate referral to a physician is warranted. Antibiotics are only effective in the early stages (before the persistent coughing spells).

HAEMOPHILUS INFLUENZAE TYPE B

Haemophilus influenzae type b (Hib) is one of the leading causes of invasive bacterial disease in children under 5 years old, and is the leading cause of meningitis in this age group. The disease can also cause pneumonia, cellulitis, septic arthritis, otitis, sinusitis, and bronchitis. The bacteria is transmitted through respiratory droplets or via other person-to-person contact. Groups at high risk include those over 65 years of age, persons with chronic disorders of the pulmonary or cardiovascular system, including those with asthma, those with chronic metabolic diseases (diabetes), renal dysfunction, or immunosuppression, and children and teenagers receiving long-term aspirin therapy (risk of Reye's syndrome). Since introduction of the Hib vaccine in 1988, infections have decreased by 95% (1).

➤ SIGNS AND SYMPTOMS

If the organism leads to meningitis, the symptoms generally include fever, chills, malaise, headache, and vomiting. As the meninges become more irritated, other signs and symptoms occur such as a stiff neck, exaggerated deep tendon reflexes, and back spasm in which the back arches backward so that the body rests on the head and heels.

➤ MANAGEMENT

When the condition is identified, immediate referral to a physician is warranted. Antibiotics are administered intravenously for at least 2 weeks, followed by oral antibiotics. Prophylactic treatment of close contacts with rifampin is also indicated.

Viral Childhood Diseases

In 1955, Jonas Salk introduced the first killed-virus vaccine for poliomyelitis, one of the most feared diseases of the time because of its potential for permanent crippling, disability, and death. Shortly thereafter, Albert B. Sabin introduced the first live-virus vaccine for polio, and because of its widespread success, it became the preferred protection from polio. By 1969, vaccines were also available for mea-

sles, mumps, and rubella. Vaccines for chicken pox and influenza soon followed.

POLIOMYELITIS (POLIO)

Polio is an inflammation of the gray matter of the spinal cord. It often results in spinal and muscle paralysis. The virus is spread by direct contact via fecal–oral and oral–oral routes.

➤ SIGNS AND SYMPTOMS

The site of paralysis depends on the location of nerve cell destruction in the spinal cord or brain stem. Only one leg may be involved, or the individual may have progressive paralysis that affects the vital organs and leads to death. In general, there are four possible outcomes of the infection (1):

- Asymptomatic illness occurs in 90% of poliovirus infections.
- Minor illness with fever, headache, malaise, sore throat, and vomiting occurs in about 5% of the population.
- Nonparalytic poliomyelitis with back pain and muscle spasms in addition to symptoms of minor illness occurs in 1 to 2% of the population.
- Paralytic polio with spinal and/or cranial paralysis occurs 3 to 4 days after minor illness has subsided in 0.1 to 2% of infected individuals.

➤ MANAGEMENT

Although the disease has been eradicated in the Western hemisphere by widespread immunization, poliomyelitis remains a potentially serious disease in developing countries. Other than analgesics to relieve pain, there is no treatment for polio.

CHICKENPOX (VARICELLA)

Most individuals have chickenpox by age 10. It is a mild, but very contagious disease in children. In adults, the disease can have severe effects. Chickenpox is caused by the human herpes virus 3 (varicella zoster). Incubation period may be 2 to 3 weeks, but generally runs 13 to 17 days. The disease is spread by direct contact with respiratory secretions and fluid from lesions of the infected person, and may be communicable from 5 days before to 5 days after the appearance of the first vesicles.

➤ SIGNS AND SYMPTOMS

Chickenpox has a sudden onset of slight fever, mild headache, malaise, and loss of appetite for about 24 to 36 hours before the skin rash appears. The rash begins as flat red spots that develop on the trunk and scalp, and in a day or two, develop into raised bumps. Finally, it leads to blisters containing a clear fluid surrounded by a red base. Within 24 to 48 hours, the blisters turn cloudy and encrusted with a granular scab. They erupt in crops so that all three stages are present at the same time, beginning first on the back and chest, and then spreading to the face, neck, and limbs.

> ▶ MANAGEMENT

 Immediate referral to a physician is warranted. Treatment is limited to relief of the symptoms because there is no cure for chickenpox. Bicarbonate of soda baths, or calamine or antihistamine lotions may help relieve the pruritis. In severe cases, an antiviral agent, acyclovir, may be used.

MUMPS

Mumps is most prevalent in the 5- to 9-year-old age group. In contrast to chickenpox, mumps is characterized by a swelling of the salivary glands near the neck. The incubation period is generally 18 days, and is communicable from 6 days before symptoms appear and up to 9 days after they appear. Mumps is spread by airborne droplets and by direct contact with the saliva of an infected person.

> ▶ SIGNS AND SYMPTOMS

Initially there is a loss of appetite, headache, discomfort, and mild fever. These signs are followed by an earache, salivary gland swelling, and temperature of 38.3° to 40°C (101° to 104°F) (3). The salivary glands may become so swollen that it hurts to drink sour liquids or chew food. Complications, which tend to occur more frequently in males, may include epididymitis, meningitis, and rarely, a number of other serious illnesses.

> ▶ MANAGEMENT

 Immediate referral to a physician is warranted. Because of the viral nature of the disease, antibiotics are ineffective. Analgesics, plenty of fluids, and rest are the main forms of treatment.

MEASLES (RUBEOLA)

Measles, in particular, is known to spread rapidly among unimmunized individuals and those who have not received booster shots against the childhood disease. It is spread by airborne droplets, direct contact with nasal or throat secretions of infected individuals, and by articles that have been freshly contaminated. The incubation period is generally 7 to 18 days, usually 14 days to onset of the rash.

> ▶ SIGNS AND SYMPTOMS

Early symptoms include fever, photophobia, malaise, conjunctivitis, runny nose, and cough. The disease is characterized by small spots (Koplik's spots) inside the cheeks, that appear 4 to 5 days after the initial symptoms, and 1 to 2 days before the onset of the rash. Koplik's spots are on the oral mucosa opposite the molars and look like tiny, bluish gray specks surrounded by a red halo. Throat swelling is present, and the temperature may rise to 39.4° to 40.6°C (103° to 105°F). The rash first appears as irregular, brownish-pink spots around the hairline, ears, and neck.

It spreads within 24 to 48 hours to the body, arms, and legs, giving the skin a blotchy appearance. Within 3 to 5 days, the fever decreases and the spots flatten, turn a brownish color, and begin to fade. Encephalitis is the most serious complication.

> ▶ MANAGEMENT

 Immediate referral to a physician is warranted. Plenty of fluids and acetaminophen for fever are recommended. Aspirin is not recommended for children because of the chance of developing Reye's syndrome.

RUBELLA (GERMAN MEASLES)

Rubella is normally a mild disease in children and adults, with one attack giving lifelong vaccination, but the disease can be extremely dangerous for an unborn child when a pregnant woman is infected during the first trimester of pregnancy. Birth defects may include heart disorders, eye clouding (cataracts), deafness, and mental retardation. The disease is transmitted by droplets or direct contact with throat and nasal secretions of infected individuals. The incubation period ranges from 14 to 23 days, and is communicable for about 1 week before and at least 4 days after the onset of the rash.

> ▶ SIGNS AND SYMPTOMS

Rubella is marked by a fever, symptoms of a mild upper respiratory tract infection, swollen lymph nodes, joint pain, and a fine, red rash on the face that spreads to the body. The symptoms usually last only 2 to 3 days except for the joint pain, which may last longer or return.

> ▶ MANAGEMENT

 Referral to a physician is warranted. Treatment is symptomatic.

INFLUENZA

The influenza virus attacks the respiratory tract. It develops rapidly, spreads quickly, and can lead to complications, most often pneumonia, which can be fatal. Influenza viruses are classified into three groups. Type A is the most prevalent and responsible for most epidemics. Type B is associated with regional epidemics every 2 to 3 years. There are also mixed A and B epidemics. Type C is endemic and has been identified in scattered cases and minor localized outbreaks. The different strains of A and B are often named according to where they were first identified (e.g., Hong Kong flu, Russian flu). Infection with one strain results in immunity to that strain, but not to other strains that may develop. The virus is spread through the air from person to person, particularly where large numbers of people are in close quarters. It may also be transmitted by airborne droplets and indirect contact with contaminated objects.

TABLE 21.1 COMMON VIRAL INFECTIONS

Disease	Transmission	Incubation Period	Clinical Symptoms	Duration
Chickenpox (varicella)	Direct contact with respiratory secretions and fluid from lesions	13–17 days	Fever, headache, rash profuse on trunk and on oral mucosa that leads to blisters that turn cloudy and become encrusted with scabs	1–2 weeks
Influenza	Airborne droplets; indirect contact with contaminated objects	1–5 days	Chills, fever, headache, muscle aches and pains, nonproductive cough, sore throat, hoarseness, rhinitis	2–7 days
German measles (rubella)	Nasopharyngeal droplets; direct contact with throat and nasal secretions of infected person	14–23 days	Light rash on face that spreads to trunk and extremities, low-grade fever and enlarged lymph nodes. Can cause congenital heart defects in an infant if acquired by the mother in the first trimester of pregnancy	1–5 days
Measles (rubeola)	Airborne droplets; direct contact with nasal and throat secretions of infected person	7–18 days	Fever, photophobia, malaise, rhinitis, Koplik's spots, swollen throat, progressive brownish-pink rash on face and body	4–7 days
Mumps	Airborne droplets; direct contact with saliva of infected person	18 days	Enlarged salivary glands, fever, headache, malaise, and males may have swollen and tender testes	10 days

➤ SIGNS AND SYMPTOMS

Typical symptoms include a sudden onset of chills, fever, headache, muscle aches and pains, fatigue, and a nonproductive cough. Occasionally, a sore throat, hoarseness, conjunctivitis, and inflammation and congestion of the nasal mucosa may be present. Most symptoms are usually self-limiting with recovery occurring in 2 to 7 days, but the cough and weakness may last for several weeks. Groups at high risk include persons over 65 years old; individuals with chronic lung and cardiovascular conditions, including asthma; persons with renal dysfunction, endocrine disorders (diabetes), and immunosuppression; and children or teenagers receiving long-term aspirin therapy.

➤ MANAGEMENT

Immediate referral to a physician is warranted. Bed rest, analgesics (acetaminophen for children), and plenty of liq-

uids are recommended. For those at risk, the vaccine, given annually, is 70 to 90% effective, and can reduce the severity and duration of the disease if given within 48 hours of the onset of symptoms (4).

Table 21.1 summarizes the incubation period, signs and symptoms, and duration of the more common viral childhood diseases. **Table 21.2** identifies the vaccines and booster shots recommended for adults, by age groups, in the United States.

 Did the swimmer's initial signs and symptoms suggest asking questions about past childhood diseases and immunizations? You may want to ask if he has had current booster shots for measles, mumps, rubella, or chickenpox. Be aware that certain religions and cultures may not approve of immunizations. Your treatment should include an immediate physician referral.

TABLE 21.2 VACCINES AND TOXOIDS RECOMMENDED FOR ADULTS IN THE UNITED STATES

Age (in years)	Vaccine/Toxoid						
	Influenza	Hepatitis B[1]	Measles	Mumps	Rubella	Varicella	Td[2]
18–24	X[3]	X	X	X	X	X	X
25–64		X	X	X	X[1]	X	X
65	X					X	X

[1] Personnel in contact with blood or blood products
[2] Booster every 10 years at middecade (25, 35, 45, etc.)
[3] Individuals at risk of exposure (military recruits, students in dorms, etc.)
Adapted from Bartlett (4), pages 105–108.

INFECTIOUS MONONUCLEOSIS

 A basketball player has been diagnosed with infectious mononucleosis. The physical examination also revealed an enlarged spleen. What implications will this have for sports participation?

The Epstein-Barr virus (EBV) in the herpes family is known to cause infectious mononucleosis, an acute viral disease manifested by a general feeling of malaise and fatigue. Mononucleosis, commonly called the kissing disease, is transmitted in saliva by the oral–pharyngeal route. It may also be spread by sharing a can of pop or other beverage with an infected individual. Infectious rates are highest among individuals between ages 15 and 25; after age 40, the condition is rare. The incubation period for infectious mononucleosis is 4 to 6 weeks. "Chronic fatigue syndrome" and EBV have similar signs and symptoms, but the association of the two continues to be debated.

➤ SIGNS AND SYMPTOMS

Initial symptoms include headache, malaise, and fatigue. After 3 to 5 days, fever, swollen lymph glands, and a sore throat develop. Athletes often describe the sore throat as "the worst sore throat I have ever had." In 10 to 15% of patients, jaundice and a rubella-like rash may also be present. Complications may arise if enlarged tonsils or adenoids obstruct the airway, or if neurologic or cardiac changes occur.

➤ MANAGEMENT

 Individuals with suspected mononucleosis should be immediately referred to a physician.

In larger individuals (football players) where palpation of the spleen is difficult, an ultrasonograph may be indicated to better assess its size. The overwhelming majority of individuals will recover uneventfully. Anti-inflammatory medication may be used to control headaches, fever, and general muscle aches and pains. Lozenges, saltwater gargles, and viscous lidocaine (xylocaine) can ease throat pain. Corticosteroid therapy (prednisone) is only used for individuals with severe cases or specific indications, such as imminent airway obstruction, severe mono-hepatitis, or in the presence of neurologic, hematologic, or cardiac complications.

Individuals with mononucleosis should not participate in any contact or collision sport where trauma could rupture the enlarged and vulnerable spleen. Enlarged spleens have been known to rupture up to 3 weeks after initial symptoms appear. If the spleen is not markedly enlarged or painful, and liver function is normal as determined by appropriate lab tests, limited physical training may be resumed 3 weeks after the onset of the illness, with strenuous exercise and return to contact sports occurring in another 1 to 2 weeks. A flak jacket can be worn to protect the spleen from injury.

💡 The basketball player's spleen was enlarged, secondary to the infectious mononucleosis. Because

of the serious risk of a splenic rupture, this individual must be excluded from sports participation. The individual will not be cleared for participation until the spleen has returned to its normal size and liver function is normal as determined by appropriate lab tests.

VIRAL MENINGITIS

Viral infections of the nervous system are rare in athletes. Athletes are, however, at a greater risk for viral meningitis when poor hygienic measures are used with drink dispensing machines, water bottles, and water buffaloes that are not kept properly clean and germ free.

➤ SIGNS AND SYMPTOMS

Signs and symptoms of viral meningitis include fever, headache, nausea, vomiting, neck pain, muscle pain (myalgia) and neck stiffness (nuchal rigidity), decreased coordination, malaise, photophobia, and altered mental status. Because the meninges are inflamed, stretching them through neck flexion produces pain.

➤ MANAGEMENT

 The most important step in treating this condition is an immediate referral to a physician for an accurate diagnosis. Drug therapy is used to control symptoms, with the condition usually resolving on its own.

The athlete should not return to activity for 2 to 3 weeks after symptoms have eased. Upon return, activity should be resumed in a gradual progression. If symptoms recur, this indicates the virus is still present, and activity should cease until the athlete is reevaluated by a physician.

SEXUALLY TRANSMITTED DISEASES

Infections of the genital tract are called sexually transmitted diseases (STDs). They affect more than 12 million Americans every year, with transmission being most common in those aged 15 to 19. Furthermore, more than 80% of college students report being sexually active, and nearly one-fifth of these report at least one past STD episode (5). Chlamydia, the most common bacterial STD in the United States, is the leading STD in college students, with a 10 to 20% incidence rate reported annually (6). In a recent study of 100 female athletes at Division 1 universities, 11% reported having an STD. Of those, 37% reported having chlamydia and 18% having gonorrhea or genital warts (7). Chlamydia, unlike herpes and the human papillomavirus (HPV), is highly preventable since transmission can be interrupted through the use of condoms, and it is easily treated with antibiotic therapy. In women, chlamydia is often asymptomatic and undiagnosed, leading to potentially dangerous health and fertility problems. Some experts suggest that chlamydia screening become a routine part of annual gynecological examinations.

Gonorrhea, the second most common STD in the

United States, is characterized in males by a pungent, thick, milky yellow or greenish discharge, and a burning sensation during urination. In women, the condition is often asymptomatic until it progresses into pelvic inflammatory disease. Genital ulcers commonly result from herpes (with herpes simplex affecting nearly 20% of young adults), syphilis, and chancroids. A summary of the modes of transmission, incubation periods, signs and symptoms, and general treatments of the more common STDs can be found in **Table 21.3**.

TABLE 21.3   COMMON SEXUALLY TRANSMITTED DISEASES (STDs)

STD	Transmission	Incubation	Symptoms	Treatment
+Bacterial vaginosis	Caused by *Gardnerella vaginalis* bacterium; primarily spread through coitus	1–3 weeks	**Women:** a pungent, fishy or musty smelling, thin, gray vaginal discharge resembling flour paste **Men:** often asymptomatic; may have inflammation of the foreskin and glans of penis, urethritis, or cystitis	Oral antibiotics
+Candidiasis (yeast infection)	Growth of the *Candida albicans* fungus may accelerate when the vaginal chemical balance is disturbed; also transmitted through coitus	2 weeks to 1 month	**Women:** thin, clear, watery discharge to a white, "cheesy" discharge. Intense itching, swelling, irritation, and burning of the vaginal and vulval tissues may lead to a dry rash that makes coitus painful	Vaginal suppositories or creams for yeast infections
+Trichomoniasis	Caused by the parasite *Trichomonas vaginalis,* it is passed through sexual contact, or less frequently by towels, toilet seats, or bathtubs used by an infected person	24 hours in men; 2–3 days in women	**Women:** a white or yellow vaginal discharge with an unpleasant odor; vulva is sore and irritated **Men:** often asymptomatic; may have mild itching and burning during urination and a whitish discharge from the penis	Anti-infective; oral antibiotics for all cases except pregnant women
+Chlamydia	Caused by *Chlamydia trachomatis,* it is passed through sexual contact, or less frequently by fingers from one body site to another	7–28 days	**Women:** asymptomatic until condition invades upper reproductive tract leading to PID (see below). Can lead to ectopic pregnancies, postpartum endometritis, spontaneous abortion, premature labor, blindness or death in a newborn **Men:** a water discharge, burning during urination, rectal pain, groin pain, fever, chills, and/or a sense of heaviness in the affected testicle(s), inflammation of scrotal skin, and a small, hard, painful swelling at the bottom of the testicle	Anti-infective broad spectrum; oral antibiotics
+Gonorrhea ("clap")	Caused by *Neisseria gonorrhea;* spread through sexual contact	1–5 days in men; 2 weeks in women	**Women:** asymptomatic until PID develops; green or yellowish discharge may be present. May lead to sterility and ectopic pregnancy **Men:** pungent, thick, milky yellow or greenish discharge, and a burning sensation during urination.	Penicillin drugs; antibiotics
+Pelvic inflammatory disease (PID)	Caused by multiple infections (chlamydia, gonorrhea). Risk factors: <25 years of age, multiple sexual partners, excessive douching and use of feminine hygiene sprays	Results from complications of other infections	Chronic lower abdominal pain that increases sharply with exercise; vaginal discharge, menstrual dysfunction, fever, headache, nausea, vomiting. May lead to ectopic pregnancy and sterility	Must treat the initial cause; may include injected or oral antibiotics
+Nongonococcal urethritis (NGU)	Most commonly caused by *Chlamydia trachomatis* and *Ureaplasma urealyticum;* passed through coitus	7–28 days, but may disappear after 2–3 months	**Women:** asymptomatic; may have mild itching, burning on urination, and slight vaginal discharge of pus **Men:** a penile discharge and burning during urination	Antibiotics

(Continued)

TABLE 21.3   *(Continued)*

STD	Transmission	Incubation	Symptoms	Treatment
+Syphilis	Caused by the spiral-shaped bacterium *Treponema pallidum,* it is spread from open lesions through penile–vaginal, oral–genital, or genital–anal contact	10–90 days, with infected individuals contagious during the early stages of the disease and during the first year of the latent stage	**Primary stage:** painless ulcer/chancre is visible at site of entry **Secondary stage** (6 weeks to 6 months): chancre disappears and low-grade fever, sore throat, swollen glands, and skin rash appear on body **Latent stage** (several months to a lifetime): may be no observable symptoms **Tertiary stage** (3–40 years): heart failure, blindness, mental disturbance, and death	In the first year, a single intramuscular injection of benzathine penicillin, doxycycline, tetracycline, or erythromycin. After 1 year, three successive weekly intramuscular injections are used
*Herpes	Oral herpes virus (HSV-1) is spread primarily by nongenital contact. Genital herpes virus (HSV-2) is transmitted by vaginal, anal, or oral–genital intercourse, but can be transmitted through autoinoculation (touching the lesion, then scratching or rubbing elsewhere)	3–5 days; occasionally less than 24 hours	Small, painful red bumps (papules) appear on the genitals (genital herpes) or mouth (oral herpes). Papules become painful blisters that will rupture to form wet, open sores that form a yellow crust and heal within 10 days. Other symptoms include vaginal discharge, fever, muscle aches, swollen lymph nodes in the groin, and headache	No known cure; oral or intravenous antiviral may reduce symptoms, promote healing, and suppress recurrent outbreaks
*Genital warts	Caused by the human papilloma virus, it spreads primarily through vaginal, anal, or orogenital sexual interaction	3 weeks to 18 months (3 months average)	On dry skin, warts appear hard and yellow-gray. In moist regions, warts appear soft pinkish red with a cauliflower-like appearance	Topical antineoplastic (antimetabolite) cream, or cauterization, freezing, surgical removal, or vaporization by carbon dioxide laser
*Viral hepatitis (See Table 21.4)				
*Acquired immunodeficiency syndrome (AIDS)	HIV has only been found to be transmitted in blood, semen, and vaginal secretions through sexual contact or needle sharing among IV drug users or steroid users	Unknown	Varies depending on the degree to which the immune system is impaired. Refer to Box 21.2	At present, there is no effective cure or vaccine. Therapy focuses on controlling the symptoms

+Can be successfully treated if recognized early
*Symptoms may be treated, but no effective cure is available

HEPATITIS

There are five major types of hepatitis, each caused by a different virus **(Table 21.4)**. The American Medical Association, the American Academy of Family Physicians (AAFP), and the American Academy of Pediatrics (AAP) advocate that all children should receive a complete series of hepatitis B virus (HBV) vaccinations during the first 18 months of life. Vaccination as a prophylactic measure is required of an employer at no cost to an employee, if the employee may be exposed to bloodborne pathogens. The vaccine is given in three doses over a 6-month period. All older children and adolescents at high risk for HBV infection, in addition to those listed in **Box 21.1**, should also receive a complete series of the vaccination. Although not specifically mentioned, coaches, referees, officials, and recreational sport supervisors should also be vaccinated,

TABLE 21.4   MAJOR VIRUSES KNOWN TO CAUSE HEPATITIS IN HUMANS

	Hepatitis A	Hepatitis B	Hepatitis C	Hepatitis D	Hepatitis E
Transmitted	Fecal–oral; contaminated food and water (epidemics)	Bloodborne; sexual contact; contaminated needles	Bloodborne; sexual contact	Bloodborne	Fecal–oral
Incubation period	15–50 days	45–160 days	15–150 days	30–60 days	20–60 days
Special features	IG-prophylaxis effective	Pre- and postexposure prophylaxis available	Asymptomatic in many; main cause of posttransfusion hepatitis; often becomes chronic	Coinfection with active HBV or infection superimposed on chronic HB	High mortality in pregnant women. Large epidemics due to contaminated water supplies

Adapted from Bartlett (4), pages 193-196, 289-291.

since they are often first on the scene of an acute injury involving hemorrhage.

Hepatitis B (HBV), the most common form of viral hepatitis, has an incubation period of 45 to 160 days, and is transmitted by blood or blood products (posttransfusion hepatitis), semen, vaginal secretions, and saliva. Manual, oral, or penile stimulation of the anus are practices strongly associated with the spread of this virus. It is possible that an individual infected with HBV will exhibit no signs or symptoms, and the virus may go undetected. However, the HBV antigen is still present, and can unknowingly be transmitted to others through exposure to blood or other body fluids or through sexual contact. The HBV virus can survive for at least 1 week in dried blood or on contaminated surfaces.

➤ SIGNS AND SYMPTOMS

Hepatitis primarily attacks the liver, severely impairing function. Early symptoms include mild flu-like symptoms such as malaise, fatigue, and loss of appetite. Progressive signs include severe fatigue, anorexia, nausea, vomiting, diarrhea, general muscle and joint pain, high fever, vomiting, severe abdominal pain, and dark urine. Among the most notable signs is a yellowing of the whites of the eyes, and a yellowish or jaundiced skin appearance in light-complexioned individuals. Hepatitis may increase the risk of developing cancer of the liver and, in rare cases, is fatal.

➤ MANAGEMENT

Immediate referral to a physician is warranted if the individual has been exposed, or suspected of being exposed, to the virus. Currently, there is no specific drug therapy to cure viral hepatitis. Postexposure vaccination is also available when individuals have come into direct contact with bodily fluids of an infected person. Bed rest and adequate fluid intake can prevent dehydration, but the disease must run its course.

ACQUIRED IMMUNODEFICIENCY SYNDROME (AIDS)

Acquired immunodeficiency syndrome (AIDS) results from infection with the human immunodeficiency virus (HIV), which falls within a special category called **retroviruses**. An individual can be HIV positive, and thus infectious to others, for years before any signs of AIDS appears. The HIV virus attacks and destroys cells in the body's immune system, particularly the lymphocyte known as the helper T-cell. In a healthy individual, these cells stimulate the immune system to fight disease. In an infected individual, a gradual deterioration of the immune system leaves the body vulnerable to a variety of infections and cancers, such as herpes, oral candidiasis, pneumonia, encephalitis, and retinitis.

Currently, HIV has only been found to be transmitted in blood, semen, and vaginal secretions. In sports, the risk of AIDS is rare. In boxing, football, or wrestling, where participants may have a bloody nose or open cuts, close contact with the competitor may pose a health risk. Uni-

---

➤➤ **Box 21.1**

Individuals at High Risk for Hepatitis B and HIV Infection

- Individuals exposed to blood, including athletic trainers, student athletic trainers, nurses, and physicians
- Staff and residents of institutions for the developmentally disabled
- Staff and patients in kidney dialysis units
- Intravenous drug users
- Gay men
- Sexually active heterosexuals with multiple partners
- Anyone who has resided in Haiti or central Africa (HIV virus)
- Heterosexual women and men who do one or more of the following:
  Have anal intercourse
  Have multiple sexual partners
  Have multiple contacts with an infected partner
  Do not use a condom

forms that become saturated with blood must be changed before returning to competition. Small amounts of bloodstain on a uniform, however, do not require removal of the participant from the game or a uniform change.

➤ SIGNS AND SYMPTOMS

Signs and symptoms of AIDS vary, depending upon the degree to which the immune system is impaired. Common symptoms include those listed in **Box 21.2**. Some researchers suggest that AIDS is more severe in women, with the HIV infection progressing much faster.

➤ MANAGEMENT

Immediate referral to a physician is warranted if the individual has been exposed, or suspected of being exposed, to the virus. To date, there is no effective cure or vaccine for AIDS.

Various drug therapies have been developed for controlling symptoms and decreasing the progression of the disease, but the success of drug therapy appears to be related to the stage of the virus and the time in which the drug therapy was initiated. Healthy HIV-positive athletes and those with AIDS may continue physical activity. The Americans with Disabilities Act of 1991 states that athletes infected with HIV cannot be discriminated against and may be excluded from participation only on sound medical grounds. At times, however, fatigue may not allow participation in intensive exercise or competition. The best defenses against the virus remain education about safe sex practices and the use of condoms, and practicing universal precautions in dealing with blood and blood products (refer to Field Strategy 5.1).

Summary

1. Childhood diseases can be prevented by early immunization given between birth and 18 months. Booster shots are given upon entry into school, and again in adolescence.

2. Childhood bacterial diseases that can be prevented through vaccinations include diphtheria, tetanus, pertussis (whooping cough), and *Haemophilus influenzae* type b (Hib). Childhood viral diseases that can be prevented through vaccinations include poliomyelitis (polio), chickenpox (varicella), mumps, measles (rubeola), rubella (German measles), influenza, and hepatitis.

3. Adults 18 to 24 should receive booster shots for measles, mumps, rubella, varicella, and tetanus. Diphtheria and tetanus shots should be repeated every 10 years.

4. Mononucleosis is transmitted in saliva. Infectious rates are highest among individuals aged 15 to 25. Signs and symptoms include headache, fatigue, loss of appetite, enlarged lymph nodes, swollen glands, and an enlarged spleen.

5. Athletes are at a greater risk of viral meningitis when poor hygienic measures are used around water bottles and watering stations.

6. Chlamydia is the most common bacterial STD in the United States, followed by gonorrhea and genital ulcers from herpes, syphilis, and chancroids. In men, common signs and symptoms of an STD include mild itching and burning during urination and a discharge from the penis. In women, a vaginal discharge may be present, but many STDs are asymptomatic until the more serious pelvic inflammatory disease occurs.

7. Hepatitis B is the most common form of viral hepatitis, yet can be prevented with proper vaccination. The condition primarily attacks the liver, severely impairing function. Signs and symptoms include severe fatigue, malaise, and loss of appetite progressing to anorexia, nausea, vomiting, high fever, and a jaundiced appearance.

8. AIDS results from infection with the HIV virus, which has been found to be transmitted in blood, semen, and vaginal secretions.

9. Most common viral diseases, including hepatitis and AIDS, can be prevented in the athletic setting by following universal precautions when dealing with blood and blood products.

10. If an athlete is suspected of contracting an infectious disease, a physician referral is always recommended so drug therapy can be prescribed along with other treatment. If the infection can be spread from person to person, athletes who are infected should be isolated from other players until the physician determines that cross-infection is no longer possible.

References

1. U.S. Department of Health and Human Services. Clinician's Handbook of Preventive Services. U.S. Department of Health and Human Services. Washington, DC: U.S. Government Printing Office, 1994.

2. Tam TWS, Bentsi-Enchill A. The return of the 100-day cough: Resurgence of pertussis in the 1990s. Can Med Assoc J 1998;159(6):695-696.

3. Benenson AS (ed.). Control of Communicable Diseases Manual. Washington, DC: American Public Health Association, 1995.

4. Bartlett JG. Pocket Book of Infectious Disease Therapy. Baltimore: Williams & Wilkins, 1997.

5. Zinner SH, McCormack WM. Three decades of research on sexual behavior, and sexually transmitted pathogens in college students. Med Health 1997;80(10):338-340.

6. Sawyer RG, Moss DJ. Sexually transmitted diseases in college men: A preliminary clinical investigation. College Health 1993;42: 111-115.

7. Watson A, Martin M, Hunt H. Incidence of sexually transmitted diseases and the need for sexual education for female collegiate athletes. J Ath Train 1998;33(2 Suppl):S-61.

8. Cleavenger RL, Juckett RG, Hobbs GR. Trends in chlamydia and other sexually transmitted diseases in a university health service. College Health 1996;44:263-265.

22

Seizure Disorders

OBJECTIVES

1. Differentiate between a seizure disorder and epilepsy.

2. Identify the causes of epilepsy.

3. List the types of generalized and partial seizures.

4. Describe characteristics of the more common seizures.

5. Name and describe the seizure situation that constitutes a medical emergency.

6. Describe the management and treatment of the more common types of seizures.

7. Explain exercise guidelines for individuals with controlled seizures.

In the past, there has been much controversy over whether or not an individual with a seizure disorder should be permitted to participate in physical activity and strenuous exercise. Recently, the American Medical Association (AMA) and other medical organizations have suggested that individuals with seizures can safely participate in physical activity as long as certain precautions are exercised. First, this chapter will identify the various types of seizure disorders. The signs and symptoms of the more common seizures will be followed by the protocol for handling a seizure. Finally, physical activity guidelines for those who suffer from a seizure disorder will be presented.

SEIZURE DISORDERS AND EPILEPSY

 A high school baseball player reports to preseason physical examination with a history of partial seizures. What guidelines might this athlete be given for athletic participation?

A **seizure** is an abnormal electrical discharge in the brain. A **seizure disorder** entails recurrent episodes of sudden excessive charges of electrical activity in the brain, whether from known or unknown (idiopathic) causes. **Epilepsy**, on the other hand, is a general term used to describe only recurrent idiopathic episodes (at least two) of sudden, excessive discharges of electrical activity in the brain (1,2). The discharge may trigger altered sensation, perception, behavior, mood, or level of consciousness, or convulsive movements. Seizures and epilepsy are often used interchangeably; however, it is important to understand their definitions.

Causes of Epilepsy

The causes of epilepsy appear to be directly related to age of onset, and are generally categorized as provoked or unprovoked (**Box 22.1**). Seizures that begin prior to age 5 are usually associated with mental or neurologic impairment. Seizures that begin between the ages of 5 and 15 are usually not associated with a known metabolic or structural cause, and are called idiopathic or unprovoked seizures. These seizures respond very well to treatment, and individuals can usually participate in activity with little to no restrictions. Trauma and tumors are responsible for most seizures in young adults; strokes become the most frequent cause in those 40 years and older (1,3).

Types of Seizures

Seizures may be divided into three basic types: partial or focal, generalized, and special epileptic syndromes. Athletic trainers tend to see only generalized and partial seizures; therefore, information on special epileptic syndromes will be minimal. **Box 22.2** summarizes the classifications of seizures.

PARTIAL SEIZURES

Partial or focal seizures have a localized onset, are focused in one particular area of the brain, and are restricted to specific areas of the body (2). Partial seizures may be subdivided into simple (where consciousness is retained) and complex (where consciousness is impaired).

> ▶▶ **Box 22.1**

Causes of Epilepsy

1. Unprovoked or idiopathic—no cause of the seizure is identified
2. Provoked
   - Posttraumatic (skull fracture, intracranial hematoma, other)
   - Metabolic (hyponatremia, hypocalcemia, hypoglycemia, hypomagnesemia, dehydration)
   - Drug and drug withdrawal (alcohol, cocaine)
   - Infections (meningitis, encephalitis, brain abscess)
   - Anoxia and hypoxia
   - Cerebrovascular (stroke, intracerebral or subarachnoid hemorrhage, sinus thrombosis)
   - Hyperthermia
   - Sleep deprivation
   - Febrile seizures
   - Neoplasms (primary intracranial, carcinomatous meningitis, metastatic, lymphoma, leukemia)
   - Perinatal or hereditary (congenital anomalies, genetic and hereditary disorders, perinatal trauma)

> ▶▶ **Box 22.2**

Classification of Seizures

1. Partial (focal) seizures
   - Simple (consciousness not impaired)
   - Complex (with impairment of consciousness)
   - Partial with secondary generalization
2. Generalized seizures
   - Tonic-clonic (grand mal)
   - Intermittent seizure
   - Continuous seizure (status epilepticus)
   - Absence (petit mal)
   - Myoclonic epilepsy
   - Posttraumatic
3. Special epileptic syndromes
   - Febrile seizures
   - Hysterical seizures
   - Reflex epilepsy

A simple partial seizure is relatively common and may be classified according to the main clinical manifestations. The symptoms include bodily sensations and discomforts, like tingling or numbness, a pins-and-needles sensation, or a loss of feeling. A motor manifestation is characterized by involuntary movements of the face, limbs, or head, and may involve an inability to speak. The seizures may be followed by localized weakness or paralysis in the body part in which the seizure occurs, lasting for minutes or hours; this is called Todd's paralysis. The individual may experience powerful emotions such as fear, anxiety, depression, or embarrassment for no apparent reason, or feeling as if the mind and body are separating. The person may see objects and people get larger or smaller or appear distorted, see things that are not there (visual hallucinations), smell things that are not there (olfactory hallucinations), and hear things that are not there (auditory hallucinations). Psychic symptoms may include disturbing memory flashbacks or frequent disconcerting feelings of déjà vu (something or someone unfamiliar seems familiar) or jamais vu (something or someone familiar seems unfamiliar). Time distortions, out-of-body experiences, sudden nausea, or stomach pain may occur. There is no impairment of consciousness; however, a partial or focal seizure may precede a generalized seizure, and serve as an aura, or warning, that consciousness is about to be altered (4).

Complex partial seizures affect a larger area of the brain and therefore impair consciousness. They are also referred to as temporal lobe epilepsy or psychomotor seizures. The seizures are characterized by attacks of purposeful movements or experiences followed by impairment in consciousness. In other words, the individual may appear conscious, but he or she will be in an altered state of consciousness, an almost trance-like state. These purposeful activities and experiences may include (3):

- Emotions (depression, fear, paranoia, crying out)
- Simple automatism (chewing, swallowing, lip smacking, chewing, saying the same words over and over)

- Complex automatism (walking into a room, undressing, arranging objects)
- Hallucinations (auditory, visual, gustatory, olfactory)

If engaged in activity, movements are usually disorganized, confused, and unfocused, but observers may find it hard to believe that the individual does not know what he or she is doing. The average seizure is 1 to 5 minutes. The individual is unresponsive to verbal stimuli and may exhibit disorientation or confusion. Afterwards, the individual is unable to recall what he or she did. Most cases start between the ages of 10 and 30.

GENERALIZED SEIZURES

Generalized seizures can affect the entire brain. These seizures may be further subdivided into convulsive and nonconvulsive types.

The tonic-clonic (grand mal) seizure, the most common and most severe seizure of the convulsive type, may occur in either an intermittent or continuous form. **Tonic** refers to prolonged contractions of skeletal muscles, while **clonic** refers to rhythmic contractions and relaxation of muscles in rapid succession.

An intermittent seizure may be tonic, clonic, or both, and is often associated with loss of consciousness. Many individuals experience a sensory phenomenon (aura), such as a particular taste or smell, prior to the seizure. The average seizure lasts from 50 to 90 seconds, but may extend up to 5 minutes. Because the unconscious seizing athlete is overtaken by the excessive electrical discharge during the seizure, he or she may lose control over bladder and bowel functions, resulting in urination or defecation. This is embarrassing and unpleasant, but not unexpected. When the seizure ends, the brain may shift into a sleep pattern. As such, the athlete may be unarousable for a brief period of time (seconds to a few minutes). The muscles relax during this period, and the person awakens. Following the seizure, the person is often disoriented, confused, and lethargic, and may not remember what happened.

 A continuous tonic-clonic seizure (status epilepticus) is a medical emergency. Continuous convulsions can last 30 minutes or longer, or recurrent generalized convulsions can occur without the person regaining full consciousness between attacks. If the convulsions exceed 60 minutes, irreversible neuronal damage may occur. Any seizure that lasts longer than 5 minutes should signal a serious problem, and the athletic trainer should immediately activate EMS.

Myoclonic seizures are characterized by sporadic or continuous clonus of muscle groups, and are associated with progressive mental deterioration. These are seldom seen in the physically active population.

Posttraumatic seizures are provoked by head trauma and are classified as impact, immediate, early, and late. Impact seizures occur at the time of trauma and are considered to be the result of electrochemical changes induced by the trauma. Immediate seizures occur within the first 24 hours of trauma. Early seizures occur within the first week after head trauma (e.g., depressed skull fracture, acute intracranial hematoma), and are often associated with prolonged posttraumatic amnesia lasting more than 24 hours. A late seizure occurs after the first week of head trauma but primarily within 1 year, and may be associated with a history of childhood epilepsy (3).

The typical absence, or petit mal, attack is characterized by a slight loss of consciousness, or blank staring into space, for 3 to 15 seconds without loss of body tone or falling. Slight twitching of the facial muscles, lip smacking, or fluttering of the eyelids may occur. Onset is usually between the ages of 4 and 8, and the condition tends to resolve by age 30.

SPECIAL EPILEPTIC SYNDROMES

A third category of seizures includes such disorders as febrile seizures of infancy and childhood. Febrile seizures have their onset during the course of a fever usually above 38.9°C (102°F) and are most likely to happen while the temperature is rising rapidly. Other seizures in this category include hysterical seizures and reflex epilepsy, a small subgroup of seizures that occur only in response to specific stimuli such as flickering lights, specific sounds, sudden movements, eating, or reading of words or numbers (2).

Immediate Management of Seizures

It is essential to note the time on your watch immediately upon observing an individual having a seizure. Seconds may seem like minutes; unless accurately timed, one may tend to exaggerate the length of the seizure. Management of any seizure is directed toward protecting the individual from injury. Nearby objects should be removed or padded so the individual does not strike them during uncontrollable muscle contractions. Protect the individual's head at all times, but do not stop or restrain the person. Although the individual may bite the tongue during the seizure, never place fingers or any object into the mouth. Because of the excessive electrical discharge during the seizure, the athlete may also lose control of bladder and bowel functions. This can be very embarrassing. If possible, remove any observers or spectators from the area to allow the athlete privacy. When the seizure ends, the individual may fall into a sleep pattern. This is normal. Ensure an adequate airway and wait until the athlete awakens.

 Document the length of time the seizure occurred, and how long the individual slept. If a single continuous seizure or a series of intermittent seizures exceeds 5 minutes, activate EMS. The athlete should be evaluated by a physician. If possible, cover the individual to maintain body heat. If the individual has a known seizure disorder, the athletic trainer should attempt to discern why the athlete seized. Inquire about whether the athlete has been taking the medication

as prescribed, whether the prescription ran out and wasn't refilled, or if the athlete simply decided to wean off the medication. This information should be provided to EMS upon their arrival.

Field Strategy 22.1 summarizes management of a seizure.

Medications and Epilepsy

Antiepileptic/anticonvulsive medications are the agents of choice for those with seizure disorders and epilepsy. These medications should be taken at least 1 to 2 hours prior to physical activity. The long-term goal is to control or eliminate seizure activity with the lowest doses of the fewest medications. Because anticonvulsive agents have long half-lives (clear the body slowly) and take time to build up to the therapeutic range, regular long-term administration (months to years to a lifetime) of medication is needed to keep the body in the therapeutic range. Failure to take medication over several days would result in falling out of the effective therapeutic range. Serum levels should be checked frequently for two reasons: (1) to ensure that the medication is within the therapeutic range, and (2) if physically active, to ensure that increased fitness levels have not altered the drug metabolism. If serum levels are too low, there is an increased risk of seizures; if levels are too high, toxic effects of the medication may depress brain activity, which may not support vital functions. Some anticonvulsive agents may cause fatigue, headache, or nausea, while others may cause ataxia (incoordination) (3,5). These agents should be avoided in competitive athletes, although many anticonvulsive agents are approved by the National Collegiate Athletic Association (NCAA) and United States Olympic Committee (USOC).

FIELD STRATEGY 22.1   MANAGEMENT ALGORITHM FOR SEIZURES

<u>During the seizure</u>

Note the time that the seizure began

↓

Help the athlete to a supine position; protect the head

↓

Remove glasses and loosen clothing

↓

Do not:
– stop or restrain the person
– place fingers or any object in the mouth

<u>After the seizure</u>

Ensure an adequate airway

↓

Turn the individual to one side to allow saliva to drain from mouth

↓

Protect the person from curious bystanders

↓

Do not leave the person until he or she is fully awake

↓

If this is:

A first-time seizure   A continuous seizure, or if another seizure
                                                     occurs in rapid succession

↓   ↓

The individual should be   ➤   *Activate EMS for immediate transport*
seen by a physician   *to the nearest medical facility*

Send documentation—a written description of:
– type of seizure; localized or generalized
– how it started
– length of time from onset until return of consciousness
– number of seizures

Physical Activity Guidelines

In nearly all instances, seizure disorders can be controlled with proper medication. Good seizure control is traditionally identified as being seizure-free for 6 months or a year. Participation in sports, particularly in those with a danger of falling, contact sports, and water sports should be carefully evaluated with a neurologist prior to participation. Several issues must be addressed in determining participation levels:

- What type of sport is being played (i.e., contact or collision versus noncontact)?
- Is there a risk of death or severe injury if the athlete has a seizure during activity?
- Is there a preexisting brain injury or any neurologic dysfunction?
- Is there a risk of potential brain injury from participation in the sport (e.g., concussion, intracranial hematoma)?
- Will exercise adversely affect seizure control?
- What are the potential effects of anticonvulsive medications on sport performance (e.g., impaired judgment, delayed reaction time)?

Head injury during sport participation can certainly precipitate seizures. Those with epilepsy, however, are no more prone to seizures after a head injury than athletes without epilepsy. In addition, it has been found that epilepsy does not increase the risk of injury while participating in sports (6). It is highly recommended that children with seizure disorders be allowed to participate in physical activity and sports, provided that good seizure control and proper supervision are available at all times. Certain activities (e.g., football, scuba diving, mountain climbing, automobile racing) may put the individual or others at risk if a seizure occurs. These activities should be discouraged. Any athlete with a history of seizures should be prohibited from boxing, regardless of seizure control. Individuals who experience frequent seizures should choose physical activities accordingly.

 If the athlete has controlled his seizure disorder with medication, and other precautionary measures are taken, he most likely will be able to participate in baseball with no limitations.

Summary

1. A seizure disorder entails recurrent episodes of sudden excessive charges of electrical activity in the brain, whether from known or unknown (idiopathic) causes. Epilepsy is a general term used to describe only recurrent idiopathic episodes (at least two) of sudden, excessive discharges of electrical activity in

the brain. The discharge may trigger altered sensation, perception, behavior, mood, level of consciousness or lead to convulsive movements.

2. Seizures are classified as partial, generalized, or special epileptic syndromes.

3. The most serious seizure is the tonic-clonic, which may occur in either an intermittent or continuous form. An intermittent seizure, which only lasts 50 to 90 seconds but may extend to 5 minutes, is often preceded by a particular taste or smell (aura).

4. The typical absence (petit mal) attack is characterized by a slight loss of consciousness or blank staring into space for 3 to 15 seconds, without loss of body tone or falling.

5. The simple partial seizure is characterized by involuntary movements of the face, limbs, or head; the individual may experience tingling or numbness. The localized motor seizures may be followed by localized weakness or paralysis in the body part in which the seizure occurs.

6. Complex partial (psychomotor) seizures are characterized by purposeful movements or experiences followed by impairment in consciousness.

7. Management of any seizure is directed toward protecting the individual from injury. Remove or pad nearby objects, and protect the individual's head at all times, but do not stop or restrain the person or try to put anything in the mouth. When the seizure is over, ensure an adequate airway. If the time of the seizure exceeds 5 minutes, activate EMS.

8. In nearly all instances, individuals with a seizure disorder can be allowed to participate in certain sports provided that good seizure control and proper supervision are available at all times.

9. Certain activities (e.g., football, scuba diving, mountain climbing, and automobile racing) may put the athlete or others at risk if a seizure occurs. These activities should be discouraged.

References

1. Lang D. Seizure disorders and physical activity. Your Patient and Fitness 1996;10(5):24e-24k.
2. Agnew CM, Nystul MS, Conner MC. Seizure disorders: An alternative explanation for students' inattention. Prof Sch Coun 1998;2(1):54-60.
3. Jordan BD. Epilepsy and the athlete. In: The Team Physicians' Handbook. Edited by Mellion MB, Walsh WM, Shelton GL. Philadelphia: Hanley & Belfus, 1997.
4. Kistner D, DeWeaver KL. Nonconvulsive seizure disorders: Importance and implications for school social workers. Soc Work Ed 1997; 19(2):73-86.
5. Martin M, Yates WN. Therapeutic Medications in Sports. Baltimore: Williams & Wilkins, 1998.
6. Nakkan KO, et al. Effect of physical training on aerobic capacity, seizure occurrence, and serum level of antiepileptic drugs in adults with epilepsy. Epilepsia 1990;31(1):88-94.

CHAPTER **23**

Blood Pressure Disorders

OBJECTIVES

1. Define hypertension and hypotension.
2. List the four stages of hypertension, and describe what predisposing factors or diseases place the individual at risk for developing hypertension.
3. Identify medications that can adversely elevate blood pressure.
4. Describe how hypertension is managed.
5. List the factors and conditions that can lead to hypotension.
6. Describe how hypotension is managed.
7. Demonstrate the measurement of blood pressure.

Blood pressure is the force per unit area exerted on the walls of an artery, generally considered to be the aorta. It is the result of two factors: cardiac output and total peripheral resistance. Cardiac output is determined by heart rate, myocardial contractility (force of contraction), blood volume, and venous return; peripheral resistance is determined by arteriolar constriction. As one of the most important vital signs, blood pressure reflects the effectiveness of the circulatory system. Although blood pressures vary between individuals, normal blood pressure is considered 120 mm Hg systolic blood pressure (SBP) and 80 mm Hg diastolic blood pressure (DBP). **Systolic blood pressure** is measured when the left ventricle contracts and expels blood into the aorta. **Diastolic blood pressure**, the residual pressure present in the aorta between heartbeats, averages 70 to 80 mm Hg in healthy adults. Blood pressure may be affected by gender, weight, race, lifestyle, and diet, and can vary throughout the day depending on the time of day and the individual's fitness level. It is not unusual for a relatively physically fit person to have a blood pressure of 90/70 mm Hg. Blood pressure is measured in the brachial artery with a sphygmomanometer and stethoscope; this was discussed in Field Strategy 2.1.

Any change in either cardiac output or peripheral resistance will result in an increase or decrease in blood pressure. **Hypertension** (high blood pressure) is defined as a sustained elevated blood pressure greater than 140 mm Hg systolic blood pressure (SBP) or greater than 90 mm Hg diastolic blood pressure (DBP). **Hypotension** is characterized by a fall of 20 mm Hg or more from a person's normal baseline systolic blood pressure.

TABLE 23.1   RISK FACTORS FOR DEVELOPING HYPERTENSION

Risk Factor	Reason
Age	Arteries lose their elasticity, and blood pressure increases with age. High incidence of hypertension after age 60.
Diabetes	High incidence in diabetics due to insulin resistance promoted by abdominal obesity.
Heredity	Higher incidence with a family history of hypertension and heart disease in women (<65) and in men (<55).
High blood lipids	High blood lipids contribute to atherosclerosis and hypertension. A high-fat diet also contributes to hypertension.
Obesity	Excess body fat, especially abdominal fat, is closely associated with hypertension.
Race	Prevalence differs among racial and ethnic groups, but incidence in African-Americans is among the highest in the world.
Sex	Higher incidence in men and postmenopausal women.
Smoking	Smoking increases the workload of the heart, thereby increases blood pressure.

Adapted from Whitney EN, Rolfes SR. Understanding Nutrition. Belmont, CA: Wadsworth Publishing, 1999:572.

HYPERTENSION

 During the preparticipation examination, a football player was found to have a blood pressure of 150/90 mm Hg. Should the athletic trainer be concerned over this measurement? What implications might this blood pressure have on his athletic participation?

Nearly a third of the entire adult population will develop hypertension, contributing to more than a million heart attacks and half a million strokes each year (1). Several factors increase the risk of developing hypertension **(Table 23.1)**. Onset is generally between the ages of 20 and 50, with the frequency greatest in African-Americans. Hypertension may also be caused by a variety of substances **(Box 23.1)**, and is classified into four stages **(Table 23.2)**. This categorization applies to adults aged 18 and older who are not taking antihypertensive medication and are not acutely ill. When systolic and diastolic pressures fall into different categories, the higher category is used to classify the athlete's blood pressure status. For more detailed standards in children and adolescents, refer to Table 2.2.

➤➤ Box 23.1

Causes of Hypertension

- Certain prescribed medications
- Oral contraceptives
- Anabolic steroids
- Amphetamines
- Chronic alcohol use
- Nasal decongestants containing sympathomimetic amines
- Some nonsteroidal anti-inflammatory drugs (NSAIDs)

Categories of Hypertension

There are two categories of hypertension. Primary, or essential hypertension, is a chronic, progressive disorder with no identifiable cause that often attacks the heart, brain, kidneys, and eyes, and is associated with increased morbidity and mortality. The condition can be successfully treated with pharmacy intervention, diet modification, and exercise. Secondary hypertension has an identified cause, which often is associated with chronic renal disease, renovascular disease, **coarctation** (constriction or stenosis of an artery), and other conditions. Secondary hypertension can also be controlled, once the cause is identified.

Sport Participation Clearance

An individual who has mild or moderate hypertension should not participate in competitive sports until cleared

TABLE 23.2   CLASSIFICATION OF HYPERTENSION

	Systolic (mm Hg)	Diastolic (mm Hg)
Normal*	<130	<85
High normal	130–139	85–89
Hypertension†		
Stage 1 (mild)	140–159	90–99
Stage 2 (moderate)	160–179	100–109
Stage 3 (severe)	180–209	110–119
Stage 4 (very severe)	>210	>120

*Optimal blood pressure with respect to cardiovascular risk is <120/80 mm Hg. However, unusually low readings should be evaluated for clinical significance.
†Based on the average of >2 readings taken at each of two or more visits after an initial screening.
Standards taken from the Fifth Report on the Joint National Committee on the Detection, Evaluation, and Treatment of High Blood Pressure (JNCV). Arch Intern Med 1993;153:153-183.

by a physician. These individuals are often allowed to play if the blood pressure is well controlled and there is no target organ damage or heart disease. The blood pressure is rechecked by the athletic trainer on a weekly basis and the physician every 2 to 4 months. For individuals in stage 3 or 4 of hypertension, play is restricted, especially in sports that have a high static component (e.g., wrestling, gymnastics, weightlifting, rock climbing, rowing) until the hypertension is well controlled.

Management of Hypertension

Treatment of hypertension is two-fold: reduce systolic and diastolic blood pressure, and prevent long-term complications. Nonpharmaceutical treatment includes lifestyle modifications and aerobic exercise. Pharmaceutical treatment may involve antihypertensive medications.

LIFESTYLE MODIFICATIONS

Because hypertension has a significant impact on risks for cardiovascular disease, individuals with hypertension will be encouraged to establish lifestyle modifications in collaboration with the exercise program. These steps may include measures to (3):

- Lose weight if overweight
- Limit alcohol intake to <1 oz/day of ethanol (24 oz of beer, 8 oz of wine, or 2 oz of 100-proof whiskey)
- Reduce sodium intake to <100 mmol/day (<2.3 g of sodium or approximately <6 g of sodium chloride)
- Maintain adequate dietary potassium, calcium, and magnesium intake
- Stop smoking and reduce dietary saturated fat and cholesterol intake for overall cardiovascular health; reducing fat intake also helps reduce caloric intake, which is important for control of weight and type 2 diabetes

Diet modifications should include a diet low in saturated fats with total dietary fat not exceeding 30% of total caloric intake, and increased potassium, calcium, and magnesium intake. In more serious cases of hypertension, more significant sodium and alcohol restrictions, weight loss, and reduction of other cardiovascular risk factors must be incorporated into the program.

EXERCISE PROGRAM

Aerobic exercise has been shown to lower resting systolic BP an average of 11 mm Hg, and diastolic BP an average of 6 mm Hg, in hypertensive individuals, but specific mechanisms are still unknown (4,5). Significant contributing factors may include:

- Reduced activity of the sympathetic nervous system, which decreases peripheral resistance and bloodflow
- Altered renal function, which facilitates the elimination of sodium by the kidneys, subsequently reducing fluid volume and BP
- Decreased body fat
- Decreased smoking and alcohol consumption that often accompany exercise conditioning
- Increased relaxation during exercise

Twenty to 30 minutes of aerobic exercise at 55 to 70% of maximum heart rate (MHR), five to six sessions per week, is recommended. In older or less fit individuals, start at 55 to 60% MHR; in more fit individuals, start at 65 to 70% MHR (6). Refer to Chapter 2 to measure maximum heart rate. Daily walking at a moderate pace is excellent, but isometric exercises and heavy resistance training should be avoided. **Field Strategy 23.1** provides an exercise program for individuals with hypertension.

 FIELD STRATEGY 23.1 HYPERTENSION EXERCISE PROGRAM

- Have a physical examination prior to beginning an exercise program.
- If taking medication, make sure the medication does not negatively interact with the exercise program.
- Initially perform aerobic exercise 3 or more times per week (walking, jogging, cycling, swimming), progressing to 5 to 6 times per week at a rate of 55 to 70% maximum heart rate.
- Begin the exercise bout with a 5-minute warm-up, followed by 25 to 30 minutes of exercise, ending with a 5-minute cool-down period.
- Progressively increase the intensity of the program, as tolerated.
- Do not perform isometric exercises or exercises using heavy resistance.

 Stop exercise immediately if you feel pain in the chest, jaw, or arm, or experience dizziness or unusual shortness of breath.

Adapted from Massie BM. To combat hypertension, increase activity. Phys Sports Med 1992;20(5):97.

PHARMACEUTICAL MEDICATIONS

When lifestyle modifications, diet, and physical activity fail to control hypertension, diuretics and antihypertensive agents may be prescribed. Diuretics lower blood pressure by increasing fluid loss; however, some diuretics can lead to a potassium deficiency. Individuals should be aware of the signs of potassium imbalance, such as weakness (particularly of the legs), unexplained numbness or tingling sensations, cramps, irregular heartbeats and excessive thirst and urination. Antihypertensive agents, such as calcium channel blockers and angiotensin-converting enzyme (ACE) inhibitors, are used to manage the condition (5,7). The ACE inhibitors are the pharmaceutical interventions least likely to interact negatively with exercise; however, they are not recommended for individuals with exercise-induced bronchospasm or pregnant women. Taking calcium channel blockers while exercising may cause orthostatic problems, but this can be prevented by a thorough cool-down following all exercise activities.

 The football player had a BP of 150/90 mm Hg, which is classified as stage 1 of hypertension. This individual should be evaluated by a physician before being cleared for participation. In most cases, he will be allowed to play if the BP is well controlled and there is no target organ damage or heart disease.

HYPOTENSION

 While working with a group of Senior-Olympic athletes, you discover that two have hypotension. What exercise precautions should be followed by these individuals?

When arterial blood pressure is lower than normal, inadequate blood is circulated to the heart, brain, and other vital

---

> ➤➤ **Box 23.2**
>
> ## Nonneurogenic Causes of Hypotension
>
> - Shock as a response to stress or trauma
> - Hemorrhage, burns
> - Diabetes mellitus
> - Allergic drug reaction
> - Dehydration
> - Low salt diets
> - Diarrhea
> - Heat (hot environments, hot showers and baths, fever)
> - Drug toxicity (alcohol, anesthesia, diuretics, analgesics, vasodilators)
> - Overtreatment of hypertension (diuretics, antihypertensives, vasodilators)
> - Orthostatic or postural hypotension (sudden change in body position, especially upon rising in the morning)
> - Straining on heavy lifting, urination, defecation
> - Vasovagal syncope (fainting)

> ➤➤ **Box 23.3**
>
> ## Nonpharmacologic Treatment of Orthostatic Hypotension
>
> - Avoid:
>   Prolonged standing
>   Vigorous exercise
>   Alcohol
>   Hot environments, and hot showers or baths
> - Do slow, careful changes in position, especially when arising in the morning
> - Eat multiple small meals
> - Schedule physical activities in the afternoon
> - Increase salt and fluid intake

organs, often resulting in a collapse of bodily functions. Hypotension, or low blood pressure, is defined as a decrease of 20 mm Hg or more in systolic blood pressure. It can be caused by a variety of factors, including shock, acute hemorrhage, dehydration, and **orthostatic** or **postural hypotension** (caused by sudden change in body position, such as moving from a lying to a standing position), or overtreatment of hypertension **(Box 23.2)**.

Orthostatic hypotension is not unusual. It is estimated to occur in about half of all elderly people, which can lead to fainting and falls (8). However, treatment is not required in the absence of symptoms. Symptoms that would indicate a medical referral is necessary include dimming or loss of vision, lightheadedness, dizziness, excessive perspiration, diminished hearing, pallor, nausea, and weakness (9). It should be noted that certain medications (e.g., vasodilators, antidepressants) may cause orthostatic hypotension. If this occurs, a physician can adjust the dose or change the medication.

Physically active people usually do not need to be concerned with hypotension. In general, the lower the blood pressure, the better, as long as the person feels well. Older athletes, however, should always check with their physician prior to performing heavy resistance exercise. Some nonpharmaceutical steps that can be taken to reduce the effects of orthostatic hypotension can be seen in **Box 23.3**.

 Under most circumstances, physically active people do not need to be concerned with hypotension. Because of the age of the senior athletes, these individuals should consult their physician prior to heavy resistance exercise.

Summary

1. Blood pressure is the force per unit area exerted on the walls of an artery, generally considered to be the aorta. It is the result of two factors: cardiac output and total peripheral resistance.

2. Blood pressure varies among individuals, but normal is considered to be 120 mm Hg systolic blood pres-

sure (SBP) over 80 mm Hg diastolic blood pressure (DBP). Hypertension is defined as a sustained elevated blood pressure greater than 140 mm Hg SBP or greater than 90 mm Hg DBP. Hypotension is characterized by a fall of 20 mm Hg or more from a person's normal baseline SBP.

3. An individual in stage 1 or 2 of hypertension should not participate in sports until cleared by a physician. These individuals can usually participate if the blood pressure is well controlled and there is no target organ damage or heart disease. The blood pressure is rechecked every week by the athletic trainer, and by the physician every 2 to 4 months.

4. For individuals in stage 3 or 4 of hypertension, play is restricted, especially in sports that have a high static component, until the hypertension is well controlled.

5. Diet modifications for hypertension include limiting sodium and saturated fats, with the total dietary fat not exceeding 30% of total caloric intake, and increasing potassium, calcium, and magnesium.

6. Aerobic exercise has been shown to reduce blood pressure in high normal and stage 1 hypertension.

7. Orthostatic hypotension is not unusual; however, if dizziness or lightheadedness becomes more frequent with a sudden change in body position, a physician should be consulted.

8. Physically active people usually do not need to be concerned with hypotension. In general, the lower the blood pressure, the better, as long as the person feels well.

References

1. Whitney EN, Rolfes SR. Understanding Nutrition. Belmont, CA: Wadsworth Publishing, 1999.

2. Joint National Committee on the Detection, Evaluation, and Treatment of High Blood Pressure. The Fifth Report on the Joint National Committee on the Detection, Evaluation, and Treatment of High Blood Pressure (JNCV). Arch Intern Med 1993;153:153-183.

3. Hollenberg NK, Braunwald E (eds.). Atlas of Heart Diseases. Hypertension: Mechanisms and Therapy. Philadelphia: Current Medicine, 1998.

4. Bove AA, Sherman C. Active control of hypertension. Phys Sport Med 1998;26(4):45-53.

5. Sachtleben TR, Mellion MB. The hypertensive athlete. In: The Team Physician's Handbook. Edited by Mellion MB, Walsh WM, Shelton GL. Philadelphia: Hanley & Belfus, 1997.

6. Massie BM. To combat hypertension, increase activity. Phys Sportsmed 1992;20(5):89-111.

7. Martin M, Yates WN. Therapeutic Medications in Sports Medicine. Baltimore: Williams & Wilkins, 1998.

8. Parson Y. Feeling faint: Sudden changes in blood pressure can lead to falls. Contemp Longterm Care 1997;220(6):13.

9. Engstrom JW. Evaluation and treatment of orthostatic hypotension. Am Fam Phys 1997;56(5):1378-1385.

24

Sudden Death

OBJECTIVES

1. List epidemiological factors associated with sudden death in the physically active population.

2. Explain the basic physiological principles of common cardiac conditions, particularly hypertrophic cardiomyopathy, that can lead to sudden death in the physically active population.

3. Differentiate between the cardiac-related causes of sudden death in individuals under age 30, and the causes in those over age 30.

4. List the risk factors for coronary artery disease and Marfan's syndrome, developed by the American College of Sports Medicine.

5. Explain the general principles of noncardiac conditions that may also lead to sudden death.

6. Describe the two-tiered approach to identifying risk factors associated with sudden death used during the preparticipation examination.

7. Explain the ethical, legal, and practical considerations that affect the medical decision-making process for determining eligibility of competitive athletes with cardiovascular abnormalities.

P articipation in physical activity and sport is known to yield positive effects on an individual's physical, mental, and social health. However, participation in any sport has inherent risks of injury. Preparticipation examinations (PPEs); (see Chapter 2) can often identify conditions that may predispose an athlete to injury. Even with the best PPE though, certain conditions may go undetected. Fortunately, most injuries are minor and require minimal management, but regardless of the intensity of physical activity, the chance for severe and even catastrophic injury exists. Sudden death has been termed the "silent killer" among athletes and physically active individuals. Although very rare, its effects are devastating and often permanent for fellow athletes, coaches, athletic trainers, family, and friends. Because of this, it is essential that every sport program have a well-established emergency procedures plan that delineates when EMS should be activated, and how the facility and its personnel can facilitate the arrival of EMS. It is also critical that all athletic trainers and coaches maintain current certification in cardiopulmonary resuscitation (CPR), as they will be the first on the scene to identify the situation and render immediate care to the athlete. For further information on developing an emergency procedures plan, refer to Chapter 4.

This chapter examines the causes of sudden death in the physically active population. After introducing epidemiological findings, a review of the physiology and pathology of common cardiac and noncardiac conditions associated with sudden death will be discussed. Recommendations for reducing the risk of sudden death in this population by means of a thorough cardiac history and preparticipation screening are then presented. Finally, issues concerning counseling athletes at risk for sudden death are discussed.

EPIDEMIOLOGY

 Think for a minute about which individuals are at risk for sudden death during physical activity. When would episodes of sudden death be most likely to occur? Are the precipitating factors that lead to sudden death preventable?

The prevalence of sudden death during physical activity is uncertain; estimates range from one in 100,000 to 300,000 in the high school–aged athlete (1). It is often precipitated by physical activity and may be caused by an array of cardiovascular conditions; the most common is hypertrophic cardiomyopathy. One study claimed that, within a 10-year period (1985–1995), 158 young competitive athletes died from sudden death. Most deaths resulted from cardiac-related causes (85%), of which 36% were a direct result of hypertrophic cardiomyopathy. Noncardiac causes included commotio cordis, heat stroke, pulmonary complications, and drug abuse (2).

The age of the athlete appears to dictate the underlying physiological pathology for the occurrence of sudden death. Congenital cardiac abnormalities are responsible for the vast majority of sudden death in athletes under the age of 30, while atherosclerotic coronary artery disease is more likely to be the cause in athletes over the age of 30 (2–4).

Sudden death appears to occur more in males (90%) than females (10%), and more in males who participate in basketball and football. Explanation for the lower rate of occurrence in female athletes is inconclusive. However, some researchers postulate that:

- Fewer females participate in sports
- Fewer participate in highly intense sports that require full-body protective equipment (football, hockey)
- There are gender differences regarding cardiac adaptations to training demands
- Females have smaller hearts

The majority of subjects in Maron's study were white (52%), but of those who died from hypertrophic cardiomyopathy, 48% were African-American, and 26% were white. Death frequently occurred immediately or shortly after physical activity, and most reported the time of death between 3:00 and 9:00 p.m. This time is not surprising since

it is the peak time for participation in most competitive sport programs. Death was instantaneous in all but 12 of the subjects. The subjects complained of chest pain, dizziness, dyspnea, and syncope prior to collapse.

 Most sudden death cases occur instantaneously in males under age 30 after vigorous activity, particularly between 3:00 and 9:00 p.m. With the use of more appropriate screening protocols, it may be possible to identify physiological factors that increase the risk of sudden death in certain individuals, and in doing so, enable appropriate measures to be taken to safeguard the health of the individual.

CARDIAC CAUSES OF SUDDEN DEATH

 What are the most common cardiac anomalies associated with sudden death? How can these anomalies be detected?

Cardiac anomalies are the most direct cause of sudden death in athletes under age 30, with hypertrophic cardiomyopathy being the most common. Other reported cardiac-related causes include mitral-valve prolapse, myocarditis, acquired valvular heart disease, coronary artery disease, and Marfan's syndrome. Other rare cardiac conditions that may contribute to sudden death involve abnormalities of the cardiac conduction system, and result in lethal cardiac rhythm problems (**Box 24.1**).

Hypertrophic Cardiomyopathy

Hypertrophic cardiomyopathy (HCM), characterized by an abnormal thickening of the left ventricle wall, develops prior to age 20, and is the leading cause of sudden death in young athletes. It typically goes undetected during routine physical examination. By definition, HCM is a hypertrophied, nondilated left ventricle in the absence of another cardiac or systemic disease capable of producing the degree of hypertrophy present. A normal left ventricle is about 1 cm thick. In HCM, the wall typically ranges from 2 to 4 cm thick, and can be greater than 15 cm thick (5). This

> ➤➤ **Box 24.1**
>
> ### Cardiac Causes of Sudden Death
> - Hypertrophic cardiomyopathy
> - Mitral-valve prolapse
> - Myocarditis
> - Acquired valvular heart disease
> - Coronary artery disease
> - Marfan's syndrome
> - Long QT syndrome
> - Wolff-Parkinson-White syndrome
> - Arrhythmogenic right ventricular dysplasia

abnormal thickness can lead to electrical problems and abnormal heart rhythms (including ventricular fibrillation, lethal rhythm).

Hypertrophic cardiomyopathy occurs in about 0.2% of the young adult population and is usually genetically transmitted (6). The features appear in childhood and adolescence, reaching full development by the time of physical maturity. Symptoms of cardiac dysfunction, which do not appear until early adulthood if they appear at all, result in impaired ventricle filling. As a result, there can be periods of **arrhythmia** (irregular heartbeats) or blood flow obstruction that may produce syncope during physical exertion.

Unfortunately, HCM often goes undetected during routine physical examinations. Athletes can compete for years without demonstrating signs or symptoms. Physical examinations should include a thorough cardiac history and cardiac examination (see Cardiovascular Preparticipation Screening near the end of this chapter).

 *Any athlete who complains of **prodromal symptoms** (an early symptom of a disease), such as syncope, dizziness, or undue fatigue during or after exercise, should be seen by a physician or cardiologist.*

Since the heart is a muscle, and muscles hypertrophy as a result of exercise, does HCM result from intense exercise? There has been concern about this issue because if a trained athlete without HCM were detrained for a rest period of 2 to 3 months, the heart muscle would decrease in size. However, training and detraining have no effect on heart size or thickness in individuals with HCM.

Mitral Valve Prolapse

Mitral valve prolapse (MVP) is not a frequent cause of sudden death, but can affect 2 to 5% of the population spanning all ages (7). MVP is a condition in which redundant tissue is found on one or both leaflets of the mitral valve. During a ventricular contraction, a portion of the redundant tissue on the mitral valve pushes back beyond the normal limit and, as a result, produces an abnormal sound. This sound is followed by a systolic murmur as blood is regurgitated back through the mitral valve into the left atrium. Because of the characteristic sound, this condition is often referred to as a "click-murmur syndrome." Individuals with MVP usually experience some degree of chest pain, dyspnea, palpitations, and fatigue with exertion (8).

Myocarditis

Myocarditis is an inflammatory condition of the muscular walls of the heart that can result from a bacterial or viral infection. The condition is characterized by the infiltration of inflammatory cells into the myocardium, leading to an abnormally enlarged left ventricle. Sudden death occurs when the inflammatory changes in the myocardium lead to degeneration or death of adjacent muscle cells, resulting in electrical instability and life-threatening arrhythmias. Although some individuals may be asymptomatic, others exhibit symptoms commonly associated with viral infections, including fever, body aches, fatigue, cough, or vomiting, which often impedes the diagnosis. Exercise intolerance, shortness of breath, and more serious cardiac symptoms including **palpitations** (rapid, forceful heartbeats) or syncope may occur without warning.

Acquired Valvular Heart Disease

Acquired valvular heart disease stems from a defect or insufficiency in a heart valve that can lead to improper blood flow through the heart. The condition is manifested as either **valvular stenosis** (a narrowing of the orifice around the cardiac valves) or **regurgitation** (backward flow of blood), and is named according to the valve affected (e.g., mitral valve, aortic valve, tricuspid valve). If more than one valve is affected, the condition is called **multivalvular disease**, which occurs in the context of rheumatic heart disease. Due to the characteristic murmurs, diagnosis is usually made during the physical examination.

Individuals with mild to moderate mitral and tricuspid valve stenosis or regurgitation may still participate in sports, although each case must be evaluated on an individual basis. Initially, experts thought that aortic stenosis was a common cause of sudden death. With new research, however, this has not been proven to be the case. Aortic stenosis, like other valve conditions, can often be detected early through physical examination. Those with mild aortic stenosis may participate in all competitive sports. Athletes with mild or moderate asymptomatic aortic stenosis with a history of **supraventricular tachycardia** (rapid heartbeats proximal to the ventricles, in the atrium or A-V node) or ventricular arrhythmias at rest should only participate in low-intensity competitive sports. Athletes with severe aortic stenosis or symptomatic, moderate stenosis should not engage in any competitive sport (9).

Coronary Artery Disease

The most common cause of sudden death in individuals over age 30 is coronary artery disease, also referred to as **atherosclerosis**. An excessive buildup of cholesterol within the coronary arteries narrows the diameter of the arteries and impedes blood flow, which in turn reduces the amount of oxygen supplied to the heart. Due to the diminished oxygen, angina or chest pain during physical exertion is a common symptom. If excessive cholesterol buildup blocks a coronary artery, the person is at risk for a **myocardial infarction** (heart attack). If the blockage is in a major coronary artery, death often occurs.

Unlike young athletes, who rarely know if they have a cardiac anomaly that may put them at risk for sudden death, athletes over the age of 30 have usually experienced prodromal cardiovascular symptoms or have a known

TABLE 24.1 **ACSM CORONARY ARTERY DISEASE RISK FACTORS**

Positive Risk Factors	Defining Criteria
Age	Men >45 years; women >55 or premature menopause without estrogen replacement therapy
Family history	Myocardial infarction or sudden death before age 55 in father or other male relative (uncle or first cousin), or before age 65 in mother or other female relative (aunt or first cousin)
Current cigarette smoker	
Hypertension	Blood pressure >140/90 on at least two occasions, or using antihypertensive medication
Hypercholesterolemia	Total serum cholesterol >200 mg/dL, or HDL <35 mg/dL
Diabetes mellitus	Persons with insulin-dependent diabetes mellitus (IDDM) who are >30 years of age, or have had IDDM for >15 years, and persons with noninsulin-dependent diabetes mellitus (NIDDM) who are >35 years of age
Sedentary lifestyle	Persons comprising the least active 25% of the population, as defined by the combination of a sedentary job involving sitting for a large part of the day and no regular exercise or active recreational pursuits
Negative Risk Factor	**Defining Criteria**
High serum HDL cholesterol	>60 mg/dL (1.6 mmol/L)

Reprinted with permission from American College of Sports Medicine. ACSM's Guidelines for Exercise Testing and Prescription. 5th ed. Baltimore: Williams & Wilkins, 1995:18.

medical history of coronary artery disease. Therefore, athletes over the age of 30 have three options. They can choose to:

- Ignore the symptoms and continue participating at the same level, placing themselves at risk for sudden death
- Change their lifestyle according to CAD recommendations and continue to participate in limited activity
- No longer participate in physical activity

The American College of Sports Medicine (ACSM) has developed a list of risk factors for CAD (10) **(Table 24.1)**. The criteria should be used to identify individuals at risk for a heart attack, and may warrant an exercise **electrocardiogram** (ECG), or treadmill stress test before beginning an exercise program. In addition, ACSM recommends that anyone who has had a history of angina, palpitations, syncope, or dyspnea during exercise should also have an exercise ECG prior to beginning a moderate or vigorous exercise program (11).

Marfan's Syndrome

Marfan's syndrome does not necessarily lead to sudden death. When sudden death does occur, it is usually caused by the condition's hallmark characteristic: a weakened aorta. Marfan's syndrome is a genetic disorder of the connective tissue that can affect the skeleton, lungs, eyes, heart, and blood vessels. It affects more than 40,000 people in the United States, both men and women of any race or ethnic group (12). A single mutant gene is linked to the condition. Although usually inherited, there is no family history in one-third of all cases.

Individuals with Marfan's are tall in stature with overly long extremities; the arm span exceeds the person's height. Joints are usually hypermobile, and the person may have a pigeon (sunken) chest, stretch marks, scoliosis, and an increased incidence of hernias. A positive thumb and wrist test begins the initial identification of Marfan's. The thumb

test involves adduction of the thumb across the palm of the hand and flexion of the fingers around the thumb. The test is positive if the thumb extends past the fifth finger. The wrist test involves the person encircling a wrist with the thumb and fifth finger of the opposite hand. The test is positive if the thumb and fifth finger overlap. In addition to orthopedic anomalies, it is not unusual to find an excessively high palate, eye defects (particularly myopia or near-sightedness), mitral valve prolapse, and defects in the connective tissue layers of the aorta. As a result of this defect, death from Marfan's is usually associated with an aortic dissection or rupture.

Screening for Marfan's syndrome includes a musculoskeletal and eye examination, and an echocardiogram to determine abnormalities of the aorta **(Box 24.2)**. There is

---

➤➤ **Box 24.2**

Screening for Marfan's Syndrome

Screen all men over 6 feet and all women over 5 feet 10 inches with an electrocardiogram and slit-lamp examination when any two of the following exist:
- Family history of Marfan's syndrome*
- Cardiac murmur or midsystolic click
- Kyphoscoliosis (kyphosis combined with scoliosis)
- Anterior thoracic deformity (i.e., pectus excavatum)
- Arm span greater than height
- Upper-to-lower body ratio more than 1 standard deviation below the mean
- Myopia
- Ectopic lens (displacement of the lens of the eye)

---

* This finding alone should prompt further investigation.
Reprinted with permission from Crown LA, Hizon JW, Rodney WM. The athlete's heart. In: The Team Physician's Handbook. Edited by Mellion MB, Walsh WM, Shelton GL. Philadelphia: Hanley & Belfus, 1997: 300.

no cure for Marfan's, but with careful medical management, most people can live a normal life.

Those with Marfan's syndrome should avoid contact sports due to the risk of injury to the eye and aorta. Athletes with a family history of premature sudden death and without evidence of aortic root dilation may participate in moderate, low-static and low-dynamic competitive sports, such as brisk walking, leisure bicycling, golf, slow jogging, and slow-paced tennis (see Table 2.1). Athletes with aortic root dilatation may only participate in low-intensity competitive sports (see Table 2.1). All isometric exercise is contraindicated, and noncompetitive, nonstrenuous aerobic activities should not exceed 50% of aerobic capacity (12,14).

Rare Cardiac Conditions

Other rare cardiac conditions may also contribute to sudden death. Long QT syndrome and right ventricular dysplasia produce serious arrhythmias, which may cause sudden death. Right ventricular dysplasia, a disorder of the right ventricle, is characterized by the formation of adipose or fibrous tissue extending from the epicardium to the endocardium. This abnormal growth of tissue increases the risk of ventricular fibrillation. Any unstable ventricular heart rhythm, such as ventricular tachycardia or ventricular fibrillation, can lead to death. In fact, most cardiac conditions resulting in sudden death are the result of an abnormal ventricular rhythm (2,7,15).

Wolff-Parkinson-White syndrome is an abnormality of cardiac rhythm that manifests as a supraventricular tachycardia. The condition is associated with an accessory electrical pathway in the heart proximal to the ventricles that can spontaneously produce episodes of rapid twitching of the atrium muscle fibers within a range of 200 to 300 heartbeats/minute. The condition is often seen in asymptomatic, healthy individuals during electrocardiographic examination. Although rarely associated with sudden death, the condition may complicate other heart conditions, such as myocarditis or ischemic heart disease.

Congenital coronary artery anomalies are another cause of sudden death in young athletes. The most common anomaly is an abnormal origin of the left coronary artery. The anomaly necessitates an acute take-off angle, forcing the artery to pass between the aorta and pulmonary artery, both of which can decrease blood flow to the heart. Other anomalies may involve an abnormal origin of the right coronary artery, presence of a right coronary artery without a left coronary artery, and abnormal coronary artery spasm. Congenital coronary artery anomalies may not be detected during exercise because symptoms such as syncope, near-syncope, and chest pain are intermittent and unpredictable (3).

 The most common cardiac condition associated with sudden death in physically active individuals is hypertrophic cardiomyopathy, an abnormal thickening of the left ventricle of the heart. This

thickening obstructs blood flow, causing an arrhythmia that can lead to myocardial infarction. Other cardiac anomalies include mitral-valve prolapse, myocarditis, and Marfan's syndrome. Cardiac conditions can be detected with a thorough cardiac history and examination. If detected, alterations in the exercise program can be made to ensure safe participation.

NONCARDIAC CAUSES OF SUDDEN DEATH

 Are there other causes of sudden death in the physically active population, not associated with cardiac anomalies? How are these conditions identified? Are they preventable?

Sudden death in athletes is usually directly related to cardiac conditions. However, there are instances where noncardiac conditions may lead to sudden death **(Box 24.3)**. Often, noncardiac conditions are more easily identifiable through physical examination and field evaluation. Once identified, the condition can be treated.

Van Camp and colleagues conducted a study to determine the frequency and causes of nontraumatic sport-related deaths in high school and college athletes. Between the years of 1983 and 1993, 160 nontraumatic deaths were reported, of which 124 were high school athletes and 34 were collegiate athletes. Of the 160 athletes, adequate information regarding cause of death was available in 136. There were five times more deaths in male than female athletes at both levels of competition. Cardiovascular conditions were the most common cause of sudden death (74%), but other causes (22%) included exertional hyperthermia, exertional rhabdomyolysis (destruction of skeletal muscles, which releases myoglobin into the blood and urine), status asthmaticus (state of prolonged asthma), and electrocution due to lightning.

Commotio Cordis

Cardiac arrest from a blunt blow to the chest in the absence of a structural cardiovascular disease is rare in sports, but it can occur. In one study, 25 subjects collapsed and died instantaneously after receiving an unexpected blow to the

> ➤➤ **Box 24.3**
>
> ## Noncardiac Causes of Sudden Death
>
> - Commotio cordis
> - Substance abuse
> - Head injuries
> - Heat illness
> - Exertional hyperthermia
> - Exercise-induced anaphylaxis
> - Exertional rhabdomyolysis
> - Sickle cell anemia

chest, usually inflicted by a projectile object (e.g., baseball or hockey puck). Subjects ranged from 3 to 19 years of age, and most were male (24:1). Most deaths occurred while participating in softball and baseball, but subjects also participated in hockey, football, and karate. Some subjects (28%) were wearing some form of chest protection, but the impact to the chest was judged not to be extraordinary for the sport involved and did not appear to have sufficient force to cause death. The majority of the chest contusions occurred directly over the left ventricle, with the force delivered during an electrically vulnerable phase of the ventricular impulse. This results in a premature heartbeat, leading to ventricular fibrillation and sudden death (16).

Mechanical observations suggest that, during rapid, high-level acceleration to the sternum, the elastic skeletal structures attain a velocity similar to that of the impacting object. Children and adolescents seem to be at a greater risk for commotio cordis since their chest walls are thinner and more compliant to impacting forces, which may enhance the transmission of force to the heart (17). Since the known forces that cause ventricular fibrillation and cardiac arrest in sport participants are not extraordinary, it is unclear if chest protection can decrease the risk of sudden death in athletes. Further research is needed to determine: (a) if chest protection would indeed reduce the risk of sudden death from blunt trauma, and (b) what type of material can be used in protective equipment to absorb and disperse projectile forces to the chest and heart.

Substance Abuse

Certain types of drug abuse can lead to cardiac changes that predispose an athlete to sudden death. Amphetamines are central nervous system stimulants that increase heart rate, respiration rate, and blood pressure. Cocaine, an anesthetic, constricts coronary arteries and has been known to lead to myocardial infarction in those with and without coronary artery disease. In addition, myocarditis has been found in autopsy reports of cocaine-related sudden death cases. It must be noted that a massive dose of cocaine is not required to produce cardiac or respiratory consequences. There have been several reported cases of sudden death in anabolic steroid users, although a direct relationship between steroid use and sudden death has not yet been established.

Erythropoietin, produced in the kidneys, is a hormone that stimulates bone marrow to increase production of red blood cells. Erythropoietin (EPO/EPOGEN) became synthetically available in the late 1980s when its use as an ergogenic aid for endurance athletes was first documented. The use of EPO is equal to blood doping, and like blood doping, can increase blood volume and viscosity of the blood, leading to decreased circulation, thrombosis, and myocardial infarction. These adverse cardiovascular effects have led to sudden death in athletes; EPO may be one of the most deadly ergogenic aids available (18).

Head Injuries

Catastrophic brain injuries that can lead to death in athletes include a skull fracture, epidural hematoma, acute and subacute subdural hematoma, second impact syndrome, or various other brain hemorrhaging conditions (19). Athletes should be observed closely after sustaining any type of head injury, regardless of the level of consciousness. Signs of rapidly increasing intracranial pressure include a dilated or irregular pupil or pupils, reduced pulse, nausea or vomiting, dyspnea, **photophobia** (sensitivity to light), mood swings, muscle weakness, and a decreased level of consciousness. **Decortication** (extension of the legs with flexion of the elbows, wrists, and fingers) or **decerebration** (extension of all four extremities) is often present in severe injuries (see Figure 4.3). An individual who is unable to remember events leading up to (retrograde amnesia), or following the injury (anterograde amnesia) should not be permitted to continue play, and should be referred immediately to a physician.

Additional information concerning head injuries can be found in Chapter 8.

Heat Illness

Heat illness is one of the most preventable causes of death in athletes, yet every year athletes die from exertional hyperthermia. In football, heat stroke is second only to head injuries as the most frequent cause of death. The condition is also seen in distance runners and wrestlers dehydrated through weight loss. Heat stroke is almost always preceded by prolonged, strenuous physical exercise in individuals who are poorly acclimatized or in situations where evaporation of sweat is inhibited.

The athlete often complains of a feeling of burning up. Deep breaths, irritability, hysterical behavior, and an unsteady gait may be present. Although traditionally it was thought that a failed sweating mechanism was present during heat stroke, it is now known that in most cases, the sweating mechanism is still functioning. As the condition deteriorates, the skin is hot and dry and appears red or flushed, and the pulse becomes rapid and strong, as high as 150 to 170 beats per minute. Brain tissue damage by excessive body heat leads to vasomotor collapse, shallow breathing, decreased blood pressure, and a rapid and weak pulse. Muscle twitching or seizures may occur just before the individual lapses into coma (20). This is a medical emergency, and EMS should be activated immediately.

Further information concerning heat illness is presented in Chapter 17.

Sickle Cell Trait

Sickle cell trait is an inherited disorder in which red blood cells tend to form into a sickle-shaped structure (see Figure

25.2). This sickling formation of red blood cells prevents an efficient transportation of oxygen to the tissues, and can lead to vascular occlusion, coagulation, and death. Eight percent of all African-Americans have sickle cell trait, and those ages 23 to 30 have a 1.3 in 1000 chance of dying from sudden death during exertional activities, particularly during extreme conditions of heat, humidity, and increased altitude (21). Unexpected death is almost always associated with severe exertional **rhabdomyolysis**, a fatal disease stemming from renal failure caused when cellular contents of damaged skeletal muscle (myoglobin) enter the circulation. Sickle cell anemia is easily screened through laboratory testing; when identified, recommendations can be made to ensure safe sport participation.

 Noncardiac-related causes of sudden death in the physically active population usually involve commotio cordis, substance abuse, head injury, heat illness, or sickle cell trait. Most of these can be prevented through prescreening protocols to identify those at risk, proper use of protective equipment, and taking certain precautions during exercise to reduce the risk.

CARDIOVASCULAR PREPARTICIPATION SCREENING

 How can athletic trainers better identify the risks associated with sudden death? When identified, what recommendations can be made for safe sport participation?

To identify the risks associated with sudden death in athletes, a two-tiered approach must be implemented. First, a standard screening examination should be done 6 to 8 weeks prior to the start of the sport season and every 2 years thereafter (22,23). Screening should be performed by a healthcare provider with the medical skills, requisite training, and clinical experience to obtain a detailed cardiovascular history, perform an extensive physical examination, and recognize potential heart disease or cardiac anomalies.

According to recommendations from a joint summit on sudden death sponsored by the NATA Research and Education Foundation (22), and the 26th Bethesda Conference (24), a cardiac history should include extensive questions on previous symptomatic episodes and family history. In addition to the medical history, the physical examination, performed by an individual with special skills in identifying heart abnormalities, should include Marfan's syndrome screening and a cardiovascular examination **(Box 24.4)**. Unfortunately, many experts believe that a personal cardiac history does little to detect abnormalities in young athletes. However, an extensive medical history has been found to be advantageous in older athletes (24,25).

Recommendations for Sudden Death Screening

1. Medical History Questions
   - Prior chest pain during physical exertion
   - Exercise-induced syncope or near syncope
   - Excessive unexplained shortness of breath, fatigue, or dizziness with exercise
   - Prior history of heart murmur or increased blood pressure
   - Family history of death from cardiovascular disease in a relative younger than age 50
   - Family history of hypertrophic cardiomyopathy, dilated cardiomyopathy, long QT syndrome, or Marfan's syndrome
2. Physical Examination
   - Marfan's syndrome screening
   - Cardiovascular examination emphasizing:
     - Brachial artery blood pressure measurement
     - Precordial auscultation in both the supine and standing positions
     - Assessment of the femoral artery pulse

Identification of a possible cardiovascular abnormality during the cardiac history or standard physical examination is the first tier of recognition. Many of these conditions were listed in Box 2.3. The second tier involves referral to a specialist (cardiologist) for more extensive screening, including an echocardiogram, particularly when seeking detection of hypertrophic cardiomyopathy. Table 24.2 identifies the various causes of sudden death and associated diagnostic tests.

The decision on whether to permit an athlete to participate after identifying a cardiovascular abnormality must be resolved on an individual basis under the Americans with Disabilities Act of 1990 (ADA), the Rehabilitation Act of 1973, and similar state statues prohibiting unjustified discrimination against physically impaired athletes. These laws permit an athlete with the physical capabilities and skills to play a sport despite the fact that a cardiovascular abnormality is present. Exclusion from participation must be based on reasonable medical judgments, given the state of scientific research on the specific condition. These laws require the careful balancing of the athlete's right to participate, the physician's evaluation of the medical risks of participation, and the team's interests in conducting a safe athletic program.

The American College of Sports Medicine, at its 26th Bethesda Conference, established guidelines for determination of athletic participation eligibility (24). These guidelines are directed to team physicians, athletes, team officials, and athletic governing bodies, as well as to the courts, regarding the acceptable medical risks of athletic participation with known cardiovascular abnormalities. In addition, the NCAA Committee on Competitive Safeguards and Medical Aspects of Sports has firmly stated that the team

TABLE 24.2 **DIAGNOSTIC TESTING FOR VARIOUS CAUSES OF SUDDEN DEATH**

Condition	Test	Possible Abnormalities
Coronary artery disease	Electrocardiogram (ECG) Exercise ECG (treadmill) Thallium scan Angiogram*	Previous myocardial infarction Myocardial ischemia (less oxygen to heart) Myocardial ischemia Coronary artery occlusion
Hypertrophic cardiomyopathy	ECG Chest x-ray Echocardiogram*	Ventricular hypertrophy Cardiomegaly (enlarged heart) Hypertrophy of ventricular walls, obstruction of blood flow
Congenital coronary artery anomalies	ECG Exercise ECG Thallium scan Angiogram*	Previous myocardial infarction Myocardial ischemia Myocardial ischemia Abnormal coronary artery anatomy
Marfan's syndrome	Physical examination Ophthalmology exam Echocardiogram	Musculoskeletal abnormalities Lens dislocation, myopia, retinal detachment Aortic enlargement, aneurysm, or dissection
Acute myocarditis	ECG Chest x-ray Blood chemistry Myocardial biopsy*	Tachycardia, other abnormalities Cardiomegaly, pulmonary edema Elevated cardiac enzymes Inflammatory cells, muscle degeneration
Arrhythmias	ECG Holter monitor/event recorder Exercise ECG	Abnormal heart rhythm Intermittent arrhythmia Exercise-induced arrhythmia

*Most definitive test. [Diagnostic tests are performed only when there is significant clinical suspicion based on the medical history and physical examination.]

Reprinted with permission from Kronisch RL. Sudden cardiac death in sports. Ath Ther Today 1996;1(4):40.

physician should be the final authority in determining whether the athlete should return to competition. It is essential that the team physician use all resources available to reach an appropriate decision. These resources may include consultation with recognized cardiologists, either locally or nationally; other ancillary administrative, medical, and coaching staffs; and input from the athlete and family. Certainly, the more elite the athlete, the more complex and difficult the decisions are regarding eligibility. However, the key players in this relationship remain the team physician and athlete. It is clearly in the best interest of the physician charged with the responsibility of determining medical clearance for athletes with known cardiovascular abnormalities to know and follow the Bethesda Conference guidelines (26).

 Athletic trainers can identify those at risk for sudden death by ensuring that PPEs are performed by a qualified healthcare provider 6 to 8 weeks prior to the start of a sport season, and every 2 years thereafter. The PPE should include an extensive cardiac medical history and cardiac physical examination, emphasizing brachial artery blood pressure measurement, assessment of femoral pulse, precordial auscultation, and screening for Marfan's syndrome. Individuals with a cardiovascular abnormality should be counseled by the team physician and a cardiologist to determine what activities could be recommended according to the ACSM guidelines.

Summary

1. Sudden death in athletes occurs infrequently. When it does, the on-site personnel should immediately activate EMS and begin cardiopulmonary resuscitation.
2. Hypertrophic cardiomyopathy is the most common cardiac-related cause of sudden death.
3. Other cardiac-related causes of sudden death include mitral-valve prolapse, myocarditis, acquired valvular heart disease, coronary artery disease, Marfan's syndrome, long QT syndrome, Wolff-Parkinson-White syndrome, and arrhythmogenic right ventricular dysplasia.
4. Noncardiac causes of sudden death include commotio cordis, heat illness, head injuries, substance abuse, exertional hyperthermia, exercise-induced anaphylaxis, exertional rhabdomyolysis, and sickle cell anemia.
5. To decrease the risk of sudden death in physically active individuals, a two-tiered system must be implemented:
   - The preparticipation physical examination should include an extensive cardiac medical history and physical examination.
   - If a cardiac abnormality is identified, the athlete should be referred to a specialist for further evaluation.
6. Determination of continued participation in sports should rest with the athlete and the team physician after consultation with expert cardiologists, family, and team officials.

7. Clearance for participation should follow the 26th Bethesda Conference ACSM's recommendations for determining eligibility for competition in athletes with cardiovascular abnormalities.

References

1. Van Camp SP, et al. Non-traumatic sports death in high school and college athletes. Med Sci Sports Exerc 1995;27(5):641-647.
2. Maron BJ, et al. Sudden death in young competitive athletes: Clinical, demographic, and pathological profiles. JAMA 1996;276(3):199-204.
3. Kronisch RL. Sudden cardiac death in sports. Ath Ther Today 1996;1(4):39-41.
4. Thompson PD. The cardiovascular complications of vigorous physical activity. Arch Intern Med 1996;156(20):2297-2302.
5. Pelliccia A, et al. Athlete's heart in women. JAMA 1996;276(3):211-215.
6. Maron BJ. Hypertrophic cardiomyopathy in athletes. Phys Sportsmed 1993;21(9):83-90.
7. Maron BJ, et al. Prevalence of hypertrophic cardiomyopathy in a general population of young adults: Echocardiographic analysis of 4111 subjects in the CARDIA Study—Coronary Artery Development in (Young) Adults. Circulation 1995;92(4):785-789.
8. Kenny A, Shapiro LM. Sudden cardiac death in athletes. Br Med Bull 1992;48(3):534-545.
9. Cheitlin MD, Douglas PS, Parmley WW. Acquired valvular heart disease. Med Sci Sports Exerc 1994;26(10):S254-S260.
10. American College of Sports Medicine. ACSM's guidelines for exercise testing and prescription. Baltimore: Williams & Wilkins, 1995.
11. Thompson PD, et al. Coronary artery disease. Med Sci Sports Exerc 1994;26(10):S271-S275
12. The Marfan Syndrome Fact Sheet. Washington, DC: National Marfan Foundation, 1997.
13. Crown LA, Hizon JW, Rodney WM. The athlete's heart. In: The Team Physician's Handbook. Edited by Mellion MB, Walsh WM, Shelton GL. Philadelphia: Hanley & Belfus, 1997.
14. Mitchell JF, Haskell W, Raven PB. Classification of sports. Med Sci Sports Exerc 1994;26(10):S242-245.
15. Sudden Death in Sports. Champaign, IL: Human Kinetic Publishers and NATA-Research and Education Foundation, 1997.
16. Maron BJ, et al. Blunt impact to the chest leading to sudden death from cardiac arrest during sports activities. N Engl J Med 1995;333(6):337-342.
17. Viano DC, et al. Mechanism of fatal chest injury by baseball impact: Development of an experimental model. Clin J Sport Med 1992;2:166-171.
18. Cowart VS. Erythropoietin: A dangerous new form of blood doping. Phys Sportsmed 1989;17(8):115-118.
19. Cantu RC. Cerebral concussion in sport management and prevention. Sports Med 1992;14(1):67-74.
20. Mellion MB, Shelton GL. Safe exercise in the heat and heat injuries. In: The Team Physician's Handbook. Edited by Mellion MB, Walsh WM, Shelton GL. Philadelphia: Hanley & Belfus, 1997.
21. Kerle KK, Nishimura KD. Exertional collapse and sudden death associated with sickle cell trait. Am Fam Phys 1996;54(1):237-240.
22. Van Camp SP, et al. Sudden death in athletes: Summit statement. Dallas: National Athletic Trainer's Association Research and Education Foundation, 1997.
23. Maron B, et al. Cardiovascular preparticipation screening of competitive athletes. Washington, DC: American Heart Association, 1996.
24. American College of Sports Medicine, American College of Cardiology 26th Bethesda Conference. Recommendations for determining eligibility for competition in athletes with cardiovascular abnormalities. Edited by Mitchell JG, Maron BJ, Raven PB. Med Sci Sports Exerc 1994;26(10):S223-S283.
25. Maron BJ, Pelliccia A, Spirito P. Cardiac disease in young trained athletes: Insights into methods for distinguishing athlete's heart from structural heat disease, with particular emphasis on hypertrophic cardiomyopathy. Circulation 1995;91(5):1596-1601.
26. Mitten MJ, Maron BJ. Legal considerations that affect medical eligibility for competitive athletes with cardiovascular abnormalities and acceptance of Bethesda conference recommendations. Med Sci Sports Exerc 1994;26(10):S238-S241.

CHAPTER 25

Conditions of the Female Athlete, Disabled Athlete, and Senior Athlete

OBJECTIVES

1. Name several menstrual irregularities and the implications they may have on sport participation.

2. Describe how female athletes may be affected by the use of oral contraceptives and other commonly used birth control methods.

3. Describe postural and musculoskeletal issues that can affect a pregnant woman, and the implications each may have on a physically active pregnant woman.

4. List indications and contraindications for sport participation during pregnancy.

5. Describe the common types of anemia and how they are identified and treated.

6. Describe the various eating disorders, and explain guidelines for safe weight loss and weight gain.

7. Describe osteoporosis and how it may be affected by physical activity and exercise.

8. Define the Female Athlete Triad, and describe how it affects health and sport performance.

9. List injuries and medical conditions more commonly seen in wheelchair athletes.

10. Discuss special considerations associated with physical activity for an amputee athlete, an athlete with cerebral palsy, and a visually impaired athlete.

11. Explain how the aging process affects skeletal and neuromuscular function.

12. List specific injuries and medical conditions more commonly seen in the senior athlete.

As more children, females, seniors, and people with varying levels of physical ability participate in exercise and sport, increasing levels of knowledge and clinical skills are required to meet the needs of these participants. This chapter focuses on considerations of these special populations. Issues specific to the female athlete will be discussed first, followed by special concerns for the disabled athlete. Finally, special considerations for the senior athlete will be presented. Because special needs of the pediatric athlete have been integrated throughout the text, they will not be repeated here.

SPECIAL CONCERNS OF THE FEMALE ATHLETE

 A female athlete complains of gastrointestinal distress. After reviewing her medical history, you discover that this athlete has repeatedly complained of GI distress and has also suffered two metatarsal stress fractures in the last year. What concerns might you have? How will you address this situation?

As more and more women of all ages participate in competitive sports and physical activity, an increasing understanding of the unique physical nature of the female athlete is required to meet the needs of this population. This section addresses menstrual irregularities, oral contraceptives and other birth control methods, pregnancy and exercise, ane-mia, dysfunctional eating disorders, osteoporosis, and the Female Athlete Triad.

The Uterine (Menstrual) Cycle

The **uterine**, or menstrual, **cycle** is a series of cyclic changes that the inner lining of the uterus (endometrium) goes through each month as it responds to varying levels of hormones in the blood. It coincides with the **ovarian cycle**, which is associated with the maturation of an egg. The ovarian cycle is divided into two phases. The **follicular phase** (days 1 to 14) is the period of follicle (spheroidal cell cluster in the ovary contain an ovum or egg) growth. **Ovulation**, or release of the egg, occurs midcycle when the ballooning ovary wall ruptures and expels the egg. The **luteal phase** (days 14 to 28) occurs after ovulation. The ruptured follicle collapses and forms a new endocrine gland called the corpus luteum, which begins to secrete progesterone and some estrogen. If pregnancy does not occur, the corpus luteum begins to degenerate in about 10 days, and its hormonal output ends. In contrast, if the egg is fertilized and pregnancy ensues, the corpus luteum persists until the placenta is ready to take over its hormone-producing responsibility in about 3 months. The menstrual cycle follows three distinctive phases, depicted in **Figure 25.1**:

1. **Days 1–5: Menstrual phase**. In this phase, the uterus sheds all but the deepest portion of the endometrium. As the endometrium detaches from the uter-

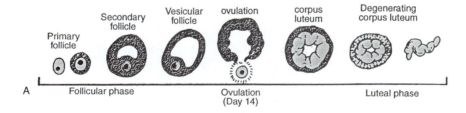

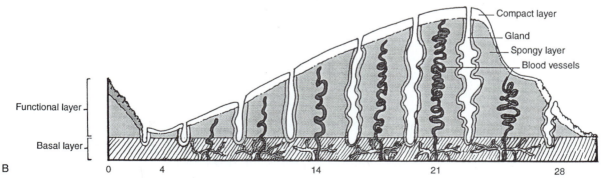

➤ **FIGURE 25.1 Ovarian and uterine cycle**. A, Structural changes in the ovarian follicles during the 28-day ovarian cycle correlate with changes in the endometrium of the uterus during the uterine cycle. B, The uterine cycle has three stages: menstrual, proliferative, and secretory. Phase one is a shedding, and the second phase rebuilds the endometrium. Both of these events occur prior to ovulation. The final phase involves enriching the blood supply and providing nutrients that prepare the endometrium to receive a fertilized egg.

ine wall, it is often accompanied by bleeding for 3 to 5 days. The tissue and blood pass out through the vagina as the menstrual flow.

2. **Days 6–14. Proliferative phase**. During this phase, the endometrium rebuilds itself. The basal layer, influenced by rising blood levels of estrogen, generates a new functional layer. As the layer thickens, its glands enlarge and its spiral arteries increase in number. As a result, the endometrium once again becomes thick, velvety, and well vascularized. Also during this phase, estrogen induces synthesis of progesterone receptors in the endometrial cells, readying them for interaction with progesterone. Ovulation occurs in the ovary at the end of this stage.

3. **Days 15–28. Secretory phase**. In this phase, the endometrium prepares for implantation of an embryo. Rising levels of progesterone act on the estrogen-primed endometrium, causing the spiral arteries to coil more tightly and convert the functional area to a secretory mucosa. The uterine glands enlarge, coil, and begin secreting nutritious glycoproteins into the uterine cavity. These nutrients can sustain an embryo until it becomes implanted into the blood-rich endometrial lining. If fertilization does not occur, the corpus luteum begins to degenerate toward the end of the secretory phase. Progesterone levels fall, depriving the endometrium of hormonal support, and the spiral arteries kink and go into spasm. Without oxygen and nutrients, the endometrial cells begin to die and the functional layer begins to self-digest, setting the stage for menstruation to begin on day 28.

Nonathletes experience **menarche** (onset of menstruation) at an average age of 12.5 years, while for athletes the average age is 13.5 to 15.5 years. The normal cycle is 28 days, but can range from 25 to 35 days. Menarche continues throughout a women's life until menopause, which is the cessation of menstrual function and the subsequent decline in ovarian hormone production. Although the average age for menopause is around 51, there is a gradual change in reproductive function, called the **climacteric phase**, that ranges from age 46 to 55. During this period, called the perimenopausal years, the menstrual cycle may shorten and become irregular in both frequency and bleeding. After 56 years of age, a woman is said to be postmenopausal (1).

Menstrual Irregularities

Many girls and women will, at one time or another, be affected by menstrual irregularities. Research is just beginning to explore the effects of conditioning and training on gynecological function, yet much needs to be done. Menstrual irregularities may include dysmenorrhea, menstrually induced leg pain, anovulatory oligomenorrhea, luteal phase deficiency, and exercise-associated amenorrhea. Although each of these conditions can be identified and managed, without early detection and proper treatment some of these irregularities can lead to long-term health problems that include chronic stress fractures, osteoporosis, endometriosis, and infertility.

DYSMENORRHEA

Dysmenorrhea, or menstrual cramps, is usually caused by an overproduction of prostaglandins, a group of chemicals acting as local hormones that are produced in the body and synthesized in all tissues. Uterine prostaglandins cause the muscles of the uterus to contract. Under most conditions, the contractions are minor and go unnoticed. More severe myometrial contractions and the resulting myometrial ischemia lead to the severe abdominal pain associated with dysmenorrhea.

Pain is usually localized in the lower abdomen but may radiate into the back, hip, and thighs. The condition usually begins with the onset of menses and continues through the first days of the menstrual cycle. Other symptoms include bloating, nausea, vomiting, diarrhea, headache, breast tenderness, fatigue, irritability, and nervousness. Signs and symptoms can last from a few hours to several days, but tend to decrease in intensity as a woman ages.

Relief from mild to moderate discomfort can be achieved with a variety of methods. Regular exercise and a diet high in fluids and fiber and low in salt can alleviate bloating and swelling caused by water retention. Over-the-counter medications such as ibuprofen, aspirin, Midol, and Tylenol can relieve pain and cramping. These medications inhibit prostaglandin synthesis, which decreases myometrial contractions. Ice massage to the low back, application of heat packs, and acupressure can also help relieve pain. Severe or persistent discomfort may necessitate physician referral to rule out pelvic inflammatory disease (PID), benign uterine tumors, obstruction of the cervical opening, and **endometriosis**, a condition in which endometrial cells from the uterine lining implant themselves in the abdominal and uterine cavities and occasionally in the ovarian lining. Hormone therapy is a common method of treatment to decrease pain, discomfort, and other unwanted signs and symptoms associated with dysmenorrhea.

MENSTRUALLY INDUCED LEG PAIN

It has been noted that some female athletes report leg pain induced by physical activity in the week prior to their menstrual cycle. This leg pain is associated with women who are ovulating and normally have premenstrual fluid retention. It is thought that the fluid retention allows less room for muscle hypertrophy during exercise, resulting in exertional compartment-like symptoms. Women with menstrually induced leg pain can be treated with oral contraceptives that suppress ovulation and decrease fluid retention.

Conversely, some women report exertional compartment leg pain after using hormonal therapy as a means of contraception. It appears that the progesterone of the birth control pill increases the likelihood of fluid retention, resulting in the induced leg pain. Changing the birth control pill to one that has lower progesterone levels often brings relief. Women with menstrually induced exertional compartment-like symptoms should be questioned about their menstrual cycle and if they are taking oral contraceptives.

ANOVULATORY OLIGOMENORRHEA

Anovulation (cessation of ovulation) is associated with chronic, unopposed estrogen production that leads to continuous endometrial stimulation and lower levels of progesterone. Several different patterns of irregular bleeding range from short (less than 21 days) to long cycles with 35 to 90 days between bleeding (1). The longer pattern is associated with **oligomenorrhea**. Oligomenorrhea refers to infrequent menstrual cycles, and is often associated with a combination of strenuous exercise and significant weight loss. As such, oligomenorrhea and amenorrhea are more prevalent among runners (10 to 50%) than the general population (2 to 5%) (1). Unlike secondary amenorrhea, which is linked with cessation of normal menstrual cycles, athletes with oligomenorrhea continue to have menstrual cycles, but may not be consistent from month to month, or may have a menstrual cycle with a minimal menstrual discharge. For example, an athlete with oligomenorrhea may have a normal cycle 1 month, not have a cycle for the following 2 months, and return to a normal cycle the fourth month. During anovulatory oligomenorrhea, bleeding can be very heavy (menorrhagia), at times leading to iron depletion and anemia, both of which may affect athletic performance.

Management includes a physician referral to rule out endometriosis. Monthly progesterone therapy is usually indicated. Progesterone therapy matures the endometrium, resulting in regular bleeding, and protects against endometrial **hyperplasia** (overgrowth of the endometrium). Oral contraceptives may also be used to control the menstrual cycle. There are no contraindications to exercise for those with anovulatory oligomenorrhea.

LUTEAL PHASE SUPPRESSION

The luteal phase of the ovarian cycle extends from ovulation until the onset of the next menstrual bleeding, normally about 12–17 days. The hormone progesterone is produced only after ovulation. During this period, both estrogen and progesterone levels are high. Luteal phase deficiency is characterized by a shortened luteal phase length and insufficient progesterone production. The menstrual cycle is usually normal but occurs more frequently. Research on this condition is scarce. While the incidence in the sedentary population is 16%, the incidence in the

athletic population is said to be 33%, but no side effects of luteal phase suppression are known (1). In runners, more miles per week paralleled greater shortening of the luteal phase.

EXERCISE-ASSOCIATED AMENORRHEA

Amenorrhea, the absence of menstruation, is more prevalent among athletes, particularly runners, than the general population. Amenorrhea is a symptom, not a disease, and has been linked to prepubertal exercise, premature ovarian failure, central nervous system tumors, infections, hypothalamic-pituitary-ovarian (HPO) hormonal imbalances, chronic diseases, osteoporosis, and malnutrition. Other related causes of athletic amenorrhea include weight loss, low body fat levels, loss of specific fat stores (particularly femoral adipose tissue stores), excessive exercise, and being a vegetarian. Several risk factors can predispose a female to the condition **(Box 25.1)**.

There are two types of amenorrhea: primary and secondary. Primary amenorrhea (delayed menarche) is the absence of menstruation by age 16 in a girl with secondary sex characteristics. Delayed menarche prolongs the hypoestrogenic state of menses, which can lead to **osteopenia** (bone mineral loss) at an age when bone density should be increasing. Scoliosis and increased risk of stress fractures

---

▶▶ Box 25.1

Risk Factors for Amenorrhea

- Young age—may have immature hypothalamic pituitary ovarian (HPO) axis
- Higher activity level—runners, cyclists, swimmers
- Higher intensity—more strenuous or longer exercise period
- History of menstrual irregularity
- Prepubertal training
- Delayed menarche
- Low body weight/weight loss; low body fat/fat loss
- Never having given birth
- Never used oral contraceptive pills—twice as likely to suffer a stress fracture than those who use them
- Diet lacking in protein and total calories. Poor nutrition may be the most important factor to increase the risk of amenorrhea
- Eating disorders
- Psychological stress studies are contradictory
- Genetic/hereditary factors may play a role in the age of menarche
- Total number of risk factors—the more risk factors an athlete has, the more likely she will have exercise-related menstrual dysfunction

---

Adapted from Joy EA, Macintyre JG. Women in sports. In: The Team Physician's Handbook. Edited by Mellion MB, Walsh WM, Shelton GL. Philadelphia: Hanley & Belfus, 1997.

may therefore result. Secondary amenorrhea is the absence of menstruation for three or more consecutive menstrual cycles after menarche. This can result from pregnancy or dysfunction in the ovaries, endometrium, pituitary gland, or hypothalamus.

Exercise-associated amenorrhea is a form of hypothalamic amenorrhea, which stems from decreased ovarian hormone production and hypoestrogenemia similar to menopause. It has been reported in women participating in virtually every sport. Amenorrhea has been shown to affect up to 50% of competitive runners and professional ballet dancers, and 12% of cyclists and swimmers (2). Amenorrheic athletes tend to have begun physical training at a younger age than those not affected by the problem.

It is commonly accepted that amenorrhea and decreased circulating levels of estrogen predispose women to reduced bone density, leading to increased risk of stress fractures, particularly in the lumbar vertebrae and lower extremities, and increased musculoskeletal injuries (3,4). Within the first 3 months of amenorrhea, a woman should be fully evaluated to rule out pregnancy, counseled on the risks of bone density loss, and encouraged to alter training regimens. Decreasing training, increasing food intake, and administrating hormone therapy have been used to manage amenorrhea.

Research suggests that menses returns in some amenorrheic women after they gain weight or decrease exercise, or both. This is accomplished by reducing the number of training days, mileage, or intensity. Diet should be evaluated to ensure adequate caloric intake to match the high energy output. Hormone therapy, including oral contraceptives and cyclic estrogen/progesterone therapy, does not increase bone mass, but prevents further bone loss, vaginal and breast atrophy, and osteopenia. However, individuals may choose not to take oral contraceptives because of the side effects, such as increased incidence of vaginitis, weight gain, acne, breast tenderness, and mood alterations. Women who remain amenorrheic should be examined annually.

GENERAL MANAGEMENT OF MENSTRUAL DYSFUNCTION

All athletes experiencing any type of menstrual dysfunction should be referred to a physician, preferably a gynecologist. The referral should include a pelvic examination and, in some cases, blood tests to determine if the menstrual dysfunction is related to exercise or some pathological condition. In addition, female athletes with oligomenorrhea or amenorrhea should have an annual history and physical examination. Management of menstrual dysfunction often depends upon the type of dysfunction. Hormone therapy, including both progesterone and estrogen protocols, is often the treatment of choice, but some side effects may result from the drug therapy. Estrogen therapy would not be indicated for women with hypertension, diabetes mellitus, migraine headaches, fibrocystic breast disease, or gall bladder disease.

Endometriosis

When endometrial tissue grows outside of the endometrial cavity, dysmenorrhea, oligomenorrhea, severe pelvic pain, and pain upon defecation can occur. Endometriosis may develop asymptomatically, leading to eventual infertility. Management consists of gynecological referral for a laparoscopic examination. Depending upon the level of severity, drug therapy or surgical intervention is often indicated. There are no contraindications to exercise for athletes who develop endometriosis.

Premenstrual Syndrome

Headaches, breast tenderness, back pain, bloating, irritability, depression, fatigue, and certain food cravings are all symptoms that may occur during the luteal phase (days 15 to 28) of the menstrual cycle. These symptoms are collectively termed **premenstrual syndrome** (PMS). PMS symptoms are frequently divided into physical and psychological, but a women must exhibit a combination of one psychological change and one physical symptom consistently during the luteal phase to be diagnosed with PMS (5) **(Box 25.2)**.

Menstruating women suffer from PMS across the life span. Symptoms can often become debilitating, interfering with an athlete's training and competition. Fatigue may result in subpar performance and an increase in injuries. Causes of PMS vary, but fluctuations in hormone levels during the menstrual cycle appears to be the most common cause.

Regular exercise, particularly aerobic activities, and an overall healthy diet with a reduction in salt intake can help alleviate some symptoms. Dysmenorrhea and headaches associated with PMS can be treated with nonsteroidal anti-inflammatory drugs (NSAIDs). Hormonal therapy may be used, but this should be done on an individual basis. If self-help techniques do not alleviate symptoms, or if symptoms

---

➤➤ **Box 25.2**

Symptoms Associated with Premenstrual Syndrome

Physical Symptoms	Psychological Symptoms
Headache	Irritability
Bloating	Depression
Breast tenderness	Fatigue
Gastrointestinal upset	Difficulty in concentrating
Changes in appetite	Forgetfulness
Vasomotor flushing	
Heart palpitations	
Dizziness	

▶▶ **Box 25.3**

Contraindications to the Use of Oral Contraceptives

- Hypertension (diastolic pressure greater than 90)
- Migraine headaches
- Depression
- Hepatitis or impaired liver function
- Oligomenorrhea or amenorrhea
- Abnormal glucose tolerance
- Recent major elective surgery (less than 4 weeks postoperative)

involve moderate to severe psychological problems, a physician referral is warranted.

Birth Control and Sport Participation

According to a recent unpublished study, 60% of Division I female college athletes are sexually active (6). Many of these women practice safe sex (81.6%), but less than one-third (32.4%) use oral contraceptives (OCs) as a birth control method. Oral contraceptives prohibit ovulation, reduce dysmenorrhea, and decrease the amount and duration of the menstrual flow. There are, however, certain contraindications to the use of oral contraceptives **(Box 25.3)**. In addition, medications such as antibiotics, analgesics, antihistamines, and drugs used to treat tuberculosis, epilepsy, and depression may interfere with the effectiveness of OCs.

The choice of birth control depends upon coital frequency, exercise habits, lifestyle, medical history, fertility plans, and potential positive side effects **(Box 25.4)**. Almost one-fourth of women in the general population between the ages of 15 and 44 use OCs. In comparison, fewer female athletes choose OCs; they rely more on barrier methods (diaphragms, condoms, spermicides). The decision to use barrier methods rather than OCs may be in response to studies that report decreased maximal oxygen uptake, decreased isometric strength and endurance time, and reduction of mitochondrial citrate (an oxidative enzyme) with OC use (7). Most side effects associated with the amount of estrogen versus progestin and other compounds found in the various OCs are counteracted by exercise. Regular

exercise is known to increase the protective high-density lipoprotein (HDL) cholesterol, reduce deleterious low-density lipoprotein (LDL) cholesterol, lower total triglyceride levels, and activate the fibrinolytic system responsible for converting fibrin to soluble products. In addition, most physically trained women have lower arterial blood pressure, lower body fat, and higher lean body weight and do not smoke, all factors that put sedentary women at risk for complications (7). As such, for healthy, active young women, benefits of OCs outweigh the risks.

Pregnancy and Sport Participation

The impact of exercise on a pregnant women and her developing fetus is an area of concern, particularly because chemicals and nutrients pass freely in placental blood flow. Certainly, any factors that compromise this fetal blood supply would be important in counseling a pregnant women regarding exercise during pregnancy. Gains in body weight and fat accumulation are obvious adaptations to pregnancy that can have some effect on weight-bearing exercise. The hormones progesterone and relaxin increase joint laxity, making articulations wider and more mobile during the later stages of pregnancy. Because of this, ballistic movements (bouncing) must be avoided during daily activities and exercise. Exercise should be an important normal part of pregnancy for the active woman, and has been shown to have several benefits **(Box 25.5)**.

POSTURAL AND MUSCULOSKELETAL ISSUES

Postural adaptations to compensate for the weight of the uterus lead to increased lordosis and upper spine extension. The woman's center of gravity shifts upward and forward, often leading to lower back pain. Exercises to strengthen the abdominal and hip extensors (hamstrings, gluteus maximus), as well as relaxing and/or stretching the erector spinae and hip flexors (iliopsoas, pectineus, rectus femoris), can relieve some of this pain. Proper lifting techniques to relieve stress on the low back should be incorpo-

▶▶ **Box 25.4**

Benefits from the Use of Oral Contraceptives

- Menstrual cycle regulation
- Prevention of iron-deficiency anemia
- Decreased risk of fibroids, endometrial cancer, and endometrial hyperplasia
- Prevention of osteoporosis
- Decreased risk of ovarian cancer and cysts
- Decreased dysmenorrhea and premenstrual tension

▶▶ **Box 25.5**

Benefits of Exercise During Pregnancy

- Maintenance or improvement of maternal fitness
- Control of excess weight gain
- Improved posture and appearance
- Increased energy
- Improved sleep
- Decreased incidence of low back pain
- Improved self-image and self-esteem
- Decreased incidence of varicose veins
- Decreased water retention
- Decreased level of tension
- Possible decrease in complications during labor and shortened labor
- More rapid postpartum recovery

rated in daily activities. For a previously active, healthy woman during an uncomplicated pregnancy, moderate aerobic exercise does not produce circulatory alterations that compromise fetal oxygen supply. In looking at fetal development, fetoplacental growth, prematurity, fetal stress/distress, and condition during labor and at birth, it was found that women who exercise regularly do not experience an increase in abortion, congenital abnormalities, abnormal placentation, premature rupture of the membranes, or preterm labor. Although increases were found in fetal heart rate after exercise, no adverse effects were seen (8).

EXERCISE CONSIDERATIONS

Pregnant women should be aware of the potential for fetal hypoglycemia during exercise. Under prolonged exercise, maternal blood sugar may decrease. The pregnant women needs to consume extra calories to meet the demands of pregnancy, and if she exercises, more calories are needed. Furthermore, after the fifth month of pregnancy, maternal hypotension can develop if exercises are performed in a supine position. In this position, the uterus compresses the vena cava, slowing venous return and leading to a decrease in fetal circulation, as well as maternal hypotension. Absolute medical conditions where exercise is contraindicated include cardiovascular disease; significant anemia; premature rupture of membranes; persistent second or third trimester bleeding; preterm labor during the prior or current pregnancy, or both; incompetent cervix or cerclage; and uncontrolled hypertension, renal disease, and diabetes mellitus.

Exercise programs need to be individualized in consultation with the supervising physician or obstetrician. The primary goal with exercise during pregnancy is safety. Recreational athletes and those who exercise regularly can participate in several aerobic activities such as walking, bicycling, aerobic dance, water aerobics, swimming, jogging, cross-country skiing, ice or roller skating, and tennis. Aerobic classes should be modified to decrease the amount of ballistic movements, and exercising in a supine position should be avoided. A 5- to 10-minute warm-up can be followed by 30 to 60 minutes of exercise at 65 to 85% of maximum heart rate (perceived exertion = moderately hard to hard), three to five times per week. Elite athletes can exercise for 60 to 90 minutes at 75 to 85% of maximum heart rate (perceived exertion = hard), four to six times per week (1). The exercise period should be followed by an appropriate cool-down and stretching period. Weight training with light weights and higher repetitions can be continued during pregnancy when the goal is strength maintenance, not gain. Proper lifting and breathing techniques, such as exhaling during exertion, must be practiced consistently. Free-weight exercises that place the joints in a traction position, thereby stressing ligamentous structures, should be avoided. In running programs, distance and intensity of workouts will need to be decreased as the pregnancy progresses. **Box 25.6** summarizes some of the problems pregnant women may encounter during exercise and suggested recommendations. Because many physiological and morphologic changes of pregnancy persist for 4 to 6 weeks postpartum, exercise routines should be resumed gradually after the 6-week postpartum medical check-up in consultation with the supervising obstetrician.

Anemia

Iron is present is all human cells and serves several functions as a carrier of oxygen from the lungs to the tissues in the form of hemoglobin (Hb), as a facilitator of oxygen use and storage in the muscles as myoglobin, as a transport medium for electrons within the cells in the form of cytochromes, and as an integral part of enzyme reactions in various tissues. Too little iron can interfere with these vital functions and lead to serious illness or death. A reduction

---

➤➤ **Box 25.6**

Recommendations for Pregnant Women with Exercise Problems

Problem	Recommendation
Poor balance	Slow down and exercise cautiously. If exercising outdoors, be alert to changes in terrain. Experiment with posture changes to identify the most stable position while exercising.
Overheating and dehydration	Drink plenty of liquids prior to the run. Do not exercise at midday in hot weather, but rather in the early morning or late evening. If exercise at midday is necessary, run shorter distances, or decrease the length and intensity of the exercise period. If dizziness or nausea occurs, stop exercising, cool down, and drink plenty of cool fluids.
Leg, hip, or abdominal pain	Always stretch and warm up prior to exercise, regardless of the activity. Wear well-cushioned shoes with a very firm midsole, a straight last, and a high degree of hindfoot stability. Stop exercising and walk for a short distance if pain occurs in a specific area.
Concern from others about safe exercise during the pregnancy	Consult the physician or obstetrician about problems that may arise. Exercise with other women who may have run or remained active during their pregnancy. Be assertive about exercise during pregnancy, but do it in a cautious, reasonable manner. Run with friends, if possible, and keep a positive attitude.

in either the red blood cell volume (hematocrit) or hemoglobin (Hb) concentration is called **anemia**. Although there are five classifications of anemia, all are caused by either impaired red blood cell (RBC) formation, excessive loss, or destruction of RBCs.

The recommended dietary allowance (RDA) for iron in adolescent girls and women of childbearing age is 15 mg per day. The average diet contains 5 to 7 mg of iron per 1000 kcal (9). Therefore, women need 3000 kcal per day to meet the RDA, yet many female athletes consume less than 2000 kcal per day, particularly in those sports that emphasize a lean physique. In addition, many female athletes eat a modified vegetarian diet low in iron content and low in iron bioavailability. Good sources of iron include lean animal meat (liver, beef roasts, tenderloin, lamb, chicken or turkey legs), tuna, oysters, shrimp, enriched raisin bran or corn flakes, bagels, bran muffins, dried apricots, baked potatoes with the skin, peas, kidney beans, chickpeas, tofu, and molasses.

In sport participation, anemia reduces maximum aerobic capacity, decreases physical work capability at submaximal levels, increases lactic acidosis, increases fatigue, and decreases exercise time to exhaustion (9,10). Although several predisposing factors may increase the risk of getting anemia **(Box 25.7)**, athletes tend to be more prone to specific anemic conditions.

STAGES OF ANEMIA

Iron status is assessed through several laboratory tests. Because each test assesses a different aspect of iron metabolism, results of one test may not always agree with results of other tests. Hemoglobin (Hb) concentration and hematocrit (Hct) are commonly tested because they measure the amount of functional iron in the body. The concentration of Hb in circulating red blood cells in the more direct and sensitive measure. Hct indicates the proportion of whole blood occupied by the red blood cells; it falls only after the Hb concentration falls. Hematological tests based on characteristics of red blood cells (hemoglobin, hematocrit, total iron-binding capacity [TIBC]) are more popular and less expensive than biochemical tests. However, the biochemical tests (free erythrocyte protoporphyrin [FEP] concentration, serum ferritin concentration, and transferrin saturation) detect earlier changes in iron status. Iron deficiency develops gradually, progressing through several stages before anemia is evident. These stages include:

- Stage I—Iron depletion is characterized by ferritin (an iron protein complex) less than 12 mg/mL, an indicator of reduced iron stores in the bone marrow. Other components of iron status remain normal: hemoglobin, hematocrit, FEP, serum iron, IBC, and transferrin saturation.
- Stage II—Iron-deficiency erythropoiesis follows several months of iron depletion and is characterized by decreased levels of circulating iron, but hemoglobin and hematocrit remain normal.
- Stage III—Iron-deficiency anemia follows several weeks of iron-deficient erythropoiesis. Hemoglobin production diminishes, and the individual develops clinically recognized iron-deficiency anemia, referred to as frank anemia.

IRON-DEFICIENCY ANEMIA

Iron deficiency is characterized by deficient hemoglobin synthesis. It is the most common nutritional deficiency in the United States, affecting 7.8 million adolescent girls and women of childbearing age, secondary to menstrual blood loss and increased iron demand during pregnancy (11). Among men (males 18 years and older) and postmenopausal women in the United States, iron-deficiency anemia is uncommon. In infancy and early childhood, inadequate diet may be an underlying factor; in older children and adults, blood loss or impaired absorption of iron should be suspected. The condition is also seen in endurance athletes and in those who maintain a low percentage of body fat.

Early symptoms include fatigue, tachycardia, blood mixed with feces, pallor, and epithelial abnormalities such as a sore tongue. Later symptoms include cardiac murmurs, congestive heart failure, loss of hair, and pearly sclera. **Box 25.8** lists the general signs and symptoms of iron-deficiency anemia. Treatment may involve dietary iron supplementation (ferrous sulfate, ferrous gluconate) and ascorbic acid (vitamin C) to enhance iron absorption. Colas, coffee, tea, chocolates, and other caffeine products should be avoided, as caffeine hampers iron absorption. Surgery may be needed if active bleeding from polyps, ulcers, malignancies, or hemorrhoids is the cause.

➤➤ **Box 25.7**

Predisposing Factors for Developing Anemia

- Personal or family history of anemia, bleeding disorders, or chronic disease
- Intermittent jaundice early in life
- Excessive menstrual flow; increased duration, frequency, or volume
- Chronic blood loss through gastrointestinal bleeding (chronic use of aspirin or NSAIDs)
- Certain drugs and toxins
- Childbirth
- Disadvantaged socioeconomic background
- Poor diet or dietary restriction (vegetarian diet, weight loss diets, or fad diets)
- Cancer
- Volunteer blood donor
- Diminished hepatic, renal, or thyroid function

Adapted from Harris (9), pages 44-46.

➤➤ **Box 25.8**

Signs and Symptoms of Iron-Deficiency Anemia

- Exercise fatigue
- Muscle burning
- Nausea
- Shortness of breath (dyspnea)
- Appetite for substances that have little or no nutritional value (starch, ice, clay)
- Pallor
- Palpitations
- Loss of hair
- Pearly sclera
- Spoon-shaped nails (koilonychia)
- Dry scaling and fissures of the lips (angular cheilosis)
- Inflammation of the tongue (glossitis)

EXERCISE-INDUCED HEMOLYTIC ANEMIA

Exercise-induced hemolytic anemia occurs during exercise when the red blood cells are destroyed and the hemoglobin is liberated into the medium in which the cells are suspended (intravascular hemolysis). Intravascular hemolysis can occur in both high- and low-impact sports. In high-impact sports such as running, it is thought that the trauma of repetitive, hard foot strikes destroys the red blood cells. The condition is sometimes referred to as foot strike hemolysis, and is more commonly observed in marathoners and middle-age distance runners, particularly those who are overweight, run on hard surfaces, wear poorly cushioned shoes, and run with a stomping gait. However, the intravascular hemolysis has also been reported in competitive swimmers and rowers. Thus, other possibilities such as muscle contraction, acidosis, or increased body temperature may account for damage to the cells.

Prevention and treatment focuses on encouraging runners to be lean, run on soft surfaces, run light on their feet, and wear well-cushioned shoes and insoles. The condition is rarely severe enough to cause appreciable iron loss. The condition may be of more concern to highly competitive, world-class athletes for whom a fractional physiological difference can result in a competitive disadvantage.

SICKLE CELL ANEMIA

Sickle cell anemia, most commonly seen in African-Americans, results from abnormalities in hemoglobin structure that produce a characteristic sickle- or crescent-shaped red blood cell that is fragile and unable to transport oxygen. The condition arises because of inheriting an autosomal recessive gene (possessing two sickle genes) as opposed to having the sickle cell trait, in which only one sickle gene is inherited. Because of their rigidity and irregular shape, sickle cells clump together and block small blood vessels, leading to vascular occlusions, or infarcts, in organs, such as the heart, lungs, kidneys, spleen, and central nervous system (**Figure 25.2**). Although individuals with sickle cell trait may be asymptomatic for their entire lives, exercising excessively in high heat, humidity, or altitude may lead to dehydration, increased body temperature, hypoxia, and acidosis, which can predispose an individual to increased protein concentration in the circulating blood cells. This high concentration of protein increases blood viscosity and impairs blood flow, which can lead to a stroke, congestive heart failure, acute renal failure, pulmonary embolism, or sudden death.

Signs and symptoms may include swollen, painful, and inflamed hands and feet, irregular heartbeat, severe fatigue, headache, pallor, muscle weakness, and severe pain due to oxygen deprivation. Currently, there is no known treatment to reverse the condition. Since dehydration can complicate the condition, individuals should hydrate maximally before, during, and after exercise or physical exertion. Liquids with caffeine should be avoided due to their diuretic effect. Individuals with sickle cell trait should limit running to no more than 1 mile without rest, and avoid activity in extremely hot humid weather, and at altitudes greater than 2500 ft (10).

Eating Disorders

Clinically, an eating disorder may entail a refusal to maintain a healthy body weight (85% of expected body weight), dramatic weight loss, fear of gaining weight even when underweight, preoccupation with food, abnormal food-consumption patterns, or recent binge eating behaviors associated with loss of control and feelings of guilt. Eating disorders are becoming more prevalent in both competitive and recreational sport participants. They typically affect females at the onset of puberty and into the late teens, but they also occur in males. Although these disorders are

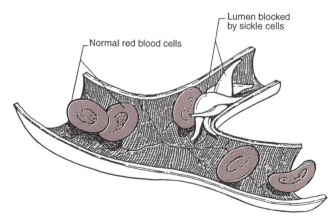

➤ **FIGURE 25.2** **Sickle cell.** Sickle cells are abnormal red blood cells that are very fragile and unable to transport oxygen. Because of their rigidity and irregular shape, they often clump together and block small blood vessels, leading to vascular occlusions in the vital organs.

often linked to sports that stress leanness (e.g., gymnastics, distance running, swimming, diving, rowing, ballet, cross-country skiing, and wrestling), no sport is exempt. The incidence of eating disorders is difficult to pinpoint because of the secretive nature of those who have the disorders. Many sport participants engage in weight-control practices to afford optimal performance. When eating habits are altered because of a distorted body image, however, serious problems result.

There are four specific eating disorders: atypical eating disorders, bulimia nervosa, anorexia nervosa, and combined disorders of anorexia and bulimia. Anorexia and bulimia account for about 66% of all eating disorders. In addition to these four, a subclinical eating disorder has recently been termed **anorexia athletica**, which classifies athletes who demonstrate significant signs and symptoms of eating disorders but do not meet the APA criteria for anorexia or bulimia (15).

ATYPICAL EATING DISORDERS

Many athletes show signs of disordered eating habits, but do not meet the criteria established for bulimia nervosa or anorexia nervosa. Many of these individuals exhibit certain physical features, and psychological and behavioral symptoms that indicate a possible eating disorder, listed in **Box 25.9**.

BULIMIA NERVOSA

Bulimia nervosa is characterized by normal body weight for age and height, and having a minimum average of two binge eating episodes per week for at least 3 months (12). The bulimic maintains a cyclical pattern of ingesting large quantities of food, often 1,000 to 10,000 calories during a few minutes to several hours. Purging may or may not occur. If purging does occur, it is referred to as the "binge-purge cycle." The individual often has significant fluid and electrolyte abnormalities that can result in cardiac arrhythmias, hypotension due to low blood volume, metabolic acidosis caused by laxative-induced diarrhea, and cardiomyopathy. Gastrointestinal complications include esophagitis, possible esophageal perforation, pancreatitis, and constipation secondary to chronic laxative abuse. Irregular menses is common, rather than amenorrhea as seen in anorexics. The three most common physical signs associated with bulimia are (13):

- Russell's sign, a lesion on the dorsum of the hand caused by repetitive trauma to the area during self-induced vomiting. This elongated ulceration, or hyper-pigmented callus or scar, is visible on the metacarpophalangeal joint.
- Hypertrophy of the salivary glands, particularly the parotid glands. The individual often has a chipmunk-like face.

➤➤ **Box 25.9**

Signs and Symptoms of a Possible Eating Disorder

Physical Features
- Weight that is too low for athletic performance, or extreme fluctuations in weight
- Swollen salivary glands (puffy cheeks or jaw just in front of the ear)
- Amenorrhea
- Sores or calluses on knuckles or back of hand from inducing vomiting
- Hypoglycemia
- Cardiac arrhythmias, bradycardia
- Gastrointestinal complaints
- Headaches, dizziness, muscle cramps, weakness due to electrolyte disturbances
- Renal dysfunction due to electrolyte disturbances
- Tendency toward stress fractures
- Loss or thinning of the hair

Psychological and Behavioral Symptoms
- Excessive dieting and guilt about eating
- Excessive eating without weight gain
- Excessive exercise that is not part of the training program
- Claiming to feel fat at normal weight despite reassurances from others
- Preoccupation with food or hoarding of food
- Avoidance of eating in public, denial of hunger
- Frequent weighing
- Evidence of binge eating or self-induced vomiting
- Use of drugs to attempt to control weight (abuse of laxatives, diet pills, diuretics, emetics)

- Dental erosion caused by acidic gastric secretions that decalcify the teeth during recurrent vomiting episodes.

ANOREXIA NERVOSA

Anorexia nervosa is defined as a refusal to maintain body weight over a minimal normal weight for age and height, with body weight being 15% below what is expected (12). The disorder is typically seen in females during adolescence, although it has been known to occur after menopause. These individuals are usually easy to identify because of severe weight loss over a period of time.

Anorexics have a distorted body image and maintain a great fear of gaining weight even though they are underweight. They view themselves as fat and equate body appearance with self-worth. An obsessive-compulsive nature for perfection and achievement leads many individuals to develop into obsessive exercisers. Amenorrhea often occurs prior to significant weight loss and continues for at least 3 consecutive months. There is a desire to control the body and eating, and remain in a prepuberty state, resulting in a near-starvation behavior. Many complain of being cold even on hot days. Others suffer from severe constipation because of poor food intake.

TABLE 25.1 COMPARISON OF BULIMIA NERVOSA AND ANOREXIA NERVOSA

Factor	Bulimia Nervosa	Anorexia Nervosa
Weight	Normal for age and height	15% below what is expected
Weight loss	Fluctuations are common	Loss is gradual
Age	Women in the teens and twenties; also seen in wrestlers	Women in the teens and twenties
Body image	Distorted for body shape and weight	Distorted, person feels fat even when emaciated
Eating habits	Recurrent binge eating, followed by fasting	Near-starvation is commonly seen
Purging	May or may not occur; laxatives, diuretics, and self-induced vomiting may be used	Not common
Self-esteem	Low; depression is common; obsessive-compulsive behavior is present	Low; obsessive-compulsive behavior for perfection
Menses	Irregular menses is common	Amenorrhea is common

Detection of anorexia is easier than bulimia nervosa because of the deteriorated physical state of the individual. **Table 25.1** compares bulimia nervosa with anorexia nervosa, and **Box 25.10** list medical complications that can result from these eating disorders.

GENERAL TREATMENT OF EATING DISORDERS

Treatment for both bulimia and anorexia nervosa involves a three-pronged approach: referral to a physician, a mental health professional (psychologist or psychiatrist), and a nutritionist. If it is determined by the mental health professional that a personality disorder is present, an extensive rehabilitation program of psychological and pharmacological intervention is necessary. If recognized early enough, behavioral and psychoeducational intervention with individual counseling can help. Nutritional supervision and guidance can help the patient overcome myths about eating and instill factual knowledge in focusing the direction of proper nutrition. Bulimia nervosa and anorexia

nervosa may not be curable, but can be managed with a well-structured and supervised rehabilitation program (14).

Osteoporosis

Osteoporosis is a serious condition of decreased bone mass and strength that often leads to fractures. These fractures commonly occur in the vertebral bodies, proximal femur, and distal radius. Cortical bone reaches its peak density at about age 40; trabecular bone (hip, spine, femur) density peaks in the midtwenties. After this, bone density decreases at a rate of 1% per year. Forty percent of postmenopausal women suffer at least one osteoporotic fracture in their lifetimes (15). Identifiable risk factors are listed in **Box 25.11**. Estrogen, as well as calcium, is needed to develop strong bone. This is why postmenopausal women are at a greater risk for developing osteoporosis than other populations.

Primary prevention of osteoporosis includes adequate calcium intake (1200 mg per day), adequate circulating estrogen levels, and adequate (but not excessive) weight-bearing exercise. The most important of these is adequate circulating estrogen. If the athlete is amenorrheic, even in the face of proper calcium intake and exercise, loss of bone density is likely. In the face of adequate circulating estrogen, excessive calcium intake does not lead to greater bone density than would be the case by ingesting only the recom-

---

➤➤ **Box 25.10**

Complications of Eating Disorders

Related to Purging
- Electrolyte disturbances caused by decreased blood volume, heart muscle metabolic alkalosis, and magnesium deficiency nausea
- Inflammation of the salivary glands and pancreas
- Erosion of the esophagus and stomach that can lead to severe GI bleeding
- Erosion and decay of dental enamel and discoloration of the teeth due to gastric juices

Related to Weight Loss
- Loss of fat and muscle mass, including bloating, constipation, abdominal pain, amenorrhea
- Osteopenia, osteonecrosis, and femoral head collapse
- Peripheral neuropathy
- Loss of scalp and pubic hair, or increased growth of pigmented baby-like hair over body

---

➤➤ **Box 25.11**

Risk Factors for Osteoporosis

- Low calcium intake
- Sedentary lifestyle
- Tobacco use
- Being underweight
- Amenorrhea related to bone density loss
- Estrogen deficiency
- Decreased bone-mass mineral content, as detected by a bone-mass density test

mended amount of calcium daily. A sedentary, but normally menstruating (eumenorrheic) woman is likely to have a higher bone density level than an active amenorrheic woman (even though both will be below the optimum of the active, eumenorrheic woman), assuming all three groups of women ingest equal amounts of calcium. The primary focus in preventing osteoporosis is to maintain estrogen levels to ensure healthy bones. Since women can only add to their bone mass between puberty and about age 40, periods of amenorrhea may produce long-term harm to the woman by introducing osteoporosis prematurely.

Inadequate estrogen levels may be caused by metabolic conditions such as athletic amenorrhea, menopause, or excessive prolactin, a protein that stimulates the secretion of milk, which normally occurs during pregnancy, but is an abnormal sign at other times. Other causes may be related to malnutrition, chronic illness, renal insufficiency, connective tissue disorders, an abnormal thyroid, connective tissue disorders, or malignancy. Too much exercise adversely affects bone remodeling and can actually increase the risk of osteoporosis. Secondary prevention is estrogen therapy started at menopause or within 5 to 6 years (15). Weight-bearing exercise and estrogen therapy can prevent bone loss in postmenopausal women.

The Female Triad

In 1992, the American College of Sports Medicine gathered a panel of experts to discuss a triad of disorders commonly seen in adolescent and young adult female athletes: disordered eating, amenorrhea, and osteoporosis (16). The Female Triad, as it is now called, is particularly common among athletes participating in sports that require an ideal body weight or optimal body fat level for achievement (e.g., gymnastics, figure skating, cross-country running, diving, swimming, and ballet) **(Figure 25.3)**.

Each of these conditions has potentially serious affects on health and sport performance. When seen together, however, they often accelerate each other, producing even more devastating affects on both the quality and longevity of life. There is still much to be known concerning this triad; what is known is that long-term affects of disordered eating often alter menstrual function, which in turn increases the onset of osteoporosis.

Studies have confirmed that athletes who have experienced stress fractures are more likely to have low bone mass density and dietary calcium intake, menstrual irregularities, and lower use of oral contraceptives (17,18). These studies suggest that amenorrhea is associated with eating disorders, low estrogen levels, and increased risk of lowered bone mass density, which brings the Female Triad to full circle. Athletes who remain amenorrheic continue to lose bone mass. However, once menses resumes, increase in bone mass also returns, particularly in the vertebra.

 In the female athlete who reported gastrointestinal distress and had suffered two metatarsal stress fractures, you should suspect that these symptoms are associated with the Female Triad. Your management plan should include physician referral and a complete medical history of diet and menstrual function.

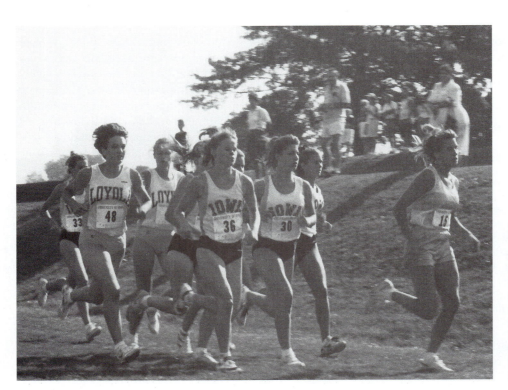

➤ **FIGURE 25.3   Female Triad.** The Female Triad is a combination of three disorders commonly seen in adolescent and young adult female athletes: disordered eating, amenorrhea, and osteoporosis. It is particularly common among athletes participating in sports that require an ideal body weight or optimal body fat level for achievement (e.g., gymnastics, figure skating, cross-country running, diving, swimming, and ballet).

THE DISABLED ATHLETE

 A wheelchair athlete is preparing to participate in a 10k road race on a warm, sunny day. What precautions, if any, should be taken to prevent injuries and dehydration for this athlete?

Two to three million people with disabilities in the United States participate in recreational and organized sports. Although one might suspect that athletes with disabilities are at a greater risk for physical injury, this is not true. In fact, the percentage of injuries is no higher in athletes with disabilities than in those without (19). For the most part, the types of injuries sustained by the disabled athlete are similar to those who are not disabled—the majority involve soft tissue injuries. The exceptions are the focus of this section, along with specific medical conditions associated with neurologic or neuromuscular involvement pertaining to the disabled athlete.

Wheelchair Athletes

Athletes with spinal cord injuries, spina bifida, postpolio paralysis, and amputations are often identified as wheelchair athletes. Wheelchair athletes most commonly participate in track, road-racing, and basketball, but others may participate in tennis, field events, bowling, archery, slalom skiing, table tennis, swimming, or any other sport. Wheelchair designs have changed dramatically over the past 2 decades **(Figure 25.4)**. The overall mass of the chair has greatly decreased, the seat and back rest lowered, the wheels cambered, and the size of the push rims modified to suit the needs of individual events.

INJURIES TO WHEELCHAIR ATHLETES

Altered patterns of muscle strength and flexibility can change the biomechanical forces applied to muscle and joints, making some athletes more susceptible to injury due to repetitive wheelchair propulsion movements. The greatest velocity of ambulation is attained with rapid, rather than long, strokes on the push rims of the chair. The arms operate with a lower mechanical efficiency than the legs, in part because effort is expended in stabilizing the trunk during arm work. Efficiency is particularly poor for individuals with high-level spinal cord injuries. For these reasons, it is common to see the majority of injuries occurring in the upper extremities. The most frequent injuries are strains and muscular injuries and other soft tissue injuries, including abrasions, blisters, and calluses on the arms and hands (20,21) **(Box 25.12)**. Constant compression of the heel of the hand on the push rim of a wheelchair can also lead to carpal tunnel syndrome. In addition, constant pressure from sitting can lead to pressure-related sores on the hips and the buttocks region. Due to the very nature of their condition, many wheelchair athletes do not have

> ### ➤➤ Box 25.12
>
> ## Common Injuries in Wheelchair Athletes
> - Soft tissue injuries (sprains, strains, tendinitis, bursitis)
> - Blisters
> - Lacerations, abrasions, and cuts (including skin infections)
> - Pressure sores
> - Arthritis and joint disorders
> - Fractures
> - Hand weakness or numbness
> - Problems with hyperthermia or hypothermia

sensation in the lower extremities (paraplegia). Extreme caution should be directed toward the feet and toes, which can become scraped or dragged on concrete or other hard surfaces during an event, resulting in abrasions or lacerations.

Many of these injuries may be related to accidents inherent in the operation of a wheelchair at high speeds. Other overuse injuries to the upper extremity are often associated with an increased training load. To prevent soft tissue injuries and pressure-related injuries to the hands, gloves should be worn. If more padding is needed, layers of athletic tape can be applied to areas of high pressure. To decrease the risk of pressure injuries or irritation occurring in the buttocks and hip area, athletes should shift their weight every 30 minutes. Those with open pressure sores should stop physical activity to prevent additional pressure damage. Training progression, along with flexibility and warm-up, are critical to decrease the incidence of musculotendinous injuries; these should be done before and after both training and competition. Some wheelchair athletes suffer from chronic pain in the upper extremities that is related to the nature of their disability. This chronic pain should not be mistaken for acute or chronic injury. When treating injuries in this population, application of cold and heat modalities must be done with caution. Most of these individuals lack sensation in various extremity areas and cannot feel when a modality is too hot or too cold, resulting in the risk of skin irritation or burning.

ENVIRONMENTAL CONSIDERATIONS

Wheelchair athletes are at a greater risk for environment-related conditions, such as heat illness and hypothermia. Spinal cord injuries (especially lesions above the first thoracic vertebra) are known to compromise the parasympathetic nervous system, which affects circulating blood volume and sweat production, and can adversely influence thermoregulation (22). As a result, quadriplegics do not perspire below the site of the spinal cord lesion and cannot effectively cool the body. Extra precautions must be used when these athletes participate in warm environments.

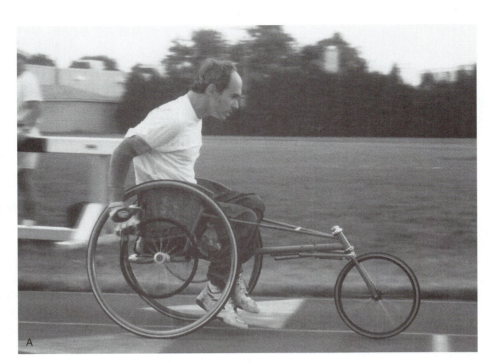

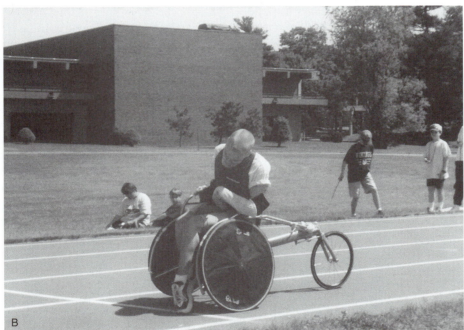

➤ FIGURE 25.4 **Wheelchair design for athletes**. The overall mass of today's wheelchair has greatly decreased, the seat and back rest are lowered, the wheels are cambered, and the size of the push rims are modified to suit the needs of individual events. A, Paraplegic athlete. B, Cerebral palsy athlete.

Practice and competitions should be limited when temperatures exceed 85°F and the humidity is 70% or greater. The same fluid hydration and rehydration guidelines for athletes without disabilities should be followed (refer to Chapter 17). Water should be sprayed frequently on the skin, and water carriers with bottles should be mounted on wheelchairs so fluids are readily available. In addition to dehydration concerns, those with spinal cord injury have decreased sensory distribution and circulatory changes, and are at a greater risk for sunburn during sun exposure. These athletes should wear appropriate sunblock and move to a shaded area before participation, during breaks, and after participation.

Just as wheelchair athletes are at greater risk for the development of heat-related conditions, they are also at increased risk for cold-induced conditions. Retaining body heat becomes problematic when the temperature drops to around 50°F. Wheelchair athletes should wear adequate insulating clothing in the winter, especially on inactive parts such as amputation stumps.

BLADDER DYSFUNCTION

Incomplete or lack of proper emptying of the bladder, bladder infections, bladder stones, and bladder obstructions occur in individuals with a neurogenic bladder. Wheelchair athletes often have to use an indwelling or intermittent catheter to drain the bladder. Catheters increase the risk of bladder and urine infections if not cleaned and used properly. To flush the bladder, athletes must drink 2 liters of water per day. It is imperative that wheelchair athletes drink plenty of water and properly care for their catheters to decrease the risk of bladder dysfunction. If an athlete does get a bladder infection, an antibiotic is usually pre-scribed. Athletes should not participate in physical activity for at least 8 hours after starting antibiotic treatment and should be free of fever for at least 24 hours.

ORTHOSTATIC HYPOTENSION

Orthostatic hypotension caused by prolonged sitting or sudden and rapid shifts in body position is due to the inability of the sympathetic nervous system to adjust to these rapid changes in body position. Athletes with or-thostatic hypotension feel lightheaded or faint. The ath-letes should be placed in a recumbent position (tipping the wheelchair backward) and should be instructed to breath deeply. This will help return blood flow to the brain. If a wheelchair athlete develops a pounding headache, flushed face, and heavy perspiration on the face and neck, he or she may be experiencing **autonomic dysreflexia**, which disturbs regulation of blood pressure and heart rate.

 Autonomic dysreflexia, a rare but dangerous condition, is commonly triggered by an obstructed bowel or bladder and is a medical emergency.

SAFETY AND THE WHEELCHAIR ATHLETE

Since many wheelchair athletes take a variety of drugs for infection, abnormal muscle tone, seizures, and other neurologic conditions, it is important to be on the alert for drug reactions. Know what medications the athlete is taking, and always refer to a physician or pharmacist before giving any over-the-counter medications to an athlete. In addition, several steps can be taken to ensure the safety of a wheelchair athlete during practice and competition (**Box 25.13**). Although many of these steps are dependent upon the athlete, the athletic trainer must emphasize safety dur-ing participation.

Amputee Athletes

The most common problem for the amputee athlete is irritation at the junction of the amputated limb and a pros-

> ➤➤ **Box 25.13**
>
> ## Safety Points When Training Wheelchair Athletes
>
> - Use protective devices (gloves, pressure wraps, cushions)
> - Monitor environmental conditions
> - Provide plenty of fluids (water bottle holders on wheelchairs)
> - Make sure there is ample opportunity for empty-ing catheters
> - Protect against sunburn
> - Protect the feet and toes from abrasions
> - Be alert for drug reactions

thetic device. This is more of a problem with limbs of the lower extremity because of weight-bearing forces. The athletic trainer should work closely with the appropriate specialist (physical therapist, orthopedist) to resolve any problems quickly. Observation of the juncture will reveal redness, skin irritation, and occasional swelling. To prevent this problem, a proper fit between the prosthetic and limb is required. If the fit is too loose, friction will occur; if it is too tight, vascular function can be impaired. Treatment of stump irritation involves properly cleansing the area and applying protective padding. If the irritation is severe, the athlete may have to limit or discontinue use of the pros-thetic and reduce physical activity.

Cerebral Palsy

Cerebral palsy (CP) involves uncontrolled muscle spas-ticity, which can range from mild to severe levels. Due to the increased load on the musculotendinous units that re-sults from the constant spasticity and a limited joint range of motion, muscle strains are a common injury. To help this condition, many CP athletes have Achilles tendon and hamstring surgery to increase range of motion and better accommodate any muscle spasticity. To decrease the inci-dence of muscular injuries, a flexibility program including proprioceptive neuromuscular facilitation (PNF) stretch-ing and a strengthening program should be initiated. The goal of the strength program should be to develop muscle balance between the agonist and antagonist muscles, to further reduce muscular injuries.

Visual Impairment

Athletes with visual impairments have a serious problem with unseen barriers. The lack of visual cues, such as visual-izing road surface conditions, walls, curbs, and other ath-letes, often puts the visually impaired athlete at a greater risk for lower extremity injuries caused by failure to respond to these varying surface conditions. In addition, it is specu-lated that visually impaired athletes expend more energy and are likely to fatigue more quickly, increasing the risk of chronic, overuse injuries in the lower extremity. It is suggested that a guide be used to provide auditory assistance to the visually impaired athlete during training sessions and competition.

 In your preparation of the wheelchair athlete, you should recommend emptying the bladder prior to the race, applying sunscreen, wearing gloves and padding in high pressure areas particularly on the hands, having plenty of water prior to and during the race, and making sure the athlete participates in a warm-up and flexibility program before and after the event. Doing these things will help the athlete reduce the risk of injury.

THE SENIOR ATHLETE

 A senior tennis athlete reports to you with chronic shoulder pain. What conditions might predispose this athlete to a shoulder injury? What signs and symptoms would indicate a subacromial impingement syndrome?

As the United States population continues to age, it is estimated that more than 60% of adults age 65 and older participate in physical activity **(Figure 25.5)**. As these individuals participate in recreational and organized sports, there will be an increasing need for strength, conditioning, and care of athletic injuries. The aging process plays a major role in skeletal and neuromuscular function. As previously mentioned, bone mass decreases with aging, though physical activity can delay this process. Aging decreases the density of collagen, which lowers tissue elasticity. On the other

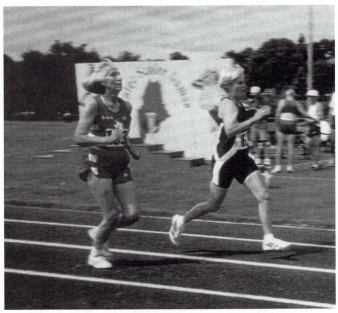

➤ **FIGURE 25.5 Senior athletes**. It is estimated that more than 60% of adults age 65 and older participate in physical activity. With regular exercise, many of the detrimental affects of aging can be offset, leading to a more healthy, longer life.

> ➤➤ **Box 25.14**
>
> ### Common Injuries in the Senior Athlete
> - Adhesive capsulitis
> - Subacromial bursitis
> - Subacromial impingement syndrome
> - Strains of the hamstrings, quadriceps, and triceps surae
> - Trochanteric bursitis
> - Degenerative meniscal tears
> - Achilles tendon rupture
> - Posttraumatic ankle instability
> - Plantar fasciitis

hand, physical activity stimulates collagen production, which in turn helps maintain elasticity. Aging also causes deterioration of type I and type II muscle fibers, but activity maintains these fibers for longer periods of time. Activity also stimulates and maintains chondrocyte activity, which helps maintain the status of menisci and cartilage tissue.

As individuals age, muscles tend to become shortened and weak, which can lead to muscle imbalance. This is often caused by chronic injury, postural adaptations to gravity, neuromuscular and neurologic dysfunction, and overall body fatigue. The very nature of the aging process increases the risk of injury for the senior athlete. In fact, most injuries in this population are a direct response to the effects of aging on the musculoskeletal system. The key to treating older athletes, just as with any athlete, is to enable them to continue participating as painlessly as possible. This section will focus on special musculoskeletal considerations for this population **(Box 25.14)**. The reader should refer to the relevant condition chapters for more information on specific injuries and conditions.

Upper Extremity Considerations

Adhesive capsulitis, subacromial bursitis, and subacromial impingement syndrome are common injuries in older athletes. These conditions are seen frequently in individuals with kyphosis, which often leads to structural alterations, biomechanical changes, and muscle imbalances in the shoulder region. All may cause referred pain to the lateral arm.

Adhesive capsulitis occurs when the glenohumeral capsular lining tightens or develops adhesions. The condition is more common in women than men, and is found with progressive rotator cuff lesions. Signs include acute, intense pain with passive and active movement in the terminal ranges of motion. Limitations in range of motion are most noticeable during glenohumeral flexion, abduction, and external rotation. Night pain is often a complaint. The first steps in managing the condition are to identify the capsular pattern of restricted movement, and then to apply thermotherapy (ultrasound), NSAID therapy, and mobilization techniques that focus on the terminal ranges. A full rehabilitation program should be developed to compliment the thermotherapy. If the person ignores the restricted range of motion and continues activity, additional damage to surrounding soft tissue will result.

Subacromial bursitis is often associated with subacromial impingement syndrome. Predisposing factors include a calcific rotator cuff tendon, and poor biomechanical alignment and function of the glenohumeral joint. Pain is reported as intense, constant, acute, or dull, and increases with terminal glenohumeral flexion and abduction. During the acute phase, subacromial bursitis should be treated with cryotherapy, NSAIDs, and application of a sling, along with controlled range-of-motion exercises. In the chronic phase, thermotherapy (ultrasound) may be used in combination with appropriate rehabilitation exercises. In some cases, an injection of corticosteroids may be administered by a physician to complement traditional therapy techniques.

A kyphotic spinal alignment, muscle imbalances of the shoulder, and past rotator cuff tears or chronic tendinitis are all predisposing factors for subacromial impingement syndrome. Pain is isolated in the anterolateral shoulder, with referred pain to the lateral arm extending distally to the elbow. The onset of pain is usually gradual and increases with glenohumeral abduction, flexion, and external rotation. Management involves rest, NSAIDs, and avoiding aggravating activities. Ultrasound and friction massage are frequently used with rehabilitative exercises. Corticosteroid injections are sometimes indicated. If the impingement is associated with degenerative lesions, healing is extremely slow, and in some cases does not occur due to poor blood flow and continued stress on the shoulder.

Lower Extremity Considerations

Poor flexibility and aging changes in soft tissue put the senior athlete at increased risk for strains of the hamstrings and quadriceps muscle groups. These injuries are most often associated with "power" sports such as running, sprinting, field events, soccer, and basketball. Acute strains occur more frequently than chronic strains. Signs, symptoms, and management are the same for strains occurring in younger populations, but because of the aging process, the injury may take longer to heal.

Weak hip abductors and lack of flexibility in the iliotibial band also increases the risk of trochanteric bursitis in this age group. Hallmark signs include an insidious onset of pain at the lateral hip extending to the lateral thigh, and pain when rolling over on the affected hip. Pain increases with resisted hip abduction, jumping, running up inclines, and climbing stairs. Management includes application of cryotherapy, use of NSAIDs, and limitation of aggravating activities. A biomechanical analysis should be conducted to determine if aspects of the individual's gait increase stress on the iliotibial band and greater trochanter. Non-weight-bearing activities (swimming) may need to be sub-

stituted during the healing phase of injury. If the condition does not improve with therapy and rest, a physician referral is warranted.

Degenerative meniscal tears of the knee (wearing away of meniscal cartilage), which result from a constant grinding motion between the tibia and femur, do not resemble injuries seen in the knees of younger athletes. Degenerative meniscal tears normally occur in individuals who participate in sports that require large weight-bearing forces (running, jumping, twisting). Pain is usually at the medial joint line. A history of "catching" or inability to extend the knee is reported, and there may be joint instability due to a lack of a full meniscal cartilage. Acute management includes cryotherapy and partial weight-bearing with crutches. If the athlete appears to have instability or limited motion, a physician referral is warranted.

Partial tears of the gastrocnemius-soleus complex (triceps surae) is the second most common muscle strain in experienced senior athletes (23). The tear normally occurs in the muscle belly, with a popping or snapping sound often heard. There is immediate intense pain, and a palpable defect in the muscle can often be found. The athlete will not be able to push off with the involved foot. Management includes ice, rest, and limited weight-bearing with crutches. Once the acute phase has passed, ultrasound is suggested with rehabilitation exercises and gradual return to activity.

Rupture of the Achilles tendon occurs during push-off while the knee is extended, as in jumping (volleyball, basketball) or sprinting (tennis, soccer). As with the triceps surae strain, the athlete will feel a popping or snapping sensation. The athlete will not be able to bear weight while standing on the toes of the affected leg. An observable and palpable defect will be present, and the Thompson test will be positive (see Chapter 16). Application of ice, a posterior splint, crutches, and a physician referral are necessary.

Repeated sprains to the collateral ligaments of the ankle, along with osteoarthritis, may predispose the senior athlete to posttraumatic ankle instability. Limited dorsiflexion is associated with osteophyte development on the anterior portion of the talus. Instability is usually in an anterior direction, and is evaluated with a positive anterior drawer test (see Chapter 16). Treatment primarily focuses on rehabilitation of the supportive musculature. If this is unsuccessful in providing enough stability, reconstructive surgery is indicated.

Plantar fasciitis occurs in all ages, but it is more common in older individuals due to a tight heel cord and calcaneal spurs. Pain is often greatest in the morning, decreases during the day, and then increases at the end of the day or during weight-bearing activities. Pain is generally localized on the plantar surface of the calcaneus. Palpation reveals a tight plantar fascia with or without defects. Acute management includes cryotherapy, NSAIDs, and a heel lift to reduce tension on the Achilles tendon. Stretching exercises of the heel cord, plantar fascia, and hamstrings are suggested, and if the individual has excessive foot prona-tion, an orthrosis may be required.

 The senior athlete with shoulder pain is predis-posed to subacromial impingement syndrome if any of the following conditions are present: ky-photic spinal alignment, muscle imbalance of the shoulder complex, or a history of chronic rotator cuff tendinitis. Additional signs and symptoms indicating the syndrome include a gradual onset of pain in the anterolateral shoulder region that increases with glenohumeral abduction, flexion, and external rotation.

Summary

1. Menstrual dysfunction of the female athlete may in-clude dysmenorrhea (menstrual cramps), menstrually induced leg pain, anovulatory oligomenorrhea (infrequent menstrual cycles), luteal phase deficiency (shortened luteal phase and insufficient progesterone production), and exercise-associated amenorrhea (ab-sence of menstruation).

2. Endometriosis involves tissue growth outside of the endometrial cavity, and can lead to dysmenorrhea, oligomenorrhea, severe pelvic pain, and pain upon defecation. In extreme situations, endometriosis can lead to infertility.

3. Premenstrual syndrome (PMS) is associated with the luteal phase (days 15 to 28) of the menstrual cycle. Signs and symptoms of PMS include headaches, breast tenderness, back pain, bloating, irritability, de-pression, fatigue, and certain food cravings.

4. Exercise programs for the pregnant woman must be individualized in consultation with the supervising physician. A 5- to 10-minute warm-up and 30 to 60 minutes at 65 to 85% maximum heart rate, three to fives times per week is recommended for a recre-ational athlete or regular fitness exercises. Each exer-cise period should be followed by a cool-down and stretching period.

5. A reduction in either the red blood cell volume (he-matocrit) or hemoglobin concentration is called ane-mia. The most common cause of anemia is iron deficiency caused by deficient hemoglobin synthesis. Early symptoms include fatigue, tachycardia, blood mixed with feces, and pallor. Treatment may involve dietary iron supplementation and ascorbic acid to en-hance iron absorption.

6. Sickle cell anemia, most commonly seen in African-Americans, results from abnormalities in hemoglo-bin structure that produce a characteristic sickle- or crescent-shaped red blood cell that is fragile and un-able to transport oxygen. Signs and symptoms in-clude swollen, painful, and inflamed hands and feet, irregular heartbeat, severe fatigue, headache, muscle weakness, and severe pain due to oxygen depriva-tion. Currently there is no known treatment to re-verse the condition. Since dehydration can compli-cate the condition, individuals should hydrate maximally before, during, and after exercise.

7. Eating disorders manifest themselves as a refusal to maintain a healthy body weight (85% of expected body weight), dramatic weight loss, fear of gaining weight even when underweight, preoccupation with food, abnormal food-consumption patterns, or re-cent binge eating behaviors associated with loss of control and feelings of guilt. Treatment involves a three-pronged approach: referral to a physician, a mental health professional, and a nutritionist.

8. Osteoporosis occurs when there is a decrease in bone mass and strength, which predisposes the indi-vidual to fractures. Primary prevention includes ade-quate calcium intake, circulating estrogen levels, and weight-bearing exercise. The most important of these is adequate circulating estrogen.

9. The combination of disordered eating habits, amen-orrhea, and osteoporosis is commonly referred as the Female Triad. When seen together, they often accelerate each other, producing even more devasta-ting affects on the quality and longevity of life.

10. Disabled athletes are no more prone to athletic injur-ies than nondisabled athletes. The most common in-juries seen in wheelchair athletes are muscle strains and sprains; bursitis of the upper extremity; soft tis-sue injuries such as blisters, abrasions, lacerations, and cuts; carpal tunnel syndrome; and pressure-related injuries of the hands, hips, and buttocks. In addition, wheelchair athletes are at a higher risk of sunburn, dehydration, hyperthermia and hypother-mia, bladder dysfunction, and hypotension.

11. Common injuries in the senior athlete include adhe-sive capsulitis, bursitis, muscles strains, plantar fasci-itis, degenerative conditions, and decreases in flexi-bility, strength, and balance.

References

1. Joy EA, Macintyre JG. Women in sports. In: The Team Physician's Handbook. Edited by Mellion MB, Walsh WM, Shelton GL. Phila-delphia: Hanley & Belfus, 1997.
2. Teitz C. The Female Athlete. Rosemont, IL: American Academy of Orthopaedic Surgeons, 1997.
3. Brukner P, Bennell K. Stress fractures in female athletes: Diagnosis, management and rehabilitation. Sports Med 1997;24(6):419-429.
4. Bennell KL, Malcolm SA, Wark JD, Brukner PD. Skeletal effects of menstrual disturbances in athletes. Scand J Med Sci Sports 1997; 7(5):261-273.
5. Ransom S, Moldenhauer J. Premenstrual syndrome: Systematic diag-nosis and individualized treatment. Phys Sportsmed 1998;26(4): 35-43.
6. Martin M, Stalans L. Unpublished. Sexual behaviors of NCAA divi-sion I female basketball, softball, and volleyball players, 1998.
7. Wells CL. Women, Sport & Performance: A Physiological Per-spective. Champaign, IL: Human Kinetics Publishers, 1991.

8. Clapp JF III. A clinical approach to exercise during pregnancy. Clin Sports Med 1994;13(2):443-458.

9. Harris SS. Helping active women avoid anemia. Phys Sportsmed 1995;23(5):35-48.

10. Fields KB. Anemia in athletes. In: The Team Physician's Handbook. Edited by Mellion MB, Walsh WM, Shelton GL. Philadelphia: Hanley & Belfus, 1997.

11. Recommendations to prevent and control iron deficiency in the United States. MMWR 1998;47(RR-3):1-29.

12. American Psychiatric Association. Diagnostic and Statistical Manual of Mental Disorders (4th ed.) (DSM-IV). Washington DC: American Psychiatric Association, 1994.

13. Daluiski A, Rahbar B, Meals RA. Russell's sign: Subtle changes in patients with bulimia nervosa. Clin Orthop 1997;343:107-109.

14. Powers PS. Initial assessment and early treatment options for anorexia nervosa and bulimia nervosa. Psych Clin North Am 1996;19(4):639-653.

15. Isenbarger DW, Chapin BL. Osteoporosis: current pharmacologic options for prevention and treatment. Postgrad Med 1997;101(1):129-143.

16. Otis CL, et al. American College of Sports Medicine position stand: The female athlete triad. Med Sci Sports Exerc 1997;29(5):i-ix.

17. Kadel NJ, Teitz CC, Kronmal RA. Stress fractures in ballet dancers. Am J Sports Med 1992;20(3):445-449.

18. Licata AA. Stress fractures in young athletic women: Case reports of unsuspected cortisol-induced osteoporosis. Med Sci Sports Exer 1992;24(8):955-957.

19. Ferrar MS, et al.. The injury experience of the competitive athlete with a disability: Prevention implications. Med Sci Sports Exerc 1992;24(2):184-188.

20. Taylor D, Williams T. Sports injuries in athletes with disabilities: Wheelchair racing. Paraplegia 1995;33(5):296-299.

21. Curtis KA. Prevention and treatment of wheelchair athletic injuries. Ath Ther Today 1997;2(1):19-25.

22. Hopman MTE, Oseburg B, Binkhorst RA. Cardiovascular responses in paraplegics to prolonged arm exercise and thermal stress. Med Sci Sports Exerc 1993;25(5):577-583.

23. Scott WA, Couzens GC. Treating injuries in active seniors. Phys Sport Med 1996;24(5):63-68.

CHAPTER 26

Pharmacology

OBJECTIVES

1. Define pharmacokinetics.

2. List the five major principles associated with pharmacokinetics.

3. Name and define the two common routes of drug administration: enteral and parenteral.

4. Explain the factors that affect a drug's absorption rate in crossing cell membranes.

5. Explain how drugs are distributed, metabolized, and excreted from the body.

6. Describe the factors that influence the therapeutic effects produced by a drug.

7. Explain the importance of potentially dangerous drug interactions, and discuss adverse side effects of therapeutic medications.

8. Describe how drugs are named.

9. List general guidelines for the documentation and storage of therapeutic medications used in sports.

10. Distinguish common therapeutic medications used to treat soft tissue injuries.

The use of therapeutic medications has always been part of sports injury management. In a 1993 NCAA national study of the substance use and abuse habits of college student-athletes, it was found that 33% of all collegiate athletes used therapeutic medications for the relief of pain and inflammation associated with a sport injury (1). The results of this survey and other data sources demonstrate how imperative it is that certified athletic trainers have an understanding of the therapeutic medications used in the treatment of injuries, including their effects, indications, and contraindications. The study also verifies the need for the profession of athletic training to establish appropriate standards regarding the use of therapeutic medications in the management of injuries.

This chapter examines the process of a drug's journey through the body. It begins with pharmacokinetics, which is the study of how drugs enter the body, and how they are absorbed, distributed, metabolized, and excreted. This is followed by information on factors that contribute to the therapeutic effect of a drug, drug interactions, drug reactions, guidelines for use of therapeutic medications, and common medications used in the management of sports injuries. With the exception of the section on non-steroidal anti-inflammatory medications (NSAIDs), only over-the-counter (OTC) therapeutic medications are presented.

PHARMACOKINETICS

 Does the manner in which a drug enters the body determine its effect on bodily functions? Once absorbed, how do drugs get to a target site to either inhibit or facilitate a response? Are all drugs metabolized and excreted by the body?

A **drug** is a chemical agent that affects living processes, whether the effects are beneficial or harmful. Drugs become effective only when they reach a particular site and interact at the cellular level. The interaction may result in either the reduction or enhancement of chemical processes in the body. This interaction can help restore an impaired body function or prevent a disease process from occurring. The effects can be local, systemic, or both. Some medications result in only a local effect, as occurs when ulcer drugs block stomach acid production. Others, such as oral decongestants, produce both positive and negative effects throughout the body (systemically) even though the desired effect is to open the nasal passages. Undesirable or negative effects are characterized as side effects of the medication.

Pharmacokinetics is the study of how a drug moves through the body to produce the desired effects. Movement of the drug through the body involves five steps: administration, absorption, distribution, metabolism, and excretion **(Figure 26.1)**. Each step can affect a drug's concentration once it reaches the desired target. The amount of the

drug's concentration when it reaches the target site within a certain time frame is referred to as the drug's **bioavailability**. The bioavailability of a drug is influenced by two of the pharmacokinetic processes: route of drug administration and absorption. Once at the target site, the drug receptor interaction either facilitates or inhibits a sequence of biological changes that ultimately alters the function of the cell, tissue, or organ. Drugs that facilitate or produce a change are called agonists; drugs that inhibit or block effects are antagonists.

Drug Administration

The means by which a drug is administered often determines its **absorption rate**, or how quickly it gets into the tissues to produce a therapeutic effect. There are two general routes of drug administration: (1) enteral and (2) parenteral. Each route is further divided into subroutes.

ENTERAL ROUTE

Enteral routes (i.e., oral, sublingual, or rectal) use the gastrointestinal tract for entry into the body, and are the most commonly used routes for drug administration. Medications that use enteral routes are combined with substances called **vehicles** that facilitate entry into the body. These vehicles include tablets, capsules, liquids, powders, suppositories, enteric coated preparations, and sustained-release preparations.

Enteric coated preparations are drugs covered by acid-resistant materials (e.g., fatty acids, waxes, shellac) that protect the drug from the acid and pepsin in the stomach. The drug passes through the stomach and is dissolved in the intestine, thus preventing stomach and duodenal irritation. An enteric coated medication such as Ecotrin (aspirin) may be used if an athlete has gastrointestinal sensitivity to aspirin. Other enteric medications are also available. **Sustained-released** preparations are capsules or tablets filled with tiny spheres that contain the drug. These spheres are coated and designed to dissolve at variable rates. Sustained-released preparations can reduce the number of daily doses and provide a relatively steady drug level for an extended period of time (usually 8 to 24 hours). Short-acting medications such as antihistamines and decongestants are offered as sustained-released preparations.

Oral medications are absorbed within the stomach, small intestine, or large intestine, and can enter the blood stream within 30 minutes after ingestion. Drugs placed under the tongue (sublingual route) are quickly absorbed through the oral mucosa into the venous system draining the mouth region. This allows the medication to avoid initial metabolism in the liver. Nitroglycerin tablets are the most commonly used sublingual medication. This route is also used when drugs, such as those in smokeless tobacco, are placed in the **buccal** region of the mouth (space between the lip and gum). Suppositories and enemas are examples of drugs that enter the body through the rectal

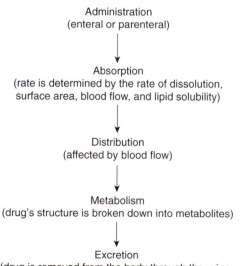

➤ **FIGURE 26.1 Pharmacokinetics.** Movement of the drug though the body involves five steps: administration, absorption, distribution, metabolism, and excretion.

TABLE 26.1   ENTERAL ROUTES OF DRUG ADMINISTRATION

Route of Administration	Advantages	Disadvantages
Oral	Easy and convenient to administer Relatively inexpensive Usually safe Avoids sudden increases in plasma levels	Rates of absorption vary Difficult to control concentrations Must undergo initial liver metabolism (first-pass effect) Requires patient compliance May cause local stomach and duodenal irritation
Sublingual	Rapid onset	Must be absorbed by oral mucosa
Rectal	Alternative to oral medications Used for unconscious patients or in those who have trouble holding down foods or liquids	Can be poorly and incompletely absorbed May cause rectal irritation

route. This route is used in individuals who have trouble holding down foods or liquids, and for unconscious patients. **Table 26.1** lists advantages and disadvantages of enteral routes of drug administration.

PARENTERAL ROUTE

Parenteral routes do not use the gastrointestinal tract as entry to the body, but rather use other methods, both invasive and noninvasive. Invasive avenues include intravenous, intra-arterial, intramuscular, and subcutaneous injections, while noninvasive methods include inhalation, topical, and transdermal application.

Intravenous and intra-arterial injections put the drug directly into the blood stream where it is instantaneously absorbed. Drugs used for anesthesia prior to surgery, and fluids given through an intravenous (IV) drip, are examples of these routes. Pain medications are often injected intramuscularly, while local anesthetics and insulin are injected subcutaneously. Drugs that are given through intramuscular or subcutaneous means are absorbed at variable rates (rapid and slow) through capillary walls.

Inhaled drugs are rapidly absorbed through the lungs or sinus passages, and should not irritate the nasal cavity, bronchial tubes, or lungs. Bronchial inhalers for exercise-induced bronchial spasms are an example of an inhaled drug. Antibiotic, antifungal, and anesthetic ointments are applied topically; they penetrate the superficial layers of the skin and underlying tissue, but they do not provide deep skin penetration. Unlike inhaled and topical drugs, drugs administered with a transdermal patch provide a more controlled, slow release of medication into the body. Similar to topical medications, transdermal drugs must be capable of penetrating the skin. Examples include nicotine patches, medicated patches for motion sickness, and drugs used in iontophoresis. **Table 26.2** lists advantages and disadvantages of parenteral routes of drug administration.

Drug Absorption

Drug absorption is the movement of a drug from its site of administration into the blood. The rate of absorption determines when the drug's effects begin, i.e., the amount of absorption determines the intensity of the effects. There

TABLE 26.2   PARENTERAL ROUTES OF DRUG ADMINISTRATION

Route of Administration	Advantages	Disadvantages
Intravenous/intra-arterial	Instantaneous/complete absorption Rapid onset (10–15 seconds) Controlled dosage Allows administration of large volumes of fluid	Irreversible once in body Can overload the body with fluids Relatively expensive
Intramuscular/subcutaneous	Complete absorption Controlled dosage	Inconvenient Can produce local soreness
Inhalation	Quick absorption Rapid onset (5–8 seconds)	Patient compliance Can produce tissue irritation
Topical	Local effects Noninvasive Easy to administer Relatively safe	Only effective in treating outer layers of skin Can produce skin irritation
Transdermal	Local effects Noninvasive Easy to administer Relatively safe	Must be capable of passing through dermal layers of skin Can produce skin irritation

are several factors that affect the absorption rate of drugs, including the rate of dissolution, surface area, blood flow, and lipid solubility (2).

FACTORS AFFECTING DRUG ABSORPTION

A drug's **rate of dissolution** simply means that the more rapidly a drug dissolves, the faster its onset of effects will be. Drugs that dissolve quickly, such as liquid medications, have a more rapid onset of effects than those that dissolve more slowly (e.g., enteric coated preparations).

The surface area in which a tablet or capsule dissolves in also plays a major role in the absorption rate. The larger the surface area, the faster the absorption rate. For example, most oral medications are absorbed in the small intestine, which has a larger surface area than the stomach. Drugs that are inhaled are absorbed into the lungs, which also have a large surface area.

Drugs are also absorbed more rapidly when administered in areas where blood flow is high. For example, drugs that are administered intravenously are absorbed more quickly than drugs taken orally.

To reach the blood, drugs must pass through various cell membranes. Membranes that surround cells are called cytoplasmic membranes, and are composed primarily of a double layer of phospholipids, or simple fats. The **blood brain barrier** (the barrier that protects the brain against toxic substances) is also composed of highly phospholipid materials. Drugs that are lipid soluble have the ability to cross cell membranes readily and enter the blood quickly, and therefore, are absorbed more quickly than other drugs. Once in the blood, drugs are carried throughout the body to the target sites. This **lipid solubility** concept explains the difference between water- and fat-soluble vitamin absorption. Fat-soluble vitamins are absorbed better than water-soluble vitamins, and can accumulate in the body, because of their increased ability to cross cell membranes.

CROSSING CELL MEMBRANES

For drugs to reach the target site, they must cross the cell membrane in one of three methods. First, drugs can cross via channels and pores, but few drugs are small enough in chemical structure for entry into the membrane by this method. Secondly, drugs may cross cell membranes using a transport system, which uses natural body chemicals as carriers to move the drugs from one side of the membrane to the other. These body chemicals are extremely selective as to which drugs they will carry, and as a result, few drugs cross cell membranes using the transport system. The most common method of crossing cell membranes is through direct penetration. As previously mentioned, cell membranes are phospholipids. Drugs that cross cell membranes through penetration must be lipid soluble and have the ability to dissolve into the lipid membrane. These drugs move from an area of high to low lipid concentration.

Drug Distribution

Once absorbed, drugs are distributed throughout the body and may be influenced by several factors. Just as blood flow affects the rate and amount of drug absorption, it also affects drug distribution. For example, blood flow to the heart, kidneys, liver, and brain is much greater than blood flow to the muscles or skin. Because tissue normally is well perfused, however, regional blood flow is rarely a limiting factor in drug distribution (3).

EXITING THE VASCULAR SYSTEM

Once blood distributes a drug to a target site, it must be capable of exiting the vascular system and entering the cell membrane via a transport system or through lipid solubility. Most drugs leave the blood at the capillary beds, which provide little or no resistance to the drug's exit. In the brain, drugs must pass from the blood through the blood brain barrier. They must be lipid soluble to cross the barrier in significant quantities. Some drugs, however, do not exit the blood. Drugs that bind to proteins, particularly albumin, cannot leave the blood because the albumin molecule is too large. Therefore, the drug never gets distributed to target sites and will remain in the blood. Only free-floating (unbound) drug molecules can exit the blood to produce a therapeutic effect.

RECEPTORLESS DRUGS

For most drugs to exert a therapeutic effect (facilitate or inhibit an action), they must be absorbed and distributed to a **receptor** or target site. A receptor is a functional macromolecule in a cell to which a drug binds to produce its effects. Some drugs, however, do not need to attach to a receptor to produce a therapeutic effect. These drugs produce their effects by acting through physical or chemical interactions. An example of a receptorless drug is an antacid, which decreases gastric acidity by direct chemical reaction with stomach acids. Antiseptics are another example, which produce their effects by direct physical and chemical reactions with the skin.

Drug Metabolism

Drug metabolism, or biotransformation, is the enzymatic alteration of a drug's structure, whereby the original drug is broken down into **metabolites** (altered products of metabolism). Most drug metabolism takes place in the liver via hepatic enzymes. This is called the **first-pass effect**. Metabolism in the liver can increase or decrease the therapeutic action as well as the toxicity of a drug. Many drugs are given by non-oral routes to avoid the first-pass effect, to avoid the loss of effectiveness once metabolized. However, not all drugs are metabolized. Aminoglycoside antibiotics (gentamycin), for example, are excreted in the urine almost unchanged. Because the body does not have a mechanism to breakdown the drug, toxicity can occur with these types of medications. Drugs that are highly lipid soluble often cannot be excreted by the kidneys. During metabolism, however, the liver can convert drugs into less lipid-soluble compounds, which can accelerate renal drug excretion. Drug metabolism can also inactivate a drug.

Medications may be active before being metabolized, after being metabolized, or both, because many drug metabolites have the same effect as the original medication. Some medications are specifically designed to become active after being metabolized; others become inactive and ineffective once metabolized. Drugs that are inactivated by the liver cannot be taken orally.

Metabolism can also be affected by the condition of the liver and other medications. Patients with hepatic diseases may metabolize drugs slower or faster than a healthy individual. Alcohol, smoking, and other medications may affect enzymes that speed or slow metabolism of specific medications.

Drug Excretion

Drug excretion is the process by which a drug is removed from the body through the urine, sweat, bile, saliva, breast milk, or lungs. Most drugs are excreted in the urine by the kidneys. The rate at which a drug is excreted is significantly determined by the quantity and frequency of the drug dosage. As it is with metabolism, kidney function is very important to the ability of the body to properly excrete the medication and/or metabolites at the proper rate. Patients with reduced kidney function run the risk of toxicity from many medications, and must either avoid certain medications or use lower dosages. Some medications (diuretics) may increase excretion, resulting in the need to alter dosage. **Box 26.1** provides two examples of the pharmacokinetic process.

➤➤ Box 26.1

Examples of the Pharmacokinetic Process

Aspirin
- Administered orally
- Quickly absorbed in stomach and small intestine
- Once in the blood: 80 to 90% binds to plasma proteins; the remaining 10 to 20% is free-floating
- Free-floating aspirin exits the blood and exerts therapeutic effects
- Metabolism begins in the blood, where it is converted into salicylic acid, and continues in the liver
- Excreted via the kidneys

Acetaminophen (Tylenol)
- Administered orally
- Quickly absorbed in the upper gastrointestinal tract
- Once in the blood: 20 to 50% binds to plasma proteins; remaining portion is left free-floating
- Free-floating acetaminophen exits the blood and exerts therapeutic effects
- Metabolized in the liver
- Excreted via the kidneys

 The route of drug administration determines how quickly a drug will be absorbed within the body. Although a drug's chemical structure does play a role in its absorption rate, the lipid solubility of a drug determines how quickly it can move across cell membranes to reach the target site. Most drugs are metabolized in the liver and broken down into metabolites that reach their target site via the blood circulation. Oral medication, therefore, must be able to pass through the liver without being inactivated during metabolism. Drugs are most commonly excreted from the body by the kidneys in urine. However, drugs can also be excreted through sweat, saliva, or breast milk.

FACTORS THAT CONTRIBUTE TO THE THERAPEUTIC EFFECT OF A DRUG

 What factors contribute to the therapeutic effect of a drug during the pharmacokinetic process? Does taking more medication increase its effectiveness?

Once a drug has been absorbed and distributed in the body, various factors will contribute to its therapeutic effects. These include the blood plasma levels, therapeutic range, a drug's half-life, dose response, and potency.

Blood Plasma Levels

For most drugs, there is a direct correlation between therapeutic and toxic responses, and a drug's concentration level in the blood plasma. As a result, drug dosing objectives (frequency and quantity of drug to be taken) are often referred to in terms of achieving specific blood plasma levels. There are two basic drug plasma levels. **Minimum effective concentration (MEC)** refers to a drug's minimum concentration that must be present for the drug to be effective. **Toxic concentrations** reflect drug levels in blood plasma that are too high, and therefore increase the risk of toxic effects.

Therapeutic Range

The range between the minimum effective concentration and toxic concentration is referred to as the **therapeutic range** of a drug. The objective of drug dosing is to maintain plasma levels within the therapeutic range. The wider this range, the safer the drug. For example, because acetaminophen has a toxic concentration range that is 30 times greater than the MEC, it is considered to be a safe drug. Lithium, on the other hand, has a much more narrow toxic concentration range of only 3 times greater than the MEC, and is not considered as safe a drug (4).

Medications with a very narrow therapeutic range often require monitoring of blood levels. The asthmatic medication theophylline is a drug with a narrow therapeutic range. If the dose is too low, the patient runs the risk of an asthma attack; if too high, the extreme result can be arrhythmias or convulsions. A slight alteration in the dose or a change in the absorption, distribution, metabolism, or excretion can easily result in the blood level falling below, or rising above, the therapeutic range of the drug.

Dosing Intervals and Plasma Concentrations

Drug concentrations in the blood rise during metabolism and decline during excretion. Because an adequate response to a drug cannot occur until plasma levels meet the MEC, there is a latency period between the time of drug administration and the onset of effects. The extent of this delay is determined by the absorption rate. For example, because injected drugs are absorbed and enter the blood rapidly, they produce more rapid effects. In contrast, drugs that are taken orally usually require about 30 minutes before the onset of effects is noted. Time-release medications are examples of drugs that keep an average plasma level over a period of time. As a result, the effects of time-release medications do not decline prior to the next dose. The effects continue throughout the dosing schedule. As long as plasma levels remain above the MEC, the therapeutic response will continue. However, once plasma levels drop below the MEC, the therapeutic response will gradually diminish. As metabolism continues, drug levels decline until excretion eliminates the drug from the body.

Maximal Efficacy

Maximal efficacy is the dose at which a response occurs, and continues to increase in magnitude before reaching a plateau, or threshold. Once the response reaches the threshold, the increase in response does not continue, even if more medication is given. Maximal efficacy serves as an index for the maximal response a drug can produce. This explains why taking more than the recommended dose of a drug does not produce increased effects. In fact, taking more than the recommended dose can lead to toxicity.

Half-life

The time required for the amount of a drug in the body to reduce by 50% is the drug's **half-life**. Half-lives can be as short as a few minutes, or as long as a week. The longer the half-life of a drug, the slower it leaves the body. Acetaminophen, for example, has a half-life of 2 hours. Every 2 hours, 50% of the acetaminophen in the body will be excreted. This means that if you ingest 200 mg, after 2 hours there will be 100 mg left, and after another 2 hours 50 mg will remain. If acetaminophen is administered with repeated doses over a period of time, it will accumulate in the blood and reach a threshold. This threshold will decline

TABLE 26.3	HALF-LIFE OF ASPIRIN
Time in Hours	mg
00.00	325.0
03.15	162.5
06.30	81.25
09.45	40.63
12.60	20.31
15.75	10.15
18.90	05.08
22.05	02.54
25.20	01.27
28.35	00.63
31.50	00.32
34.65	00.16
37.80	00.08
40.95	00.04
44.10	00.02
47.25	00.01

if the dosing is diminished or discontinued. It must be noted that not all drugs have a half-life. Alcohol, for example, is excreted by the body at a constant rate regardless of the amount present. **Table 26.3** demonstrates the half-life of a single aspirin tablet. One aspirin tablet is generally 5 grains or 325 mg with a half-life of approximately 3.15 hours. Although the half-life of a drug depends on its volume distribution as well as its clearance, a single aspirin can remain in the body for several hours after ingestion.

Potency

When comparing two similar drugs, the drug that is more potent requires a lower dosage to produce the same effects. Potency serves as an index for how much of a drug can be administered to elicit a desired response; it is not synonymous with maximal efficacy. Achieving pain relief with acetaminophen requires a higher dosage than morphine, because morphine is much more potent than acetaminophen, requiring less dosage to elicit a given response. The more potent medication, however, is not necessarily the best medication. All factors must be considered, such as side effects, dosing, other available medications, and the patient's specific health factors.

 For a drug to exert a therapeutic effect, it must reach certain blood plasma concentration levels. This level is considered the therapeutic range, or the range between minimal effective concentration and toxic concentration levels. Maximal efficacy is the maximal response of a drug, no matter how much more of the drug is taken. Some drugs are more potent than others. A drug that requires a lower dosage for desired effects is more potent than a similar drug that requires a higher dosage.

DRUG INTERACTIONS

 Is it important to know if an athlete is taking more than one drug at a given time? Does taking certain drugs simultaneously pose a health or performance risk for the athlete?

It is not unusual that an athlete will use two or more drugs simultaneously, leading to the potential for a drug interaction. **Drug interaction** refers to the ability of one drug to alter the effects of another drug; it may either intensify (synergistic action), or reduce (inhibit) the effects of the drug. In some cases, drug interaction may become life threatening. Individual response to a drug interaction can be influenced by several factors, many of which alter pharmacokinetic processes (absorption, distribution, metabolism, excretion) **(Box 26.2)**.

For example, if an athlete is taking a muscle relaxant for a low back spasm and drinks alcohol, the depressant effects of both the muscle relaxant and the alcohol will intensify, leading to increased drowsiness. In contrast, if two stimulants are combined, such as a nasal decongestant and caffeine, an increased central nervous system stimulation effect may result in nervousness, heart palpitations, and even insomnia. Some drugs, such as the H2 antagonist cimetidine (Tagamet) used to promote stomach ulcer healing by suppressing secretion of gastric acid, can reduce the hepatic (liver) metabolism of many drugs. Taken with NSAIDs, Tagamet may intensify the side effects of the NSAIDs.

While most medications are not affected by food, drug interactions with food may also occur. Some drugs (e.g., tetracycline antibiotics) should not be taken with milk or milk products, because calcium combines with the medication and inactivates it. Other medications such as NSAIDs should be taken with food or plenty of fluids to reduce stomach irritation. Some antifungal medications require food to increase absorption of the medication. As such, it is always important to ask the physician or pharmacist how a medication should be taken.

 Athletes often will be in situations where they will be taking more than one drug at a time; however, a combination of drugs may intensify or diminish the therapeutic response of a drug. Occasionally, the drug combination may be toxic. Combining alcohol with almost any drug is contraindicated.

▶▶ Box 26.2

Influencing Factors in Drug Interaction
- Genetics and age
- Current illness or disease
- Quantity of drug ingested
- Duration of the drug therapy
- Time interval between taking two or more drugs
- Which drug is taken first

ADVERSE DRUG REACTIONS

 A baseball player is taking a prescription medication. While practicing on a sunny, hot day he suddenly complains of a headache, hot skin, and heat illness—like symptoms. What factor(s) might explain these symptoms?

All prescription and OTC medications have the potential of producing adverse reactions. Adverse drug reactions range from mild to severe. Mild reactions are often described as side effects; these include drowsiness, nausea, and an upset stomach. These reactions are often temporary and can be tolerated for short periods of time. If the reactions do not dissipate in a few days, a physician should be contacted immediately.

 Severe reactions are life threatening and are characterized by respiratory depression, rash (hives, urticaria), allergic reactions (anaphylaxis), and shock.

Adverse drug reactions are often immediate (acute), and may be either local or systemic. Local reactions are isolated to a limited area and are often associated with topical medications. Systemic reactions affect the entire body, such as heart palpitations and acute bronchospasm. Adverse drug reactions that are not immediate are usually associated with long-term use of a drug, such as gastrointestinal irritation from long-term use of some NSAIDs.

Certain drugs such as tetracycline, sulfa drugs, and even NSAIDs may make an individual more susceptible to ultraviolet rays from the sun, resulting in a decreased exposure interval needed to develop a sunburn, rash, or allergy to the sun. These reactions can occur with the first dose, or may occur up to 1 week after taking the medication. Other drugs may increase an athlete's risk of heat illness or dehydration. Diuretics can also lead to dehydration in an exercising athlete. Prior to participation in physical activity, it is important to know if a medication increases the risk of sun sensitivity, heat illness, or other complications. This information is available from a pharmacist.

Unlike prescription medications, most OTC medications labels identify the risk of adverse drug reactions. However, a physician or pharmacist should be consulted before taking two or more drugs simultaneously.

 Depending upon the severity of the adverse reaction, the athlete should be taken to the nearest medical facility.

Most adverse reactions subside once the medication is discontinued.

 The baseball player is most likely exhibiting signs and symptoms associated with adverse effects while taking prescription medication and participating in sunny, hot weather conditions. All drugs, including OTC medications, can potentially produce local or systemic adverse effects or reac-

tions. Most adverse effects are medication specific, but general effects often include skin or gastrointestinal irritation. These adverse effects usually subside once the medication has been discontinued. It is imperative that an individual read the label and be aware of possible adverse drug reactions prior to taking any medication.

DRUG NAMES

 What does it mean when you are prescribed a medication and the pharmacist asks if you want a brand or generic product? Are there differences in their effectiveness?

The Food and Drug Administration (FDA) is responsible for supervising the manufacturing, labeling, and distribution of chemical substances, including therapeutic medications. Drugs are classified either as prescription (Rx) or nonprescription/over-the-counter (OTC) products. Prescription medications must be prescribed by a licensed practitioner and are generally dispensed by pharmacists. OTC, which can be purchased directly by the consumer, are usually used to treat minor problems. Unlike prescription medication, containers holding OTC medication provide a variety of critical information **(Box 26.3)**.

Every medication has a chemical, generic, and brand name. The *chemical name* describes the actual scientific compound. Due to the complexity of chemical names, they are seldom used. The *generic name* is considered to be a drug's official name, and is preferred over brand names for general use. *Trade* or *brand names* are specific names used

---

> **➤➤ Box 26.3**
>
> ### Information Found on Medication Containers
>
> **Prescription Medication Container**
> - Patient's name
> - Pharmacy name, address, and telephone number
> - Name of medication
> - Dose information and directions for use
> - Number of refills (if any)
> - Warnings for use (if any)
> - Date prescription was filled
> - Name of practitioner who prescribed the medication
> - Additional information may be on the container depending upon individual state laws
>
> **Over-the-Counter Medication Container**
> - Name of product
> - Name and address of manufacturer
> - Net contents
> - Directions for safe and effective use
> - Name of habit-forming drugs
> - Cautions and warnings
> - Name and quantity of active ingredients
>
> ---
> Adapted from Martin M, Yates W. Therapeutic Medications in Sports Medicine. Baltimore: Williams & Wilkins, 1998.

---

by the individual manufacturer. They are created by drug companies for ease of use by consumers and physicians, and are generally shorter than the generic name, are capitalized, or carry the registered trademark symbol (®). In addition, generic drugs can appear under more than one trade name. For example, the common OTC medication acetaminophen can be identified with the following names:

Chemical name	4'-hydroxyacetanilide
Generic name	acetaminophen
Trade or brand name	Tylenol, Panadol

Generally, but not always, the OTC products are of lower strength than their counter prescription products. Use of higher doses than what is indicated on OTC medications labels is not wise unless prescribed by a physician or other licensed practitioner, as this increases the risk of side effects and adverse reactions. In most cases, the prescription generic drug is therapeutically equivalent to the primary brand-name drug, but less expensive.

Drugs differ not by generic or brand names, but by the route of administration, and rate and extent of absorption. Drug names are used for written and verbal communication, and for verifying the contents of drug containers.

 A drug's generic name is its official name. In most cases, a generic drug provides the same therapeutic effects as the brand-name equivalent, and the generic form is usually less expensive.

GUIDELINES FOR THE USE OF THERAPEUTIC MEDICATIONS

 What responsibilities does an athletic trainer have when using therapeutic medications for the treatment of sport-related injuries? When indications are used as part of the treatment protocol, how can athletic trainers protect themselves from possible litigation?

State laws vary tremendously on who can prescribe, administer, and dispense medications; therefore, legal ramifications also vary. In general, prescription medications can only be prescribed by a licensed practitioner and can only be dispensed by a registered pharmacist. Depending upon individual state regulations, only authorized persons (e.g., nurse, physician assistant, physicians) can administer medications. **Administration of medication** is defined as providing one dose of a medication to an individual. **Drug dispensing** is providing more than one individual dose.

Certified athletic trainers cannot administer or dispense prescription medications, nor should they be assigned duties that may put them in a situation to do so. Physicians cannot delegate the duties associated with prescription drug control or prescription dispensing to certified athletic trainers. These duties extend beyond the role delineation and employment requirements of a certified athletic trainer and put the athletic trainer at risk for legal liability (6).

Depending on individual state regulations, however, athletic trainers may be authorized to administer OTC medications. Prior to providing an athlete with an individual dose, the athletic trainer should have reason for doing so based on written protocol provided by a physician. Preceding any administration of OTC medication, it is important to ask if the athlete is allergic to any type of medication and document the response. Some athletes may be allergic to aspirin and aspirin products. When furnishing medication, both written and oral directions for the use of the medication should be provided. After administering the medication, the athletic trainer should keep a written record of the transaction, including the date, athlete's name, sport, medication, and why the medication was administered (5,6). All drug distribution records should be maintained in accordance with appropriate legal guidelines.

In addition, it is important to follow-up with the athlete to make sure the medication is effective, and to ensure compliance with the drug dosing regimen. It is important that the athlete follows directions and completes the prescribed dosage **(Box 26.4)**. This is especially important when taking antibiotic and antifungal agents. Incomplete therapy can result in developing a resistance to the medication, or in a recurrence of the infection. Just because an athlete is feeling great does not mean the infection is completely gone. The entire course of the prescribed treatment must be completed.

Traveling with Medications

It is important to plan ahead when traveling, to ensure that an adequate supply of a particular medication is available in case of emergency **(Box 26.5)**. If an athlete forgets a

---

> ▶▶ **Box 26.4**

Tips For Proper Use of Medications

- Use only as directed
- Keep medication in the original container; do not alter the label
- Do not use if the container has been tampered with
- Do not use the medication if discolored or if the expiration date has passed
- Measuring spoons or cups should be used when measuring liquid medication
- Never share your medication with another person
- When directed, oral medications should be taken with food
- If a corticosteroid is injected into a joint, do not stress the joint too soon following the injection, because pain will be masked
- If an overdose occurs, immediately contact the nearest poison control center and transport the individual to the nearest medical facility

Adapted from Martin M, Yates W. Therapeutic Medications in Sports Medicine. Baltimore: Williams & Wilkins, 1998.

> ▶▶ **Box 26.5**

Tips While Traveling with Prescription Medications

- Medications should not be placed in checked luggage
- Plan ahead and make sure there is a source of medication while traveling
- A large enough supply should be taken to cover emergency situations
- Take a copy of any written prescriptions
- Keep medications in the original container for identification purposes
- Keep medications in a safe and secure location

---

medication or a medication is depleted, it is not easy to obtain a refill. Each individual state has specific rules and regulations concerning the prescription and refilling of medications. Physicians usually cannot prescribe medications from state to state, nor can pharmacists fill out-of-state prescriptions. If an athlete needs prescription medication while traveling, it is wise to seek assistance from a team physician of the host team. Another solution is to have the athlete's personal physician call the team physician of the host team to discuss the situation. In either case, prescription medications should remain in the original containers and be kept either by the athlete or the athletic trainer. Medications should not be placed in checked baggage.

Storing Medications

All Rx and OTC medications should be kept in the original container and stored in a locked cabinet or other secure place. They should be kept away from heat, direct light, dampness, and freezing temperatures. A dry environment with temperatures between 15° to 31.7°C (59° to 89°F) is suggested (6). All stocked medications should be examined at regular intervals, and expired medications should be discarded. If medications are kept in athletic training, emergency, or travel kits, they should be routinely inspected for medication quality and security. When stocking medications, do not overstock. Overstocking is often determined by (a) the quantity of expired medications in stock, and (b) the quantity of medications in stock and how many were actually used in a given period. Overstocking wastes medication and money.

 Depending on individual state regulations, an athletic trainer can administer single doses of over-the-counter medications provided the team physician has documented standard orders for the process. With any administration of an OTC medication, a drug distribution form should be completed. In addition, all medications should be stored in a locked cabinet.

COMMON MEDICATIONS USED TO TREAT SPORT-RELATED INJURIES

 Think for a minute about common soft tissue injuries or conditions that are sport related. If an athlete complains of chronic pain over the patellar tendon, what type of therapeutic medication might be used to relieve the pain and inflammation associated with this condition?

A variety of different types of medications are used to treat soft tissue injuries in sports. The more common medications include **analgesics** (pain relievers) and **antipyretics** (fever reducers), nonsteroidal anti-inflammatories (NSAIDs), corticosteroids, anesthetics, antiseptics, topical antibiotics, and antifungal agents.

Analgesics and Antipyretics

Two of the more common analgesic–antipyretic medications are acetaminophen (Tylenol) and aspirin. Acetaminophen inhibits the synthesis of prostaglandins in the central nervous system but does not inhibit their synthesis in peripheral tissues. As a result, it acts as an analgesic and reduces fever, but has no anti-inflammatory or antiplatelet (anticlotting) properties. It is often used as a replacement for aspirin because it does not cause gastrointestinal irritation. Overdosage of this medication can lead to liver damage and death.

Aspirin (acetylsalicylic acid) is a commonly used analgesic, antipyretic, and anti-inflammatory medication. Unfortunately, its use can lead to gastrointestinal bleeding, nausea, vomiting, and the development of gastric ulcers. In high doses, **tinnitus** (ringing in the ears) and dizziness may result. It is important to note that most practitioners prefer that no individual under the age of 18 receive aspirin, regardless of the circumstances, although there may be some controversy about the actual level of risk. If aspirin is used in a child under age 18 during chickenpox or influenza, the risk of **Reye's syndrome** increases. This is a severe disorder characterized by recurrent vomiting beginning a week after onset of the condition, from which the child either recovers rapidly or lapses into a coma with the possibility of death. Individuals who have an intolerance to aspirin, particularly asthmatics, may have an anaphylactic reaction to it. Because aspirin also prolongs blood clotting time, it should not be used by athletes in contact sports.

Nonsteroidal Anti-inflammatory Drugs (NSAIDs)

NSAIDs are aspirin-like drugs that suppress inflammation and pain, produce analgesia, and reduce fever. They are among the most commonly used drugs in the treatment of soft tissue injuries, and are distributed as both OTC and Rx medications (refer to Table 6.4).

NSAIDs were developed in an attempt to decrease the gastrointestinal and hemorrhagic effects produced by aspirin. They produce the same effects as aspirin without many of the side effects. Individuals may respond differently to different types of NSAIDs. The various types of NSAIDs differ chemically and pharmacokinetically based on their duration of action, potency level, over-the-counter and prescription status, and dosing regimen.

THERAPEUTIC EFFECTS

Therapeutically, NSAIDs interfere with the biosynthesis of prostaglandins and other related compounds by inhibiting cyclooxygenase, an enzyme responsible for the synthesis of prostaglandins. Prostaglandins are lipid-like compounds produced by almost every living cell, with the exception of red blood cells. Under normal conditions, these lipid-like compounds regulate cell function. During inflammation of a soft tissue, increased prostaglandin activity seems to mediate inflammation by increasing blood flow, capillary permeability, and the permeability effects of histamine and bradykinin. Because NSAIDs inhibit prostaglandin activity, they reduce inflammation and pain. NSAIDs also provide analgesia without sedation or the euphoria that is often associated with narcotic analgesics such as morphine, meperidine (Demerol), codeine, oxycodone (Percodan, Tylox), and propoxyphene (Darvon, Darvocet). Narcotic analgesics potentially produce physical dependence and tolerance; nonnarcotic analgesics, such as NSAIDs, normally do not (3).

NSAIDs, may also reduce fever without reducing normal body temperature. The hypothalamus (part of the brain that regulates body temperature) has a set point, which determines body temperature. If this set point is elevated by fever-promoting substances (e.g., endogenous pyrogens), fever develops. NSAIDs inhibit prostaglandins and, as a result, lower the set point of the hypothalamus and reduce fever. In addition, NSAIDs have some antiplatelet (anticlotting) properties. In contrast to aspirin's strong antiplatelet properties, however, NSAIDs' effects are much lower in intensity. They are considered safe when used to treat acute soft tissue injuries.

ADVERSE EFFECTS

Side effects of NSAIDs include gastrointestinal irritation, renal impairment, and hypersensitivity reactions (e.g., asthma, urticaria, rhinitis), or toxicity. To decrease the risk of gastrointestinal irritation, NSAIDs should be taken with food, milk, or a glass of water. Alcohol should never be taken with NSAIDs as it increases the risk of gastrointestinal irritation and the development of gastric ulcers.

The risk of renal impairment is relatively low with most NSAIDs. Signs of renal impairment include reduced urine output, and rapid increase in serum creatinine and blood urea nitrogen. Hypersensitivity reactions or toxicity to NSAIDs occurs in about 0.3% of consumers, more often in individuals with asthma, nasal polyps, hay fever, chronic urticaria, and other chronic diseases (7,8). Signs and symptoms of a hypersensitive reaction or toxicity include dyspnea, rapid and irregular heartbeat, hematuria (blood in urine), upper abdominal tenderness, and jaundice.

 If any of these develop, immediate medical attention is required.

USE AND AVAILABILITY

NSAIDs are used to treat mild to moderate pain associated with joints, muscles, and headaches. They are often used to treat inflammation associated with rheumatoid arthritis, tendinitis, and bursitis conditions. However, they are not effective for the relief of severe pain.

NSAIDs are available in both OTC and Rx strengths, and are routinely taken orally. **Table 26.4** lists the more common NSAIDs used in treating soft tissue injuries in sports. Prescription strength can only be prescribed by a licensed practitioner. They are prescribed on a case-by-case basis and should not be shared among athletes with similar soft tissue injuries or conditions. For example, Anaprox is prescribed to treat dysmenorrhea, and is often shared by female athletes. Sharing medication is not recommended because individuals respond differently to the same medication. Nonprescription NSAIDs include ibuprofen (Advil, Motrin, Nuprin), ketoprofen (Orudis KT, Actron), and naproxen sodium (Aleve).

Pain relief is usually noted within 30 minutes after ingestion and lasts for several hours, depending on the dosage and duration of the particular NSAID taken. Both OTC and Rx products should be used for only short-term (10 days maximum) treatment of inflammation and pain associated with soft tissue injuries. When used as an antipyretic, they should only be used for 3 days (7,8).

 If pain, inflammation, or fever does not subside or increases within these time periods, a physician should be consulted immediately.

As with most medications, NSAIDs should not be used in combination with alcohol, and a physician or pharmacist should be consulted before combining NSAIDs with other medications.

Corticosteroids

Corticosteroids are steroid hormones produced naturally within the adrenal cortex, but that can also be synthetically produced. They are powerful drugs that affect nearly the entire body.

THERAPEUTIC EFFECTS

Corticosteroids are lipid soluble and block the body's natural response to inflammation by inhibiting the synthesis of chemical mediators (prostaglandins, leukotrienes, histamine). As a result, swelling, warmth, redness, and pain associated with inflammation are decreased. It should be noted that the manner in which corticosteroids suppress inflammation is much broader in scope than the manner

TABLE 26.4	**COMMON NONSTEROIDAL ANTI-INFLAMMATORY MEDICATIONS**			
Generic Name **Brand Name**	Side Effects	Warning		Dosing Notes
Diclofenac *Cataflan, Voltarin* Rx	Upset stomach, ulceration, drowsiness, blurred vision, dizziness, photophobia	Avoid aspirin and alcoholic beverages		Take with food
Ibuprofen *Advil, Motrin* OTC *Motrin, Rufen* Rx	Upset stomach, ulceration, drowsiness, blurred vision, dizziness, photophobia	Avoid aspirin and alcoholic beverages		Take with food
Idomethacin *Indocin* Rx	Headaches, upset stomach, blurred vision, ulceration, drowsiness, dizziness, photophobia	Avoid aspirin and alcoholic beverages		Take with food
Ketoprofen *Acron, Orudis KT* OTC *Oruvail* Rx	Upset stomach, ulceration, drowsiness, blurred vision, dizziness, photophobia	Avoid aspirin and alcoholic beverages		Take with food
Nabumetone *Ralafen* Rx	Upset stomach, ulceration, drowsiness, blurred vision, dizziness, photophobia	Avoid aspirin and alcoholic beverages		Take with food
Naproxen *Naproxyn* Rx	Upset stomach, ulceration, drowsiness, blurred vision, dizziness, photophobia	Avoid aspirin and alcoholic beverages		Take with food
Naproxen Sodium *Aleve* OTC *Anaparox* Rx	Upset stomach, ulceration, drowsiness, blurred vision, dizziness, photophobia	Avoid aspirin and alcoholic beverages		Take with food
Piroxicam *Feldene* Rx	Upset stomach, ulceration, drowsiness, blurred vision, dizziness, photophobia	Avoid aspirin and alcoholic beverages		Take with food
Sulindac *Clinoril* Rx	Upset stomach, ulceration, drowsiness, dizziness, blurred vision, photophobia	Avoid aspirin and alcoholic beverages		Take with food
Tolemetin *Tolectin* Rx	Upset stomach, ulceration, drowsiness, dizziness, blurred vision, photophobia	Avoid aspirin and alcoholic beverages		Take with food

in which NSAIDs do so. Corticosteroids inhibit prostaglandin synthesis as do NSAIDs, but they also act in several other ways to decrease inflammation.

ADVERSE EFFECTS

Side effects of corticosteroids, which often resemble the condition they are prescribed to treat, include itching, burning, dry skin, and fluid retention. Other more rare side effects are an increase or decrease in appetite, dizziness, restlessness, facial or body hair growth, gastrointestinal irritation, menstrual irregularities, and optic pain. Most of these side effects disappear soon after the medication is discontinued. Because oral NSAIDs and corticosteroids have similar effects on the gastrointestinal tract, concurrent use severely increases the risk of GI irritation and ulceration. In addition, chronic use of corticosteroids can suppress the body's immune system, making the user more susceptible to infection.

AVAILABILITY AND USE

Corticosteroids are indicated for skin disorders, nasal inflammation, rheumatic disorders (bursitis, arthritis, and tendinitis), and skin infections. They are administered through oral and nasal inhalation, intra-articular injection, subcutaneous injection, intravenous injection, topically, and orally. **Table 26.5** lists the more common corticosteroids administered through oral and nasal inhalation, or injections.

Corticosteroids should not be used by individuals who have HIV/AIDS, heart disease, hypertension, diabetes, gastritis, peptic ulcers, lupus, or any infections (e.g., bronchitis, flu). By reducing inflammation and pain, corticosteroids may also delay exercise-induced pain, placing an athlete at an increased risk for further injury. Corticosteroids are not banned by the NCAA, but the USOC bans all types with the exception of most topical (ear, eye, and skin) agents. With written permission, the USOC will allow inhaled, local, or intra-articular injections (6,9).

Route of Administration	Generic Name	Brand Name
Oral Inhalation	beclomethasone	Beclovent, Vanceril
	dexamethasone	Decadron Respihaler
	flunisolide	Aerobid
Nasal Inhalation	beclomethosone	Benconase, Vancanase
	budesonide	Rhinocort
	dexamethasone	Decadron Turbinaire
	flunisolide	Nasalide
	fluticasone	Flonase
Injectable	betamethasone	Celestone
	dexamethasone	Decadron
	hydrocortisone	Solu-Cortef
	prednisolone	Hydeltrasol

TABLE 26.5 COMMON CORTICOSTEROIDS

Adapted from Martin M, Yates W. Therapeutic Medications in Sports Medicine. Baltimore: Williams & Wilkins, 1998.

Local Anesthetics

Anesthetics, frequently called "pain killers," inhibit the activity of sensory nerve receptors in the skin. Under normal conditions, the skin does not respond well to aspirin or other oral analgesics. When irritated, the same sensory nerve endings in the skin can lead to **pruritis** (itching) from a weak stimulation, or skin pain from a strong stimulation. The skin responds more readily to topical medications. Local anesthetics are categorized by route of administration, and may be injectable, topical, or sprayed. Injectable anesthetics are prescription medications that can only be administered by a licensed professional (physician, physician assistant, nurse practitioner, or nurse).

INJECTABLE ANESTHETICS

In the treatment of sports-related injuries, injectable anesthetics are most commonly used for **infiltrative anesthesia**, a process that produces numbness by interfering with nerve function in a localized subcutaneous soft tissue area. Infiltrative anesthesia is commonly used for the treatment of soft tissue injuries such as hip pointers and turf toe, and for reduction of phalangeal fractures. In addition, they are used as an anesthetic prior to minor surgical procedures, such as suturing or aspiration of bursa or joint fluid. They are classified by the duration of action: short-, intermediate-, and long-term acting. Side effects are minimal when used as directed. Large quantities of the drugs must be absorbed to produce any associated side effects, such as tremors, drowsiness, hypotension, or hypersensitivity and anaphylactic reactions.

TOPICAL ANESTHETICS

Topical anesthetics are OTC and Rx medications that are applied to the skin as needed. Topical anesthetics or analgesics are often used to relieve pain associated with musculoskeletal injury (strains, sprains, tendinitis, bursitis). When used for these purposes, topical medications are called **counterirritants**. They stimulate skin nerve endings that respond to pain, and warm and cold sensations, which in theory distracts the user from the original pain or itching. In other words, these products irritate the skin in order to relieve pain and itching. Counterirritants come in various forms, including lotions, rubs, liniments, and creams. Popular examples include: Ben-Gay, Mineral Ice, Flex-All 454, Menthol, Absorbine Jr., wintergreen oil, and Icy Hot. The FDA suggests that these drugs are safe when applied three to four times per day, but they are not suggested for long-term use.

If pain persists after 7 days, a physician should be consulted immediately (5).

In addition to the counterirritant properties, topical anesthetics can further be classified according to whether they reduce itching, pain, or both. Most topical anesthetics are easily identified in their brand names by the suffix -caine (e.g., Americaine, Lanacaine, Xylocaine, and Solarcaine).

SPRAY ANESTHETICS

In addition to creams, lotions, and liniments, there are a few spray anesthetics on the market (Aerofreeze, ethyl chloride, flurimethane). These products temporarily freeze the skin in an effort to decrease pain. The duration of action, however, is quite limited and only lasts about one minute. These products are not recommended for use because the freezing action can damage the skin and delay healing (6).

ADVERSE EFFECTS

Topical anesthetics are relatively safe when used as directed. Common side effects are limited to skin irritation (rashes or hives). These normally disappear once use of the product is stopped. Systemic absorption can occur if large amounts of these products are used over a large surface area, or if used on deep wounds. Systemic absorption is toxic and may produce convulsions and paralysis of the central nervous system.

Individuals allergic to aspirin should not use methyl salicylate products because the body may absorb the salicylate, the major ingredient in aspirin. In addition, products that produce warm sensations should never be used in combination with a heating pad or occlusive dressing. This may increase systemic absorption and result in skin and muscle necrosis. These products also should never be used prior to exercise in hot, humid conditions, or immediately following exercise. Application is appropriate after the body cools down. The NCAA and USOC permit the use of topical anesthetics. The NCAA also permits intra-articular injections of local anesthesia when medically justified (6).

Muscle Relaxants

Unlike local anesthetics that inhibit sensory nerve receptors in the skin and subcutaneous tissue, muscle relaxants actually block afferent messages that travel from the muscles to the brain. Skeletal muscle relaxants are classified as either central or direct acting. Central agents exert their effects within the spinal cord, while direct-acting muscle relaxants affect the skeletal muscle cell. Both types are available by prescription only. Muscle relaxants prescribed for muscle spasms associated with athletic injury are central acting. They decrease local pain, spasm, and tenderness, and thus allow increased range of motion. Examples of common muscle relaxants are chlorzoxazone (Parafon Forte, Paraflex), cyclobenzaprine (Flexeril), diazepam (Valium), methocarbamol (Robaxin), and orphenadrine (Norflex). Often these drugs are used in combination with rest and physical therapy methods (thermotherapy, cryotherapy, and electrotherapy) to relieve pain from acute muscle spasms associated with musculoskeletal conditions. Because central acting muscle relaxants produce their effects by acting on the central nervous system, they often produce general depression of CNS functions. As a result, common side effects include dizziness, drowsiness, and sedation. Muscle relaxants are not banned by either the NCAA or USOC. They may, however, be prohibited by international federations of certain sports. **Table 26.6** lists the more common muscle relaxant medications with possible side effects.

Topical Antibiotics

Antibiotics are substances that kill disease-producing bacteria, and are used to prevent and treat infections. Two basic types of bacteria cause most skin infections: *streptococcus* and *staphylococcus*. Because it is difficult to predict which type of bacteria may be producing a skin infection, most topical antibiotics contain several active ingredients that treat both organisms. Topical antibiotics are used on small

TABLE 26.6	COMMON MUSCLE RELAXANT MEDICATIONS			
Generic Name **Brand Name**	**Side Effects**	**Warning**	**Dosing Notes**
Carisoprodol *Soma* Rx	Constipation, nausea, tremors, increased heart rate, dizziness, sleeplessness, confusion	May cause drowsiness. Caution should be used when performing tasks that require alertness	Take with food
Chlorzoxazone *Paraflex, Parafon Forte* Rx	Constipation, nausea, tremors, increased heart rate, dizziness, sleeplessness, confusion	May cause drowsiness. Caution should be used when performing tasks that require alertness	Take with food
Cyclobenzaprine *Flexeril* Rx	Constipation, nausea, tremors, increased heart rate, dizziness, sleeplessness, confusion	May cause drowsiness. Caution should be used when performing tasks that require alertness	Take with food
Methocarbamol *Robaxin* Rx	Constipation, nausea, tremors, increased heart rate, dizziness, sleeplessness, confusion	May cause drowsiness. Caution should be used when performing tasks that require alertness	Take with food
Orphenadrine Citrate *Norflex* Rx	Constipation, nausea, tremors, increased heart rate, dizziness, sleeplessness, confusion	May cause drowsiness. Caution should be used when performing tasks that require alertness	Take with food

TABLE 26.7 COMMON TOPICAL ANTIBIOTICS

Generic Name / *Brand Name*	Side Effects	Warning	Dosing Notes
Bacitracin / *Baciquent* OTC	Rash, itching, burning, redness, localized swelling	Avoid contact with eyes	Use thin layer
Polymyxin B Sulfate / *Neosporin* OTC	Rash, itching, burning, redness, localized swelling	Avoid contact with eyes	Use thin layer
Polymysix B Sulfate Neomycin Base, Bacitracin / *Triple Antibiotic, Mycitracin* OTC	Rash, itching, burning, redness, localized swelling	Avoid contact with eyes	Use thin layer
Polymyxin B Sulfate Zinc Bacitracin / *Polysporin* OTC	Rash, itching, burning, redness, localized swelling	Avoid contact with eyes	Use thin layer

open wounds, such as abrasions; these can be purchased as creams, ointments, or powders. Bacitracin, Neosporin, Neomycin, and Polysporin are examples of OTC topical antibiotics. These products are not designed to be used over deep wounds, as internal absorption of some of these antibiotics can be toxic. Topical antibiotics should be used in small amounts, generally three times daily, and for not more than 1 week (2,5). Topical antibiotics are not banned by the NCAA or USOC. **Table 26.7** lists the more common topical antibiotics and their side effects.

Antiseptics and Disinfectants

The terms antiseptic and disinfectant are sometimes used interchangeably, but they are not the same. **Antiseptics** are applied to living tissue to stop growth of microorganisms or destroy bacteria on contact and prevent infection. They are most appropriate in the cleansing and treatment of large, open skin wounds, and come in sprays, powders, and swab-on liquids. Isopropyl alcohol, betadine, and tincture of iodine are common OTC antiseptics. Antiseptics are for external use only, and are not banned by the NCAA or USOC. **Disinfectants** are chemical agents applied to nonliving objects. They are most commonly used to disinfect surgical instruments and cleanse medical equipment and facilities. Common disinfectants used in athletic training are alcohol products, Vira-Quat, and Iso-quin. Refer to Field Strategy 5.1 for information on disinfecting techniques used in the athletic training room to prevent the spread of infections diseases related to bloodborne pathogens.

Antifungal Agents

Tolnaftate (Tinactin), miconazole nitrate (Micitin), and clotrimazole (Lotrimin and Mycelex) are all agents that treat infections caused by fungal cells. In humans, fungal cells are either molds or yeasts. Tinea pedis, tinea curis, and tinea corporis are caused by fungal molds, while candidiasis and moniliasis are caused by fungal yeasts. Products used to treat fungal molds are usually applied twice daily with symptoms disappearing within a few days of initial treatment. After symptoms disappear, the molds can often still be found within skin cracks and nail beds. For this reason, physicians suggest regular, continued application of antifungal agents as part of a preventive protocol. Prior to applying antifungal agents, the infected area should be cleansed thoroughly with mild soap and water. If the infec-

TABLE 26.8 COMMON ANTIFUNGAL AGENTS

Generic Name / *Brand Name*	Side Effects	Warning	Dosing Notes
Ciclopirox / *Loprox* Rx	Irritation, burning, redness	Do not use with an occlusive dressing	Clean and dry the skin prior to application
Clotrimazole / *Lotrimin AF, Mycelex* OTC *Lotrimin lotion* OTC or Rx	Erythema, stinging, edema, blistering, pruritis	Keep out of the eyes	Clean and dry the skin prior to application
Miconazole Nitrate / *Micatin* OTC *Monistat-Derm* OTC	Burning, itching, stinging	Keep out of the eyes	Used for tinea pedis and versicolor
Tolnftate / *Tinactin* OTC	Mild irritation	Keep out of the eyes	Used for tinea pedis and versicolor
Undecylenic Acid / *Cruex, Desenex* OTC	Burning, irritation, rash, stinging	Keep out of the eyes	Used for tinea pedis and versicolor

tion does not clear within a week (tinea curis) or 1 month (tinea pedis and corporis), another antifungal agent should be used, or a physician should be consulted.

Historically, drugs used to treat vaginal yeast infections were by prescription only, but today, various antiyeast agents can be purchased over-the-counter; clotrimazole (Gyne-Lotrimin, Mycelex-7, Mycelex-G), minconazole nitrate (Monistat), and tioconazole (Vagistat-1) are examples. Approximately 25% of women of childbearing age will develop a yeast infection. Predisposing factors include pregnancy, obesity, diabetes, debilitation, and the use of certain drugs (oral contraceptives, systemic antibiotics). Depending on the product, it should be used once daily for 1 to 14 days (2).

If a course of treatment does not resolve the problem, the possibility exits that some other microorganism is present, and a physician should be consulted immediately.

Antifungal agents are relatively safe when used as directed. Some can be toxic if absorbed systemically, and should thus be for external use only. Side effects that do occur usually resemble worsening of the condition being treated: increased redness, irritation, and itching. These products are not banned by the NCAA or USOC. **Table 26.8** lists the more common antifungal agents and their side effects.

Nonsteroidal anti-inflammatory drugs (NSAIDs) are the most common therapeutic medication used for the treatment of pain and inflammation associated with acute and chronic soft tissue injures. NSAIDs are available in over-the-counter and prescription forms.

Summary

1. Medications have chemical, generic, and brand names.
2. Pharmacokinetics is the process that explains how a drug enters the body, and is absorbed, distributed, metabolized, and excreted.
3. The pharmacokinetic process determines how a drug reaches a target site to either facilitate or inhibit an action.
4. A drug's half-life, lipid solubility, therapeutic range, dosage, potency, and maximal efficacy all play roles in determining the drug's action and effect.

5. Common medications for the treatment of soft tissue injuries include analgesics and antipyretics, nonsteroidal anti-inflammatory drugs (NSAIDs), corticosteroids, muscle relaxants, topical antibiotics, antiseptics, and antifungal agents. All of these drugs come in both prescription and over-the-counter forms.
6. Athletic trainers are not allowed to prescribe or dispense prescription medication to athletes.
7. Depending on state regulations, athletic trainers may be authorized to administer a one-dose pack of an OTC medication when approved protocols by the team physician warrant their use.
8. When providing OTC medications, a record log should be kept indicating the athlete's name, date, name of medication administered, reasons for administering the medication, and signature of the athletic trainer who administered the medication.
9. All OTC medications should be stored as directed on packaging labels, and placed in a secure, locked cabinet.
10. Prescription medications should be kept in a secured and locked location under the direct supervision of a licensed physician or pharmacist.
11. Therapeutic medications, if not used as directed, can cause adverse reactions and in some cases toxicity and death.

References

1. Anderson WA, Albrecht R, McKeag D. A national study of the substance use and abuse habits of college student-athletes. Kansas City, MO: National Collegiate Athletic Association, 1993.
2. Pharmacology for Athletic Trainers: Therapeutic Medications. Champaign, IL: Human Kinetics, 1997.
3. Ciccone CD. Pharmacology in Rehabilitation. Philadelphia: FA Davis, 1995.
4. Longenecker GL. How Drugs Work: Drug Abuse and the Human Body. Emeryville, CA: Ziff-Davis Press, 1994.
5. Martin M, Yates W. Therapeutic Medications in Sports Medicine. Baltimore: Williams & Wilkins, 1998.
6. Benson, M (ed.). Dispensing prescription medication. In: 1997-98 NCAA Sports Medicine Handbook. Overland Park, KA: National Collegiate Athletic Association, 1997.
7. Martin M, Yates W. The use of over-the-counter non-steroidal anti-inflammatory drugs in athletic training. NATA News 1997;(Dec): 12-13.
8. Martin M, Yates W. The use of prescription non-steroidal anti-inflammatory drugs in athletic training. NATA News 1998;(Jan): 13-14.
9. United States Olympic Committee. Drug Education Handbook. Colorado Springs: United States Olympic Committee, 1996.

CHAPTER 27

Dermatology

OBJECTIVES

1. Describe common skin lesions.

2. List the more common bacterial, fungal, and viral skin infections.

3. Describe the signs and symptoms of acne, onychia, paronychia, folliculitis, furuncles, carbuncles, cellulitis, and impetigo contagiosa.

4. Describe the signs and symptoms of tinea unguium, tinea pedis, tinea cruris, tinea corporis, tinea capitis, tinea versicolor, and candidiasis.

5. Describe the signs and symptoms of herpes gladiatorum, herpes zoster, verrucae, and molluscum contagiosum.

6. Explain the general management of bacterial, fungal, and viral skin infections.

7. List common skin irritations due to mechanical reactions.

8. Describe the signs and symptoms of sunburn, pernio, miliaria, eczema, and hyperhidrosis, and explain the management of each condition.

9. Describe the signs and symptoms of a bite or sting from a mosquito, bee, wasp, ant, spider, flea, and tick.

10. Explain the management of an insect bite or sting.

11. Differentiate between allergic contact dermatitis and irritant contact dermatitis, and explain the management of both conditions.

12. Describe the three different types of urticaria and explain the management of each type.

Dermatology is the study of the skin. Athletes, just as nonathletes, occasionally contract skin conditions, but several are more commonly seen in the physically active population. Skin infections may be caused by bacteria, fungi, or viruses; related inflammatory skin conditions may be due to mechanical, environmental, allergic, or chemical skin reactions. Early identification of the ensuing lesions and specific treatment minimizes the healing time and prevents the spread and recurrence of the condition.

This chapter will first provide an overview of the various types of skin lesions, and will then discuss the more common skin infections and skin conditions seen in the physically active population. Many of these conditions can be seen in the color plates included with this chapter. It is important to note that many systemic diseases are manifested in skin lesions or rashes.

Therefore, it is critical for the athletic trainer to identify potentially serious lesions and refer the individual immediately to a physician, particularly if there is any uncertainty as to the nature of the skin lesion.

TYPES OF SKIN LESIONS

A football player has what appears to be a raised, pus-filled skin irritation on the underside of his jaw. Based on the location and appearance, what type of skin lesion may be present?

The skin, the largest organ of the body, serves three major functions. It:

- Protects the body from bacteria, fungi, various viruses, and other germs in the outside environment.
- Helps regulate body temperature.
- Aids in the transmission of information from the outside environment to the brain.

The outer layer of skin, called the **epidermis**, contains the germinal layer where production of new skin cells (epidermal cells) occurs, and **sebum** (oily substance that binds epidermal cells) is produced. The underlying **dermis** contains the sweat glands, hair follicles, sebaceous glands, blood vessels, and a complex array of nerve endings (see Figure 5.8). The deepest layer, the subcutaneous tissue, is primarily composed of fat for insulation and energy storage.

The skin can be damaged by direct trauma, allergic reactions, chemical irritants, heat, cold, bacteria, fungi, and viruses. Whenever the skin is damaged, a lesion appears. These lesions are identified by their size and depth **(Table 27.1).**

The skin lesion had a raised pus-filled appearance and was located in the facial hair, indicating a possible pustule.

SKIN INFECTIONS

A lacrosse athlete is complaining of an irritating itch on the bottom of the feet and between the toes. The skin appears red and scaly. What condition might you suspect? How could this condition be prevented?

TABLE 27.1	CLASSIFICATION OF SKIN LESIONS
Macule	Flat, discolored spot of varied size and shape (freckle, mole, rubella)
Papule	Solid, elevated lesion <10 mm in diameter (wart, psoriasis)
Plaque	Plateau-like lesion >10 mm, or a group of papules joined together
Nodule	Palpable lesion >5 mm in diameter that may be elevated (lipoma, cysts, tumors)
Vesicle	Circumscribed, elevated lesion <5 mm in diameter containing serous fluid (contact dermatitis, herpes simplex, herpes zoster)
Bulla	Vesicle >5 mm in diameter
Pustule	Elevated lesion containing pus (acne, furuncle [boil], carbuncle)
Wheal	Transient, elevated lesion caused by local edema; common allergic reaction from insect bites, sunlight, or pressure
Scales	Heaped up particles of horny epithelium (psoriasis, tinea versicolor)
Crust	Dried serum, pus, or blood seen in infectious and inflammatory disease (scab)
Erosion	Loss of part of the epidermis, commonly seen in herpetic infections
Ulcer	Loss of epidermis and part of dermis, commonly seen in trauma, peripheral vascular disease, and diseases that manifest themselves with tumors
Excoriation	Linear, hollowed-out, crusted area caused by digital trauma (rubbing)
Scar	Result of healing after partial destruction of the dermis

Skin infections may stem from bacteria, fungi, or viruses. Bacterial or fungal infections can cause pustules on or within the skin or its associated structures, such as the sweat glands and hair follicles. While most infections tend to be painful, superficial irritations can also be extremely itchy (pruritis). The three main bacteria are staphylococcus, streptococcus, and bacillus. Staphylococcus commonly appears in clumps on the skin, in upper respiratory tract infections, and in lesions in which pus is present. Streptococcus is associated with serious systemic diseases, such as scarlet fever. Many bacillus are not pathological, but some can lead to major systemic diseases, such as tetanus. Fungi, such as yeast and molds, often attack the skin, hair, and nails. Fungi fall into three basic categories: dermatophytes, candidiasis (moniliasis), and tinea versicolor. Viruses invade the living cells and may multiply until they kill the cell, burst out to reinfect other cells, or lie dormant within the cell without ever causing an infection.

Bacterial Skin Conditions

Bacterial lesions are typically caused by a staphylococcal or streptococcal infection. Hot tubs or whirlpools that are not adequately chlorinated may harbor *Pseudomonas*; most infections are self-limiting and need no treatment, other than regulating pool chlorination. The more common bacterial infections in the physically active population are acne vulgaris, onychia and paronychia, folliculitis, furuncles (boils) and carbuncles, cellulitis, and impetigo contagiosa.

ACNE

Nearly all adolescents will experience acne at one time or another, but a few will develop a more serious case. Although the etiology is unknown, it is believed to be due to a sex hormonal imbalance. At age 8 or 9 years, the adrenal glands begin to produce increasing amounts of an androgen that causes the sebaceous glands to enlarge and produce more sebum. Sebum secretion peaks during adolescence and declines after age 20 (1). Acne develops when the sebaceous glands become clogged with sebum and cellular debris, and become infected by common skin bacteria. The obstructed follicle may become apparent as a blackhead (open follicle) or a whitehead (closed follicle). The blackhead is not dirt, so scrubbing or washing will not remove it. Whiteheads represent follicles that have become dilated with cellular debris but possess only a microscopic opening to the skin surface. When the oil (sebum) and other material in the whitehead breaks through the pore wall and causes irritation under the skin, a pimple results. Pimples can range from erythematous papules, pustules, or nodules, and are commonly seen on the face, neck, and back. Papules and pustules are small, measuring <5 mm in diameter, while nodules are larger. The superficial pustules will eventually dry, whereas the deeper nodules may become chronic and form disfiguring scars.

There is no cure for acne, but it can be controlled with medication. Management is usually symptomatic with routine cleansing of the inflamed area once or twice a day with a mild soap. The skin is allowed to dry for 20 to 30 minutes before applying any medication to prevent drying and redness on the skin. Medications are divided into topical and systemic preparations. Topical therapies include benzoyl peroxide, antibiotics, retinoids, and salicylic acid. Common systemic preparations include oral antibiotics and hormonal therapy. The type of medication used is based on the type and number of lesions present, the severity of the disease, the extent of the acne, the patient's past experiences with medications, and the physician's personal preference. Most acne treatment is a long-term process, taking 6 to 8 weeks before any therapeutic benefit is seen (1). Serious cases may necessitate referral to a dermatologist for treatment.

During the treatment phase, it is important not to pinch, pop, or pick at the acne, as this may cause the pimples to become larger, taking longer to disappear, or the area may scar. Protective equipment such as a helmet or chinstrap, and tight clothing may put added pressure on the skin, making acne worse in this area. Cosmetics and moisturizers that contain oils can also aggravate the condition. Young women may notice premenstrual flare-ups. These are often caused by androgenic effects of progesterone that is dominant during the second half of the menstrual cycle.

ONYCHIA AND PARONYCHIA

Onychia is inflammation of the matrix of the nail plate, while **paronychia** involves only the lateral border or nail fold. The conditions may develop from staphylococcal, streptococcal, or fungal organisms; if fungal, the infection is called onychomycosis. Paronychia follows a hangnail and is seen in individuals whose hands are frequently immersed in water or mud, such as football linemen. The nail fold becomes red, swollen, and painful, and can produce purulent drainage. The condition is treated with warm water soaks and germicide. In more severe cases, a physician may recommend systemic antibiotics and drainage of localized pus. The area is then protected with a dry, sterile dressing. If left unchecked, onychia may lead to yellowing, onycholysis (separation of the nail plate from the bed), and an accumulation of subungual debris under the nail.

This condition requires immediate physician referral for possible removal of the nail.

FOLLICULITIS

Folliculitis is an infection of a hair follicle caused by staphylococcus. Commonly referred to as an "ingrown" hair, the hair grows inward and curls up to form an infected nodule. It tends to occur wherever there is short, coarse hair (e.g., facial hair, nape of the neck, chest, back, buttocks, thighs, or on skin under protective padding), and develops from friction with pads or during shaving. Pustular rashes on the trunk have been reported where occlusive bathing suits are worn (2). Chemical irritants, inadequate chlorination, and superhydration of the skin caused by high water temperatures (i.e., hot tubs) are also causative factors. The inflammation begins with a pustule forming at the mouth of the hair follicle; a crust forms later, which will eventually slough off, along with the hair. Treatment involves eliminating the friction-causing agent and applying antibiotic medication. If the face is involved, shaving should be avoided for several days.

FURUNCLES AND CARBUNCLES

Furuncles (boils) and carbuncles are complications of folliculitis that result from friction or repeated blunt trauma. A furuncle is a deep, red, inflamed nodule that progresses into a pustule, turning large, hard, and tender when staphylococci invade subcutaneous tissue. A carbuncle is several furuncles that have merged. Common sites include the buttocks, back of the neck, face, and axillae.

Treatment requires an immediate physician referral for several weeks of systemic antibiotic therapy, and may also include immobilization, incision, and drainage, and, in severe cases, hospitalization.

During treatment, it is best to keep the athlete isolated from other team members while the boil is draining. Picking, squeezing, or cutting a boil is not recommended. Physical activity is contraindicated until the infection no longer exists, as trauma can lead to cellulitis or thrombophlebitis.

CELLULITIS

Cellulitis is a painful infection of the deep dermis and subcutaneous tissues caused by β-hemolytic streptococci or *Staphylococcus aureus*. The lesion appears as an ill-defined area of tender erythema on the trunk or extremities, usually around a break in the skin from trauma or a fissure caused by athlete's foot. Intense pain may be present, as well as malaise, fever, and **lymphangitis** (inflammation of the lymphatic vessels). Sport participation is contraindicated because trauma to the site can cause **bacteremia** (presence of bacteria in the blood). Of particular concern in children is periorbital cellulitis, because of the potential meningeal seeding by *Haemophilus influenzae* following bacteremia. However, with the introduction of the *H. influenzae* type b (Hib) vaccine in 1985, the prevalence of *H. influenzae* bacteremia in children has decreased.

Mild cases of cellulitis are managed with oral antibiotics, warm tap water compresses for 15 minutes three times a day, elevation, and bed rest.

In severe cases, immediate referral to a physician for hospitalization and intravenous antibiotics may be necessary.

IMPETIGO CONTAGIOSA

Impetigo is a highly contagious bacterial inflammation of the skin most often seen in wrestlers, swimmers, and gymnasts. Caused by *Staphylococcus aureus* alone, or in combination with β-hemolytic streptococci, it is characterized by honey-colored crusts with little surrounding redness. Bacterial toxins cause a split near the skin surface. Symptoms include itching or burning, and crust removal leaves a raw, often weeping, base. Impetigo favors body folds and areas that are subject to friction and occlusion, such as thighs and axillae, and may complicate several conditions (**Box 27.1**). The condition can be transmitted by direct contact or through sharing towels, clothing, and equipment. Lack of personal hygiene, including inadequate cleansing of clothing and equipment, can also aid in the spread of this condition.

MANAGEMENT OF BACTERIAL INFECTIONS

Most infectious bacterial skin conditions (e.g., folliculitis, acne, cellulitis, furuncles, carbuncles) should be

> ▶▶ **B o x   2 7 . 1**
>
> ### Conditions Complicated by Impetigo
> - Abrasions
> - Atopic dermatitis:
>   - Individuals with a history of asthma, hay fever, or eczema
>   - Crusts will frequently be on the face, popliteal region, or antecubital fossae
> - Contact dermatitis (especially from shoe materials and rubberized pads)
> - Irritant dermatitis (hands chapped from frequent immersion in or handling of irritating substances)

cleansed with soap, water, and **astringents** (substances that cause constriction of the tissues), and are initially treated with over-the-counter (OTC) topical antibacterial agents applied several times per day. A physician referral may be necessary for incision, drainage, and in some instances, debridement. If the condition is more severe, systemic antibiotics may need to be prescribed.

Localized impetigo can be treated with mupirocin ointment applied to the skin three times a day. This is appropriate at the end of the season for athletes in contact sports and may be used during the season for athletes in noncontact sports (3). With diffuse or multiple areas of impetigo, treatment consists of systemic antibiotics, rather than topical therapy. Gentle cleansing with soap and water helps to remove the crusts. It should be emphasized that the entire course of antibiotics should be taken even if the lesions seem to have resolved. With prompt treatment, impetigo usually clears within 7 to 10 days after the initiation of antibiotics.

The presence of satellite lesions, cellulitis, purulent conjunctivitis, large or multiple honey-crested lesions, and weeping lesions warrants withholding the athlete from competition. With impetigo, athletes should not participate until the crusts have dried to a thick, coagulated crust. Individuals who have cellulitis, furuncles, or carbuncles are not significantly contagious to others, but they should not participate in sports because continued trauma to the involved areas can lead to systemic complications, such as bacteremia and progressive soft-tissue infections. **Field Strategy 27.1** summarizes the general treatment of bacterial infections.

Fungal Skin Conditions

Fungal skin infections are quite common among physically active individuals. Fungus grows and thrives in dark, warm, moist environments, such as the areas between the toes or between the skin of the groin and scrotum. During activity, perspiration often accumulates in these areas. Augmented with wearing constrictive clothing such as an athletic supporter, tight shorts, or spandex, the perspiration often enhances and encourages fungal growth. In addition, tight garments often cause chafing and irritation. Fungal infec-

NONINFECTIOUS BACTERIAL SKIN CONDITIONS

- Wash the region 4 to 5 times daily and after physical exertion.
- Rinse all soap residue from the region and completely dry the area by patting gently.
- When dry, apply OTC topical antibacterial agents 2 to 3 times daily.
- If the condition is more severe, refer to a physician. Incision, drainage, or debridement may be necessary. Systemic antibiotics may be prescribed for 7 to 10 days.

SUSPECTED IMPETIGO

- Isolate the infected individual from other players, including athletic clothing and towels, to prevent the spread of the disease.
- Localized impetigo can be treated with mupirocin ointment applied to the skin 3 times a day.
- With diffuse or multiple areas of impetigo, refer to a physician. Systemic antibiotics may be indicated for 5 to 7 days.
- Gentle cleansing with soap and water will help to remove the crusts.

PARTICIPATION GUIDELINES

- Presence of satellite lesions, cellulitis, purulent conjunctivitis, large or multiple honey-crested lesions, and weeping lesions warrants withholding the athlete from competition.
- With impetigo: no participation until the crusts have dried to a thick, coagulated crust.
- Individuals with cellulitis, furuncles, or carbuncles should not participate in sports due to possible systemic complications, such as bacteremia and progressive soft-tissue infections.

---

tions are identified by small patches of erythema, scaling, and severe itching. Dematophytes, also known as ringworm (*tinea*) fungi, and yeasts cause most fungal infections, including tinea unguium (nails), tinea pedis (feet), tinea cruris (groin), tinea corporis (body), and tinea capitis (scalp), candidiasis, and tinea versicolor. All but tinea versicolor are contagious and spread from person to person by sharing towels or socks, and walking with no shoes in the locker room and shower stalls. Fungal infections can be prevented by taking several precautionary measures (**Box 27.2**).

> ➤➤ Box 27.2

Prevention of Fungal Infections

- Shower after every practice and competition.
- Thoroughly dry the feet, groin, and areas between the toes and under the arms and breasts, after each shower.
- Apply absorbent antifungal powder to the shoes, socks, feet, between the toes, under the arms and breast, and in the groin area.
- Change socks and underwear daily, and allow wet shoes to dry thoroughly before wearing them.
- Wear street shoes that allow some ventilation to the feet.
- Clean and disinfect the floors in the shower room, dressing room, and athletic training room daily.
- Never go barefoot in a shower or locker room.

TINEA UNGUIUM

Tinea unguium (nail), or onychomycosis as it is more properly known, is a fungal infection of the toenails and fingernails. The fungi first invade the hyponychium (most distal attachment of the nail plate), or a lateral nail fold, to reach the undersurface of the nail plate. Distal subungual onychomycosis (DSO), the most common form, is usually associated with athlete's foot (tinea pedis). Infection leads to yellowing of the nail, separation of the nail plate from the bed (onycholysis), and accumulation of subungual debris.

The fingernails are more commonly affected by the fungus *Candida albicans*, which leads to *Candida* onychomycosis. Although the fungus can cause primary nail infection in people who have chronic mucocutaneous candidiasis or other immunologic disorders, it usually occurs as a secondary infection in otherwise healthy nails. Clinically, *Candida* onychomycosis may appear similar to DSO, except that the entire thickness of the nail plate is affected and appears yellow, green, or opaque (4).

Treatment will vary depending on the type of infection, severity of the nail changes, and the personal preference of the supervising physician and patient. DSO may be treated with topical creams only in its early, mild stage. The affected portion of the nail is trimmed away as much as possible, and then a topical antifungal agent is applied several times daily. Treatment usually takes 6 to 12 months or longer for a toenail infection. Oral griseofulvin is more commonly used to treat DSO, and is typically taken twice daily for 6 to 12 months. *Candida* onychomycosis does not respond to griseofulvin; therefore, oral ketaconazole is used, though it has a greater potential for toxicity. If topical or systemic drug therapy does not resolve the condition, surgical nail avulsion is performed (4).

TINEA PEDIS

Tinea pedis (athlete's foot) is the most frequent fungal infection in the physically active population. It can spread in the locker room during casual handling of contaminated socks, or can be picked up by another player on the floor or shower stall. It is based on individual susceptibility, however, and may not affect certain people. Although 1 to 3% of the population are carriers of tinea pedis, prepubertal children are rarely affected. Tinea pedis is recognized by extreme **pruritus** (itching), redness, and scaling on the sole of the feet and between the toes. When the toe webs are **macerated** (soften skin due to moisture) and infected, a *Candida* yeast is usually present in addition to the original dermatophyte. Dry vesicular lesions may exude a yellowish serum. Scratching the area will lead to scaling, peeling, and cracking fissures in the skin, particularly between the toes, and can spread the problem to other parts of the body.

TINEA CRURIS

Tinea cruris (jock itch) involves the genitalia, but often originates in the feet; therefore the feet should always be examined when this condition is present. Although typically seen in men, women are reporting an increase in the incidence of the condition due to the increased use of panty hose, spandex, and other tight, restricting clothing. Perspiration can accumulate between the genitals and skin of the thigh. The crural or perineal folds between the scrotum and inner thighs are usually the first areas to exhibit small patches of erythema and scaling. Other signs and symptoms include diffuse, thick, dark lesions; weeping vesicles or pustules on the margins of inflammation; and severe itching. The infection can spread to the thighs, perineal area, buttocks, and abdomen. When scrotal redness or scaling occurs, it typically results from an allergic reaction to skin medications used prior to seeing a physician, or from chronic skin inflammation caused by scratching or long-term irritation. It is important to note that an individual with tinea cruris can infect bedding, towels, and clothing. These should be changed daily and thoroughly washed in hot water.

TINEA CORPORIS

Tinea corporis gladiatorum (tinea of the body) is caused by dermatophytes, usually of the genus *Trichophyton*. It affects both humans and animals, and is characterized by circular, pruritic patches that are well demarcated and scaly with raised borders and a central healing zone. A well-defined central ring is generally found on the upper extremities, axillae, and trunk. Certain individuals can carry the spores without the rash; the degree of rash will depend on the host's cellular-based immune response, which can vary widely. Tinea corporis is common in prepubertal children, as they often contract the condition from infected pets. Wrestlers are also at a high risk for outbreaks because of improper or inadequate cleansing of the mats and uniforms.

TINEA CAPITIS

Tinea capitis, or ringworm of the scalp, begins as a small papule on the scalp and spreads peripherally. It is very common among children. The lesions appear as small gray scales, resulting in scattered bald patches. The primary sources of the infection are contaminated hair brushes and combs, and animals. Oral griseofulvin is the treatment of choice.

TINEA VERSICOLOR

Tinea versicolor is a yeast infection common to active individuals because the causative agent (*Pityrosporum obliculare*) is a normal inhabitant of hair follicles and sebaceous glands that grows rapidly on warm, moist skin. It is most often seen on the trunk, upper arms, neck, abdomen, groin, and thighs. Referred to as "sun spots," tinea versicolor is best noticed after exposure to the sun. While the rest of the skin tans, the area with tinea versicolor will not. In addition to being visible after sun exposure, the lesions are easily identified by the widespread, rust-colored dermatitis of varied sizes and shapes. On dark-skinned individuals, the infection appears as well-defined white patches. The area may be asymptomatic or mildly pruritic. Tinea versicolor often resembles freckles. Unlike other fungal infections, it is not contagious.

Treatment involves a topical selenium sulfide shampoo daily for 1 week, or imidazole antifungal agents, either topical or oral. For extensive infections, systemic ketoconazole is recommended. The individual takes a single dose of two 200 mg tablets with a carbonated beverage or cranberry juice to increase absorption. The athlete works out for an hour or more, then delays showering for an hour to facilitate drug excretion in the sweat. Treatment is repeated in 1 week if diagnostic tests remain positive (5). Tinea versicolor often recurs; therefore, periodic treatment is recommended.

CANDIDIASIS

Candidiasis, caused by the yeast fungus *Candida albicans*, can produce infections on the skin or mucous membranes, or in the vagina. Skin infections tend to occur in skinfolds, such as the axillae, groin, and below the breasts, when friction occurs within a hot, moist, humid environment. The condition is more common in female athletes who wear a swimsuit or competition uniform for long periods of time. The lesion appears as a deep, beefy-red color, and is bordered with small, red satellite pustules. In skinfolds, a white, macerated border may surround the red area. Later, deep, painful fissures may develop where the skin creases. If left untreated, the infection can lead to a life-threatening systemic disease. The condition can be prevented by showering immediately after exercise, wearing clean sports briefs made of absorbent fabric, and using absorbent powder in the groin and axillae before workouts. A candidal infection of the mucous membranes of the mouth is called thrush, and is treated with oral nystatin. This infection is seen in immunocompromised hosts and in those using inhaled corticosteroids for asthma.

MANAGEMENT OF FUNGAL SKIN INFECTIONS

Treatment of fungal skin infections involves antifungal medication and changing the warm, moist environment. Dry infections of athlete's foot, jock itch, and tinea capitis respond well to OTC topical imidazoles, such as miconazole, clotrimazole, or tolnaftate. These are typically applied twice daily for at least 1 month. For reluctant fungal scaling, a two- to five-week regimen of prescription medication is warranted; this may induce longer fungus-free periods than do the imidazoles. For individuals who continue the type of activity that led to the infection, topical treatment should continue for 2 weeks after signs of the infection are gone. During treatment, the area should be kept clean and dry. Loose, absorbent clothing (cotton socks and underwear) should be worn, and shower and locker rooms kept clean **(Field Strategy 27.2)**.

Individuals with widespread fungal infections (tinea corporis or tinea capitis) should be treated with griseofulvin, but it is not always effective. Resistant cases may respond better to systemic ketoconazole, fluconazole, and itraconazole; however, long-term use of these drugs, especially ketoconazole, may cause liver toxicity.

Viral Skin Conditions

Skin lesions caused by viruses, such as herpes gladiatorum, herpes zoster (shingles), verrucae (warts), and molluscum contagiosum, can be difficult to treat because they often require long-term therapy and activity restrictions. Routine hygienic measures such as showering immediately after a game or workout, and keeping athletes with open lesions on exposed skin from participating in contact sports, may reduce or eliminate transmission of these pathogens.

HERPES GLADIATORUM

Herpes gladiatorum is a cutaneous infection caused by the herpes simplex virus type I (HSV-1). It is spread by direct skin-to-skin contact in contact sports, such as wrestling and rugby. The lesions, characterized by grouped vesicles on an erythematous base, are capable of latency with a tendency to recur regularly, even monthly, at the site of the primary lesion. The infection may cause no other symptoms or may involve fever, localized lymphadenopathy, malaise, **myalgia** (muscle pain), pharyngitis, or, rarely, keratoconjunctivitis. Preexisting abrasions or other underlying skin conditions will increase the likelihood of transmission. Common sites for infection include the head, upper extremities, and trunk.

The incubation period for primary infection, which is 2 to 14 days, usually begins with a prodome of burning, stinging pain, tenderness, or itching at the infected site, followed by clusters of vesicles on an erythematous base.

 It is critical to identify the condition at this stage and refer the athlete to a physician immediately for care. When seen later during the ulceration and crusting stage, the rash is often confused with impetigo.

To treat the primary infection by arresting viral replication, 200 to 400 mg of acyclovir three times a day for 10 days is usually required. Acyclovir is very effective early in the course of the virus when it is multiplying rapidly. Once the vesicles are fully formed and ulcerating, the medication is no longer effective. If ulceration has occurred, topical benzoyl peroxide and gentle use of a hair dryer may dry the crusts more rapidly and minimize secondary bacterial infection. Wrestlers with a history of recurrent HSV infection may be supplied with a prophylactic course of acyclovir (1 to 2 capsules of 400 mg acyclovir daily for 5 days) so they can start at the first sign of vesicle formation. With active infections, however, wrestlers should be barred from physical contact during practice until their scabs are dry and they have no further vesicles, open ulcers, or drainage (5).

 FIELD STRATEGY 27.2 **MANAGEMENT OF FUNGAL SKIN CONDITIONS**

- Wash the region 4 to 5 times daily and after physical exertion.
- Rinse all soap residue from the region and completely dry the area. With tinea cruris, apply antifungal powder liberally.
- Apply topical antifungal agents, such Halotex, Lotrimin, Micatin, and Tinactin, twice daily for 1 month.
- If the condition does not clear up, refer to a physician to rule out candidiasis, dermatitis, psoriasis, or other skin disorders.
- In resistant infections, oral griseofulvin can be used for 4 to 8 weeks.
- Follow proper personal hygiene as listed in Box 27.2.

HERPES ZOSTER

Herpes zoster, or shingles as it is more commonly known, is rare but can affect young athletes. Local trauma in contact sports can occasionally precipitate reactivation of the varicella (chickenpox) virus. Acyclovir, valacyclovir, or famciclovir, if given early five times a day for 7 days, will shorten the course. Participation should be prohibited, both for pain relief and to lessen transmission to others who have never had chickenpox. Because human immuno-deficiency virus (HIV) can precipitate herpes zoster in a young person, an HIV test is appropriate.

VERRUCAE VIRUS

Dozens of varieties of the human papilloma virus can cause warts; verrucae plana (flat wart) and verrucae plantaris (plantar wart) are only two of the more common ones. Incubation is several weeks to 5 years after exposure. The common wart is prevalent on the hands, and appears as a small, round, elevated lesion with a rough, dry surface. Pressure on the wart increases the pain. Because of its location, the common wart is often subjected to secondary bacterial infection. A plantar wart, which grows into the thick stratum corneum of the foot, has tiny, dark red or black dots representing capillaries that have been penetrated by the root of the wart. Verrucae plantaris is likely transmitted from swimming pool decks or shower rooms.

Recurrences are frequent and no single method of treatment is effective for all lesions. Within 6 months, most young people develop an immunologic reaction to the virus, and the wart may disappear with or without treatment. For others, any treatment will be ineffective. During the competitive season, a doughnut pad can be worn to alleviate some of the pressure to the area. After the season, under the direction of a physician or podiatrist, treatment may involve chemical therapy including salicylic acid pads applied every few days following bathing, injections or application of an antimetabolite including intralesional bleomycin or 5-fluorouracil (5-FU) to destroy the wart, cryosurgery (liquid nitrogen), electrosurgery, scalpel excision, or carbon dioxide laser excision.

MOLLUSCUM CONTAGIOSUM

A pox virus, molluscum contagiosum, is commonly reported by wrestlers and in younger athletes who have immature immune systems. The virus is spread by personal contact, and contaminated swimming pools and gymnastic equipment. Lesions, which are multiple pearly papules, flesh-colored to yellow, have a tiny, round spot on the surface and can be found on the trunk, axilla, face, perineum, and thighs. The condition is primarily a cosmetic problem; however, blunt trauma can rupture a papule, causing a disabling local inflammatory reaction that can mimic cellulitis. Treatment involves immediate referral to a physician who may employ a destructive modality, such as curet-

tage, light hyfrecation, liquid nitrogen cryotherapy, laser surgery, or topical 50% trichloroacetic acid over the lesion surface. Full activity can be resumed in 2 to 4 days.

 The lacrosse athlete has tinea pedis. Prevention involves keeping the feet and toes dry, and wearing clean cotton socks; applying an antifungal ointment, cream, or powder; and wearing footwear while walking in showers and locker rooms.

OTHER SKIN REACTIONS

 A gymnast notices small itching bumps covering her lower leg and foot after removing tape applied to her ankle to support a sprain. The area is extremely red, and it itches. What condition may be present, and what treatment should be recommended?

Unlike skin infections caused by bacteria, fungi, and viruses, other skin problems caused by mechanical, environmental, allergic, or chemical reactions are not infectious and are generally mild in nature. Once identified, they can easily be treated with topical medications.

Chafing of the Skin

Chafing of the skin (intertrigo) is a superficial dermatitis more often caused by the friction of fabric rubbing against moist, warm, skin than by skin rubbing on skin. The condition may occur between the creases of the neck, in the axillary and buttocks area, or beneath large breasts, but is primarily seen in the groin region in individuals with muscular thighs or in obese individuals. The condition is characterized by erythema, maceration, burning, and itching. In severe cases, the skin becomes eroded and weeping. The condition can be prevented by wearing loose, soft, cotton underwear to keep the skin dry, clean, and friction free, or by wearing shorts with longer legs made of low-friction fabric. Treatment involves initial application of a cold compress. The area should be cleansed daily with mild soap and water, followed by an application of a soothing ointment. Talcum powders should be avoided as they can be abrasive and do not absorb moisture well.

Athlete's Nodules

Also referred to as surfer's nodules, athlete's nodules are asymptomatic dermal nodules found at various sites of the body that encounter repeated minor trauma, such as the feet of surfers and runners, knees of canoeists, and the knuckles of boxers. Protective pads at the trauma sites can help decrease pain. Otherwise, high-potency topical or intralesional corticosteroids can be applied. If this does not provide relief, the nodules can be incised.

Acne Mechanica

Characterized by a local exacerbation of acne vulgaris due to heat, occlusion, pressure, and friction, **acne mechanica** presents with erythematous crops of papules and pustules in areas of mechanical trauma. Sometimes referred to as "football acne," the acne develops wherever skin is exposed to prolonged causative factors, such as under chin straps, forehead bands, shirt collars, football shoulder pads, backpack straps, automobile seats, bras, wide belts, and orthopedic casts and braces. If left unattended, the acne may develop into a cyst. Treatment and prevention includes thoroughly cleansing the area after a workout with a mild abrasive cleanser and back brush. Application of a topical astringent or 10% benzoyl peroxide agent, topical antibiotic, and in severe cases, a systemic antibiotic may be prescribed. The condition usually improves or resolves after the season. Prevention involves wearing a clean, absorbent T-shirt under the football pads, and treating any underlying acne vulgaris. If an exercise leotard is worn during exercise, it should be removed immediately after the workout.

Striae Distensae

Stretch marks or **striae distensae** are characterized by linear pink or flesh-colored patches most often seen on the chest, shoulders, and upper outer arms. They are often seen in athletes who do high-intensity weight training. Even though the origin is unclear, it is most often seen after rapid growth of a body part, which is believed to result in fragmented elastic skin fibers. There is no treatment for striae distensae.

Sunburn

Sunscreens applied to the skin prior to sun exposure can prevent many of the damaging effects of ultraviolet radiation. The effectiveness of the sunscreen is based on the sun protection factor (SPF). For example, an SPF of 15 indicates that an individual can be exposed to ultraviolet light 15 times longer than without a sunscreen before the skin will begin to burn. Higher numbers provide better protection; SPF 15 is good, SPF 30 is better, and SPF 50 provides a complete sunblock. Acute sunburn (actinic dermatitis) can be painful and disfiguring, and—depending upon the degree—can prevent participation in sport activities. The degree of sunburn depends upon the length of exposure to the sun, the sun's relative level of intensity, and personal skin type.

Sunburns are classified as first, second, and third degree. The full extent of the injury may not be assessed until 24 to 48 hours after exposure. First-degree burns have mild erythema throughout the area of exposure. Second-degree burns have vesicles or blisters in addition to the erythema. Third-degree burns will exhibit skin ulcerations. Systemic

> ### ➤➤ Box 27.3
>
> ## Prevention of Sunburn
>
> - Use a sunscreen with an appropriate sun protection factor (SPF) for your skin type, preferably a 15 or higher.
> - Apply sunscreen 20 to 30 minutes prior to exposure.
> - Apply evenly over all exposed skin to avoid isolated areas of sunburn.
> - Reapply every 2 to 4 hours, especially if sweating profusely.
> - Select sunscreen that has a high rate of efficacy when subjected to moisture.
> - Be careful when applying the sunscreen around the eyes.
> - Sunscreen sprays work well for the top of the head; lip protectors should also be used.
> - Avoid midday exposure to the sun (10:00 AM to 3:00 PM)
> - While in the sun, wear loose, woven, light cotton clothing.
> - Hats with brims are much better than caps or visors.
> - Sunburn can occur on cloudy days, so sunscreen should be worn at all times.
> - Be aware of reflectant photoenergy potential when around water or snow.
> - Several medications (antibiotics, antiseptics, anesthetics, certain NSAIDs) increase sensitivity to the sun. Read the instructions for use of any mediations prior to sun exposure. If there are questions, consult a pharmacist or physician.
> - Drink plenty of nonalcoholic beverages to prevent dehydration.

symptoms of all three degree burns include fever, chills, nausea, and exhaustion. Although sunburns are easily treated, it is best to prevent them from occurring (**Box 27.3**).

If sunburn occurs, apply a cold compress, topical hydrocortisone 1% cream or spray, and aloe vera to decrease pain and discomfort. If systemic aspirin or NSAIDs are used, they must be taken immediately after sun exposure to be effective.

With serious second- and third-degree burns, immediate referral to a physician is warranted to ensure proper treatment and prevention of infection.

Oral corticosteroids may be prescribed to relieve the pain.

Pernio (Chilblains)

Excessive exposure to cold can lead to pernio, in which the tissue does not freeze, but rather reacts with erythema, itching, and burning. This happens especially on the dorsa of the fingers and toes, and on the heels, nose, and ears. More commonly seen in young women, the condition often occurs with the first exposure to lower temperatures in highly humid conditions. Lesions may be single or multiple, and in severe cases, may appear blistered or ulcerated. Treatment involves gradual warming of the body part. Topical steroids will help reduce the inflammation, but the potency must be low enough to prevent further vasoconstriction. Heavy woolen socks may need to worn at all times, including indoors and while sleeping.

Miliaria

Miliaria, or "prickly heat," is caused when active sweat glands become blocked by organic debris, leading to an inflamed, pruritic skin eruption. It was discussed in detail in Chapter 17. Treatment involves cooling and drying the skin, controlling the itching, and watching for infection. Individuals should avoid occlusive topical ointments and close-fitting, poorly absorbent fabrics on the skin.

Dry (Xerotic) Skin

Dry skin is commonly seen during the winter months. Athletes, who must shower frequently, are particularly prone to this condition. Xerotic skin can be caused by a number of factors, but decreased skin lipids appears to be the major one **(Box 27.4)**. In the winter, dry, cold winds increase evaporation from convection, and low temperatures decrease skin flexibility, thus exacerbating the condition. The skin appears dry, with variable erythema and scale. Usually appearing first on the shins, it is also common on the forearms and dorsal hands. For individuals who exercise outdoors in the winter, the face can also be affected. Localized or generalized pruritus is the most common symptom. When severe, the dry skin loses its suppleness, and cracks, fissures, and erythema appear.

Treatment is focused on preventing excessive water loss and replacing water already lost. Tepid water, rather than hot, should be used for bathing, and time spent in the shower should be limited. Moisturizing soaps should be used; however, avoid the xerotic areas. If possible, soap use should be limited to the genitalia, underarms, hands, feet, and face. Bubblebaths and brisk scrubbing should be avoided. Emollient lotions that contain high concentrations of lipids increase and maintain hydration by occluding the skin surface, and help insulate against the cold. They should be applied frequently and liberally, especially after each hand washing and immediately after bathing, to minimize water loss from evaporation. Swimmers should moisturize the whole body after bathing. In severe cases, antipruritics may be used to decrease pruritis and scratching, thus enabling the outer skin layer to heal. Alphahydroxy acids and topical corticosteroids can be used to decrease the inflammation associated with severely dry skin with fissures.

Eczema

Eczema can be an acute or chronic inflammatory condition of the skin characterized by poorly marginated erythema with scaling and exudate. Persistent itching and burning can lead to evidence of **excoriation** (scratch marks usually covered with blood or serious crusts). The condition is aggravated by an increase in body heat and perspiration, both of which occur during physical activity. Treatment involves topical corticosteroids in an emollient cream or ointment base. Antihistamines may provide relief for the itching; however, systemic corticosteroids are most often used during acute flares.

Hyperhidrosis

A condition involving excessive perspiration, particularly on the palms and axillary region, is called **hyperhidrosis**. The condition can interfere with sports that require holding various objects (balls, discus, bars, oars, sticks), or require gripping (tennis, racquetball). The plantar sweat glands are often stimulated when the extremities are used, and during times of emotional excitement, which also stimulates the axillary apocrine glands. Little can be done for the condition. Athletes may choose to participate in activities that do not require a prolonged hand grip; they may also apply aluminum chloride in anhydrous ethyl alcohol to the hands, or wear gloves to help absorb the sweat.

Bites and Stings

Bites and stings come from a variety of insects, including mosquitoes, flies, spiders, ants, bees, fleas, and ticks. Although many are just annoying pests that can be discouraged with standard insect repellent, their bites and stings can be painful, and even life threatening if the individual develops an allergic reaction to the venom (anaphylaxis). **Anaphylaxis** is an immediate shock-like, frequently fatal

---

➤➤ **Box 27.4**

Causes of Dry (Xerotic) Skin

- Genetic predisposition to dry skin
- Decreased skin lipids due to:
  - Age
  - Chronic illness
  - Malnutrition
  - Use of industrial or domestic cleansers or solvents
  - Frequent bathing
- Repetitive trauma from scratching already dry skin
- Environmental factors, such as:
  - Decreased humidity
  - Winter weather (dry, cold winds)
  - Indoor heating and air conditioning
  - Dry environments (airplanes)

hypersensitive reaction that occurs within minutes of administration of an allergen unless appropriate first aid measures are taken immediately. The condition is characterized by contraction of smooth muscle and dilation of capillaries due to the release of pharmacologically active substances (histamine, bradykinin, serotonin). Signs and symptoms of anaphylactic shock include respiratory distress, cyanosis, weakness, rapid and weak pulse, low blood pressure, localized urticaria or edema, paresthesia, dilated pupils, choking, wheezing, sudden collapse, involuntary loss of bowel and bladder control, headache, dizziness, seizures, and unconsciousness. The individual may have a history of such reactions, may wear a medical identification tag, and may have a self-administered epinephrine device (Epipen®).

 Immediate treatment involves activation of EMS and is covered in more detail in Field Strategy 27.3 later in the chapter.

MOSQUITOES, GNATS, AND FLIES

Mosquitoes, gnats, and a variety of flies feed on human blood, and are considered biting insects. Most bites appear as erythematous, macular or papular, pruritic, painful lesions. The lesion may not be apparent immediately, but rather may appear as a delayed hypersensitive response to the saliva of the biting organism. Immediate application of a cold compress can relieve pain, or an OTC topical corticosteroid or systemic antihistamine may be utilized. Systemic corticosteroids are used in severe cases. Once a lesion has appeared, it should be monitored closely for secondary infection.

BEES, WASPS, AND ANTS

It is estimated that more than 20% of the population is allergic to the hymenopteran venom from bees, wasps, and ants, which in turn carries a higher risk of allergic and anaphylactic reactions. Athletes involved in outdoor activities are at special risk for insect stings. Yellow jackets and honeybees, for example, are fond of sweets and can be drawn to rehydration stations stocked with sugar-containing sports drinks. Fire ants, found especially in the southern United States, can be found on practice and game fields where athletes may sit on the ground.

The sting results in a painful wheal or hive caused by the venom. The site rapidly becomes pruritic, and the itching can last for several hours. Occasionally, an exaggerated local reaction can occur in which the swelling and itching extend beyond the sting site to the involved extremity, and may be associated with dyspnea, tachycardia, hypotension, and anaphylaxis.

 This may result in a medical emergency.

When a sting occurs, follow the guidelines outlined in **Field Strategy 27.3**.

SPIDERS

The venom from several spiders can also lead to painful lesions. Black widow spiders are found throughout the United States; however, only the female, a dark black, globular-shaped spider with the characteristic ventral, reddish marking (typically an "hourglass") on her abdomen, is large enough to bite through human skin. Because the webs are typically built in relatively undisturbed, protected areas, most sport-related bites occur in equipment storage areas (6). The bite is often felt as a "pinprick" and may be slightly red. Significant symptoms usually start 1 hour after the bite, with the most common being spasmodic muscle pain. The spasms may progress to regional muscle groups of the trunk, with pain and spasm lasting from 12 to 48 hours. Other reactions may include an increased respiratory rate, tachycardia, hypertension, fever, headache, nausea, vomiting, restlessness, and anxiety.

Bites from a brown recluse spider are relatively painless and may go undetected. In the ensuing hours, the site becomes pruritic, red, and mildly swollen. Local pain, due to vasospasm and ischemia, begins within 2 to 8 hours. After 12 to 18 hours, a small, central vesicle develops, surrounded by an irregular border of erythema, ecchymosis, and edema. If the blister ruptures, the erythema will darken and may spread distally. After 5 to 7 days of progressive aseptic necrosis, the bite area becomes depressed and covered with a black crust, that eventually sloughs off, leaving an open ulcer that tends to heal over several weeks (6).

The bark scorpion, native to Arizona and adjacent regions, is a nocturnal spider that tends to hide in dark areas during the day. The small tooth at the base of its stinger distinguishes itself from less toxic species. Athletes involved in outdoor activities are most at risk. Rock climbers often put their hands into blind spots on overhead ledges. Campers and hikers need to be cautious about turning over stones and logs. They should also inspect footwear before slipping their feet into the shoes, since scorpions may hide in the shoes during the night. Individuals stung by a scorpion will feel immediate, intense pain that significantly worsens with light pressure over the site. The pain may radiate throughout the extremity. Systemic reactions include restlessness, hypersalivation, dysphagia, visual changes, roving eye movements, respiratory distress (with stridor or wheezing), hypertension, fever, loss of bowel or bladder continence, muscle spasms, and paralysis.

The majority of stings occurring in healthy young adults can be managed on-site. Management includes cleaning the site with soap and water, application of ice, elevation of the affected limb to approximately heart level, and administration of aspirin or Tylenol as needed for minor discomfort.

FIELD STRATEGY 27.3   MANAGEMENT ALGORITHM FOR A BEE STING

<u>Prevention Note</u>
For sensitive athletes who participate outdoors, suggest that they:
-refrain from wearing bright, colorful, or floral clothing
-refrain from using scented soaps, lotions, or aftershaves

<u>After Sustaining a Bee Sting</u>
Immediately refrain from strenuous exercise

↓

Remove the stinger with a fingernail;
do not squeeze it, as this will inject more venom

↓

Apply ice to the site

↓

Systemic antihistamines may help with local reactions

↓

Observe closely for signs of anaphylactic shock:

-faintness, deteriorating consciousness, or other signs of shock	-generalized urticaria or edema
-paresthesia	-choking or signs of laryngeal edema
-pupillary dilation	-wheezing, coughing, or difficulty breathing

<u>If Anaphylaxis Occurs</u>

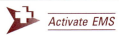
Activate EMS

↓

Place the athlete supine with feet elevated

↓

Apply a constricting band a few inches proximal to the sting site that:
-occludes superficial venous and lymphatic return
-does not obstruct arterial flow

↓

Continue ice application to further reduce venom absorption

↓

Check for a medical identification tag

↓

If the person has an Epipen® or other allergy kit,
inject the epinephrine into the thigh as instructed

↓

If respiratory or cardiac arrest occurs, begin CPR

↓

Transport immediately to the nearest medical facility

Stings occurring in children or any individual experiencing severe symptoms such as respiratory distress, should be transported immediately to the nearest medical facility for evaluation and management.

FLEAS AND TICKS

Bites from fleas cause only minor discomfort. Most fleas bite in patterns of three, and tend to attack the ankle and foot. Scratching the area could complicate the condition by developing a secondary infection. Treatment is limited to applying an antipruritic lotion over the area.

Ticks are parasites that attach their heads onto people or animals, and absorb blood. They are frequent carriers of Rocky Mountain spotted fever and Lyme disease (LD), which can produce headache, low grade fever, fatigue, and muscle pain. A characteristic sign of Lyme disease is a bulls-eye rash appearing 3 days to 1 month after infection.

It is a round ring with central clearing. Sometimes many patches appear, varying in shape, depending on their location. Common sites are the thigh, groin, trunk, and the armpits. As the rash enlarges, the center of the rash may clear, resulting in a bulls-eye appearance. The rash may be warm, but it is usually not painful. The rash can disappear and return several weeks later. For dark complected individuals, the rash will look like a bruise. If a rash is present, it is wise to take a picture of it, as some physicians require evidence of the rash prior to prescribing medication. Not all rashes occurring at the site of a tick bite are indicators of LD. An allergic reaction to tick saliva often occurs at the bite site. The resulting rash usually occurs within hours to a few days after the tick bite, usually does not expand, and disappears within a few days.

Management involves safely removing a tick by applying a substance that blocks access to air (petroleum jelly, mineral oil, or fingernail polish). The tick should withdraw the head. Do not attempt to pull the tick from the body; doing so may leave the head embedded under the skin.

If signs and symptoms of Rocky Mountain spotted fever or Lyme disease appear, immediately refer the individual to a physician for treatment.

Antibiotics are usually recommended for a minimum of 4 to 6 weeks.

SCABIES

Scabies is a skin disease caused by the mite sarcoptes scabiei, which produces severe, intense itching. It appears as small dark burrows and tiny vesicles in a linear distribution between the finger webs, or on the elbows, periumbilical skin, and genitalia. The condition can lead to a "mini-epidemic" in sports such as wrestling. The mite can be spread on towels, uniforms, or equipment.

Immediate referral to a physician is essential.

Treatment must be aggressive and persistent. Any individual in contact with the person should also be examined. For those with symptoms, a prescribed lindane lotion should be applied over the entire body from the neck down the first night at bedtime; then to affected areas only, every 3 nights until resolved. The locker room and game equipment should be disinfected; bedding and clothing must be washed daily in hot water. If asymptomatic, individuals are still treated with the prescribed lindane lotion over the entire body at bedtime, with two applications, 1 week apart.

LICE (PEDICULOSIS)

Pediculosis, a louse infestation, can infect the head, pubic region, or any location on the body. Head lice live in the hair of the scalp and cause itching when they bite the skin of the scalp and neck. Egg sacks, or nits, can adhere firmly to the hair shafts. Body lice, 2 to 4 mm long, are clearly visible, living in the folds of clothing, and tend to bite in areas of close contact with clothing. Pubic lice (crab lice, 1 to 2 mm long) are typically seen in the genitals and lower abdomen, but can be found on the chest or axillary hair. Signs and symptoms of lice mimic those of an insect bite: pruritis and, through subsequent scratching, pustules and excoriation. Treatment of head and pubic lice is done with medicated shampoos or cream rinses containing lindane or pyrethrins. Products containing pryethrins are available over-the-counter, but lindane is available only through a physician's prescription. Dose and duration of shampoo treatment should be followed according to label instructions. Retreatment should occur 7 to 10 days after the initial treatment to assure that no eggs have survived. Nit combs are available to help remove nits from hair. Body lice treatment also requires the boiling and ironing of clothing.

Contact Dermatitis

Contact dermatitis is classified as either allergic or irritant dermatitis. **Allergic contact dermatitis** results when a substance comes in direct contact with the skin and leads to a simple inflammatory reaction. In contrast, **irritant contact dermatitis** results when the substance causes direct skin damage, pain, or ulceration. Contact dermatitis affects only the area in direct contact with the causative agent, leading to a sharp line of demarcation between normal skin and the affected skin. For example, reacting to a watch band or to swimming goggles will lead to characteristic patterns of erythema and irritation.

ALLERGIC CONTACT DERMATITIS

Allergic dermatitis, which accounts for 20 to 30% of all contact dermatitis, is identified by dry vesicles accompanied by pain, erythema, and pruritic conditions (7). Heat, whether internal or external, intensifies symptoms. Common agents that contribute to the condition include adhesive tape, rubber articles (e.g., straps, pads, swim goggles, swim fins, swim caps, shoes), tape adherent and remover, soap, detergent, and deodorant. Allergic dermatitis remains localized to the affected area, and does not spread in water, although hot baths may accelerate the skin's reaction.

IRRITANT CONTACT DERMATITIS

Irritant dermatitis also presents with erythema, pruritis, pain, and swelling. It often occurs secondary to physical and mechanical agents, such as dry ice burns, abrasions from Astroturf®, poorly fitted equipment that causes friction burns, striae (bands of thin wrinkled skin), or increased sweating between skinfolds (groin, under breast tissue), and during skin loss secondary to an application of a causative agent (adhesive tape). Diagnosis of either type of contact dermatitis relies on the history and distribution of the rash.

GENERAL MANAGEMENT OF CONTACT DERMATITIS

During acute reactions, a cold compress should be applied to the affected area. Systemic antihistamines are used to reduce itching and inflammation, along with topical agents (corticosteroids). Topical antihistamines and benzocaine products should never be used for these conditions (7). The causative agent should be identified and contact with the agent eliminated. Disqualification from activity is dependent upon the degree of skin involvement, severity of symptoms, and the specific sport (i.e., contact versus noncontact).

Chronic contact dermatitis requires avoiding contact with or establishing a barrier against the causative agent, application of topical corticosteroids, and use of antibiotics if a secondary bacterial infection develops. The skin should be kept clean during both acute and chronic cases.

Urticaria

Urticaria (hives) is usually systemic in origin, and is caused by a hypersensitivity to foods or drugs, infection, physical agents (heat, cold, light, friction), or psychic stimuli. The resulting wheal is a smooth, slightly elevated area on the body that appears red or white, and is accompanied by severe itching. It is commonly seen in allergies to mechanical or chemical irritants.

CHOLINERGIC URTICARIA

Cholinergic urticaria, also known as generalized heat urticaria, is the most common type of urticaria. It is acetylcholine mediated and provoked by heat, exercise, or fever. Clinical presentation reveals small papules that appear first in the upper thorax and neck, spreading inferiorly to involve the entire body. Systemic symptoms, although rare, include generalized sweating, abdominal cramps, dizziness, wheezing, and bradycardia. The inner aspects of the arms, legs, and lateral flanks are common sites. Currently, there is no cure, but antihistamines such as hydroxyzine and cyproheptadine are generally used to relieve symptoms. While symptomatic, the athlete may wish to avoid physical activity and sports participation.

EXERCISE-INDUCED URTICARIA

Some medical experts believe that **exercise-induced urticaria** may be a variation of cholinergic urticaria, but the lesions are much larger. Systemic signs are limited to wheezing and hypotension. Unlike cholinergic urticaria, exercise-induced urticaria can be successfully treated with prescribed antihistamines, anticholinergics, or beta-ago-

nists. Epinephrine is generally the treatment of choice when systemic signs are present.

COLD URTICARIA

Cold urticaria is very common in athletes, is nonallergic, and is characterized by localized or generalized wheals that develop in response to cold exposure. The condition often becomes apparent when a cold pack is placed on an individual who is hypersensitive to cold (see Figure 6.3). The condition responds well to small doses of oral corticosteroids.

 The gymnast has allergic contact dermatitis and might be allergic to the adhesive tape or tape adherent. Treatment should include application of a cold compress and topical agent, and trying an alternative to tape for support of the ankle.

Summary

1. Whenever skin is damaged, a lesion appears. Skin lesions are identified by their size and depth. Recognizing the type of lesion can help identify the cause of the skin damage.

2. Skin infections may stem from fungi, bacteria, or viruses.

3. Bacterial lesions are typically caused by a staphylococcal or streptococcal infection. Impetigo is highly contagious and is characterized by small vesicles that form pustules and eventually honey-colored weeping crustations. Bacterial skin conditions are treated with OTC antibacterial topical agents.

4. Fungi thrive in dark, warm, moist environments, and often attack the fingernails, toenails, foot, groin, body, and scalp. Common signs and symptoms include pruritis, redness, and scaling. Antifungal medication is used to treat the condition.

5. Viral skin conditions can range from the common wart to the highly contagious herpes gladiatorum and molluscum contagiosum, which can infect an entire team. Any lesions on the trunk, axilla, face, and thigh should be immediately referred to a physician.

6. Sunburns are classified as first, second, and third degree. Prevention involves using a sunscreen with an SPF of 15 or higher, and avoiding exposure to the sun during the midday.

7. Miliaria, or prickly heat, occurs when active sweat glands become blocked by organic debris. Treatment involves cooling and drying the skin, controlling the itching, and watching for secondary infection.

8. Bites and stings from insects can be painful and itchy. Immediate cold application can relieve pain, or a topical corticosteroid or systemic antihistamine may be used. Systemic corticosteroids are used in severe cases. The individual should be watched carefully for signs of anaphylactic shock.

9. Allergic contact dermatitis results when a substance comes in direct contact with the skin and causes a simple inflammatory reaction; irritant contact dermatitis results when the substance causes direct skin damage, pain, or ulceration. Treatment involves removing the substance, applying a cold compress, possible topical corticosteroids, and systemic antihistamines to reduce itching and inflammation.

10. Urticaria, or hives, is caused by hypersensitivity to foods or drugs, infection, physical agents, or psychi stimuli. The resulting wheal is accompanied by severe itching and is treated with antihistamines, anticholinergics, or beta-agonists.

References

1. Krowchuk DP. Treating acne: A practical guide for pediatricians. Am Acad Ped 1998;11(1):1-10.
2. Basler RS. Skin problems in athletes. In: The Team Physician's Handbook. Edited by Mellion MB, Walsh WM, Shelton GL. Philadelphia: Hanley and Belfus, 1997.
3. Martin M, Colluchi T. Impetigo in high school football: A case review. Ath Ther Today 1997;(Jan):47-48.
4. Ramsey ML. Clearing up fungal infection of the nail plate. Phys Sportsmed 1993;21(2):70-80.
5. Dienst WL, Jr., et al. Pinning down skin infections: Diagnosis, treatment, and prevention in wrestlers. Phys Sportsmed 1997;25(12):45-56.
6. Norris RL. Managing arthropod bites and stings. Phys Sportsmed 1998;26(7):47-58.
7. Fisher AA. Sports-related allergic dermatitis. Cutis 1992;50(2):95-97.

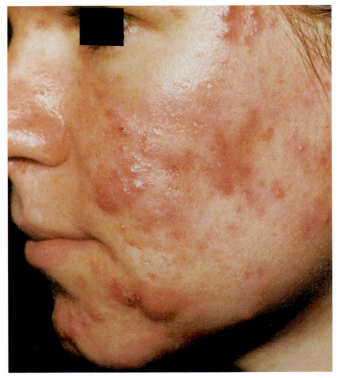

➤ COLOR PLATE 1 Acne

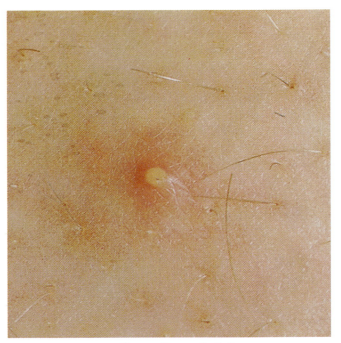

➤ COLOR PLATE 2 Boil

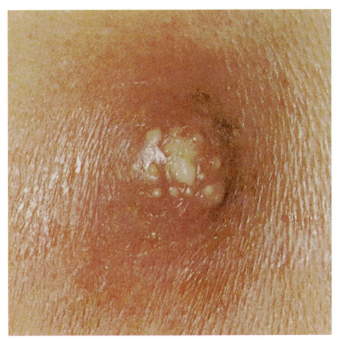

➤ COLOR PLATE 3 A group of interconnected boils is called
a carbuncle

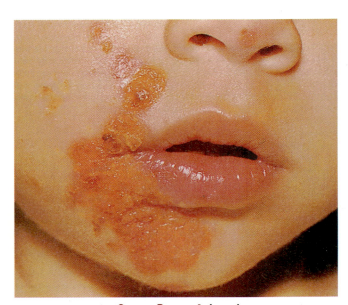

➤ COLOR PLATE 4 Impetigo

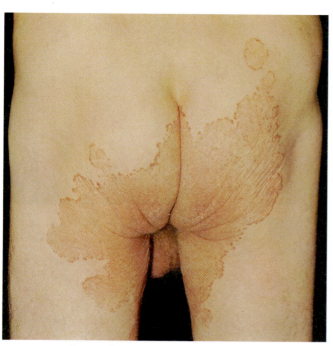

➤ COLOR PLATE 5 Tinea cruris (jock itch)

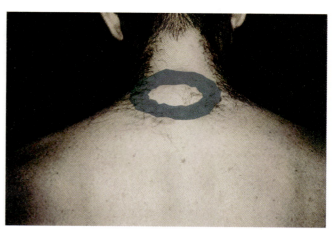

➤ COLOR PLATE 6 Tinea corporis (body ringworm)

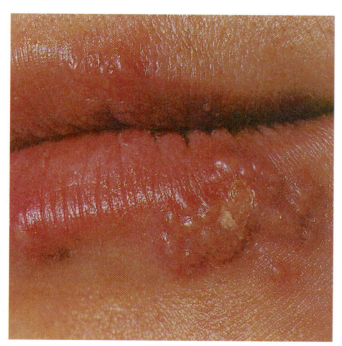

➤ COLOR PLATE 7 Herpes simplex

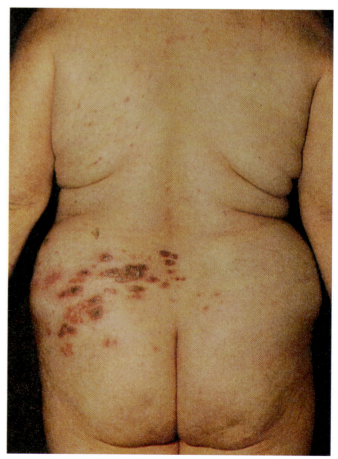

➤ COLOR PLATE 8 Herpes zoster

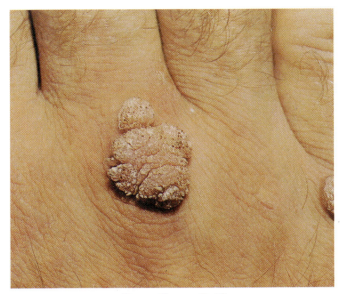

➤ COLOR PLATE 9 Wart

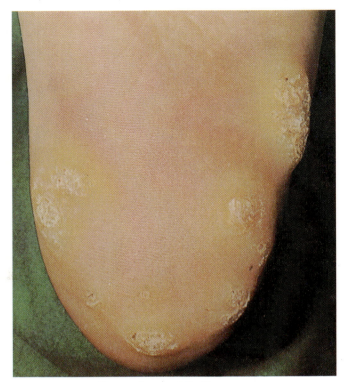

➤ COLOR PLATE 10 Plantar warts

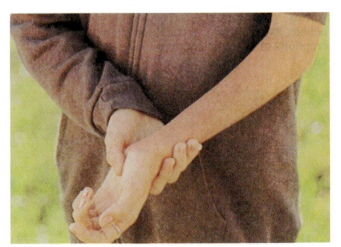

➤ COLOR PLATE 11 First-degree burn (sunburn)

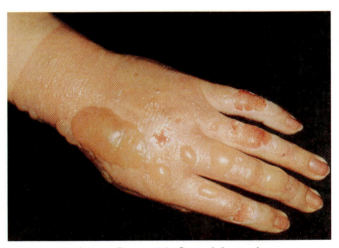

➤ COLOR PLATE 12 Second-degree burn

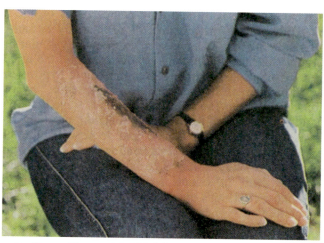

➤ COLOR PLATE 13 Third degree burn with scar tissue

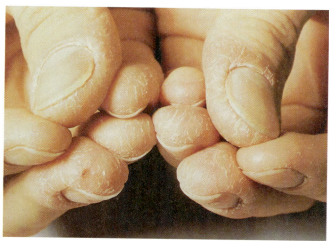

➤ COLOR PLATE 14 Eczema

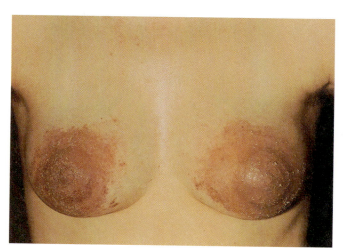

➤ COLOR PLATE 15 Dermatitis

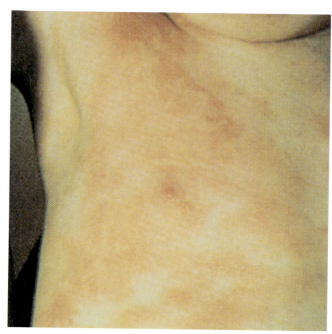

➤ COLOR PLATE 16 Urticaria (hives)

Appendix of Medical Terminology

Glossary of Prefixes, Suffixes, and Combining Forms

Term Component to English

a-	without
ab-	away from
abdomin/o	abdomen
-ac	pertaining to
acous/o	hearing
acr/o	extremity or topmost
-acusis	hearing condition
ad-	to, toward, or near
aden/o	gland
adip/o	fat
adren/o	adrenal gland
aer/o	air or gas
-al	pertaining to
albumin/o	protein
-algia	pain
alveol/o	alveolus (air sac)
ambi-	both
an-	without
an/o	anus
andr/o	male
angi/o	vessel
ankyl/o	crooked or stiff
ante-	before
anti-	against or opposed to
aort/o	aorta
appendic/o	appendix
aque/o	water
-ar	pertaining to
-arche	beginning
arteri/o	artery
arthr/o	joint
articul/o	joint

-ary	pertaining to
-ase	enzyme
-asthenia	weakness
ather/o	fat
-ation	process
-atri/o	atrium
audi/o	hearing
aur/i	ear
bacteri/o	bacteria
balan/o	glans penis
bi-	two or both
bil/i	bile
-blast	germ or bud
blast/o	germ or bud
blephar/o	eyelid
brachi/o	arm
brady-	slow
bronch/o	bronchus (airway)
bronchiol/o	bronchiole (little airway)
bucc/o	cheek
capn/o	carbon dioxide
carb/o	carbon dioxide
carcin/o	cancer
cardi/o	heart
-cele	pouching or hernia
celi/o	abdomen
-centesis	puncture for aspiration
cephal/o	head
cerebell/o	cerebellum (little brain)
cerebr/o	brain
cerumin/o	wax
cervic/o	neck or cervix
cheil/o	lip
chol/e	bile

choledoch/o	common bile duct
chondr/o	cartilage (gristle)
chrom/o	color
chyl/o	juice
circum-	around
col/o	colon
colon/o	colon
colp/o	vagina (sheath)
con-	together or with
conjunctiv/o	conjunctiva (to join together)
contra-	against or opposed to
corne/o	cornea
coron/o	circle or crown
cost/o	rib
crani/o	skull
crin/o	to secrete
cutane/o	skin
cyan/o	blue
cyst/o	bladder or sac
cyt/o	cell
dacry/o	tear
dactyl/o	digit (finger or toe)
de-	from, down, or not
dent/i	teeth
derm/o	skin
dermat/o	skin
-desis	binding
dextr/o	right, or on the right side
dia-	across or through

diaphor/o	profuse sweat
dips/o	thirst
dis-	separate from or apart
duoden/o	duodenum
-dynia	pain
dys-	painful, difficult, or faulty
-e	noun marker
e-	out or away
-eal	pertaining to
ec-	out or away
-ectasis	expansion or dilation
ecto-	outside
-ectomy	excision (removal)
-emesis	vomiting
-emia	blood condition
en-	within
encephal/o	brain
endo-	within
enter/o	small intestine
epi-	upon
epididym/o	epididymis
episi/o	vulva (covering)
erythr/o	red
esophag/o	esophagus
esthesi/o	sensation
eu-	good or normal
ex-	out or away
exo-	outside
extra-	outside
fasci/o	fascia (a band)
femor/o	femur

fibr/o .... fiber
gangli/o .... ganglion (knot)
gastr/o .... stomach
-gen .... origin or production
-genesis .... origin or production
-genic .... origin or production
gingiv/o .... gums
gli/o .... glue
glomerul/o .... glomerulus (little ball)
gloss/o .... tongue
glott/o .... opening
gluc/o .... sugar
glyc/o .... sugar
gnos/o .... knowing
-gram .... record
-graph .... instrument for recording
-graphy .... process of recording
gynec/o .... woman
hem/o .... blood
hemat/o .... blood
hemi- .... half
hepat/o,
hepatic/o .... liver
herni/o .... hernia
hidr/o .... sweat
hist/o .... tissue
histi/o .... tissue
hormon/o .... hormone (an urging on)
hydr/o .... water
hyper- .... above or excessive
hypo- .... below or deficient
hyster/o .... uterus
-ia .... condition of
-iasis .... formation of or presence of
-iatrics .... treatment
-iatry .... treatment
-ic .... pertaining to
-icle .... small
ile/o .... ileum
immun/o .... safe
infra- .... below or under
inguin/o .... groin
inter- .... between
intra- .... within
ir/o .... colored circle
irid/o .... colored circle
-ism .... condition of
iso- .... equal, like
-ist .... one who specializes in

-itis .... inflammation
-ium .... structure or tissue
jejun/o .... jejunum (empty)
kerat/o .... hard or cornea
ket/o .... ketone bodies
keton/o .... ketone bodies
kinesi/o .... movement
kyph/o .... humped
lacrim/o .... tear
lact/o .... milk
lapar/o .... abdomen
laryng/o .... larynx (voice box)
lei/o .... smooth
-lepsy .... seizure
leuc/o .... white
leuk/o .... white
lingu/o .... tongue
lip/o .... fat
lith/o .... stone or calculus
lob/o .... lobe (a portion)
-logist .... one who specialized in the study or treatment of
-logy .... study of
lord/o .... bent
lumb/o .... loin (lower back)
lymph/o .... clear fluid
-lysis .... breaking down or dissolution
macr/o .... large or long
-malacia .... softening
mamm/o .... breast
mast/o .... breast
meat/o .... opening
-megaly .... enlargement
melan/o .... black
men/o .... menstruation
mening/o .... meninges (membrane)
meningi/o .... meninges (membrane)
meso- .... middle
meta- .... beyond, after, or change
-meter .... instrument for measuring
metr/o .... uterus
-metry .... process of measuring
micro- .... small
mono- .... one
morph/o .... form
multi- .... many
muscul/o .... muscle
my/o .... muscle

myc/o .... fungus
myel/o .... bone marrow or spinal cord
myring/o .... eardrum
narc/o .... stupor
nas/o .... nose
nat/i .... birth
necr/o .... death
neo- .... new
nephr/o .... kidney
neur/o .... nerve
ocul/o .... eye
-oid .... resembling
-ole .... small
olig/o .... few or deficient
-oma .... tumor
onych/o .... nail
oophor/o .... ovary
ophthalm/o .... eye
opt/o .... eye
orch/o .... testis (testicle)
orchi/o .... testis (testicle)
orchid/o .... testis (testicle)
or/o .... mouth
orth/o .... straight, normal, or correct
-osis .... condition or increase
oste/o .... bone
ot/o .... ear
-ous .... pertaining to
ovari/o .... ovary
ov/i .... egg
ov/o .... egg
ox/o .... oxygen
pachy- .... thick
pan- .... all
pancreat/o .... pancreas
para- .... alongside of or abnormal
-paresis .... slight paralysis
patell/o .... knee cap
path/o .... disease
pector/o .... chest
ped/o .... child or foot
pelv/i, pelv/o .... hip bone
-penia .... abnormal reduction
per- .... through
peri- .... around
perine/o .... perineum
peritone/o .... peritoneum
-pexy .... suspension or fixation
phac/o .... lens (lentil)
phag/o .... eat or swallow
phak/o .... lens (lentil)
pharyng/o .... pharynx (throat)
phas/o .... speech

-phil .... attraction for
-philia .... attraction for
phleb/o .... vein
phob/o .... exaggerated fear or sensitivity
phon/o .... voice or speech
phot/o .... light
phren/o .... diaphragm (also mind)
plas/o .... formation
-plasia .... formation
-plasty .... surgical repair or reconstruction
-plegia .... paralysis
pleur/o .... pleura
-pnea .... breathing
pneum/o .... air or lung
pneumon/o .... air or lung
pod/o .... foot
-poiesis .... formation
poly- .... many
post- .... after or behind
pre- .... before
presby/o .... old age
pro- .... before
proct/o .... rectum
prostat/o .... prostate
psych/o .... mind
-ptosis .... falling or downward displacement
pulmon/o .... lung
purpur/o .... purple
py/o .... pus
pyel/o .... basin
pylor/o .... pylorus (gatekeeper)
quadr/i .... four
radi/o .... radius (a bone of the forearm); radiation (especially x-ray)
re- .... again or back
rect/o .... rectum
ren/o .... kidney
reticul/o .... a net
retro- .... backward or behind
rhabd/o .... rod shaped or striated (skeletal)
rhin/o .... nose
-rrhage .... to burst forth
-rrhagia .... to burst forth
-rrhaphy .... suture
-rrhea .... discharge
-rrhexis .... rupture

salping/o	uterine (fallopian) tube; also eustachian tube
sarc/o	flesh
schiz/o	split, division
scler/o	hard or sclera
scoli/o	twisted
-scope	instrument for examination
-scopy	examination
seb/o	sebum (oil)
semi-	half
sial/o	saliva
sigmoid/o	sigmoid colon
sinistr/o	left, or on the left side
sinus/o	hollow (cavity)
somat/o	body
somn/o	sleep
son/o	sound
-spasm	involuntary contraction
sperm/o	sperm (seed)
spermat/o	sperm (seed)
sphygm/o	pulse
spin/o	spine (thorn)
spir/o	breathing
splen/o	spleen
spondyl/o	vertebra
squam/o	scale
-stasis	stop or stand
steat/o	fat
sten/o	narrow
stere/o	three dimensional or solid
stern/o	sternum (breastbone)
steth/o	chest
stomat/o	mouth
-stomy	creation of an opening
sub-	below or under
super-	above or excessive
supra-	above or excessive
sym-	together or with
syn-	together or with
tachy-	fast
tax/o	order or coordination
ten/o	tendon (to stretch)
tend/o	tendon (to stretch)

tendin/o	tendon (to stretch)
test/o	testis (testicle)
thalam/o	thalamus (a room)
thorac/o	chest
thromb/o	clot
thym/o	thymus gland
thyr/o	thyroid gland (shield)
-tic	pertaining to
toc/o	labor
tom/o	to cut
-tomy	incision
ton/o	tone or tension
tonsill/o	tonsil (almond)
top/o	place
tox/o	poison
toxic/o	poison
trache/o	trachea (windpipe)
trans-	across or through
tri-	three
trich/o	hair
-tripsy	crushing
troph/o	nourishment or development
tympan/o	eardrum
-ula, -ule	small
uln/o	ulna (a bone of the forearm)
ultra-	beyond or excessive
uni-	one
ur/o	urine
ureter/o	ureter
urethr/o	urethra
urin/o	urine
uter/o	uterus
vagin/o	vagina (sheath)
varic/o	swollen or twisted vein
vas/o	vessel
vascul/o	vessel
ven/o	vein
ventricul/o	ventricle (belly or pouch)
vertebr/o	vertebra
vesic/o	bladder or sac
vesicul/o	bladder or sac
vitre/o	glassy
vulv/o	vulva (covering)
xanth/o	yellow
xer/o	dry
-y	condition or process of

English to Term Component

abdomen	abdomin/o, celi/o, lapar/o
abnormal	-para-
abnormal reduction	-penia
above	hyper-, super-, supra-
across	dia-, trans-
adrenal gland	adren/o
after	post-, meta-
again	re-
against	anti-, contra-
air	aer/o, pneum/o, pneumon/o
air sac	alveol/o
airway	bronch/o, bronchi/o
all	pan-
alongside of	para-
alveolus	alveol/o
anus	an/o
aorta	aort/o
apart	dis-
appendix	appendic/o
arm	brachi/o
around	circum-, peri-
artery	arteri/o
atrium	atri/o
attraction for	-phil, -philia
away	e-, ec-, ex-
away from	ab-
back	re-
backward	retro-
bacteria	bacteri/o
basin	pyel/o
before	ante-, pre-, pro-
beginning	-arche
behind	post-, retro-
below	hypo-, infra-, sub-
bent	lord/o
between	inter-
beyond	meta-, ultra-
bile	bil/i, chol/e
bile duct	choledoch/o
binding	-desis
birth	nat/i
black	melan/o
bladder	cyst/o, vesic/o, vesicul/o
blood	hem/o, hemat/o,
blood condition	-emia
blue	cyan/o
body	somat/o
bone	oste/o
bone marrow	myel/o

both	ambi-, bi-
brain	cerebr/o, encephal/o
breaking down	-lysis
breast	mamm/o, mast/o
breathing	-pnea, spir/o
bronchus	bronch/o, bronchi/o
bud	-blast, blast/o
burst forth	-rrhage, -rrhagia
calculus	lith/o
cancer	carcin/o
carbon dioxide	capn/o, carb/o
cartilage	chondr/o
cavity (sinus)	atri/o, sin/o
cell	cyt/o
cerebellum	cerebell/o
cerebrum	cerebr/o
cervix	cervic/o
change	meta-
cheek	bucc/o
chest	pectoro, steth/o, thorac/o
child	ped/o
circle	coron/o
clear fluid	lymph/o
clot	thromb/o
colon	col/o, colon/o
colon, sigmoid	sigmoid/o
color	chrom/o
colored circle	irid/o, ir/o
condition	-osis
condition of	-ia, -ism, -ium, -y
contraction, involuntary	-spasm
coordination	tax/o
cornea	corne/o, kerat/o
correct	ortho-
creation of an opening	-stomy
crooked	ankyl/o
crown	coron/o
crushing	-tripsy
to cut	tom/o
death	necr/o
deficient	hypo-, olig/o
development	troph/o
diaphragm	phren/o
difficult	dys-
digit (finger or toe)	dactyl/o
dilation or expansion	-ectasis
discharge	-rrhea
disease	path/o

dissolution	-lysis	glomerulus	glomerul/o	measuring, instrument for	-meter	pharyn/x	pharyng/o

dissolution .... -lysis
division .... schiz/o
down .... de-
downward
   displacement ..... -ptosis
dry .... xer/o
duodenum .... duoden/o
ear .... aur/i, ot/o
eardrum .... myring/o,
   tympan/o
eat, swallow .... phag/o
egg .... ov/i, ov/o
enlargement .... -megaly
enzyme .... -ase
epididymis .... epididym/o
equal .... iso-
esophagus .... esophag/o
eustachian tube ..... salping/o
examination .... -scopy
excessive .... hyper-, super-,
   supra-, ultra-
excision
   (removal) .... -ectomy
expansion or
   dilation .... -ectasis
extremity .... acr/o
eye .... ocul/o,
   ophthalm/o,
   opt/o
eyelid .... blephar/o
falling .... -ptosis
fallopian tube .... salping/o
fascia .... fasci/o
fast .... tachy-
fat .... adip/o,
   ather/o,
   lip/o,
   steat/o
faulty .... dys-
fear,
   exaggerated ...... phob/o
femur .... femor/o
few .... olig/o
fiber .... fibr/o
fixation .... -pexy
flesh .... sarc/o
foot .... pod/o, ped/o
form .... morph/o
formation .... -plasia,
   plas/o,
   -poiesis
formation of .... -iasis
four .... quadri-
from .... de-
fungus .... myc/o
ganglion .... gangli/o
gas .... aer/o
germ or bud .... -blast, blast/o
gland .... aden/o
glans penis .... balan/o
glassy .... vitre/o

glomerulus .... glomerul/o
glue .... gli/o
good .... eu-
groin .... inguin/o
gums .... gingiv/o
hair .... trich/o
half .... hemi-, semi-
hard .... kerat/o,
   scler/o
head .... cephal/o
hearing .... acous/o,
   audi/o
hearing
   condition .... -acusis
heart .... cardio/o
hernia .... -celae, herni/o
hip bone .... pelv/i, pelv/o
hormone .... hormon/o
humped .... kyph/o
ileum .... ile/o
incision .... -tomy
increase .... -osis
inflammation .... -itis
instrument for
   examination .... -scope
instrument for
   measuring .... -meter
instrument for
   recording .... -graph
jejunum
   (empty) .... jejun/o
joint .... arthr/o,
   articul/o
juice .... chyl/o
ketone bodies .... ket/o, keton/o
kidney .... nephr/o,
   ren/o
kneecap .... patell/o
knowing .... gnos/o
labor .... toc/o
large .... macr/o
larynx .... laryng/o
left or on left
   side .... sinistr/o
lens .... phac/o,
   phak/o
light .... phot/o
like .... iso-
lip .... cheil/o
liver .... hepat/o,
   hepatic/o
lobe .... lob/o
loin (lower
   back) .... lumb/o
long .... macr/o
lung .... pneum/o,
   pneumon/o,
   pulmon/o
male .... andr/o
many .... multi-, poly-

measuring,
  instrument
  for .... -meter
measuring,
  process of .... -metry
meninges .... mening/o,
   meningi/o
menstruation .... men/o
milk .... lact/o
mind .... psych/o,
   phren/o
mouth .... or/o, stomat/o
movement .... kinesi/o
muscle .... muscul/o,
   my/o
nail .... onych/o
narrow .... sten/o
near .... ad-
neck .... cervic/o
nerve .... neur/o
net .... reticul/o
new .... neo-
normal .... eu-, ortho-
nose .... nas/o,
   rhin/o
not .... de-
nourishment .... troph/o
oil .... seb/o
old age .... presb/o
one .... mono-
one who
  specializes in ..... -ist
one who
  specializes in
  the study or
  treatment of ...... -logist
opening .... glott/o,
   meat/o
opening, creation
  of .... -stomy
opposed to .... anti-, contra-
order .... tax/o
origin .... -gen,
   -genesis,
   -genic
out .... e-, ec-, ex-
outside .... ecto-, exo-,
   extra-
ovary .... oophor/o,
   ovari/o
oxygen .... ox/o
pain .... -algia, -dynia
painful .... dys-
pancreas .... pancreat/o
paralysis .... -plegia
paralysis, slight ..... -paresis
perineum .... perine/o
peritoneum .... peritone/o
pertaining to .... -ac, -al, -ar,
   -ary, -eal, -ic,
   -ous, -tic

pharyn/x .... pharyng/o
place .... top/o
pleura .... pleur/o
poison .... tox/o,
   toxic/o
portion .... lob/o
pouching .... -cele
presence of .... -iasis
process .... -ation
process of .... -y
production .... -gen, -genic,
   -genesis
prostate .... prostat/o
protein .... albumin/o
pulse .... sphygm/o
puncture for
  aspiration .... -centesis
purple .... purpur/o
pus .... py/o
pylorus .... pylor/o
radius .... radi/o
record .... -gram
recording,
  process of .... -graphy
rectum .... proct/o, rect/o
red .... erythr/o
resembling .... -oid
reticulum .... reticul/o
rib .... cost/o
right or on the
  right side .... dextr/o
rod shaped .... rhabd/o
rupture .... -rrhexis
sac .... cyst/o,
   vesic/o,
   vesicul/o
safe .... immun/o
saliva .... sial/o
scale .... squam/o
sclera .... scler/o
sebum .... seb/o
secrete .... crin/o
seizure .... -lepsy
sensation .... esthesi/o
sensitivity,
  exaggerated .... phob/o
separate from .... dis-
sigmoid colon .... sigmoid/o
sinus .... sinus/o
skeletal .... rhabd/o
skin .... cutane/o,
   derm/o,
   dermat/o
skull .... crani/o
sleep .... somn/o
slow .... brady-
small .... -icle, micro-,
   -ole, -ula, -ule
small intestine .... enter/o
smooth .... lei/o
softening .... -malacia

sound	son/o	suspension	-pexy
specializes, one who	-ist	suture	-rrhaphy
speech	phas/o, phon/o	swallow	phag/o
sperm	sperm/o, spermat/o	sweat	hidr/o
spinal cord	myel/o	sweat, profuse	diaphor/o
spine	spin/o	tear	dacry/o, lacrim/o
spleen	splen/o	teeth	dent/i
split	schiz/o	tendon	ten/o, tend/o, tendin/o
sternum	stern/o	tension	ton/o
stiff	ankyl/o	testis (testicle)	orch/o, orchi/o, orchid/o, test/o
stomach	gastr/o	thalamus	thalam/o
stone	lith/o	thick	pachy-
stop or stand	-stasis	thirst	dips/o
straight	orth/o	three	tri-
striated	rhabd/o	three dimensional or solid	stere/o
structure	-ium	throat	pharyng/o
study of	-logy	through	dia-, per-, trans-
study of, one who specializes in	-logist	thymus gland	thym/o
stupor	narc/o	thyroid gland	thyr/o
sugar	gluc/o, glyc/o		
surgical repair or reconstruction	-plasty		

tissue	hist/o, -ium	vagina	colp/o, vagin/o
to or toward	ad-	vein	phleb/o, ven/o
together	con-, sym-, syn-	vein, swollen or twisted	varic/o
tone	ton/o	ventricle	ventricul/o
tongue	gloss/o, lingu/o	vertebra	vertebr/o, spondyl/o
tonsil	tonsill/o	vessel	angi/o, vas/o, vascul/o
topmost	acr/o	voice	phon/o
trachea	trache/o	voice box	laryng/o
treatment	-iatrics, -iatry	vomiting	-emesis
treatment, one who specializes in	-logist	vulva	vulv/o, episi/o
tumor	-oma	water	aque/o, hydr/o
twisted	scoli/o	wax	cerumin/o
two	bi-	weakness	-asthenia
ulna	uln/o	white	leuc/o, leuk/o
under	infra-, sub-	windpipe	trache/o
upon	epi-	with	con-, sym-, syn-
ureter	ureter/o	within	en-, endo-, intra-
urethra	urethr/o	without	a-, an-
urine	ur/o, urin/o	woman	gynec/o
uterine tube	salping/o	yellow	xanth/o
uterus	hyster/o, metr/o, uter/o		

APPENDIX B

Abbreviations and Symbols

ā	before	CAD	coronary artery disease	ECHO	echocardiogram
A	anterior; assessment	cap	capsule	ECU	emergency care unit
A&P	auscultation and percussion	CAT	computerized axial tomography	EDC	estimated date of confinement
A&W	alive and well			EEG	electroencephalogram
AB	abortion	CBC	complete blood count	EGD	esophagogastroduodenoscopy
ABG	arterial blood gas	cc	cubic centimeter	EIA	enzyme immunoassay
ABMS	American Board of Medical Specialists	CC	chief complaint; cardiac catheterization	EKG	electrocardiogram
				EMG	electromyogram
a.c.	before meals	CCU	coronary (cardiac) care unit	ENT	ear, nose, throat
ACE	angiotensin-converting enzyme	CHF	congestive heart failure	ER	emergency room
ACP	American College of Physicians	CIN	cervical intraepithelial neoplasia	ERCP	endoscopic retrograde cholangiopancreatography
ACS	American College of Surgeons	CIS	carcinoma in situ	ESR	erythrocyte sedimentation rate
ACTH	adrenocorticotrophic hormone	cm	centimeter	ESWL	extracorporeal shock wave lithotripsy
AD	right ear	CNS	central nervous system		
ad lib.	as desired	CO	cardiac output	ETOH	ethyl alcohol
AIDS	acquired immunodeficiency syndrome	c/o	complains of	F	Fahrenheit
		COPD	chronic obstructive pulmonary disease	F.A.C.P.	fellow of the American College of Physicians
alb	albumin				
a.m.	morning	CP	cerebral palsy; chest pain	F.A.C.S.	fellow of the American College of Surgeons
amt	amount	CPD	cephalopelvic disproportion		
ANS	autonomic nervous system	CPR	cardiopulmonary resuscitation	FBS	fasting blood sugar
AP	anterior posterior	CSF	cerebrospinal fluid	FH	family history
aq	water	CT	computed tomography	fl oz	fluid ounce
AS	left ear	cu mm	cubic millimeter	FS	frozen section
ASD	atrial septal defect	CVA	cerebrovascular accident	FSH	follicle-stimulating hormone
ASHD	arteriosclerotic heart disease	CVS	chorionic villus sampling	Fx	fracture
AU	both ears	CXR	chest x-ray	g	gram
AV	atrioventricular	d	day	GERD	gastroesophageal reflux disease
Ⓑ	bilateral	D&C	dilation and curettage	GH	growth hormone
BCP	biochemistry panel	DC,		GI	gastrointestinal
b.i.d.	twice a day	D/C	discharge; discontinue	gm	gram
BM	black male; bowel movement	D.C.	doctor of chiropractic medicine	gr	grain
BP	blood pressure			gt	drop
BPH	benign prostatic hypertrophy/ hyperplasia	D.D.S.	doctor of dental surgery	gtt	drops
		DJD	degenerative joint disease	GTT	glucose tolerance test
BRP	bathroom privileges	D.O.	doctor of osteopathic medicine	GYN	gynecology
BS	blood sugar	D.P.M.	doctor of podiatric medicine	h	hour
BUN	blood urea nitrogen	dr	dram	H&P	history and physical
Bx	biopsy	DRE	digital rectal examination	HBV	hepatitis B virus
c̄	with	DTR	deep tendon reflex	HCT or	
C	Celsius; centigrade	DVT	deep vein thrombosis	Hct	hematocrit
C&S	culture and sensitivity	Dx	diagnosis	HEENT	head, eyes, ears, nose, throat
CABG	coronary artery bypass graft	ECG	electrocardiogram	HGB or	
				Hgb	hemoglobin

663

HIV	human immunodeficiency virus	NIDDM	non-insulin-dependent diabetes mellitus	PTH	parathyroid hormone
HPI	history of present illness	NKA	no known allergy	PTT	partial thromboplastin time
HPV	human papilloma virus	NKDA	no known drug allergy	PV	per vagina
HRT	hormone replacement therapy	noc.	night	PVC	premature ventricular contraction
h.s.	bedtime (hour of sleep)	NPO	nothing by mouth	Px	physical examination
HSV-1	herpes simplex virus Type 1	NSR	normal sinus rhythm	q	every
		O	objective	qd	every day
HSV-2	herpes simplex virus Type 2	OB	obstetrics	qh	every hour
Ht	height	OD	right eye; doctor of optometry	q2h	every two hours
HTN	hypertension	OH	occupational history	q.i.d.	four times a day
Hx	history	OP	outpatient	q.n.s.	quantity not sufficient
I&D	incision and drainage	OR	operating room	q.o.d.	every other day
ICD	implantable cardioverter-defibrillator	ORIF	open reduction, internal fixation	q.s.	quantity sufficient
ICU	intensive care unit	OS	left eye	qt	quart
ID	intradermal	OU	both eyes	R	right; respiration
IDDM	insulin-dependent diabetes mellitus	oz	ounce	RBC	red blood cell; red blood count
		p̄	after	RIA	radioimmunoassay
IM	intramuscular	P	plan; posterior; pulse	RLQ	right lower quadrant
IMP	impression	PA	posterior anterior	R/O	rule out
IOL	intraocular lens implant	PaCO$_2$	arterial partial pressure of carbon dioxide	ROM	range of motion
IP	inpatient			ROS	review of symptoms
IUD	intrauterine device	PaO$_2$	arterial partial pressure of oxygen	RP	retrograde pyelogram
IV	intravenous			RRR	regular rate and rhythm
IVP	intravenous pyelogram	PAP	Papanicolaou test (smear)	RTC	return to clinic
kg	kilogram	PAR	postanesthetic recovery	RTO	return to office
KUB	kidney, ureter, bladder	p.c.	after meals	RUQ	right upper quadrant
L	left, liter	PDA	patent ductus arteriosus	Rx	recipe; take thou
L&W	living and well	PE	physical examination	s̄	without
lb	pound	PEFR	peak expiratory flow rate	S	subjective
LEEP	loop electrosurgical excision procedure	per	by	SA	sinoatrial
		PERRLA	pupils equal, round, and reactive to light and accommodation	SH	social history
LH	luteinizing hormone			Sig:	instruction to patient
LLQ	left lower quadrant			SLE	systemic lupus erythematosus
LP	lumbar puncture	PET	positron emission tomography	SMA	sequential multiple analyzer
LTB	laryngotracheobronchitis	PF	peak flow	SOB	shortness of breath
LUQ	left upper quadrant	PFT	pulmonary function testing	SPECT	single photon emission computed tomography
ⓜ	murmur	PH	past history		
m	meter	Ph.D.	doctor of philosophy	SpGr	specific gravity
MCH	mean corpuscular hemoglobin	PI	present illness	sq	subcutaneous
MCHC	mean corpuscular hemoglobin concentration	PID	pelvic inflammatory disease	SR	systems review
		PIH	pregnancy-induced hypertension	s̄s̄	one-half
MCV	mean corpuscular volume			STAT	immediately
MD	muscular dystrophy; medical doctor	p.m.	afternoon	STD	sexually transmitted disease
		PMH	past medical history	suppos	suppository
mg	milligram	PNS	peripheral nervous system	SV	stroke volume
MI	myocardial infarction	p.o.	by mouth	Sx	symptom
mL	milliliter	post op	postoperation	T	temperature
mm	millimeter	PPBS	postprandial blood sugar	T&A	tonsillectomy and adenoidectomy
MRA	magnetic resonance angiography	PR	per rectum		
		pre op	preoperation	tab	tablet
MRI	magnetic resonance imaging	p.r.n.	as needed	TAB	therapeutic abortion
MS	multiple sclerosis; musculoskeletal	PSA	prostate-specific antigen	TB	tuberculosis
		PSG	polysomnography	TEDS	thromboembolic disease stockings
MSH	melanocyte-stimulating hormone	pt	patient		
		PT	physical therapy; prothrombin time	TEE	transesophageal echocardiogram
MVP	mitral valve prolapse			TIA	transient ischemic attack
NCV	nerve conduction velocity	PTCA	percutaneous transluminal coronary angioplasty	t.i.d.	three times a day
NG	nasogastric			TM	tympanic membrane
				TPR	temperature, pulse, respiration

Tr	treatment	WBC	white blood cell, white blood count	♀	sitting	
TSH	thyroid-stimulating hormone			○—	lying	
TURP	transurethral resection of the prostate	WDWN	well developed, well nourished	×	times or for	
TV	tidal volume	wk	week	>	greater than	
Tx	treatment; traction	WNL	within normal limits	<	less than	
UA	urinalysis	wt	weight	i̇	one	
UCHD	usual childhood diseases	y.o.	year old	ïï	two	
URI	upper respiratory infection	yr	year	ïïï	three	
UTI	urinary tract infection	♀	female	ïⱽ	four	
VC	vital capacity	♂	male	I, II, III,		
VCU	voiding cystourethrogram	#	number or pound	IV, V,		
VS	vital signs	°	degree or hour	VI,		
VSD	ventricular septal defect	↑	increased; above	VII,		
V_T	tidal volume	↓	decreased; below	VIII,		
w.a.	while awake	∅	none or negative	IX, X	uppercase Roman numerals 1–10	
		♀	standing			

A-Angle Angle between a vertical line dividing the patella into half and a second line drawn from the tibial tubercle to the apex of the inferior pole of the patella. An angle of 35° or greater has been linked to increased patellofemoral pain.

Absorption Occurs when an electrical wave passes through a medium and its kinetic energy is partially or totally assimilated by the tissue.

Absorption rate How quickly a drug gets into the tissues to produce a therapeutic effect

Accessory movements Movements within a joint that cannot be voluntarily performed by the individual.

Acclimatization Physiological adaptations of an individual to a different environment, especially climate or altitude.

Acne mechanica A local exacerbation of acne vulgaris due to heat, occlusion, pressure, and friction.

Active inhibition Technique whereby an individual consciously relaxes a muscle prior to stretching.

Active movement Joint motion performed voluntarily by the individual through muscular contraction.

Acute injury Injury with rapid onset due to traumatic episode, but with short duration.

Adhesions Tissues that bind the healing tissue to adjacent structures, such as other ligaments or bone.

ADLs Activities of daily living.

Administration of medication Providing one dose of a medication to an individual.

Affective Pertaining to feelings or a mental state.

Afferent nerves Nerves carrying sensory input from receptors in the skin, muscles, tendons, and ligaments to the central nervous system.

Agonist muscles Muscles that perform the desired movement; primary movers.

Albuminuria Protein in the urine.

Allergic contact dermatitis Results when a substance comes in direct contact with the skin and leads to a simple inflammatory reaction.

Alveoli Air sacs at the terminal ends of the bronchial tree where oxygen and carbon dioxide are exchanged between the lungs and surrounding capillaries.

Amenorrhea Absence or abnormal cessation of menstruation.

Amplitude A measure of the force, or intensity, that drives an electrical current, the maximum amplitude being the top or highest point of each phase.

Analgesia Conscious state in which normal pain is not perceived, such as a numbing or sedative effect.

Analgesic Agent that produces analgesia.

Anaphylaxis An immediate shock-like, frequently fatal, hypersensitive reaction that occurs within minutes of administration of an allergen unless appropriate first aid measures are taken immediately.

Anastomosis A network of communicating blood vessels that supply a joint.

Androgen A class of hormones that promotes development of male genitals, secondary sex characteristics, and influences sexual motivation.

Anemia Abnormal reduction in red blood cell volume or hemoglobin concentration.

Anesthesia Partial or total loss of sensation.

Anesthetic Agents that produce anesthesia.

Angle of inclination Angle of depression formed by the meeting of a line drawn through the shaft of the femur with one passing through the long axis of the femoral neck; normally about 125° in the frontal plane.

Angle of torsion In the transverse plane, the relationship between the femoral head and femoral shaft, which is normally rotated 15°.

Anisocoria A condition in which the two pupils are not of equal size.

Anisotropic Having different strengths in response to loads from different directions.

Annulus fibrosus The ring of fibrocartilage and fibrous tissue forming the circumference of the intervertebral disc.

Anorexia athletica Classification of athletes who demonstrate significant signs and symptoms of eating disorders but do not meet the APA criteria for anorexia or bulimia.

Anorexia nervosa Personality disorder manifested by extreme aversion toward food, resulting in extreme weight loss, amenorrhea, and other physical disorders.

Anovulation Suspension or cessation of ovulation.

Antacids An antacid or agent that neutralizes stomach acid.

Antagonist muscles Muscles that oppose or reverse a particular movement.

Anterograde amnesia Loss of memory of events following a head injury.

Anteversion Forward displacement or turning forward of a body segment without bending.

Antibiotics A soluble substance derived from a mold or bacterium that inhibits the growth of other microorganisms.

Antihistamine Medication used to counteract the effects of histamine; one that relieves the symptoms of an allergic reaction.

Antipyretic Medication used to relieve or reduce a fever.

Antiseptics Substances that inhibit the growth of infectious agents.

Apnea Temporary cessation of breathing.

Appendicitis Inflammation of the appendix.

Arrhythmia Disturbance in the heartbeat rhythm.

Arthralgia Severe joint pain.

Arthrogram Diagnostic tool whereby a radiopaque material is injected into a joint to facilitate an x-ray.

Arthrokinematics Accessory motion, or an involuntary joint motion, that occurs simultaneously with physiological motion, but cannot be measured precisely.

Arthroscopy Diagnostic tool whereby the inside of a joint is viewed through a small camera lens (arthroscope) to facilitate surgical repair of the joint and/or joint structures.

Aseptic necrosis The death or decay of tissue due to a poor blood supply in the area.

Asthma Disease of the lungs characterized by constriction of the bronchial muscles, increased bronchial secretions, and mucosa swelling, all leading to airway narrowing and inadequate airflow during respiration.

Astringent Agents that cause contraction of the tissues, arrest secretion, or control bleeding.

Ataxia Inability to coordinate the muscles in the execution of voluntary movement.

Atherosclerosis Condition whereby irregularly distributed lipid deposits are found in the large and medium-sized arteries.

Atrophy A wasting away or deterioration of tissue due to disease, disuse, or malnutrition.

Aura A peculiar sensation that precedes an epileptic attack.

Auscultation Listening for sounds, often with a stethoscope, to denote the condition of the lungs, heart, pleura, abdomen, and other organs.

Autoinoculation Spreading of an infection from one body part to another by touching the lesion, then scratching or rubbing somewhere else.

Autonomic dysreflexia A rare but dangerous condition in wheelchair athletes, commonly triggered by an obstructed bowel or bladder, which disturbs the regulation of blood pressure and heart rate.

Axial force Loading directed along the long axis of a body.

Axonotmesis Damage to the axons of a nerve followed by complete degeneration of the peripheral segment, without severance of the supporting structure of the nerve.

Bacteremia The presence of viable bacteria in the circulating blood.

Ballistic stretch Increasing flexibility by utilizing repetitive bouncing motions at the end of the available range of motion.

Bankart lesion Avulsion or damage to the anterior lip of the glenoid as the humerus slides forward in an anterior dislocation.

Battery Unpermitted or intentional contact with another individual without their consent.

Battle's sign Delayed discoloration behind the ear due to basilar skull fracture.

Bending Loading that produces tension on one side of an object and compression on the other side.

Benign pain Pain characterized as dull, generalized, not lasting long after exertion, and not associated with swelling, localized tenderness, or long-term soreness.

Bennett's fracture Fracture-dislocation to the proximal end of the first metacarpal at the carpal-metacarpal joint.

Bimalleolar fracture Fractures of both the medial and lateral malleolus.

Bioavailability The amount of the drug's concentration when it reaches the target site within a certain time frame.

Bipartite Having two parts.

Blood brain barrier The barrier that protects the brain against toxic substances.

Boutonniere deformity Rupture of the central slip of the extensor tendon at the middle phalanx, resulting in no active extensor mechanism at the PIP joint.

Bowler's thumb Compression of the digital nerve on the medial aspect of the thumb, leading to paresthesia in the thumb.

Boxer's fracture Fracture of the fifth metacarpal, resulting in a flexion deformity due to rotation of the head of the metacarpal over the neck.

Brachial plexus A complex web of spinal nerves (C_5–T_1) that innervate the upper extremity.

Break test Used to test resistance, an overload pressure is applied in a stationary or static position.

Bronchitis Inflammation of the mucosal lining of the tracheobronchial tree characterized by bronchial swelling, mucus secretions, and dysfunction of the cilia.

Bronchospasm Contraction of the smooth muscles of the bronchial tubes, causing narrowing of the airway.

Buccal Pertaining to, or adjacent to, or in the direction of the cheek.

Bucket-handle tear Longitudinal meniscal tear of the central segment that can displace into the joint, leading to locking of the knee.

Bulimia nervosa Personality disorder manifested by episodic bouts of bingeing large amounts of food followed by purging and feelings of guilt, self-disgust, and depression.

Burner Burning or stinging sensation characteristic of a brachial plexus injury.

Bursa A fibrous sac membrane containing synovial fluid typically found between tendons and bones; acts to decrease friction during motion.

Bursitis Inflammation of a bursae.

Calcific tendinitis Accumulation of mineral deposits in a tendon.

Call person During an emergency, the person responsible for providing assistance, relaying messages to the sideline, and obtaining additional help if necessary.

Callus Localized thickening of skin epidermis due to physical trauma. Fibrous tissue containing immature bone tissue that forms at fracture sites during repair and regeneration.

Cancellous tissue Bone tissue of relatively low density.

Cardiac asystole Cardiac standstill.

Cardiac tamponade Acute compression of the heart due to effusion of fluid or blood into the pericardium from rupture of the heart or penetrating trauma.

Carpal tunnel syndrome Compression of the median nerve as it passes through the carpal tunnel, leading to pain and tingling in the hand.

Carrying angle The angle between the humerus and ulna when the arm is in anatomical position.

CAT scan Computerized axial tomography scan. A computer-assisted x-ray tomogram that provides detailed images of tissue based on their density.

Cathode Negatively charged electrode in a direct current system.

Cauda equina Lower spinal nerves that course through the lumbar spinal canal; resembles a horse's tail.

Cavitation Gas bubble formation due to nonthermal effects of ultrasound.

Celiac plexus Nerve plexus that innervates the abdominal region.

Charge person During an emergency, the most medically trained individual who controls the scene and supervises the care of the athlete until the assessment is complete and the athlete is safely moved.

Chemosensitive Sensitive to chemical stimulation.

Chondral fracture Fracture involving the articular cartilage at a joint.

Chondromalacia patellae Degenerative condition in the articular cartilage of the patella caused by abnormal compression or shearing forces.

Chronic injury An injury with long onset and long duration.

Chyme A semifluid mass of partly digested food passed from the stomach into the duodenum.

Cirrhosis Progressive inflammation of the liver usually caused by alcoholism.

Claw toe Toe deformity characterized by hyperextension of the metatarsophalangeal (MP) joint and hyperflexion of the interphalangeal (IP) joints.

Climacteric phase The perimenopausal years, ranging from age 46 to 55, when the menstrual cycle may shorten, and become irregular in frequency and irregular in bleeding.

Clonic Movement marked by repetitive muscle contractions and relaxation in rapid succession.

Close-packed position Joint position in which contact between the articulation structures is maximal.

Closed-cell foam Foam material in which air cannot pass from one cell to another, allowing the material to rebound and return to its original shape quickly, but offering less cushioning at low levels of impact.

Coach's finger Fixed flexion deformity of the finger resulting from dislocation at the PIP joint.

Coarctation A constriction, stricture, or stenosis.

Coccygodynia Prolonged or chronic pain in the coccygeal region due to irritation of the coccygeal nerve plexus.

Cognitive The quality of knowing or perceiving.

Cognitive model Model that seeks to explain how an athlete approaches the rehabilitation process, encompassing personal factors, such as performance anxiety, self-esteem/motivation, extroversion/introver-

sion, psychological investment in the sport, coping resources, a history of past stressors, and previous intervention strategies.

Cold diuresis Excretion of urine in cold weather due to blood being shunted away from the skin to the core to maintain vascular volume.

Cold urticaria Condition characterized by redness, itching, and large blister-like wheals on skin that is exposed to cold.

Collateral ligaments Major ligaments that cross the medial and lateral aspects of a hinge joint to provide stability from valgus and varus forces.

Colles fracture Fracture involving a dorsally angulated and displaced, and a radially angulated and displaced fracture within $1\frac{1}{2}$ inches of the wrist.

Compartment syndrome Condition which increased intramuscular pressure brought on by activity impedes blood flow and function of tissues within that compartment.

Compression A pressure or squeezing force direct through a body in such a way as to increase density.

Concussion Violent shaking or jarring action of the brain, resulting in immediate or transient impairment of neurologic function.

Conduction The direct transfer of energy between two objects in physical contact with each other.

Conductors Mediums that facilitate movement of the ions such as water, blood, and electrolyte solutions such as sweat.

Congenital Existing at birth.

Conjunctivitis Bacterial infection leading to itching, burning, watering, and inflamed eye; pinkeye.

Constipation Infrequent or incomplete bowel movements.

Contracture Permanent muscular contraction due to tonic spasm, fibrosis, loss of muscular equilibrium, or paralysis.

Contraindication A condition adversely affected if a particular action is taken.

Contralateral Pertaining to the opposite side.

Contranutation Anterior rotation of the ilium on the sacrum indicating anterior torsion of the joint, or posterior rotation of the sacrum on the ilium on one side; the limb on that side will probably be medially rotated.

Contrecoup injuries Injuries away from the actual injury site due to rotational components during acceleration.

Contusion Compression injury involving accumulation of blood and lymph within a muscle; a bruise.

Convection The transfer of energy between two objects via a medium, such as air or water, as it moves across the body creating temperature variations.

Conversion Involves the changing of another energy form (e.g., sound, electricity, or a chemical agent) into heat.

Coordination The body's ability to execute smooth, fluid, accurate, and controlled movements.

Cortical tissue Compact bone tissue of relatively high density.

Cosine law As the angle deviates from 90°, the energy varies with the cosine of the angle: effective energy = energy × cosine of the angle of incidence.

Counterirritant A substance causing irritation of superficial sensory nerves so as to reduce pain transmission from another underlying irritation.

Coxa valga Alteration of the angle made by the axis of the femoral neck to the axis of the femoral shaft, so that the angle exceeds 135°; the femoral neck is in more of a straight line relationship to the shaft of the femur.

Coxa varum Alteration of the angle made by the axis of the femoral neck to the axis of the femoral shaft so that the angle is less than 135°; the neck becomes more horizontal.

Cramp Painful involuntary muscle contraction either clonic or tonic.

Crepitation Crackling sound or sensation characteristic of a fracture when the bone ends are moved.

Cruciate ligaments Major ligaments that crisscross the knee in the anteroposterior direction, providing stability in that plane.

Cryokinetics Use of cold treatments prior to an exercise session.

Cryotherapy Cold application.

Cubital recurvatum Extension beyond 0° at the elbow.

Cubital valgus At the elbow, a valgus angle greater than 20°.

Cubital varus At the elbow, a valgus angle less than 10°.

Current The actual movement of ions.

Cyanosis A dark bluish or purple skin color due to deficient oxygen in the blood.

Cyclist's nipples Nipple irritation due to the combined effects of perspiration and wind-chill producing cold, painful nipples.

Cyclist's palsy Seen when bikers lean on the handlebar for an extended period of time, resulting in paresthesia in the ulnar nerve distribution.

Dead arm syndrome Common sensation felt with a recurrent anterior shoulder dislocation.

Decerebrate rigidity Extension of all four extremities.

Decompression Surgical release of pressure from fluid or blood accumulation.

Decorticate rigidity Extension of the legs with flexion of the elbows, wrists, and fingers.

de Quervain's tenosynovitis An inflammatory stenosing tenosynovitis of the abductor pollicis longus and extensor pollicis brevis tendons.

Dermatome Region of skin supplied by cutaneous branches of a single spinal nerve.

Dermis Corium of the skin that contains blood and lymphatic vessels, nerves and nerve endings, glands, and, except for glabrous skin, hair follicles.

Detached retina Neurosensory retina is separated from the retinal epithelium by swelling.

Detraining Loss of the benefits gained in physical training, which can occur after only 1 to 2 weeks of nonactivity, with significant decreases measured in both metabolic and working capacity.

Diabetes mellitus Metabolic disorder characterized by near or absolute lack of the hormone insulin, or insulin resistance, or both.

Diabetic ketoacidosis Condition where an excess of ketoacids in the blood can lower the blood pH to 7.0 and is manifested by ketones in the breath, blood, and in the urine.

Diagnosis Definitive determination of the nature of the injury or illness made only by physicians.

Diarrhea Loose or watery stools.

Diathermy Local elevation of temperature in the tissues produced by therapeutic application of high-frequency electric current, ultrasound, or microwave radiation.

Diffuse injuries Injury over a large body area, usually due to low velocity–high mass forces.

Diplopia Double vision.

Disinfectants Chemical agents applied to nonliving objects; they are most commonly used to disinfect surgical instruments and cleanse medical equipment and facilities.

Diuretics Chemicals that promote the excretion of urine.

Drug A therapeutic agent used in the prevention, diagnosis, cure, treatment, or rehabilitation of a disease, condition, or injury.

Drug dispensing Providing more than one individual dose to a person.

Drug interaction The ability of one drug to alter the effects of another drug; it may either intensify (synergistic action) or reduce (inhibit) the effects of the drug.

Drug metabolism The enzymatic alteration of a drug's structure, whereby the original drug is broken down into metabolites (an altered product of metabolism).

Dural sinuses Formed by tubular separations in the inner and outer layers of the dura mater, these sinuses function as small veins for the brain.

Dysesthesia A disagreeable sensation, or a sensation short of anesthesia.

Dysmenorrhea Difficult or painful menstruation; menstrual cramps.

Dyspepsia Gastric indigestion.

Dysphagia Difficulty in swallowing.

Dysplasia Abnormal tissue development.

Dyspnea Labored or difficult breathing.

Dysrhythmia Serious irregularity of the heart rate.

Ecchymosis Superficial tissue discoloration.

Echocardiogram Ultrasonic record obtained by echocardiography in the investigation of the heart and great vessels.

Ectopic bone Proliferation of bone ossification in an abnormal place.

Edema Swelling resulting from a collection of exuded lymph fluid in interstitial tissues.

Effective radiating area In ultrasound, the portion of the transducer's surface area that actually produces the ultrasound wave.

Efferent nerves Nerves carrying motor impulses from the central nervous system to the muscles.

Effusion The escape of fluid from the blood vessels into the surrounding tissues or joint cavity.

Elastic limit A material's yield point.

Electrocardiogram Graphic record of the heart's action currents obtained with an electrocardiograph.

Electromagnetic radiation Energy emitted by an object.

Electromagnetic spectrum Graphic presentation of electromagnetic radiation based on its wavelength or frequency.

Embolism Obstruction or occlusion of a vessel by bacteria or other foreign body.

Emergency medical services A well-developed process that activates the emergency health care services of the athletic training facility and community to provide immediate health care to an injured individual.

Emesis Vomiting.

End feel The sensation felt in the joint as it reaches the end of the available range of motion.

Endometriosis Ectopic occurrence of endometrial tissue, frequently forming cysts containing altered blood.

Enteric coated Drugs covered by acid-resistant materials (e.g., fatty acids, waxes, shellac) that protect the drug from the acid and pepsin in the stomach.

Epicondylitis Inflammation and micro-rupturing of the soft tissues on the epicondyles of the distal humerus.

Epidermis The outer epithelial portion of the skin.

Epilepsy Disorder of the brain characterized by recurrent episodes of sudden, excessive discharges of electrical activity in the brain.

Epiphyseal fracture Injury to the growth plate of a long bone in children and adolescents; may lead to arrested bone growth.

Epistaxis Profuse bleeding from the nose; nosebleed.

Erythema Inflammatory redness of the skin.

Erythropoietin A hormone produced in the kidneys that stimulates bone marrow to increase production of red blood cells.

Estrogens Hormones that produce female secondary sex characteristics and affect the menstrual cycle.

Excoriation A scratch mark; a linear break in the skin surface, usually covered with blood or serous crusts.

Exculpatory waiver Based on the athlete's assumption of risk, a release that is signed by the athlete or parent of an athlete under the age of 18, that releases the physician from liability of negligence.

Exercise-induced urticaria Hives brought on by exercise; a variation of cholinergic urticaria, but the lesions are much larger.

Expressed warranty Written guarantee that states the product is safe for consumer use.

Extensor mechanism Complex interaction of muscles, ligaments, and tendons that stabilize and provide motion at the patellofemoral joint.

Extrasynovial Structures found outside of the synovial cavity and synovial fluid.

Extruded Tooth driven in an outwardly direction.

Extruded disc Condition in which the nuclear material bulges into the spinal canal and runs the risk of impinging on adjacent nerve roots.

Exudate Material composed of fluid, pus, or cells that has escaped from blood vessels into surrounding tissues following injury or inflammation.

Failure Loss of continuity; rupturing of soft tissue or fracture of bone.

Fasciitis Inflammation of the fascia surrounding portions of a muscle.

Female Athlete Triad A combination of three disorders commonly seen in adolescent and young adult female athletes: disordered eating, amenorrhea, and osteoporosis.

Fibrositis Inflammation of fibrous tissue.

First-pass effect Drug metabolism that takes place first in the liver via hepatic enzymes.

Flatulence Presence of an excessive amount of gas in the stomach and intestines.

Flexibility Total range of motion at a joint dependent on normal joint mechanics, mobility of soft tissues, and muscle extensibility.

Focal injuries Injury in a small concentrated area, usually due to high velocity–low mass forces.

Focus The ability to perceive and address various internal (thoughts, emotions, physical responses) and external (sights, sounds) cues and, when needed, to shift one's attention to other cues in a natural, effortless manner.

Follicular phase Days 1 to 14 of the ovarian cycle in which the follicle (spheroidal cell cluster in the ovary containing an ovum or egg) grows.

Foreseeability of harm Condition in which danger is apparent, or should have been apparent, resulting in an unreasonably unsafe condition.

Fracture A disruption in the continuity of a bone.

Frieberg's disease Avascular necrosis that occurs to the second metatarsal head in some adolescents.

Ganglion cyst Benign tumor mass commonly seen on the dorsal aspect of the wrist.

Gangrene Necrosis due to obstruction, loss, or diminution of blood supply; may be localized to a small area or involve an entire extremity or organ.

Gastritis Inflammation, especially mucosal, of the stomach.

Gastrocolic reflex Propulsive reflex in the colon that stimulates defecation.

Gastroenteritis Inflammation of the mucous membrane of the stomach and/or small intestine.

Genu recurvatum A condition of hyperextension of the knee.

Genu valgum A deformity marked by abduction of the leg in relation to the thigh; knock-knee.

Genu varum A deformity marked by adduction of the leg in relation to the thigh; bowleg.

Gestation Pregnancy.

Glenoid labrum Soft tissue lip around the periphery of the glenoid fossa that widens and deepens the socket to add stability to the joint.

Glucagon A polypeptide hormone secreted by pancreatic alpha cells. It activates hepatic phosphorylase, thereby increasing glycogenolysis; decreases gastric motility and gastric and pancreatic secretions; and increases urinary excretion of nitrogen and potassium.

Goniometer Protractor used to measure joint position and available joint motion (ROM).

Gross negligence Committing, or not committing an act with total disregard for the health and safety of others.

Grottus-Draper law A law stating that there is an inverse relationship between the amount of penetration and absorption. The more energy absorbed by superficial tissues, the less is available to be transmitted to the underlying tissues.

Gynecomastia Excessive development of the male mammary glands.

Hallux The first, or great, toe.

Hammer toes A flexion deformity of the distal interphalangeal (DIP) joint of the toes.

Harmful pain Pain that is sharp, localized to the injury site, experienced during and persisting after exertion, and is usually associated with swelling, localized tenderness, and prolonged soreness.

Heat cramps Painful involuntary muscle spasms caused by excessive water and electrolyte loss.

Heel bruise Contusion to the subcutaneous fat pad located over the inferior aspect of the calcaneus.

Hemarthrosis Collection of blood within a joint or cavity.

Hematocele A rapid accumulation of blood and fluid in the scrotum around the testicle and cord.

Hematoma A localized mass of blood and lymph confined within a space or tissue.

Hematuria Blood or red blood cells in the urine.

Hemoglobinuria Presence of hemoglobin in the urine; in sufficient quantities, they result in the urine being colored from light red-yellow to fairly dark red.

Hemorrhoids Dilations of the venous plexus surrounding the rectal and anal area that can become exposed if they protrude internally or externally.

Hemothorax Condition involving the loss of blood into the pleural cavity, but outside the lung.

Hepatitis Inflammation of the liver.

Hernia Protrusion of abdominal viscera through a weakened portion of the abdominal wall.

High-density material Material that absorbs more energy from higher impact intensity levels through deformation, thus transferring less stress to a body part.

Hill-Sachs lesion A small defect usually located on the posterior aspect of the articular cartilage of the humeral head caused by the impact of the humeral head on the glenoid fossa as the humerus dislocates.

Hip pointer Contusions caused by direct compression to an unprotected iliac crest that crushes soft tissue, and sometimes the bone itself.

Homeostasis The state of a balanced equilibrium in the body's various tissues and systems.

Hydrocele Swelling in the tunica vaginalis of the testes.

Hyperemia Presence of increased blood flow into a region or body part once treatment has ended.

Hyperesthesia Excessive tactile sensation.

Hyperglycemia Abnormally high levels of glucose in the circulating blood that can lead to diabetic coma.

Hyperhidrosis Excessive or profuse sweating.

Hyperhydrated Overhydration; excess water consumption of the body.

Hypermobile patella Movement of the patella equal to three or more quadrants of the patella, indicating laxity of the restraints, which can predispose an athlete to a laterally subluxating or dislocating patella.

Hypermobility Increased motion at a joint; joint laxity.

Hyperplasia An increase in the number of cells in a tissue or organ, excluding tumor formation; overgrowth of the endometrium.

Hypertension Sustained elevated blood pressure above the norms of 140 mm Hg systolic or 90 mm Hg diastolic.

Hyperthermia Elevated body temperature.

Hypertrophic cardiomyopathy Excessive hypertrophy of the heart, often of obscure or unknown origin.

Hypertrophy General increase in bulk or size of an individual tissue not due to tumor formation.

Hyphema Hemorrhage into the anterior chamber of the eye.

Hypoesthesia Decreased tactile sensation.

Hypoglycemia Abnormally low levels of glucose in the circulating blood that can lead to insulin shock.

Hypomobile patella Movement of the patella equal to one quadrant or less.

Hypomobility Decreased motion at a joint.

Hypotension Characterized by a fall of 20 mm Hg or more from a person's normal baseline systolic blood pressure.

Hypothalamus A region of the diencephalon that forms the floor of the third ventricle of the brain and is responsible for thermoregulation and other autonomic nervous mechanisms underlying moods and motivational states.

Hypothermia Decreased body temperature.

Hypoxia Having a reduced concentration of oxygen in air, blood, or tissue, short of anoxia.

Impetigo A highly contagious bacterial infection characterized by small vesicles that form pustules and eventually honey-colored weeping crustations.

Impingement syndrome Chronic condition caused by repetitive overhead activity that damages the glenoid labrum, long head of the biceps brachii, and subacromial bursa.

Implied warranty Unwritten guarantee that the product is reasonably safe when used for its intended purpose.

Indication A condition that could benefit from a specific action.

Infarcts Clumping together of cells that block small blood vessels, leading to vascular occlusion, ischemia, and necrosis in organs.

Infiltrative anesthesia A process that produces numbness by interfering with nerve function in a localized subcutaneous soft tissue area. Commonly used for the treatment of soft tissue injuries or as an anesthetic prior to minor surgical procedures.

Inflammation Pain, swelling, redness, heat, and loss of function that accompany musculoskeletal injuries.

Influenza Acute infectious respiratory tract condition characterized by malaise, headache, dry cough, and general muscle aches.

Informed consent Consent given by a person of legal age who understands the nature and extent of any treatment, and available alternative treatments prior to agreeing to receiving treatment.

Interpulse interval The period within a discrete pulse when the current is not flowing. The duration of the intrapulse interval cannot exceed the duration of the interpulse interval.

Intersection syndrome A tendinitis or friction tendinitis in the first and second dorsal compartments of the wrist.

Intracapsular Structures found within the articular capsule; intra-articular.

Intruded tooth Tooth driven deep into the socket in an inwardly direction.

Ion An atom or group of atoms carrying a charge of electricity by virtue of having gained or lost one or more electrons.

Iontophoresis Technique whereby direct current is used to drive charged molecules from certain medications into damaged tissue.

Ipsilateral Situated on, pertaining to, or affecting the same side, as opposed to contralateral.

Irritant contact dermatitis Results when a substance causes direct skin damage, pain, or ulceration.

Ischemia Local anemia due to decreased blood supply.

Jaundice A yellowish discoloration of the skin, sclera, and deeper tissues often due to liver damage.

Jersey finger Rupture of the flexor digitorum profundus tendon from the distal phalanx due to rapid extension of the finger while actively flexed.

Jones fracture A transverse stress fracture of the proximal shaft of the fifth metatarsal.

Joule's law A law that states that the greater the resistance or impedance, the more heat will be developed. Tissues with a high fluid content, such as skeletal muscle and areas surrounding joints, absorb more of the energy and are heated to a greater extent, whereas fat is not heated as much.

Kehr's sign Referred pain down the left shoulder indicative of a ruptured spleen.

Ketoacidosis Condition caused by excess accumulation of acid or loss of base in the body; characteristic of diabetes mellitus.

Ketonemia Presence of recognizable concentration of ketone bodies in the blood plasma.

Ketonuria Enhanced urinary excretion of ketone bodies.

Kinebock's disease Avascular necrosis of the lunate often seen in young athletes thought to be caused by repetitive trauma or an unrecognized lunate fracture.

Kinematic chain Series of interrelated joints that constitute a complex motor unit so that motion at one joint will produce motion at the other joints in a predictable manner.

Kinematics Study of the spatial and temporal aspects of movement.

Kinesthesia The sensation of position, movement, tension, etc. of parts of the body perceived through nerve end organs in the muscles, tendons, and joints.

Kinetics Study of the forces causing and resulting from motion.

Kyphosis Excessive curve in the thoracic region of the spine.

Laryngospasm Spasmodic closure of the glottic aperture leading to shortness of breath, coughing, cyanosis, and even loss of consciousness.

Legg-Calvé-Perthes disease Avascular necrosis of the proximal femoral epiphysis seen especially in young males ages 3 to 8.

Lipid solubility Fat-soluble; denoting the ability of fat-soluble vitamins to be absorbed better than water-soluble vitamins, and to accumulate in the body because of their increased ability to cross cell membranes.

Lisfranc injury Involves disruption of the tarsometatarsal joint, with or without an associated fracture caused by a severe twisting injury. The first metatarsal is typically dislocated from the first cuneiform, while the other four metatarsals are displaced laterally, usually in combination with a fracture at the base of the second metatarsal.

Little league shoulder Fracture of the proximal humeral growth plate in adolescents caused by repetitive rotational stresses during the act of pitching.

Little leaguer elbow Tension stress injury of the medial epicondyle seen in adolescents.

Loose-packed position Resting position where the joint is under the least amount of strain.

Lordosis Excessive convex curve in the lumbar region of the spine.

Low-density material Material that absorbs energy from low-impact intensity levels.

Lumbar plexus Interconnected roots of the first four lumbar spinal nerves.

Luteal phase Phase of the ovarian cycle extending from ovulation until the onset of the next menstrual bleeding, normally about 12–17 days. During this period, both estrogen and progesterone levels are high.

Lymphangitis Inflammation of the lymphatic vessels.

Macerated To soften skin with moisture by steeping or soaking.

Macrotrauma When a single force produces an acute injury.

Magnetic resonance imaging (MRI) Diagnostic technique using magnetism to produce high-quality cross-sectional images of organs or structures within the body without x-rays or other radiation.

Maisonneuve fracture An external rotation injury of the ankle with an associated fracture of the proximal third of the fibula.

Malaise Lethargic feeling of general discomfort; out-of-sorts feeling.

Malfeasance Committing an act that is not your responsibility to perform.

Mallet finger Rupture of the extensor tendon from the distal phalanx due to forceful flexion of the phalanx.

Mallet toe A toe in neutral position at the MTP and PIP joints, but flexed at the DIP joint.

Malocclusion Inability to bring the teeth together in a normal bite.

Malpractice Committing a negligent act while providing care.

Marfan's syndrome Inherited connective tissue disorder affecting many organs, but commonly resulting in the dilation and weakening of the thoracic aorta.

Mast cells Connective tissue cells that carry heparin, which prolongs clotting, and histamine.

Maximal efficacy The drug dose at which a response occurs, and continues to increase in magnitude before reaching a plateau, or threshold.

McBurney's point A site one-third the distance between the ASIS and umbilicus that with deep palpation produces rebound tenderness, indicating appendicitis.

Mechanosensitive Sensitive to mechanical stimulation.

Menarche The onset of menses.

Meninges Three protective membranes that surround the brain and spinal cord.

Meningitis Inflammation of the meninges of the brain and spinal column.

Menisci Fibrocartilaginous discs found within a joint that serve to reduce joint stress.

Menstrual phase Phase in the menstrual cycle when the thickened vascular walls of the uterus, the unfertilized ova, and blood from damaged vessels are lost during the menstrual flow.

Metabolites Any altered product of metabolism, especially of catabolism.

Metatarsalgia A condition involving general discomfort around the metatarsal heads.

Microtrauma Injury to a small number of cells due to accumulative effects of repetitive forces.

Miliaria An eruption of minute vesicles and papules caused when active sweat glands become blocked by organic debris; prickly heat.

Minimum effective concentration Refers to a drug's minimum concentration that must be present for the drug to be effective.

Misfeasance Committing an act that is your responsibility to perform, but the wrong procedure is followed, or the right procedure is done in an improper manner.

Mitral valve prolapse A condition in which redundant tissue is found on one or both leaflets of the mitral valve. During a ventricular contraction, a portion of the redundant tissue on the mitral valve pushes back beyond the normal limit and, as a result, produces an abnormal sound followed by a systolic murmur as blood is regurgitated back through the mitral valve into the left atrium; often called a click-murmur syndrome.

Modality Therapeutic agent that promotes optimal healing while reducing pain and disability.

Multivalvular disease Acquired valvular heart disease stemming from a defect or insufficiency in more than one heart valve manifested as either valvular stenosis or regurgitation.

Myalgia Pain in a muscle.

Myocardial infarction Heart attack.

Myocarditis An inflammatory condition of the muscular walls of the heart that can result from a bacterial or viral infection.

Myopia Nearsightedness.

Myositis Inflammation of connective tissue within a muscle.

Myositis ossificans Accumulation of mineral deposits within muscle tissue.

Myotome A group of muscles primarily innervated by a single nerve root.

Necrosis Death of a tissue due to deprivation of a blood supply.

Negligence Breach of one's duty of care that causes harm to another individual.

Neoplasm Mass of tissue that grows more rapidly than normal and may be benign or malignant.

Nephropathy Any disease of the kidney.

Neuralgia Pain of a severe throbbing or stabbing nature in the course or distribution of a nerve.

Neurapraxia Injury to a nerve that results in temporary neurologic deficits followed by complete recovery of function.

Neuroma A nerve tumor.

Neurotmesis Complete severance of a nerve.

Nightstick fracture Fracture to the ulna due to a direct blow; commonly seen in football players.

Nonfeasance Failing to perform your legal duty of care.

Nuchal rigidity Stiffness in the nape or back of the neck.

Nucleus pulposus The soft fibrocartilage central portion of the intervertebral disc.

Nutation The backward rotation of the ilium on the sacrum. When occurring on only one side, the ASIS is higher and the PSIS is lower on that side, resulting in an apparent or functional short leg on the same side.

Nystagmus Abnormal jerking or involuntary eye movement.

Ohm's law A law that states that current (I) in a conductor increases as the driving force (V) becomes larger, or resistance (R) is decreased; I = V/R.

Oligomenorrhea Infrequent menstrual cycles or menstruation involving scant blood flow.

Onychia Inflammation of the nail matrix.

Organomegaly Abnormal enlargement of an organ.

Open-cell foam Foam with cells that are connected to allow air passage from cell to cell, allowing the foam to deform quickly

under stress, which limits the shock-absorbing qualities.

Orthostatic hypotension Low blood pressure caused by a sudden change in body position, such as moving from a lying to a standing position.

Osgood-Schlatter disease Inflammation or partial avulsion of the tibial apophysis due to traction forces.

Osteitis pubis Stress fracture to the pubic symphysis caused by repeated overload of the adductor muscles or repetitive stress activities.

Osteochondral fracture Fracture involving the articular cartilage and underlying bone.

Osteochondritis dissecans Localized area of avascular necrosis resulting in complete or incomplete separation of joint cartilage and subchondral bone.

Osteochondrosis Any condition characterized by degeneration or aseptic necrosis of the articular cartilage due to limited blood supply.

Osteomyelitis Inflammation or infection of the bone and bone marrow.

Osteopenia Condition of reduced bone mineral density that predisposes the individual to fractures.

Osteoporosis Pathological condition of reduced bone mass and strength.

Otitis externa Bacterial infection involving the lining of the auditory canal; swimmer's ear.

Otitis media Localized infection in the middle ear secondary to upper respiratory infections.

Ovarian cycle Cycle associated with the maturation of an egg.

Overload principle Physiological improvements occur only when an individual physically demands more of the muscles than is normally required.

Ovulation Release of the egg occurring midcyle when the ballooning ovary wall ruptures and expels the egg.

Painful arc Pain located within a limited number of degrees in the range of motion.

Palpitations Perceptible forcible pulsation of the heart, usually with an increase in frequency or force, with or without irregularity in rhythm.

Papules Small, red, elevated painful bumps on the skin.

Paresis Partial paralysis of a muscle, leading to a weakened contraction.

Paresthesia Abnormal sensations such as tingling, burning, itching, or prickling.

Paronychia A fungal/bacterial infection in the folds of skin surrounding a fingernail or toenail.

Parrot-beak tear Horizontal meniscal tear typically in the middle segment of the lateral meniscus.

Patella plica A fold in the synovial lining that may cause medial knee pain without associated trauma.

Patellofemoral joint Gliding joint between the patella and patellar groove of the femur.

Patellofemoral stress syndrome Condition in which the lateral retinaculum is tight, or the vastus medialis oblique is weak, leading to lateral excursion and pres-

sure on the lateral facet of the patella, causing a painful condition.

Pathology The cause of an injury, its development, and functional changes due to the injury process.

Periorbital ecchymosis Swelling and hemorrhage into the surrounding eyelids; black eye.

Periostitis Inflammation of the periosteum (outer membrane covering the bone).

Peristalsis Periodic waves of smooth muscle contraction that propel food through the digestive system.

Pes cavus High arch.

Pes planus Flat feet.

Phagocytosis Process by which white blood cells surround and digest foreign particles, such as bacteria, necrotic tissue, and foreign particles.

Pharmacokinetics The study of how a drug moves through the body to produce the desired effects.

Pharyngitis Viral, bacterial, or fungal infection of the pharynx leading to a sore throat.

Phlebothrombosis Thrombosis, or clotting, in a vein without overt inflammatory signs and symptoms.

Phonophoresis The introduction of anti-inflammatory drugs through the skin with the use of ultrasound.

Photophobia Abnormal sensitivity to light.

Plantar fascia Specialized band of fascia that covers the plantar surface of the foot and helps support the longitudinal arch.

Plyometric training Type of explosive exercise that maximizes the myotatic on-stretch reflex.

Pneumothorax Condition in which air is trapped in the pleural space, causing a portion of a lung to collapse.

Polydipsia Frequent drinking because of extreme thirst.

Polyphagia Excessive hunger and food consumption; gluttony.

Polyuria Excessive excretion of urine, leading to a huge urine output of water and electrolytes that leads to decreased blood volume and further dehydration.

Postconcussion syndrome Delayed condition characterized by persistent headaches, blurred vision, irritability, and inability to concentrate.

Premenstrual syndrome A series of physical and psychological symptoms, such as headaches, breast tenderness, back pain, bloating, irritability, depression, fatigue, and certain food cravings occurring during the luteal phase (days 15–28) of the menstrual cycle.

Prodromal symptom An early symptom of a disease.

Progesterone Hormone responsible for thickening the uterine lining in preparation for the fertilized ovum.

Progressive-resistance exercise A method to improve strength by increasing resistance using the overload principles as the individual's strength increases.

Prolapsed disc Condition in which the eccentric nucleus produces a definite deformity as it works its way through the fibers of the annulus fibrosus.

Proliferation phase In the menstrual cycle, days 6–14, when the endometrium rebuilds itself.

Pronation Inward rotation of the forearm; palms face posteriorly. At the foot, combined motions of calcaneal eversion, foot abduction, and dorsiflexion.

Pronator syndrome Median nerve is entrapped by the pronator teres, leading to pain on activities involving pronation.

Prophylactic To prevent or protect.

Proprioceptive neuromuscular facilitation (PNF) Exercises that stimulate proprioceptors in muscles, tendons, and joints to improve flexibility and strength.

Proteinuria Abnormal concentrations of protein in the urine.

Pruritus Intense itching.

Pulmonary contusion Contusion to the lungs due to compressive force.

Pulmonary embolism A blood clot that travels through the circulatory system to lodge in the lungs.

Pupillary light reflex Rapid constriction of pupils when exposed to intense light.

Pyarthrosis Suppurative pus within a joint cavity.

Q-angle Angle between the line of quadriceps force and the patellar tendon.

Raccoon eyes Delayed discoloration around the eyes from anterior cranial fossa fracture.

Radial tunnel syndrome Condition caused by direct trauma or entrapment at the elbow as the radial nerve passes anterior to the cubital fossa, pierces the supinator muscle, and runs posterior again into the forearm.

Radiation The transfer of energy in the form of infrared waves (radiant energy) without physical contact.

Rales Abnormal breath sounds.

Rate of dissolution Condition by which the more rapidly a drug dissolves, the faster its onset of effects will be, as in drugs that dissolve quickly (liquid medications) have a more rapid onset of effects than those that dissolve more slowly (enteric coated preparations).

Raynaud's disease Condition characterized by intermittent bilateral attacks of ischemia of the fingers or toes, marked by severe pallor, numbness, and pain.

Receptor The functional macromolecule, or target site, to which a drug binds to produce its effects.

Reciprocal inhibition Technique using an active contraction of the agonist to cause a reflex relaxation in the antagonist, allowing it to stretch; a phenomenon resulting from reciprocal innervation.

Reflection Occurs when an energy wave strikes an object and is bent back away from the material, as in an echo.

Reflex Action involving stimulation of a motor neuron by a sensory neuron in the spinal cord without involvement of the brain.

Refraction The deflection of an energy wave due to a change in the speed of absorption as the wave passes between mediums of different densities.

Regurgitation A backward flow, as of blood through an incompetent heart valve; the return of contents in small amounts from the stomach.

Resilience The ability to bounce or spring back into shape or position after being stretched, bent, or impacted.

Resistors Mediums that inhibit the movement of ions, such as skin, fat, and lotion.

Resting position Slightly flexed position of a joint that allows for maximal volume to accommodate any intra-articular swelling.

Retrograde amnesia Forgetting events prior to an injury.

Retroversion A turning backward; a decreased angle between the femoral condyles and femoral head, usually <15°.

Retroviruses Any virus of the family Retroviridae known to reverse the usual order of reproduction within the cells they infect.

Reverse piezoelectric effect In ultrasound, the conversion of electrical current into mechanical energy as is passes through a piezoelectric crystal (e.g., quartz, barium titanate, lead zirconate, or titanate) housed in the transducer head.

Reye's syndrome A severe disorder of young children following an acute illness, usually influenza or varicella infection, characterized by recurrent vomiting beginning within a week after onset of the condition, from which the child either recovers rapidly or lapses into a coma with intracranial hypertension; death may result from edema of the brain and resulting cerebral herniation.

Rhabdomyolysis An acute, fulminating, potentially fatal disease of skeletal muscles, which entails destruction of skeletal muscles evidenced by the release of myoglobin into the blood and urine.

Rhinitis Inflammation of the nasal membranes with excessive mucus production resulting in nasal congestion and postnasal drip.

Rhinorrhea Clear nasal discharge.

Rotator cuff The SITS muscles (supraspinatus, infraspinatus, teres minor, and subscapularis) hold the head of the humerus in the glenoid fossa and produce humeral rotation.

Runner's nipples Nipple irritation due to friction as the shirt rubs over the nipples.

Sacral plexus Interconnected roots of the L4–S4 spinal nerves that innervate the lower extremities.

Salicylates Any salt of salicylic acid; used in aspirin.

Scapulohumeral rhythm Coordinated rotational movement of the scapula that accompanies abduction and adduction of the humerus.

Scheuermann's disease Osteochondrosis of the spine due to abnormal epiphyseal plate behavior that allows herniation of the disc into the vertebral body, giving a characteristic wedge-shaped appearance.

Sciatica Compression of a spinal nerve due to a herniated disc, annular tear, myogenic or muscle-related disease, spinal stenosis, facet joint arthropathy, or compression from the piriformis muscle.

Scoliosis Lateral rotational spinal curvature.

Scope of care The roles and responsibilities of an individual in a profession, which delineates what should be learned in the professional preparation of that individual.

Screwing-home mechanism Rotation of the tibia on the femur at the end of extension to produce a "locking" of the knee in a close-packed position.

Sebum Secretions of the sebaceous glands; oily substance that binds epidermal cells.

Secretory phase Phase in the menstrual cycle, usually days 15–28, in which the endometrium prepares for implantation of an embryo.

Seizure Abnormal electrical discharge in the brain.

Seizure disorder Recurrent episodes of sudden excessive charges of electrical activity in the brain, whether from known or unknown (idiopathic) causes.

Serous otitis Fluid buildup behind the eardrum associated with otitis media and upper respiratory infections.

Sever's disease A traction-type injury, or osteochondrosis, of the calcaneal apophysis seen in young adolescents.

Shear force A force directed parallel to a surface.

Shin bruise A contusion to the tibia; sometimes referred to as tibial periostitis.

Sickle cell anemia Abnormalities in hemoglobin structure resulting in a characteristic sickle- or crescent-shaped red blood cell that is fragile and unable to transport oxygen.

Sinding-Larsen-Johansson disease Inflammation or partial avulsion of the apex of the patella due to traction forces.

Sinusitis Inflammation of the paranasal sinuses.

SLAP lesion An injury to the superior labrum that typically begins posteriorly and extends anteriorly, disrupting the attachment of the long head of the biceps tendon to the superior glenoid tubercle.

Snapping hip syndrome A snapping sensation either heard or felt during motion at the hip.

Snowball crepitation Sound similar to that heard when crunching snow into a snowball indicative of tenosynovitis.

Spasm Transitory muscle contractions.

Spear tackler's spine A condition caused by a history of using a spear-tackling technique, whereby the athlete used the top or crown of the helmet as the initial point of contact, placing the cervical spine at risk for serious injury due to excessive axial loading.

Spinal stenosis A loss of cerebrospinal fluid around the spinal cord due to deformation of the spinal cord, or a narrowing of the neural canal.

Spondylolisthesis Anterior slippage of a vertebrae resulting from complete bilateral fracture of the pars interarticularis.

Spondylolysis A stress fracture of the pars interarticularis.

Sports medicine Area of health and special services that applies medical and scientific knowledge to prevent, recognize, manage, and rehabilitate injuries related to sport, exercise, or recreational activity.

Stage model Emotional stages that an individual progresses through when confronted with grief, including denial and isolation, anger, bargaining, depression, and acceptance.

Standard of care What another minimally competent professional educated and practicing in the same profession would have done in the same or similar circumstance to protect an individual from harm.

Static stretch Slow and deliberate muscle stretching used to increase range of motion.

Status epilepticus A condition in which one major attack of epilepsy succeeds another with little or no intermission.

Stenosing Narrowing of an opening or stricture of a canal; stenosis.

Steroids A large family of chemical substances including endocrine secretions and hormones.

Sticking point Presence of insufficient strength to move a body segment through a particular angle.

Strain Amount of deformation with respect to the original dimensions of the structure.

Stress The distribution of force within a body; quantified as force divided by the area over which the force acts.

Stress fracture Fracture resulting from repeated loading with relatively low magnitude forces.

Striae distensae Bands of thin wrinkled skin, initially red but becoming purple and white, which occur commonly on the abdomen, buttocks, and thighs during and following pregnancy, and result from atrophy of the dermis and overextension of the skin.

Strict liability Manufacturer's absolute liability for any and all defective or hazardous equipment that unduly threatens an individual's personal safety.

Subconjunctival hemorrhage Minor capillary ruptures in the eye globe.

Subcutaneous emphysema Presence of air or gas in subcutaneous tissue, characterized by a crackling sensation on palpation.

Subungual hematoma Hematoma beneath a finger- or toe-nail.

Sudden death A nontraumatic, unexpected death occurring instantaneously or within a few minutes of an abrupt change in an individual's previous clinical state.

Supination Outward rotation of the forearm; palms facing forward. At the foot, combined motions of calcaneal inversion, foot adduction, and plantar flexion.

Supraventricular tachycardia Rapid heartbeats proximal to the ventricles, in the atrium or A-V node.

Sustained-release Capsules or tablets filled with tiny spheres that contain a drug. The sphere is coated and designed to dissolve at variable rates ranging from 8 to 24 hours.

Sustentaculum tali The anteromedial surface of the calcaneus that largely supports the talus.

Syncope Fainting or lightheadedness.

Syndrome An accumulation of common signs and symptoms characteristic of a particular injury or disease.

Tachycardia Rapid beating of the heart, usually applied to rates greater than 100 beats per minute.

Tachypnea Rapid breathing.

Tackler's exostosis Irritative exostosis on the anterior or lateral humerus.

Tendinitis Inflammation of a tendon.

Tendinosis A tendinous condition associated with degeneration, rather than inflammation.

Tenosynovitis Inflammation of a tendon sheath.

Tensile force A pulling or stretching force directed axially through a body or body part.

Tension pneumothorax Condition in which air continuously leaks into the pleural space, causing the mediastinum to displace to the opposite side, compressing the uninjured lung and thoracic aorta.

Therapeutic drugs Prescription or over-the-counter medications used to treat an injury or illness.

Therapeutic range The range between the minimum effective concentration and toxic concentration.

Thermoregulation The process by which the body maintains body temperature; primarily controlled by the hypothalamus.

Thermotherapy Heat application.

Thoracic outlet syndrome Condition in which nerves and/or vessels become compressed in the root of the neck or axilla, leading to numbness in the arm.

Thrombophlebitis Acute inflammation of a vein.

Tibiofemoral joint Dual condyloid joints between the tibial and femoral condyles that function primarily as a modified hinge joint.

Tidal volume The amount of air inspired and expired in a single breath.

Tinea Ringworm; fungal infection of the hair, skin, or nails characterized by small vesicles, itching, and scaling; tinea pedis—athlete's foot; tinea cruris—jock itch; tinea capitis—ringworm of the scalp.

Tinnitus Ringing or other noises in the ear due to trauma or disease.

Tomograms Cross-sectional image of an organ or body part at various depths of field produced by an x-ray technique.

Tonic Steady rigid muscle contractions with no relaxation.

Torque A rotary force; the product of a force and its moment arm, or moment.

Torsion force Twisting around an object's longitudinal axis in response to an applied torque.

Tort A wrong done to an individual whereby the injured party seeks a remedy for damages suffered.

Toxic concentration Concentration of drug levels in the blood plasma that are too high, and therefore increase the risk of toxic effects.

Toxic synovitis Occurring largely in children, a transient inflammatory condition characterized by a painful hip joint accompanied by an antalgic gait and limp.

Translation Refers to anterior gliding of the tibial plateau on the femur.

Traumatic asphyxia Condition involving extravasation of blood into the skin and conjunctivae due to a sudden increase in venous pressure.

Trigger finger Condition in which the finger flexors contract but are unable to re-extend due to a nodule within the tendon sheath or the sheath being too constricted to allow free motion.

Tunics Three layers of protected tissues that surround the eye.

Urticaria Hives; an eruption of itching wheals, usually of systemic origin; may be due to a state of hypersensitivity to foods or drugs, infection, physical agents, or psychic stimuli.

Uterine cycle The menstrual cycle; a series of cyclic changes that the inner lining of the uterus (endometrium) goes through each month as it responds to varying levels of hormones in the blood.

Valgus An opening on the medial side of a joint caused by the distal segment moving laterally.

Valsalva effect Holding one's breath against a closed glottis, resulting in sharp increases in blood pressure.

Valvular stenosis A narrowing of the orifice around the cardiac valves.

Varicocele Abnormal dilation of the veins of the spermatic cord, leading to engorgement of blood into the spermatic cord veins when standing.

Varus An opening on the lateral side of a joint caused by the distal segment moving medially.

Vehicles Substances combined with medications that use enteral routes to facilitate entry into the body; may include tablets, capsules, liquids, powders, suppositories, enteric coated preparations, and sustained-release preparations.

Vertigo Balance disturbance characterized by a whirling sensation of one's self or external objects.

Viscoelastic Responding to loading over time with changing rates of deformation.

Volkmann's contracture Ischemic necrosis of the forearm muscles and tissues caused by damage to the blood flow.

Voltage The force that causes ions to move.

Watt A unit of electrical power. For an electrical current: Watts = Voltage × Amperage.

Wedge fracture A crushing compression fracture that leaves a vertebra narrowed anteriorly.

Wheal A smooth, slightly elevated area on the body that appears red or white, and is accompanied by severe itching; commonly seen in allergies to mechanical or chemical irritants.

Wolff's law A law that states that bone and soft tissue will respond to the physical demands placed on them, causing the formation of collagen to remodel or realign along the lines of stress, thus promoting healthy joint biomechanics.

Wrist drop Weakness and/or paralysis of the wrist and finger extensors due to radial nerve damage.

Yield point (elastic limit) The maximum load that a material can sustain without permanent deformation.

Zone of primary injury Region of injured tissue prior to vasodilation.

Zone of secondary injury Region of damaged tissue following vasodilation.

Page numbers in italics denote figures; those followed by a t denote tables.